McKENNA'S PHARMACOLOGY FOR NURSING AND HEALTH PROFESSIONALS

SECOND EDITION REVISED

Lisa McKenna RN, RM, BEdSt, MEdSt, GD Health Admin & InfoSys, GDLFAH, PhD, FACN
Professor, School of Nursing and Midwifery,
La Trobe University, Bundoora, Australia

Anecita Gigi Lim RN, BSc (Nursing), MHSc, GD Science Pharmacology, PGD Social Science, PhD, FCN
Senior Lecturer, School of Nursing, University of Auckland,
Auckland, New Zealand

Original US edition

Focus on Nursing Pharmacology

Amy M. Karch RN, MS
Associate Professor of Clinical Nursing,
University of Rochester School of Nursing, Rochester, New York

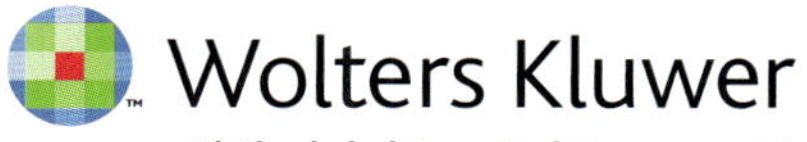

Philadelphia • Baltimore • New York • London
Buenos Aires • Hong Kong • Sydney • Tokyo

Wolters Kluwer Health Australia Pty Limited
Ground floor, 66 Talavera Road, Macquarie Park, NSW 2113

Wolters Kluwer Health
Two Commerce Square, 2001 Market Street, Philadelphia, PA 19103

Publishing Director – Asia Pacific: Vaughn Curtis
Senior Project & Program Manager: Helena Klijn
Technical checking: Lynne Perkins BPharm (Syd) BVA (Syd); Jerry Perkins BPharm (Syd) BSc (UNSW); Sanja Mirkov BPharm, PGDipPH, MPS
Editor: Julian McAllan BSc
Proofreader: Marnie Firipis
Indexer: Puddingburn Publishing Services; revised by Mary Coe
Typesetter: Toppan Best-set Premedia Limited
Cover design: XouCreative; revised by Lisa Petroff Design
Printer: RR Donnelley, Shenzhen, China

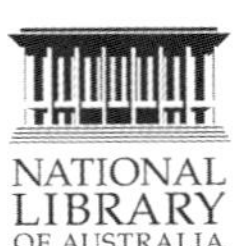

A catalogue record for this book is available from the National Library of Australia

RRS1910

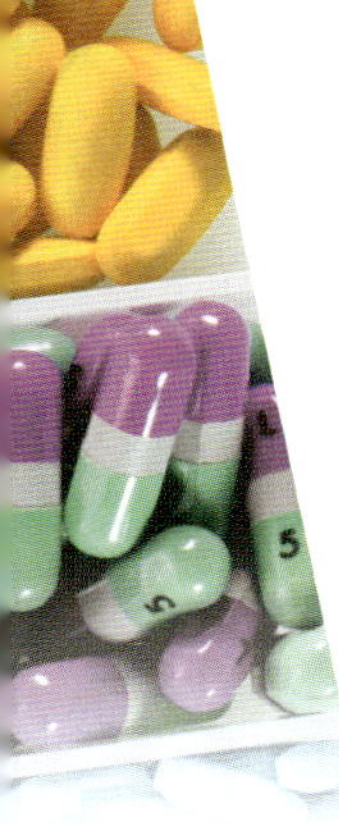

Reviewers, Australia and New Zealand

Genevieve BRIDESON RN, RM, BN (Hons), PhD (cand.)
Lecturer, School of Nursing and Midwifery, Flinders University, Adelaide, South Australia

Petra CZARNIAK BPharm, MPharm, DipTeach, GCert (DiabEd), MPS, AACPA
Senior Lecturer, School of Pharmacy, Curtin University, Perth, Western Australia

Julie HANSON RN, BN, PGCert (Advanced Nursing Practice), PhD (cand.)
Lecturer, School of Nursing and Midwifery, University of the Sunshine Coast, Maroochydore, Queensland

Karole HOGARTH RN, BSc (Hons), PGCert (Tertiary Teaching), PhD
Senior Lecturer, School of Nursing, Otago Polytechnic Te Kura Matatini ki Otago, Dunedin, New Zealand

Heather JOSLAND RN, BN, MA (Hlth Sci), PGCert (Clin Tchg)
Senior Nursing Lecturer, Department of Nursing and Human Services, Christchurch Polytechnic Institute of Technology, Christchurch, New Zealand

Snezana KUSLJIC BSci (Hons), PhD
Senior Lecturer, Pharmacologist, Department of Nursing, The University of Melbourne, Melbourne, Victoria; Honorary Senior Research Fellow, The Florey Institute of Neuroscience and Mental Health, Melbourne, Victoria

Victoria KAIN RN, MN, PhD
Senior Lecturer, School of Nursing and Midwifery, Griffith University, Brisbane, Queensland

Catherine KING MPharm, PhD
Senior Lecturer, School of Pharmacy and Medical Sciences, University of South Australia, Adelaide, South Australia

Patricia LOGAN BSc, MAppSc, GCert (Uni Tech & Learn), PhD, ANMT
Lecturer in Health Science, School of Biomedical Science, Charles Sturt University, New South Wales

Rosie MacLEAVY RN, BN, GDip (Paediatrics), MCN (Paediatrics)
Lecturer, Unit Coordinator, School of Health Sciences, University of Tasmania, Hobart, Tasmania; Board of Directors, Australian College of Children and Young People's Nurses (ACCYPN)

Michael J. McGIVERN RGN, RMN, BN, DipHE, PGDipHSc (Advanced Nursing), NCAET, Cert Mgmt
Clinical Nursing Tutor, NorthTec School of Nursing Tai Tokerau Wānanga, Whangarei, Northland, New Zealand

Andrea MILLER BN (Hons), MCN, MEd
Clinical Lecturer, School of Health Sciences, University of Tasmania, Hobart, Tasmania

Sanja MIRKOV BPharm, PGDipPH, MPS
Professional Teaching Fellow, School of Pharmacy, The University of Auckland, New Zealand; Quality Use of Medicines Pharmacist
Ramsay Health Care, Australia

Kate NORRIS RN, BN, MA (Nursing), PGCert (HlthSci), CAT
Senior Nursing Lecturer, Department of Nursing and Human Services, Christchurch Polytechnic Institute of Technology, Christchurch, New Zealand

Nadim RAHMAN RN, BN, MBBS, AMC (Primary Assessment), PGT (General Practice), GCHPE
Lecturer, Faculty of Medicine, Nursing and Health Sciences, Monash University, Melbourne, Victoria

Joanne RAMSBOTHAM RN, EM, Cert Adult Ed, MN Child Health, PhD
Lecturer, School of Nursing, Queensland University of Technology, Brisbane, Queensland

David STANLEY RN, RM, NursD, BA Ng, MSc HS, Dip HE (Nursing), GCert (HPE)
Associate Professor, School of Population Health, The University of Western Australia, Perth, Western Australia

Jenny WILKINSON BSc (Hons), GradDip (FET), MHEd, PhD
Associate Professor, School of Biomedical Sciences, Charles Sturt University, Wagga Wagga, New South Wales

Cecilia YEBOAH RN, RM, MN, PhD, MRCNA
Lecturer/International Academic Advisor – Nursing, School of Nursing, Midwifery and Paramedicine (Melbourne Campus), Australian Catholic University, Victoria

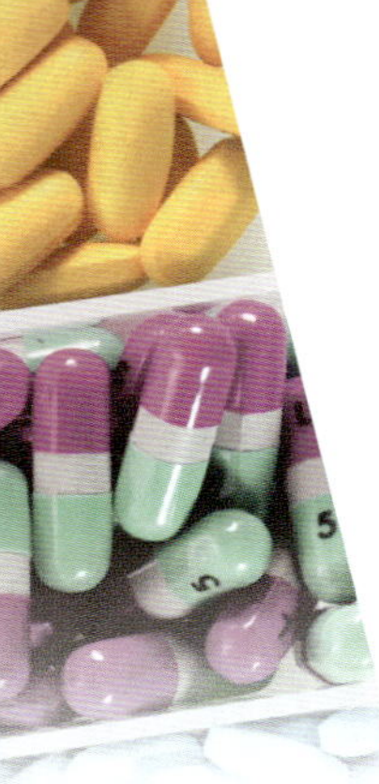

Contents

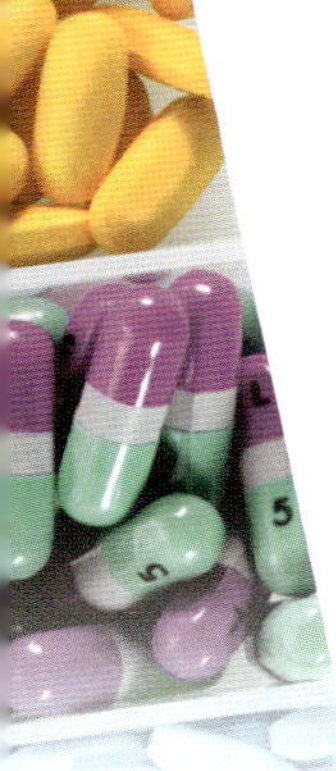

Preface

Pharmacology is regarded by some as a difficult area to teach in standard nursing, midwifery and professional health care curricula, whether it be at the diploma, undergraduate or graduate level. Many related pharmacology texts are large and burdensome, mainly because they need to cover not only the basic pharmacology, but also the particulars included in each area considered. Teachers are scarce, and time and money often dictate that the invaluable content is incorporated into other courses. As a result, the content is often lost.

At the same time, changes in health care delivery – more outpatient and home-based care, shorter hospital stays and more self-care – have resulted in additional legal and professional responsibilities for nurses, midwives and other health professionals, making them ever more responsible for the safe and effective delivery of drug therapy.

Pharmacology should not be seen as such a formidable obstacle in nursing and professional health care curricula. The study of drug therapy incorporates physiology, pathophysiology, chemistry and clinical fundamentals – subjects that are already incorporated into curricula in most schools.

OUR PHILOSOPHY

McKenna's Pharmacology for Nursing and Health Professionals is a text for nursing and professional health care students that approaches pharmacology as an understandable, teachable and learnable subject. It is based on the premise that students first need to have a solid and clearly focused concept of the principles of drug therapy before they can easily grasp the myriad details associated with individual drugs. Armed in advance with this fundamental knowledge of pharmacology, the student can then appreciate and use the specific details that are so readily available in many annually updated and published drug guides, such as Wolters Kluwer Health's *McKenna's Drug Handbook for Nursing and Midwifery.*

With this goal in mind, *McKenna's Pharmacology for Nursing and Health Professionals* provides a concise and uncluttered text for today's student, presenting the subject in a user-friendly and understandable manner. Because this text is designed to be used in conjunction with a handbook of current drug information, it remains streamlined.

Thoroughly revised and updated, the second edition of *McKenna's Pharmacology for Nursing and Health Professionals* emphasises 'need-to-know' concepts. The text reviews and integrates previously learned knowledge of physiology, chemistry and clinical fundamentals into chapters focused on helping students to conceptualise what is important to know about each group of drugs. Illustrations and tables sum up concepts to enhance learning.

Carefully designed pedagogical features further focus student learning on clinical application, critical thinking, safety, lifespan issues related to drug therapy, evidence-based practice, individual and family teaching, and case-study-based critical thinking exercises that incorporate clinical reasoning principles. *Check your understanding* sections at the end of each chapter provide review questions to help the student master the material and prepare for examinations.

ORGANISATION

McKenna's Pharmacology for Nursing and Health Professionals is organised following a 'simple-to-complex' approach, much like the syllabus for a basic pharmacology course. Because students learn best 'from the bottom up', the text is divided into 11 distinct parts.

Part 1 begins with an overview of basic pharmacology, including challenges such as street drugs, herbal therapies and information overload. Each of the other parts begins with a review of the physiology of the system affected by the specific drugs being discussed. This review refreshes the information for students and provides a quick and easy reference when they are reading about drug actions.

Part 2 introduces the drug classes, starting with chemotherapeutic agents – both antimicrobial and antineoplastic drugs. Because the effectiveness of these drugs depends on their interference with the most basic element of body physiology – the cell – students can easily understand the pharmacology of this class. Mastering the pharmacotherapeutic effects of this drug class helps students to establish a firm grasp of the basic principles taught in Part 1. Once the easiest pharmacological concepts are understood, students are enabled to move on to the more challenging physiological and pharmacological concepts.

Part 3 focuses on drugs affecting the immune system, because recent knowledge about the immune system has made it the cornerstone of modern therapy. All of the immune system drugs act in ways in which the immune system would act if it were able. Recent immunological research has contributed to a much greater understanding of this system, making it important to position information about drugs affecting this system close to the beginning of the text instead of at the end, as has been the custom.

Parts 4 and 5 address drugs that affect the nervous system, the basic functioning system of the body. Following the discussion of the nervous system, and closely linked with it in **Part 6**, is the endocrine system. The sequence of these parts introduces students to the concept of control, teaches them about the interrelatedness of these two systems and prepares them for understanding many aspects of shared physiological function and the inevitable linking of the two systems into one: the neuro-endocrine system.

Parts 7, 8 and 9 discuss drugs affecting the reproductive, cardiovascular and renal systems, respectively. The sequencing of cardiovascular and renal drugs is logical because most of the augmenting cardiovascular drugs, such as diuretics, affect the renal system.

Part 10 covers drugs that act on the respiratory system, which provides the link between the left and right ventricles of the heart.

Part 11 addresses drugs acting on the gastrointestinal system. The gastrointestinal system stands on its own; it does not share any actions with any other system.

FEATURES OF THIS EDITION

The text's features are skilfully designed to support the text discussion, encouraging the student to look at the whole person and to focus on the essential information about each drug class. Important features focus on incorporating basic clinical skills, person safety, critical thinking and application of the material learned to the clinical scenario, helping the student to understand the pharmacology material.

Chapter structure

Each chapter opens with a list of *learning objectives* for that chapter, helping the student to understand what the key learning points will be.

Learning objectives

On completing this chapter you should be able to:

1. Define the word pharmacology.
2. Outline the steps involved in developing and approving a ne
3. Describe the legislative controls on drugs that have abuse po

Chapter openings also include a *glossary of key terms* and a *list of featured drugs.*

Glossary of key terms

adverse effects: drug effects that are not the desired therapeut
brand name: name given to a drug by the pharmaceutical com
chemical name: name that reflects the chemical structure of a
drugs: chemicals that are introduced into the body to bring abo
drugs with the same active ingredient as an orig

SYSTEMIC ANTIFUNGALS

Azole antifungals
fluconazole
itraconazole
posaconazole
voriconazole

Echinocandin antifungals
anidulafungin
caspofungin

Other antifungals
amphotericin B
flucytosine

Key points appear periodically throughout each chapter to summarise important concepts.

KEY POINTS

- Clinical pharmacology is the study of drugs used to treat, diagnose or prevent a disease.
- Drugs are chemicals that are introduced into the body and affect the body's chemical processes.

The text of each chapter ends with a *summary of important concepts.*

CHAPTER SUMMARY

- Drugs are chemicals that are introduced into the body to bring about some sort of change.
- Drugs can come from many sources: plants, animals, inorganic elements and synthetic preparations.

This is followed by a series of review exercises in the *Check your understanding* section, to help focus student learning on the seminal information presented in the chapter. This section assists students in testing their knowledge and preparing for examinations.

CHECK YOUR UNDERSTAND

Answers to the questions in this chapter can be found in Appendix A at the back of this book.

MULTIPLE CHOICE

Select the best response to the following.

1. Laxatives are drugs that are used to:
   a. increase the quantity of wastes excreted.
   b. speed the passage of the intestinal contents through the GI tract.
2. The laxative of ch needed to prevent
   a. senna.
   b. castor oil.
   c. bisacodyl.
   d. magnesium su
3. Cathartic depend
   a. people do not experience sev
   b. chronic laxativ intense stimula

Links to *Laerdal clinical simulations* enable students to link theory to practice, prepare for clinical placement and acquire the knowledge and skills essential for professional practice.

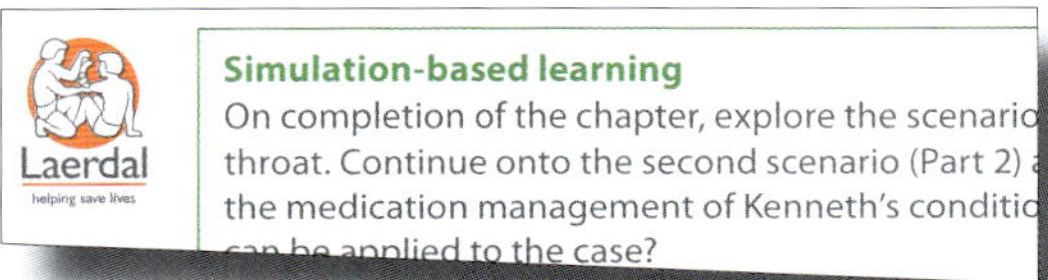

Icons for *Concepts in action* animations depicting pharmacological concepts, *Watch and learn* video clips, *Practice and learn* activities and clinical simulation case studies guide students to online resources to further enhance understanding of complex topics.

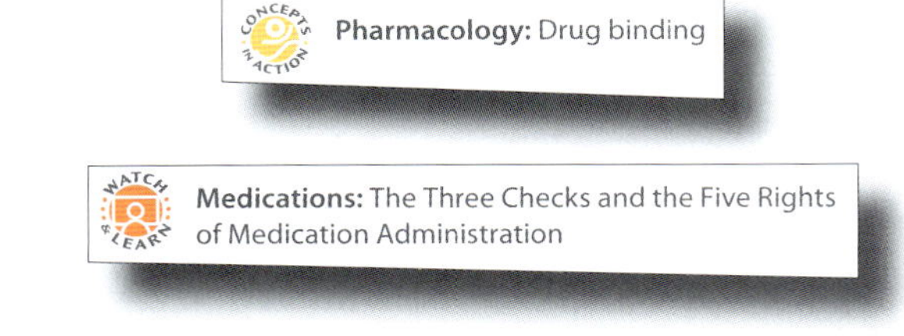

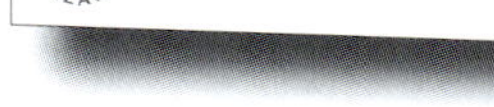

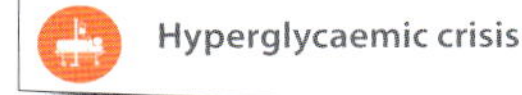

Text highlights

- In the *Care considerations* section of each chapter, italics highlight the rationale for each care intervention, helping the student to apply the information in a clinical situation. Elsewhere in the text, the rationale is consistently provided for therapeutic drug actions, contraindications and adverse effects.

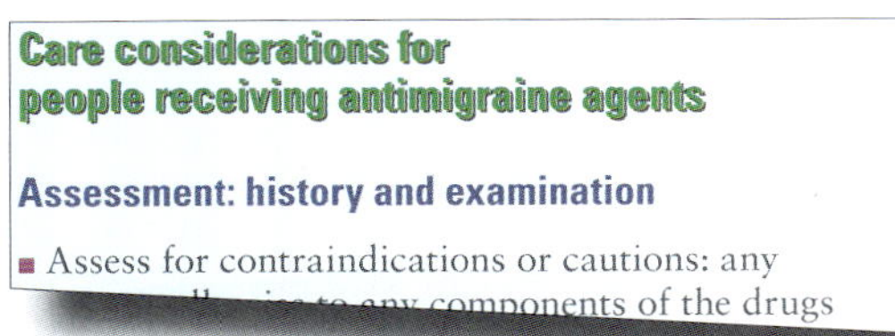

- In the *Drug list* at the beginning of each chapter, a special icon appears next to the drug that is considered the prototype drug of each class. In each chapter, prototype summary boxes spotlight need-to-know information for each prototype drug.

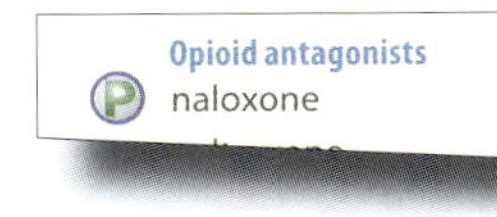

Prototype summary: naloxone

Indications: complete or partial reversal of opioid depression; diagnosis of suspected opioid

- ***Drugs in focus*** tables clearly summarise and identify the drugs within a class, highlighting them by generic and trade names, usual dosage and indications. The icon appears in these tables next to each drug that is considered to be the prototype for its specific class.

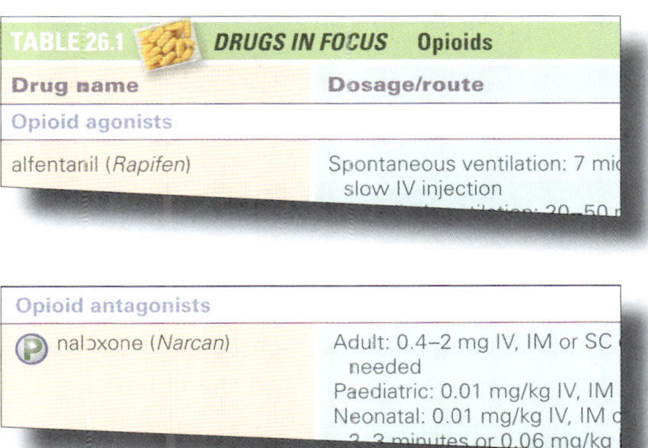

- ***Focus on safe medication administration*** boxes present important safety information to help keep the person safe, prevent medication errors and increase the therapeutic effectiveness of the drugs.

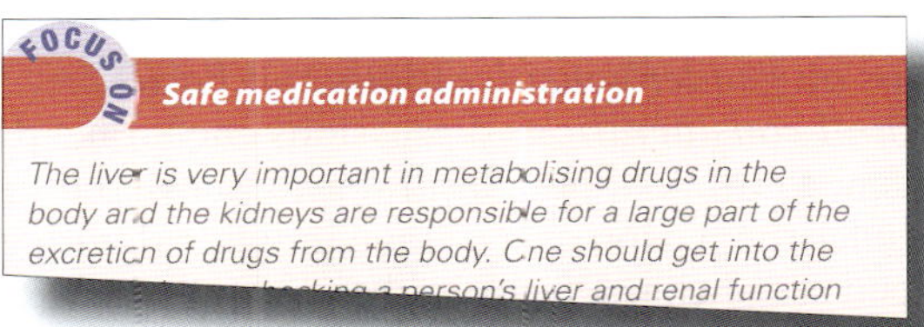

- ***Focus on the evidence*** boxes compile information based on research to identify the best clinical practices associated with specific drug therapy.

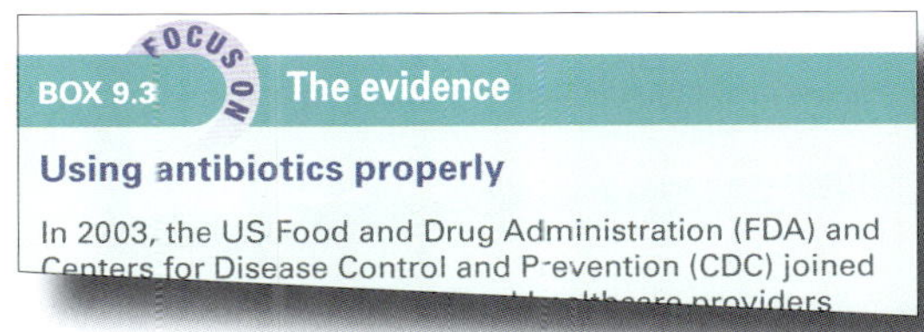

- ***Focus on herbal and alternative therapies*** boxes highlight known interactions with specific herbs or alternative therapies that could affect the actions of the drugs being discussed.

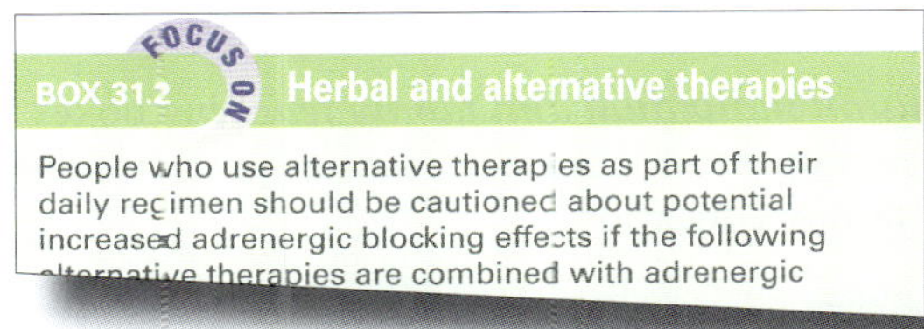

- ***Focus on calculations*** reviews are designed to help the student hone calculation and measurement skills while learning about the drugs for which doses might need to be calculated.

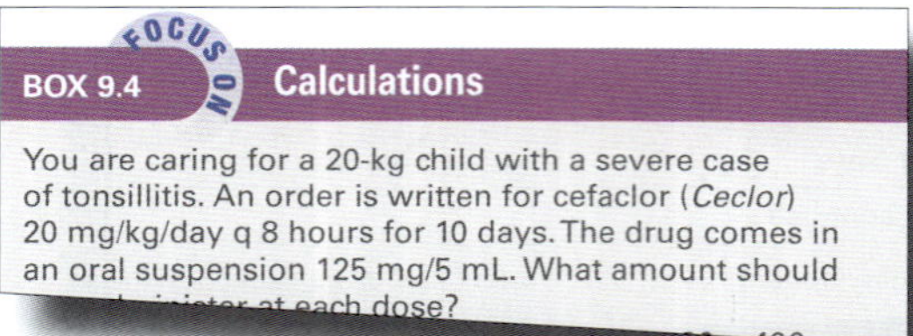
BOX 9.4 FOCUS ON Calculations

You are caring for a 20-kg child with a severe case of tonsillitis. An order is written for cefaclor (*Ceclor*) 20 mg/kg/day q 8 hours for 10 days. The drug comes in an oral suspension 125 mg/5 mL. What amount should

- ***Focus on drug therapy across the lifespan*** boxes concisely summarise points to consider when using the drugs of each class with children, adults, pregnant and breastfeeding women, and the elderly.

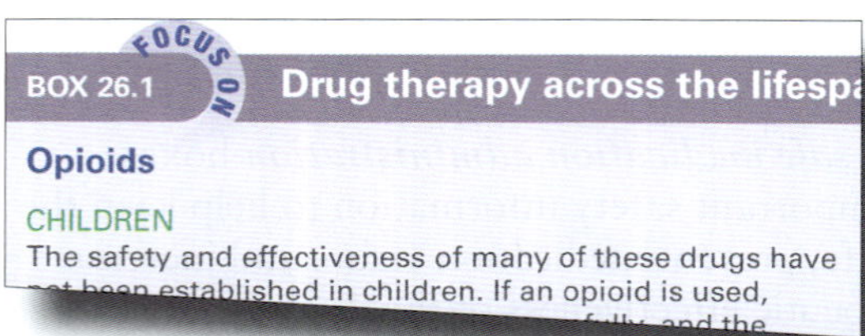
BOX 26.1 FOCUS ON Drug therapy across the lifespa

Opioids

CHILDREN

The safety and effectiveness of many of these drugs have not been established in children. If an opioid is used,

- ***Focus on gender considerations*** and ***Focus on cultural considerations*** discussions encourage the student to think about cultural awareness and to consider the person as a unique individual with a special set of characteristics that not only influences variations in drug effectiveness, but also could influence a person's perspective on drug therapy.

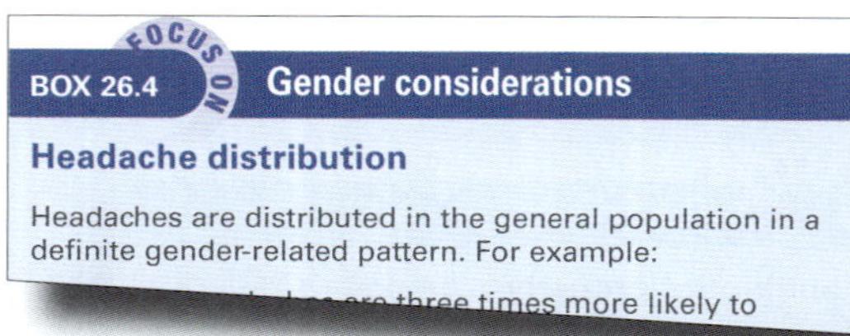
BOX 26.4 FOCUS ON Gender considerations

Headache distribution

Headaches are distributed in the general population in a definite gender-related pattern. For example:

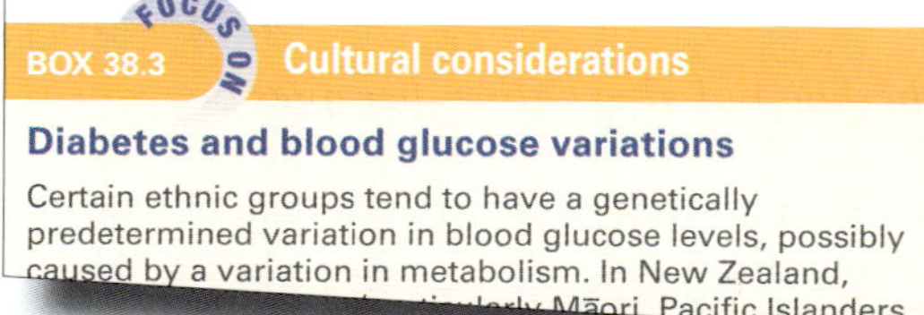
BOX 38.3 FOCUS ON Cultural considerations

Diabetes and blood glucose variations

Certain ethnic groups tend to have a genetically predetermined variation in blood glucose levels, possibly caused by a variation in metabolism. In New Zealand,

- ***Focus on individual and family teaching*** boxes review important points to cover as part of individual and family education.

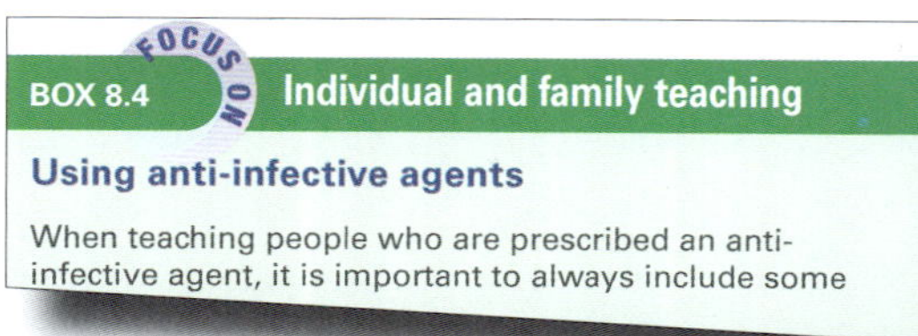
BOX 8.4 FOCUS ON Individual and family teaching

Using anti-infective agents

When teaching people who are prescribed an anti-infective agent, it is important to always include some

- ***Critical thinking scenarios*** tie each chapter's content together by presenting clinical scenarios about a person using a particular drug from the class being discussed. Included in the case study are hints to guide critical thinking about the case and a discussion of drug- and nondrug-related care considerations for that particular person and situation. Most importantly, the case study also provides a plan of care specifically developed for that person.

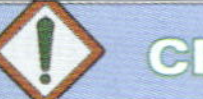 CRITICAL THINKING SCE

Non-selective beta-blockers (pro

THE SITUATION

M.R., a 59-year-old man, has been seen several times complaining of tremor in his hands that eventually made it very difficult for him to work as a computer programmer. A diagnosis of essential tremor was made, and he was prescribed propranolol (*Inderal*) 40 mg twice daily. M.R. had

CRITICAL THIN

Why did M.R. hav measures sho fully and does

What sort of sup going throug about the chil

CARE GUIDE FOR M.R.: PROPRANOLOL

Assessment: history and examination

Review the person's history for allergy to propranolol, HF, shock, bradycardia, heart block, hypotension, COPD, thyroid disease, diabetes, respiratory impairment, and concurrent use of barbiturates, NSAIDs,

The care plan is followed by a checklist of teaching points designed for the person presented in the case study. This approach helps the student to see how assessment and the collected data are applied in the clinical situation.

TEACHING FOR M.R.

- The drug that has been prescribed for you, propranolol, is a non-selective beta adrenergic–blocking agent. This agent works to prevent certain stimulating activities that normally occur in the body in response to such factors as stress, injury or excitement. It stabilises certain nerve

- ***Web links*** alert the student to electronic sources of drug information and sources of drug therapy information for specific diseases.

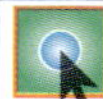 WEB LINKS

Health care providers and students may want to consult the following web resources:

www.anztpa.org
The Australia New Zealand Therapeutic Product Agency (ANZTPA).

A COMPREHENSIVE PACKAGE FOR LEARNING AND TEACHING

Online resources

To further facilitate learning and teaching, an extensive suite of online resources is available for lecturers and students whose institutions have adopted this text. These may be accessed at the text's accompanying website located on thePoint* (http://thePoint.lww.com).

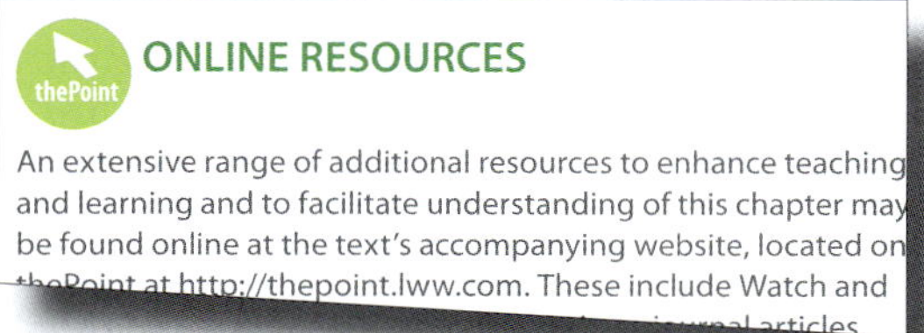

Students can access journal articles, learning objectives and a wide range of concepts in action animations, watch and learn videos, and clinical simulation case studies. Instructors can access journal articles, PowerPoint presentations, image banks, guided lecture notes, case studies, pre-lecture quizzes, assignments, discussion topics and testbank questions.

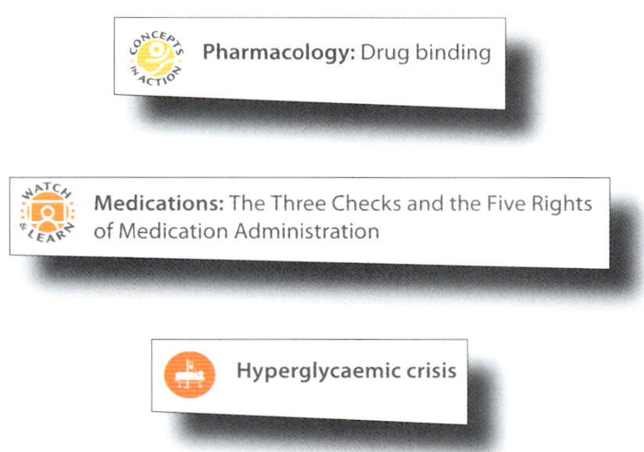

Simulation-based learning

Interactive, simulation-based learning is a vital component in nursing education today. It empowers students to develop their knowledge and skills and to integrate theory with practice in realistic clinical settings, and it offers a rich, content-based immersive learning experience in a risk-free environment. This fully revised edition of *McKenna's Pharmacology for Nursing and Health Professionals* offers students and lecturers an abundant and diverse learning and teaching experience through unique access to Laerdal scenarios.

Wolters Kluwer Health's partnership with leading health care simulation experts **Laerdal** enables this edition to provide references to the Australian and New Zealand Nursing Education scenarios developed by Laerdal Australia, The Council of Deans of Nursing and Midwifery (Australia & New Zealand) and the National League for Nursing.

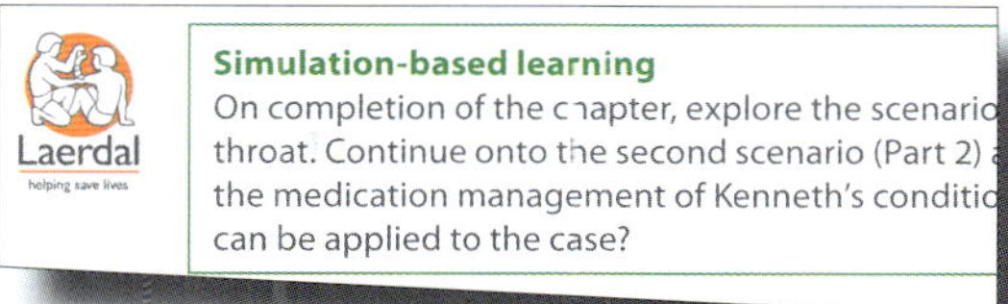

The simulation scenarios address major learning objectives and different levels of complexity. They are pedagogically designed to facilitate acquisition of knowledge and skills in all key aspects of nursing care, from assessment to patient management, prioritisation of patient problems and identification of nursing interventions. The scenarios form the basis of the extensive learning experience that case-based learning in a simulated environment provides to nursing students, enabling them to link theory to practice, prepare for clinical placement and acquire the knowledge and skills essential for professional registration and practice in today's complex health care environment. These scenarios are available to subscribers.

PrepU

PrepU* is an adaptive quizzing engine consisting of a database of calibrated questions, with a difficulty level based on actual student responses. Built by teachers and tested in the classroom, PrepU offers students personalised quizzes that help them learn, and that enable educators to gain insight into student progress. PrepU is available to subscribers.

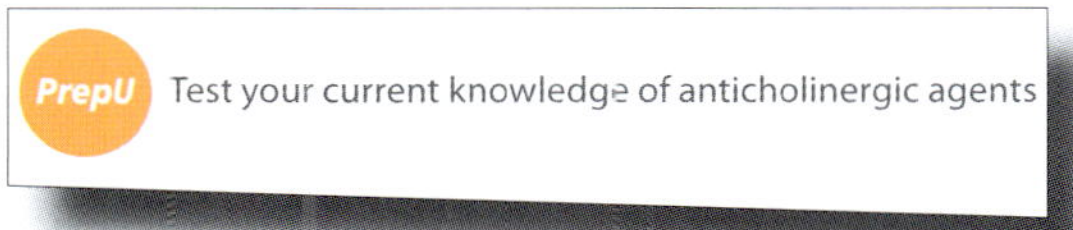

A POWERFUL RESOURCE FOR STUDENTS AND INSTRUCTORS

With this new edition of *McKenna's Pharmacology for Nursing and Health Professionals*, lecturers and students alike can rely on a dynamic teaching and learning resource – a unique combination of the authoritative text, complemented by an extensive suite of resources in every format, all designed to extend the student learner's understanding and to assist the instructor in teaching preparation.

*thePoint and PrepU are trademarks of Wolters Kluwer Health

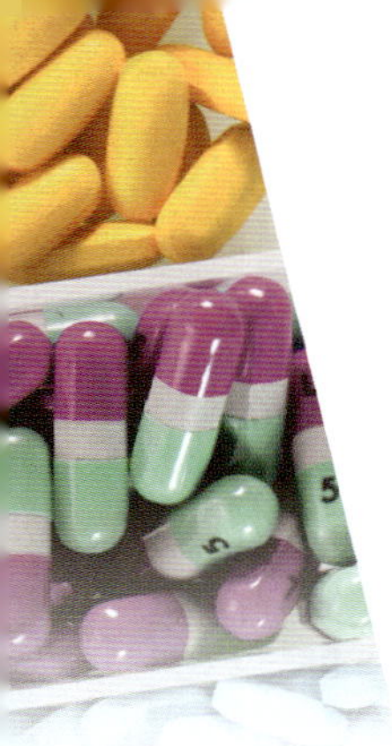

To the student using this text

As you begin your study of pharmacology, don't be overwhelmed or confused by all of the details. The study of drugs fits perfectly into your study of the human body – anatomy, physiology, chemistry, nutrition, psychology and sociology.

Approach the study of pharmacology from the perspective of putting all of the pieces together; this can be not only fun, but also challenging! Work to understand the concepts and all of the details will fall into place and be easy to remember and apply to the clinical situation. This understanding will help you in creating the picture of the whole person as you are learning to provide comprehensive care. This text is designed to help you accomplish all of this in a simple and concise manner. Good luck!

Lisa McKenna and Anecita Gigi Lim

Acknowledgements

Focus on Nursing Pharmacology by Amy Karch provided the foundation for the development of the first edition of this text, which was titled *Pharmacology for Nursing and Midwifery*. We are grateful to Amy for the exciting opportunity to further develop her work in an Australian and New Zealand context in this second edition. Reflecting the local nature, we have been mindful in the adaptation of the needs of nursing, midwifery and other professional health care students.

Pharmacology knowledge is vital for safe and effective nursing and midwifery care. This text aims to provide evidence-based information to support optimal learning and ease of knowledge application to practice for students, and ultimately, to promote high levels of care delivery.

We are grateful to the many reviewers who provided valuable feedback. We are also incredibly thankful to Penny Martin and Caroline Hunter from Wolters Kluwer Health and to the editors at Puddingburn Publishing Services for their continued encouragement, support and guidance across all stages of development.

Finally, we are especially grateful to our respective families, Hayley and Lachlan, and Gerald and Morteza for their patience and support during the process of developing this book.

Lisa McKenna and Anecita Gigi Lim

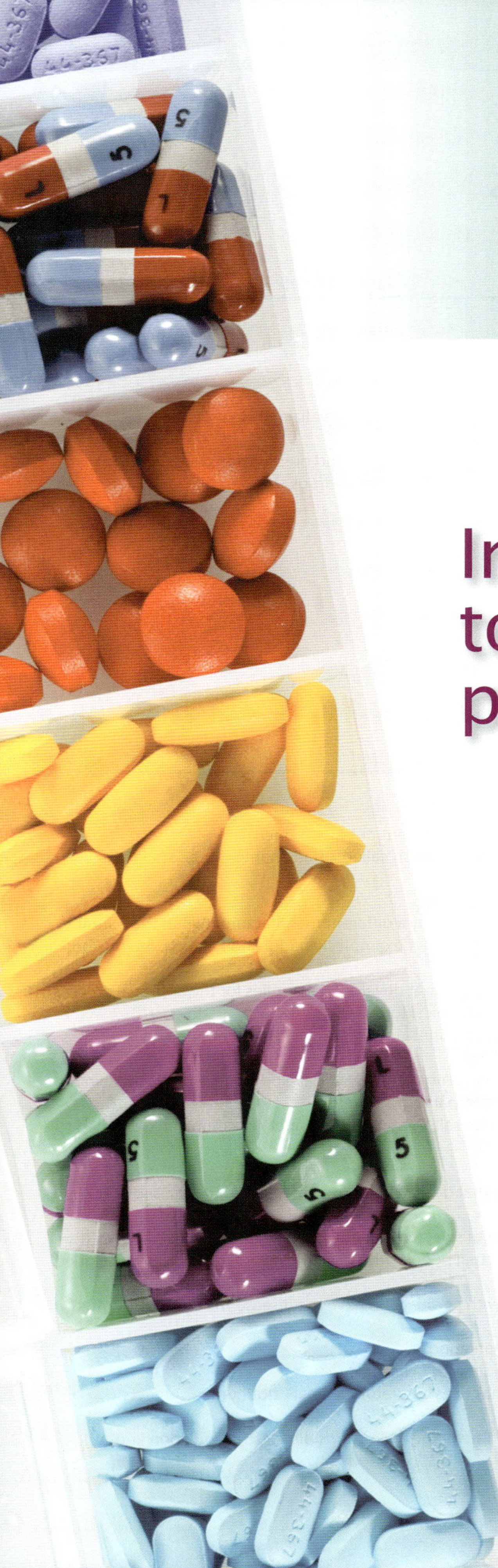

PART 1

Introduction to nursing pharmacology

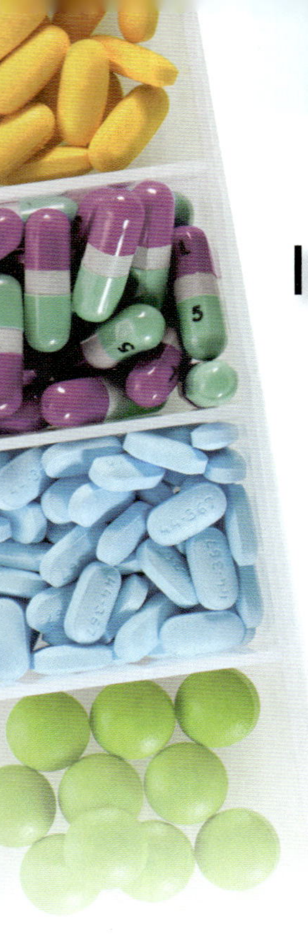

1 Introduction to drugs

Learning objectives

On completing this chapter you should be able to:

1. Define the word pharmacology.
2. Outline the steps involved in developing and approving a new drug in Australia and New Zealand.
3. Describe the legislative controls on drugs that have abuse potential.
4. Differentiate between generic and brand-name drugs, over-the-counter and prescription drugs.
5. Explain the benefits and risks associated with the use of over-the-counter drugs.

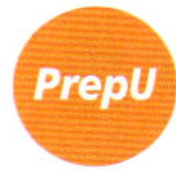

PrepU Test your current knowledge of drugs with a PrepU Practice Quiz!

Glossary of key terms

adverse effects: drug effects that are not the desired therapeutic effects; may be unpleasant or even dangerous
brand name: name given to a drug by the pharmaceutical company that developed it; also called a trade name
chemical name: name that reflects the chemical structure of a drug
drugs: chemicals that are introduced into the body to bring about some sort of change
generic drugs: drugs with the same active ingredient as an originator drug, but made by a different manufacturer (when the patent on the originator drug expires) and with a different brand name from the originator; for example, Panadol and Panamax brands both contain the active ingredient paracetamol.
generic name: the original designation that a drug is given when the drug company that developed it applies for the approval process
genetic engineering: process of altering DNA, usually of bacteria, to produce a chemical to be used as a drug
New Zealand Medicines and Medical Devices Safety Authority (MEDSAFE): a business unit of the Ministry of Health and the authority responsible for the regulation of therapeutic products in New Zealand
orphan drugs: drugs that have been discovered but would not be profitable for a drug company to develop; usually drugs that would treat only a small number of people; these orphans can be adopted by drug companies to develop
over-the-counter (OTC) drugs: drugs that are available without a prescription for self-treatment of a variety of complaints; deemed to be safe when used as directed
pharmacology: the study of the biological effects of chemicals
pharmacotherapeutics: clinical pharmacology – the branch of pharmacology that deals with drugs; chemicals that are used in medicine for the treatment, prevention and diagnosis of disease in humans
phase I study: a pilot study of a potential drug conducted with a small number of selected, healthy human volunteers
phase II study: a clinical study of a proposed drug by selected doctors using actual people who have the disorder the drug is designed to treat; the subjects must provide informed consent
phase III study: use of a proposed drug on a wide scale in the clinical setting with people who have the disease the drug is designed to treat
phase IV study: continual evaluation of a drug after it has been released for marketing
postmarketing surveillance: monitoring the safety of medicines and medical devices in use
preclinical trials: initial trial of a chemical thought to have therapeutic potential; uses laboratory animals, not human subjects
teratogenic: having adverse effects on the fetus
Therapeutic Goods Administration (TGA): Australian Commonwealth Government agency responsible for the regulation and enforcement of drug evaluation and distribution policies

The human body works through a complicated series of chemical reactions and processes. **Pharmacology** is the study of the biological effects of chemicals. **Drugs** are chemicals that are introduced into the body to cause some sort of change. When drugs are administered, the body begins a sequence of processes designed to handle the new chemicals. These processes, which involve breaking down and eliminating the drugs, in turn affect the body's complex series of chemical reactions. In clinical practice, health care providers focus on how chemicals act on living organisms.

Nurses and midwives deal with **pharmacotherapeutics**, or clinical pharmacology, the branch of pharmacology that uses drugs to treat, prevent and diagnose disease. Clinical pharmacology addresses two key concerns: the drug's effects on the body and the body's response to the drug.

For many reasons, understanding how drugs act on the body to cause changes and applying that knowledge in the clinical setting are important aspects of practice. For example, people today often follow complicated drug regimens and receive potentially toxic drugs. Many also manage their care at home. A drug can have many effects, and the nurse or midwife must know which ones may occur when a particular drug is administered. Some drug effects are therapeutic, or helpful, but others are undesirable or potentially dangerous. These negative effects are called **adverse effects**. (See Chapter 3 for a detailed discussion of adverse effects.)

The nurse and midwife are in a unique position regarding drug therapy because care responsibilities include the following:

- Administering drugs
- Assessing drug effects
- Intervening to make the drug regimen more tolerable
- Providing individual and family teaching about drugs and the drug regimen
- Monitoring the overall care plan to prevent medication errors

Knowing how drugs work makes these tasks easier to handle, thus enhancing the effectiveness of drug therapy.

This text is designed to provide the pharmacological basis for understanding drug therapy. The physiology of a body system and the related actions of many drugs on that system are presented in a way that allows clear understanding of how drugs work and what to anticipate when giving a particular type of drug.

Thousands of drugs are available for use, and it is impossible to memorise all the individual differences among drugs in a class. This text addresses *general* drug information. It is useful to refer to *McKenna's Drug Handbook for Nursing and Midwifery* or to another drug guide to obtain *specific* details required for safe and effective drug administration. Drug details are changing constantly. Practising nurses and midwives must be knowledgeable about these changes and rely on an up-to-date and comprehensive drug guide in the clinical setting.

A section related to care considerations for individuals receiving particular drugs can be found in each chapter of this book. This includes assessment points, implementation or particular interventions that should be considered, and evaluation points will provide a guide for using clinical decision making to effectively incorporate drug therapy into care. This information can be used to develop an individual care plan for each individual. The monographs in *McKenna's Drug Handbook for Nursing and Midwifery* can be used to provide the specific information that you need to plan care for each particular drug you might be giving. The various sections of each drug monograph (Figure 1.1) can provide information to help in the development of appropriate teaching guides and drug cards for reference in the clinical setting.

SOURCES OF DRUGS

Drugs are available from varied sources, both natural and synthetic. Natural sources include plants, animals and inorganic compounds.

Natural sources

Chemicals that might prove useful as drugs can come from many natural sources, such as plants, animals or inorganic compounds. To become a drug, a chemical must have a demonstrated therapeutic value or efficacy without severe toxicity or damaging properties.

Plants

Plants and plant parts have been used as medicines since prehistoric times. Even today, plants are an important source of chemicals that are developed into drugs. For example, digitalis products used to treat cardiac disorders and various opiates used for sedation are still derived from plants. Table 1.1 provides examples of drugs derived from plant sources.

Drugs also may be processed using a synthetic version of the active chemical found in a plant. An example of this type of drug is dronabinol, which contains the active ingredient delta-9-tetrahydrocannabinol found in marijuana. This drug helps prevent nausea and vomiting in people with cancer but does not have all the adverse effects that occur when the marijuana leaf is smoked. Marijuana leaf is a controlled substance with high abuse potential and has no legal or accepted medical use. The synthetic version of the active ingredient allows for an accepted form to achieve

nivolumab

Opdivo

Pregnancy risk category D
Use in sport: permitted

AVAILABLE FORMS

Solution for infusion 40 mg/4 mL, 100 mg/10 mL

INDICATIONS & DOSAGES

➤ *Adjuvant treatment for melanoma with involvement of lymph nodes, or metastatic disease that has undergone complete resection*

Adults Initially 1 mg/kg IV over 60 min q3w for first 4 doses in combination with ipilimumab 3 mg/kg IV over 90 min. Followed by single-agent nivolumab therapy at 3 mg/kg IV over 60 min q2w.

IV ADMINISTRATION

- Can be administered with or without dilution.
- Diluted with 0.9% NaCl or 5% dextrose solution to a concentration of 1–10 mg/mL.
- Do not shake solution, gently rotate to combine.
- Inspect solution for particulate matter or discolouration before administering. If present, do not use.
- Transfer solution to sterile glass bottle or PVC, non-PVC or polyolefin container and administer over 60 h.
- Unused solution should be carefully discarded according to local guidelines.

ACTION

Immunological agent: human IgG4 monoclonal antibody. Inhibits signal of programmed death ligand 1 (PD-L1) and PD-L2 that promotes T-cell activation, proliferation and lymphocyte infiltration into tumour cells, resulting in tumour cell death.

Route	Onset	Peak	Half-life
IV	Unknown	Unknown	25 days

ADVERSE REACTIONS

CNS Autoimmune neuropathy, ***encephalitis,*** Guillain–Barré syndrome, dizziness, headache, neuritis, peripheral neuropathy, polyneuropathy.
CV Arrhythmia, atrial fibrillation, hypertension, myocarditis, tachycardia, vasculitis.
ENT Nasal disorder, oropharyngeal pain, sinus congestion.
Eye Blurred vision, dry eye, uveitis.
GI Abdominal pain, colitis, constipation, *diarrhoea,* dry mouth, duodenal ulcer, gastritis, *nausea,* pancreatitis, stomatitis, vomiting.
GU ***Renal failure,*** tubulointerstitial nephritis.
Haematological *Anaemia,* eosinophilia, **leukopenia, lymphopenia, neutropenia, thrombocytopenia.**
Hepatic Cholestatis, *elevated liver enzyme levels,* hepatitis.
Metabolic Dehydration, diabetes mellitus, ***diabetic ketoacidosis,*** *hypercalcaemia, hyperglycaemia, hyperkalaemia, hypermagnesaemia, hypernatraemia,* hyperpituitarism, *hypokalaemia, hypomagnesaemia, hyponatraemia,* hypoglycaemia, hypopituitarism, hyperthyroidism, *hypocalcaemia, hypothyroidism,* ***metabolic acidosis,*** reduced appetite, thyroiditis.
Musculoskeletal *Arthralgia,* arthritis, musculoskeletal pain, myalgia, myopathy, polymyalgia rheumatica, ***rhabdomyolysis,*** spondyloarthropathy.
Psychiatric Anxiety, confusion, decreased libido, depression.
Respiratory Cough, dyspnoea, lung infiltration, pleural effusion, pneumonia, pneumonitis.
Skin Alopecia, dry skin, erythema, erythema multiforme, *pruritus,* psoriasis, *rash,* rosacea, ***Stevens–Johnson syndrome, toxic epidermal necrolysis,*** urticaria, vitiligo.
Other ***Anaphylaxis,*** histiolytic necrotising lymphadenitis, ***hypersensitivity,*** *infusion related reaction.*

INTERACTIONS

None reported.

CONTRAINDICATIONS

Contraindicated in people with hypersensitivity to drug or other component of preparation.

CARE CONSIDERATIONS

- Monitor vital signs, renal function, liver function, blood glucose levels and mental status closely.
- Monitor closely for signs and symptoms of GI events such as alteration in bowel function.
- LFTs, FBC and serum creatinine level test should be performed before starting treatment and regularly throughout.
- Monitor for signs of infection.

PATIENT TEACHING

- Instruct person to report symptoms of hypersensitivity, such as itching, rash, chills or rigors, during and after infusion.
- Urge person to watch for signs and symptoms of infection (fever, sore throat, fatigue) or allergic reaction.
- Caution women to avoid pregnancy during treatment.
- Caution person against driving or operating machinery until drug's effects are known.
- Advise not to take any other drugs or OTC preparations without consulting with medical practitioner.
- Advise that some adverse effects are delayed and may develop weeks or months after completing treatment.

FIGURE 1.1 Example of a drug monograph from *McKenna's Drug Handbook for Nursing and Midwifery* (8th edn).

the desired therapeutic effect in people with cancer. It is only available in Australia through the Australian Government's Special Access Scheme.

Ingestion of a plant-derived food can sometimes lead to a drug effect. For example, the body converts natural liquorice to a false aldosterone – a hormone found in the body – resulting in fluid retention and hypokalaemia (low serum potassium levels) if large amounts of liquorice are eaten. However, people seldom think of liquorice as a drug.

Finally, plants have become the main component of the growing complementary and alternative therapy movement. Chapter 6 discusses this movement and its impact on today's drug regimens.

Animal products

Animal products are used to replace human chemicals that fail to be produced because of disease or genetic problems. Until recently, insulin for treating diabetes was obtained exclusively from the pancreas of cows and

TABLE 1.1 Drugs derived from plants

Plant	Product
Ricinus communis	Seed Oil Castor oil
Digitalis purpurea (foxglove plant)	Leaves Dried leaves Digitalis leaf
Papaver somniferum (poppy plant)	Unripe capsule Juice Opium Morphine (*MS Contin, Ordine*) Codeine Papaverine

pigs. Now **genetic engineering** – the process of altering DNA – permits scientists to produce human insulin by altering *Escherichia coli* bacteria, making insulin a better product without some of the impurities that come with animal products.

Thyroid drugs and growth hormone preparations also may be obtained from animal thyroid and hypothalamic tissues. Many of these preparations are now created synthetically, however, and the synthetic preparations are considered to be purer and safer than preparations derived from animals.

Inorganic compounds

Salts of various chemical elements can have therapeutic effects in the human body. Aluminium, fluoride, iron and even gold are used to treat various conditions. The effects of these elements were usually discovered accidentally when a cause–effect relationship was observed. Table 1.2 shows examples of some elements used for their therapeutic effects.

Synthetic sources

Today, many drugs are developed synthetically after chemicals in plants, animals or the environment have been tested and found to have therapeutic activity. Scientists use genetic engineering to alter bacteria to produce chemicals that are therapeutic and effective. Other technical advances allow scientists to alter a chemical with proven therapeutic effectiveness to make it better. Sometimes, a small change in a chemical's structure can make that chemical more useful as a drug – more potent, more stable, less toxic. These technological advances have led to the development of groups of similar drugs, all of which are derived from an original prototype, but each of which has slightly different properties, making a particular drug more desirable in a specific situation. Throughout this book, the icon (P) will be used to designate drugs of a class that are considered the prototype of the class, the original drug in the class or the drug that has emerged as the most effective. For example, the cefalosporins are a large group of antibiotics derived from the same chemical structure. Alterations in the chemical rings or attachments to that structure make it possible for some of these drugs to be absorbed orally, whereas others must be given parenterally. Some of these drugs cause severe toxic effects (eg, renal toxicity), but others do not.

TABLE 1.2 Elements used for their therapeutic effects

Element	Therapeutic use
Aluminium	Antacid to decrease gastric acidity Management of hyperphosphataemia Prevention of the formation of phosphate urinary stones
Fluorine (as fluoride)	Prevention of dental cavities Prevention of osteoporosis
Gold	Treatment of rheumatoid arthritis
Iron	Treatment of iron deficiency anaemia

KEY POINTS

- Clinical pharmacology is the study of drugs used to treat, diagnose or prevent a disease.
- Drugs are chemicals that are introduced into the body and affect the body's chemical processes.
- Drugs can come from plants, foods, animals, salts of inorganic compounds or synthetic sources.

DRUG EVALUATION

After a chemical that might have therapeutic value is identified, it must undergo a series of scientific tests to evaluate its actual therapeutic and toxic effects. This process is tightly controlled by the **Therapeutic Goods Administration** (**TGA**), an agency of the Australian Government Department of Health that regulates the development and sale of drugs. TGA-regulated tests are designed to ensure the safety and reliability of any drug approved in this country. For every 100,000 chemicals that are identified as being potential drugs, only about five end up being marketed. Before receiving final TGA

TABLE 1.3 Comparison of generic, chemical, and brand names of drugs

thyroxine sodium	←	**generic name**	→	poractant alfa
L-thyroxine, T_4	←	**chemical name**	→	dipalmitoylphosphatidylcholine
Eutroxsig, Oroxine	←	**brand names**	→	*Curosurf*

approval to be marketed to the public, drugs must pass through several stages of development. These include **preclinical trials** and phase I, II and III studies. The drugs listed in this book have been through rigorous testing and are approved for sale to the public, either with or without a prescription from a health care provider.

In New Zealand, the **New Zealand Medicines and Medical Devices Safety Authority (MEDSAFE)** is responsible for administering the Medicines Act 1981 and Regulations 1984. MEDSAFE is responsible for applying a framework of controls designed to ensure that the therapeutic products available in New Zealand are those that can be expected to have greater benefits than risks if used appropriately. This is achieved through the premarketing and the **postmarketing surveillance** processes that are set-up by the Ministry of Health.

The premarket approval system for medicines is managed by MEDSAFE. The subsidisation of medicines is managed by PHARMAC (the Pharmaceutical Management Agency). PHARMAC is a Crown Entity whose primary objective is to secure, for eligible people in need of pharmaceuticals, the best health outcomes that are reasonably achievable from pharmaceutical treatment from within the funding provided. MEDSAFE and PHARMAC work independently, and MEDSAFE is not involved in funding issues. Postmarketing surveillance monitors the safety of medicines and medical devices in use. Products shown to be unsafe are removed from use, and prescribers are advised about new safety information for products.

Preclinical trials

In preclinical trials, chemicals that may have therapeutic value are tested on laboratory animals for two main purposes: (1) to determine whether they have the presumed effects in living tissue, and (2) to evaluate any adverse effects. Animal testing is important because unique biological differences can cause very different reactions to the chemical. These differences can be found only in living organisms, so computer-generated models alone are often inadequate.

At the end of the preclinical trials, some chemicals are discarded for the following reasons:

- The chemical lacks therapeutic activity when used with living animals.
- The chemical is too toxic to living animals to be worth the risk of developing into a drug.
- The chemical is highly **teratogenic** (causing adverse effects to the fetus).
- The safety margins are so small that the chemical would not be useful in the clinical setting.

Some chemicals, however, are found to have therapeutic effects and reasonable safety margins. This means that the chemicals are therapeutic at doses that are reasonably different from doses that cause toxic effects. Such chemicals will pass the preclinical trials and advance to phase I studies.

Phase I studies

A **phase I study** uses human volunteers to test the drugs. These studies are more tightly controlled than preclinical trials and are performed by specially trained clinical investigators. The volunteers are fully informed of possible risks and may be paid for their participation. Usually, the volunteers are healthy young men. Women are not good candidates for phase I studies because the chemicals may exert unknown and harmful effects on a woman's ova, and too much risk is involved in taking a drug that might destroy or alter the ova. Women do not make new ova after birth. Men produce sperm daily, so there is less potential for complete destruction or alteration of sperm.

Some chemicals are therapeutic in other animals but have no effects in humans. Investigators in phase I studies scrutinise the drugs being tested for effects in humans. They also look for adverse effects and toxicity. At the end of phase I studies, many chemicals are dropped from the process for the following reasons:

- They lack therapeutic effect in humans.
- They cause unacceptable adverse effects.
- They are highly teratogenic.
- They are too toxic.

Some chemicals move to the next stage of testing despite undesirable effects. For example, the antihypertensive drug minoxidil (*Loniten*) was found to effectively treat malignant hypertension, but it caused unusual hair growth on the palms and other body areas. However, because it was so much more effective for treating malignant hypertension at the time of its development than any other antihypertensive drug, it proceeded to phase II studies. (Now, its hair-growing effect has been channelled for therapeutic use into various hair-growth preparations such as *Rogaine*.)

Phase II studies

A **phase II study** allows clinical investigators to try out the drug on individuals who have the disease that the drug is designed to treat. People are told about the possible benefits of the drug and are invited to participate in the study. Those who consent to participate are fully informed about possible risks and are monitored very closely, often at no charge to them, to evaluate the drug's effects. Usually, phase II studies are performed at various sites across the country – in hospitals, clinics and doctors' offices – and are monitored by representatives of the pharmaceutical company studying the drug. At the end of phase II studies, a drug may be removed from further investigation for the following reasons:

- It is less effective than anticipated.
- It is too toxic when used with people.
- It produces unacceptable adverse effects.
- It has a low benefit-to-risk ratio, meaning that the therapeutic benefit it provides does not outweigh the risk of potential adverse effects that it causes.
- It is no more effective than other drugs already on the market, making the cost of continued research and production less attractive to the drug company.

A drug that continues to show promise as a therapeutic agent receives additional scrutiny in phase III studies.

Phase III studies

A **phase III study** involves use of the drug in a vast clinical market. Prescribers are informed of all the known reactions to the drug and precautions required for its safe use. Prescribers observe individuals very closely, monitoring them for any adverse effects. Sometimes, prescribers ask people to keep journals and record any symptoms they experience. Prescribers then evaluate the reported effects to determine whether they are caused by the disease or by the drug. This information is collected by the drug company that is developing the drug and is shared with the TGA. When a drug is used widely, totally unexpected responses may occur. A drug that produces unacceptable adverse effects or unforeseen reactions is usually removed from further study by the drug company. In some cases, the TGA may have to request that a drug be removed from the market.

Therapeutic Goods Administration approval

Drugs that finish phase III studies are evaluated by the TGA, which relies on committees of experts familiar with the specialty area in which the drugs will be used. Only drugs that receive TGA committee approval may be marketed. Figure 1.2 recaps the various phases of drug development discussed.

An approved drug is given a **brand name** (trade name) by the pharmaceutical company that developed it. The **generic name** of a drug is the original designation that the drug was given when the drug company applied for the approval process. **Chemical names** are names that reflect the chemical structure of a drug. Some drugs are known by all three names. It can be confusing to study drugs when so many different names are used for the same compound. In this text, the generic and chemical names always appear in straight print, and the brand name is always italicised (eg, minoxidil *[Rogaine]*). Table 1.3 compares examples of drug names.

The entire drug development and approval process can take 5–6 years, resulting in a so-called drug lag in Australia and New Zealand. In some instances, a drug that is available in another country may not become available here for years. The TGA regards public safety as primary in drug approval, so the process remains strict; however, it can be accelerated in certain instances involving the treatment of deadly diseases. For example, some drugs (eg, delavirdine [*Rescriptor*] and efavirenz [*Stocrin*]) that were thought to offer a benefit to individuals with acquired immune deficiency syndrome (AIDS), a potentially fatal immune disorder, were pushed through because of the progressive nature of AIDS and

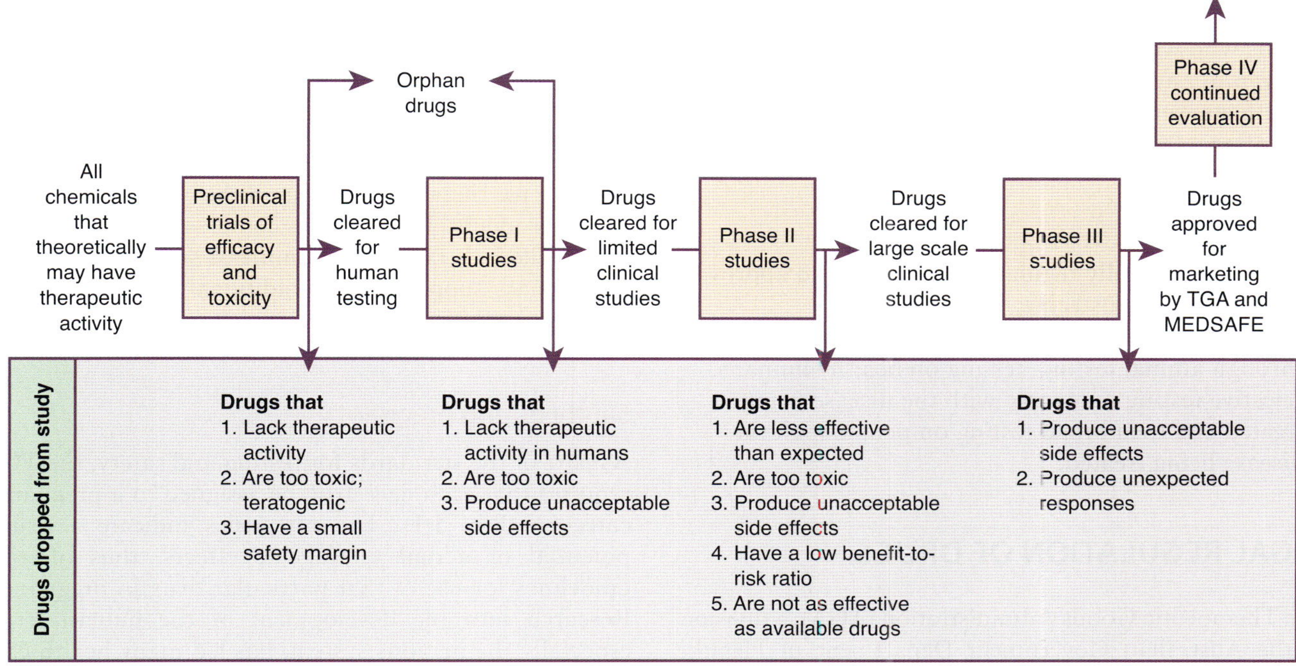

FIGURE 1.2 Phases of drug development.

the lack of a cure. All literature associated with these drugs indicates that long-term effects and other information about the drug may not yet be known.

In addition to the drug lag issue, there also are concerns about the high cost of drug approval. In 2011, *Morgan et al.* published a systematic review on the costs of drug development. These authors found that the estimated cost of taking a chemical from discovery to marketing as a drug could be as high as $US 1.8 billion. Because of this kind of financial investment, pharmaceutical companies are unwilling to risk approval of a drug that might cause serious problems and prompt lawsuits.

Phase IV studies

After a drug is approved for marketing, it enters a phase of continual evaluation, or **phase IV study**. Prescribers are obligated to report to the TGA any untoward or unexpected adverse effects associated with drugs they are using, and the TGA continually evaluates this information. Some drugs cause unexpected effects that are not seen until wide distribution occurs. Sometimes, those effects are therapeutic. For example, individuals taking the antiparkinsonism drug amantadine (*Symmetrel*) were found to have fewer cases of influenza than other people, leading to the discovery that amantadine is an effective antiviral agent.

In other instances, the unexpected effects are dangerous. In 1997 the diet drug dexfenfluramine (*Ponderax*) was removed from the market only months after its release because people taking it developed serious heart problems. In 2004, the drug company Merck withdrew its cyclo-oxygenase-2 (Cox-2) specific non-steroidal anti-inflammatory drug rofecoxib (*Vioxx*) from the market when postmarketing studies seemed to show a significant increase in cardiovascular mortality in individuals who were taking the drug. These problems were not seen in any of the premarketing studies of the drug. The effects were only seen with a much wider use of the drug after it had been marketed.

KEY POINTS

- The TGA carefully regulates the testing and approval of all drugs in Australia.
- To be approved for marketing, a drug must pass through animal testing, testing on healthy humans, selective testing on people with the disease being treated and then broad testing on people with the disease being treated.

LEGAL REGULATION OF DRUGS

The Therapeutic Goods Administration (TGA), a division of the Australian Government Department of Health, is responsible for administering the provisions of the *Therapeutic Goods Act 1989* in Australia that regulates the manufacture, availability and supply of drugs. Each state and territory also has Acts and Regulations that deal with control and administration of drugs. In most cases, the strictest law is the one that prevails. Nurses and midwives should become familiar with the rules and regulations in the area in which they practise. They have a professional responsibility to be informed of the legislation underpinning administration and supply of drugs.

MEDSAFE is New Zealand's Medicines and Medical Devices Safety Authority. MEDSAFE is a business unit of the Ministry of Health (Acts and Regulations; Medicine Management) and is the authority responsible for the regulation of therapeutic products in New Zealand. This includes medicines, related products, herbal medicines, medical devices, controlled drugs used as medicines, etc, through the *Medicines Act 1981* and *Medicines Regulations 1984*, and parts of the *Misuse of Drugs Act 1975* and *Misuse of Drugs Regulations 1977*. The overall objective of these Acts is to ensure the quality, safety and efficacy of therapeutic goods, including medicines and medical devices, available to the Australian and New Zealand public.

The Australian and New Zealand Governments are currently working to harmonise the regulatory arrangements for therapeutic products between both countries. Both governments signed a Treaty in Wellington in December 2003 to establish a single, bi-national agency to regulate therapeutic products, including medical devices and prescription medicines, and over-the-counter, complementary and alternative medicines. Transition to the new agency, Australia New Zealand Therapeutic Products Agency (ANZTPA) is underway. This agency will eventually replace the Australian TGA and the New Zealand MEDSAFE, will be accountable to both Australian and New Zealand Governments and will have a fully functional office in both countries. Under the joint Australia–New Zealand therapeutic products agency (the joint agency), products represented as being for therapeutic use are to be regulated as therapeutic products. This includes complementary medicines such as herbal, vitamin and mineral supplements, other nutritional supplements, traditional medicines and aromatherapy oils. Table 1.4 provides a summary of Australian and New Zealand legislation around medications.

Safety during pregnancy

As part of the standards for testing and safety, the TGA requires that each new drug be assigned to a pregnancy category (Box 1.1). The categories indicate a drug's potential or actual teratogenic effects, thus offering guidelines for use of that particular drug in pregnancy. Research into the development of the human fetus, especially the nervous system, has led many health care providers to recommend that no drug should be used

TABLE 1.4 Australian and New Zealand legislation affecting the clinical use of drugs

Commonwealth of Australia	Therapeutic Goods Act 1989 Therapeutic Goods Regulation National Health Act 1953 Narcotic Drugs Act 1967
Australian Capital Territory	Drugs of Dependence Act 1989 Drugs of Dependence Regulations Poisons and Drugs Act 1978 Poisons Act 1933 Poisons Regulations
New South Wales	Poisons and Therapeutic Goods Act 1966 Poisons and Therapeutic Goods Regulation 2002
Northern Territory	Poisons and Dangerous Drugs Act 2007 Poisons and Dangerous Drugs Regulations
Queensland	Health Act 1937 Health (Drugs and Poisons) Regulation 1996
South Australia	Controlled Substances Act 1984 Controlled Substances (Poisons) Regulations 1996
Tasmania	Poisons Act 1971 Poisons Regulations
Victoria	Drugs, Poisons and Controlled Substances Act 1981 Drugs, Poisons and Controlled Substances Regulations 2006
Western Australia	Poisons Act 1964 Poisons Regulations
New Zealand	Medicines Act 1981 Medicines Act Amended 2005 Medicine Regulations 1984 Misuse of Drugs Act 1975 Misuse of Drugs Regulation

during pregnancy because of potential effects on the developing fetus. In cases in which a drug is needed, it is recommended that the drug of choice be one for which the benefit outweighs the potential risk.

Drugs and poisons schedules

In 2003, the Australian Health Minister's Advisory Council established categories for ranking the abuse potential of various drugs and management of poisons in the Uniform Scheduling of Drugs and Poisons. There are nine schedules under which drugs are classified. Box 1.2 contains descriptions of each category or schedule. Those of specific relevance to nurses and midwives are schedules 2, 3, 4, 8 and occasionally 9. It is important that all health professionals involved in dispensing, prescribing and administering medicines are aware of their responsibilities in regard to each of the relevant schedules.

Each prescriber has a prescriber number, which allows for monitoring of prescription patterns and possible abuse.

BOX 1.1 Australian Drug Evaluation Committee (ADEC) – Classification of drugs in pregnancy

Category	Description
A	These drugs have been taken by a large number of pregnant women without identified risk to the fetus.
B1	These drugs have been taken by limited numbers of women without evidence of increased fetal malformation. Animal studies have not indicated a higher than normal incidence of fetal impairment.
B2	These drugs have been taken by limited numbers of women without evidence of increased fetal malformation or other harmful effect. Animal studies are inadequate. There are no data to suggest increased risk.
B3	These drugs have been taken by limited numbers of women without evidence of increased fetal malformation or other harmful effect. Animal studies have shown increased incidence of fetal effects.
C	These drugs have caused or been suspected to cause fetal or neonatal effects, but the effects are often reversible and not congenital malformations.
D	These drugs have caused, or have been suspected as causing, fetal malformation or irreversible damage.
X	These drugs are not recommended for use in pregnancy due to a high risk of causing permanent damage to the fetus.

Taken from Dempsey et al. p.749

Nurses and midwives should be familiar with not only the guidelines for controlled substances, but also the local policies and procedures within their state, territory or even their workplace, which might be even more rigorous.

Generic drugs

When a drug receives approval for marketing from the TGA, the drug formula is given a time-limited patent, in much the same way as an invention is patented. The length of time for which the patent is extant depends on the type of chemical involved. When the patent runs out on a brand-name drug, the drug can be produced by other manufacturers. **Generic drugs** are chemicals that are produced by companies involved solely in the manufacturing of drugs. Their pharmacological effects are exactly the same as those of their brand name counterparts, and clinical trials to demonstrate comparable quality, clinical efficacy and safety are not required. Because they do not have the research, the advertising or, sometimes, the quality control departments that

BOX 1.2 Uniform scheduling of drugs and poisons in Australia

Schedule		Description
1		This schedule is left blank
2	Pharmacy medicine	Substances available from pharmacies, or from people licensed to sell these drugs
3	Pharmacist only medicine	Substances that require professional advice but are available from a pharmacist
4	Prescription available	Substances that are prescribed by a person permitted under state or territory legislation to prescribe, and only medicine from a pharmacy by prescription
5	Caution	Hazardous substances that are available to the public but require care with handling
6	Poison	Substances that are readily available to the public but are more hazardous, requiring strong warnings
7	Dangerous poison	Substances that are highly harmful and require special manufacture, handling and use precautions
8	Controlled drug	Substances with potential for dependence
9	Prohibited substance	Substances that are prohibited due to the potential for abuse; use is limited to approved medical or scientific research purposes

Taken from Dempsey et al. p.748

pharmaceutical companies have, they can produce the generic drugs more cheaply. In the past, some quality-control problems were found with generic products. For example, the binders used in a generic drug might not be the same as those used in the brand-name product. As a result, the way the body breaks down and uses the generic drug may differ from that of the brand-name product. In that case, the bioavailability of the drug is different from that of the brand name product.

It is often recommended that a drug be dispensed in the generic form if one is available. This requirement helps to keep down the cost of drugs and health care. Some prescribers, however, specify that a drug prescription be 'dispensed as written' (DAW), that is, that the brand-name product be used. By doing so, the prescriber ensures the quality control and the action and effect expected with that drug. These elements may be most important in drugs that have narrow safety margins, such as digoxin (*Lanoxin*), a heart drug, and warfarin (*Coumadin*), an anticoagulant. The initial cost may be higher, but some prescribers believe that, in the long run, the cost to the individual will be less.

Orphan drugs

Orphan drugs are drugs that have been discovered but are not financially viable and therefore have not been 'adopted' by any drug company. Orphan drugs may be useful in treating a rare disease or they may have potentially dangerous adverse effects. Orphan drugs are often abandoned after preclinical trials or phase I studies. Some drugs in this book have orphan drug uses listed. More information about orphan drugs, and current listings, can be found at www.tga.gov.au/industry/pm-orphan-drugs.htm.

Over-the-counter drugs

Over-the-counter (OTC) drugs are products that are available without prescription for self-treatment of a variety of complaints. Some of these agents were approved as prescription drugs but later were found to be very safe and useful for individuals without the need of a prescription. Some were not rigorously screened and tested by the current drug evaluation protocols because they were developed and marketed before the current laws were put into effect. Many of these drugs were 'grandfathered' into use because they had been used for so long. The TGA is currently testing the effectiveness of many of these products and, in time, will evaluate all of them. Although OTC drugs have been found to be safe when taken as directed, nurses and midwives should consider several problems related to OTC drug use:

- Taking these drugs could mask signs and symptoms of underlying disease, making diagnosis difficult.
- Taking these drugs with prescription medications could result in drug interactions and interfere with drug therapy.
- Not taking these drugs as directed could result in serious overdoses.

Many people do not consider OTC drugs to be medications and therefore do not report their use. Nurses and midwives must always include specific questions about OTC drug use when taking a drug history and should provide information in all drug-teaching protocols about avoiding OTC drug use while taking prescription drugs.

KEY POINTS

- Generic drugs are drugs no longer protected by patent and can be produced by companies other than the one that developed them.
- OTC drugs are available without a prescription and are deemed safe when used as directed.
- Orphan drugs are drugs that have been discovered but are not financially viable because they have a limited market or a narrow margin of safety. These drugs may have then been adopted for development by a drug company in exchange for tax incentives.

SOURCES OF DRUG INFORMATION

The fields of pharmacology and drug therapy change so quickly that it is important to have access to sources of information about drug doses, therapeutic and adverse effects and nursing-related implications. Textbooks provide valuable background and basic information to help in the understanding of pharmacology, but in clinical practice it is important to have access to up-to-the-minute information. Several sources of drug information are readily available. Nurses and midwives often need to consult more than one source.

Drug labels

Drug labels have specific information that identifies a specific drug. For example, a drug label identifies the brand and generic names for the drug, the drug dosage, the expiration date and special drug warnings. Some labels also indicate the route and dose for administration. Figure 1.3 illustrates an example of a drug label.

Understanding how to read a drug label is essential. Nurses and midwives need to become familiar with each aspect of the label.

Package inserts

All drugs come with a package insert prepared by the manufacturer according to strict TGA regulations. The package insert contains all the chemical and study information that led to the drug's approval. Package inserts sometimes are difficult to understand and are almost always in very small print, making them difficult to read. The TGA (www.tga.gov.au), MEDSAFE (www.medsafe.govt.nz) and New Zealand Formulary websites are good resources for finding the prescribing information or package insert for most drugs.

Reference books

A wide variety of reference books are available for drug information. The *Monthly Index of Medical Supplements* (MIMS) is a compilation of package insert information from drugs used in Australia. As the content can be quite technical, the book may be difficult to use.

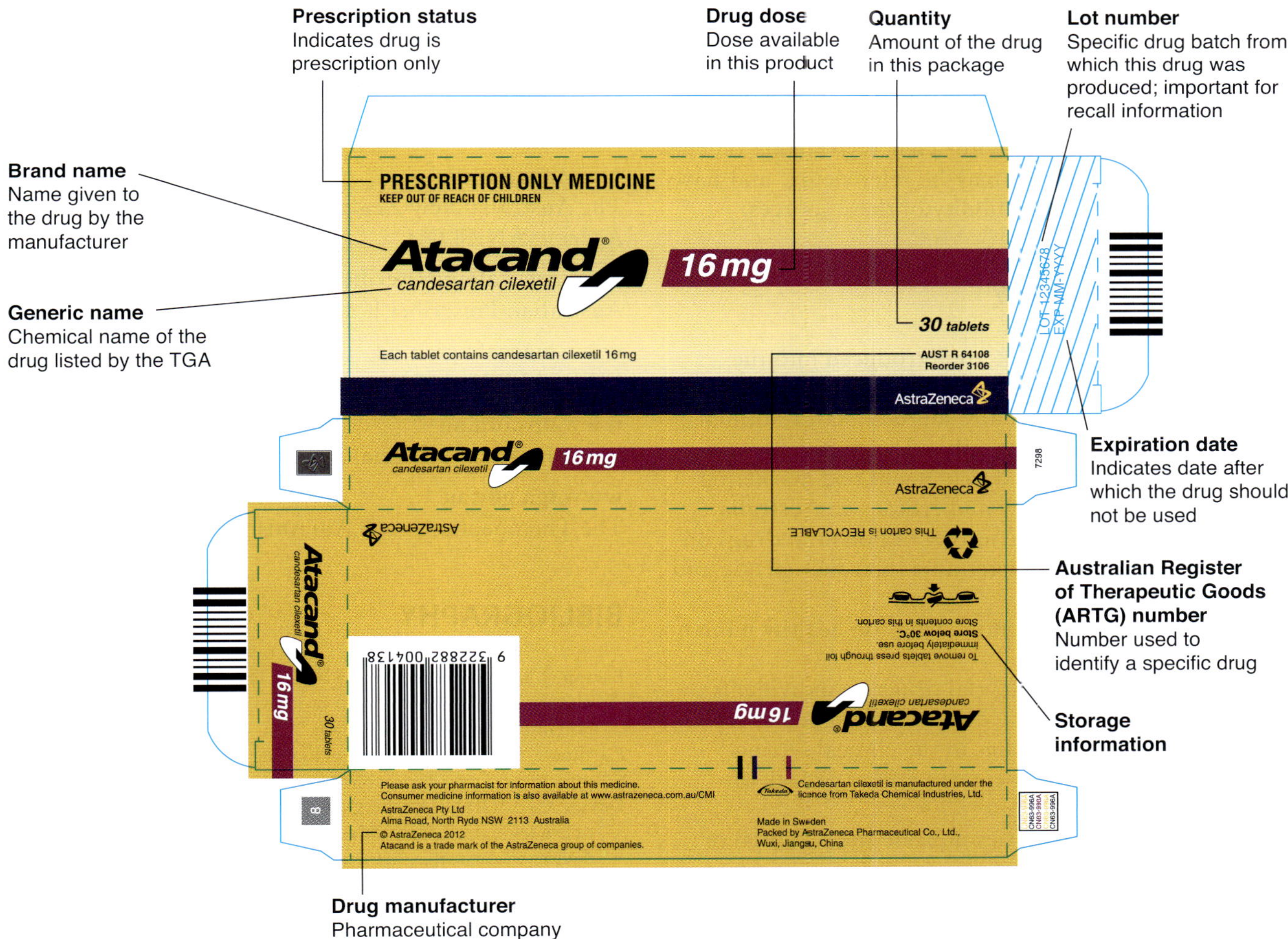

FIGURE 1.3 A sample drug label. (Used with permission from AstraZeneca Pty Ltd.)

Therapeutic Guidelines provides a wide range of drug information in a series of systematic guides, such as antibiotics and gastrointestinal pharmacology. These guidelines draw upon a range of evaluated literature and research.

McKenna's Drug Handbook for Nursing and Midwifery has drug monographs organised alphabetically and includes care implications and important teaching points specifically relevant to nursing and midwifery practice.

Numerous other drug handbooks are also on the market and readily available for nurses and midwives to use.

Journals

Various journals can be used to obtain drug information. For example, the *Medical Letter* is a monthly review of new drugs, drug classes and specific treatment protocols. Many clinical nursing and midwifery journals offer information on new drugs, drug errors and care implications. *Australian Prescriber* is a useful source of easily interpreted pharmacology information and is freely available online.

Online information

Many individuals now use the Internet as a source of medical information and advice. Nurses and midwives need to become familiar with what is available on the Internet and what people may be referencing, and have skills in critiquing the credibility of these sources.

CHAPTER SUMMARY

- Drugs are chemicals that are introduced into the body to bring about some sort of change.
- Drugs can come from many sources: plants, animals, inorganic elements and synthetic preparations.
- The TGA regulates the development and marketing of drugs to ensure safety and efficacy in Australia.
- Preclinical trials involve testing of potential drugs on laboratory animals to determine their therapeutic and adverse effects.
- Phase I studies test potential drugs on healthy human subjects.
- Phase II studies test potential drugs on individuals who have the disease the drugs are designed to treat.
- Phase III studies test drugs in the clinical setting to determine any unanticipated effects or lack of effectiveness.
- TGA pregnancy categories indicate the potential or actual teratogenic effects of a drug.
- Generic drugs are sold under their chemical names, not brand names; they may be cheaper but are not necessarily as safe as brand-name drugs.
- Orphan drugs are chemicals that have been discovered to have some therapeutic effect but that are not financially advantageous to develop into drugs.
- OTC drugs are available without prescription for the self-treatment of various complaints.
- Information about drugs can be obtained from a variety of sources, including the drug label, reference books, journals and Internet sites.

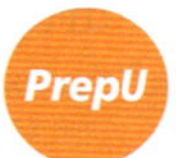

Knowing your strengths and weaknesses helps you to study more effectively. Take a PrepU Practice Quiz to find out how you measure up!

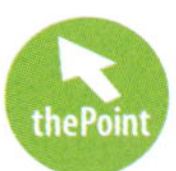

ONLINE RESOURCES

An extensive range of additional resources to enhance teaching and learning and to facilitate understanding of this chapter may be found online at the text's accompanying website, located on thePoint at http://thepoint.lww.com. These include Watch and Learn videos, Concepts in Action animations, journal articles, review questions, case studies, discussion topics and quizzes.

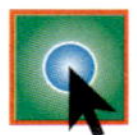

WEB LINKS

Health care providers and students may want to consult the following web resources:

www.anztpa.org
The Australia New Zealand Therapeutic Product Agency (ANZTPA).

www.australianprescriber.com
Australian Prescriber home page.

www.medsafe.govt.nz
MEDSAFE New Zealand.

www.nps.org.au
MedicineWise, National Prescribing Service.

www.tga.gov.au
The Therapeutic Goods Administration.

BIBLIOGRAPHY

Barton, J. H. & Emanuel, E. J. (2005). The patient-based pharmaceutical development process: rationale, problems and potential reforms. *JAMA, 294,* 2075–2082.

Cardinale, V. (1998). Consumers looking for more answers, clearer directions. *Drug Topics Supplement, 142*(11), 23a.

Davies, C. A. (2004). Keeping advertisers honest—An overview of the regulation of the advertising of medicines and medical devices in Australia. *Australian Prescriber, 27,* 124–127.

Dempsey, J., Hillege, S. & Hill, R. (2014). *Fundamentals of Nursing and Midwifery: A Person-centred Approach to Care* (2nd Australian and New Zealand edn). Sydney: Lippincott Williams & Wilkins.

Drug Enforcement Agency. (2000). *Guidelines for prescription of narcotics for physicians*. Washington, DC: U.S. Government Printing Office.

Gilman, A., Hardman, J. G. & Limbird, L. E. (Eds). (2006). *Goodman and Gilman's the Pharmacological Basis of Therapeutics* (11th edn). New York: McGraw-Hill.

Koo, M. M., Krass, I. & Aslani, P. (2003). Factors influencing consumer use of written drug information. *Annals of Pharmacotherapy, 37*(2), 259–267.

Kuo, G. M. (2003). Pharmacodynamic basis of herbal medications. *Annals of Pharmacotherapy, 37*(2), 308.

McKenna, L. & Mirkov, S. (2019). *McKenna's Drug Handbook for Nursing and Midwifery* (8th edn). Sydney: Wolters Kluwer Health Australia.

Morgan, S., Grootendorst, P., Lexchin, J., Cunningham, C. & Greyson, D. (2011). The cost of drug development: A systematic review. *Health Policy, 100*(1), 4–17.

Sun, S. X., Lee, K. Y., Bertram, C. T. & Goldstein, J. L. (2007). Withdrawal of COX-2 selective inhibitors rofecoxib and valdecoxib: Impact on NSAID and gastroprotective drug prescribing and utilization. *Current Medical Research and Opinion, 23*(8), 1859–1866.

CHECK YOUR UNDERSTANDING

Answers to the questions in this chapter can be found in Appendix A at the back of this book.

MULTIPLE CHOICE

Select the best answer to the following.

1. Clinical pharmacology is the study of:
   a. the biological effects of chemicals.
   b. drugs used to treat, prevent or diagnose disease.
   c. plant components that can be used as medicines.
   d. binders and other vehicles for delivering medication.

2. Phase I drug studies involve:
   a. the use of laboratory animals to test chemicals.
   b. people with the disease the drug is designed to treat.
   c. mass marketing surveys of drug effects in large numbers of people.
   d. healthy human volunteers who are often paid for their participation.

3. The generic name of a drug is:
   a. the name assigned to the drug by the pharmaceutical company developing it.
   b. the chemical name of the drug based on its chemical structure.
   c. the original name assigned to the drug at the beginning of the evaluation process.
   d. the name that is often used in advertising campaigns.

4. An orphan drug is a drug that:
   a. has failed to go through the approval process.
   b. is available in a foreign country but not in this country.
   c. has been tested but is not considered to be financially viable.
   d. is available without a prescription.

5. The ADEC pregnancy categories:
   a. indicate a drug's potential or actual teratogenic effects.
   b. are used for research purposes only.
   c. list drugs that are more likely to have addicting properties.
   d. are tightly regulated by the TGA.

6. Healthy young women are not usually involved in phase I studies of drugs because:
   a. male bodies are more predictable and responsive to chemicals.
   b. females are more apt to suffer problems with ova, which are formed only before birth.
   c. males can tolerate the unknown adverse effects of many drugs better than females.
   d. there are no standards to use to evaluate the female response.

7. A person has been taking fluoxetine (*Prozac*) for several years, but when picking up the prescription this month, found that the tablets looked different and became concerned. The health professional, checking with the pharmacist, found that fluoxetine had just become available in the generic form and the prescription had been filled with the generic product. The nurse should tell the person:
   a. that the new tablet may not work at all and the person should carefully monitor response.
   b. that generic drugs are available without a prescription and they are just as safe as the brand-name medication.
   c. that the law allows for prescriptions to be filled with the generic form if available, to cut down the cost of medications.
   d. that the pharmacist filled the prescription with the wrong drug and it should be returned to the pharmacy for a refund.

MULTIPLE RESPONSE

Select all that apply.

1. When teaching a person about over-the-counter (OTC) drugs, which points should the nurse or midwife include?
   a. These drugs are very safe and can be used freely to relieve your complaints.
   b. These compounds are called drugs, but they aren't really drugs.
   c. Some of these drugs were once prescription drugs, but are now thought to be safe when used as directed.
   d. Reading the label of these drugs is very important; the active ingredient is very prominent; you should always check the ingredient name.
   e. It is important to read the label and to see what the recommended dose of the drug is; some of these drugs can cause serious problems if too much of the drug is taken.
   f. It is important to report the use of any OTC drug to your health care provider because many of them can interact with drugs that might be prescribed for you.

2. A person asks what generic drugs are and if he should be using them to treat his infection. Which of the following statements should be included in the nurse's explanation?
   a. A generic drug is a drug that is dispensed by the name of the active ingredient, not the brand name.
   b. Generic drugs are always the best drugs to use because they are never any different from the familiar brand names.
   c. Generic drugs are not available until the patent on the originator drug expires.
   d. Generic drugs are usually cheaper than the well-known brand names, and some insurance companies require that you receive the generic drug if one is available.
   e. Generic drugs are forms of a drug that are available over the counter and do not require a prescription.
   f. Your doctor may want you to have a specific brand of a drug, not the generic form, and 'DAW', or 'dispense as written', will be on your prescription form.
   g. Generic drugs are less likely to cause adverse effects than brand-name drugs.

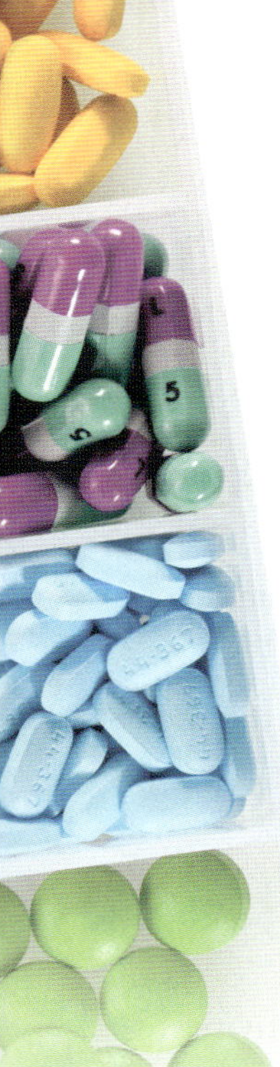

Drugs and the body

2

Learning objectives

On completing this chapter you should be able to:

1. Describe how body cells respond to the presence of drugs that are capable of altering their function.
2. Outline the process of dynamic equilibrium that determines the actual concentration of a drug in the body.
3. Explain the meaning of half-life of a drug and calculate the half-life of given drugs.
4. List at least six factors that can influence the actual effectiveness of drugs in the body.
5. Define drug–drug, drug–alternative therapy, drug–food and drug–laboratory test interactions.

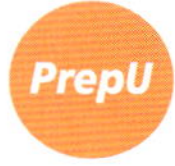

Test your current knowledge of drugs and the body with a PrepU Practice Quiz!

Glossary of key terms

absorption: what happens to a drug from the time it enters the body until it enters the circulating fluid; intravenous administration causes the drug to directly enter the circulating blood, bypassing the many complications of absorption from other routes

active transport: the movement of substances across a cell membrane against the concentration gradient; this process requires the use of energy biotransformation

agonist: drug that interacts directly with a receptor site to cause an effect

antagonist: drug that interacts with a receptor but does not cause an effect, instead blocks it

biotransformation: the process by which drugs are changed into new, less active chemicals

chemotherapeutic agents: synthetic chemicals used to interfere with the functioning of foreign cell populations; this term is frequently used to refer to the drug therapy of neoplasms, but it also refers to drug therapy affecting any foreign cell

competitive antagonist: drug that interacts with a receptor, blocking the ability of another drug to combine with it

distribution: movement of a drug to body tissues; the places where a drug may be distributed depend on the drug's solubility, perfusion of the area, cardiac output and binding of the drug to plasma proteins

effective concentration: the concentration a drug must reach in the tissues that respond to the particular drug to cause the desired effect

endocytosis: the process through which cells absorb molecules by engulfing them

endogenous substances: naturally occurring chemicals that are vital to the normal functioning of the body, eg, neurotransmitters, hormones and paracrines

enzyme induction: process by which the presence of a chemical that is biotransformed by a particular enzyme system in the liver causes increased activity of that enzyme system

excretion: removal of a drug from the body; primarily occurs in the kidneys, but can also occur through the skin, lungs, bile or faeces

first-pass effect: a phenomenon in which drugs given orally are carried directly to the liver after absorption, where they may be largely inactivated by liver enzymes before they can enter the general circulation; oral drugs are frequently given in higher doses than drugs given by other routes because of this early breakdown

glomerular filtration: the passage of water and water-soluble components from the plasma into the renal tubule

half-life: the time it takes for the amount of drug in the body to decrease to half of the peak level it previously achieved

hepatic microsomal system: liver enzymes tightly packed together in the hepatic intracellular structure, responsible for the biotransformation of chemicals, including drugs

loading dose: use of a higher dose than that which is usually used for treatment to allow the drug to reach the effective concentration sooner

passive diffusion: movement of substances across a semipermeable membrane with the concentration gradient; this process does not require energy

pharmacodynamics: the science that deals with the interactions between the chemical components of living systems and the foreign chemicals, including drugs, that enter living organisms; the way a drug affects a body

pharmacogenomics: the study of genetically determined variations in the response to drugs

pharmacokinetics: the way the body deals with a drug, including absorption, distribution, biotransformation and excretion

placebo effect: documented effect of the mind on drug therapy; if a person perceives that a drug will be effective, the drug is much more likely to actually be effective

receptor sites: specific areas on cell membranes that react with certain chemicals to cause an effect within the cell

selective toxicity: property of a chemotherapeutic agent that affects only systems found in foreign cells without affecting healthy human cells (eg, specific antibiotics can affect certain proteins or enzyme systems used by bacteria but not by human cells)

therapeutic concentration: *see* effective concentration

transmitter: an endogenous chemical usually released from nerve terminals to transfer nerve impulse from one neuron to the next or from a neuron to an effector cell such as muscle

To understand what happens when a drug is administered, the health professional must understand **pharmacodynamics** – how the drug affects the body – and **pharmacokinetics** – how the body acts on the drug. These processes form the basis for the guidelines that have been established regarding drug administration – for example, why certain agents are given intramuscularly (IM) and not intravenously (IV), why some drugs are taken with food and others are not, and the standard dose that should be used to achieve the desired effect. Knowing the basic principles of pharmacodynamics and pharmacokinetics helps the nurse or midwife to anticipate therapeutic and adverse drug effects and to intervene in ways that ensure the most effective drug regimen for the person.

Chemicals control many physiological processes in the body. Drugs are chemicals used for their therapeutic benefits. These chemicals are **endogenous substances** and are vital to the physiological functioning of the body. For example, acetylcholine, a neurotransmitter is necessary to contract the muscle as well as for neuronal functioning. Drugs mimic these endogenous substances. Many drugs are therefore designed to have similar chemical groups to those of naturally occurring chemicals. So for drugs to work, interaction with bodily process is necessary.

PHARMACODYNAMICS

Pharmacodynamics is the science dealing with interactions between the chemical components of living systems and the foreign chemicals, including drugs, which enter those systems. All living organisms function by a series of complicated, continual chemical reactions. When a new chemical enters the system, multiple changes in, and interferences with, cell functioning may occur. To avoid adverse effects, drug development works to provide the most effective and least toxic chemicals for therapeutic use.

Drugs usually work in one of four ways:

1. To replace or act as substitutes for missing substances, such as transmitters.
2. To increase or stimulate certain cellular activities.
3. To depress or slow cellular activities.
4. To interfere with the functioning of foreign cells, such as invading microorganisms or neoplasms. (Such drugs are called **chemotherapeutic agents.**)

Drug molecules do not confer any new functions on a tissue or organ in the body; they modify existing physiological, biochemical or biophysical functions. They can act in several different ways to achieve these results. They can combine with a small molecule (eg, antacids neutralise gastric acid) or produce an alteration of cell membrane activity (eg, local anaesthetics). Many drugs act by binding to a protein target, which is called the molecular target or site of action. Four kinds of regulatory proteins are commonly involved as primary drug targets, because they mediate the actions of hormones, neurotransmitters and autocoids. These regulatory proteins are:

- Enzymes
- Carrier molecules
- Ion channels
- Receptors

Drug–enzyme interactions

Enzymes are proteins and biological catalysts, which speed up the rate of chemical reactions. Drugs also can cause effects by interfering with the enzyme systems that act as catalysts for various chemical reactions. Enzyme systems work in a cascade fashion, with one enzyme activating another and then that enzyme activating another, until a cellular reaction eventually occurs. If a single step in one of the many enzyme systems is blocked, normal cell function is disrupted. Acetazolamide (*Diamox*) is a diuretic that blocks the enzyme carbonic anhydrase, which subsequently causes alterations in the hydrogen ion and water exchange system in the kidney, as well as in the eye.

Drug–carrier molecules (ion transporters) interactions

Some drugs are transported inside the cell through an ion transporter or an ion molecule. Ion or drug molecules that are not lipid soluble enough to diffuse across the biological cell membrane must be transported. Examples of transporters include those that transport glucose and move sodium and calcium ions out of cells. Other important transporters include those that are involved in the uptake of chemicals acting at nerve terminals, such as noradrenaline, 5-hydroxytryptamine (5-HT, serotonin) and glutamate.

Drug–ion channel interactions

Ion channels are selective pores in the cell membrane that allow the movement of ions in and out of the cell. Some drugs will block these channels, which ultimately interferes with ion transport and causes an altered physiological response. Drugs working in this way include nifedipine, verapamil and lidocaine (lignocaine).

Drug–receptor interactions

Receptors are target molecules that a drug molecule has to combine with to elicit a specific effect. The drug molecule combines with and affects the function of the protein receptor molecule, thus producing its effect. This is called *receptor activation*. However, occupation of a receptor by a drug molecule may or may not result in *activation* of the receptor. The tendency of a drug to bind to receptors is governed by *affinity*, whereas the tendency for a drug molecule, once bound, to activate the receptor is denoted by its *efficacy*. More importantly, in order to produce a therapeutic effect, a drug molecule must act *selectively* on particular cells and tissues. This means that individual drug molecules will only bind to certain targets and individual targets will only recognise certain classes of drug molecules.

Receptor sites

Many drugs are thought to act at specific areas on cell membranes called **receptor sites**. The receptor sites react with certain endogenous chemicals (**transmitters** and hormones) to cause an effect within the cell. In many situations, nearby enzymes break down the reacting chemicals and make the receptor site ready for further stimulation.

To better understand this process, think of how a key works in a lock. The specific chemical (the key) approaches a cell membrane and finds a perfect fit (the lock) at a receptor site (Figure 2.1). The interaction between the chemical and the receptor site affects enzyme systems within the cell. The activated enzyme systems then produce certain effects, such as increased or decreased cellular activity, changes in cell membrane permeability or alterations in cellular metabolism.

Some drugs interact directly with receptor sites to cause the same activity that natural or endogenous chemicals would cause at that site. These drugs are called ***agonists*** (Figure 2.1A). For example, insulin reacts with specific insulin-receptor sites to change cell membrane permeability, thus promoting the movement of glucose into the cell. Therefore, agonists are drug molecules that bind to receptors *(affinity)* and once bound activate receptors (*efficacy*). This ability to initiate a response after binding with the receptor is referred to as intrinsic activity.

Some drugs bind with receptor sites to block normal stimulation, producing no effect. These drugs are called antagonists (Figure 2.1C). **Antagonists** are drug molecules that bind to receptors (*affinity*) without causing activation (*efficacy*). For example, curare (a drug used on the tips of spears by inhabitants of the Amazon basin to paralyse prey and cause death) occupies receptor sites for acetylcholine, which is necessary for muscle contraction and movement. Curare prevents muscle stimulation, causing paralysis. Curare is said to be a *competitive antagonist* of acetylcholine (Figure 2.1B).

Still other drugs react with specific receptor sites on a cell and, by reacting there, prevent the reaction of another chemical with a different receptor site on that cell. Such drugs are called *non-competitive antagonists* (Figure 2.1C). For some drugs, the actual mechanisms of action are unknown. Speculation exists, however, that many drugs use receptor-site mechanisms to bring about their effects.

Other drugs act to prevent the breakdown of natural chemicals that are stimulating the receptor site. For example, monoamine oxidase (MAO) inhibitors block the breakdown of noradrenaline by the enzyme MAO. (Normally, MAO breaks down noradrenaline, removes it from the receptor site and recycles the components to form new noradrenaline.) The blocking action of MAO inhibitors allows noradrenaline to stay on the receptor site, stimulating the cell longer and leading to prolonged noradrenaline effects. Those effects can be therapeutic (eg, relieving depression) or adverse (eg, increasing heart rate and blood pressure). Selective serotonin reuptake inhibitors (SSRIs) work similarly to MAO inhibitors in that they also exert a blocking action. Specifically, they block removal of serotonin from receptor sites. This action leads to prolonged stimulation of certain brain cells, which is thought to provide relief from depression.

Loss of receptor response

Prolonged exposure of receptors to drug molecules can result in gradual decrease in the number of receptors. This is often referred to as *desensitisation* and *tachyphylaxis*. There are several mechanisms that give rise

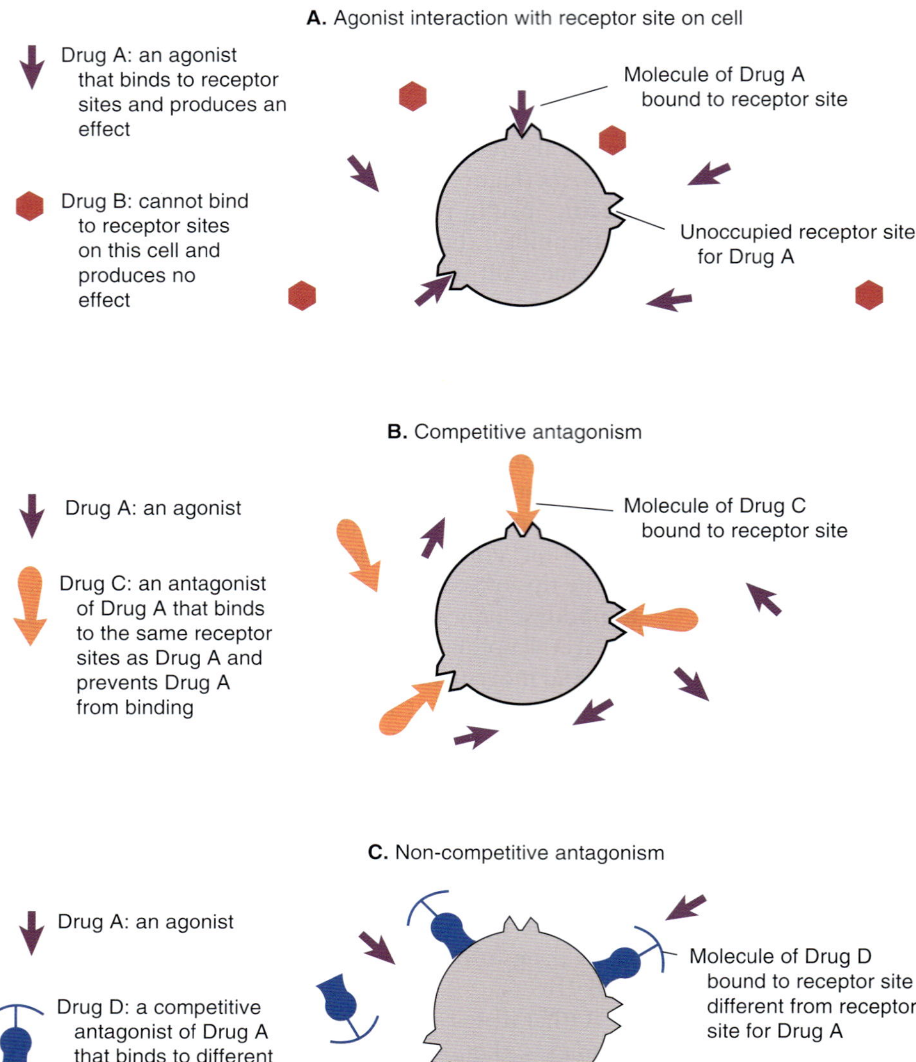

FIGURE 2.1 Receptor theory of drug action. **A.** Agonist interaction with receptor site on cell. Molecules of drug A react with specific receptor sites on cells of effector organs and change the cells' activity. **B.** Competitive antagonism. Drug A and drug C have an affinity for the same receptor sites and compete for these sites; drug C has a greater affinity, occupies more of the sites and antagonises drug A. **C.** Non-competitive antagonism. Drug D reacts with a receptor site that is different from the receptor site for drug A but still somehow prevents drug A from binding with its receptor sites. Drugs that act by inhibiting enzymes can be pictured as acting similarly to the receptor site antagonists illustrated in panels B and C. Enzyme inhibitors block the binding of molecules of normal substrate to active sites on the enzyme.

to this phenomenon. A change in receptors or loss of receptors can develop when a drug is given repeatedly or continuously. Prolonged exposure to an *agonist* drug can often result in a gradual decrease in the number of receptors expressed on the cell's surface or *receptor downregulation*. This has often been shown for beta-adrenergic receptors. The vanishing receptors are taken into the cells by **endocytosis**. By contrast, prolonged use of an *antagonist* drug can result in *receptor upregulation*. Upregulation of receptor numbers is an increase in the number of receptors on the surface of target cells, making the cells more sensitive to a hormone or another agent.

Selective toxicity

Ideally, all chemotherapeutic agents would act only on receptors, structures or enzyme systems that are essential for the life of a pathogen or neoplastic cell and would not affect healthy cells. The ability of a drug to attack only those systems found in foreign cells is known as **selective toxicity**. Penicillin, an antibiotic used to treat bacterial infections, has selective toxicity. It affects an enzyme system unique to bacteria, causing bacterial cell death without disrupting normal human cell functioning.

Unfortunately, most other chemotherapeutic agents also destroy normal human cells, causing many of the adverse effects associated with antipathogen and antineoplastic chemotherapy. Cells that reproduce or are replaced rapidly (eg, bone marrow cells, gastrointestinal [GI] cells, hair follicles) are more easily affected by these agents. Consequently, the goal of many chemotherapeutic regimens is to deliver a dose that will be toxic to the invading cells yet cause the lowest toxic effect to the host.

KEY POINTS

- Pharmacodynamics is the process by which a drug works or affects the body.
- Drugs may work by replacing a missing body chemical, by stimulating or depressing cellular activity or by interfering with the functioning of foreign cells.
- There are four primary drug targets: enzymes, ion channels, carrier molecules and receptors.
- Drugs are thought to work by interacting with specific receptor sites or by interfering with enzyme systems in the body.

PHARMACOKINETICS

Pharmacokinetics involves the study of absorption, distribution, metabolism (biotransformation) and excretion of drugs. In clinical practice, pharmacokinetic considerations include the onset of drug action, half-life of a drug, timing of the peak effect, duration of drug effects, metabolism or biotransformation of the drug and the site of excretion. Figure 2.2 outlines these processes, which are described in the following sections.

Effective concentration

After a drug is administered, its molecules must first be absorbed into the body; then they make their way to the site of action in the responding tissues. If a drug is going to work properly on these tissues and thereby have a therapeutic effect, it must attain a sufficiently high concentration in the body. The amount of a drug that is needed to cause a therapeutic effect has to be high enough to result in an **effective** or a **therapeutic concentration.**

Drug evaluation studies determine the effective concentration required to cause a desired therapeutic effect. The recommended dose of a drug is based on the amount that must be given to eventually reach the effective concentration. Too much of a drug will produce toxic (poisonous) effects and too little will not produce the desired therapeutic effects.

Therapeutic index

Most drugs produce multiple effects. The relationship between a drug's desired therapeutic effects and its adverse effects is called the drug's *therapeutic index*. It is also referred to as its *margin of safety*.

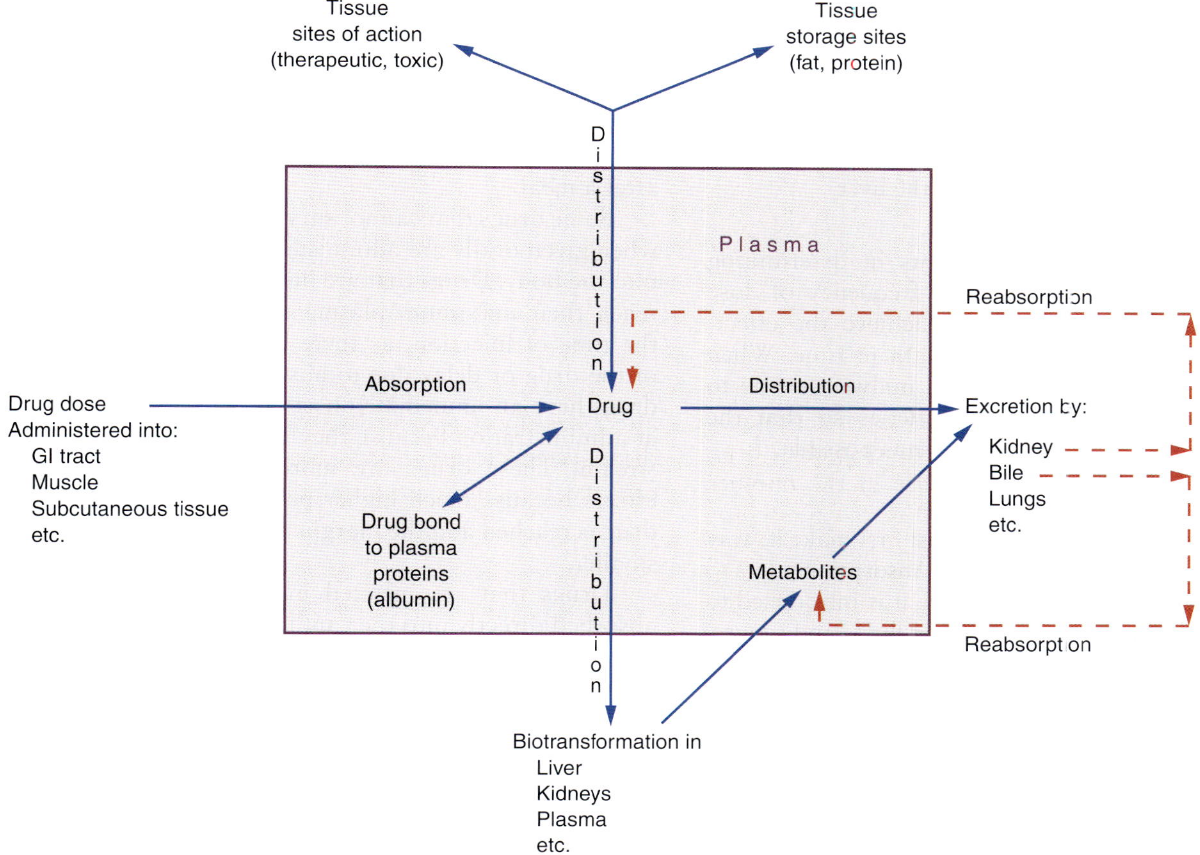

FIGURE 2.2 The processes by which a drug is handled by the body. Dashed lines indicate that some portion of a drug and its metabolites may be reabsorbed from the excretory organs. The dynamic equilibrium of pharmacokinetics is shown.

The therapeutic index usually measures the difference between:

- an effective dose for 50% of the people treated
- the minimal dose at which adverse reactions occur.

A drug with a low or narrow therapeutic index has a narrow range of safety between an effective dose and a lethal one. Examples of drugs with narrow margins of safety are warfarin, digoxin and gentamycin. On the other hand, a drug with a high therapeutic index has a wide range of safety and less risk of toxic effects.

Loading dose

Some drugs may take a prolonged period to reach an effective concentration. If their effects are needed quickly, a loading dose is recommended. Digoxin (*Lanoxin*) – a drug used to increase the strength of heart contractions – and many of the xanthine broncho-dilators (eg, aminophylline, theophylline) used to treat asthma attacks are often started with a **loading dose** (a higher dose than that usually used for treatment) to reach the effective concentration. The effective concentration is then maintained by using the recommended dosing schedule.

Dynamic equilibrium

The actual concentration (generally this concentration refers to blood or plasma concentration) that a drug reaches in the body results from a dynamic equilibrium involving several processes:

- absorption from the site of entry
- distribution to the active site
- biotransformation (metabolism) in the liver
- excretion from the body.

These processes are key elements in determining the amount of drug (dose) and the frequency of dose repetition (scheduling) required to achieve the effective concentration for the desired length of time. When administering a drug, the nurse or midwife needs to consider the phases of pharmacokinetics so that the drug regimen can be made as effective as possible.

Absorption

To reach responsive tissues, a drug must first make its way into the circulating fluids of the body. **Absorption** refers to what happens to a drug from the time it is introduced to the body until it reaches the circulating fluids and tissues. Drugs can be absorbed from many different areas in the body: through the GI tract either orally or rectally, through mucous membranes, through the skin, through the lung, or through muscle or subcutaneous tissues (Figure 2.2).

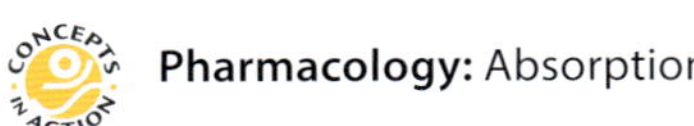

Pharmacology: Absorption

Routes of administration

Drug absorption is influenced by the route of administration. Generally, drugs given by the oral route are absorbed more slowly than those given parenterally. Of the parenteral route, intravenously administered drugs are 'absorbed' the fastest.[1]

The oral route is the most frequently used drug administration route in clinical practice. Oral administration is not invasive and, as a rule, is less expensive than drug administration by other routes. It is also the safest way to deliver drugs. People can easily continue their drug regimen at home when they are taking oral medications.

Oral administration subjects the drug to a number of barriers aimed at destroying ingested foreign compounds, including drugs. The acidic environment of the stomach is one of the first barriers to foreign chemicals. The acid breaks down many compounds and inactivates others. This fact is taken into account by pharmaceutical companies when preparing drugs in capsule or tablet form. The binders that are used are often designed to break down in a certain acidity and release the active drug to be absorbed.

When food is present, stomach acidity is higher and the stomach empties more slowly, thus exposing the drug to the acidic environment for a longer period. Certain foods that increase stomach acidity, such as milk products, alcohol and protein, also speed the breakdown of many drugs. Other foods may chemically bind drugs or block their absorption. To decrease the effects of this acid barrier and the direct effects of certain foods, oral drugs ideally are to be given 1 hour before or 2 hours after a meal.

Some drugs that cannot survive in sufficient quantity when given orally are administered by injection directly into the body. Drugs that are injected intravenously (IV) reach their maximum plasma concentration almost at the time of injection, as there is no initial breakdown of the drug or delay due to absorption. Basically, these drugs have an immediate onset and are fully 'absorbed' at administration because they directly enter the bloodstream. These drugs are more likely to cause toxic effects because much higher peak concentration of the drug is reached and the margin for error in dose is much smaller.

Drugs that are injected intramuscularly (IM) are absorbed directly into the capillaries in the muscle. This takes time because the drug must be picked up by the capillaries and transferred into the veins and the general circulation. Men have more vascular muscles than women do. As a result, drugs administered to men via the IM route reach a peak level faster than they do in women. Subcutaneous injections deposit the drug just

1 In case of intravenous administration the drug does not need to be absorbed through any membranes, thus using the term absorption in relation to intravenous administration of a drug is somewhat of a misnomer.

under the skin, where it is slowly absorbed into circulation. Timing of absorption varies with subcutaneous injection, depending on the fat content of the injection site and the state of local circulation. Table 2.1 outlines the various factors that affect drug absorption for different routes of administration.

Absorption processes

Drugs can be absorbed into cells through various processes, which include passive diffusion, active transport and filtration. **Passive diffusion** is the major process by which drugs are absorbed into the body. Passive diffusion occurs across a concentration gradient. When there is a greater concentration of drug on one side of a cell membrane, the drug will move through the membrane to the area of lower concentration. This process does not require any cellular energy. It occurs more quickly if the drug molecule is small, is soluble in water and in lipids (cell membranes are made of lipids and proteins – see Chapter 7) and has no electrical charge that could repel it from the cell membrane.

Unlike passive diffusion, **active transport** is a process that uses energy to actively move a molecule across a cell membrane. The molecule may be large, or it may be moving against a concentration gradient. This process is not very important in the absorption of most drugs, but it is often a very important process in drug excretion in the kidney.

Filtration involves movement through pores in the cell membrane, either down a concentration gradient or as a result of the pull of plasma proteins (when pushed by hydrostatic, blood or osmotic pressure). Filtration is another process the body commonly uses in drug excretion.

TABLE 2.1 Factors that affect absorption of drugs

Route	Factors affecting absorption
IV (intravenous)	None: direct entry into the venous system
IM (intramuscular)	Perfusion or blood flow to the muscle Fat content of the muscle Temperature of the muscle: cold causes vasoconstriction and decreases absorption; heat causes vasodilation and increases absorption
Subcutaneous	Perfusion or blood flow to the tissue Fat content of the tissue Temperature of the tissue: cold causes vasoconstriction and decreases absorption; heat causes vasodilation and increases absorption
PO (oral)	Acidity of stomach Length of time in stomach Blood flow to gastrointestinal tract Presence of interacting foods or drugs
PR (rectal)	Perfusion or blood flow to the rectum Lesions in the rectum Length of time retained for absorption
Mucous membranes (sublingual, buccal)	Perfusion or blood flow to the area Integrity of the mucous membranes Presence of food or smoking Length of time retained in area
Topical (skin)	Perfusion or blood flow to the area Integrity of skin
Inhalation	Perfusion or blood flow to the area Integrity of lung lining Ability to administer drug properly

Factors affecting gastrointestinal absorption

Numerous factors can affect or alter the absorption of oral drugs. Some are physiological barriers and some are due to the formulation of the drug. The main factors are:

- GI motility
- splanchnic blood flow
- particle size and formulation
- physicochemical factors.

Many disease conditions can slow down drug absorption. For example, diabetic neuropathy and migraine are conditions that affect gastric stasis. There are also drug treatments that can affect gastric motility. Drugs that block the muscarinic receptors reduce gastric motility and some drugs such as metoclopromide increase gastric motility. A drug taken after a meal is often more slowly absorbed because its movement to the small intestines is delayed in the presence of food. However, not all drugs taken after a meal can result in slow absorption of the drug. Propanol when taken with meals reaches higher plasma concentration because the drug increases splanchnic blood flow. In clinical situations in which a person is hypovolaemic, splanchnic blood flow is slow and results in a slowing of absorption of oral drugs.

Formulation and particle size have major effects in the absorption of oral drugs. Capsules may be designed to remain intact for some hours after the person takes the drug in order to delay absorption. In some cases, tablets may have a resistant coating to give the same effect. Slow-release capsules and sustained-release capsules are formulated to produce rapid but sustained absorption of the drug. Physicochemical factors such as changes in gastric pH due to ageing and presence of other drugs can all affect drug absorption. Tetracycline, an antibiotic, binds strongly to $Ca^{2}+$. Absorption of this drug is prevented if administered with calcium rich foods (especially milk).

First-pass effect

Drugs that are taken orally are usually absorbed from the small intestine directly into the portal venous system (the blood vessels that flow through the liver on their way back to the heart). Aspirin and alcohol are two drugs that are known to be absorbed from the lower end of the stomach. The portal veins deliver these absorbed molecules into the liver, which immediately transforms most of the chemicals delivered to it by the action of a series of liver enzymes. These enzymes break the drug into metabolites, some of which are active and cause effects in the body and some of which are deactivated and can be readily excreted. As a result, a large percentage of the oral dose is destroyed at this point and never reaches the tissues. This phenomenon is known as the **first-pass effect**. The portion of the drug that gets through the first-pass effect is delivered to the circulatory system for transport throughout the body.

Injected drugs and drugs absorbed from sites other than the GI tract undergo a similar biotransformation when they pass through the liver. Because some of the active drug already has had a chance to reach the responsive tissues before reaching the liver, the injected drug is often more effective at a lower dose than the oral equivalent. Thus, the recommended dose for oral drugs can be considerably higher than the recommended dose for parenteral drugs, taking the first-pass effect into account.

Bioavailability and bioequivalence

Bioavailability refers to the proportion of drug that passes through to systemic circulation after oral administration, taking into account both absorption and metabolic degradation. It relates to the total proportion of drug that reaches the systemic circulation. The use of the concept of bioavailability is limited, as it relates only to the total proportion of the drug that reaches the systemic circulation and neglects the rate of absorption. Regulatory authorities make decisions about the 'generic equivalence' of patented products. The concept of bioavailability may be used to provide evidence that a new product behaves sufficiently similarly to the existing one to be substituted for without causing clinical problems *(bioequivalence)*.

Distribution

Distribution involves the movement of a drug to the body's tissues (Figure 2.2). As with absorption, factors that can affect distribution include the drug's lipid solubility and ionisation, and the perfusion of the responsive tissue.

For example, tissue perfusion is a factor in caring for a person with diabetes who has a lower-leg infection and needs antibiotics to destroy the bacteria in the area. In this case, systemic drugs may not be effective because part of the disease process involves changes in the vasculature and decreased blood flow to some areas, particularly the lower limbs. If there is not adequate blood flow to the area, little antibiotic can be delivered to the tissues and little antibiotic effect will be seen.

In the same way, people in a cold environment may have constricted blood vessels (vasoconstriction) in the extremities, which would prevent blood flow to those areas. The circulating blood would be unable to deliver drugs to those areas and the person would receive little therapeutic effect from drugs intended to react with those tissues.

Many drugs are bound to proteins and are not lipid soluble. These drugs cannot be distributed to the central nervous system (CNS) because of the effective blood–brain barrier (see later discussion), which is highly selective in allowing lipid soluble substances to pass into the CNS.

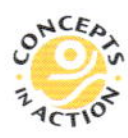

Pharmacology: Distribution

Protein binding

Most drugs are bound to some extent to proteins in the blood to be carried into circulation. The protein–drug complex is relatively large and cannot enter into capillaries and then into tissues to react. The drug must be freed from the protein's binding site at the tissues.

Many drugs are extensively bound to proteins and it should be noted that only the unbound fraction of the drug can reach the site of action in responsive tissues. Some drugs compete with each other for protein binding sites, altering effectiveness or causing toxicity when the two drugs are given together. The toxicity is attributed to sudden increase in the fraction of the previously protein-bound drug that is now free.

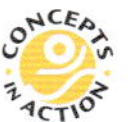

Pharmacology: Drug binding

Blood–brain barrier

The blood–brain barrier is a protective system of cellular membranes that keep many things (eg, foreign invaders, poisons) away from the CNS. The fundamental structural difference of the membranes forming the blood–brain barrier is the use of so-called tight-junctions between cells, leaving no gaps between the cells. Drugs that are highly lipid soluble are more likely to pass through the blood–brain barrier and reach the CNS. Drugs that are not lipid soluble are not able to pass the blood–brain barrier. This is clinically significant in treating a brain infection with antibiotics. Almost all antibiotics are not lipid soluble and cannot cross the blood–brain barrier. Effective antibiotic treatment can occur only when the infection is severe enough to damage the blood–brain barrier and allow antibiotics to cross.

Although many drugs can cause adverse CNS effects, these are often the result of indirect drug effects and not the actual reaction of the drug with CNS tissue. For example, alterations in glucose levels and electrolyte changes can interfere with nerve functioning and produce CNS effects such as dizziness, confusion or changes in thinking ability.

Placenta and breast milk

Many drugs readily pass through the placenta and affect the developing fetus in pregnant women. As stated earlier, it is best not to administer any drugs to pregnant women because of the possible risk to the fetus. Drugs should be given only when the benefit clearly outweighs any risk. Many other drugs are secreted into breast milk and therefore have the potential to affect the neonate. Because of this possibility, the midwife or nurse must always check the ability of a drug to pass into breast milk when giving a drug to a breastfeeding mother.

Biotransformation (metabolism)

The body is well prepared to deal with a myriad of foreign chemicals. Enzymes in the liver, in many cells, in the lining of the GI tract and even circulating in the body detoxify foreign chemicals to protect the fragile homeostasis that keeps the body functioning (Figure 2.2). Almost all the chemical reactions that the body uses to convert drugs and other chemicals into non-toxic substances are based on a few processes that work to make the chemical less active and more easily excreted from the body.

The liver is the most important site of drug metabolism, or **biotransformation**, the process by which drugs are changed into new, less active chemicals. Think of the liver as a sewage treatment plant. Everything that is absorbed from the GI tract first enters the liver to be 'treated'. The liver detoxifies many chemicals and uses others to produce needed enzymes and structures.

Hepatic enzyme system

The intracellular structures of the hepatic cells are lined with enzymes packed together in what is called the **hepatic microsomal system**. Because orally administered drugs enter the liver first, the enzyme systems immediately work on the absorbed drug to biotransform it. As explained earlier, this first-pass effect can be responsible for neutralising most of the drug that is taken.

Phase I biotransformation involves oxidation, reduction or hydrolysis of the drug and the main oxidising enzyme is the cytochrome P450 system. These enzymes are found in most cells but are especially abundant in the liver. A majority of useful drugs are metabolised by the cytochrome P450 enzyme system, consequently interfering with this enzyme system can markedly alter the effectiveness of drug therapy. The cytochrome P450 system in particular is subject to inhibition (reduced activity) and induction (increased activity) by drugs and other chemicals as well as natural constituents of foods. Table 2.2 gives some examples of drugs that induce or inhibit the cytochrome P450 system. Phase II biotransformation usually involves a conjugation reaction that makes the drug more polar and more readily excreted by the kidneys.

The presence of a chemical that is metabolised by a particular enzyme system often increases the activity of that enzyme system. This process is referred to as **enzyme induction.** Only a few basic enzyme systems are responsible for metabolising most of the chemicals that pass through the liver. Increased activity in an enzyme system speeds the metabolism of the drug that caused the enzyme induction, as well as any other drug that is metabolised by that same enzyme system. This explains why some drugs cannot be taken together effectively. The presence of one drug speeds the metabolism of others, preventing them from reaching their therapeutic levels.

Some drugs inhibit an enzyme system, making it less effective. As a consequence, any drug that is metabolised by that system will not be broken down for excretion and the blood levels of that drug will increase, often to toxic levels. These actions also explain why liver disease is often a contraindication or a reason to use caution when administering certain drugs. If the liver is not functioning effectively, the drug will not be metabolised as it should be and toxic levels could develop rather quickly.

Excretion

Excretion is the removal of a drug from the body. Skin, sweat, lungs, bile and faeces are some of the routes used to excrete drugs. Drugs are also excreted into saliva and milk. The kidneys, however, play the most important role in drug excretion (Figure 2.2).

Drugs that have been made water-soluble in the liver are often readily excreted from the kidney by **glomerular filtration** – the passage of water and water-soluble components from the plasma into the renal tubule. Other drugs are secreted or reabsorbed through the renal tubule by active transport systems. The active transport systems that move the drug into the tubule often do so by exchanging it for acid or bicarbonate molecules. Therefore the acidity of urine can play an important role in drug excretion. This concept is important to remember when trying to clear a drug rapidly from the system or trying to understand why a drug is being given at the usual dose but is reaching toxic levels in the system. One should always consider the person's kidney function and urine acidity before administering a drug. Kidney

TABLE 2.2 Examples of drugs that alter the effects of the cytochrome P450 hepatic enzyme system

Drugs that induce or increase activity	Drugs that inhibit or decrease activity
Alcohol (drinking)	Clarithromycin
Carbamazepine	Diltiazem
Nicotine (cigarette smoking)	Erythromycin
Glucocorticoids (Cortisone, others)	Itraconazole
Phenobarbital (phenobarbitone)	Ritonavir
Phenytoin	Verapamil
Rifampicin	

dysfunction can lead to toxic levels of a drug in the body because the drug cannot be excreted. Figure 2.3 outlines the pharmacokinetic processes that occur when a drug is administered orally.

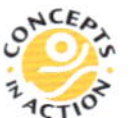

Pharmacology: Excretion

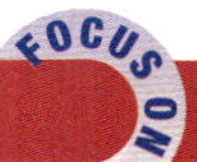

Safe medication administration

The liver is very important in metabolising drugs in the body and the kidneys are responsible for a large part of the excretion of drugs from the body. One should get into the habit of always checking a person's liver and renal function before they start a drug regimen. If the liver is not functioning properly, the drug may not be metabolised correctly and may reach toxic levels in the body. If the kidneys are not functioning properly, the drug may not be excreted properly and could accumulate in the body. Dose adjustment needs to be considered if a person has problems with either the liver or the kidneys.

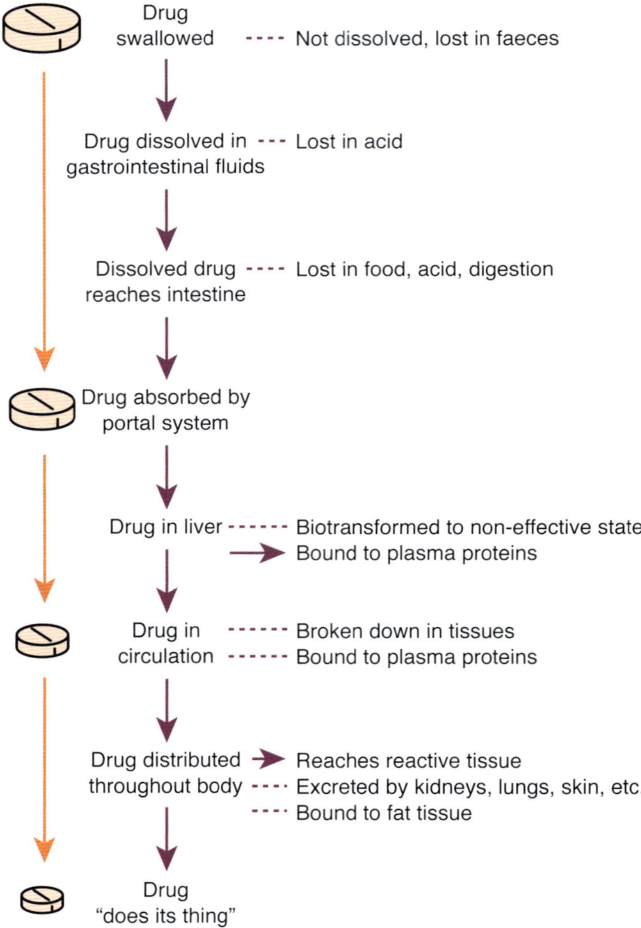

FIGURE 2.3 Pharmacokinetics affects the amount of a drug that reaches reactive tissues. Very little of an oral dose of a drug actually reaches reactive sites.

Half-life

The **half-life** of a drug is the time it takes for the amount of drug in the body to decrease to half of the peak level it previously achieved. For example, if a person takes 20 mg of a drug with a half-life of 2 hours, 10 mg of the drug will remain 2 hours after administration. Two hours later, 5 mg will be left (half of the previous level); in 2 more hours, only 2.5 mg will remain. This information is important in determining the appropriate timing for a drug dose or determining the duration of a drug's effect on the body. (See Box 2.1 Focus on calculations.)

The absorption rate, the distribution to the tissues, the speed of biotransformation and how fast a drug is excreted are all taken into consideration when determining the half-life of a drug. The half-life that is indicated in any drug monograph is the half-life for a healthy person. Using this information, one can estimate the half-life of a drug for a person with kidney or liver dysfunction (which could prolong the biotransformation and the time required for excretion of a drug), allowing the prescriber to make changes in the dosing schedule.

The timing of drug administration is important to achieve the most effective drug therapy. Nurses and midwives can use their knowledge of drug half-life to explain the importance of following a schedule of drug administration in the hospital or at home. Figure 2.4 shows the effects of drug administration on the effective concentration of a drug.

BOX 2.1 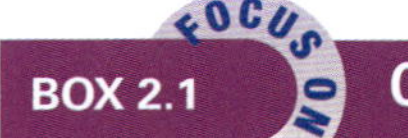 **Calculations**

Determining the impact of half-life on drug levels

A person is taking a drug that has a half-life of 12 hours. You are trying to determine when a 50 mg dose of the drug will be gone from the body:

- In 12 hours, half of the 50 mg (25 mg) would remain in the body.
- In another 12 hours (24 hours), half of 25 mg (12.5 mg) would remain in the body.
- After 36 hours, half of 12.5 mg (6.25 mg) would remain.
- After 48 hours, half of 6.25 mg (3.125 mg) would remain.
- After 60 hours, half of 3.125 (1.56 mg) would remain.
- After 72 hours, half of 1.56 (0.78 mg) would remain.
- After 84 hours, half of 0.78 (0.39 mg) would remain.
- Twelve more hours (for a total of 96 hours) would reduce the drug amount to 0.195 mg.
- Finally, 12 more hours (108 hours) would reduce the amount of the drug in the body to 0.097 mg, which would be quite negligible.
- Therefore, it would take 4½–5 days to clear the drug from the body.

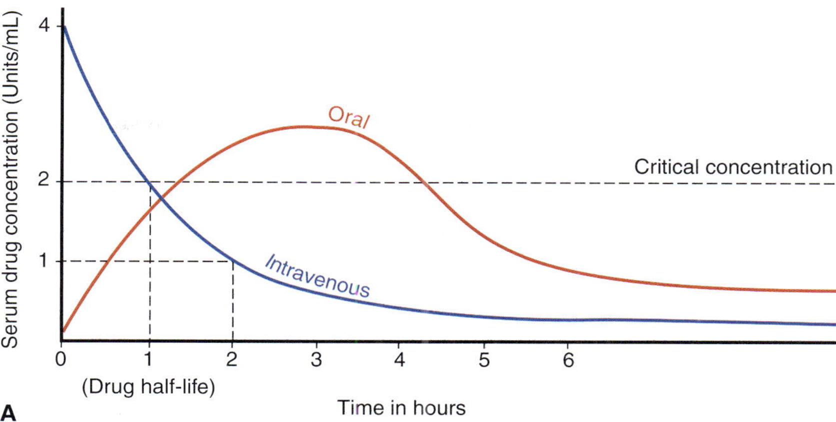

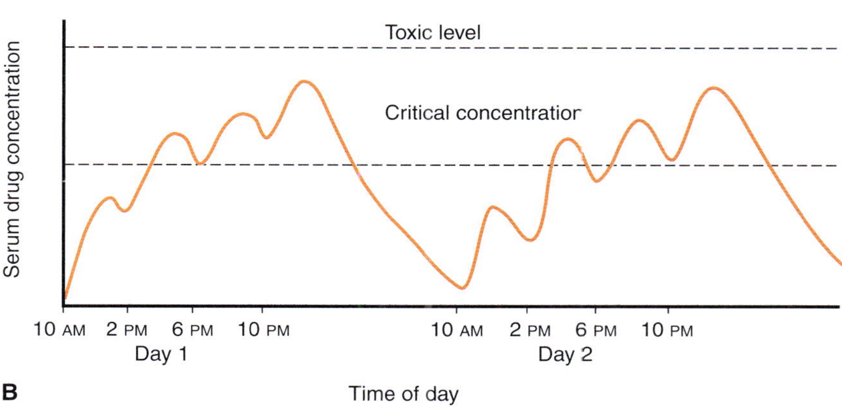

FIGURE 2.4 Influence of biological half-life, route of administration, and dosing regimen on serum drug levels. **A.** Influence of route of administration on the time course of drug levels after administration of a single dose of a drug. The dashed lines indicate how the biological half-life of the drug may be determined from the curve of drug concentration after an intravenous dose. At time 0, immediately after the injection, there were 4 units of the drug in each millilitre of serum. The drug concentration fell to half of this amount, 2 units/mL, after 1 hour, the drug's biological half-life. **B.** Influence of dosing regimen on serum drug levels (drug given four times daily, at 10 AM and at 2, 6, and 10 PM). The drug accumulates as successive doses are given throughout each day; the drug is being given at a rate greater than the person's body can eliminate it. This dosing regimen has been chosen so that the person will have a therapeutic level of the drug for a significant portion of the day yet never have a toxic level of the drug.

KEY POINTS

- Pharmacokinetics is the study of how the body deals with a drug.
- The concentration of a drug in the body is determined by the balance of absorption, distribution, metabolism and excretion of the drug.
- In determining the amount, route and appropriate timing of a drug dose, the pharmacokinetics of that drug has to be considered.

FACTORS INFLUENCING DRUG EFFECTS

When administering a drug to a person, the professional must be aware that the human factor has a tremendous influence on what actually happens to a drug when it enters the body. No two people react in exactly the same way to any given drug. Even though textbooks and drug guides explain the pharmacodynamics and pharmacokinetics of a drug, it must be remembered that such information is usually based on studies of healthy adult males. Things may be very different in the clinical setting. Consequently, before administering any drug, it is vital to consider a number of factors. These are discussed in detail in the following sections and summarised in Box 2.2.

BOX 2.2 Factors affecting the body's response to a drug

Weight
Age
Gender
Physiological factors – diurnal rhythm, electrolyte balance, acid–base balance, hydration
Pathological factors – disease, hepatic dysfunction, renal dysfunction, gastrointestinal dysfunction, vascular disorders, low blood pressure
Genetic factors
Immunological factors – allergy
Psychological factors – placebo effect, health beliefs, compliance
Environmental factors – temperature, light, noise
Drug tolerance
Cumulation effects
Interactions

Weight

The recommended dose of a drug is based on drug evaluation studies and is targeted at a 70 kg person. People who are much heavier may require larger doses to get a therapeutic effect from a drug because they have increased tissues to perfuse and increased receptor sites in some responsive tissue. People who weigh less than the norm may require smaller doses of a drug. Toxic effects may occur at the recommended dose if the person is very small.

Age

Age is a factor primarily in children and older adults. Children metabolise many drugs differently than adults do and they have immature systems for handling drugs. Many drugs come with recommended paediatric doses and others can be converted to paediatric doses using one of several conversion formulas.

Older adults undergo many physical changes that are a part of the ageing process. Their bodies may respond very differently in all aspects of pharmacokinetics – less effective absorption, less efficient distribution because of less efficient perfusion, altered protein binding and altered biotransformation or metabolism of drugs because of age-related liver changes, and less effective excretion owing to less efficient kidneys. Many drugs now come with recommended doses for people who are older. The doses of other drugs may also need to be decreased for the older adult.

When administering drugs to a person at either end of the age spectrum, one should monitor the person closely for the desired effects. If the effects are not what would normally be expected, one should consider the need for a dose adjustment.

Gender

Physiological differences between men and women can influence a drug's effect. When giving IM injections, for example, it is important to remember that men have more vascular muscles, so the effects of the drug will be seen sooner in men than in women.

Women have more fat cells than men do, so drugs that deposit in fat may be slowly released and cause effects for a prolonged period. For example, gaseous anaesthetics have an affinity for depositing in fat and can cause drowsiness and sedation sometimes weeks after surgery. Women who are given any drug should always be questioned about the possibility of pregnancy because, as stated previously, the use of drugs in pregnant women is not recommended unless the benefit clearly outweighs the potential risk to the fetus.

Physiological factors

Physiological differences such as diurnal rhythm of the nervous and endocrine systems, acid–base balance, hydration and electrolyte balance can affect the way that a drug works on the body and the way that the body handles the drug. If a drug does not produce the desired effect, one should review the person's acid–base and electrolyte profiles, and the timing of the drug administration.

Pathological factors

Drugs are usually used to treat disease or pathology. However, the disease that the drug is intended to treat can change the pharmacodynamic responses of a drug within the body and thus change the response to the drug.

Other pathological conditions can change the basic pharmacokinetic behaviour of a drug. For example, GI disorders can affect the absorption of many oral drugs. Vascular diseases and low blood pressure alter the distribution of a drug, preventing it from being delivered to the responsive tissue, thus rendering the drug non-therapeutic. Liver or kidney diseases affect the way that a drug is biotransformed and excreted and can lead to toxic reactions when the usual dose is given.

Genetic factors

Genetic differences can sometimes explain people's varied responses to a given drug. Some lack certain enzyme systems necessary for metabolising a drug, whereas others have overactive enzyme systems that cause drugs to be broken down more quickly. Still others have differing metabolisms or slightly different enzymatic makeups that alter their chemical reactions and the effects of a given drug.

Predictable differences in the pharmacokinetics and pharmacodynamic effects of drugs can be anticipated with people of particular ethnic backgrounds because of their genetic makeup. **Pharmacogenomics** is a new area of study that explores the unique differences in response to drugs that each individual possesses based on genetic makeup. The mapping of the human genome has accelerated research in this area. It is thought that in the future, medical care and drug regimens could be individually designed based on each person's unique genetic makeup. Trastuzumab (*Herceptin*) (see Chapter 17) is a drug that was developed to treat breast cancer when the tumour expresses human epidermal growth factor receptor 2 – a genetic defect seen in some tumours. The drug has no effect on tumours that do not express that genetic defect. This drug was developed as a personalised or targeted medicine based on genetic factors. Such differences are highlighted throughout this book. In late 2007, the U.S. Food and Drug Administration (FDA) approved a blood test to check for specific genetic markers that would indicate that a person would metabolise warfarin (*Coumadin*, *Marevan*), an oral anticoagulant, differently than the standard person. However, there is some debate about whether this fully covers a person's response.

Immunological factors

People can develop an allergy to a drug. After exposure to its proteins, a person can develop antibodies to a drug.

With future exposure to the same drug, that person may experience a full-blown allergic reaction. Sensitivity to a drug can range from mild (eg, dermatological reactions such as a rash) to more severe (eg, anaphylaxis, shock and death). (Drug allergies are discussed in detail in Chapter 3.)

Psychological factors

The person's attitude about a drug has been shown to have an effect on how that drug works. A drug is more likely to be effective if the person thinks it will work than if the person believes it will not work. This is called the **placebo effect**.

The person's personality also influences compliance with the drug regimen. Some people who believe that they can influence their health actively seek health care and willingly follow a prescribed regimen. These people usually trust the medical system and believe that their efforts will be positive. Other people do not trust the medical system. They may believe that they have no control over their health and may be unwilling to comply with any prescribed therapy. Knowing a person's health-seeking history and feelings about health care is important in planning an educational program that will work for that person. It is also important to know this information when arranging for necessary follow-up procedures and evaluations.

As carers most often involved in drug administration, nurses and midwives are in a position to influence the person's attitude about drug effectiveness. Frequently, the professional's positive attitude, combined with additional comfort measures, can improve the response to a medication.

Environmental factors

The environment can affect the success of drug therapy. Some drug effects are enhanced by a quiet, cool, non-stimulating environment. For example, sedating drugs are given to help a person relax or to decrease tension. Reducing external stimuli to decrease tension and stimulation help the drug be more effective. Other drug effects may be influenced by temperature. For example, antihypertensives that work well during cold winter months may become too effective in warmer environments, when natural vasodilation may lead to a release of heat that tends to lower the blood pressure. If a person's response to a medication is not as expected, look for possible changes in environmental conditions.

Tolerance

The body may develop a tolerance to some drugs over time. Tolerance may arise because of increased biotransformation of the drug, increased resistance to its effects or other pharmacokinetic factors. When tolerance occurs, the drug no long causes the same reaction. Therefore, increasingly larger doses are needed to achieve a therapeutic effect. An example is morphine, an opiate used for pain relief. The longer morphine is taken, the more tolerant the body becomes to the drug, so that larger and larger doses are needed to relieve pain. Clinically, this situation can be avoided by giving the drug in smaller doses or in combination with other drugs that may also relieve pain. Cross-tolerance – or resistance to drugs within the same class – may also occur in some situations.

Cumulation

If a drug is taken in successive doses at intervals that are shorter than recommended, or if the body is unable to eliminate a drug properly, that drug can accumulate in the body, leading to toxic levels and adverse effects. This can be avoided by following the drug regimen precisely. In reality, with many people managing their therapy at home, strict compliance with a drug regimen seldom occurs. Some people take all of their medications first thing in the morning, so that they won't forget to take the pills later in the day. Others realise that they forgot a dose and then take two to make up for it. Many interruptions of everyday life can interfere with strict adherence to a drug regimen. If a drug is causing serious adverse effects, review the drug regimen with the person to find out how the drug is being taken and then educate them appropriately.

Interactions

When two or more drugs or substances are taken together, there is a possibility that an interaction can occur, causing unanticipated effects in the body. Alternative therapies, such as herbal products, act as drugs in the body and can cause these same interactions. Certain foods can interact with drugs in much the same way. Usually this is an increase or decrease in the desired therapeutic effect of one or all of the drugs or an increase in adverse effects.

Drug–drug or drug–alternative therapy interactions

Clinically significant drug–drug interactions occur with drugs that have small margins of safety. If there is very little difference between a therapeutic dose and a toxic dose of the drug, interference with the drug's pharmacokinetics or pharmacodynamics can produce serious problems. For example, drug–drug interactions can occur in the following situations:

- *At the site of absorption:* one drug prevents or accelerates absorption of the other drug. For example, the antibiotic tetracycline is not absorbed from the GI tract if calcium or calcium products (milk) are present in the stomach.

- *During distribution:* one drug competes for the protein binding site of another drug, so the second drug cannot be transported to the responsive tissue. For example, aspirin competes with the drug methotrexate for protein-binding sites. Because aspirin is more competitive for the sites, the methotrexate is bumped off, resulting in increased release of methotrexate and increased toxicity to the tissues.
- *During biotransformation:* one drug stimulates or blocks the metabolism of the other drug. For example, warfarin, an oral anticoagulant, is biotransformed more quickly if it is taken at the same time as barbiturates, rifampicin or many other drugs. Because the warfarin is biotransformed to an inactive state more quickly, higher doses will be needed to achieve the desired effect. People who use St John's wort may experience altered effectiveness of several drugs that are affected by that herb's effects on the liver. Ciclosporin, digoxin, theophylline, oral contraceptives, anticancer drugs, drugs used to treat HIV and antidepressants are all reported to have serious interactions with St John's wort.
- *During excretion:* one drug competes for excretion with the other drug, leading to accumulation and toxic effects of one of the drugs. For example, digoxin and clarithromycin are both excreted from the same sites in the kidney via P-glycoprotein transporter. Clarithromycin may inhibit the P-glycoprotein-mediated tubular secretion of digoxin. If they are given together, the clarithromycin is more competitive for these sites and is excreted, resulting in increased serum levels of digoxin, which cannot be excreted.
- *At the site of action:* one drug may be an antagonist of the other drug or may cause effects that oppose those of the other drug, leading to no therapeutic effect. This is seen, for example, when an antihypertensive drug is taken with an antiallergy drug that increases blood pressure. The effects on blood pressure are negated and there is a loss of the antihypertensive effectiveness of the drug. If a person is taking antidiabetic medication and also takes the herb ginseng, which lowers blood glucose levels, they may experience episodes of hypoglycaemia and loss of blood glucose control.

Whenever two or more drugs are being given together, first consult a drug guide for a listing of clinically significant drug–drug interactions. Sometimes problems can be avoided by staggering the administration of the drugs or adjusting their doses.

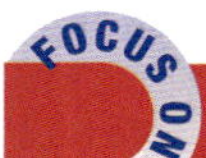

Safe medication administration

Always check the monograph of any drug that is being given to monitor for clinically important drug–drug, drug–alternative therapy or drug–food interactions.

Drug–food interactions

For the most part, a drug–food interaction occurs when the drug and the food are in direct contact in the stomach. Some foods increase acid production, speeding the breakdown of the drug molecule and preventing absorption and distribution of the drug. Some foods chemically react with certain drugs and prevent their absorption into the body. The antibiotic tetracycline cannot be taken with iron products for this reason. Tetracycline also binds with calcium to some extent and should not be taken with foods or other drugs containing calcium. Grapefruit juice has been found to affect liver enzyme systems for up to 48 hours after it has been ingested. This can result in increased or decreased serum levels of certain drugs. Many drugs come with the warning that they should not be combined with grapefruit juice. This drug–food interaction does not take place in the stomach, so the grapefruit juice needs to be avoided the entire time the drug is being used, not just while the drug is in the stomach.

In most cases, oral drugs are best taken on an empty stomach. If the person cannot tolerate the drug on an empty stomach, the food selected for ingestion with the drug should be something that is known not to interact with it. Drug monographs usually list important drug–food interactions and give guidelines for avoiding problems and optimising the drug's therapeutic effects.

Drug–laboratory test interactions

As explained previously, the body works through a series of chemical reactions. Because of this, administration of a particular drug may alter results of clinical tests that are done as part of a diagnostic study. This drug–laboratory test interaction is caused by the drug being given and not necessarily by a change in the body's responses or actions. Keep these interactions in mind when evaluating a person's diagnostic tests. If one test result is altered and does not fit in with the clinical picture or other test results, consider the possibility of a drug–laboratory test interference. For example, dalteparin (*Fragmin*), a low-molecular-weight heparin used to prevent deep vein thrombosis after abdominal surgery, may cause increased levels of the liver enzymes aspartate aminotransferase (AST) and alanine aminotransferase (ALT) with no injury to liver cells or hepatitis.

OPTIMAL THERAPEUTIC EFFECT

As overwhelming as all of this information may seem, most people can follow a drug regimen to achieve optimal therapeutic effects without serious adverse effects. Avoiding problems is the best way to treat adverse or ineffective drug effects. One should incorporate basic history and physical assessment factors into any plan of care so that obvious problems can be spotted and handled promptly. If a drug just does not do what it is expected to do, further examine the factors that are known to influence drug effects (Box 2.2). Frequently the drug regimen can be modified to deal with that influence. Rarely is it necessary to completely stop a needed drug regimen because of adverse or intolerable effects. In many cases, the nurse is the carer in the best position to assess problems early.

CHAPTER SUMMARY

- Pharmacodynamics is the study of the way that drugs affect the body.
- Most drugs work by replacing natural (endogenous) chemicals, by stimulating normal cell activity or by depressing normal cell activity.
- Chemotherapeutic agents work by interfering with normal cell functioning, causing cell death. The most desirable chemotherapeutic agents are those with selective toxicity to foreign cells and foreign cell activities.
- Drugs frequently act at specific receptor sites on cell membranes to stimulate enzyme systems within the cell and to alter the cell's activities.
- Pharmacokinetics – the study of the way the body deals with drugs – includes absorption, distribution, biotransformation and excretion of drugs.
- The goal of established dosing schedules is to achieve an effective concentration of the drug in the body. This effective concentration is the amount of the drug necessary to achieve the drug's therapeutic effects.
- Arriving at an effective concentration involves a dynamic equilibrium among the processes of drug absorption, distribution, metabolism or biotransformation and excretion.
- Absorption involves moving a drug into the body for circulation. Oral drugs are absorbed from the small intestine, undergo many changes and are affected by many things in the process. IV drugs are injected directly into the circulation and do not need additional absorption.
- Drugs are distributed to various tissues throughout the body depending on their solubility and ionisation. Most drugs are bound to plasma proteins for transport to responsive tissues.
- Drugs are metabolised or biotransformed into less toxic chemicals by various enzyme systems in the body. The liver is the primary site of drug metabolism or biotransformation. The liver uses the cytochrome P450 enzyme system to alter the drug and start its biotransformation.
- The first-pass effect is the breakdown of oral drugs in the liver immediately after absorption. Drugs given by other routes often reach responsive tissues before passing through the liver for biotransformation.
- Drug excretion is removal of the drug from the body. This occurs mainly through the kidneys.
- The half-life of a drug is the period of time it takes for an amount of drug in the body to decrease to half of the peak level it previously achieved. The half-life is affected by all aspects of pharmacokinetics. Knowing the half-life of a drug helps in predicting dosing schedules and duration of effects.
- The actual effects of a drug are determined by its pharmacokinetics, its pharmacodynamics and many human factors that can change the drug's effectiveness.
- To provide the safest and most effective drug therapy, the nurse or midwife must consider all the possible factors that influence drug concentration and effectiveness.

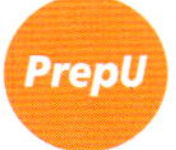

Knowing your strengths and weaknesses helps you to study more effectively. Take a PrepU Practice Quiz to find out how you measure up!

ONLINE RESOURCES

An extensive range of additional resources to enhance teaching and learning and to facilitate understanding of this chapter may be found online at the text's accompanying website, located on thePoint at http://thepoint.lww.com. These include Watch and Learn videos, Concepts in Action animations, journal articles, review questions, case studies, discussion topics and quizzes.

BIBLIOGRAPHY

Barrett, K. E. & Ganong, W. F. (2010). *Ganong's Review of Medical Physiology* (23rd edn). New York: McGraw-Hill.

Dale, M. M. & Rang, H.P. (2012). *Pharmacology* (7th edn). Edinburgh: Elsevier, Churchill Livingstone.

Dempsey, J., Hillege, S. & Hill, R. (2014). *Fundamentals of Nursing and Midwifery: A Person-centred Approach to Care* (2nd Australian and New Zealand edn). Sydney: Lippincott Williams & Wilkins.

Goodman, L. S., Brunton, L. L., Chabner, B. & Knollmann, B. C. (2011). *Goodman and Gilman's Pharmacological Basis of Therapeutics* (12th edn). New York: McGraw-Hill.

Gudin, J. & Gudin, J. (2012). "Opioid therapies and cytochrome P450 interactions." *Journal of Pain & Symptom Management, 44(6 Suppl)*, S4–14.

Guyton, A. & Hall, J. (2011). *Textbook of Medical Physiology* (12th edn). Philadelphia: Saunders Elsevier.

Martin, J. H. (2009). Pharmacogenetics of warfarin—Is testing clinically indicated? *Australian Prescriber, 32*, 76–80.

Miksys, S. & Tyndale, R. F. (2013). Cytochrome P450-mediated drug metabolism in the brain: 2011 CCNP Heinz Lehmann Award paper. *Journal of Psychiatry & Neuroscience, 38(3)*, 152–163.

Porth, C. M. (2011). *Essentials of Pathophysiology: Concepts of Altered Health States* (3rd edn). Philadelphia: Lippincott Williams & Wilkins.

Porth, C. M. (2009). *Pathophysiology: Concepts of Altered Health States* (8th edn). Philadelphia: Lippincott Williams & Wilkins.

CHECK YOUR UNDERSTANDING

Answers to the questions in this chapter can be found in Appendix A at the back of this book.

MULTIPLE CHOICE

Select the best answer to the following.

1. Chemotherapeutic agents are drugs that:
   a. are used only to treat cancers.
   b. replace normal body chemicals that are missing because of disease.
   c. interfere with foreign cell functioning, such as invading microorganisms or neoplasms.
   d. stimulate the normal functioning of a cell.
2. Receptor sites:
   a. are a normal part of enzyme substrates.
   b. are protein areas on cell membranes that react with specific chemicals.
   c. can usually be stimulated by many different chemicals.
   d. are responsible for all drug effects in the body.
3. Selective toxicity is:
   a. the ability of a drug to seek out a specific bacterial species or microorganism.
   b. the ability of a drug to cause only specific adverse effects.
   c. the ability of a drug to cause fetal damage.
   d. the ability of a drug to attack only those systems found in foreign or abnormal cells.
4. When trying to determine why the desired therapeutic effect is not being seen with an oral drug, the nurse or midwife should consider:
   a. the blood flow to muscle beds.
   b. food altering the makeup of gastric juices.
   c. the weight of the person.
   d. the temperature of the peripheral environment.
5. Much of the biotransformation that occurs when a drug is taken occurs as part of:
   a. the protein-binding effect of the drug.
   b. the functioning of the renal system.
   c. the first-pass effect through the liver.
   d. the distribution of the drug to the reactive tissues.
6. The half-life of a drug:
   a. is determined by a balance of all pharmacokinetic processes.
   b. is a constant factor for all drugs taken by a person.
   c. is influenced by the fat distribution of the person.
   d. can be calculated with the use of a body surface nomogram.
7. Jack B. has Parkinson disease that has been controlled for several years with levodopa. After he begins a health food regimen with lots of vitamin B6, his tremors return, and he develops a rapid heart rate, hypertension and anxiety. The nurse investigating the problem discovers that vitamin B6 can speed the conversion of levodopa to dopamine in the periphery, leading to these problems. The nurse would consider this problem:
   a. a drug–laboratory test interaction.
   b. a drug–drug interaction.
   c. a cumulation effect.
   d. a sensitivity reaction.

MULTIPLE RESPONSE

Select all that apply.

1. When reviewing a drug to be given, the nurse or midwife notes that the drug is excreted in the urine. What points should be included in the nurse's assessment of the person?
   a. the person's liver function tests
   b. the person's bladder tone
   c. the person's renal function tests
   d. the person's fluid intake
   e. other drugs being taken that could affect the kidney
   f. the person's intake and output for the day
2. When considering the pharmacokinetics of a drug, what points would the health care professional need to consider?
   a. how the drug will be absorbed
   b. the way the drug affects the body
   c. receptor-site activation and suppression
   d. how the drug will be excreted
   e. how the drug will be metabolised
   f. the half-life of the drug
3. Drug–drug interactions are important considerations in clinical practice. When evaluating a person for potential drug–drug interactions, what would the nurse or midwife expect to address?
   a. bizarre drug effects on the body
   b. the need to adjust drug dose or timing of administration
   c. the need for more drugs to balance the effects of the drugs being given
   d. a new therapeutic effect not encountered with either drug alone
   e. increased adverse effects
   f. the use of herbal or alternative therapies

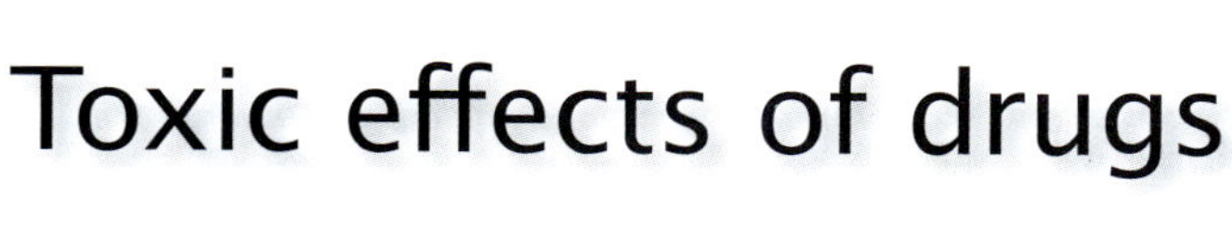

3 Toxic effects of drugs

Learning objectives

On completing this chapter you should be able to:

1. Define the term adverse drug reaction and explain the clinical significance of this reaction.
2. List four types of allergic responses to drug therapy.
3. Discuss five common examples of drug-induced tissue damage.
4. Define the term poison.
5. Outline the important factors to consider when applying the clinical decision-making process to selected situations of drug poisoning.

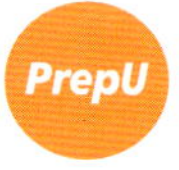

Test your current knowledge of the toxic effects of drugs with a PrepU Practice Quiz!

Glossary of key terms

blood dyscrasia: bone marrow depression caused by drug effects on the rapidly multiplying cells of the bone marrow; lower-than-normal levels of blood components can be seen

dermatological reactions: skin reactions commonly seen as adverse effects of drugs; can range from simple rash to potentially fatal exfoliative dermatitis

drug allergy: formation of antibodies to a drug or drug protein; causes an immune response when the person is next exposed to that drug

hypersensitivity: excessive responsiveness to either the primary or the secondary effects of a drug; may be caused by a pathological condition or, in the absence of one, by a particular person's individual response

iatrogenesis/iatrogenic artefact: inadvertent adverse effects or complications caused by, or as a result of, medical treatment or advice

poisoning: overdose of a drug that causes damage to multiple body systems and has the potential for fatal reactions

stomatitis: inflammation of the mucous membranes related to drug effects; can lead to alterations in nutrition and dental problems

superinfections: infections caused by the destruction of bacteria of the normal body flora by certain drugs, which allow other bacteria to enter the body and cause infection; may occur during the course of antibiotic therapy

All drugs are potentially dangerous. Even though chemicals are carefully screened and tested in animals and in people before they are released as drugs, drug products often cause unexpected or unacceptable reactions when they are administered. Drugs are chemicals, and the human body operates by a vast series of chemical reactions. Consequently, many effects can be seen when just one chemical factor is altered. Today's potent and amazing drugs can cause a great variety of reactions, many of which are more severe than those seen before.

ADVERSE EVENTS, ADVERSE DRUG EVENTS AND ADVERSE DRUG REACTIONS

An adverse event (AE) is a drug-related harm in a person administered the drug but not necessarily caused by the drug. An adverse drug event (ADE) is harm that is caused by the use of a drug, or inappropriate use of a drug, while an adverse drug reaction (ADR) is harm directly caused by a drug at normal doses and is usually preventable.

These terms were first introduced from the field of *pharmacovigilance*, the study of drug related injury. Several studies have reported adverse drug reactions to be among leading causes of morbidity and mortality. An adverse drug reaction is defined as 'an appreciably harmful or unpleasant reaction, resulting from an intervention related to the dose of a medicinal product, which predicts hazards from future administration and warrants prevention or specific treatment, or alteration of the dosage regimen or withdrawal of the product' (Edwards & Aronson, 2000).

The nurse or midwife, as the carers who most frequently administer medications, must be constantly alert for signs of drug reactions of various types. People and their families need to be taught what to look for when taking drugs at home. Some adverse drug effects can be countered with specific comfort measures or precautions. Knowing that these effects may occur and what actions can be taken to prevent or cope with them may be the most critical factor in helping the person to comply with drug therapy. Adverse effects can be one of several types: primary actions, secondary actions and hypersensitivity reactions.

The Australian Commission on Safety and Quality in Health Care (ACSQHC) has developed 10 National Safety and Quality Health Service Standards. These Standards aim to improve the quality of health service provision across Australia and provide a national statement of the level of care consumers should be able to expect from health services. Awareness and knowledge of Standard 4 on Medication Safety is an important part of the nurse's and midwife's clinical repertoire. For more information, see www.safetyandquality.gov.au/standards/nsqhs-standards/medication-safety-standard.

ADVERSE DRUG EFFECTS

Adverse drug effects are undesired effects that may be unpleasant or even dangerous. They can occur for many reasons, including the following:

- The drug may have other effects on the body besides the therapeutic effect.
- The person may be sensitive to the drug being given.
- The drug's action on the body may cause other responses that are undesirable or unpleasant.
- The person may be taking too much or too little of the drug, leading to adverse effects.
- The person may be taking a complementary product interacting with the drug, leading to adverse effects.
- The person may be taking many drugs (polypharmacy).

Primary actions

One of the most common occurrences in drug therapy is the development of adverse drug effects from simple overdose. In such cases, the person suffers from effects that are merely an extension of the desired effect. This is sometimes known as 'predictable side effects'. For example, an anticoagulant may act so effectively that the person experiences excessive and spontaneous bleeding. This type of adverse drug effect can be avoided by monitoring the person carefully and adjusting the prescribed dose to fit that particular person's needs.

In the same way, a person taking an antihypertensive drug may become dizzy, weak or faint when taking the 'recommended dose' but will be able to adjust to the drug therapy with a reduced dose. These effects can be caused by individual response to the drug, high or low body weight, age or underlying pathology that alters the effects of the drug.

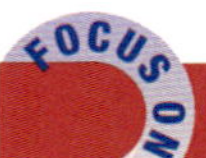

Safe medication administration

Before administering any drug to a person, it is important to review the contraindications and cautions associated with that drug, as well as the anticipated adverse effects of the drug. This information will direct your assessment of the person, helping you to focus on particular signs and symptoms that would alert you to contraindications or to proceed cautiously, and help you to establish a baseline for that person so that you will be able to identify adverse effects that occur. When teaching the person about a drug, you should list the adverse drug effects that should be anticipated, along with appropriate actions that can be taken to alleviate any discomfort associated with these effects. Being alert to adverse drug effects – what to assess and how to intervene appropriately – can increase the effectiveness of a drug regimen, provide for a person's safety and improve their compliance.

Secondary actions

Drugs can produce a wide variety of effects in addition to the desired pharmacological effect. Sometimes the drug dose can be adjusted so that the desired effect is achieved without producing undesired secondary reactions. Sometimes this is not possible and the adverse effects are almost inevitable. In such cases, the person needs to be informed that these effects may occur and counselled about ways to cope with the undesired effects. For example, many antihistamines are very effective in drying up secretions and helping breathing, but they also cause drowsiness. The person who is taking antihistamines needs to know that driving a car or operating power tools or machinery should be avoided because the drowsiness could pose a serious problem. A person taking an oral antibiotic needs to know that frequently the effects of the antibiotic on the gastrointestinal tract result in diarrhoea, nausea and sometimes vomiting. The person should be advised to eat small, frequent meals to help alleviate this problem.

Hypersensitivity

Some people are excessively responsive to either the primary or the secondary effects of a drug. This is known as **hypersensitivity** and it may result from a pathological or underlying condition. For example, many drugs are excreted through the kidneys; a person who has kidney problems may not be able to excrete the drug and may accumulate the drug in the body, causing toxic effects. The person will exhibit exaggerated adverse effects from a standard dose of the medication because of the accumulation of the drug. In some cases, individuals exhibit increased therapeutic and adverse effects with no definite pathological condition. Each person has slightly different receptors and cellular responses. Frequently older people will react to narcotics with increased stimulation and hyperactivity, not with the sedation that is expected. It is thought that this response is related to a change in receptors with age, leading to an increased sensitivity to a drug's effects.

Hypersensitivity can also occur if a person has an underlying condition that makes the drug's effects especially unpleasant or dangerous. For example, a person with an enlarged prostate who takes an anticholinergic drug may develop urinary retention or even bladder paralysis when the drug's effects block the urinary sphincters. This person needs to be taught to empty the bladder before taking the drug. A reduced dose may also be required to avoid potentially serious effects on the urinary system.

DRUG ALLERGY

A **drug allergy** occurs when the body forms antibodies to a particular drug, causing an immune response when the person is re-exposed to the drug. This is considered an 'unpredictable side effect'. A person cannot be allergic to a drug that has never been taken, although people can have cross-allergies to drugs within the same drug class as one formerly taken. Many people state that they have a drug allergy because of the effects of a drug. For example, one woman stated that she was allergic to the diuretic furosemide (frusemide) *(Lasix)*. On further questioning, the nurse or midwife discovered that the woman was 'allergic' to the drug because it made her urinate frequently – the desired drug effect, but one that the woman thought was a reaction to the drug. Ask additional questions of people who state that they have a drug 'allergy' to ascertain the exact nature of the response and whether or not it is a true drug allergy. Many people do not receive needed treatment because the response to the drug is not understood.

Drug allergies fall into four main classifications: anaphylactic reactions, cytotoxic reactions, serum sickness and delayed reactions (see Table 3.1). Nurses and midwives involved in administering drugs must constantly assess for potential drug allergies and must be prepared to intervene appropriately.

KEY POINTS

- All drugs have effects other than the desired therapeutic effect.
- Primary actions of the drug can be extensions of the desired effect.
- Secondary actions of a drug are effects that the drug causes in the body that are not related to the therapeutic effect.
- Hypersensitivity reactions to a drug are individual reactions that may be caused by increased sensitivity to the drug's therapeutic or adverse effects.
- Drug allergies occur when a person develops antibodies to a drug after exposure to the drug.

DRUG-INDUCED TISSUE AND ORGAN DAMAGE

Drugs can act directly or indirectly to cause many types of adverse effects in various tissues, structures and organs (see Figure 3.1). These drug effects account for many of the cautions that are noted before drug administration begins. The possibility that these effects can occur also accounts for the contraindications for the use of some drugs in people with a particular history or underlying pathology. The specific contraindications and cautions for the administration of a given drug are noted with each drug type discussed in this book and in the individual monographs found in various drug guides. These effects occur frequently enough that the nurse or midwife should be knowledgeable about the presentation of the drug-induced damage and about appropriate interventions to be used should they occur.

Dermatological reactions

Dermatological reactions are adverse reactions involving the skin. These can range from a simple rash to potentially fatal exfoliative dermatitis. Many adverse reactions involve the skin because many drugs can deposit there or cause direct irritation to the tissue. In dark-skinned people, including Indigenous Australians, Māori people and dark-skinned Africans, careful skin assessment is needed, as such reactions may not be as evident due to differences in pigmentation. For example, redness is not often evident so assessment will be based upon skin temperature, localised swelling or tightness.

Rashes, hives

Many drugs are known to cause skin reactions. Older drugs such as procainamide, used in the past to treat

TABLE 3.1 Interventions for types of drug allergies

Allergy type	Assessment	Interventions
Anaphylactic reaction This allergy involves an antibody that reacts with specific sites in the body to cause the release of chemicals, including histamine, that produce immediate reactions (mucous membrane swelling and constricting bronchi) that can lead to respiratory distress and even respiratory arrest	Hives, rash, difficulty breathing, increased BP, dilated pupils, diaphoresis, 'panic' feeling, increased heart rate, respiratory arrest	Administer adrenaline (epinephrine), 0.3 mL of a 1:1000 solution, IM for adults or 0.01 mg/kg of 1:1000 IM for children. Massage the site to speed absorption rate. Repeat the dose every 15–20 minutes, as appropriate. Notify the prescriber and/or primary carer and discontinue the drug. Be aware that prevention is the best treatment. Counsel the people with known allergies to wear Medic-Alert identification and, if appropriate, to carry an emergency adrenaline kit
Cytotoxic reaction This allergy involves antibodies that circulate in the blood and attack antigens (the drug) on cell sites, causing death of that cell. This reaction is not immediate but may be seen over a few days	Full blood count showing damage to blood-forming cells (decreased haematocrit, white blood cell count and platelets); liver function tests show elevated liver enzyme levels; renal function test shows decreased renal function	Notify the prescriber and/or primary carer and discontinue the drug. Support the person to prevent infection and conserve energy until the allergic response is over
Serum sickness reaction This allergy involves antibodies that circulate in the blood and cause damage to various tissues by depositing in blood vessels. This reaction may occur up to 1 week or more after exposure to the drug	Itchy rash, high fever, swollen lymph nodes, swollen and painful joints, oedema of the face and limbs	Notify the prescriber and/or primary carer and discontinue the drug. Provide comfort measures to help the person cope with the signs and symptoms (cool environment, skin care, positioning, ice to joints, administer antipyretics or anti-inflammatory agents, as appropriate)
Delayed allergic reaction This reaction occurs several hours after exposure and involves antibodies that are bound to specific white blood cells	Rash, hives, swollen joints	Notify the prescriber and/or primary carer and discontinue the drug. Provide skin care and comfort measures that may include antihistamines or topical corticosteroids

cardiac arrhythmias, caused in many people a characteristic skin rash that appeared like a bright red blood vessel pattern under the skin. Although people may report that they are allergic to a drug because they develop a skin rash when taking the drug, it is important to determine whether a rash is a commonly associated adverse effect of the drug.

Assessment

Hives, rashes and other dermatological lesions may be seen. Severe reactions may include exfoliative dermatitis, which is characterised by rash and scaling, fever, enlarged lymph nodes, enlarged liver and the potentially fatal erythema multiforme exudativum (Stevens–Johnson syndrome), which is characterised by dark red papules appearing on the extremities with no pain or itching, often in rings or disc-shaped patches.

Interventions

In mild cases, or when the benefit of the drug outweighs the discomfort of the skin lesion, provide frequent skin care; instruct the person to avoid rubbing, wearing tight or rough clothing and using harsh soaps or perfumed lotions; and administer antihistamines, as appropriate. In severe cases, discontinue the drug and notify the prescriber and/or primary carer. Be aware that, in addition to these interventions, topical corticosteroids, antihistamines and emollients are frequently used.

Stomatitis

Stomatitis, or inflammation of the mucous membranes, can occur because of a direct toxic reaction to the drug or because the drug deposits in the end capillaries in the mucous membranes, leading to inflammation. Many drugs are known to cause stomatitis. The antineoplastic drugs commonly cause these problems because they are toxic to rapidly turning-over cells, like those found in the gastrointestinal tract. People receiving antineoplastic drugs are usually given instructions for proper mouth care when the drugs are started.

Assessment

Symptoms can include swollen gums, inflamed gums (gingivitis), and a swollen and red tongue (glossitis).

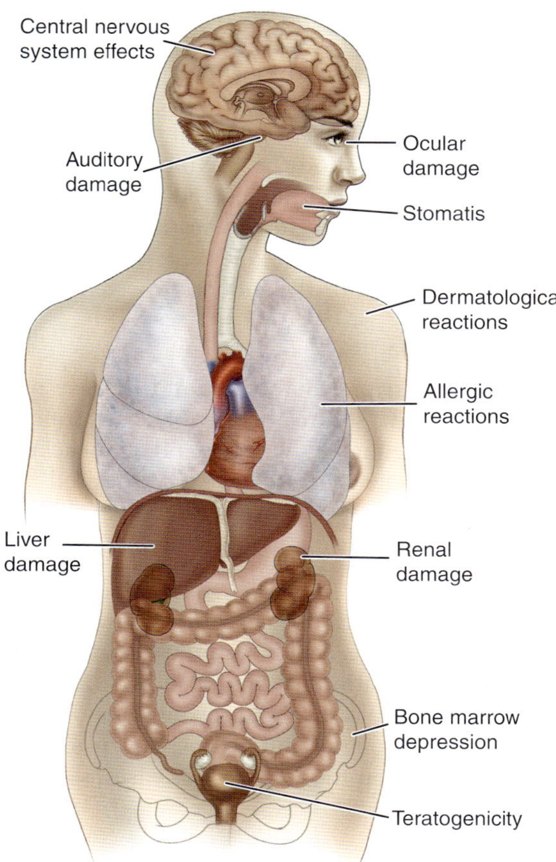

FIGURE 3.1 Variety of adverse effects and toxicities associated with drug use.

Other symptoms include difficulty swallowing, bad breath, and pain in the mouth and throat.

Interventions

Provide frequent mouth care with a non-irritating solution. Offer nutrition evaluation and development of a tolerated diet, which usually involves frequent small meals. If necessary, arrange for a dental consultation. Note that antifungal agents and/or local anaesthetics are sometimes used.

Superinfections

One of the body's protective mechanisms is provided by the wide variety of bacteria that live within or on the surface of the body. This bacterial growth is called the *normal flora*. Normal flora protect the body from invasion by other bacteria, viruses, fungi and so on. Several kinds of drugs (especially antibiotics) destroy the normal flora, leading to the development of **superinfections**, or infections caused by organisms that are usually controlled by the normal flora.

Assessment

Symptoms can include fever, diarrhoea, a black or hairy tongue, an inflamed and swollen tongue (glossitis), mucous membrane lesions and vaginal discharge with or without itching.

Interventions

Provide supportive measures (frequent mouth care, skin care, access to bathroom facilities, small and frequent meals). Administer antifungal therapy as appropriate. In severe cases, discontinue the drug responsible for the superinfection.

Blood dyscrasia

Blood dyscrasia is bone marrow suppression caused by drug effects. This occurs when drugs that can cause cell death (eg, antineoplastics, antibiotics) are used. Bone marrow cells multiply rapidly; they are said to be rapidly turning over. Because they go through cell division and multiply so often, they are highly susceptible to any agent that disrupts cell function.

Assessment

Symptoms include fever, chills, sore throat, weakness, back pain, dark urine, decreased haematocrit (anaemia), low platelet count (thrombocytopenia), low white blood cell count (leucopenia) and a reduction of all cellular elements of the full blood count (pancytopenia).

Interventions

Monitor blood counts. Provide supportive measures (rest, protection from exposure to infections, protection from injury, avoidance of activities that might result in injury or bleeding). In severe cases, discontinue the drug or stop administration until the bone marrow recovers to a safe level.

KEY POINTS

- Adverse drug effects can include skin irritation ranging from rashes and hives to potentially fatal Stevens–Johnson syndrome. Adverse effects can be predictable or unpredictable based on the mechanism of action of the drug to its drug profile.
- Other adverse drug effects include superinfections, or infections caused by destruction of protective normal flora bacteria; blood dyscrasias caused by bone marrow suppression of the blood-forming cells; and stomatitis or mucous membrane eruptions.

Toxicity

Introducing chemicals into the body can sometimes affect the body very severely. These effects are not acceptable adverse effects but are potentially serious reactions to a drug. When a drug is known to have toxic effects, the benefit of the drug to the person must be weighed against the possibility of toxic effects causing harm.

Liver injury (hepatotoxicity)

Oral drugs are absorbed and passed directly into the liver in the first-pass effect. This exposes the liver cells to the full impact of the drug before it is broken down or distributed throughout the body. Most drugs are metabolised in the liver, so any active metabolites that are toxic will also affect the integrity of the liver cells (hepatocytes).

Assessment

Symptoms may include fever, malaise, nausea, vomiting, jaundice, change in colour of urine or stools, abdominal pain or colic, elevated liver enzyme levels (eg, aspartate aminotransferase [AST], alanine aminotransferase [ALT]), alterations in bilirubin levels and changes in clotting factor activity (eg, partial thromboplastin time).

Interventions

Discontinue the drug and notify the prescriber and/or primary carer. Offer supportive measures such as small, frequent meals, skin care, a cool environment and rest periods.

Renal injury (nephrotoxicity)

The glomerulus in the kidney has a very small capillary network that filters the blood into the renal tubule. Some drug molecules can precipitate in the renal tubules causing acute inflammation and severe renal problems. Some drugs are excreted from the kidney unchanged; they have the potential to directly affect the renal tubule and alter normal absorption and secretion processes. Gentamicin, a potent antibiotic, is frequently associated with renal toxicity.

Assessment

Elevated blood urea nitrogen (BUN) level, elevated creatinine concentration, decreased haematocrit, electrolyte imbalances, fatigue, malaise, oedema, irritability and skin rash may be seen.

Interventions

Notify the prescriber and/or primary carer and discontinue the drug as needed. Offer supportive measures – for example, positioning, diet and fluid restrictions, skin care, electrolyte therapy, rest periods, a controlled environment. In severe cases, be aware that dialysis may be required for survival.

Poisoning

Poisoning occurs when an overdose of a drug damages multiple body systems, leading to the potential for fatal reactions. Assessment parameters vary with the particular drug. Treatment of drug poisoning also varies, depending on the drug. Throughout this book, specific treatments for poisoning are identified, if known. Emergency and life support measures are often needed in severe cases.

Alterations in glucose metabolism

All cells need glucose for energy; the cells of the central nervous system (CNS) are especially dependent on constant glucose levels to function properly. The control of glucose in the body is an integrated process that involves a series of hormones and enzymes that use the liver as the place for glucose storage or release. Many drugs have an impact on glucose levels because of their effects on the liver or the endocrine system.

Hypoglycaemia

Some drugs affect metabolism and the use of glucose, causing a low serum blood glucose concentration, or hypoglycaemia. Glipizide and glibenclamide are antidiabetic agents that have the desired action of lowering the blood glucose level but can lower blood glucose too far, causing hypoglycaemia.

Assessment

Symptoms may include fatigue; drowsiness; hunger; anxiety; headache; cold, clammy skin; shaking and lack of coordination (tremulousness); increased heart rate; increased blood pressure; numbness and tingling of the mouth, tongue and/or lips; confusion; and rapid and shallow respirations. In severe cases, seizures and/or coma may occur.

Interventions

Restore glucose – orally, if possible, or intravenously (IV). Provide supportive measures (eg, skin care, environmental control of light and temperature, rest). Institute safety measures to prevent injury or falls. Monitor blood glucose levels to help stabilise the situation. Offer reassurance to help the person cope with the experience.

Hyperglycaemia

Some drugs stimulate the breakdown of glycogen or alter metabolism in such a way as to cause high serum glucose levels, or hyperglycaemia. Ephedrine (generic), a drug used as a bronchodilator and antiasthma drug and to relieve nasal congestion, can break down stored glycogen and cause an elevation of blood glucose by its effects on the sympathetic nervous system. Diazoxide, a drug used for treatment of malignant hypertension, causes a decrease in insulin release, leading to an increase in blood glucose levels.

Assessment

Fatigue, increased urination (polyuria), increased thirst (polydipsia), deep respirations (Kussmaul respirations), restlessness, increased hunger (polyphagia), nausea, hot or flushed skin and fruity breath odour may be observed.

Interventions

Administer insulin therapy to decrease blood glucose as appropriate, while carefully monitoring glucose levels.

Provide support to help the person deal with signs and symptoms (eg, provide access to bathroom facilities, control the temperature of the room, decrease stimulation while the person is in crisis, offer reassurance, provide mouth care – [the person will experience dry mouth and bad breath with the ensuing acidosis and mouth care will help to make this more tolerable]).

Electrolyte imbalances

Drugs can have an effect on various electrolyte levels in the body. These effects can have serious consequences, as many physiological functions are intricately dependent on certain electrolyte levels. The electrolyte that can cause the most serious effects when it is altered, even a little, is potassium.

Hypokalaemia

Some drugs affecting the kidney can cause low serum potassium levels (hypokalaemia) by altering the renal exchange system. For example, loop diuretics function by causing the loss of potassium, as well as of sodium and water. Potassium is essential for the normal functioning of nerves and muscles.

Assessment

Symptoms include a serum potassium concentration ($[K^+]$) lower than 3.5 mmol/L, weakness, numbness and tingling in the extremities, muscle cramps, nausea, vomiting, diarrhoea, decreased bowel sounds, irregular pulse, weak pulse, orthostatic hypotension and disorientation. In severe cases, paralytic ileus (absent bowel sounds, abdominal distension and acute abdomen) may occur.

Interventions

Replace serum potassium and carefully monitor serum levels and the person's response; achieving the desired level can take time and the person may experience high potassium levels in the process. Provide supportive therapy (eg, safety precautions to prevent injury or falls, reorientation of the person, comfort measures for pain and discomfort). Cardiac monitoring may be needed to evaluate the effect of the fluctuating potassium levels on heart rhythm.

Hyperkalaemia

Some drugs that affect the kidney, such as the potassium-sparing diuretics, can lead to potassium retention and a resultant increase in serum potassium levels (hyperkalaemia). Other drugs that cause cell death or injury, such as many antineoplastic agents, can also cause the cells to release potassium, leading to hyperkalaemia.

Assessment

Symptoms include a serum potassium level higher than 5.0 mmol/L, weakness, muscle cramps, diarrhoea, numbness and tingling, slow heart rate, low blood pressure, decreased urine output and difficulty breathing.

Interventions

Institute measures to decrease the serum potassium concentration, including use of sodium polystyrene sulfonate. When trying to stabilise the potassium level, it is possible that the person may experience low potassium levels. Careful monitoring is important until the person's potassium levels are stable. Offer supportive measures to cope with discomfort. Institute safety measures to prevent injury or falls. Monitor for cardiac irregularities because potassium is an important electrolyte in the action potential, which is needed for cell membrane stability. When potassium levels are too high, the cells of the heart become very irritable and rhythm disturbances can occur. Be prepared for a possible cardiac emergency. In severe cases, be aware that dialysis may be needed.

Sensory effects

Drugs can affect the senses, including the eyes and ears. Alterations in seeing and hearing can pose safety problems for people.

Ocular damage

The blood vessels in the retina are very tiny and are called 'end arteries', that is, they stop and do not interconnect with other arteries feeding the same cells. Some drugs are deposited into these tiny arteries, causing inflammation and tissue damage. Hydroxychloroquine *(Plaquenil)*, a drug used to treat some rheumatoid diseases, can cause retinal damage and even blindness.

Assessment

Blurring of vision, vision changes, corneal damage and blindness may be noted.

Interventions

Monitor the person's vision carefully when they are receiving known oculotoxic drugs. Consult with the prescriber and/or primary carer and discontinue the drug as appropriate. Provide supportive measures, especially if vision loss is not reversible. Monitor lighting and exposure to sunlight.

Auditory damage (ototoxicity)

Tiny vessels and nerves in the eighth cranial nerve are easily affected and damaged by certain drugs. The macrolide antibiotics can cause severe auditory nerve damage. Aspirin, one of the most commonly used drugs, is often linked to auditory ringing and eighth cranial nerve effects.

Assessment

Dizziness, ringing in the ears (tinnitus), loss of balance and loss of hearing may be assessed.

Interventions

Monitor the person's perceptual losses or changes. Provide protective measures to prevent falling or injury. Consult with the prescriber to decrease the dose or discontinue the drug. Provide supportive measures to cope with drug effects.

Neurological effects (neurotoxicity)

Many drugs can affect the functioning of the nerves in the periphery and the CNS. Nerves function by using a constant source of energy to maintain the resting membrane potential and allow excitation. This requires glucose, oxygen and maintenance of electrolyte balance.

General central nervous system effects

Although the brain is fairly well protected from many drug effects by the blood–brain barrier, some drugs do affect neurological function, either directly or by altering electrolyte or glucose levels. Beta blockers, which are used to treat hypertension, angina and many other conditions, can cause feelings of anxiety, insomnia and nightmares.

Assessment

Symptoms may include confusion, delirium, insomnia, drowsiness, hyperreflexia or hyporeflexia, bizarre dreams, hallucinations, numbness, tingling and paraesthesias.

Interventions

Provide safety measures to prevent injury. Caution the person to avoid dangerous situations such as driving a car or operating dangerous machinery. Orient the person and provide support. Consult with the prescriber to decrease drug dose or discontinue the drug.

Atropine-like (anticholinergic) effects

Some drugs block the effects of the parasympathetic nervous system by directly or indirectly blocking cholinergic receptors. Atropine, a drug used preoperatively to dry up secretions and any other indications, is the prototype anticholinergic drug. Many cold remedies and antihistamines also cause anticholinergic effects.

Assessment

Dry mouth, altered taste perception, dysphagia, heartburn, constipation, bloating, paralytic ileus, urinary hesitancy and retention, impotence, blurred vision, cycloplegia, photophobia, headache, mental confusion, nasal congestion, palpitations, decreased sweating and dry skin may be noted.

Interventions

Provide sugarless lozenges and mouth care to help relieve dryness of the mouth. Arrange for a bowel program as appropriate. Have the person void before taking the drug, to aid voiding. Provide safety measures if vision changes occur. Arrange for medication for headache and nasal congestion as appropriate. Advise the person to avoid hot environments and to take protective measures to prevent falling and also dehydration, which may be caused by exposure to heat, owing to decreased sweating.

Parkinson-like syndrome (parkinsonism)

Drugs that directly or indirectly affect dopamine levels in the brain can cause a syndrome that resembles Parkinson disease. Many of the antipsychotic and neuroleptic drugs can cause this effect. In most cases, the effects go away when the drug is withdrawn.

Assessment

Lack of activity, akinesia, muscular tremors, drooling, changes in gait, rigidity, extreme restlessness or 'jitters' (akathisia), or spasms (dyskinesia) may be observed.

Interventions

Discontinue the drug, if necessary. Know that treatment with anticholinergics or antiparkinson drugs may be recommended if the benefit of the drug outweighs the discomfort of its adverse effects. Provide small, frequent meals if swallowing becomes difficult. Provide safety measures if ambulation becomes a problem.

Neuroleptic malignant syndrome

General anaesthetics and other drugs that have direct CNS effects can cause neuroleptic malignant syndrome, a generalised syndrome that includes high fever.

Assessment

Extrapyramidal symptoms, including slowed reflexes, rigidity, involuntary movements; hyperthermia; and autonomic disturbances, such as hypertension, fast heart rate and fever, may be noted.

Interventions

Discontinue the drug if necessary. Know that treatment with anticholinergics or antiparkinson drugs may be required. Provide supportive care to lower the body temperature. Institute safety precautions as needed.

Teratogenicity

Many drugs that reach the developing fetus or embryo can cause death or congenital defects, which can include skeletal and limb abnormalities, CNS alterations, heart defects and the like. The exact effects of a drug on the fetus may not be known. In some cases, a predictable syndrome occurs when a drug is given to a pregnant woman. In any situation, inform any pregnant woman who requires drug therapy about the possible effects on the baby. Before a drug is administered to a pregnant woman, the actual benefits should be weighed against the potential risks. All pregnant women should be

BOX 3.1 Summary of types of adverse drug effects

- Extension of primary action
- Occurrence of secondary action
- Allergic reactions
  - Anaphylactic reactions
  - Cytotoxic reactions
  - Serum sickness reactions
  - Delayed allergic reactions
- Tissue and organ damage
  - Dermatological reactions
  - Stomatitis
  - Superinfections
  - Blood dyscrasia
- Toxicity
  - Liver injury
  - Renal injury
  - Poisoning
- Alterations in glucose metabolism
  - Hypoglycaemia
  - Hyperglycaemia
- Electrolyte imbalances
  - Hypokalaemia
  - Hyperkalaemia
- Sensory effects
  - Ocular toxicity
  - Auditory damage
- Neurological effects
  - General central nervous system effects
  - Atropine-like (anticholinergic) effects
  - Parkinson-like syndrome
  - Neuroleptic malignant syndrome
- Teratogenicity
- Iatrogenicity

advised not to self-medicate during the pregnancy. Emotional and physical support is needed to assist the woman in dealing with the possibility of fetal death or birth defects.

Box 3.1 summarises all of the adverse effects that have been described throughout this chapter.

Iatrogenicity

The terms **iatrogenesis** and **iatrogenic artefact** refer to inadvertent adverse effects or complications caused by, or as a result of, medical treatment or advice. In addition to harmful consequences of actions by doctors, iatrogenesis can also refer to actions by other health care professionals, such as psychologists, therapists, pharmacists, nurses, dentists, midwives and others. Iatrogenesis is not restricted to conventional medicine, as iatrogenesis can also result from complementary and alternative medicine treatments. Causes of iatrogenesis include chance, medical error, negligence, social control, anxiety or annoyance related to medical procedures, and the adverse effects or interactions of medications.

CHAPTER SUMMARY

- No drug does only what is desired of it. All drugs have adverse effects associated with them.
- Adverse drug effects can range from allergic reactions to tissue and cellular damage. The nurse or midwife, as the health care provider associated with drug administration, needs to assess each situation for potential adverse effects and intervene appropriately to minimise those effects.
- Adverse effects can be extensions of the primary action of a drug or secondary effects that are not necessarily desirable, but are unavoidable.
- Allergic reactions can occur when a person's body makes antibodies to a drug or drug–protein complex. If the person is exposed to that drug at another time, an immune response may occur. Allergic reactions can be of various types. The exact response should be noted to avoid future confusion in care provision.
- Tissue damage can include skin problems, mucous membrane inflammation, blood dyscrasia, superinfections, liver or renal toxicity, poisoning, hypoglycaemia or hyperglycaemia, electrolyte disturbances, various CNS problems (ocular damage, auditory damage, atropine-like effects, Parkinson-like syndrome, neuroleptic malignant syndrome) and teratogenicity.

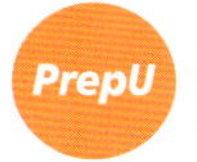

Knowing your strengths and weaknesses helps you to study more effectively. Take a PrepU Practice Quiz to find out how you measure up!

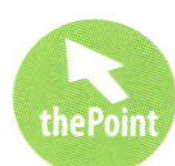

ONLINE RESOURCES

An extensive range of additional resources to enhance teaching and learning and to facilitate understanding of this chapter may be found online at the text's accompanying website, located on thePoint at http://thepoint.lww.com. These include Watch and Learn videos, Concepts in Action animations, journal articles, review questions, case studies, discussion topics and quizzes.

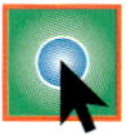

WEBLINKS

Health care providers and students may want to consult the following web resources:

www.who.int/patientsafety/events/05/Reporting_Guidelines.pdf
World Health Organization (2005) World Alliance for Patient Safety – WHO Draft Guidelines for Adverse Event Reporting and Learning Systems – from information to action.

BIBLIOGRAPHY

Dempsey, J., Hillege, S. & Hill, R. (2014). *Fundamentals of Nursing and Midwifery: A Person-centred Approach to Care* (2nd Australian and New Zealand edn). Sydney: Lippincott Williams & Wilkins.

Edwards, R. & Aronson, J. K. (2000). Adverse drug reactions: Definitions, diagnosis, and management. *Lancet, 356*, 1255–1259.

Gabe, M. E., Davies, G. A., Murphy, F., Davies, M., Johnstone, L. & Jordan, S. (2011). Adverse drug reactions: treatment burdens and nurse-led medication monitoring. *Journal of Nursing Management, 19(3)*, 377–392.

Goodman, L. S., Brunton, L. L., Chabner, B. & Knollmann, B. C. (2011). *Goodman and Gilman's Pharmacological Basis of Therapeutics* (12th edn). New York: McGraw-Hill.

Hakkarainen, K. M., Hedna, K., Petzold, M. et al. (2012). Percentage of patients with preventable adverse drug reactions and preventability of adverse drug reactions—A meta-analysis. *PLoS ONE, 7(3)*, 1–9.

Kalisch, L. M., Caughey, G. E., Roughead, E. E. & Gilbert, A. L. (2011). The prescribing cascade. *Australian Prescriber, 34(6)*, 162–166.

McKenna, L. & Mirkov, S. (2019). *McKenna's Drug Handbook for Nursing and Midwifery* (8th edn). Sydney: Wolters Kluwer Health Australia.

Mercier, E., Giraudeau, B., Ginies, G., Perrotin, D. & Dequin, P. (2010). Iatrogenic events contributing to ICU admission: a prospective study. *Intensive care medicine, 36(6)*, 1033–1037.

CHECK YOUR UNDERSTANDING

Answers to the questions in this chapter can be found in Appendix A at the back of this book.

MULTIPLE CHOICE

Select the best answer to the following.

1. An example of a drug allergy is:
   a. dry mouth occurring with use of an antihistamine.
   b. increased urination occurring with use of a thiazide diuretic.
   c. breathing difficulty after an injection of penicillin.
   d. skin rash associated with procainamide use.
2. A person taking glyburide (an antidiabetic drug) has his morning dose and then does not have a chance to eat for several hours. An adverse effect that might be expected from this would be:
   a. a teratogenic effect.
   b. a skin rash.
   c. an anticholinergic effect.
   d. hypoglycaemia.
3. A person with a severe infection is given gentamicin, the only antibiotic shown to be effective in culture and sensitivity tests. A few hours after the drug is started intravenously, the person becomes very restless and develops oedema. Blood tests reveal abnormal electrolyte levels and elevated BUN. This reaction was most likely caused by:
   a. an anaphylactic reaction.
   b. renal toxicity associated with gentamicin.
   c. superinfection related to the antibiotic.
   d. hypoglycaemia.
4. Persons receiving antineoplastic drugs that disrupt cell function often have adverse effects involving cells that turn over rapidly in the body. These cells include:
   a. ovarian cells.
   b. liver cells.
   c. cardiac cells.
   d. bone marrow cells.
5. A woman has had repeated bouts of bronchitis throughout the autumn and has been taking antibiotics. She calls the clinic with complaints of vaginal pain and itching. When she is seen, it is discovered that she has developed a yeast infection. You would explain to her that:
   a. her bronchitis has moved to the vaginal area.
   b. she has developed a superinfection because the antibiotics kill bacteria that normally provide protection.
   c. she probably has developed a sexually transmitted disease related to her lifestyle.
   d. she will need to take even more antibiotics to treat this new infection.
6. Knowing that a person is taking a loop diuretic and is at risk for developing hypokalaemia, the health care provider would assess the person for:
   a. hypertension, headache and cold and clammy skin.
   b. decreased urinary output and yellowing of the sclera.
   c. weak pulse, low blood pressure and muscle cramping.
   d. diarrhoea and flatulence.

MULTIPLE RESPONSE

Select all that apply.

1. A person is taking a drug that is known to be toxic to the liver. The person is being discharged home. What teaching points related to liver toxicity and the drug should the health care provider teach the person to report to the doctor?
   a. fever; changes in the colour of urine
   b. changes in the colour of stool; malaise
   c. rapid, deep respirations; increased sweating
   d. dizziness; drowsiness; dry mouth
   e. rash; black or hairy tongue; white spots in the mouth or throat
   f. yellowing of the skin or the whites of the eyes
2. Pregnant women should be advised of the potential risk to the fetus any time they take a drug during pregnancy. What fetal problems can be related to drug exposure in utero?
   a. fetal death
   b. nervous system disruption
   c. skeletal and limb abnormalities
   d. cardiac defects
   e. low-set ears
   f. deafness
3. A person is experiencing a reaction to the penicillin injection that was administered approximately 30 minutes ago. The health care provider is concerned that it might be an anaphylactic reaction. What signs and symptoms would validate her suspicion?
   a. rapid heart rate
   b. diaphoresis
   c. constricted pupils
   d. hypotension
   e. rash
   f. the person reporting a panic feeling
4. A person is experiencing a serum sickness reaction to a recent rubella vaccination. Which of the following interventions would be appropriate when caring for this person?
   a. administration of adrenaline
   b. cool environment
   c. positioning to provide comfort
   d. ice to joints as needed
   e. administration of anti-inflammatory agents
   f. administration of topical corticosteroids

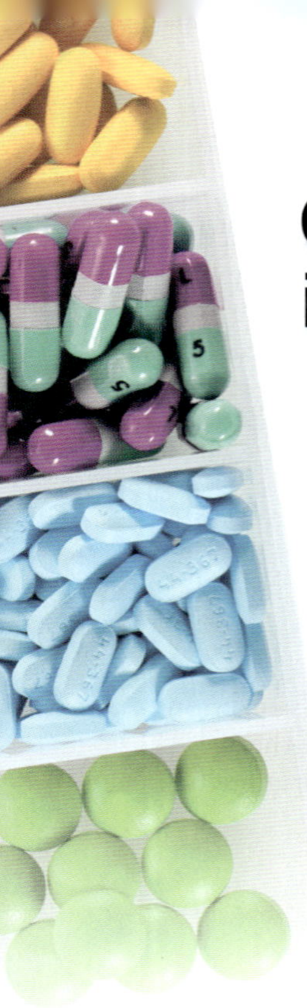

Clinical decision making in drug therapy

4

Learning objectives

On completing this chapter you should be able to:

1. List the responsibilities of the nurse and midwife in relation to drug therapy.
2. Explain what is involved in clinical decision making as it relates to drug therapy.
3. Describe key points that must be incorporated into the assessment of a person receiving drug therapy.
4. Describe the essential elements of a medication order.
5. Outline the important points that must be assessed and considered before administering a drug, combining knowledge about the drug with knowledge of the person and the environment.
6. Describe the role of the nurse or midwife and the individual in preventing medication errors.
7. Identify what is meant by pharmacovigilance.

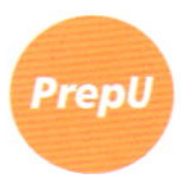

PrepU Test your current knowledge of clinical decision making in drug therapy with a PrepU Practice Quiz!

Glossary of key terms

assessment: information gathering regarding the current status of a particular person, including evaluation of past history and physical examination; provides a baseline of information and clues to effectiveness of therapy

clinical decision making: problem solving process that underpins formulation and evaluation of care

evaluation: determining the effects of the interventions that were instituted for the person and leading to further assessment and intervention

implementation: actions undertaken to meet a person's needs, such as administration of drugs, comfort measures or teaching

midwifery: art and science of working with women and their families throughout the childbearing process, combining scientific application of chemistry, anatomy, physiology, biology, nutrition, psychology and pharmacology to the individual woman's situation

nursing: the art of nurturing and administering to the sick, combined with the scientific application of chemistry, anatomy, physiology, biology, nutrition, psychology and pharmacology to the particular clinical situation

pharmacovigilance: monitoring and preventing adverse effects of medication to promote safe use

The delivery of health care today is in a constant state of change, at times reaching crisis levels. The population is ageing, resulting in an increased incidence and prevalence of chronic disease and more complex care issues. The population is also more transient, with individuals and families more mobile, often resulting in unstable support systems and fewer at-home care providers and helpers. At the same time, health care is undergoing a technological boom, including greater use of more sophisticated diagnostic methods and treatments, new specialised drugs, including experimental drugs, and so on. Moreover, people are being discharged earlier from acute care facilities or are not being admitted at all for procedures that once were treated in hospital with follow-up support and monitoring.

People are also becoming more responsible for their care and for adhering to complicated medical regimens at home. The wide use of the Internet and an emphasis in the media on the need to question all aspects of health care has led to more knowledgeable and challenging care provision. People may no longer accept a drug regimen or therapy without question and often feel confident in adjusting it on their own because of information that they have found on the Internet. Such information might not be accurate or even relevant to their particular situation. Nurses and midwives are often central to clarifying people's understandings of their medications and health conditions, and providing evidence-based, accurate information.

NURSING: ART AND SCIENCE

Nursing is a unique and complex science, as well as a nurturing and caring art. In the traditional sense, nursing has been viewed as ministering to and soothing the sick through the provision of person-centred care. In the current state of medical changes, nursing also has become increasingly technical and scientific. Nurses are assuming increasing responsibilities that involve not only nurturing and caring, but also assessing, diagnosing and intervening with people to treat, to prevent and to educate as they assist people in coping with various health states.

The nurse deals with the whole person, including physical, emotional, intellectual, social and spiritual aspects. Nurses must consider how a person responds to disease and its treatment, including the changes in lifestyle that may be required. Therefore, a nurse is a key health care provider who is in a position to assess the whole person, to administer therapy as well as medications, to teach the person how best to cope with the therapy so as to ensure the most favourable outcome and to evaluate the effectiveness of the therapy. Nurses accomplish these tasks by integrating knowledge of the basic sciences (anatomy, physiology, nutrition, chemistry, pharmacology), the social sciences (sociology, psychology), education and many other disciplines and by applying clinical decision-making approaches.

MIDWIFERY: ART AND SCIENCE

Midwifery, too, is a unique discipline that combines both art and science. The midwife primarily provides person-centred care for women and their families throughout childbearing as well as promoting their health across the lifespan. This includes care before conception; during antenatal, labour and postnatal phases; and beyond. Midwives are increasingly becoming involved in public health and health promotion for women throughout the lifespan, including during adolescence and menopause.

The midwife, like the nurse, provides care that incorporates physical, emotional, intellectual, social and spiritual aspects. Such care may incorporate an array of medications, both supporting normal physiological processes, as well as managing underlying health problems or health problems arising during childbearing, as well as health promotion such as in family planning. Midwives, too, provide such care through integrating knowledge of basic sciences (anatomy, physiology nutrition, chemistry, pharmacology), the social sciences (sociology, psychology), education and many other disciplines and by applying clinical decision-making approaches.

THE CLINICAL DECISION-MAKING PROCESS

Nurses and midwives use the **clinical decision-making process** – a problem-solving process based on person-centredness – to provide efficient and effective care. Application of the process with drug therapy ensures that people receive the best, safest, most efficient, scientifically based, holistic care. Clinical decision making is a complex activity that requires practitioners to be knowledgeable in relevant aspects of care and to have access to reliable and appropriate sources of information.

The process of making judgements and decisions involves the person making a judgement or decision using information; how individuals use information and where that information comes from are key to successful decision making. Many clinical decisions occur in situations of uncertainty. Each judgement and decision a clinician makes will require them to think about an uncertain future, in the present, using evidence that comes from a (more) certain past. There are many uncertainties in delivering health care, such as uncertainty about illness and health, as there is no clear definition of a 'disease'.

Assessment

Assessment (gathering information) involves systematic, organised collection of data about the person. Because the nurse or midwife is responsible for holistic care, data must include information about physical, intellectual, emotional, social and environmental factors. When viewed together, this information provides the nurse or midwife with the facts needed to plan educational and discharge programs, arrange for appropriate consultations and monitor physical response to treatment, to disease or to pregnancy. The process of assessment never ends because the person is in a dynamic state, continuously adjusting to physical, emotional and environmental influences.

Drug therapy is a complex and important part of health care, and the principles of drug therapy must be incorporated into every person's assessment plan. The particular information that is needed varies with each drug, but the concepts involved are similar. Two major aspects associated with assessment are the person's history (past illnesses and the current problem) and examination of their physical status.

History

The person's history is an important element of assessment related to drug therapy because their past experiences and illnesses can influence a drug's effect. Knowledge of this important information before beginning drug therapy will help to promote safe and effective use of the drug and prevent adverse effects, clinically important drug–drug, drug–food or drug–alternative therapy interactions and medication errors. Relevant aspects of the person's history specifically related to drug therapy are discussed in the following text.

Chronic conditions

Chronic conditions can affect the pharmacokinetics and pharmacodynamics of a drug. For example, certain conditions (eg, renal disease, liver disease, heart disease, diabetes, chronic lung disease) may be contraindications to the use of a drug. In addition, these conditions may require cautious use or dose adjustment when administering a certain drug. For example, a person with renal disease may require a decreased dose of a drug because of the way the drug is eliminated. The nurse or midwife should be aware of the person's renal function to determine the person's ability to eliminate the drug. Therefore, if renal disease is mentioned in the person's history, the nurse or midwife should consider this factor to evaluate the dose of the drug that is prescribed.

Drug use

Prescription drugs, over-the-counter (OTC) drugs, recreational drugs, alcohol, nicotine, alternative therapies and caffeine may have an impact on a drug's effect. People often neglect to mention OTC drugs or alternative therapies because they do not consider them to be actual drugs or they may be unwilling to admit their use to the health care provider. Ask people specifically about OTC drug or alternative therapy use. Drug–drug interactions with OTC and prescribed drugs are highly likely and can be dangerous, resulting in ineffective drug therapy for some at-risk people. People might also forget to mention prescription drugs that they routinely take, for example, oral contraceptives. Always ask specifically about all types of medications that the person might use.

Allergies

A person's history of allergies can affect drug therapy. Past exposure to a drug or other allergens can provoke a future reaction or necessitate the need for cautious use of the drug, food or animal product. Obtain specific information about the person's allergic reaction to determine whether the person has experienced a true drug allergy or was experiencing an actual effect or adverse effect of the drug.

Level of education and understanding

Information about the person's education level provides a baseline from which the nurse or midwife can determine the appropriate types of teaching information to use. A person with a secondary school education may require materials at a different level from the person with a university degree. Gathering information about the person's level of understanding about their condition, illness or drug therapy helps the health care provider to determine where the person is in terms of their status and the level of explanation that will be required. It also provides additional baseline information for developing a person-focused education program. It is important not to assume anything about the person's ability to understand based on their reported education level. Stress, disease and environmental factors can all affect a person's learning readiness and ability. Direct assessment of actual learning abilities is critical for good education.

Social supports

People are being discharged from health care facilities earlier than ever before, often with continuing health care needs. In addition, earlier discharges leave minimal time for teaching. Often people need help at home with care and drug therapy. A key aspect of discharge planning involves determining what support, if any, is available to the person at home. In many situations, it also involves referral to appropriate community resources.

Financial supports

The high cost of health care in general, and of medications in particular, must be considered when initiating drug therapy and promoting compliance. Financial constraints may cause a person not to follow through with a prescribed drug regimen. For example, the drug may be too expensive or the person may lack the means to get to a pharmacy to obtain the drug. In some situations, a less expensive drug might be appropriate in place of a very expensive drug. In addition, the nurse or midwife may need to refer the person to appropriate resources that might offer financial assistance.

Pattern of health care

Knowing how a person seeks health care provides the care provider with valuable information to include when preparing the person's teaching plan. Does this person routinely seek follow-up care, or do they wait for emergency situations? Does the person tend to self-treat many complaints, or is every problem brought to a health care provider? Information about patterns of health care also provides insight into conditions that the person may have but has not reported or medication use that has not been stated.

Physical examination

It is important to assess the person's physical status before beginning drug therapy to determine if any conditions exist that would be contraindications or cautions for using the drug and to develop a baseline for evaluating the effectiveness of the drug and the occurrence of any adverse effects. Relevant aspects of the person's physical examination specifically related to drug therapy are discussed in the following text.

Weight

A person's weight helps to determine whether the recommended drug dose is appropriate. Because the recommended dose typically is based on a 70 kg adult man, people who are much lighter or much heavier often need a dose adjustment.

Age

People at the extremes of the age spectrum – children and older adults – often require dose adjustments based on the functional level of the liver and kidneys and the responsiveness of other organs. The child's age and developmental level will also alert the health care provider to possible problems with drug delivery, such as the ability to swallow pills or follow directions related to other delivery methods. The child's developmental age will also influence pharmacokinetics and pharmacodynamics; the immature liver may not metabolise drugs in the same way as in the adult or the kidneys may not be as efficient as those of an adult.

As people age, the body undergoes many normal changes that can affect drug therapy, such as a decreased blood volume, decreased gastrointestinal (GI) absorption, reduced blood flow to muscles or skin and changes in receptor-site responsiveness. Older adults often have a variety of chronic medical conditions and can be receiving a number of medications that need to be evaluated for possible interactions. Older adults with various central nervous system disorders, such as Alzheimer disease or Parkinson disease, may develop difficulty swallowing and might require liquid forms of medication. Throughout this book, Drug Therapy Across the Lifespan features present information related to the drug class being discussed as it pertains specifically to children, adults and the older adult population. These boxes highlight points that the nurse and midwife should consider to assure safe and effective therapy in each age group.

Physical parameters related to disease or drug effects

The specific parameters that need to be assessed depend on the disease process being treated and the expected therapeutic and adverse effects of the drug therapy. Assessing these factors before drug therapy begins provides a baseline level to which future assessments can be compared to determine the effects of drug therapy. For example, if a person is being treated for chronic pulmonary disease, their respiratory status and reserve need to be assessed, especially if a drug is being given that is known to affect the respiratory tract. In contrast, a thorough respiratory evaluation would not be warranted in a person with no known pulmonary disease who is taking a drug with little or no known effects on the respiratory system. The nurse or midwife has the greatest direct and continued contact with the person and is in the best position to detect minute changes that ultimately determine the course of drug therapy – therapeutic success or discontinuation because of adverse or unacceptable responses.

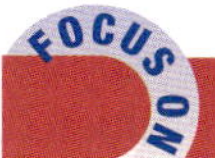

Safe medication administration

Review the monographs in a drug guide or handbook for specific parameters to be assessed in relation to the particular drug being discussed. This assessment provides not only the baseline information needed before giving that drug, but also the data required to evaluate the effects of that drug on the person. This information should supplement the overall assessment of the person, which includes social, intellectual, financial, environmental and other factors.

Identifying health problems

Information gathered during assessment is analysed to arrive at some conclusions that lead to a particular goal and set of interventions. Health care priorities reflect identified alterations in a person's function based on the assessment of the clinical situation. Because drug therapy is only a small part of the overall person's situation, priorities that are related to drug therapy must be incorporated into a total picture of the person.

Implementation involves taking the information gathered and synthesised to plan care. This process includes setting goals and desired outcomes to assure safe and effective drug therapy. These outcomes usually involve ensuring effective response to drug therapy, minimising adverse effects and understanding the drug regimen. Three types of interventions are frequently involved in drug therapy: drug administration, provision of comfort measures and education of the person and their family.

Proper drug administration

Nurses and midwives must consider a series of points, or 'rights', to ensure safe and effective drug administration. These are:

- correct drug and person
- correct storage of drug
- correct and most effective route
- correct dose
- correct preparation
- correct timing
- correct recording of administration.

See the later section on the prevention of medication errors for a detailed explanation of the nurse's and midwife's role in implementing these rights. Remembering to review each point before administering a drug will help to prevent medication errors and improve care outcomes.

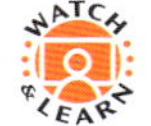

Medications: The Three Checks and the Five Rights of Medication Administration

Comfort measures

Nurses and midwives are in a unique position to help people cope with the effects of drug therapy. A person is more likely to be compliant with a drug regimen if the effects of the regimen are not too uncomfortable or overwhelming.

Placebo effect

The anticipation that a drug will be helpful (placebo effect) has proved to have tremendous impact on the actual success of drug therapy. Therefore, the health care provider's attitude and support can be a critical part of drug therapy. For example, a back rub, a kind word and a positive approach may be as beneficial as the drug itself.

Managing adverse effects

Interventions can be directed at promoting safety and decreasing the impact of the anticipated adverse effects of a drug. Such interventions include environmental control (eg, temperature, light), safety measures (eg, avoiding driving, avoiding the sun, using side rails) and physical comfort measures (eg, skin care, laxatives, frequent meals).

Lifestyle adjustment

Some medications and their effects require that a person make changes in their lifestyle. For example, people taking diuretics may have to rearrange their day so as to be near toilet facilities when the drug action peaks. People taking bisphosphonates will need to plan their morning so they can take the drug on an empty stomach, stay upright for at least half an hour and plan their first food of the day at least half an hour after taking the drug. Many drugs come with similar guidelines for assuring effectiveness and decreasing adverse effects. People taking monoamine oxidase (MAO) inhibitors must adjust their diet to prevent serious adverse effects due to potential drug–food interactions. In some cases the change in lifestyle that is needed can have a tremendous impact on the person and can affect their ability to cope and comply with any medical regimen.

Education of the person and family

With people becoming increasingly responsible for their own care, it is essential that they have all the information necessary to ensure safe and effective drug therapy at home. Many health care agencies require that people be given written information. Box 4.1 includes key elements for any drug education program. Also see the later section on prevention of medication errors for teaching tips related to the person's role in preventing medication errors.

> **FOCUS ON Safe medication administration**
>
> *Special points regarding drug administration and related comfort measures are noted with each drug class discussed in this book. Refer to the individual drug monographs in a drug guide or handbook for more detailed interventions regarding a specific drug.*

Evaluation

Evaluation is part of the continuing process of care that leads to changes in assessment, diagnosis and intervention. The person is continually evaluated for therapeutic response, the occurrence of adverse drug effects and the occurrence of drug–drug, drug–food, drug–alternative therapy or drug–laboratory test interactions. Some drug therapy requires evaluation of specific therapeutic drug levels. In addition, the efficacy of care interventions and the education program are also evaluated. In some situations, the nurse or midwife evaluates the person simply by reapplying the beginning steps of the assessment process and then analysing for changes, either positive or negative. The process of evaluation may lead to changes in the care interventions being used to provide better and safer care.

KEY POINTS

- Nurses and midwives use decision-making frameworks to organise the information that is needed to provide safe and effective care.
- The steps of the decision-making process (assessment, implementation and evaluation) are constantly being repeated to meet the ever-changing needs of the person.
- The systematic approach provides an effective method for handling all the scientific and technical information, as well as the unique emotional, social and physical factors that each person brings to a given situation.

PREVENTION OF MEDICATION ERRORS

With the increase in the older adult population, the increase in the number of available drugs and OTC and complementary and alternative therapy preparations, and the reduced length of hospital stays for people, the risk for medication errors is ever-increasing. In a report conducted for the Australian Commission on Safety and Quality in Health Care (ACSQHC) (Roughead, 2008), it was estimated that 2%–3% of Australian hospital incidents are related to medications, either through the reason for admission or arising during a hospital stay. In addition, of the incidents reported by nurses and midwives, medication events rate the second most common. Hence, they place additional burden on health services. Ensuring prevention of these errors must be foremost in medication administration by nurses and midwives.

BOX 4.1 FOCUS ON Individual and family teaching

Include the following key elements in any drug education program.

Name, dose, and action of drug. Ensure that people know this information. Many people see more than one health care provider; this knowledge is crucial to ensuring safe and effective drug therapy and avoiding drug–drug interactions. Urge people to keep a written list of the drugs that they are taking to show to any health care provider taking care of them, and in case of an emergency when they are not able to report their drug history.

Timing of administration. Teach people when to take the drug with respect to frequency, other drugs and meals.

Special storage and preparation instructions. Inform people about any special handling or storing required. Some drugs may require refrigeration; others may need to be mixed with a specific liquid such as water or fruit juice. Be sure that people know how to carry out these requirements.

Specific OTC drugs or alternative therapies to avoid. Prevent possible interactions between prescribed drugs and other drugs or remedies the person may be using or taking. Many people do not consider OTC drugs or herbal or complementary/alternative therapies to be actual drugs and may inadvertently take them along with their prescribed medications, causing unwanted or even dangerous drug–drug interactions. Prevent these situations by explaining which drugs or therapies should be avoided. Encourage people to always report all the drugs or therapies that they are using to health care providers to reduce the risk of possible inadvertent adverse effects.

Special comfort measures. Teach people how to cope with anticipated adverse effects to ease anxiety and avoid non-compliance with drug therapy. If a person knows that a diuretic is going to lead to increased urination, the day can be scheduled so that bathrooms are nearby when they might be needed. Also educate people about the importance of follow-up tests or evaluation.

Safety measures. Instruct all people to keep drugs out of the reach of children. Remind all people to inform any health care provider they see about the drugs they are taking; this can prevent drug–drug interactions and misdiagnoses based on drug effects. Also alert people to possible safety issues that could arise as a result of drug therapy. For example, teach people to avoid driving or performing hazardous tasks if they are taking drugs that can make them dizzy or alter their thinking or response time.

Specific points about drug toxicity. Give people a list of warning signs of drug toxicity. Advise people to notify their health care provider if any of these effects occur.

Specific warnings about drug discontinuation. Remember that some drugs with a small margin of safety and drugs with particular systemic effects cannot be stopped abruptly without dangerous effects. Alert people who are taking these types of drugs to this problem and encourage them to call their health care provider immediately if they cannot take their medication for any reason (eg. illness, financial constraints).

NOTE: refer to thePoint for teaching guides that can be used for people in the actual clinical setting.

In 2000, the Australian government established the National Medicines Policy. This policy sought to ensure that all parties involved in medications, including health professionals, consumers and manufacturers, worked together to ensure better health outcomes for the Australian public, through responsible, timely, safe and appropriate medication production and management. The Quality Use of Medicines arm of the policy seeks to promote:

- *judicious use* by ensuring use only when indicated and after other options have been considered
- *appropriate use*, considering the health issue, potential effects, dosage and duration of treatment
- *safe use* to avoid underuse, overuse or misuse
- *efficacious use* in ensuring a drug achieves its intended goals.

Within the Quality Use of Medicines framework, nurses and midwives play a key role through monitoring and managing medication use, providing education and advocating for people and their families.

The drug regimen process, which includes prescribing, dispensing and administering a drug to a person, has a series of checks along the way to help to catch errors before they occur. These include the doctor or nurse or midwife practitioner who prescribes a drug, the pharmacist who dispenses the drug and the nurse or midwife who administers the drug. Each serves as a check within the system to catch errors – the wrong drug, the wrong person, the wrong dose, the wrong route or the wrong time. Often the nurse or midwife is the final check in the process, being the one who administers the drug and the one responsible for education before the person is discharged.

In addition, the ACSQHC has developed 10 Standards to improve the quality of health service provision across Australia. These Standards provide a national statement of the level of care consumers should be able to expect from health services. Awareness and knowledge of Standard 4 on Medication Safety is an important part of the nurse's and midwife's clinical repertoire. For more information, see www.safetyandquality.gov.au/standards/nsqhs-standards/medication-safety-standard.

The nurse and midwife's role

The monumental task of ensuring medication safety with all of the potential problems that could confront the person can best be managed by consistently using the eight 'rights' of medication administration. These 'rights' are described in Box 4.2.

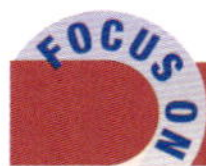

Safe medication administration

1. **Right patient.** *Use the three unique patient identifiers to ensure that you are giving the medication to the patient it is intended for. Ask the patient to tell you their full name while you check their unit record number (URN) and verify their date of birth and address. Then check the patient history you have matches the URN on their wrist.*
2. **Right drug.** *To prevent medication errors, always check to make sure the drug you are going to administer is the one that was prescribed. Many drugs may look alike and/or have sound-alike names. Ask for the generic as well as the brand name if you are unsure. Never assume the computer is correct; always double-check. Avoid abbreviations, and if you are not sure about abbreviations that were used, ask. Make sure the drug makes sense for the person for whom it is ordered.*
3. **Right dose.** *Always double-check calculations, and always do the calculations if the drug is not available in the dose ordered. Calculate the drug dose appropriately, based on the available drug form, the person's body weight or surface area or the person's kidney function. Do not assume that the computer or the pharmacy is always right; you are one more check in the system. Do not cut tablets to get to a correct dose without checking to make sure the tablet can be cut, crushed or chewed. Many of the new tablets cannot. Be very cautious if you see an order that starts with a decimal point; these orders are often the cause of medication errors. You should never see .5 mg as an order because it could be interpreted as 5 mg, 10 times the ordered dose. The proper dose would be 0.5 mg. If you see an order for 5.0 mg, be cautious; it could be interpreted as 50 mg. If a dose seems too big, question it. Throughout this book, Focus on Calculations boxes provide reviews for calculating dose properly.*
4. **Right route.** *Determine the best route of administration; this is frequently established by the formulation of the drug. Nurses and midwives can often have an impact in modifying the route to arrive at the most efficient, comfortable method for the person based on the person's specific situation. For example, perhaps a person is having trouble swallowing, and a large capsule would be very difficult for the person to handle. The health care provider could check and see if the drug is available in a liquid form and bring this information to the attention of the person prescribing the drug. When establishing the prescribed route, check the proper method of administering a drug by that route. Review drug administration methods periodically to make sure you have not forgotten important techniques. If you have instructed a person in the proper administration of a drug, be sure to have them explain it back to you and demonstrate the proper technique. This should be done not only when the person first learns this technique, but also periodically to make sure they have not forgotten any important points. Throughout this book, Focus on Safe Medication Administration boxes provide reviews of proper medication administration technique.*

   Know the specific preparation required before administering any drug. For example, oral drugs may need to be crushed or shaken; parenteral drugs may need to be reconstituted or diluted with specific solutions; and topical drugs may require specific handling, such as the use of gloves during administration or shaving of a body area before application. Many current oral drugs cannot be cut, crushed or chewed. Checking that information can help to prevent serious adverse effects. If a drug needs to be diluted or reconstituted, check the manufacturer's instructions to make sure that this is done correctly.
5. **Right time.** *When drugs are studied and evaluated, a suggested timing of administration is established. This timing takes into account all aspects of pharmacokinetics to determine a dosing schedule that will provide the needed therapeutic dose of the drug. Recognise that the administration of one drug may require coordination with the administration of other drugs, foods or physical parameters. In a busy hospital setting, getting the drug to the person at the prescribed time can be a real challenge. As carers most frequently involved in administering drugs, nurses and midwives must be aware of and manipulate all these factors, as well as educate people to do this on their own. Organising the day and the drug regimen to make it the least intrusive on a person's lifestyle can help to prevent errors and improve compliance.*
6. **Right documentation.** *Always document drug administration. If it isn't written, it didn't happen. Document the information in accordance with the local requirements for recording medication administration after assessing the person, making the appropriate care decisions and delivering the correct drug by the correct route, in the correct dose and at the correct time. Accurately record the drug given and the time given only after you have given the drug, to avoid inadvertent overdoses or missing doses, which would lead to a lack of therapeutic effect. Encourage people to keep track of their drugs at home, what they take and when they take it, especially if they could be confused.*
7. **Right reason.** *You should also make sure that the medication is being given for the right indication.*
8. **Right response.** *Check that the patient has had the correct and intended response to the medicine. For example, if you gave an antihypertensive medication to your patient with hypertension, check the patient's blood pressure to determine if the blood pressure decreased.*

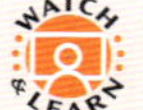

Medications: Preparing Unit Dose-Packaged Medications

Medications: Administering Oral Medications

Medications: Administering a Subcutaneous Injection

Medications: Administering an Intramuscular Injection

Medications: Administering IV Medication by Piggyback Infusion via an Electronic Infusion Device

Medications: Administering Eye Drops

Medications: Administering Ear Drops

The person's role

With so many people managing their drug regimens at home, one other very important check in the system also exists: the person being treated. Only the person really knows what is being taken and when, and only the person can report the actual, as opposed to the prescribed, drug regimen being followed. Education of the person and their family plays a vital role in the prevention of medication errors. Encourage people to be their own advocates and to speak up and ask questions. Doing so helps to prevent medication errors. The following teaching points help to reduce the risk of medication errors in the home setting:

- *Keep a written list of all medications you are taking, including prescription, OTC and herbal medications.* Keep this list with you at all times in case you are in an emergency situation and to keep your health care providers up to date. This list can be essential if you are travelling and need to refill a prescription while away from home.
- *Know what each of your drugs is being used to treat.* If you know why you are taking each drug, you will have a better understanding of what to report, what to watch for and when to report to your health care provider if the drug is not working.
- *Read the labels and follow the directions.* It is easy to make up your own schedule or to just take everything all at once in the morning. Always check the labels to see if there are specific times you should be taking your drugs. Make a calendar if you take drugs on alternating days. Using a weekly pillbox may also help with correct drug administration.
- *Store drugs in a dry place, away from children and pets.* Humid and hot storage areas (like the bathroom) tend to cause drugs to break down faster. Storing drugs away from children and pets can prevent possible toxic effects if these drugs are inadvertently ingested by children or your family pet.
- *Speak up.* You are the most important member of the health care team and you have information to share that no one else knows.

Children present unique challenges related to medication errors. Children often cannot speak for themselves and rely on a carer or carers to manage their drug regimen. Because their bodies are still developing and respond differently from those of adults to many drugs, the risk of serious adverse reactions is greater with children. The margin of safety with many drugs is very small when dealing with a child. When teaching parents about their children's drug regimens, be sure to include the following instructions:

- *Keep a list of all medications you are giving your child, including prescription, OTC and herbal medications.* Share this list with any health care provider who cares for your child. Never assume that a health care provider already knows what your child is taking.
- *Never use adult medications to treat a child.* The body organs and systems of children, primarily their livers and kidneys, are very different from those of an adult. As a result, children respond differently to drugs.
- *Read all labels before giving your child a drug.* Many OTC drugs contain the same ingredients, and you could accidentally overdose your child if you are not careful. In addition, some OTC drugs are not to be used with children younger than a certain age. Doses may also differ for children.
- *Measure liquid medications using appropriate measuring devices.* Never use a kitchen teaspoon or tablespoon to measure your child's drugs. Always use a measured dosing device or the spoon from a measuring set.
- *Call your health care provider immediately if your child seems to get worse or seems to be having trouble with a drug.* Do not hesitate; many drugs can cause serious or life-threatening problems with children and you should act immediately.
- *When in doubt, do not hesitate to ask questions.* You are your child's best advocate.

Reporting medication errors

Medication errors must be reported on a national level as well as on an institutional level. National reporting programs in Australia are coordinated by the Therapeutic Goods Administration (TGA), and they help to gather information about errors to prevent their recurrence at other health care sites and by other health care providers. These reports might prompt the issuing of health care provider warnings, which point out potential or actual medication errors and suggest ways to avoid these errors in the future. They may also lead to public warnings about look-alike or sound-alike drug names and common dosing errors and transcribing issues (see Box 4.2 for further information about reporting).

In New Zealand, the New Zealand Medicines and Medical Devices Safety Authority (MEDSAFE)

BOX 4.2 Reporting adverse drugs events

In Australia, adverse drug events are reported to the Australian Government, Department of Health, Therapeutic Goods Administration. These can be reported either electronically or by mail. Go online to: www.tga.gov.au/safety/problem.htm

Consumers can report directly by telephone on 1300 134 237.

is a business unit of the Ministry of Health and the authority responsible for regulation of therapeutic products in New Zealand. MEDSAFE is responsible for administering the *Medicines Act 1981* and *Regulations 1984* and regulates product for therapeutic uses. MEDSAFE collects information on the safety and quality of medicines from the Centre for Adverse Reaction and Monitoring (CARM) and other regulatory authorities such as the U.S. Food and Drug Administration (FDA), the European Medicines Association and TGA after they have been approved. This is called pharmacovigilance.

Pharmacovigilance involves:

- monitoring the use of medicines in everyday practice to identify previously unrecognised adverse effects or changes in the patterns of adverse effects.
- assessing the risks and benefits of medicines to determine if action is required to improve their safe use.
- providing information to health care professionals and consumers to promote safe use of medicines.
- monitoring the impact of any action taken and assessing whether further action is required.

Institutions also have their own policies for reporting medication errors that protect people and staff and identify particular areas in which education or system changes may be needed. Always be aware of the policies of your employing institution or agency. If you see or participate in a medication error, report it to your institution, then report it to the national reporting program. Your report will be shared with all the appropriate agencies – the TGA and the drug manufacturer. Health care providers working together and sharing information can make a big impact in decreasing the occurrence of medication errors.

CHAPTER SUMMARY

- Nursing is a complex art and science that provides for nurturing and care of the sick, as well as prevention and education services.
- Midwifery is also a complex art and science providing care for childbearing women and their families, as well as promotion of women's health across the lifespan.
- Components of health assessment (history of past illnesses and the current complaint, as well as a physical examination) provide a database of baseline information to ensure safe administration of a drug and to evaluate the drug's effectiveness and adverse effects.
- Assessment must include information on the history of past illnesses and the current complaint, as well as a physical examination; this provides a database of baseline information to ensure safe administration of a drug and to evaluate the drug's effectiveness and adverse effects.
- Care priorities are developed from the information gathered during health assessment. Implementation involves taking the information gathered and synthesised into care priorities to plan appropriate care. This process includes determining desired outcomes, setting goals for safe and effective drug administration, providing comfort measures to help the person cope with the therapeutic or adverse effects of a drug and providing education for the person and their family to ensure safe and effective drug therapy.
- Evaluation is part of the continuing process of care provision that leads to changes in assessment, diagnosis and intervention. The person is continually evaluated for therapeutic response, the occurrence of adverse drug effects and the occurrence of drug–drug, drug–food, drug–alternative therapy or drug–laboratory test interactions.
- Care plans and educational materials can be prepared for each drug being given, using information about a drug's therapeutic effects, adverse effects and special considerations.
- Prevention of medication errors is a complicated task that involves the prescriber, the pharmacist, the nurse or midwife administering the drugs and the person receiving them. Nurses and midwives need to be vigilant in administering drugs and to check the eight 'rights' of drug administration. The person needs to be educated to be their own advocate and to take steps to avoid medication errors.

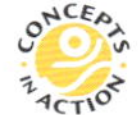

Pharmacology: Intramuscular injection

Pharmacology: Intravenous injection

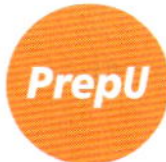

Knowing your strengths and weaknesses helps you to study more effectively. Take a PrepU Practice Quiz to find out how you measure up!

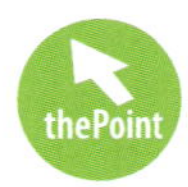

ONLINE RESOURCES

An extensive range of additional resources to enhance teaching and learning and to facilitate understanding of this chapter may be found online at the text's accompanying website, located on thePoint at http://thepoint.lww.com. These include Watch and Learn videos, Concepts in Action animations, journal articles, review questions, case studies, discussion topics and quizzes.

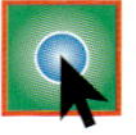

WEB LINKS

Health care providers and students may want to consult the following web resources:

www.health.gov.au/internet/main/publishing.nsf/content/nmp-quality.htm
Australian National Medicines Policy and Quality Use of Medicines (QUM).

www.nps.org.au
MedicineWise, National Prescribing Service.

nzphvc.otago.ac.nz/report
New Zealand's national monitoring centre for adverse reactions.

www.safetyandquality.gov.au/our-work/medication-safety
Australian Commission on Safety and Quality in Health Care guidelines and processes for medication safety.

www.tga.gov.au/safety/problem-medicines-forms-bluecard.htm
Guidelines for preventing medication errors in Australia.

BIBLIOGRAPHY

Carpenito, L. J. (2005). *Nursing Care Plans and Documentation* (4th edn). Philadelphia: Lippincott Williams & Wilkins.

Dempsey, J., Hillege, S. & Hill, R. (2014). *Fundamentals of Nursing and Midwifery: A Person-centred Approach to Care* (2nd Australian and New Zealand edn). Sydney: Lippincott Williams & Wilkins.

Karch, A. (2003). *Lippincott's Guide to Preventing Medication Errors*. Philadelphia: Lippincott Williams & Wilkins.

Kumac, D. L. & Tatley, M. V. (2011). Detecting medication errors in the New Zealand Pharmacovigilance Database. *Drug Safety, 34*, 59–71.

Lewis, P. & Foley, D. (2011). *Weber & Kelley's Health Assessment in Nursing* (1st Australian and New Zealand edn). Sydney: Lippincott Williams & Wilkins.

McCloskey, J. & Bulechek, G. (Eds.). (2008). *Nursing Interventions Classification* (5th edn). St Louis: Elsevier Mosby.

McKay, K. (2005). Showing the blue card: Reporting adverse reactions. *Australian Prescriber, 28*, 140–142.

McKenna, L. & Mirkov, S. (2019). *McKenna's Drug Handbook for Nursing and Midwifery* (8th edn). Sydney: Wolters Kluwer Health Australia.

Nichols, P., Copeland, T-S., Craib, I. A., Hopkins, P. & Bruce, D. G. (2008). Learning from error: Identifying contributory causes of medication error in an Australian hospital. *Medical Journal of Australia, 188*, 276–279.

Redman, B. (2007). *The Practice of Patient Education* (10th edn). St Louis: Elsevier/Mosby-Year Book.

Roughead, L. (2008). *Literature review: Medication safety in acute care in Australia*. Adelaide: University of South Australia.

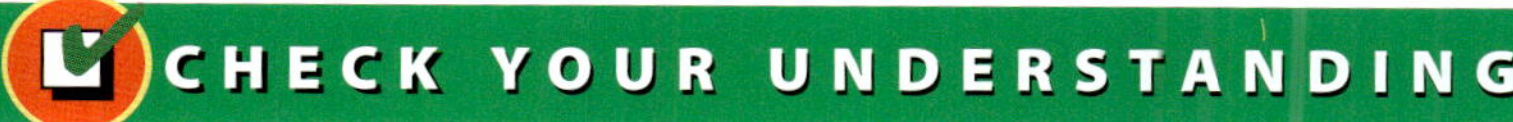

Answers to the questions in this chapter can be found in Appendix A at the back of this book.

MULTIPLE CHOICE

Select the best answer to the following.

1. A woman reports that she has a drug allergy. In exploring the allergic reaction with the woman, which of the following might indicate an allergic response?
   a. increased urination
   b. dry mouth
   c. rash
   d. drowsiness
2. The nurse or midwife obtains a medical history from a person before beginning drug therapy based on an understanding of which of the following?
   a. Medical conditions can alter a drug's pharmacokinetics and pharmacodynamics.
   b. A medical history is a key component of any nursing protocol.
   c. A baseline of information is necessary to evaluate a drug's effects.
   d. The medical history is the first step in the nursing process.

3. A person receiving an antihistamine complains of dry mouth and nose. An appropriate comfort measure for this person would be to:
   a. suggest that the person use a humidifier.
   b. encourage voiding before taking the drug.
   c. have the person avoid sun exposure.
   d. give the person a back rub.

4. When establishing the health care interventions appropriate for a given person:
   a. the person should not be actively involved.
   b. the support systems for the person should be included only at discharge.
   c. teaching should be done when the person states they are ready to learn.
   d. an evaluation of all of the data accumulated should be incorporated to achieve an effective care plan.

5. The evaluation step of the clinical decision making process:
   a. is often used as a last resort.
   b. is important primarily in the acute setting.
   c. is a continuous process.
   d. includes making care priorities.

6. After teaching a person about digoxin (*Lanoxin*) – a drug used to increase the effectiveness of the heart's contractions – which statement would indicate that the teaching was effective?
   a. 'I need to take my pulse every morning before I take my pill.'
   b. 'If I forget my pills, I usually make up the missed dose once I remember.'
   c. 'This pill might help my hay fever when it becomes a problem.'
   d. 'I don't remember the name of it, but it is the white one.'

MULTIPLE RESPONSE

Select all that apply.

1. A person is being started on a laxative regimen. Before beginning the regimen, the nurse or midwife would perform which of the following assessments?
   a. liver function test
   b. abdominal examination
   c. skin colour and lesion evaluation
   d. lung auscultation
   e. 24-hour urine analysis
   f. cardiac assessment

2. The care of a person receiving drug therapy should include measures to decrease the anticipated adverse effects of the drug. Which of the following measures would be considered?
   a. a positive approach
   b. environmental temperature control
   c. safety measures
   d. skin care
   e. refrigeration of the drug
   f. involvement of the family

3. A nurse or midwife is preparing to administer a drug to a person for the first time. What questions should the nurse or midwife consider before actually administering the drug?
   a. Is this the right person?
   b. Is this the right drug?
   c. Is there a generic drug available?
   d. Is this the right route for this person?
   e. Is this the right dose, as ordered?
   f. Did I record this properly?

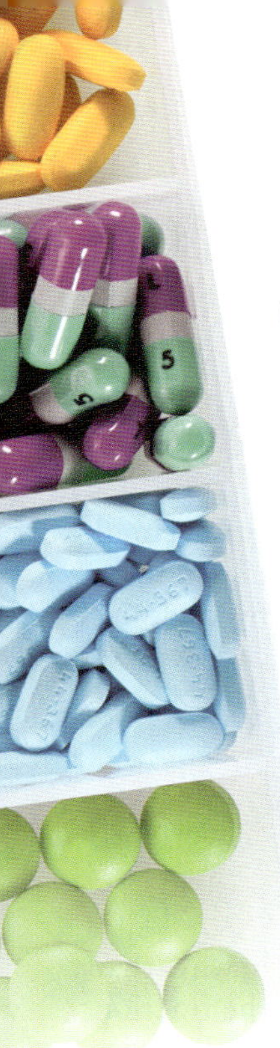

Mathematics and dosage calculations

5

Learning objectives

On completing this chapter you should be able to:

1. Perform basic mathematical calculations.
2. Calculate the correct dose of a drug when given examples of drug orders and available forms of the drugs ordered.
3. Discuss why children require different dosages of drugs to adults.
4. Explain the calculations used to determine a safe paediatric dose of a drug.

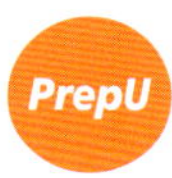

Test your current knowledge of mathematics and dosage calculations with a PrepU Practice Quiz!

Glossary of key terms

decimal: number that contains a decimal point
denominator: bottom number in a fraction
fraction: part of a whole number
improper fraction: fraction where the numerator is larger than the denominator
metric system: the most widely used system of measure, based on the decimal system; all units in the system are determined as multiples of 10
nomogram: tool for calculating body surface area
numerator: top number in a fraction
proper fraction: fraction where the numerator is lower than the denominator
whole number: a complete number

To determine the correct dose of a particular drug for an individual, it is necessary to consider the person's gender, weight, age and physical condition, as well as the other drugs that the person is taking. Frequently, the dose that is needed for a person is not the dose that is available, and it is necessary to convert the dose form available into the prescribed dose. Doing the necessary mathematical calculations to determine what should be given is the responsibility of the prescriber who orders the drug, the pharmacist who dispenses the drug and the nurse or midwife who administers the drug. This allows the necessary checks on the dose being given before the person actually receives the drug.

Another check to help prevent medication errors is that, in many institutions, drugs arrive at the ward area in unit-dose form, pre-packaged for each individual person. The nurse or midwife who will administer the drug may come to rely on this pre-packaged system, forgoing any recalculation or rechecking of the dose to match the written order. Unfortunately, mistakes still happen, and the nurse or midwife, as the person who is administering the drug, is legally and professionally responsible for any error that might occur. Practising nurses and midwives must know how to convert drug dosing orders into appropriate doses of available forms of a drug to ensure that the right person is getting the right dose of a drug.

BASIC MATHEMATICAL CALCULATIONS

Accurate and safe medication administration relies on accurate mathematic skills, including addition, subtraction, multiplication and division. In this area, an error can be potentially fatal. Nurses and midwives, therefore, have a responsibility to calculate medication doses exactly, and this relies on sound mathematical skills. Calculators are commonly used in clinical practice to aid calculations of drug dosages. Calculation errors with calculators can result in large miscalculations. Nurses and midwives choosing to use calculators also need to undertake mental calculations in conjunction with using the calculator to check the reasonableness of the calculated answer and avoid potentially disastrous outcomes.

Key mathematical concepts

Whole numbers and fractions

A **whole number** is a number that is complete. On the other hand, a **fraction** is a part of a number. For example, $^1/_2$ is a fraction that is part of the whole number 1. Fractions contain a **numerator** (top number) and **denominator** (bottom number), for example, in $^1/_2$, the numerator is 1, and the denominator is 2.

Proper fractions are those where the numerator is less than the denominator, while **improper fractions** are the reverse where the numerator is larger than the denominator. For example: $^1/_4$ is a proper fraction while $^6/_4$ is an improper fraction. Finally, a mixed number is one that contains both a whole number and a fraction, for example, $5^1/_4$. Mixed numbers can be converted into improper fractions. For example, $5^1/_4$ can also be expressed as $^{21}/_4$.

When calculating drug doses, it is common to have to simplify fractions into smaller numbers. In order to do this, both the numerator and the denominator need to be divided by the same (common) number. For example: if simplifying $^{20}/_{100}$, it can be seen that 20 can be divided into both numbers. By doing this, the fraction can be simplified to $^1/_5$ and cannot be further simplified.

Multiplying fractions

Sometimes it is necessary to multiply two different fractions. To do this, multiply both numerators and both denominators, then simplify use the common factor. For example:

$$\frac{2}{3} \times \frac{5}{8} = \frac{10}{24} = \frac{5}{12}$$

Decimals and decimal places

Decimals are numbers that contain a decimal point and are a different way to present fractions. In these numbers the digits after the decimal point represent parts of the number 10, 100, 1000, and so on. Such numbers are most commonly used in liquid drug preparation. We refer to decimal places as the number of places after the decimal point. For example,

65.4 has one decimal place
1.23 has two decimal places
2.387 has three decimal places

Converting decimals to fractions

It is important to be able to convert between decimal numbers and fractions. For example, 7.5 can be expressed as $7^5/_{10}$. Simplifying this further by dividing the fraction by the common factor of 5, we can express this as $7^1/_2$.

Examples: $5.4 = 5^4/_{10} = 5^2/_5$
$1.25 = 1^{25}/_{100} = 1^1/_4$
$53.6 = 53^6/_{10} = 53^3/_5$

Converting fractions to decimals

Sometimes we also need to convert the other way, that is, fractions to decimals. For example, using the fraction $5^1/_4$, expressing this as a decimal would be 5.25. In order to convert the fraction to a number out of 10, it is necessary to divide the numerator by the denominator.

Examples: $23^2/_3 = 23.67$
$10^1/_2 = 10.5$
$56^7/_8 = 56.875$

Rounding decimal numbers

Sometimes it is necessary to round decimal numbers containing many decimal places to one or two. The general principle in rounding decimals is that if the number in the last decimal place is 5 or more, we round the next decimal place up by one. If it is 4 or less, we round this number down. For example, rounding 5.436 to two decimal places becomes 5.44. Rounding 6.33 to one decimal place becomes 6.3, while rounding 2.35 to one decimal place becomes 2.4.

Examples:		
	One decimal place	2.54 = 2.5 3.98 = 4.0
	Two decimal places	2.453 = 2.45 0.656 = 0.66
	Three decimal places	0.2134 = 0.213 8.7935 = 8.794

Multiplying decimals

Sometimes it is necessary to multiply two decimal numbers. Multiplying decimals by 10, 100, 1000 etc. is easy and requires moving decimal points to the right. For example:

Multiplying by 10, the decimal place is moved one decimal place, eg, 3.45 × 10 = 34.5

Multiplying by 100, the decimal place is moved two decimal places, eg, 4.931 × 100 = 493.1

TABLE 5.1 Metric conversions

System	Solid measure	Liquid measure
Metric	gram (g) 1 milligram (mg) = 0.001 g 1 microgram (mcg) = 0.000001 g 1 kilogram (kg) = 1000 g	litre (L) 1 millilitre (mL) = 0.001 L 1 mL = 1 cubic centimetre = 1 cc
Household	kilogram (kg) 1 kg = 1000 grams (g or gm)	litre (L) 1000 mL = 1 L = 3.5 cups (c) 7 tablespoons (approx) = 100 mL 3 teaspoons (tsp) = 1 tbsp 60 drops (gtt) = 1 tsp

Multiplying by 1000, the decimal place is moved three decimal places, eg, 5.124 × 1000 = 5124

Multiplying two decimal numbers is a little more complex. Here it is important to add all the decimal places from both numbers then apply that number of decimal places to the product. For example:

Multiplying 3.42 × 24.76, we can do a normal multiplication with the numbers as whole numbers 342 and 2476 which is 846,792, then insert four decimal places which gives the final answer of 84.6792.

Review the following examples:

22.7 × 0.342 = 7.7634
0.87 × 0.54 = 0.4698
4.85 × 91.2 = 442.320 = 442.32

Dividing decimals

Dividing decimals is less commonly used. However, similar to multiplying, dividing decimals by 10, 100, 1000 etc. also requires moving decimal points but to the left. For example:

Dividing by 10, the decimal place is moved one decimal place, eg, 3.45 ÷ 10 = 0.345

Dividing by 100, the decimal place is moved two decimal places, eg, 534.2 ÷ 100 = 5.342

Dividing by 1000, the decimal place is moved three decimal places, eg, 3298 ÷ 1000 = 3.298

MEASURING SYSTEMS

The **metric system** is currently used in drug preparation and delivery in Australia and New Zealand and is the most widely used system of measure internationally. It is based on the decimal system, so all units are determined as multiples of 10. This system makes the sharing of knowledge and research information easier. The metric system uses the gram as the basic unit of solid measure and the litre as the basic unit of liquid measure (see Table 5.1).

Converting between different metric components is often required in calculating drug doses. Such conversions are similar to multiplying and dividing decimals. There are a number of key components to remember:

1000 micrograms (mcg) = 1 milligram (mg)
1000 mg = 1 gram (g)
1000 g = 1 kilogram (kg)
1000 millilitre (mL) = 1 litre (L)

Other systems

Some drugs are measured in 'units'. These measures may reflect chemical activity or biological equivalence. A unit usually reflects the biological activity of the drug in 1 mL of solution. The unit is unique for the drug it measures; a unit of heparin is not comparable to a unit of insulin. Milliequivalents (mEq) or millimoles (mmol) are used to measure electrolytes (eg, potassium, sodium, calcium, fluoride). The milliequivalent refers to the ionic activity of the drug in question; the order is usually written for a number of milliequivalents instead of a volume of drug. International units (IU) are sometimes used to measure certain vitamins or enzymes. These are also unique to each drug and cannot be converted to another measuring form.

KEY POINTS

- Safe and accurate drug administration requires sound mathematical skills.
- The metric system is the most widely used system of measure.
- Some drugs are measured in units.

CALCULATING DOSE

Drugs are made available only in certain forms or doses. Every time a nurse or midwife is required to administer any medication, the dose must be calculated to ensure the correct amount of drug is given.

Oral drugs

Frequently, tablets or capsules for oral administration are not available in the exact dose that has been ordered. In these situations, the person who is administering the drug must calculate the number of tablets or capsules to give for the ordered dose. In order to calculate this, we use the following formula:

$$\textit{number of tablets or capsules} = \frac{\text{Strength required}}{\text{Strength in stock}}$$

Try an example: an order is written for 0.05 g *Aldactone* (spironolactone) to be given orally (PO). The *Aldactone* is available in 25 mg tablets. How many tablets would you have to give? First, you will need to convert the grams to milligrams so that the units of the prescribed amount and the available tablets are the same:

So 0.05 g of *Aldactone* is equal to 50 mg of *Aldactone*.

Now solve for the number of tablets that you will need:

$$\frac{\text{Strength required}}{\text{Strength in stock}} = \frac{50\text{ mg}}{25\text{ mg}} = 2\text{ tablets}$$

Sometimes the desired dose will be a fraction of a tablet or capsule, $^1/_2$ or $^1/_4$. Some tablets come with scored markings that allow them to be cut. Pill cutters are readily available in most pharmacies to help people cut tablets appropriately. However, one must use caution when advising a person to cut a tablet. Many tablets come in a matrix system that allows for slow and steady release of the active drug. These drugs cannot be cut, crushed or chewed. Always consult a drug reference before cutting a tablet. However, as a quick reference, any tablet that is designated as having slow, modified or sustained release may very well be one that cannot be cut. Capsules can be very difficult to divide precisely, and some of them also come with warnings that they cannot be cut, crushed or chewed. If the only way to deliver the correct dose to a person is by cutting one of these preparations, a different formulation of the drug, a different drug or a different approach to treating the person should be tried.

Other oral drugs come in liquid preparations. Many of the drugs used in paediatrics and for adults who might have difficulty swallowing a pill or tablet are prepared in a liquid form. Some drugs that do not come in a standard liquid form can be prepared as a liquid by the pharmacist. If the person is not able to swallow a tablet or capsule, check for other available forms and consult with the pharmacist about the possibility of preparing the drug in a liquid as a suspension or a solution. The formula for calculating liquid volumes is as follows:

$$\frac{\text{Strength required}}{\text{Strength in stock}} \times \text{volume of stock solution}$$

Try this example: an order has been written for 120 mg of phenytoin. The bottle states that the solution contains 30 mg/5 mL. How much of the liquid should you give?

$$\begin{array}{c}\textit{volume of}\\ \textit{oral solution}\end{array} = \frac{\text{Strength required}}{\text{Strength in stock}} \times \begin{array}{c}\text{volume of}\\ \text{stock solution}\end{array}$$

$$= \frac{120}{30} \times 5 = \frac{60}{3} = 20\text{ mL}$$

Even if you are working in an institution that provides unit-dose medications, practise your calculation skills to keep them sharp. Power can be lost, computers can go down and the ability to determine calculations is a skill that anyone who administers drugs should have in reserve. Periodically throughout this text you will find a Focus on Calculations box to help you refresh your dose calculation skills as they apply to the drugs being discussed.

Parenteral drugs

All drugs administered parenterally must be administered in liquid form. The person administering the drug needs to calculate the volume of the liquid that must be given to administer the prescribed dose. The same formula can be used for this determination that was used for determining the dose of an oral liquid drug:

$$\begin{array}{c}\textit{volume of}\\ \textit{parenteral solution}\end{array} = \frac{\text{Strength required}}{\text{Strength in stock}} \times \begin{array}{c}\text{volume of}\\ \text{stock solution}\end{array}$$

Try this example: an order has been written for 75 mg of pethidine to be given intramuscularly (IM). The vial states that it contains pethidine 50 mg in 1.0 mL. Set up the equation just as before:

$$\frac{75\text{ mg}}{50\text{ mg}} \times 1\text{ mL}$$

$$= {}^{75}/_{50}$$

$$= 1.5\text{ mL to be administered}$$

Intravenous solutions

Intravenous (IV) solutions are used to deliver a prescribed amount of fluid, electrolytes, vitamins, nutrients or drugs directly into the bloodstream. For infusions, most institutions now use electronically monitored delivery systems. However, it is still important to be able to determine the amount of an IV solution that should be given, using standard calculations. Most IV delivery systems come with a standard control, by which each millilitre delivered contains 20 drops.

Microdrip systems, which usually deliver 60 drops/mL, are also available; they are usually used in paediatric settings. Always check the packaging of the IV tubing to see how many drops/mL are delivered by that particular device if you have any doubts or are unfamiliar with the system.

Use the following formula to determine how many drops of fluid to administer per minute:

$$\textit{drops per minute (rate)} = \frac{\text{volume} \times \text{drop factor (drops/mL)}}{\text{time (hours)} \times 60}$$

That is, the number of drops per minute, or the rate that you will set by adjusting the roller clamp on the IV tubing, is equal to the amount of solution that has been prescribed per hour times the number of drops delivered per millilitre (mL), divided by 60 minutes in an hour.

Try this example. An order has been written for a person to receive 400 mL of 5% dextrose in water over a period of 4 hours in a standard system (i.e. 20 drops/mL). Calculate the correct setting (drops per minute):

$$\textit{rate} = \frac{\text{volume} \times \text{drop factor (drops/mL)}}{\text{time (hours)} \times 60} = \frac{400}{4} \times \frac{20}{60}$$

Simplify:

$$\textit{rate} = \frac{\text{volume} \times \text{drop factor (drops/mL)}}{\text{time (hours)} \times 60} = \frac{400}{12} = 33.3$$

$= 33$ drops/min

(Note: drops must be in whole numbers as it is not possible to deliver part of a drop)

Now calculate the same order for an IV set that delivers 60 drops/mL:

$$\textit{rate} = \frac{\text{volume} \times \text{drop factor (drops/mL)}}{\text{time (hours)} \times 60} = \frac{400}{4} \times \frac{60}{60}$$

$= 100$ drops/min

If a person has an order for an IV drug, the same principle can be used to calculate the speed of the delivery. For example, an order is written for a person to receive 60 mL of an antibiotic over 30 minutes. The IV set used dispenses 20 drops/mL, which allows greater control. Calculate how fast the delivery should be:

$$\textit{rate} = \frac{\text{volume} \times \text{drop factor (drops/mL)}}{\text{time (hours)} \times 60}$$

$$= \frac{60}{0.5} \times \frac{20}{60} = \frac{1200}{30}$$

$= 40$ drops/min

Paediatric considerations

For most drugs, children require doses different to those given to adults. The 'standard' drug dose that is listed on package inserts and in many references refers to the dose that has been found to be most effective in a 70 kg adult male. An adult's body handles drugs differently and may respond to drugs differently to a child's. A child's body may handle a drug differently in all areas of pharmacokinetics – absorption, distribution, metabolism and excretion. The responses of the child's organs to the effects of the drug also may vary because of immaturity of the organs. Most of the time a child requires a smaller dose of a drug to achieve the comparable critical concentration. On rare occasions, a child may require a higher dose of a drug.

For ethical reasons, drug research is not done on children. Over time, however, enough information can be accumulated from experience with the drug to have a recommended paediatric dose. The drug guide that you select to use in the clinical setting will have the paediatric dose listed if this information is available. Unfortunately, there may be times when no recommended dose for a child is available but that particular drug is needed. In these situations, established formulae can be used to estimate the appropriate dose. Determining a paediatric dose takes into consideration the child's weight, or body surface. The **nomogram** that uses body surface area is more accurate for determining doses (see Figure 5.1).

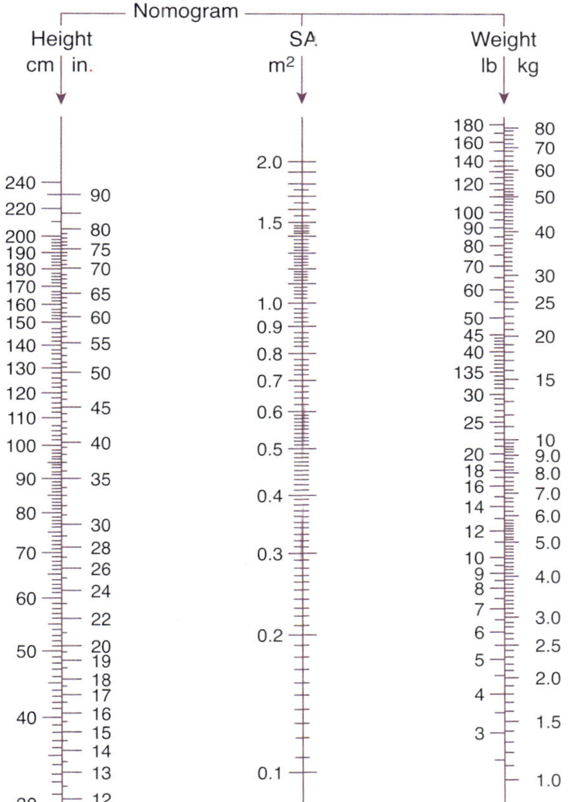

FIGURE 5.1 The West nomogram for calculating body surface area (BSA). Draw a straight line connecting the child's height (left scale) to the child's weight (right scale). The BSA value, which is calculated in square metres, is found at the point where the line intersects the SA column.

Regardless of the calculation method used for children, even a tiny dose error can be critical. When working in paediatrics, one needs to be familiar with at least one of these methods of determining the drug dose. Many institutions require that two nurses check critical paediatric doses. This is a good practice when working with small children.

Body surface area

The surface area of a child's body may also be used to determine the approximate dose that should be used. To do this, the child's surface area is determined with the use of a nomogram (Figure 5.1). The height and weight of the child are taken into consideration in this chart. The following formula is then used:

$$\text{child's dose} = \frac{\text{surface area (m}^2\text{)}}{1.73} \times \text{average adult dose}$$

This method is more precise than the formula methods, but you have to have a nomogram available to determine the surface area.

Milligrams/kilograms of body weight

When a safe and effective paediatric dose has been established, the orders for the drug dose are often written in milligrams/kilograms. This method of prescribing takes into consideration the varying weights of children and the need for a higher dose of the drug when the weight increases. For example, if a child with postoperative nausea is to be treated with ondansetron the recommended dose is 0.1 mg/kg by IV injection. If the child weighs 22 kg, the dose for this child would be 0.1 mg/kg × 22 kg, or 2.2 mg. If a child weighed only 8 kg, the recommended dose would be 0.1 mg/kg × 8 kg, or 0.8 mg. Note that this is only the dosage for the drug. Before administration, the volume required still needs to be calculated. The established guidelines allow the drug to be used safely within a large range of children. Some adult doses will also be written in this way. This is usually found in drugs with a small margin of safety or high potential for toxic effects, such as antineoplastic drugs.

CHAPTER SUMMARY

- The metric system is the most widely used system of measure. All drugs are dispensed in quantities defined using the metric system.
- Children require doses of most drugs different to those of adults because of the way their bodies handle drugs and the way that drugs affect their tissues and organs.
- Paediatric doses are based on body surface area, which requires the use of a nomogram, and milligrams per kilogram of body weight.

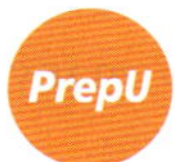

Knowing your strengths and weaknesses helps you to study more effectively. Take a PrepU Practice Quiz to find out how you measure up!

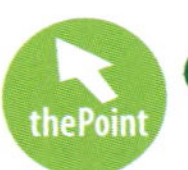

ONLINE RESOURCES

An extensive range of additional resources to enhance teaching and learning and to facilitate understanding of this chapter may be found online at the text's accompanying website, located on thePoint at http://thepoint.lww.com. These include Watch and Learn videos, Concepts in Action animations, journal articles, review questions, case studies, discussion topics and quizzes.

BIBLIOGRAPHY

Atik, A. (2013). Adherence to the Australian National Inpatient Medication Chart: the efficacy of a uniform national drug chart on improving prescription error. *Journal of Evaluation in Clinical Practice, 19(5)*, 769–772.

Boyer, M. J. (2009). *Math for Nurses: A Pocket Guide to Dosage Calculation and Drug Preparation*. Philadelphia: Lippincott, Williams & Wilkins.

Brotto, V. & Rafferty, K. (2012). *Clinical Dosage Calculations for Australia & New Zealand*. Melbourne: Cengage.

Craig, G. (2008). *Clinical Calculations Made Easy*. Philadelphia: Lippincott Williams & Wilkins.

DeCastillo, S. & Werner-McCullough, M. (2007). *Calculating Drug Dosages: An Interactive Approach* (7th edn). Philadelphia: Davis.

Dempsey, J., Hillege, S. & Hill, R. (2014). *Fundamentals of Nursing and Midwifery: A Person-centred Approach to Care* (2nd Australian and New Zealand edn). Sydney: Lippincott Williams & Wilkins.

Gatford, J. D. & Phillips, N. (2011). *Nursing Calculations* (8th edn). Edinburgh: Churchill Livingstone.

Morrison, G. (2007). Drug dosing in the intensive care unit: The patient with renal failure. In Rippe, J. M., Irwin, R. S. & Fink, M. P. (Eds.), *Intensive Care Medicine* (3rd edn) (pp. 951–986). Boston: Little, Brown.

Ogden, S. (2007). *Calculation of Drug Dosages* (7th edn). St Louis: Mosby. Springhouse, Corp.

McKenna, L. & Mirkov, S. (2019). *McKenna's Drug Handbook for Nursing and Midwifery* (8th edn). Sydney: Wolters Kluwer Health Australia.

Tzeng, H-M., Yin, C. & Schneider, T. E. (2013). Medication error-related issues in nursing practice. *MEDSURG Nursing, 22(1)*, 13–50.

CHECK YOUR UNDERSTANDING

Answers to the questions in this chapter can be found in Appendix A at the back of this book.

MULTIPLE CHOICE

Select the best answer to the following.

1. A dose of 0.125 mg of a medication is ordered for a person who is having trouble swallowing. The bottle of medication elixir reads 0.5 mg/2 mL. How much would you give?
   a. 5 mL
   b. 0.5 mL
   c. 1.5 mL
   d. 1 mL
2. An order is written for 700 mg of a medication PO. The drug is supplied in liquid form as 1 g/3.5 mL. How much of the liquid should be given?
   a. 5 mL
   b. 2.5 mL
   c. 6.2 mL
   d. 2.45 mL
3. An order is written for 1000 mL of normal saline to be administered IV over 10 hours. The drop factor on the IV tubing states 15 drops/mL. What is the IV flow rate?
   a. 50 mL/h at 50 drops/minute
   b. 100 mL/h at 25 drops/minute
   c. 100 mL/h at 100 drops/minute
   d. 100 mL/h at 15 drops/minute
4. A person needs to take 0.75 g of a medication PO. The drug comes in 250 mg tablets. How many tablets should the person take?
   a. 2 tablets
   b. 3 tablets
   c. 4 tablets
   d. 30 tablets
5. A medication is supplied in a 500 mg/2.5 mL solution. How much would be given if an order were written for 100 mg IV?
   a. 5 mL
   b. 1.5 mL
   c. 2.5 mL
   d. 0.5 mL
6. 800 units of a medication are ordered for a person. The drug is supplied in a multidose vial that is labelled 10,000 units/mL. How many millilitres of the medication would be needed to treat this person?
   a. 0.8 mL
   b. 0.08 mL
   c. 8.0 mL
   d. 0.4 mL

COMPLETE THE FOLLOWING PROBLEMS

1. Change to equivalents within the system:
   a. 100 mg = ______ g
   b. 1500 g = ______ kg
   c. 0.1 L = ______ mL
   d. 500 mL = ______ L
2. Convert to units in the household system:
   a. 5 mL = ______ tsp
   b. 30 mL = ______ tbsp
3. Robitussin cough syrup 225 mg PO is ordered. The bottle reads: 600 mg in 30 mL. How much cough syrup should be given? ______ mL
4. Ordered: 6.5 mg. Available: 10 mg/mL. Proper dose: ______ mL
5. Ordered: 0.35 mg. Available: 1.2 mg/2 mL. Proper dose: ______ mL
6. Ordered: 80 mg. Available: 50 mg/mL. Proper dose: ______ mL
7. Ordered: 150,000 units. Available: 400,000 units/5 mL. Proper dose: ______ mL

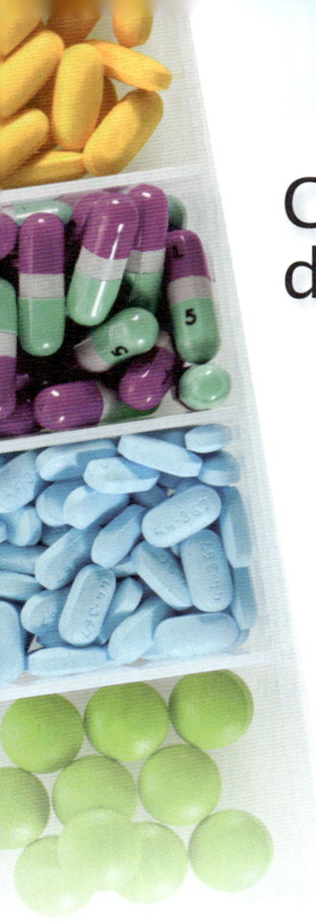

Challenges to effective drug therapy

Learning objectives

On completing this chapter you should be able to:

1. Discuss the impact of the media, the Internet and direct-to-consumer advertising on drug sales and prescriptions.
2. Discuss the importance of quality use of medicines and the role of nurses and midwives.
3. Explain the growing use of over-the-counter drugs and the impact they have on safe medical care.
4. Discuss the lack of controls on herbal or alternative therapies and the impact this has on safe drug therapy.
5. Define the off-label use of a drug.

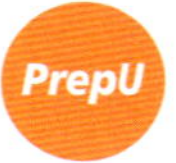

Test your current knowledge of challenges to effective drug therapy with a PrepU Practice Quiz!

Glossary of key terms

alternative therapy: includes herbs and other 'natural' products as often found in ancient records; these products are not controlled or tested by the TGA and MEDSAFE (NZ); however, they are often the basis for discovery of an active ingredient that is later developed into a regulated medication

cost comparison: a comparison of the relative cost of the same drug provided by different manufacturers to determine the cost to the consumer

off-label use: use of a drug that is not part of the stated therapeutic indications for which the drug was approved by the TGA and MEDSAFE (NZ); off-label use may lead to new indications for a drug

self-care: tendency for people to self-diagnose and determine their own treatment needs

street drugs: a loose term that refers to legal and illegal drugs that are used without medical supervision, There are four categories of recreational drugs: analgesics, depressants, stimulants, and hallucinogens. 'Recreational drugs' is a bad and misleading term as it suggests that drugs can be fun and safe. In fact, all these drugs are dangerous because they can create psychological and physical dependence.

The dawn of the 21st century arrived with myriad new considerations and pressures in the health care industry. For the first time, consumers have access to medical and pharmacological information from many sources. Consumers are taking steps to demand specific treatments and considerations. Alternative therapies are being offered and advertised at a record pace, and this is causing people to rethink their approach to medical care and the medical system. At the same time, financial pressures have led to early discharge of people from health care facilities and to provision of outpatient care for people who, in the past, would have been hospitalised and monitored closely. Health care providers are being pushed to make decisions about care and prescriptions based on finances in addition to medical judgement. Illicit drug use is at an all-time high, bringing increased health risks and safety concerns. There are increasing concerns about the environment and the need to protect it from contamination. Nurses and midwives are often caught in the middle of all of this change. People, as consumers of health care, are demanding information but may not understand it when they get it. Health teaching and home care provisions are vital to the success of any health regimen. The nurse or midwife is frequently in the best position to listen, teach and explain some of this confusing information to people and to facilitate the care of the person in the health system.

CONSUMER AWARENESS

Access to information has become so broad over the last decade that consumers are often overwhelmed with details, facts and choices that affect their health care. Gone is the era when the health care provider was seen as omniscient and always right. The person now comes into the health care system burdened with the influence of advertising, the Internet and a growing alternative therapy industry. Many people no longer calmly accept whatever medication is selected for them. They often come with requests and demands, and they partake of a complex array of over-the-counter (OTC) and alternative medicines that further complicate the safety and efficacy of standard drug therapy.

Media influence

The last 20 years have seen an explosion of drug advertising in the mass media. It became legal to advertise prescription drugs directly to the public in the US in the 1990s, and it is now impossible to watch television, listen to the radio or flip through a magazine without encountering numerous drug advertisements. This is more restricted in Australia and New Zealand. Legislation, in both countries, determines what can be said in an advertisement, but in some cases this further confuses the issue for many consumers. Because, in many cases, listing the possible adverse effects is not a good selling point, many advertisements are pure business ploys intended to interest consumers in the drug and to have them request it from their health care providers (even if it is unclear what the drug is used for). It is not unusual to see an ad featuring a smiling, healthy-looking person romping through a field of beautiful flowers on a sunny day with a cute baby or puppy in tow. The ad might simply state how wonderful it is to be outside on a day like today – contact your health care provider if you too would like to take drug X. Although most people now know what the erectile dysfunction drug *Viagra* is used for, some of the ads for this drug simply show a happy older couple smiling and dancing the night away and then encourage viewers to ask their health care providers about *Viagra*. What older person wouldn't want a drug that makes him or her feel young, happy and energetic?

Parenting magazines, which are often found in paediatricians' offices, are full of advertisements for medications that can improve the health of children. These ads picture smiling, cute children and encourage readers to check with their paediatricians about the use of these drugs. Even if the words are legible, they frequently don't have any meaning for the reader. The paediatrician or nurse may spend a great deal of time explaining why a particular drug is not indicated for a particular child and may actually experience resistance on the part of the parent who wants the drug for their child. As the marketing power for prescription drugs continues to grow, the health care provider must be constantly aware of what people are seeing, what the ads are promising and the real data behind the indications and contraindications for these 'hot' drugs. It is a continuing challenge to stay up-to-date and knowledgeable about drug therapy.

The media also look for headlines in current medical research or reports. It is not unusual for the media to take a headline or research title and make it into news. Sometimes the interpretation of the medical report is not accurate, and this can influence a person's response to suggested therapy or provide a whole new set of demands or requests for the health care provider. Many television talk shows include a medical segment that presents just a tiny bit of information, frequently out of context, which opens a whole new area of interest for the viewer. Some health care providers have learned to deal with the 'disease of the week' as seen on these shows; others can be unprepared to deal with what was presented and may lose credibility.

The Internet

The Internet, the worldwide digital information system accessed through computer systems, and World Wide Web are now readily accessible for most consumers. People who do not have Internet access at home can find it readily available at the local library, at work or even in cafés that allow community access. The information available over the Internet is completely overwhelming to most people. A person can spend hours looking up information on a drug – including pharmaceutical company information sites, chat rooms with other people who are taking the drug, online pharmacies, lists of government regulations, and research reports about the drug and its effectiveness. Many people do not know how to evaluate the information that they can access. Is it accurate or anecdotal? People often come into the health care system with pages of information downloaded from the Internet that they think pertains to their particular situation. The nurse, midwife, doctor or other health professional can spend a tremendous amount of time deciphering and interpreting the information and then explaining it. Some tips that might be helpful in determining the usefulness or accuracy of information found on the Internet are given in Box 6.1.

BOX 6.1 Evaluating Internet sites

Address identification

- *.com or .co:* commercial, advertising, selling, business site
- *.edu:* education site – school system, university, college
- *.gov:* government site
- *.net:* part of a linked network system, may include any of the above
- *.org:* sponsored by an organisation, including professional, charitable and educational groups

Site evaluation

- Navigation – Is the site easy to access and navigate or confusing?
- Contributors – Who prepared the site? Is it reviewed? Is it purely commercial? What are the qualifications of the person(s) maintaining the site? Is there a mechanism for feedback or interaction with the site?
- Dates – Is the site updated frequently? When was the site last updated?
- Accuracy/reliability – Is the information supported by other sites? Is the information accurate and in agreement with other sources you have reviewed? Does the site list other links that are reasonable and reliable?

KEY POINTS

- An overwhelming amount of readily accessible information is available to consumers. This information has changed the way people approach the health care system.
- Consumer advertising of prescription drugs, mass media health reports and suggestions, and the Internet influence some people to request specific treatments, to question therapy and to challenge the health care provider.

OVER-THE-COUNTER DRUGS

OTC medications allow people to take care of simple medical problems without seeking advice from their health care providers. Although OTC drugs have been deemed to be safe when used as directed, many of these medications were 'grandfathered in' as drugs when stringent testing and evaluation systems became law and have not been tested or evaluated to the extent that new drugs are today. Aspirin, one of the non-prescription standbys for many years, falls into this category. Slowly, the TGA in Australia and MEDSAFE in New Zealand are looking at all of these drugs to determine their effectiveness and safety. Increasingly, drugs that were available only by prescription are becoming available OTC. Some well-known approved OTC drugs are ranitidine (*Zantac*) for decreasing gastric upset and heartburn; various vaginal antifungal medications for treating yeast infections; and chloromycetin eye drops (*Chlorsig*).

Each year several prescription drugs are reviewed for possible OTC status. One factor involved in the review process is the ability of the person for **self-care,** which is the act of self-diagnosing and determining one's treatment needs. OTC drugs can also mask the signs and symptoms of an underlying problem, making it difficult to arrive at an accurate diagnosis if the condition persists. These drugs are safe when used as directed, but many times the directions are not followed or even read. The idea that 'if one makes me feel better, two will make me feel really good' is not always safe in the use of these drugs. Many people are not aware of the drugs contained in these preparations and can inadvertently overdose when taking one preparation for each symptom they have. Table 6.1 gives an example of the ingredients that are found in some common cold and allergy preparations. People who take doses of different preparations to cover their various symptoms could easily wind up with an unintended overdose or toxic reaction.

TABLE 6.1 Ingredients found in some common cold and flu OTC preparations*

Drug name	Ingredients	Use
Codral Original Cold & Flu	paracetamol, pseudoephedrine, codeine phosphate	Fever control, nasal congestion, aches
Demazin Cough Cold & Flu	pseudoephedrine, paracetamol, dextromethorphan	Cough, nasal congestion, aches
Dimetapp Cough Cold & Flu	pseudoephedrine, paracetamol, dextromethorphan	Cough, nasal congestion, aches
Nurofen Cold & Flu	ibuprofen, pseudoephedrine	Nasal congestion, aches
Panadol Cold & Flu + Decongestant	paracetamol, phenylephrine	Fever control, nasal congestion, aches
Sudafed Sinus Day & Night Relief	pseudoephedrine, paracetamol, triprolidine	Aches, nasal congestion, sinus pressure

*Safety Precautions: a person, if poorly advised, could take one preparation for cough, a second to cover sinus pressure, a third to cover aches and pains and a fourth to stay awake or fall asleep – when the total amounts of the drugs contained in these products are calculated, a serious overdosage of certain ingredients could easily occur.

Because many OTC drugs interact with prescription drugs, with possibly serious adverse or toxic effects, it is important that the health care provider ask specifically when taking a drug history whether the person is taking any OTC drugs or other medications. Many people do not consider OTC drugs to be 'real' drugs and do not mention their use when reporting a drug history to their health care provider. Every drug-teaching session should include information on which particular OTC drugs must be avoided or advice to check with the health care provider before taking any other medications or OTC products.

COMPLEMENTARY AND ALTERNATIVE THERAPIES

Another aspect of the increasing self-care movement is the rapidly growing market of alternative therapies and herbal medicines. Herbal medicines, both commercial and traditional (such as Rongoā Māori or Indigenous Australian) and **alternative therapies** are found in ancient records and have often been the basis for the discovery of an active ingredient that is later developed into a regulated medication. Today, alternative therapies can also include non-drug measures, such as imaging and relaxation.

There is a considered element of the placebo effect in using some of these therapies. The power of believing that something will work and that there is some control over the problem is often very beneficial in achieving relief from pain and suffering. The challenge for the health care provider is to balance the therapies that the person wishes to use with the medical regimen that is prescribed. This may involve altering doses or timing of various drugs.

Currently, these products are not controlled or tested by the TGA or MEDSAFE; they are considered to be dietary supplements, and therefore the advertising surrounding these products is not as restricted or as accurate as with classic drugs. Consumers are urged to use the 'natural' approach to medical care and to self-treat with a wide variety of products. Numerous Internet sites point out natural treatments that can be used to cure various disorders. Television ads and magazine spreads push the use of these products in place of prescribed medications. Many people who want to gain control of their medical care or who do not want to take 'drugs' for their diabetes, depression or fatigue are drawn to these products.

Several issues are of concern to the health care provider when a person elects to self-treat with alternative therapies. The active ingredients in these products have not been tested; when test results are available, often the tests were for only a very small number of people with no reproducible results. When a person decides to take bilberry to control diabetes, for example, the reaction that will occur is not really known. In some people, the blood glucose level might decrease; in others, it might increase. The incidental ingredients in many of these products are unknown. Many ingredients come directly from plants or from the conditions under which they grow, such as the fertiliser used for the plant, or depend on the time of the year when the plant was harvested. The other ingredients that are compounded with the product have a direct effect on its efficacy. Saw palmetto, a herb that has been used successfully to alleviate the symptoms of benign prostatic hypertrophy, is available in a wide variety of preparations from different manufacturers. A random sampling of these products performed in 2000 revealed that the contents of the identified active ingredient varied from 20% to 400% of the recommended dose. It is difficult to guide people to the correct product with such a wide range of variability.

People often do not mention the use of alternative therapies to the health care provider. Some people believe that the health care provider will disapprove of the use of these products and do not want to discuss it; others believe that these are just natural products and do not need to be mentioned. With the increasing use of these products, however, several drug interactions that can cause serious complications for people taking prescription medication have been reported. People with diabetes who decide to use juniper berries, ginseng, garlic, fenugreek, coriander, dandelion root or celery to 'maintain their blood glucose level' may run into serious problems with hypoglycaemia when they also use their prescription antidiabetic drugs. If the person does not report the use of these alternative therapies to the health care provider, extensive medical tests and dose adjustments might be done to no avail.

St John's wort, a highly advertised and popular alternative therapy, has been found to interact with oral contraceptives, digoxin (a heart medication), the selective serotonin reuptake inhibitors (used for depression), theophylline (a drug used to treat lung disease), various antineoplastic drugs used to treat cancer and the antivirals used to treat acquired immune deficiency syndrome (AIDS). People using St John's wort for the symptoms of depression who are also taking *Prozac* (fluoxetine) for depression may experience serious side effects and toxic reactions. If the health care provider is not told about the use of St John's wort, treatment of the toxicity can become very complicated.

Asking people specifically about the use of any herbal or alternative therapies should become a routine part of any health history. If a person presents with an unexpected reaction to a medication, ask them about any herbal or natural remedies they may be using. See Appendix F for an extensive listing of interactions of pharmaceutical drugs with complementary and alternative therapies. If a person reports the use of an unusual or difficult-to-find remedy, try looking it up on the Internet at http://nccam.nih.gov, the National Center for Complementary and Alternative Medicine (NCCAM) in the US, a site with general information about complementary and alternative medicines.

KEY POINTS

- OTC drugs have been deemed safe when used as directed and do not require a prescription or advice from a health care provider.
- OTC drugs can mask the signs and symptoms of disease, can interact with prescription drugs and can be taken in greater than the recommended dose, leading to toxicity.
- Herbal or alternative therapies are considered to be dietary supplements and are not tightly regulated by the TGA.
- Herbal therapies can produce unexpected effects and toxic reactions, can interact with prescription drugs and can contain various unknown ingredients that alter their effectiveness and toxicity.

OFF-LABEL USES

When a drug is approved by the TGA or MEDSAFE, the therapeutic indications for which the drug is approved are stated. **Off-label use** refers to use of a drug that is not part of the stated therapeutic indications for which the drug was approved. Once a drug becomes available for use, it may be found to be effective in a situation not on the approved list. Using it for this indication may eventually lead to a new approval of the drug for that new indication. Off-label use is commonly done for groups of people for which there is little premarketing testing, particularly paediatric and geriatric groups. With the ethical issues involved in testing drugs on children, the use of particular drugs in children often occurs by trial and error when the drug is released with adult indications. Dosing calculations and nomograms become very important in determining the approximate dose that should be used for a child. Drugs often used for off-label indications include the drugs used to treat various psychiatric problems. The fact that little is really known about the way the brain works and what happens when chemicals in the brain are altered has led to a polypharmacy approach in psychiatry – mixing and juggling drugs until the wanted effect is achieved. That same combination might not work in another person with the same diagnosis because of brain and chemical differences in that person.

Off-label use of drugs is widespread and often leads to discovery of a new use for a drug. The nurse and midwife need to be cognisant of off-label uses, and know when to question the use of a drug before administering it. Liability issues surrounding many of these uses are very fuzzy, and the care provider should be clear about the intended use, why the drug is being tried and its potential for problems.

COSTS OF HEALTH CARE AND THE IMPORTANCE OF TEACHING

Costs of medical care and drugs have increased in the last few years. This is partly due to the demand to have the best possible, most up-to-date, safest care and drug therapies. The research and equipment requirements to meet these demands are huge. At the same time, the rising cost of health insurance to pay for all of this is a major complaint for employers and consumers. To save costs, people are being discharged from hospitals far earlier than ever before, and many are not even admitted to hospitals for surgical or invasive procedures that once required several days of hospitalisation and monitoring. As a result, there is less monitoring of the person, and more responsibility for care falls on the person or their significant others. Teaching the person about self-care, drug therapies and what to expect is even more crucial now. The nurse and midwife are most often responsible for this teaching.

Role of the Pharmaceutical Management Agency (PHARMAC) in New Zealand

In an effort to contain the cost of medicines and medical devices, PHARMAC, the Pharmaceutical Management Agency, was introduced as part of the New Zealand Medicines System that works to ensure New Zealanders have affordable access to medicines. PHARMAC's central role is to manage the pharmaceutical budget on behalf of District Health Boards, and to decide which medicines are government funded. The list of funded medicines is published in the Pharmaceutical Schedule.

PHARMAC also play an important role in helping New Zealanders understand how to make the optimal use of their medicines. They have an Access and Optimal Use team which runs information campaigns and other promotions to encourage people to use medicines well, or to improve their health through better and healthier lifestyles.

Pharmaceutical Benefits Scheme (PBS) in Australia

The Australian Commonwealth Department of Health operates the Pharmaceutical Benefit Scheme (PBS) which is administered by Medicare. The Scheme lists medicines that are available at prices subsidised by the government to reduce costs to the public. It is eligible to be used by Australians and visitors from a number of countries where there are reciprocal arrangements, including New Zealand, the Republic of Ireland and the United Kingdom. Within the scheme, there exists a safety net which is set each year. Upon reaching the safety net for that year, an individual or family is eligible to receive subsequent medicines at either a concessional rate or for free, depending on their circumstances.

Quality use of medicines

The Australian Government, through the National Medicines Policy, operates the Quality Use of Medicines (QUM) program. The program is underpinned by four main principles. *Judicious use* requires that medicines are used when appropriate and after all options have been considered. Secondly, there should be *appropriate use* of medicines to treat the condition with all factors, such as risks and costs, considered. Thirdly, *safe use* of medicines is required to avoid misuse, while *efficacious use* requires that medicines used have beneficial health outcomes. Nurses and midwives play a central role in enacting this program as they are often the closest to people and their medicines.

In New Zealand, the New Zealand Medicines and Medical Devices Safety Authority collects information on the safety and quality of medicines and vaccines through a variety of sources. These activities are called pharmacovigilance. There are different pharmacovigilance centres in New Zealand that nurses and midwives need to be familiar with. The Centre for Adverse Reaction and Monitoring Centre (CARM) in Otago, the Intensive Medicines Monitoring Programme (IMMP), the Medicines Adverse Reaction Committee (MARC) and a new scheme called the Medicines Monitoring (M2). This scheme's aim is to highlight potential safety issues identified from reports of suspected adverse medicine reactions sent to CARM, to stimulate further reports and to increase the information on these potential safety signals.

Home care

The home care industry is one of the most rapidly growing responses to the changes in costs and medical care delivery. People now routinely go home directly from surgery with the responsibility for changing their own dressings, assessing wounds and monitoring their recovery. People are also being discharged from hospitals because the funded hospital days allowed for a particular diagnosis have run out. These people may be responsible for their own monitoring, rehabilitation and drug regimens. At the same time, the population is ageing and may be less accepting of all of this responsibility. Community nurses and midwives as well as hospital in the home programs are taking over some of the responsibilities that used to be handled in hospitals.

The responsibility for meeting the tremendous increase in teaching needs of people frequently resides with the nurse or midwife. People need to know exactly what medications they are taking (generic and brand names), the dose of each medication and what each is supposed to do. They also need to know what they can do to alleviate some of the adverse effects that are expected with each drug (eg, small meals if gastrointestinal upset is common, use of a humidifier if secretions will be dried and make breathing difficult); which OTC drugs or alternative therapies they need to avoid while taking their prescribed drugs; and what to watch for that would indicate a need to call the health care provider. With people who are taking many drugs at the same time, this information should be provided in writing, in language that is clear and understandable. Many pharmacies provide written information with each drug that is dispensed, but trying to organise these sheets of information into a usable and understandable form is difficult for many people. The nurse or midwife often needs to sort through the provided information to organise, simplify, and make sense of it for the person. The cost of dealing with toxic or adverse effects is often much higher, in the long run, than the cost of the time spent teaching and explaining things.

The projections for trends in health care indicate even greater expansion of home health care provision, with hospitals being used for only the most critically ill people. The role of the nurse and midwife in this home health system is crucial – as teacher, assessor, diagnostician and advocate.

Cost considerations

Despite the insurance cover a person may have for prescription medications, it is often necessary for the health care provider to choose drug therapy based on the costs of the drugs available. With more and more of the population reaching retirement age and depending on a fixed income, costs are a real issue. Sometimes this may mean not selecting a first-choice drug but settling for a drug that should be effective. People who take antibiotics must be reminded to take the full course and not to stop the drug when they feel better. People may be tempted to stop taking the antibiotic in order to save the remaining pills for the next time they feel sick and to also save the cost of another health care visit and a new prescription. This practice has contributed to the problem of resistant bacteria, which is becoming more dangerous all the time.

People also need to be advised not to split tablets in half unless specifically advised to do so. Some drugs can be split, and it is cheaper to order the larger size and have the person cut the tablet. Some people think that by cutting the drug in half they will have coverage for twice the time allowed by the prescription and will not be as dependent on the drug. With the new matrix delivery systems used for many medications, however, splitting the drug can cause it to become toxic or ineffective. People should be specifically alerted to avoid cutting drugs when it could be dangerous, especially if they are being advised to cut other tablets to be economical. The cost of treating the toxic reactions may far exceed the cost of the original drug.

Generic drug availability in many cases reduces the cost of a drug. Generic drugs are preparations that are off patent and therefore can be sold by their generic name, without the cost associated with brand-name products. Generic drugs are tested for bioequivalence with the brand-name product, and resulting information is available to prescribers. When a drug has a small margin of safety (a small difference between the therapeutic and the toxic dose), a prescriber may feel more comfortable ordering the drug by brand name to ensure that the dose and binders are what the prescriber expects. When 'brand substitution not permitted' is on a prescription, the prescription is filled with the brand-name drug – such as *Lanoxin* instead of digoxin, or *Coumadin* instead of warfarin. In some situations the generic drug is not less expensive than the brand-name drug, so using only generic drugs does not guarantee that the person is getting the least expensive preparation. Some pharmacies post the costs of commonly used drugs, and people may do a **cost comparison** to compare the relative cost of the same drug among various pharmacies or the cost differences among manufacturers of drugs and request that a different drug be prescribed. The nurse or midwife is often the person who is in the middle of this issue and must be able to explain the reason for the drug choice or request that the prescriber consider an alternative treatment.

In the last few years, with the cost of drugs becoming a political as well as a social issue, many people have begun ordering drugs on the Internet, often from other countries. These drugs may be cheaper, do not require the person to see a health care provider (many of these sites simply have customers fill out a questionnaire that is reviewed by a doctor) and are delivered right to the person's door. On checking, many discrepancies have been identified between what was ordered and what is in the product, as well as problems in the storage of these products. Some foreign brand names are the same as brand names in this country but are associated with different generic drugs. Many medications are substandard or counterfeit products and may cause harm to patients and fail to treat the diseases for which they were intended. The World Health Organization estimates that 1 in 10 medical products in low- and middle-income countries is substandard or falsified. Many warnings have been issued to consumers about the risk of taking some of these drugs without medical supervision, reminding consumers that they are not protected by Australian or New Zealand laws or regulations when they purchase drugs from other countries. The TGA website, www.tga.gov.au/consumers/import.htm provides important information and guidelines for people who elect to use the Internet to get cheaper drugs.

PHARMAC is part of New Zealand's medicines system. The medicines system of New Zealand includes the Ministry of Health, MEDSAFE and District Health Boards, all working together to improve New Zealanders access to and optimal use of medicines. The central role of PHARMAC is to manage the pharmaceutical budget on behalf of District Health Boards and to decide which medicines are funded by the Government. For more information about PHARMAC, please access the website: www.pharmac.health.nz/about/your-guide-to-pharmac.

TABLE 6.2 Generic or trade-name drugs?

Drug name	30-day supply	Approximate cost of daily dose
atenolol (generic)	50–100 mg	$11.80
Tenormin		$15.98
labetalol (generic)	200–800 mg	$13.50
Trandate		$21.40
metoprolol (generic)	50–200 mg	$5.90
Betaloc		$9.99
pindolol (generic)	10–30 mg	$9.40
		$7.39
propranolol (generic)	40–320 mg	$17.70
Inderal		$31.50

This table shows general prescription prices for common beta-blockers used to treat hypertension. It is presented to illustrate the difference in pricing between generic and trade-name drugs.

DRUG ABUSE

Illicit drug use is a growing problem. Professional athletes are cited regularly for abusing anabolic steroids. High profile television and movie stars are often part of the drug scene, using **street drugs** – non-prescription drugs with no known therapeutic use – to enhance their mood and increase pleasure. Alcohol and nicotine are two commonly abused drugs that cause serious problems for the abuser or can interact with various drugs and alter a person's response to a prescribed drug but that are often not seen as drug addiction issues. Parents are often very concerned that their children will use street drugs. The 'everyone is doing it' argument is hard to counter when today's heroes are thought to be heavily involved. Some people abuse and become addicted to prescription drugs following an injury, when confronted with chronic pain, when their occupation puts them in contact with readily available drugs or when someone else in the home is using a prescription drug. Many of the drugs used

TABLE 6.3 Frequently abused 'recreational' drugs and their potential health consequences

Drug	Recreational drug names	Class	Health consequences
Amphetamines	Uppers, whites, dexies	Stimulant	Hypertension, tachycardia, insomnia, restlessness
Amyl nitrate	Boppers, pearls	Stimulant	Tachycardia, restlessness, hypotension, vertigo
Anabolic steroids	Roids, muscle	Steroid	Hypertension, hyperlipidaemia, acne, cancer, cardiomyopathy
Barbiturates	Downers, reds	Depressant	Bradycardia, hypotension, laryngospasm, ataxia, impaired thinking
Benzodiazepines	M&Ms, Uncle Milty	Depressant	Confusion, fatigue, impaired memory, impaired coordination
Cannabis with formaldehyde; with cocaine	Pot, grass, weed, THC; fry sticks; primo	Mixed CNS	Drowsiness, elation, dizziness, memory lapse, hallucinations
Cocaine	Snow, blow, crack	Stimulant	Tachycardia, hypertension, hallucinations, confused thinking
Fentanyl	Jackpot, China white	Opioid	Sedation, arrhythmias, shock, cardiac arrest, decreased respirations, constipation
Gamma-hydroxybutyrate	GHB, G, grievous bodily harm (GBH), liquid ecstasy, 4-hydroxybutanoic acid fantasy, liquid X, liquid E, 'date rape' drug	Depressant	Memory loss, hypotension, somnolence
Heroin	Brown sugar, joy, crank, fairy dust, horse, smack	Opioid	Sedation, arrhythmias, shock, cardiac arrest, decreased respirations, constipation
Kava	kawa, waka, lewena, yaqona, grog, sakau, 'awa, 'ava, wati, Piper methysticum	Depressant	Increased risks of serious infectious disease, liver and kidney dysfunction, neurological and cardiac events, malnutrition
Ketamine	Super acid, special K	Depressant	Paralysis, loss of sensation, disorientation, psychic changes
LSD	Acid, sunshine, blotter acid	Hallucinogen	Hallucinations, hypotension, changes in thinking, loss of social control
MDMA	Ecstasy, b-bombs, Scooby, snacks, E, pills, eccy, XTC, pingas, Adam, X	Hallucinogen	Hallucinations, psychic change, loss of memory, hypotension, cardiac arrest
Methamphetamine	Crystal, glass, speed, crystal meth, ice, base mother's cocaine shabu, ox blood, whiz, goey	Stimulant	Hypertension, tachycardia, restlessness, changes in thinking
Methylphenidate	Ritalin	Stimulant	Agitation, tachycardia, hypertension, hyperreflexia, fever
Morphine	Mort, Miss Emma	Opioid	Sedation, arrhythmias, shock, cardiac arrest, decreased respirations, constipation
OxyContin	Oxy, Oxycotton, Oxy 80s, hillbilly heroin, poor man's heroin, cotton	Opioid	Sedation, arrhythmias, shock, cardiac arrest, decreased respirations, constipation
PCP with steroids	Angel dust, zombie; juices	Hallucinogen	Acute psychosis, HF, death, seizures, memory loss
Peyote	Button, mesc	Hallucinogen	Acute psychosis, tremor, altered perception, death
Rohypnol	Roofies	Amnesiac	Date rape drug, loss of memory, immobility
Viagra/MDMA	Sextasy	Hallucinogen, ED drug	Severe hypotension, hallucinations, increased sexual function

CNS, central nervous system; ED, erectile dysfunction; HF, heart failure; LSD, lysergic acid diethylamide; MDMA, methy enedioxymethamphetamine; PCP, phencyclidine; THC, tetrahydrocannabinol.

illicitly are addictive and can change a person's entire life, with drug-seeking behaviour becoming a major factor. Researchers have identified actual changes in the brain and neurotransmitter patterns of people who abuse and become addicted to such drugs. Trying to reverse these changes and return the person to a non-addicted state is a physiological, as well as a psychological, challenge. The use of these drugs can have severe consequences for health, can mask underlying signs and symptoms of medical problems and can interact with other medications that the user may need.

Being informed about drugs available in the community, current trends among teenagers or young adults and community resources available to help people can guide parents and health care professionals while dealing with this drug culture problem. Education provides a crucial defence against drug abuse and helps the public and health care professionals recognise the problem and deal with it when it occurs. Funded by the Australian Government Department of Health and Ageing as part of the National Drug Strategy, the Australian Drug Information Network provides a central point for information on drug and alcohol. Go to www.adin.com.au to find information for teens, parents and health care professionals; the latest information on the hottest fads in illicit drugs; research on dealing with drug abuse problems; and links to sites for identifying unknown drugs, community resources and laws. For the New Zealand National Drug Policy and available information, go to www.ndp.govt.nz/moh.nsf/indexcm/ndp-policyactionplans-policy.

PROTECTING THE ENVIRONMENT

In March 2008, news services across the US reported studies showing that many prescription drugs had been found in the drinking water of various large cities. These studies showed ground and watershed contamination with many pharmaceutical products. The levels of these drugs were small, but the question was raised about what this would mean for the future and for the people, animals and crops that were being affected by the presence of these drugs. The problem is quite real. People get a prescription and then get switched to a different drug. Some people end up with extra pills at the end of a prescription because they did not follow the dosing guidelines exactly. Many people store these extra pills and end up with a medicine cabinet full of prescription drugs. In the past, people would often just flush these extras down the toilet, where they would enter the water system. Some people just threw them out, where they would eventually enter the ground of various landfills or would be diverted for illicit use by drug seekers going through garbage sites. With these things in mind and the push to protect the environment, the National Return and Disposal of Unwanted Medicines Limited was established in Australia. Go to www.returnmed.com.au for more information. Medicines New Zealand (www.medicinesnz.co.nz) provides the overarching framework for desired outcomes for the medicines system in New Zealand. It provides a common strategic direction to draw together the agencies and stakeholders that make its medicines system. This strategy is intended to inform decision making over the long-term and to deliver a world-class medicines system for New Zealanders and includes policies relating to proper drug disposal. It is important to teach people how to dispose of drugs properly. Encourage people to return unused medications to their community pharmacy for free disposal. The information about the safe disposal of unwanted medications is available at https://www.tga.gov.au/safe-disposal-unwanted-medicines.

CHAPTER SUMMARY

- In the 21st century, drugs pose new challenges for people and health care providers, including information overload, demands for specific treatments, increased access to self-care systems and financial pressure to provide cost-effective care.
- The mass media bombard consumers with medical reviews, research updates and advertising for prescription drugs. If the use of a drug is stated, the adverse effects and cautions must also be stated. If the use is not stated, the drug advertisement is free to use any images and suggestions to sell the drug.
- Increased access to the Internet and World Wide Web has increased consumer access to drug information, advertising and even purchasing without a mediator of this information. Determining the reliability of an Internet site is a challenge for the consumer and the health care provider.
- OTC drugs and herbal and alternative therapies allow people to make medical decisions and self-treat many common signs and symptoms. Problems arise when they are used inappropriately, when they interact with prescription drugs or when they mask signs and symptoms, making diagnosis difficult.
- Off-label uses of drugs occur when a drug has been released and is available for use. The use of a drug for an indication that is not approved by the TGA or MEDSAFE commonly occurs in paediatric and in psychiatric medicine, in which testing is limited or made ineffective by individual differences.
- Cost comparison is a major consideration in the use of many drugs.
- Home-based care is one of the most rapidly growing areas of medical care. People are increasingly more responsible for managing their medical regimens from home with dependence on home

health providers and teaching and support from knowledgeable nurses and midwives.

- Illicit drug use can lead to dependence on the drug and physiological changes, causing health problems and changing the body's response to traditional drugs.
- Proper disposal of unused or expired medications can help to protect the environment and may decrease drug-searching behaviours in some situations.

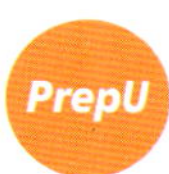

Knowing your strengths and weaknesses helps you to study more effectively. Take a PrepU Practice Quiz to find out how you measure up!

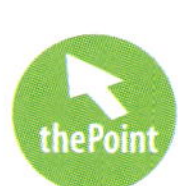

ONLINE RESOURCES

An extensive range of additional resources to enhance teaching and learning and to facilitate understanding of this chapter may be found online at the text's accompanying website, located on thePoint at http://thepoint.lww.com. These include Watch and Learn videos, Concepts in Action animations, journal articles, review questions, case studies, discussion topics and quizzes.

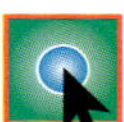

WEB LINKS

Health care providers and students may want to consult the following web resources:

www.anztpa.org
Australia New Zealand Therapeutic Products Agency (ANZTPA).

www.health.gov.au/internet/main/publishing.nsf/content/nmp-quality.htm
Quality Use of Medicines, Department of Health and Ageing, Australia.

www.medicinesnz.co.nz
Medicines New Zealand.

www.medsafe.govt.nz
Medsafe, New Zealand.

http://nccam.nih.gov
National Center for Complementary and Alternative Medicine, USA.

www.ndp.govt.nz/moh.nsf/indexcm/ndp-policyactionplans-policy
New Zealand National Drug Policy.

www.pbs.gov.au/pbs/home
Pharmaceutical Benefits Scheme, Department of Health and Ageing, Australia.

www.pharmac.health.nz
PHARMAC, New Zealand.

www.returnmed.com.au
Returning Unwanted Medicine program.

www.tga.gov.au
Therapeutic Goods Administration, Australia.

BIBLIOGRAPHY

Braun, L. & Cohen, M. (2010). *Herbs & Natural Supplements: An Evidence-based Guide*. Sydney: Churchill Livingstone, Elsevier.

Ghosh, D., Skinner, M. & Fergusson, L. (2006). The role of the Therapeutic Goods Administration and the Medicine and Medical Devices Safety Authority in evaluating complementary and alternative medicines in Australia and New Zealand. *Toxicology, 221*, 88–94

Goodman, L. S., Brunton, L. L., Chabner, B. & Knollmann, B. C. (2011). *Goodman and Gilman's Pharmacological Basis of Therapeutics* (12th edn). New York: McGraw-Hill.

Kuo, G. M. (2003). Pharmcodynamic basis of herbal medicine. *Annals of Pharmacotherapy, 37(2)*, 308.

Lucas, C. & Martin, J. (2013). Smoking and drug interactions. *Australian Prescriber, 36(3)*, 102–104.

McFadden, R. & Peterson, N. (2011). Interactions between drugs and four common medicinal herbs. *Nursing Standard, 25(19)*, 65–68.

McKenna, L. & Mirkov, S. (2019). *McKenna's Drug Handbook for Nursing and Midwifery* (8th edn). Sydney: Wolters Kluwer Health Australia.

Moses, G. M. & McGuire, T. M. (2010). Drug interactions with complementary medicines. *Australian Prescriber, 33*, 177–180.

Pizzorno, J. E. & Murray, M. T. (2013). *Textbook of Natural Medicine* (4th edn) St Louis: Elsevier.

Vernon, G. M. (2013). Sex, drugs and alcohol: Drug interactions of concern to consumers. *Australian Prescriber, 36(2)*, 46–48.

CHECK YOUR UNDERSTANDING

Answers to the questions in this chapter can be found in Appendix A at the back of this book.

MULTIPLE CHOICE

Select the best answer to the following.

1. Herbal treatments and alternative therapies:
   a. are considered drugs and regulated by the TGA.
   b. are considered dietary supplements and are not regulated by the TGA.
   c. have no restrictions on claims and advertising.
   d. contain no drugs, only natural substances.
2. OTC drugs are drugs that are:
   a. deemed to be safe when used as directed.
   b. harmless to the public.
   c. too old to be tested.
   d. cheaper to use than prescription drugs.
3. The home-based health care industry is booming because:
   a. there is a shortage of hospital beds.
   b. people feel safer at home and prefer to be cared for at home.
   c. people are going home sooner and becoming responsible for their own care sooner than in the past.
   d. staffing shortages make it difficult to care for people in hospitals.
4. The cost of drug therapy is a major consideration in most areas because:
   a. generic drugs are always cheaper.
   b. the high cost of drugs combined with more fixed-income consumers puts constraints on drug use.
   c. pharmacies usually carry only one drug from each class.
   d. people like to shop around and get the best drug for their money.
5. An off-label use of a drug means that the drug:
   a. was found without a label and its actual contents are not known.
   b. has been found to be safe when used as directed and no restrictions are needed.
   c. is being used for an indication not listed in the approved indications noted by the TGA.
   d. has expired but is still found to be useful when used as directed.

MULTIPLE RESPONSE

Select all that apply.

1. When taking a health history, the nurse or midwife should include specific questions about the use of OTC drugs and alternative therapies. This is an important aspect of the health history because:
   a. many insurance policies cover these drugs.
   b. people should be reprimanded about the use of these products.
   c. people often do not consider them to be drugs and do not report their use.
   d. people should never use these products when taking prescription drugs.
   e. these products can mask or alter presenting signs and symptoms.
   f. many of these products interact with traditional prescription drugs.
2. A health professional is caring for a person who has been diagnosed with type 2 diabetes. The person has reported that he frequently uses herbal remedies. Before administering any antidiabetic medications, the health professional should caution the person about the use of which of the following herbal therapies?
   a. glucosamine
   b. ginseng
   c. St John's wort
   d. juniper berries
   e. garlic
   f. kava

PART 2

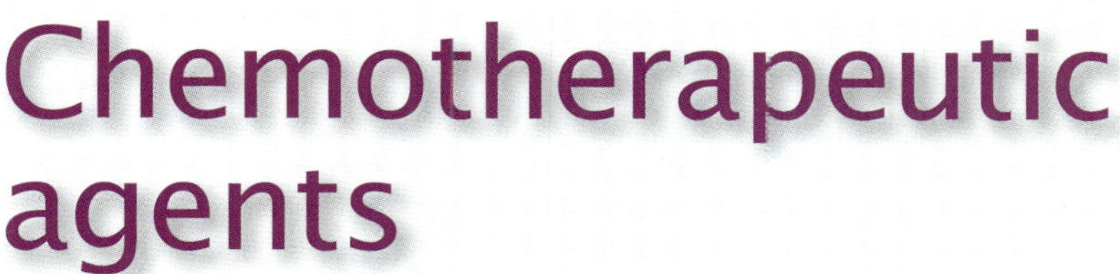

Chemotherapeutic agents

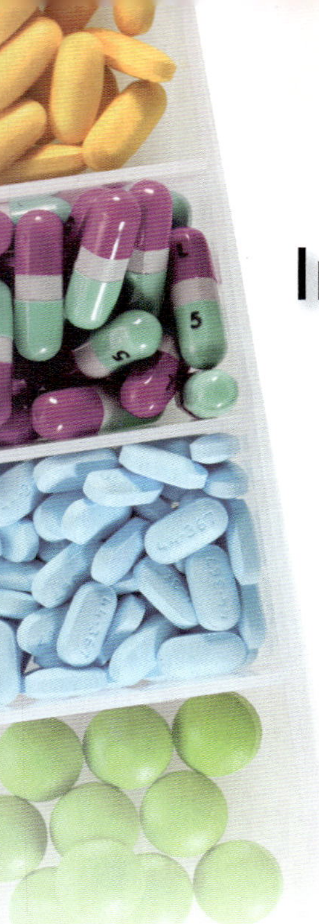

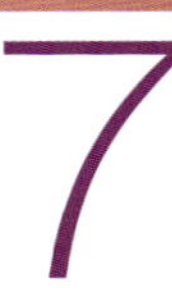

Introduction to cell physiology

Learning objectives

On completing this chapter you should be able to:

1. Identify the parts of the human cell.
2. Describe the role of each organelle found within the cell cytoplasm.
3. Explain the unique properties of the cell membrane.
4. Describe three processes used by the cell to move things across the cell membrane.
5. Outline the cell cycle, including the activities going on within the cell in each phase.

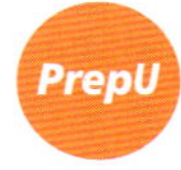

Test your current knowledge of cell physiology with a PrepU Practice Quiz!

Glossary of key terms

cell cycle: life cycle of a cell, which includes the phases G_0, G_1, S, G_2 and M; during the M phase, the cell divides into two identical daughter cells

cell membrane: lipoprotein structure that separates the interior of a cell from the external environment; regulates what can enter and leave a cell

cytoplasm: lies within the cell membrane; contains organelles for producing proteins, energy and so on

diffusion: movement of solutes from an area of high concentration to an area of low concentration across a concentration gradient

endocytosis: the process of engulfing substances and moving them into a cell by extending the cell membrane around the substance; pinocytosis and phagocytosis are two kinds of endocytosis

endoplasmic reticulum: fine network of interconnected channels known as cisternae found in the cytoplasm; site of chemical reactions within the cell

exocytosis: removal of substances from a cell by pushing them through the cell membrane

genes: sequences of DNA that control basic cell functions and allow for cell division

Golgi apparatus: a series of flattened sacs in the cytoplasm that prepare hormones or other substances for secretion and may produce lysosomes and store other synthesised proteins

histocompatibility antigens: proteins found on the surface of the cell membrane; they are determined by the genetic code and provide cellular identity as a self-cell (i.e. a cell belonging to that individual)

lipoprotein: structure composed of proteins and lipids; the bipolar arrangement of the lipids monitors substances passing in and out of the cell

lysosomes: encapsulated digestive enzymes found within a cell; they digest old or damaged areas of the cell and are responsible for destroying the cell when the membrane ruptures and the cell dies

mitochondria: rod-shaped organelles that produce energy within the cell in the form of adenosine triphosphate (ATP)

nucleus: the part of a cell that contains the DNA and genetic material; regulates cellular protein production and cellular properties

organelles: distinct structures found within the cell cytoplasm

osmosis: movement of water from an area of low solute concentration to an area of high solute concentration to equalise the concentrations

phagocytosis: the engulfing of pathogens or other particles by phagocytes (white blood cells)

pinocytosis: the introduction of fluids into a cell by invagination of the cell membrane, followed by formation of vesicles within the cells

ribosomes: membranous structures that are the sites of protein production within a cell

selective toxicity: ability of a chemical or drug to kill a microorganism without harming its host. See Chapter 2

Chemotherapeutic drugs are used to destroy both organisms that invade the body (eg, bacteria, viruses, parasites, protozoa, fungi) and abnormal cells within the body (eg, neoplasms, cancers). These drugs affect cells by altering cellular function or disrupting cellular integrity, causing cell death, or by preventing cellular reproduction, eventually leading to cell death. Because most chemotherapeutic agents do not possess complete **selective toxicity**, they also, to some extent, affect the normal cells of people. To understand the actions and adverse effects caused by chemotherapeutic agents and to determine interventions that increase therapeutic effectiveness, it is important to understand the various properties and the basic structure and function of the cell.

THE CELL

The cell is the basic structural unit of the body. The cells that make up living organisms, which are arranged into tissues and organs, all have the same basic structure. Each cell has a nucleus, a cell membrane and cytoplasm, which contains a variety of organelles (Figure 7.1).

Cell nucleus

Each cell is 'programmed' by the **genes**, or sequences of DNA, that allow for cell division, produce specific proteins that allow the cell to carry out its functions and maintain cell homeostasis or stability. The **nucleus** is the part of a cell that contains all genetic material necessary for cell reproduction and for the regulation of cellular production of proteins. The nucleus is encapsulated in its own membrane and remains distinct from the rest of the cytoplasm. A small spherical mass, called the nucleolus, is located within the nucleus. Within this mass are dense fibres and proteins that will eventually become **ribosomes**, the sites of protein synthesis within the cell. Genes are responsible for the formation of messenger RNA and transcription RNA, which are involved in production of the proteins unique to the cell. The DNA necessary for cell division is found on long strains called chromatin. These structures line up and enlarge during the process of cell division.

Cell membrane

The cell is surrounded by a thin barrier called the **cell membrane**, which separates intracellular fluid from extracellular fluid. The membrane is essential for cellular integrity and is equipped with many mechanisms for maintaining cell homeostasis.

Lipoproteins

The cell membrane is a **lipoprotein** structure, meaning that it is mainly composed of proteins and lipids –

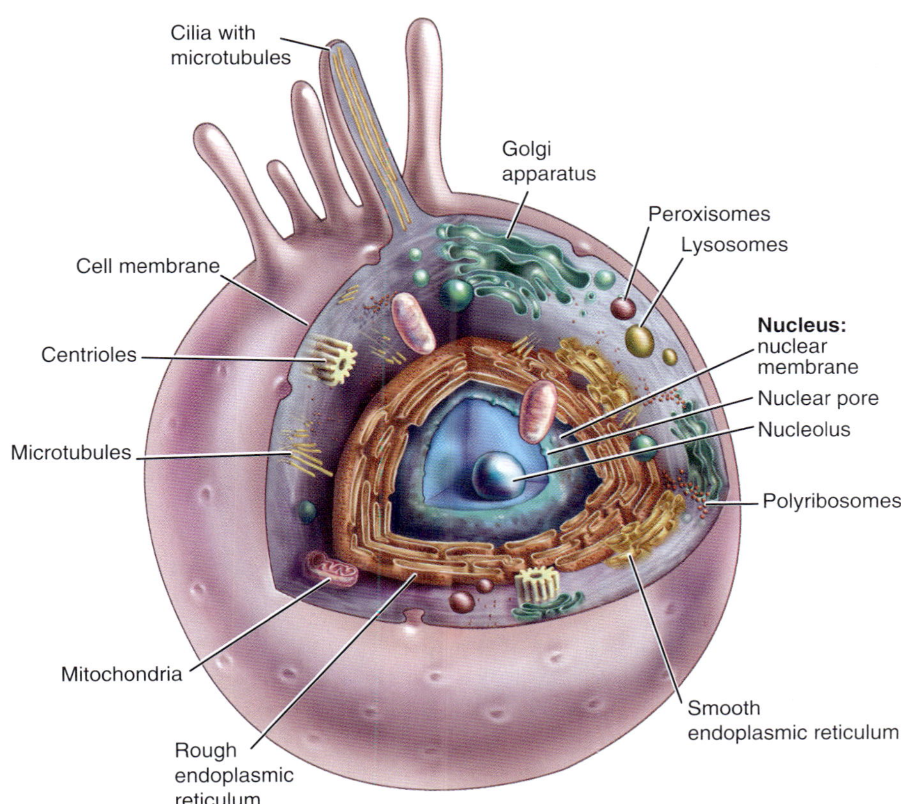

FIGURE 7.1 General structure of a cell and the location of its organelles.

phospholipids, glycolipids and cholesterol; the bipolar arrangement of the lipids monitors substances passing into and out of the cell. The phospholipids, which are bipolar in nature, line up with their polar regions pointing towards the interior or exterior of the cell and their non-polar region lying within the cell membrane. The polar regions mix well with water, and the non-polar region repels water. These properties allow the membrane to act as a barrier to regulate what can enter the cell (see Figure 7.2). The freely-moving nature of the membrane allows it to adjust to the changing shape of the cell so that areas of the membrane can move together to repair itself if it becomes torn or injured. Some of the outward-facing phospholipids have a sugar group attached to them; these are called glycolipids. Cholesterol is found in large quantities in the membrane, and it works to keep the phospholipids in place and the cell membrane stable.

Receptor sites

Embedded in the cell membrane are a series of peripheral proteins with several functions. As discussed in Chapter 2, one type of protein located on the cell membrane is known as a receptor site. This protein reacts with specific chemicals outside the cell to stimulate a reaction within the cell. For example, the receptor site for insulin reacts with the hormone insulin to cause activation of adenosine triphosphate (ATP) within the cell. This reaction alters the cell's permeability to glucose. Receptor sites are very important in the functioning of neurons, muscle cells, endocrine glands and other cell types, and they play a very important role in clinical pharmacology.

Identifying markers

Other surface proteins are surface antigens, or genetically determined identifying markers. These proteins are called **histocompatibility antigens** or human leucocyte antigens (HLAs), which the body uses to identify a cell as a self-cell (i.e. a cell belonging to that individual). The body's immune system recognises these proteins and acts to protect self-cells and to destroy non-self-cells. When an organ is transplanted from one person to another, a great effort is made to match as many histocompatibility antigens as possible to reduce the chance that the 'new' body will reject the transplanted organ.

Histocompatibility antigens can be changed in several ways: by cell injury, with viral invasion of a cell, with age, and so on. If the markers are altered, the body's immune system reacts to the change and can ignore it, allowing neoplasms to grow and develop. The immune system may also attack the cell, leading to many of the problems associated with autoimmune disorders and chronic inflammatory conditions.

Channels

Channels or pores within the cell membrane are made by proteins in the cell wall that allow the passage of small substances into or out of the cell. Specific channels have been identified for sodium, potassium, calcium, chloride, bicarbonate and water; other channels may also exist. Some drugs are designed to affect certain channels specifically. For example, calcium-channel blockers prevent the movement of calcium into a cell through calcium channels.

KEY POINTS

- The cell is the basic structure of all living organisms.
- The cell membrane features specific receptor sites that allow interaction with various chemicals, histocompatibility proteins that allow for self-identification, and channels or pores that allow for the passage of substances into and out of the cell.

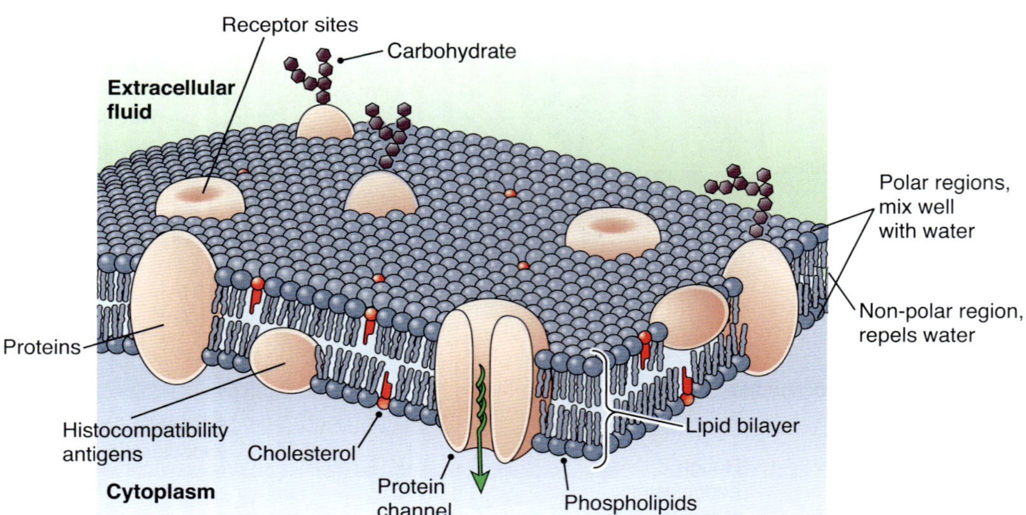

FIGURE 7.2 Structure of the lipid bilayer of the cell membrane.

Cytoplasm

The cell **cytoplasm** lies within the cell membrane and outside the nucleus and is the site of activities of cellular metabolism and special cellular functions. The cytoplasm contains many **organelles**, which are structures with specific functions such as producing proteins and energy. The organelles within the cytoplasm include the mitochondria, the endoplasmic reticulum, free ribosomes, the Golgi apparatus and the lysosomes.

Mitochondria

Mitochondria are rod-shaped 'power plants' within each cell that produce energy in the form of ATP, which allows the cell to function. Mitochondria are plentiful in very active cells such as muscle cells and are relatively scarce in inactive cells such as bone cells. Mitochondria, which can reproduce when a cell is very active, are always very abundant in cells that consume energy. For example, cardiac muscle cells, which must work continually to keep the heart contracting, contain a great number of mitochondria. Milk-producing cells in breast tissue, which are normally quite dormant, contain very few mitochondria. If a woman is breastfeeding, however, the mitochondria become more abundant to meet the demands of the milk-producing cells. The mitochondria can take carbohydrates, fats and proteins from the cytoplasm and make ATP via the Krebs cycle, which depends on oxygen. Cells use the ATP to maintain homeostasis, produce proteins and carry out specific functions. If oxygen is not available, lactic acid builds up as a byproduct of cellular respiration. Lactic acid leaves the cell and is transported to the liver for conversion to glycogen and carbon dioxide.

Endoplasmic reticulum

Much of the cytoplasm of a cell is made up of a fine network of interconnected channels known as cisternae, which form the **endoplasmic reticulum**. The undulating surface of the endoplasmic reticulum provides a large surface for chemical reactions within the cell. Many granules that contain enzymes and ribosomes, which produce protein, are scattered over the surface of the rough endoplasmic reticulum. Production of proteins, phospholipids and cholesterol takes place in the rough endoplasmic reticulum. The smooth endoplasmic reticulum is the site of further lipid and cholesterol production and the production of cell products, such as hormones. The breakdown of many toxic substances may also occur here in particular cells.

Free ribosomes

Other ribosomes that are not bound to the surface of the endoplasmic reticulum exist throughout the cytoplasm. These free-floating ribosomes produce proteins that are important to the structure of the cell and some of the enzymes that are necessary for cellular activity.

Golgi apparatus

The **Golgi apparatus** is a series of flattened sacs that may be part of the endoplasmic reticulum. These structures prepare hormones or other substances for secretion by processing them and packaging them in vesicles to be moved to the cell membrane for excretion from the cell. In addition, the Golgi apparatus may produce lysosomes and store other synthesised proteins and enzymes until they are needed.

Lysosomes

Lysosomes are membrane-covered organelles that contain specific digestive enzymes that can break down proteins, nucleic acids, carbohydrates and lipids and are responsible for digesting worn or damaged sections of a cell when the membrane ruptures and the cell dies. Lysosomes form a membrane around any substance that needs to be digested and secrete the digestive enzymes directly into the isolated area, protecting the rest of the cytoplasm from injury. This phenomenon can be seen with old lettuce in the refrigerator. The side of the lettuce head that has been 'lying down' for a prolonged period becomes brown and wet as the lettuce cells die and self-digest when their lysosomes are released. If the lettuce is not used, the released lysosomes begin to digest any healthy lettuce that remains, with eventual destruction of the entire head. Lysosomes are important in ecology. Dead trees, animals and other organisms self-digest.

KEY POINTS

- The cytoplasm of the cell contains various organelles that are important for cellular function.
- The mitochondria produce energy for the cell; the endoplasmic reticulum contains ribosomes that produce proteins; the Golgi apparatus packages proteins; and lysosomes contain protein-dissolving enzymes that are important for digestion and the recycling of organisms in nature.

CELL PROPERTIES

Cells have certain properties that allow them to survive. **Endocytosis** involves incorporation of material into the cell by extending the cell membrane around the substance. **Pinocytosis**, a form of endocytosis, refers to the engulfing of specific substances that have reacted with a receptor site on the cell membrane. This process allows cells to absorb nutrients, enzymes and other materials. **Phagocytosis** is a similar process; it allows the cell (white blood cell), usually a neutrophil or macrophage, to engulf a bacterium or a foreign protein and destroy it within the cell by secreting digestive enzymes into the area. **Exocytosis** is the opposite of endocytosis and involves removing substances from a cell by pushing them through the cell membrane. Hormones, neurotransmitters, enzymes and other substances produced within a cell are excreted into the body by this process (see Figure 7.3).

Release of stored material
Extracellular fluid
Plasma membrane
Cytoplasm
Vesicle
Fusion with plasma membrane
Stored material
A

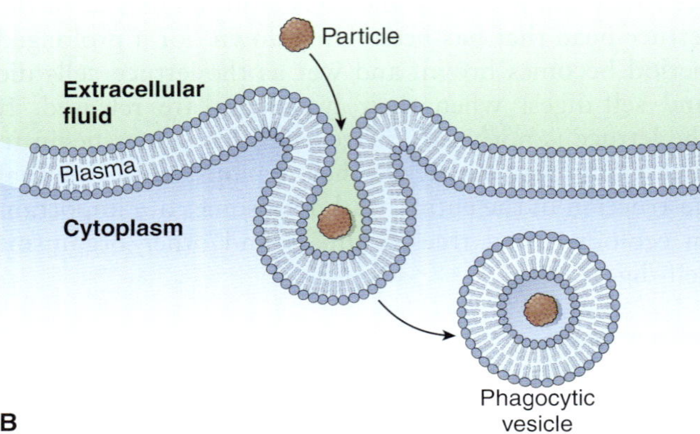

FIGURE 7.3 Schematic representation of endocytosis and exocytosis. **A.** Exocytosis is the movement of substances (waste products, hormones, neurotransmitters) out of the cell. **B.** Endocytosis involves the destruction of engulfed proteins or bacteria.

Homeostasis

The main goal of a cell is to maintain homeostasis, which means keeping the cytoplasm stable within the cell membrane. Each cell uses a series of active and passive transport systems to achieve homeostasis; the exact system used depends on the type of cell and its reactions with the immediate environment. For a cell to produce the energy needed to carry out cellular metabolism and other processes, the cell must have a means to obtain necessary elements from the outside environment. In addition, it must have a way to dispose of waste products that could be toxic to its cytoplasm. To accomplish this, the cell moves substances across the cell membrane, either by passive transport or by active (energy-requiring) transport (see Figure 7.4).

Passive transport

Passive transport happens without the expenditure of energy and can occur across any semipermeable membrane. There are essentially three types of passive transport: diffusion, osmosis and facilitated diffusion.

Diffusion

Diffusion is the movement of a substance from a region of higher concentration to a region of lower concentration. The difference between the concentrations of the substance in the two regions is called the *concentration gradient* of the substance; usually, the greater the concentration gradient, the faster the substance moves. Movement into and out of a cell is regulated by the cell membrane. Some substances move through channels or pores in the cell membrane. Small substances and

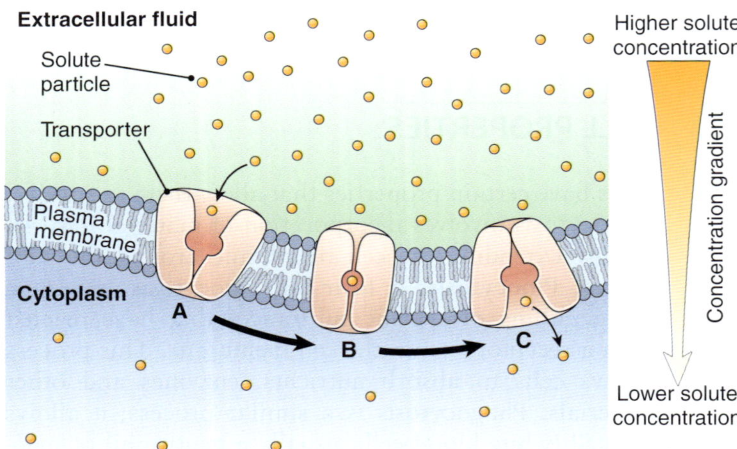

FIGURE 7.4 Schematic representation of transport across a cell membrane (**A**), which includes *diffusion* through the cell membrane (**B**) and *pore diffusion* through a protein channel (**C**).

materials with no ionic charge move most freely through the channels. Substances with a negative charge move more freely than substances with a positive charge. Substances that move into and out of a cell by diffusion include sodium, potassium, calcium, carbonate, oxygen, bicarbonate and water.

When a cell is very active and is using energy and oxygen, the concentration of oxygen within the cell decreases. The concentration of oxygen outside the cell remains relatively high, so oxygen moves across the cell membrane (down the concentration gradient) to supply needed oxygen to the inside of the cell. Cells use this process to maintain homeostasis during many activities that occur during their life.

Osmosis

Osmosis, a special form of diffusion, is the movement of water across a semipermeable membrane from an area that is low in dissolved solutes to one that is high in dissolved solutes. The water is attempting to equalise the dilution of the solutes. This diffusion of water across a cell membrane from an area of high concentration (of water) to an area of low concentration creates pressure on the cell membrane called *osmotic pressure*. The greater the concentration of solutes in the solution to which the water is flowing, the higher is the osmotic pressure.

A fluid that contains the same concentration of solutes as human plasma is called an *isotonic* solution. A fluid that contains a higher concentration of solutes than human plasma is a *hypertonic* solution; it draws water from cells. A fluid that contains a lower concentration of solutes than human plasma is *hypotonic*; it loses water to cells. If a human red blood cell, which has a cytoplasm that is isotonic with human plasma, is placed into a hypertonic solution, it shrinks and shrivels because the water inside the cell diffuses out of the cell into the solution. If the same cell is placed into a hypotonic solution, the cell swells and bursts because water moves from the solution into the cell (see Figure 7.5).

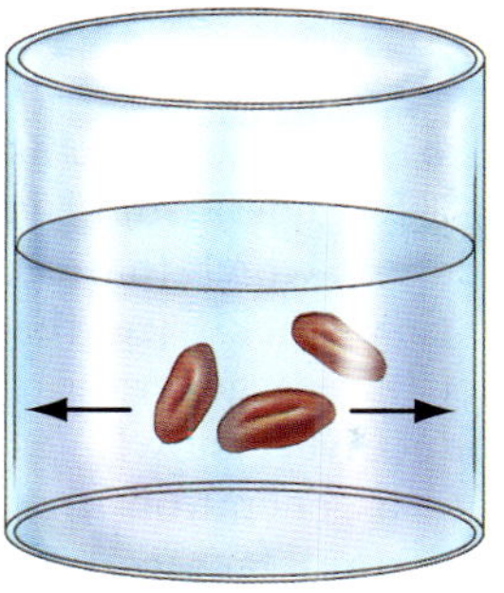

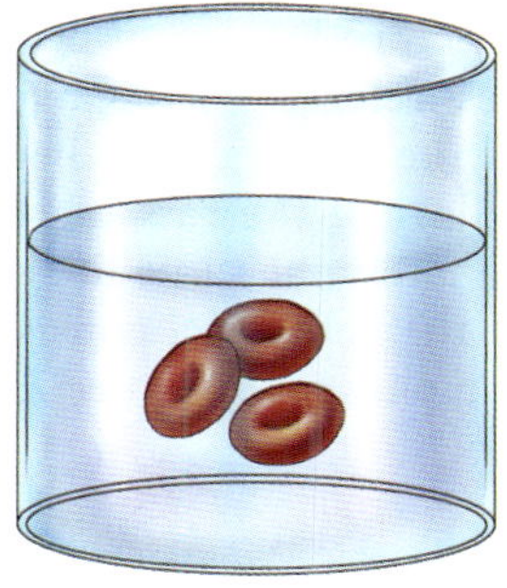

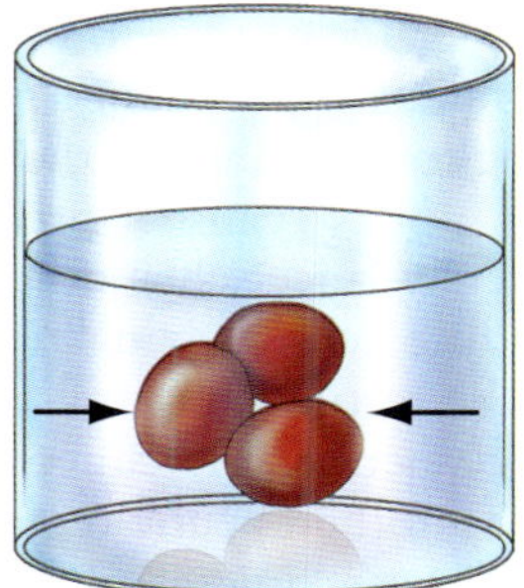

FIGURE 7.5 Red blood cell, showing the cell's response to hypertonic, isotonic and hypotonic solutions.

Facilitated diffusion

Sometimes a substance cannot move freely on its own into or out of a cell. Such a substance may attach to another molecule, called a carrier, to be diffused. This form of diffusion, known as *facilitated diffusion*, does not require energy, just the presence of the carrier. Carriers may be hormones, enzymes or proteins. Because the carrier required for facilitated diffusion is usually present in a finite amount, this type of diffusion is limited.

Active transport

Sometimes a cell requires a substance in greater concentration than is found in the environment around it or needs to maintain its cytoplasm in a situation that would normally allow chemicals to leave the cell. When this happens, the cell must move substances against the concentration gradient using active transport, which requires energy. When a cell is deprived of oxygen because of a blood supply problem or insufficient oxygenation of the blood, systems of active transport begin to malfunction, placing the cell's integrity in jeopardy.

One of the best-known systems of active transport is the sodium–potassium pump. Cells use active transport to maintain their cytoplasm with a higher level of potassium and a lower level of sodium than the extracellular fluid contains. This allows the cell to maintain an electrical charge on the cell membrane, which gives many cells the electrical properties of excitation (the ability to generate a movement of electrons) and conduction (the ability to send this stimulus to other areas of the membrane). Some drugs use energy to move into cells by active transport. Drugs are frequently bonded with a carrier when they are moved into the cell. Cells in the kidney use active transport to excrete drugs from the body, as well as to maintain electrolyte and acid–base balances.

CELL CYCLE

Most cells have the ability to reproduce themselves through the process of mitosis. The genetic makeup of a particular cell determines the rate at which that cell can multiply. Some cells reproduce very quickly (eg, the cells lining the gastrointestinal tract have a generation time of 72 hours), and some reproduce very slowly (eg, the cells found in breast tissue have a generation time of a few months). In some cases, certain factors influence cell reproduction. Erythropoietin, a hormone produced by the kidney, can stimulate the production of new red blood cells. Active leucocytes release chemicals that stimulate the production of white blood cells when the body needs new ones. Regardless of the rate of reproduction, each cell has approximately the same life cycle. The life cycle of a cell, called the **cell cycle**, consists of four active phases and a resting phase (see Figure 7.6).

G_0 phase

During the G_0 phase, or resting phase, the cell is stable. It is not making any proteins associated with cell division and is basically dormant as far as reproduction goes. These cells are just functioning to do whatever they are supposed to do. Cells in the G_0 phase cause a problem in the treatment of some cancers. Cancer chemotherapy usually works on active, dividing cells, leaving resting cells fairly untouched. When the resting cells are stimulated to become active and regenerate, the cancer can return, which is why cancer chemotherapeutic regimens are complicated and extended over time, and why a 5-year cancer-free period is usually the basic guide for considering a cancer to be cured.

G_1 phase

When a cell is stimulated to emerge from its resting phase, it enters what is called the G_1 phase, which lasts from the time of stimulation from the resting phase until the formation of DNA. During this period, the cell synthesises substances needed for DNA formation. The cell is actively collecting materials to make these substances and producing the building blocks for DNA.

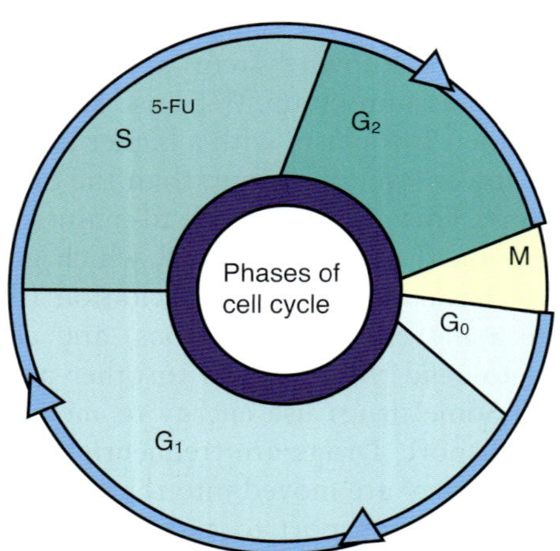

FIGURE 7.6 Diagram of the cell cycle, showing G_0, G_1, S, G_2 and M phases.

S phase

The next phase, called the S phase, involves the actual synthesis of DNA, which is an energy-consuming activity. The cell remains in this phase until the amount of cellular DNA has doubled.

G_2 phase

After the cellular DNA has doubled in preparation for replication, the G_2 phase begins. During this phase, the cell produces all the substances required for the manufacture of the mitotic spindles.

M phase

After the cell has produced all the substances necessary for formation of a new cell, or daughter cell, it undergoes cell division. This occurs during the M phase of the cell cycle. During this phase, the cell splits to form two identical daughter cells, a process called mitosis.

KEY POINTS

- All cells progress through a cell cycle, which allows them to reproduce.
- Each cell goes through a resting phase (G_0); a gathering phase (G_1), when the components needed for cell division are collected by the cell; a synthesising phase (S), when DNA and other components are produced; a final gathering phase (G_2), when the last substances needed for division are collected and produced; and an M phase, when actual cell division occurs, producing two identical daughter cells.

CHAPTER SUMMARY

- The cell is composed of a nucleus, which contains genetic material and controls the production of proteins by the cell; a cell membrane, which separates the inside of the cell from the outside environment; and a cytoplasm, which contains various organelles important to cell function.
- The cell membrane functions as a fluid barrier made of lipids and proteins. The arrangement of the lipoprotein membrane controls what enters and leaves the cell.
- Proteins on the cell membrane surface can act either as receptor sites for specific substances or as histocompatibility markers that identify the cell as a self-cell (i.e. a cell belonging to that individual).

- Channels or pores in the cell membrane allow for easier movement of specific substances needed by the cell for normal functioning.
- Mitochondria are rod-shaped organelles that produce energy in the form of ATP for use by cells.
- Ribosomes are sites of protein production within the cell cytoplasm. The specific proteins produced by a cell are determined by the genetic material within the cell nucleus.
- The Golgi apparatus packages particular substances for removal from the cell (eg, neurotransmitters, hormones).
- Lysosomes are packets of digestive enzymes located in the cell cytoplasm. These enzymes are responsible for destroying injured or non-functioning parts of the cell and for promoting cellular disintegration when the cell dies.
- Endocytosis is the process of moving substances into a cell by extending the cell membrane around the substance and engulfing it. Pinocytosis refers to the engulfing of necessary materials, and phagocytosis refers to the engulfing and destroying of bacteria or other proteins by white blood cells.
- Exocytosis is the process of removing substances from a cell by moving them towards the cell membrane and then changing the cell membrane to allow passage of the substance out of the cell.
- Cells maintain homeostasis by regulating the movement of solutes and water into and out of the cell.
- Diffusion, which does not require energy, is the movement of solutes from a region of high concentration to a region of lower concentration across a concentration gradient.
- Osmosis, which, like diffusion, does not require energy, is the movement of water from an area low in solutes to an area high in solutes. Osmosis exerts a pressure against the cell membrane that is called osmotic pressure.
- Active transport, an energy-requiring process, is the movement of particular substances against a concentration gradient. Active transport is important in maintaining cell homeostasis.
- Cells replicate at differing rates, depending on the genetic programming of the cell. All cells go through a life cycle consisting of the following phases: G_0, the resting phase; G_1, which involves the production of proteins for DNA synthesis; S, which involves the synthesis of DNA; G_2, which involves the manufacture of the materials needed for mitotic spindle production; and M, the mitotic phase, in which the cell splits to form two identical daughter cells.
- Chemotherapeutic drugs act on cells to cause cell death or alteration. All properties of the drug that affect cells should be considered when administering a chemotherapeutic agent.

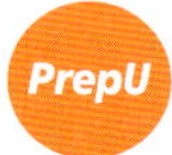

Knowing your strengths and weaknesses helps you to study more effectively. Take a PrepU Practice Quiz to find out how you measure up!

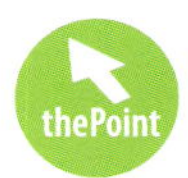

ONLINE RESOURCES

An extensive range of additional resources to enhance teaching and learning and to facilitate understanding of this chapter may be found online at the text's accompanying website, located on thePoint at http://thepoint.lww.com. These include Watch and Learn videos, Concepts in Action animations, journal articles, review questions, case studies, discussion topics and quizzes.

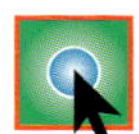

WEB LINKS

Health care providers and students may want to consult the following web resource:

www.life.uiuc.edu/plantbio/cell
Information on cell structure, properties and division.

BIBLIOGRAPHY

Alberts, B. (2008). *Molecular Biology of the Cell* (5th edn). New York: Garland Science.

Cartwright, K. (2007). Cell markers. *Australian Prescriber, 30(5)*, 128–129.

Cooper, G. & Hausman, R. (2013). *The Cell: A Molecular Approach* (6th edn). Sunderland MA: Sinauer Associates.

Goodman, L. S., Brunton, L. L., Chabner, B. & Knollmann, B. C. (2011). *Goodman and Gilman's Pharmacological Basis of Therapeutics* (12th edn). New York: McGraw-Hill.

Guyton, A. & Hall, J. (2011). *Textbook of Medical Physiology* (12th edn). Philadelphia: Saunders Elsevier.

Landowne, D. (2006). *Cell Physiology*. New York: McGraw-Hill.

Lodish, H. F. (2013). *Molecular Cell Biology* (7th edn). New York: W. H. Freeman.

Morgan, D. (2007). *The Cell Cycle: Principles of Control*. London: New Science Press.

Nair, M. & Peate, I. (2013). *Fundamentals of Applied Pathophysiology: An Essential Guide for Nursing and Healthcare Students* (2nd edn). Ames, Iowa: Wiley-Blackwell.

Porth, C. M. (2011). *Essentials of Pathophysiology: Concepts of Altered Health States* (3rd edn). Philadelphia: Lippincott Williams & Wilkins.

Porth, C. M. (2009). *Pathophysiology: Concepts of Altered Health States* (8th edn). Philadelphia: Lippincott Williams & Wilkins.

Sherwood, L. (2013). *Human Physiology from Cells to Systems* (8th edn). Belmont CA: Brooks Cole Cengage Learning.

CHECK YOUR UNDERSTANDING

Answers to the questions in this chapter can be found in Appendix A at the back of this book.

MULTIPLE CHOICE

Select the best answer to the following.

1. The basic unit of human structure is:
   a. the mitochondrion.
   b. the nucleus.
   c. the nucleolus.
   d. the cell.
2. The cell membrane is composed of:
   a. a phospholipid structure.
   b. channels of protein.
   c. a cholesterol-based membrane.
   d. Golgi apparatus.
3. The saying, 'One rotten apple can spoil the whole barrel', can be used to refer to the cell-degrading properties of:
   a. calcium channels.
   b. lysosomes.
   c. histocompatibility receptors.
   d. nuclear spindles.
4. The ribosomes are important sites for:
   a. digestion of nutrients.
   b. excretion of waste products.
   c. production of proteins.
   d. hormone receptors.
5. A human cell placed in salty seawater will:
   a. burst from water entering the cell.
   b. shrivel and die from water leaving the cell.
   c. not be affected in any way.
   d. break apart from the salt effect.
6. The sodium–potassium pump maintains a negative charge on the cell membrane by:
   a. osmosis.
   b. diffusion.
   c. active transport.
   d. facilitated diffusion.
7. All cells progress through basically the same cell cycle, including:
   a. two phases.
   b. four active phases and a resting phase.
   c. three periods of rest and a splitting phase.
   d. four active phases.

MULTIPLE RESPONSE

Select all that apply.

1. The amount of time that a cell takes to progress through the cell cycle is determined by which of the following?
   a. the acidity of the environment
   b. the genetic makeup of the cell
   c. the location of the cell in the body
   d. the number of ribosomes in the cell
   e. the cell response to contact inhibition
   f. the availability of nutrients and oxygen
2. Some substances will pass into the human cell by simple diffusion. Which of the following substances diffuse into the cell?
   a. calcium
   b. nitrogen
   c. sodium
   d. carbon dioxide
   e. oxygen
   f. potassium
3. Some substances require a channel or pore to enter a cell membrane. Which of the following substances use a channel to enter the cell?
   a. calcium
   b. urea
   c. fat-soluble vitamins
   d. sodium
   e. oxygen
   f. potassium

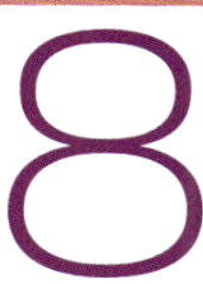

Anti-infective agents

Learning objectives

On completing this chapter you should be able to:

1. Explain what is meant by selective toxicity and discuss its importance in anti-infective therapies.
2. Differentiate between broad-spectrum and narrow-spectrum drugs.
3. Define bacterial resistance to antibiotics and discuss the emergence of resistant strains.
4. Explain three ways to minimise bacterial resistance.
5. Describe three common adverse reactions associated with the use of antibiotics.

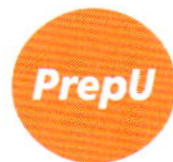

Test your current knowledge of anti-infective agents with a PrepU Practice Quiz!

Glossary of key terms

bactericidal: substance that causes the death of bacteria, usually by interfering with cell membrane stability or with proteins or enzymes necessary to maintain the cellular integrity of the bacteria

bacteriostatic: substance that prevents the replication of bacteria, usually by interfering with proteins or enzyme systems necessary for reproduction of the bacteria

culture: sample of the bacteria (eg, from sputum, cell scrapings, urine) to be grown in a laboratory to determine the species of bacteria that is causing an infection

prophylaxis: treatment to prevent an infection before it occurs, as in the use of antibiotics to prevent bacterial endocarditis or antiprotozoals to prevent malaria

resistance: ability of bacteria over time to adapt to an antibiotic and produce cells that are no longer affected by a particular drug

selective toxicity: the ability to affect certain proteins or enzyme systems that are used by the infecting organism but not by human cells

sensitivity testing: evaluation of bacteria obtained in a culture to determine the antibiotics to which the organisms are sensitive and which agent would be appropriate for treatment of a particular infection

spectrum: range of bacteria against which an antibiotic is effective (eg, broad-spectrum antibiotics are effective against a wide range of bacteria)

superinfection: infections that occur when opportunistic pathogens that were kept in check by the 'normal' bacteria have the opportunity to invade tissues and cause infections because the normal flora bacteria have been destroyed by antibiotic therapy

DRUG LIST

chloramphenicol	meropenem	teicoplanin	vancomycin

Anti-infective agents are drugs designed to target foreign organisms that have invaded and infected the body of a human host. For centuries, people have used various naturally occurring chemicals in an effort to treat disease. Often this was a random act that proved useful. For example, the ancient Chinese found that applying mouldy soybean curds to boils and infected wounds helped prevent infection or hastened cure. Their finding was, perhaps, a forerunner to the penicillins used today.

The use of drugs to treat systemic infections is a relatively new concept, beginning with Paul Ehrlich in the 1920s. Ehrlich's research to develop a synthetic chemical that would be effective only against infection-causing cells, not human cells, led the way for the scientific investigation of anti-infective agents. In the late 1920s, scientists discovered penicillin in a mould sample; in 1935, the sulfonamides were introduced. Since then, the number of anti-infectives available for use has grown tremendously. However, many of the organisms these drugs were designed to treat are rapidly adapting to repel the effects of anti-infectives, and, therefore, much work remains to deal with these emergent strains.

ANTI-INFECTIVE AGENTS

Although anti-infective agents target foreign organisms infecting the body of a human host, they do not possess **selective toxicity**, which is the ability to affect certain proteins or enzyme systems used by the infecting organism but not by human cells. Because all living cells are somewhat similar, however, no anti-infective drug has yet been developed that does not affect the host.

This chapter focuses on the principles involved in the use of anti-infective therapy, and presents some anti-infectives as examples of these principles. The following chapters discuss specific agents used to treat particular infections: antibiotics for bacterial infections; antivirals; antifungals; antiprotozoals for infections caused by specific protozoa, including malaria; and anthelmintics for infections caused by worms. The final chapter in this section discusses antineoplastics – drugs used for treating diseases caused by abnormal cells such as cancers. Antineoplastics specifically affect human cells to cause cell death or prevent cell growth and reproduction. The effects of anti-infectives on various age groups are discussed in Box 8.1.

Therapeutic actions

Anti-infective agents may act on the cells of invading organisms in several different ways. The goal is interference with the normal function of the invading organism to prevent it from reproducing and to cause cell death without affecting host cells. Various mechanisms of action are briefly described here and shown in Figure 8.1. The specific mechanism of action for each drug class is discussed in the chapters that follow.

- Some anti-infectives interfere with biosynthesis of the bacterial cell wall. Because bacterial cells have a slightly different composition than human cells, this is an effective way to destroy the bacteria without

---

BOX 8.1 FOCUS ON Drug therapy across the lifespan

This box presents general principles of use of anti-infectives across the lifespan. Specifics for each type of anti-infective agent are discussed in their respective chapters within this unit.

Anti-infective agents

CHILDREN
Use anti-infectives with caution; early exposure can lead to early sensitivity.

Controversy is widespread regarding the use of antibiotics to treat ear infections, a common paediatric problem. Some believe that the habitual use of antibiotics for what might well be a viral infection has contributed greatly to the development of resistant strains.

Because children can have increased susceptibility to the gastrointestinal and nervous system effects of anti-infectives, monitor hydration and nutritional status carefully.

ADULTS
Adults often demand anti-infectives for a 'quick cure' of various signs and symptoms. Drug allergies and the emergence of resistant strains can be a big problem with this group.

PREGNANCY AND BREASTFEEDING
Women who are pregnant or breastfeeding must exercise extreme caution in the use of anti-infectives. Many anti-infectives can affect the fetus and also cross into breast milk, leading to toxic effects in the neonate.

OLDER ADULTS
Older people often do not present with the same signs and symptoms of infection that are seen in younger people.

Culture and sensitivity tests are important to determine the type and extent of many infections.

The older person is susceptible to severe adverse gastrointestinal, renal and neurological effects and must be monitored for nutritional status and hydration during drug therapy.

Anti-infectives that adversely affect the liver and kidneys must be used with caution in older people, who may have decreased organ function.

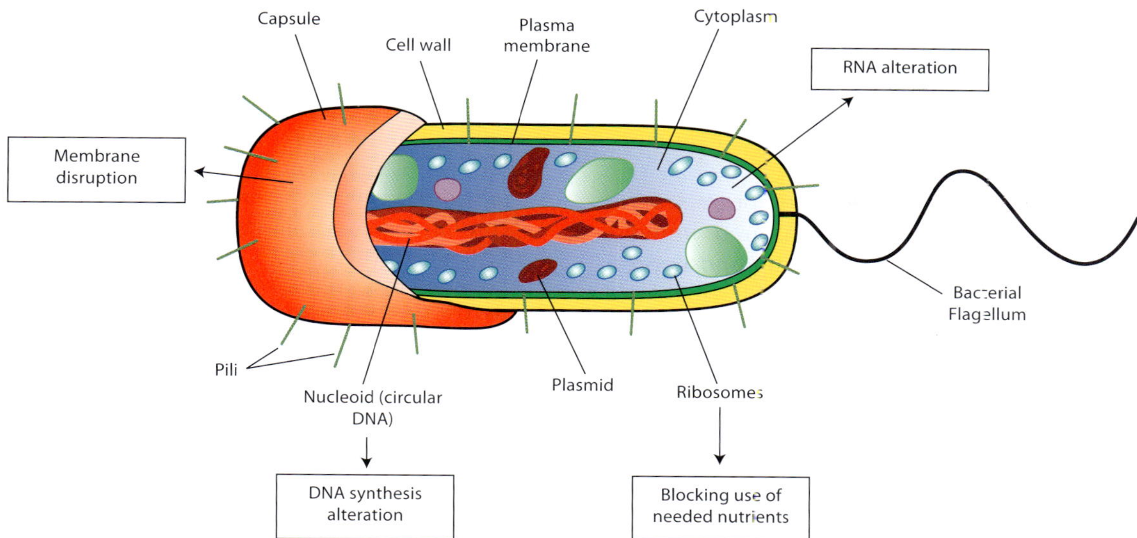

FIGURE 8.1 Anti-infectives can affect cells by disrupting the cell membrane interfering with DNA synthesis, altering RNA or blocking the use of essential nutrients.

interfering with the host (see Box 8.2). The penicillins work in this way.

- Some anti-infectives prevent the cells of the invading organism from using substances essential to their growth and development, leading to an inability to divide and eventually to cell death. The sulfonamides, the antimycobacterial drugs and trimethoprim with sulfamethoxazole (a combination drug frequently used to treat urinary tract infections) work in this way.
- Many anti-infectives interfere with the steps involved in protein synthesis, a function necessary to maintain the cell and allow for cell division. The aminoglycosides, the macrolides and chloramphenicol (see the section on adverse effects for information on chloramphenicol) work in this way.
- Some anti-infectives interfere with DNA synthesis in the cell, leading to inability to divide and cell death. The fluoroquinolones work in this way.
- Other anti-infectives alter the permeability of the cell membrane to allow essential cellular components to leak out, causing cell death. Some antibiotics, antifungals and antiprotozoal drugs work in this manner.

Anti-infective activity

The anti-infectives used today vary in their **spectrum** of activity; that is, they vary in their effectiveness against invading organisms. Some anti-infectives are so selective in their action that they are effective against only a few microorganisms with a very specific metabolic pathway or enzyme. These drugs are said to have a narrow spectrum of activity. Other drugs interfere with biochemical reactions in many different kinds of microorganisms, making them useful in the treatment of a wide variety of infections. Such drugs are said to have a broad spectrum of activity.

Some anti-infectives are so active against the infective microorganisms that they actually cause the death of the cells they affect. These drugs are said to be **bactericidal**. Some anti-infectives are not as aggressive against invading organisms; they interfere with the ability of the cells to reproduce or divide. These drugs are said to be **bacteriostatic**. Several drugs are both bactericidal and bacteriostatic, often depending on the concentration of the drug that is present. Many of the adverse effects noted with the use of anti-infectives are associated with the aggressive properties of the drugs and their effect on the cells of the host in addition to those of the pathogen.

Human immune response

The goal of anti-infective therapy is reduction of the population of the invading organism to a point at which the human immune response can take care of the infection. If a drug were aggressive enough to eliminate all traces of any invading pathogen, it also might be toxic to the host. The immune response (see Chapter 15) involves a complex interaction among

BOX 8.2 Anti-infective mechanism: interference with cell wall synthesis

Teicoplanin *(Targocid)* is an antibiotic that interferes with the cell wall synthesis of susceptible staphylococcal bacteria. Adverse effects include phlebitis, bronchospasm, pruritus and fever. Because of the development of resistant strains and more potent antibiotics, teicoplanin is only indicated for serious infections that cannot be treated by other less toxic drugs, such as osteomyelitis, bacteraemia and septicaemia. It is given by intravenous or intramuscular administration.

chemical mediators, leucocytes, lymphocytes, antibodies and locally released enzymes and chemicals. When this response is completely functional and all the necessary proteins, cells and chemicals are being produced by the body, it can isolate and eliminate foreign proteins, including bacteria, fungi and viruses.

However, if a person is immunocompromised for any reason (eg, malnutrition, age, acquired immune deficiency syndrome [AIDS], use of immunosuppressant drugs), the immune system may be incapable of dealing effectively with the invading organisms. It is difficult to treat any infections in such people for two reasons: (1) anti-infective drugs cannot totally eliminate the pathogen without causing severe toxicity in the host; and (2) these people do not have the immune response in place to deal with even a few invading organisms. Immunocompromised people present a significant challenge to health care providers. In helping these people cope with infections, prevention of infection and proper nutrition are often as important as drug therapy.

Resistance

Resistance can be natural or acquired, and refers to the ability over time to adapt to an antibiotic and produce cells that are no longer affected by a particular drug. Because anti-infectives act on specific enzyme systems or biological processes, many microorganisms that do not use that system or process are not affected by a particular anti-infective drug and are said to have a natural or intrinsic resistance. When prescribing a drug for treatment of an infection, this innate resistance should be anticipated. The selected drug should be one that is known to affect the specific microorganism causing the infection.

Since the advent of anti-infective drugs, microorganisms that were once very sensitive to the effects of particular drugs have begun to develop acquired resistance to the agents (see Box 8.3). This can result in a serious clinical problem. The emergence of resistant strains of bacteria and other organisms poses a threat. Anti-infective drugs may no longer control potentially life-threatening diseases and uncontrollable epidemics may occur.

Acquiring resistance

Microorganisms develop resistance in a number of ways, including the following:

- Producing an enzyme that deactivates the antimicrobial drug. For example, some strains of bacteria that were once controlled by penicillin now produce an enzyme called penicillinase, which inactivates penicillin before it can affect the bacteria. This occurrence led to the development of new drugs that are resistant to penicillinase.
- Changing cellular permeability to prevent the drug from entering the cell or altering transport systems to exclude the drug from active transport into the cell.
- Altering binding sites on the membranes or ribosomes, which then no longer accept the drug.
- Producing a chemical that acts as an antagonist to the drug.

Most commonly, the development of resistance depends on the degree to which the drug acts to eliminate the invading microorganisms that are most sensitive to its effects. The cells that remain may be somewhat resistant to the effects of the drug, and, with time, these cells form the majority in the population. These cells differ from the general population of the species because of slight variations in their biochemical processes or biochemicals. The drug does not cause a mutation of these cells; it simply allows the somewhat different cells to become the majority or dominant group after elimination of the sensitive cells. Other microbes may develop resistance through actual genetic mutation. A mutant cell survives the effects of an antibiotic and divides, forming a new colony of resistant microbes with a genetic composition that provides resistance to the anti-infective agent.

BOX 8.3 Bacterial resistance to an anti-infective drug

Vancomycin *(Vancocin)* is an antibiotic that interferes with cell wall synthesis in susceptible bacteria. It was developed as a result of a need for a drug that could be used both in people who are intolerant of, or allergic to, penicillin and/or cephalosporins and in the treatment of people with staphylococcal infections that no longer respond to penicillin or cephalosporins. This anti-infective drug can be used orally or intravenously to treat life-threatening infections when less toxic drugs cannot be used. It is used orally as prophylaxis against bacterial endocarditis in people who cannot take penicillins or cephalosporins and to treat staphylococcal infections in people who cannot take these groups of drugs.

Because vancomycin may be highly toxic, its use is reserved for very special situations. It can cause renal failure, ototoxicity, superinfections and a condition known as 'red man syndrome', which is characterised by sudden and severe hypotension, fever, chills, paraesthesias and erythema or redness of the neck and back. When it is the only antibiotic that is effective against a specific bacterium, however, the benefits outweigh the risks.

Usual dosage

Adult: oral administration: 500 mg PO q 6 hours for 7–10 days; intravenous administration: 500 mg IV q 6 hours; dose adjustment is required in people with impaired renal function. Monitor serum vancomycin levels.
Paediatric: 40 mg/kg/day PO or IV in four divided doses; do not exceed 2 g/day.

Preventing resistance

Because the emergence of resistant strains of microbes is a serious public health problem that continues to grow, health care providers must work together to prevent the emergence of resistant pathogens. Exposure to an antimicrobial agent leads to the development of resistance, so it is important to limit the use of antimicrobial agents to the treatment of specific pathogens known to be sensitive to the drug being used.

Drug dosing is important in preventing the development of resistance. Doses should be high enough and the duration of drug therapy should be long enough to eradicate even slightly resistant microorganisms. The recommended dosage for a specific anti-infective agent takes this issue into account. Around-the-clock dosing eliminates the peaks and valleys in drug concentration and helps to maintain a constant therapeutic level to prevent the emergence of resistant microbes during times of low concentration. The duration of drug use is critical to ensure that the microbes are completely, not partially, eliminated and are not given the chance to grow and develop resistant strains. It has proved to be difficult to convince people who are taking anti-infective drugs that the timing of doses and the length of time they continue to take the drug are important. Many people stop taking a drug once they start to feel better and then keep the remaining pills to treat themselves at some time in the future when they do not feel well. This practice favours the emergence of resistant strains. Box 8.4 gives tips on teaching about this.

Health care providers should also be cautious about the indiscriminate use of anti-infectives. Antibiotics are not effective in the treatment of viral infections or illnesses such as the common cold. However, many people seek prescriptions for these drugs when they visit practitioners because they are convinced that they need to take something to feel better. Health care providers who prescribe anti-infectives without knowing the causative organism and which drugs might be appropriate are promoting the emergence of resistant strains of microbes. With many serious illnesses, including pneumonias for which the causative organism is suspected, antibiotic therapy may be started as soon as a sample of the bacteria, or **culture**, is taken and before the results are known. Health care providers also tend to try newly introduced, more powerful drugs when a more established drug may be just as effective. Use of a powerful drug in this way leads to the rapid emergence of resistant strains to that drug, perhaps limiting its potential usefulness when it might be truly necessary.

BOX 8.4 FOCUS ON **Individual and family teaching**

Using anti-infective agents

When teaching people who are prescribed an anti-infective agent, it is important to always include some general points:

- This drug is prescribed for treating the particular infection that you have now. Do not use this drug to treat other infections.
- This drug needs to be taken as prescribed – for the correct number of times each day and for the full number of days. Do not stop taking the drug if you start feeling better. You need to take the drug for the full number of treatment days to ensure that the infection has been destroyed.

KEY POINTS

- The goal of anti-infective therapy is the reduction of the invading organisms to a point at which the human immune response can take care of the infection.
- Anti-infectives can act to destroy an infective pathogen (bactericidal) or to prevent the pathogen from reproducing (bacteriostatic).
- Anti-infectives can have a small group of pathogens against which they are effective (narrow spectrum), or they can be effective against many pathogens (broad spectrum).

Using anti-infective agents

Anti-infective agents are used to treat systemic infections and sometimes as a means of prophylaxis (to prevent infections before they occur).

Treatment of systemic infections

Many infections that once led to lengthy, organ-damaging or even fatal illnesses are now managed quickly and efficiently with the use of systemic anti-infective agents. Before the introduction of penicillin to treat streptococcal infections, many people developed rheumatic fever with serious cardiac complications. Today, rheumatic fever and the resultant cardiac valve defects are seldom seen. Several factors should be considered before beginning one of these chemotherapeutic regimens to ensure that the person obtains the greatest benefit possible with the fewest adverse effects. These factors include identification of the correct pathogen and selection of a drug that is most likely to (1) cause the least complications for that person and (2) be most effective against the pathogen involved.

Identification of the pathogen

Identification of the infecting pathogen is done by culturing a tissue sample from the infected area. Bacterial cultures are performed in a laboratory, in which a swab of infected tissue is allowed to grow on an agar plate. Staining techniques and microscopic examination are used to identify the offending bacterium. When investigators search for parasitic sources of infection, they may examine stool for ova and parasites. Microscopic examination of other samples is also used to detect fungal and protozoal infections. The correct identification of the organism causing the infection is an important first step in determining which anti-infective drug should be used.

Sensitivity of the pathogen

In many situations, health care providers use a broad-spectrum anti-infective agent that has been shown likely to be most effective in treating an infection with certain presenting signs and symptoms. In other cases of severe infection, a broad-spectrum antibiotic is started after a culture is taken but before the exact causative organism has been identified. Again, experience influences selection of the drug, based on the presenting signs and symptoms. In many cases, it is necessary to perform **sensitivity testing** on the cultured microbes to evaluate bacteria and determine which drugs are capable of controlling the particular microorganism. This testing is especially important with microorganisms that have known resistant strains. In these cases, culture and sensitivity testing identify the causal pathogen and the most appropriate drug for treating the infection.

Combination therapy

In some situations, a combination of two or more types of drugs effectively treats the infection. When the offending pathogen is known, combination drugs may be effective in interfering with its cellular structure in different areas or developmental phases.

Combination therapy may be used for several reasons:

- The health care provider may be encouraged to use a smaller dose of each drug, leading to fewer adverse effects but still having a therapeutic impact on the pathogen.
- Some drugs are synergistic, which means that they are more powerful when given in combination.
- Many microbial infections are caused by more than one organism, and each pathogen may react to a different anti-infective agent.
- Sometimes, the combined effects of the different drugs delay the emergence of resistant strains. This is important in the treatment of tuberculosis (a mycobacterial infection), malaria (a protozoal infection), HIV infection (a viral infection) and some bacterial infections. Resistant strains may be more likely to emerge when fixed combinations are used over time; however, this may be prevented by individualising the combination.

Prophylaxis

Sometimes it is clinically useful to use anti-infectives as a means of **prophylaxis** to prevent infections before they occur. For example, when people anticipate travelling to an area where malaria is endemic, they may begin taking antimalarial drugs before the journey and periodically during the trip. People who are undergoing gastrointestinal (GI) or genitourinary surgery, which might introduce bacteria from those areas into the system, often have antibiotics ordered immediately after the surgery and periodically thereafter, as appropriate, to prevent infection. People with known cardiac valve disease, valve replacements and other conditions are especially prone to the development of subacute bacterial endocarditis because of the vulnerability of their heart valves. These people use prophylactic antibiotic therapy as a precaution when undergoing invasive procedures, including dental work. Refer to Rheumatic Heart Disease Australia, National Heart Foundation of Australia and the Cardiac Society of Australia and New Zealand recommended schedule for this prophylaxis.

KEY POINTS

- Resistance of a pathogen to an anti-infective agent can be natural (the pathogen does not use the process on which the anti-infective works) or acquired (the pathogen develops a process to oppose the anti-infective agent).
- The emergence of resistant strains is a serious public health problem. Health care providers need to be alert to prevent the emergence of resistant strains by not using antibiotics inappropriately, assuring that the anti-infective is taken at a high enough dose for a long enough period of time, and avoiding the use of newer, powerful anti-infectives if other drugs would be just as effective.

Adverse reactions to anti-infective therapy

Because anti-infective agents affect cells, it is always possible that the host cells will also be damaged (see Box 8.5). No anti-infective agent has been developed that is completely free of adverse effects. The most commonly encountered adverse effects associated with the use of anti-infective agents are direct toxic effects on the kidney, GI tract and nervous system. Hypersensitivity reactions and superinfections can also occur.

Kidney damage

Kidney damage occurs most frequently with drugs that are metabolised by the kidney and then eliminated in the urine. Such drugs, which have a direct toxic effect on the fragile cells in the kidney, can cause conditions ranging from renal dysfunction to full-blown renal failure. When people are taking these drugs (eg, aminoglycosides), they should be monitored closely for any sign of renal dysfunction. To prevent any accumulation of the drug in the kidney, people should be well hydrated throughout the course of the drug therapy.

BOX 8.5 Serious adverse effects of antibiotic treatment

Chloramphenicol *(Chloromycetin)*, an older antibiotic, prevents bacterial cell division in susceptible bacteria. Because of the potential toxic effects of this drug, its use is limited to serious infections for which no other antibiotic is effective. Chloramphenicol produces a 'grey syndrome' in neonates and premature babies, which is characterised by abdominal distension, pallid cyanosis, vasomotor collapse, irregular respiration and even death. In addition, the drug may cause bone marrow depression, including aplastic anaemia that can result in death. These effects are seen even with the use of the ophthalmic and otic forms of the drug. Although the use of chloramphenicol is severely limited, it has stayed on the market because it is used to treat serious infections caused by bacteria that are not sensitive to any other antibiotic. It is available in oral, IV, ophthalmic and otic forms.

Gastrointestinal toxicity

GI toxicity is very common with many of the anti-infectives. Many of these agents have direct toxic effects on the cells lining the GI tract, causing nausea, vomiting, stomach upset or diarrhoea, and such effects are sometimes severe (see Box 8.6). There is also some evidence that the death of the microorganisms releases chemicals and toxins into the body, which can stimulate the chemoreceptor trigger zone (CTZ) in the medulla and induce nausea and vomiting.

In addition, some anti-infectives are toxic to the liver. These drugs can cause hepatitis and even liver failure. When people are taking drugs known to be toxic to the liver (eg, many of the cephalosporins) they should be monitored closely and the drug should be stopped at any sign of liver dysfunction.

BOX 8.6 Severe gastrointestinal toxicity resulting from anti-infective treatment

Meropenem *(Merrem IV)*, an IV antibiotic, inhibits the synthesis of bacterial cell walls in susceptible bacteria. It is used to treat intra-abdominal infections and some cases of meningitis caused by susceptible bacteria. Meropenem almost always causes very uncomfortable gastrointestinal effects; in fact, use of this drug has been associated with potentially fatal pseudomembranous colitis. It also results in headache, dizziness, rash and superinfections. Because of its toxic effect on gastrointestinal cells, it is used only in those infections with proven sensitivity to meropenem and reduced sensitivity to less toxic antibiotics.

Neurotoxicity

Some anti-infectives can damage or interfere with the function of nerve tissue, usually in areas where drugs tend to accumulate in high concentrations. For example, the aminoglycoside antibiotics collect in the eighth cranial nerve and can cause dizziness, vertigo and loss of hearing. Hydroxychloroquine, which is used to treat malaria and some other rheumatoid disorders, can accumulate in the retina and optic nerve and cause blindness. Other anti-infectives can cause dizziness, drowsiness, lethargy, changes in reflexes and even hallucinations when they irritate specific nerve tissues.

Hypersensitivity reactions

Allergic or hypersensitivity reactions reportedly occur with many antimicrobial agents. Most of these agents, which are protein bound for transfer through the cardiovascular system, are able to induce antibody formation in susceptible people. With the next exposure to the drug, immediate or delayed allergic responses may occur. In severe cases, anaphylaxis can occur, which can be life-threatening. Some of these drugs have demonstrated cross-sensitivity (eg, penicillins, cephalosporins), and care must be taken to obtain a complete health history before administering one of these drugs. It is important to determine what the allergic reaction was and when the person experienced it (eg, after first use of the drug, or after years of use). Some people report having a drug allergy, but closer investigation indicates that their reaction actually constituted an anticipated effect or a known adverse effect of the drug. Proper interpretation of this information is important to allow treatment of a person with a drug to which the person reported a supposed allergic reaction but which would be very effective against a known pathogen.

Superinfections

One offshoot of the use of anti-infectives, especially broad-spectrum anti-infectives, is destruction of the normal flora. **Superinfections** are infections that occur when opportunistic pathogens that were kept in check by the 'normal' bacteria have the opportunity to invade tissues. Common superinfections include vaginal or GI yeast infections, which are associated with antibiotic therapy, and infections caused by *Proteus* and *Pseudomonas* throughout the body, which are a result of broad-spectrum antibiotic use. If people receive drugs that are known to induce superinfections, they should be monitored closely for any signs of a new infection – sore patches in the mouth, vaginal itching, diarrhoea – and the appropriate treatment for any superinfection should be started as soon as possible.

CHAPTER SUMMARY

- Anti-infectives are drugs designed to act on foreign organisms that have invaded and infected the human host with selective toxicity, which means that they affect biological systems or structures found in the invading organisms but not in the host.
- Anti-infectives include antibiotics, antivirals, antifungals, antiprotozoals and anthelmintic agents.
- The goal of anti-infective therapy is interference with the normal function of invading organisms to prevent them from reproducing and promotion of cell death without negative effects on the host cells. The infection should be eradicated with the least toxicity to the host and the least likelihood for development of resistance.
- Anti-infectives can work by altering the cell membrane of the pathogen, by interfering with protein synthesis or by interfering with the ability of the pathogen to obtain needed nutrients.
- Anti-infectives also work to kill invading organisms or to prevent them from reproducing, thus depleting the size of the invasion to one that can be dealt with by the human immune system.
- Pathogens can develop resistance to the effects of anti-infectives over time when (1) mutant organisms that do not respond to the anti-infective become the majority of the pathogen population or (2) the pathogen develops enzymes to block the anti-infectives or alternative routes to obtain nutrients or maintain the cell membrane.
- An important aspect of clinical care involving anti-infective agents is preventing or delaying the development of resistance. This can be done by ensuring that the particular anti-infective agent is the drug of choice for the specific pathogen involved and that it is given in high enough doses for sufficiently long periods to rid the body of the pathogen.
- Culture and sensitivity testing of a suspected infection ensures that the correct drug is being used to treat the infection effectively. Culture and sensitivity testing should be performed before an anti-infective agent is prescribed.
- Anti-infectives can have several adverse effects on the human host, including renal toxicity, multiple GI effects, neurotoxicity, hypersensitivity reactions and superinfections.
- Some anti-infectives are used as a means of prophylaxis when people expect to be in situations that will expose them to a known pathogen, such as travel to an area where malaria is endemic, or oral or invasive GI surgery in a person who is susceptible to subacute bacterial endocarditis.

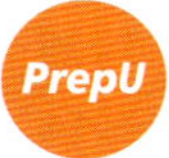

Knowing your strengths and weaknesses helps you to study more effectively. Take a PrepU Practice Quiz to find out how you measure up!

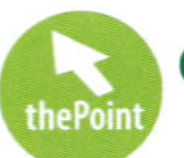

ONLINE RESOURCES

An extensive range of additional resources to enhance teaching and learning and to facilitate understanding of this chapter may be found online at the text's accompanying website, located on thePoint at http://thepoint.lww.com. These include Watch and Learn videos, Concepts in Action animations, journal articles, review questions, case studies, discussion topics and quizzes.

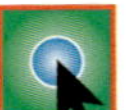

WEB LINKS

Health care providers and students may want to consult the following web resources:

www.health.gov.au/internet/main/publishing.nsf/content/cda-cdi3303e.htm
Australian Government Department of Health. Tuberculosis in Australia.

https://www.nps.org.au/professionals/reducing-antibiotic-resistance
NPS MedicineWise. Reducing antibiotic resistance.

www.who.int/mediacentre/factsheets/fs194/en
World Health Organization. Antimicrobial Resistance.

BIBLIOGRAPHY

Bassler, B. & Winans, S. C. (2008). *Chemical Communication Among Bacteria*. Hoboken, New Jersey: John Wiley & Sons.

Farrell, M. & Dempsey, J. (2014). *Smeltzer & Bare's Textbook of Medical-Surgical Nursing* (3rd edn). Sydney: Lippincott, Williams & Wilkins.

Gillespie, E., Rodrigues, A., Wright, L., Williams, N. & Stuart, R. L. (2013). Improving antibiotic stewardship by involving nurses. *American Journal of Infection Control, 41(4)*, 365–367.

McKenna, L. & Mirkov, S. (2019). *McKenna's Drug Handbook for Nursing and Midwifery* (8th edn). Sydney: Wolters Kluwer Health Australia.

McKenzie, D., Rawlins, M. & Del Mar, C. (2013). Antimicrobial stewardship: What's it all about? *Australian Prescriber, 36(4)*, 116–120.

Porth, C. M. (2011). *Essentials of Pathophysiology: Concepts of Altered Health States* (3rd edn). Philadelphia: Lippincott Williams & Wilkins.

Porth, C. M. (2009). *Pathophysiology: Concepts of Altered Health States* (8th edn). Philadelphia: Lippincott Williams & Wilkins.

RHD Australia, National Heart Foundation of Australia and the Cardiac Society of Australia and New Zealand. (2012). *Australian Guideline for Prevention, Diagnosis and Management of Acute Rheumatic Fever and Rheumatic Heart Disease* (2nd edn). www.rhdaustralia.org.au/resources/australian-guideline-prevention-diagnosis-and-management-acute-rheumatic-fever-and

Turnidge, J. (2010). Multiresistant organisms at the front line. *Australian Prescriber, 33(3)*, 68–71.

World Health Organization. (2013). *Antimicrobial resistance. Fact Sheet No. 194*. www.who.int/mediacentre/factsheets/fs194/en.

CHECK YOUR UNDERSTANDING

Answers to the questions in this chapter can be found in Appendix A at the back of this book.

MULTIPLE CHOICE

Select the best answer to the following.

1. The spectrum of activity of an anti-infective indicates:
   a. the acidity of the environment in which they are most effective.
   b. the cell membrane type that the anti-infective affects.
   c. the anti-infective's effectiveness against different invading organisms.
   d. the resistance factor that bacteria have developed to this anti-infective.
2. The emergence of resistant strains of microbes is a serious public health problem. Health care providers can work to prevent the emergence of resistant strains by:
   a. encouraging the person to stop the antibiotic as soon as the symptoms are resolved to prevent overexposure to the drug.
   b. encouraging the use of antibiotics when people feel they will help.
   c. limiting the use of antimicrobial agents to the treatment of specific pathogens known to be sensitive to the drug being used.
   d. using the most recent powerful drug available to treat an infection to ensure eradication of the microbe.
3. Sensitivity testing of a culture shows:
   a. drugs that are capable of controlling that particular microorganism.
   b. the person's potential for allergic reactions to a drug.
   c. the offending microorganism.
   d. an immune reaction to the infecting organism.
4. Combination therapy is often used in treating infections. An important consideration for using combination therapy would be that:
   a. it is cheaper to use two drugs in one tablet than one drug alone.
   b. most infections are caused by multiple organisms.
   c. the combination of drugs can delay the emergence of resistant strains.
   d. combining anti-infectives will prevent adverse effects from occurring.
5. Superinfections can occur when anti-infective agents destroy the normal flora of the body. *Candida* infections are commonly associated with antibiotic use. A person with this type of superinfection would exhibit:
   a. difficulty breathing.
   b. vaginal discharge or white patches in the mouth.
   c. elevated blood urea nitrogen.
   d. dark lesions on the skin.
6. An example of an anti-infective used as a means of prophylaxis would be:
   a. amoxicillin used for tonsillitis.
   b. penicillin used to treat an abscess.
   c. an antibiotic used before dental surgery.
   d. norfloxacin used for a bladder infection.
7. A broad-spectrum antibiotic would be the drug of choice when:
   a. the person has many known allergies.
   b. one is waiting for culture and sensitivity results.
   c. the infection is caused by one specific bacterium.
   d. treatment is being given for an upper respiratory infection of unknown cause.

MULTIPLE RESPONSE

Select all that apply.

1. Bacterial resistance to an anti-infective could be the result of which of the following?
   a. natural or intrinsic properties of the bacteria
   b. changes in cellular permeability or cellular transport systems
   c. the production of chemicals that antagonise the drug
   d. initial exposure to the anti-infective
   e. combination of too many antibiotics for one infection
   f. narrow spectrum of activity
2. Anti-infective drugs destroy cells that have invaded the body. However, they do not specifically destroy only the cell of the invader, and because of this, many adverse effects can be anticipated when an anti-infective is used. Which of the following adverse effects are often associated with anti-infective use?
   a. superinfections
   b. hypotension
   c. renal toxicity
   d. diarrhoea
   e. loss of hearing
   f. constipation

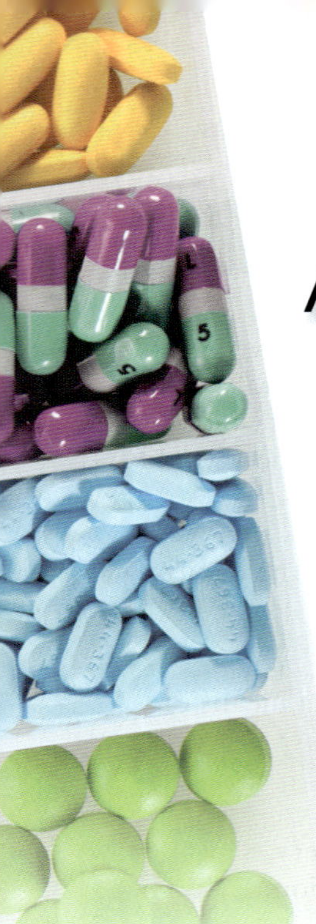

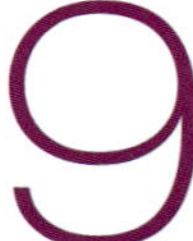

Antibiotics

Learning objectives

On completing this chapter you should be able to:

1. Explain how an antibiotic is selected for use in a particular clinical situation.
2. Describe therapeutic actions, pharmacokinetics, indications, contraindications, most common adverse reactions and important drug–drug interactions associated with each of the classes of antibiotics.
3. Discuss the use of antibiotics as they are used across the lifespan.
4. Compare and contrast key drugs for each class of antibiotics with other drugs in that class.
5. Outline care considerations for people receiving each class of antibiotic.

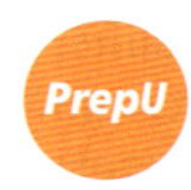

Test your current knowledge of antibiotics with a PrepU Practice Quiz!

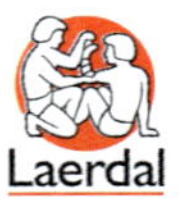

Simulation-based learning

On completion of the chapter, explore the scenario of Kenneth Bronson (Part 1) who has been diagnosed with a strep throat. Continue onto the second scenario (Part 2) as his condition deteriorates into an emergency situation. Consider the medication management of Kenneth's condition throughout his episode of care. What learning from the chapter, can be applied to the case?

Glossary of key terms

aerobic: bacteria that depend on oxygen for survival
anaerobic: bacteria that survive without oxygen, which are often seen when blood flow is cut off to an area of the body
antibiotic: chemical that is able to inhibit the growth of specific bacteria or cause the death of susceptible bacteria
Gram positive: bacteria that stain positive (purple) with Gram stain and are frequently associated with infections of the respiratory tract and soft tissues
Gram negative: bacteria that stain negative (red) with Gram stain and are frequently associated with infections of the genitourinary or gastrointestinal tract
synergistic: drugs that work together to increase drug effectiveness

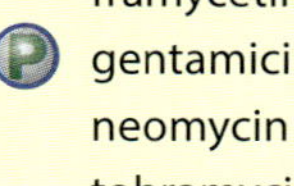

AMINOGLYCOSIDES
- amikacin
- framycetin
- Ⓟ gentamicin
- neomycin
- tobramycin

CARBAPENEMS
- Ⓟ ertapenem
- imipenem with cilastatin
- meropenem

CEFALOSPORINS

First-generation
- cefalotin
- cefalexin
- cefazolin

Second-generation
- Ⓟ cefaclor
- cefoxitin
- cefuroxime

Third-generation
- cefotaxime
- ceftazidime
- ceftriaxone

Fourth-generation
- cefepime

Fifth-generation
- ceftaroline

FLUOROQUINOLONES
- Ⓟ ciprofloxacin
- moxifloxacin

FLUOROQUINOLONES *continued*
norfloxacin
ofloxacin

PENICILLINS AND PENICILLINASE-RESISTANT ANTIBIOTICS
Penicillins
benzathine penicillin
benzylpenicillin
dicloxacillin
flucloxacillin
phenoxymethylpenicillin benzathine
phenoxymethylpenicillin potassium
procaine penicillin

Broad-spectrum penicillins
(P) amoxicillin
ampicillin
piperacillin
ticarcillin

SULFONAMIDES
sulfadiazine
sulfamethoxazole
sulfasalazine

TETRACYCLINES
(P) doxycycline
minocycline
tetracycline
tigecycline

ANTIMYCOBACTERIALS
Antituberculosis drugs
ethambutol
(P) isoniazid
rifampicin

Leprostatic drugs
clofazimine
dapsone

OTHER ANTIBIOTICS
Lincosamides
(P) clindamycin
lincomycin

Macrolides
azithromycin
clarithromycin
(P) erythromycin
roxithromycin

Monobactams
(P) aztreonam

NEW CLASSES OF ANTIBIOTICS AND ADJUNCTS
New classes of antibiotics
daptomycin
linezolid

Adjuncts to antibiotic therapy
clavulanic acid
thalidomide

Many new strains of bacteria appear each year, and researchers are challenged to develop new **antibiotics** – chemicals that inhibit specific bacteria – to deal with each new threat. Antibiotics are made in three ways: by living microorganisms, by synthetic manufacture, and, in some cases, through genetic engineering. Antibiotics may either be bacteriostatic (preventing the growth of bacteria) or bactericidal (killing bacteria directly), although several antibiotics are both bactericidal and bacteriostatic, depending on the concentration of the particular drug. This chapter discusses the major classes of antibiotics: aminoglycosides, carbapenems, cefalosporins, fluoroquinolones, penicillins and penicillinase-resistant drugs, sulfonamides, tetracyclines and the disease-specific antimycobacterials, including the antitubercular and leprostatic drugs. Antibiotics that do not fit into the large antibiotic classes include lincosamides, macrolides and monobactams. Figures 9.1 and 9.2 show sites of cellular action of these classes of antibiotics.

Safe medication administration

Many antibiotics used to treat childhood infections, such as otitis media and other upper respiratory tract infections (URTIs), come in an oral suspension, suitable for children. The order for these solutions is usually written in millilitres (mL) for the convenience of the parent who will be dispensing the medication. It is very important to make sure that the parent understands that the teaspoon in the prescription refers to a measuring teaspoon (5 mL). Inadvertent overdoses have been reported when parents used a kitchen teaspoon to measure out the child's dose. Kitchen teaspoons vary greatly in volume. If a parent calls to report that the medicine is all gone on day 4 and it was supposed to be given for 7 days, check to see how the medicine is being measured. Teaching the parent when the drug is first ordered can prevent problems during the course of treatment.

BACTERIA AND ANTIBIOTICS

Bacteria can invade the human body through many routes: for example, respiratory, gastrointestinal (GI) and skin. Once the bacteria invade the body, the human immune response is activated, and signs and symptoms of an infection occur as the body tries to rid itself of the foreign cells. Fever, lethargy, slow-wave sleep induction and the classic signs of inflammation (eg, redness, swelling, heat and pain) all indicate that the body is responding to an invader. The body becomes the host for the bacteria and supplies proteins and enzymes the bacteria need for reproduction. Unchallenged, the invading bacteria can multiply and send out other bacteria to further invade tissue.

The goal of antibiotic therapy is to decrease the population of invading bacteria to a point at which the human immune system can effectively deal with the invader. To determine which antibiotic will effectively interfere with the specific proteins or enzyme systems for treatment of a specific infection, the causative organism must be identified through a bacterial culture. Sensitivity testing is also done to determine the antibiotic to which that particular organism is most sensitive (eg, which antibiotic best kills or controls the bacteria).

Gram-positive bacteria are those whose cell walls retain a stain known as Gram's stain or resist decolourisation with alcohol during culture and sensitivity testing. Gram-positive bacteria are commonly associated with infections of the respiratory tract and soft tissues. An example of a Gram-positive bacterium is

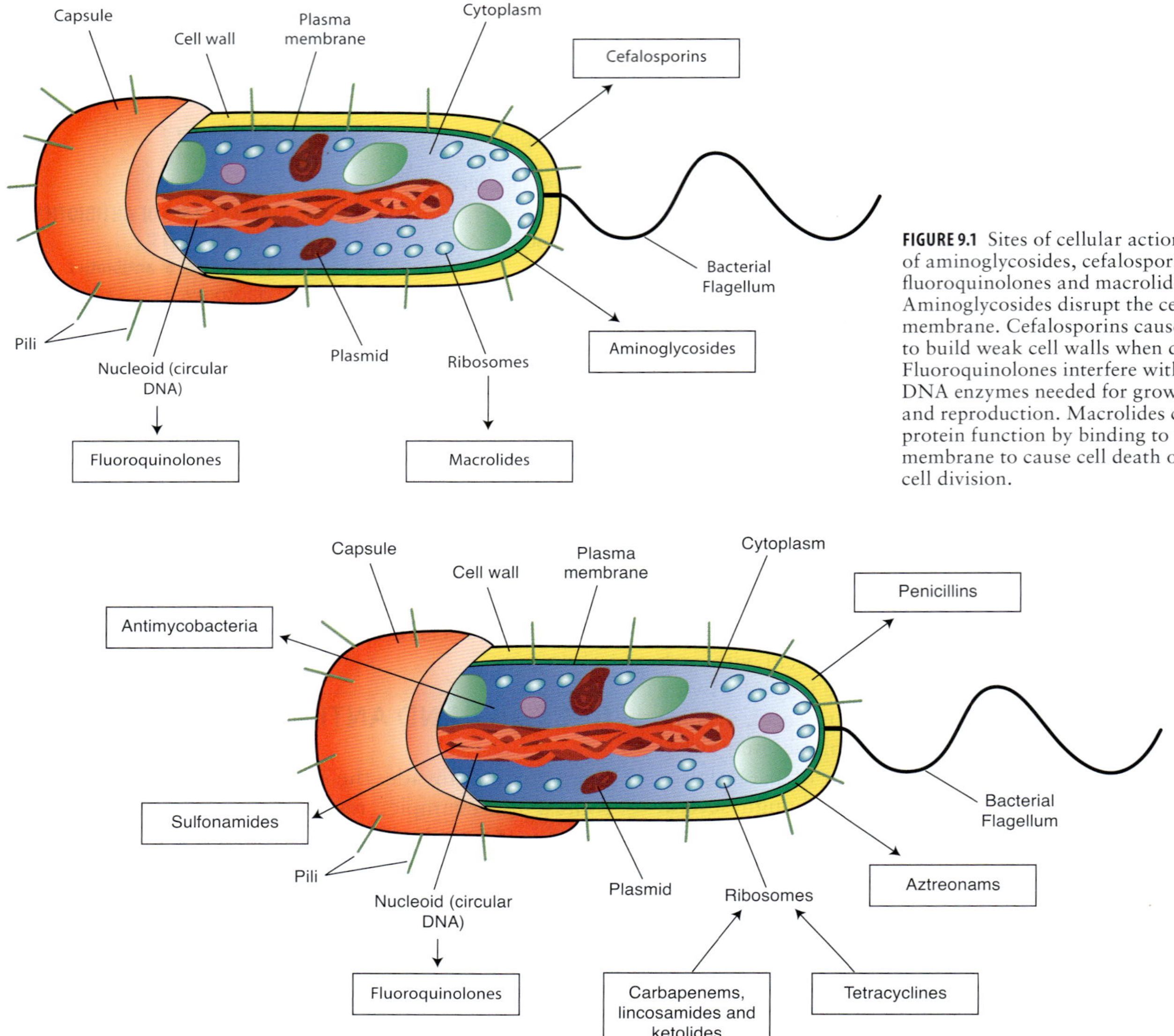

FIGURE 9.1 Sites of cellular action of aminoglycosides, cefalosporins, fluoroquinolones and macrolides. Aminoglycosides disrupt the cell membrane. Cefalosporins cause bacteria to build weak cell walls when dividing. Fluoroquinolones interfere with the DNA enzymes needed for growth and reproduction. Macrolides change protein function by binding to the cell membrane to cause cell death or prevent cell division.

FIGURE 9.2 Sites of cellular action of carbapenems, lincosamides, aztreonams, penicillins, sulfonamides, tetracyclines and antimycobacterials. Carbapenems and lincosamides change protein function and prevent cell division or cause cell death. Aztreonam alters cell membranes to allow leakage of intracellular substances and causes cell death. Penicillins prevent bacteria from building their cells during division. Sulfonamides inhibit folic acid synthesis for bacterial RNA and DNA production. Tetracyclines inhibit protein synthesis, thereby preventing reproduction. Antimycobacterial drugs affect mycobacteria in three ways: they (1) affect the mycotic coat of the bacteria, (2) alter DNA and RNA and (3) prevent cell division.

Streptococcus pneumoniae, a common cause of pneumonia. In contrast, the cell walls of **Gram-negative** bacteria lose a Gram stain or are decolourised by alcohol. These bacteria are frequently associated with infections of the genitourinary (GU) or GI tract. An example of a Gram-negative bacterium is *Escherichia coli*, a common cause of cystitis. **Aerobic** bacteria depend on oxygen for survival, whereas **anaerobic** bacteria (eg, those bacteria associated with gangrene) do not use oxygen.

If culture and sensitivity testing is not possible, either because the source of the infection is not identifiable or because the person is too sick to wait for test results to determine the best treatment, clinicians attempt to administer a drug with a broad spectrum of activity against Gram-positive or Gram-negative bacteria or against anaerobic bacteria. Antibiotics that interfere with a biochemical reaction common to many organisms are known as broad-spectrum antibiotics. These drugs are often given at the beginning of treatment until the exact organism and sensitivity can be established. Because these antibiotics have such a wide range of effects, they are frequently associated with adverse effects. Human cells have many of the same properties as bacterial cells and can be affected in much the same way, so damage may occur to the human cells, as well as to the bacterial cells.

Because there is no perfect antibiotic that is without effect on the human host, clinicians try to select an antibiotic with selective toxicity, or the ability to strike foreign cells with little or no effect on human cells. Certain antibiotics may be contraindicated in some people because of known adverse effects; this includes those people who are immunocompromised, who have severe GI disease or who are debilitated. (See Box 9.1 for effects of antibiotics across the lifespan.) The antibiotic of choice is one that affects the causative organism and leads to the fewest adverse effects for the person involved.

In some cases, antibiotics are given in combination because they are **synergistic**; meaning their combined effect is greater than their effect if they are given individually (Box 9.2). Use of synergistic antibiotics also

BOX 9.2 Using combination drugs to fight resistant bacteria

Clavulanic acid protects certain beta-lactam antibiotics from breakdown in the presence of penicillinase enzymes.

A combination of amoxicillin and clavulanic acid *(Augmentin)* is commonly used to allow the amoxicillin to remain effective against certain strains of resistant bacteria (usual dosage, 250–500 mg PO q 8 hours for adults or 20–40 mg/kg/day PO in divided doses for children). The theory behind the combination of ticarcillin and clavulanic acid *(Timentin)* is similar (usual dosage 3.1 g IM q 4–6 hours for adults; safety not established for children).

BOX 9.1 FOCUS ON Drug therapy across the lifespan

Antibiotics

CHILDREN

Children are very sensitive to the gastrointestinal and central nervous system (CNS) effects of most antibiotics, and more severe reactions can be expected when these drugs are used in children. It is important to monitor the hydration and nutritional status of children who are adversely affected by drug-induced diarrhoea, anorexia, nausea and vomiting. Superinfections can be a problem for small children as well. For example, thrush (oral candidiasis) is a common superinfection that makes eating and drinking difficult.

Many antibiotics do not have proven safety and efficacy in paediatric use, and extreme caution should be used when giving them to children. The fluoroquinolones, for example, are associated with damage to developing cartilage and are not recommended for growing children.

Paediatric dosages of antibiotics should be independently checked to make sure that the child is receiving the correct dose, thereby improving the chance of eradicating the infection and decreasing the risk of adverse effects.

Antibiotic treatment of ear infections, a common paediatric problem, is controversial. Ongoing research suggests that judicious use of decongestants and anti-inflammatories may be just as successful as the use of antibiotics without the risk of development of resistant bacterial strains.

Parents, not wanting to see their child sick, may demand antibiotics as a cure-all whenever their child is fussy or feverish. Parent education is very important in helping to cut down the unnecessary use of antibiotics in children.

ADULTS

Many adults believe that antibiotics are a cure-all for any discomfort and fever. It is very important to explain that antibiotics are useful against only specific bacteria and actually can cause problems when used unnecessarily for viral infections, such as the common cold.

Adults need to be cautioned to take the entire course of the medication as prescribed and not to store unused pills for future infections or share antibiotics with symptomatic friends.

PREGNANCY AND BREASTFEEDING

Women who are pregnant or breastfeeding should not take antibiotics unless the benefit clearly outweighs the potential risk to the fetus or neonate. Tetracyclines, for example, are associated with pitting of enamel in developing teeth and with calcium deposits in growing bones. These drugs can cause serious problems for neonates. Women of childbearing age should be advised to use barrier contraceptives if any of these drugs are used.

Many antibiotics interfere with the effectiveness of oral contraceptives and unplanned pregnancies can occur.

OLDER ADULTS

In many instances, older adults do not present with the same signs and symptoms of infections as other people. Therefore, assessing the problem and obtaining appropriate specimens for culture is especially important with this population.

Older people may be more susceptible to the adverse effects associated with antibiotic therapy. Their hydration and nutritional status should be monitored closely, as should the need for safety precautions if CNS effects occur. If hepatic or renal dysfunction is expected (particularly in very old people, in those who may have alcohol dependence, and in those who are taking other hepatotoxic or nephrotoxic drugs), the dose may need to be lowered and the person should be monitored more frequently.

Elderly people also need to be cautioned to complete the full course of drug therapy, even when they feel better, and not to save pills for self-medication at a future time.

allows the person to take a lower dose of each antibiotic to achieve the desired effect, which helps to reduce the adverse effects that a particular drug may have.

In some situations, antibiotics are used as a means of prophylaxis, or prevention of potential infection. People who will soon be in a situation that commonly results in a specific infection (eg, people undergoing GI surgical procedures, which may introduce GI bacteria into the bloodstream or peritoneum) may be given antibiotics before they are exposed to the bacteria. Usually a large, one-time dose of an antibiotic is given to destroy any bacteria that enters the host immediately and thereby prevent a serious infection.

BACTERIA AND RESISTANCE TO ANTIBIOTICS

Bacteria have survived for millions of years because they can adapt to their environment. They do this by altering their cell wall or enzyme systems to become resistant to (i.e. protect themselves from) unfavourable conditions or situations. Many species of bacteria have developed resistance to certain antibiotics. For example, bacteria that were once very sensitive to penicillin have developed an enzyme called penicillinase, which effectively inactivates many of the penicillin-type drugs. New drugs have had to be developed to effectively treat infections involving these once-controlled bacteria. It is very important to use these drugs only when the identity and sensitivity of the offending bacterium have been established. Indiscriminate use of these new drugs can lead to the development of more resistant strains for which there is no effective antibiotic (see later discussion of new antibiotics for additional information on linezolid).

The longer an antibiotic has been in use, the greater is the chance that the bacteria will develop into a resistant strain. Efforts to control the emergence of resistant strains involve intensive educational programs that advocate the use of antibiotics only when necessary and effective and not for the treatment of viral infections such as the common cold (Box 9.3).

In addition, the use of antibiotics may result in the development of superinfections or overgrowth of resistant pathogens, such as bacteria, fungi or yeasts, because antibiotics (particularly broad-spectrum agents) destroy bacteria in the flora that normally work to keep these opportunistic invaders in check. When 'normal' bacteria are destroyed or greatly reduced in number, there is nothing to prevent the invaders from occupying the host. In most cases the superinfection is an irritating adverse effect (eg, vaginal yeast infection, candidiasis, diarrhoea), but in some cases, the superinfection can be more severe than the infection that was originally being treated. Treatment of the superinfection leads to new adverse effects and the potential for different superinfections. A vicious cycle of treatment and resistance is the result.

BOX 9.3 FOCUS ON **The evidence**

Using antibiotics properly

In 2003, the U.S. Food and Drug Administration (FDA) and Centers for Disease Control and Prevention (CDC) joined efforts to educate the public and health care providers about the dangers of inappropriate use of antibiotics. The evidence-based practice guidelines combine data from many studies to outline the most efficacious use of antibiotics. To review some of the studies, review the references listed in the Bibliography. Nurses and midwives should include some of the following points about the risks and dangers of antibiotic abuse in each person's education plan:

- Explain clearly that a particular antibiotic is effective against only certain bacteria and that a culture needs to be taken to identify the bacteria.
- Explain that bacteria can develop resistant strains that will not be affected by antibiotics in the future, so use of antibiotics now may make them less effective in situations in which they are really necessary.
- Ensure that people understand the importance of taking the full course of medication as prescribed, even if they feel better. Stopping an antibiotic midway through a regimen often leads to the development of resistant bacteria. Using all the medication will also prevent people saving unused medication to self-treat future infections or to share with other family members.
- Tell people that allergies may develop with repeated exposures to certain antibiotics. In addition, explain to people that saving antibiotics to take later, when they think they need them again, may lead to earlier development of an allergy, which will negate important tests that could identify the bacteria making them sick.
- Offer other medications, such as antihistamines, decongestants, or even chicken soup, to people who request antibiotics; this may satisfy their need for something to take. Explaining that viral infections do not respond to antibiotics usually offers little consolation to people who are suffering from a cold or the flu.

The publicity that many emergent, resistant strains of bacteria have received in recent years may help to get the message across to people about the need to take the full course of an antibiotic and to use antibiotics only when they are appropriate.

KEY POINTS

- The goal of antibiotic therapy is to reduce the population of invading bacteria to a size that the human immune response can deal with.
- Bacteria can be classified as Gram-positive (frequently found in respiratory infections) or Gram-negative (frequently found in GI and GU infections). They can also be classified as anaerobic (not needing oxygen) or aerobic (dependent on oxygen).
- Culture and sensitivity testing ensures that the correct antibiotic is chosen for each infection, a practice that may help to decrease the number of emerging resistant-strain bacteria.

AMINOGLYCOSIDES

The aminoglycosides (Table 9.1) are a group of powerful antibiotics used to treat serious infections caused by Gram-negative aerobic bacilli. Because most of these drugs have potentially serious adverse effects, newer, less toxic drugs have replaced aminoglycosides in the treatment of less serious infections. Aminoglycosides include amikacin (*Amikin*), gentamicin, neomycin and tobramycin (*Tobra-Day*).

Therapeutic actions and indications

The aminoglycosides are bactericidal. They inhibit protein synthesis in susceptible strains of Gram-negative bacteria. They irreversibly bind to a unit of the bacteria ribosomes, leading to misreading of the genetic code and cell death (Figure 9.1). These drugs are used to treat serious infections caused by susceptible strains of Gram-negative bacteria, including *Pseudomonas aeruginosa*, *E. coli*, *Proteus* species, the *Klebsiella–Enterobacter–Serratia* group, *Citrobacter* species, and *Staphylococcus* species such as *S. aureus*. Aminoglycosides are indicated for the treatment of serious infections that are susceptible to penicillin when penicillin is contraindicated, and they can be used in severe infections before culture and sensitivity tests have been completed. See Table 9.1 for usual indications for each of these drugs.

Pharmacokinetics

The aminoglycosides are poorly absorbed from the GI tract but rapidly absorbed after intramuscular (IM) injection, reaching peak levels within 1 hour. These drugs have an average half-life of 2–3 hours. They are widely distributed throughout the body, cross the placenta and enter breast milk, and are excreted unchanged in the urine (see contraindications and cautions).

Amikacin is available for short-term IM or intravenous (IV) use.

Gentamicin is available in many forms: ophthalmic, topical, IV, intrathecal, impregnated beads on surgical wire and liposomal injection.

Neomycin is available in topical and oral forms.

Tobramycin is used for short-term IM or IV treatment, ophthalmic use and by inhalation.

Contraindications and cautions

Aminoglycosides are contraindicated in:

- known allergy to any of the aminoglycosides
- renal or hepatic disease *that could be exacerbated by toxic aminoglycoside effects and that could interfere with drug metabolism and excretion, leading to higher toxicity*

TABLE 9.1 DRUGS IN FOCUS Aminoglycosides

Drug name	Dosage/route	Usual indications
amikacin (generic)	15 mg/kg/day IM or IV divided into 2–3 equal doses; reduce dose in renal failure	Treatment of serious Gram-negative infections
framycetin *(Soframycin)*	Ear: 2–3 drops into the ear tds or qid Eye: 2 drops q 1–2 hours initially, then bd or tds	Treatment of ear and eye infections
(P) gentamicin (generic)	Adult: 3 mg/kg/day IM or IV in three equal doses q 8 hours; reduce dose in renal failure Paediatric: 2–2.5 mg/kg/day q 8 hours IV or IM	Treatment of *Pseudomonas* infections and a wide variety of Gram-negative infections
neomycin *(Kenacomb, Neosulf)*	Adult: 4–12 g/day in divided doses PO for 5–6 days Paediatric: 50–100 mg/kg/day in divided doses PO for hepatic coma	Suppression of GI normal flora preoperatively; treatment of hepatic coma; topical treatment of skin wounds
tobramycin *(Tobi, Tobrex)*	Adult: 3 mg/kg/day in three equal doses IM or IV q 8 hours; reduce dose in renal failure Paediatric: 300 mg bd by nebuliser	Short-term IV or IM treatment of serious infections; ocular infections caused by susceptible bacteria

- pre-existing hearing loss, *which could be intensified by toxic drug effects on the auditory nerve*
- active infection with herpes or mycobacterial infections *that could be worsened by the effects of an aminoglycoside on normal defence mechanisms*
- myasthenia gravis or parkinsonism, *which are often exacerbated by the effects of a particular aminoglycoside on the nervous system*
- breastfeeding, *because aminoglycosides are excreted in breast milk and potentially could cause serious effects in the infant.*

Caution is necessary when these agents are administered during pregnancy *because aminoglycosides are used to treat only severe infections, and the benefits of the drug must be carefully weighed against potential adverse effects on the fetus.* It is necessary to test urine function frequently when these drugs are used *because they depend on the kidney for excretion and are toxic to the kidney.*

The potential for nephrotoxicity and ototoxicity with amikacin is very high, so the drug is used only as long as absolutely necessary.

Adverse effects

The many serious adverse effects associated with aminoglycosides limit their usefulness. The drugs come with a black box warning, alerting health care professionals to the serious risk of ototoxicity and nephrotoxicity. Central nervous system (CNS) effects include:

- ototoxicity, possibly leading to irreversible deafness
- vestibular paralysis resulting from drug effects on the auditory nerve
- confusion
- depression
- disorientation
- numbness, tingling and weakness related to drug effects on other nerves.

Renal toxicity, which may progress to renal failure, is caused by direct drug toxicity in the glomerulus, meaning that the drug molecules cause damage (eg, obstruction) directly to the kidney. Bone marrow depression may result from direct drug effects on the rapidly dividing cells in the bone marrow, leading, for example, to immune suppression and resultant superinfections.

GI effects include nausea, vomiting, diarrhoea, weight loss, stomatitis and hepatic toxicity. These effects are a result of direct GI irritation, loss of bacteria of the normal flora with resultant superinfections, and toxic effects in the mucous membranes and liver as the drug is metabolised.

Cardiac effects can include palpitations, hypotension and hypertension. Hypersensitivity reactions include purpura, rash, urticaria and exfoliative dermatitis.

Clinically important drug–drug interactions

Most aminoglycosides have a synergistic bactericidal effect when given with penicillins, cefalosporins or ticarcillin. In certain conditions, this synergism is used therapeutically to increase the effectiveness of treatment. Avoid combining aminoglycosides with potent diuretics; this increases the incidence of ototoxicity, nephrotoxicity and neurotoxicity. If these antibiotics are given with anaesthetics, non-depolarising neuromuscular blockers, succinylcholine or citrate-anticoagulated blood, increased neuromuscular blockade with paralysis is possible. If a person who has been receiving an aminoglycoside requires surgery, indicate prominently on the person's chart the fact that the aminoglycoside has been given. Provide extended monitoring and support after surgery.

Prototype summary: gentamicin

Indications: treatment of serious infections caused by susceptible bacteria.

Actions: inhibits protein synthesis in susceptible strains of Gram-negative bacteria, disrupting functional integrity of the cell membrane and causing cell death.

Pharmacokinetics:

Route	Onset	Peak
IM, IV	Rapid	30–90 minutes

$T_{1/2}$: 2–3 hours; metabolised in the liver and excreted in the urine.

Adverse effects: sinusitis, dizziness, rash, fever, risk of nephrotoxicity.

Care considerations for people receiving aminoglycosides

Assessment: history and examination

- Assess for *possible contraindications or cautions:*
  - known allergy to any aminoglycoside (obtain specific information about the nature and occurrence of allergic reactions)
  - history of renal or hepatic disease
  - pre-existing hearing loss
  - active infection with herpes, vaccinia, varicella or fungal or mycobacterial organisms
  - myasthenia gravis
  - parkinsonism
  - infant botulism
  - current pregnancy or breastfeeding status.
- Perform a physical assessment *to establish baseline data for assessing the effectiveness of the drug and*

the occurrence of any adverse effects associated with drug therapy.

- Perform culture and sensitivity tests at the site of infection.
- Conduct orientation and reflex assessment, as well as auditory testing, *to evaluate any CNS effects of the drug.*
- Assess vital signs: respiratory rate and adventitious sounds *to monitor for signs of infection or hypersensitivity reactions*; temperature *to assess for signs and symptoms of infection*; blood pressure *to monitor for cardiovascular effects of the drug.*
- Perform renal and liver function tests *to determine baseline function of these organs and, possibly, the need to adjust dose.*

Implementation with rationale

- Check culture and sensitivity reports *to ensure that this is the drug of choice for this person.*
- Ensure that the person receives a full course of aminoglycoside as prescribed, divided around the clock, *to increase effectiveness and decrease the risk for development of resistant strains of bacteria.*
- Monitor the infection site and presenting signs and symptoms (eg, fever, lethargy) throughout the course of drug therapy. *Failure of these signs and symptoms to resolve may indicate the need to reculture the site.* Arrange to continue drug therapy for at least 2 days after all signs and symptoms resolve *to decrease the development of resistant strains of bacteria.*
- Monitor regularly for signs of nephrotoxicity, neurotoxicity and bone marrow suppression *to effectively arrange for discontinuation of drug or decreased dose, as appropriate, if any of these toxicities occurs.* Provide safety measures *to protect the person if CNS effects, such as confusion, disorientation or numbness and tingling, occur.*
- Provide small, frequent meals as tolerated; frequent mouth care; and ice chips or sugarless lollies to suck if stomatitis and sore mouth are problems *to relieve discomfort.*
- Provide *adequate fluids to replace fluid lost through diarrhoea.*
- Ensure that the person is hydrated at all times during drug therapy *to minimise renal toxicity from drug exposure.*
- Instruct the person about the appropriate dosage regimen and possible adverse effects *to enhance knowledge about drug therapy and to promote compliance.*
- Provide the following teaching:
  - Take safety precautions, such as changing position slowly and avoiding driving and hazardous tasks, if CNS effects occur.
  - Try to drink a lot of fluids and to maintain nutrition (very important) even though nausea, vomiting and diarrhoea may occur.
  - Avoid exposure to sources of other infections (eg, crowded areas, people with known infectious diseases).
  - Report difficulty breathing, severe headache, loss of hearing or ringing in the ears, or changes in urine output.

Evaluation

- Monitor response to the drug (resolution of bacterial infection).
- Monitor for adverse effects (orientation and affect, hearing changes, bone marrow suppression, renal toxicity, hepatic dysfunction, GI effects).
- Evaluate effectiveness of the teaching plan (person can name drug, dosage, possible adverse effects to watch for and specific measures to help avoid adverse effects).
- Monitor effectiveness of comfort and safety measures and compliance with the therapeutic regimen.

KEY POINTS

- Aminoglycosides inhibit protein synthesis in susceptible strains of Gram-negative bacteria.
- These drugs are reserved for use in serious infections because of potentially serious adverse effects. Monitor for ototoxicity, renal toxicity, GI disturbances, bone marrow depression and superinfections.

CARBAPENEMS

The carbapenems (Table 9.2) are a relatively new class of broad-spectrum antibiotics effective against Gram-positive and Gram-negative bacteria. Meropenem, the first drug of the class, was discussed in Chapter 8 and has limited use because of the severe risk for potentially fatal GI toxicities. Newer carbapenems are not as toxic. Carbapenems discussed here include ertapenem (*Invanz*) and imipenem with cilastatin (*Primaxin*).

Therapeutic actions and indications

The carbapenems are bactericidal. They inhibit cell membrane synthesis in susceptible bacteria, leading to cell death (Figure 9.2). These drugs are used to treat

TABLE 9.2 **DRUGS IN FOCUS** Carbapenems

Drug name	Dosage/route	Usual indications
(P) ertapenem *(Invanz)*	1 g/day IV or IM for 5–14 days	Treatment of community acquired pneumonia, complicated GU infections, acute pelvic infections, complicated intra-abdominal infections, skin and skin structure infections
imipenem-cilastatin *(Primaxin)*	250–500 mg IV q 6–8 hours or 500–750 mg IM q 12 hours Paediatric: < 40 kg and > 3 months: 15 mg/kg/day IV q 6 hours	Treatment of serious respiratory, intra-abdominal, urinary tract, gynaecological, bone and joint, skin and skin structure infections; septicaemia, endocarditis, bone and joint infections, and polymicrobic infections
meropenem *(Merrem I.V.)*	500 mg–1 g IV, q 8 hours	Treatment of respiratory tract infection, complicated urinary tract infection, febrile neutropenia, intra-abdominal and gynaecological infections, complicated skin infections, meningitis, septicaemia when there is resistance to commonly used antibiotics

serious infections caused by susceptible strains of *Streptococcus pneumoniae*, *Haemophilus influenzae*, *Moraxella catarrhalis*, *Staphylococcus aureus*, *Streptococcus pyogenes*, *Escherichia coli*, *Peptostreptococcus*, *Klebsiella pneumoniae*, *Clostridium clostridioforme*, *Eubacterium lentum*, *Bacteroides fragilis*, *Bacteroides distasonis*, *Bacteroides ovatus*, *Bacteroides thetaiotamicron*, *Bacteroides uniformis*, *Proteus mirabilis*, *Pseudomonas aeruginosa*, *Acinetobacter baumannii*, *Streptococcus agalactiae*, *Porphyromonas asaccharolytica*, *Prevotella bivia* and other susceptible bacteria. They are indicated for treating serious intra-abdominal, urinary tract, skin and skin structure, bone and joint and gynaecological infections. See Table 9.2 for usual indications for each of these drugs.

Pharmacokinetics

These drugs are rapidly absorbed if given IM and reach peak levels at the end of the infusion if given IV. They are widely distributed throughout the body, although it is not known whether they cross the placenta or enter breast milk (see contraindications and cautions). Carbapenems are excreted unchanged in the urine and have an average half-life of 1–4 hours.

Ertapenem can be given IV or IM. It is given once a day for 5–14 days, depending on the infection.

Imipenem–cilastatin is a combination of imipenem, which interferes with cell wall synthesis and causes bacterial cell death, and cilastin, which inactivates the imipenem and leads to increased urinary excretion of the drug and decreased renal toxicity. It can be given IM or IV and is approved for use in children.

Meropenem is given IV every 8 hours by either bolus over 5 minutes or IV infusion over 15–30 minutes.

Contraindications and cautions

Carbapenems are contraindicated in:

- known allergy to any of the carbapenems or beta-lactams
- seizure disorders, *which could be exacerbated by the drug*
- meningitis, *because safety in people with meningitis has not been established*
- breastfeeding, *because it is not known whether these drugs enter breast milk, and potentially they could cause serious effects in the infant.*

Use caution during pregnancy *because carbapenems are used to treat only severe infections, and the benefits of the drug must be carefully weighed against potential adverse effects on the fetus.* Test renal function regularly when these drugs are used *because they depend on the kidney for excretion and are toxic to the kidney.*

Adverse effects

Toxic effects on the GI tract can limit the use of carbapenems in some people. Pseudomembranous colitis, *Clostridium difficile* diarrhoea and nausea and vomiting can lead to serious dehydration and electrolyte imbalances, as well as to new serious infections.

Superinfections can occur with any of the carbapenems. Closely monitor to deal with the new infection before it becomes overwhelming.

CNS effects can include headache, dizziness and altered mental state. Seizures have been reported when carbapenems are combined with other drugs. Monitor people to provide safety measures if any of these occur.

Prototype summary: ertapenem

Indications: treatment of community-acquired pneumonia, complicated GU infections, complicated intra-abdominal infections, skin and skin structure infections, and acute pelvic infections caused by susceptible bacteria.

Actions: inhibits protein synthesis in susceptible strains of Gram-negative bacteria, disrupting functional integrity of the cell membrane and causing cell death.

Pharmacokinetics:

Route	Onset	Peak
IM, IV	Rapid	30–120 minutes

$T_{1/2}$: 4 hours; excreted unchanged in the urine.

Adverse effects: headache, dizziness, nausea, vomiting, pseudomembranous colitis, rash, pain at injection site.

Clinically important drug–drug interactions

Consider an alternative antibiotic treatment if a person is on sodium valproate. Combination of these drugs can cause serum valproic acid levels to fall and increase the risk of seizures. Avoid concurrent use of imipenem with ganciclovir because this combination may also cause seizures.

Care considerations for people receiving carbapenems

Assessment: history and examination

- Assess for *possible contraindications or cautions*: known allergy to any carbapenem or beta-lactam (obtain specific information about the nature and occurrence of allergic reactions); history of renal disease; history of seizures and current pregnancy or breastfeeding status.
- Perform physical assessment *to establish baseline data for assessing the effectiveness of the drug and the occurrence of any adverse effects associated with drug therapy.*
- Perform culture and sensitivity tests at the site of infection.
- Conduct orientation and reflex assessment *to evaluate any CNS effects of the drug.*
- Assess vital signs: respiratory rate and adventitious sounds *to monitor for signs of infection or hypersensitivity reactions*; temperature *to assess for signs and symptoms of infection.*
- Perform renal function tests *to determine baseline function of the kidneys and, possibly, the need to adjust dose.*

Implementation with rationale

- Check culture and sensitivity reports *to ensure that this is the drug of choice for this person.*
- Ensure that the person receives the full course of the carbapenem as prescribed *to increase effectiveness and decrease the risk for the development of resistant strains of bacteria.*
- Monitor the site of infection and presenting signs and symptoms (eg, fever, lethargy) throughout the course of drug therapy. *Failure of these signs and symptoms to resolve may indicate the need to reculture the site.* Arrange to continue drug therapy for at least 2 days after all signs and symptoms resolve *to decrease the development of resistant strains of bacteria.*
- Monitor the person regularly for signs of pseudomembranous colitis, severe diarrhoea or superinfections *to effectively arrange for discontinuation of drug or decreased dose, as appropriate, if any of these toxicities occurs.*
- Provide safety measures *to protect the person if CNS effects, such as confusion, dizziness or seizures, occur.*
- Provide small, frequent meals as tolerated *to relieve GI discomfort. Also provide adequate fluids to replace fluid lost through diarrhoea, if appropriate.*
- Ensure that the person is hydrated at all times during drug therapy *to minimise renal toxicity from drug exposure.*
- Instruct the person about the appropriate dosage regimen and possible adverse effects *to enhance knowledge about drug therapy and to promote compliance.*
- Provide the following teaching:
  - Take safety precautions, such as changing position slowly and avoiding driving and hazardous tasks, if CNS effects occur.
  - Try to drink a lot of fluids and to maintain nutrition (very important) even though nausea, vomiting and diarrhoea may occur.
  - Report difficulty breathing, severe headache, severe diarrhoea, fever and signs of infection.

Evaluation

- Monitor person's response to the drug (resolution of bacterial infection).
- Monitor for adverse effects (orientation and affect, superinfections, GI toxicity, severe diarrhoea effects).

- Evaluate effectiveness of the teaching plan (person can name drug, dosage, possible adverse effects to watch for and specific measures to help avoid adverse effects).
- Monitor effectiveness of comfort and safety measures and compliance with the therapeutic regimen.

KEY POINTS

- Carbapenems are used to treat serious infections caused by a wide range of bacteria.
- Monitor for GI effects, serious diarrhoea, dizziness and superinfections.

CEFALOSPORINS

The cefalosporins (Table 9.3) were first introduced in the 1960s. These drugs are similar to the penicillins in structure and in activity. Over time, four generations of cefalosporins have been introduced, each group with its own spectrum of activity.

First-generation cefalosporins are largely effective against the same Gram-positive bacteria that are affected by penicillin G, as well as the Gram-negative bacteria *Proteus mirabilis*, *E. coli* and *Klebsiella pneumoniae* (use the letters *PEcK* as a mnemonic device to remember which bacteria are susceptible to the first-generation cefalosporins). First-generation drugs include cefazolin (*Kefzol*) and cefalexin (*Cilex*, *Keflex*, *Rancef*).

Second-generation cefalosporins are effective against the previously mentioned strains, as well as *Haemophilus influenzae*, *Enterobacter aerogenes* and *Neisseria* species (remember *HENPeCK*). Second-generation drugs are less effective against Gram-positive bacteria. These include cefaclor (*Ceclor*), cefoxitin and cefuroxime (*Zinnat*).

Third-generation cefalosporins, which are effective against all the previously mentioned strains, are relatively weak against Gram-positive bacteria but are more potent against the Gram-negative bacilli, as well as against *Serratia marcescens* (remember *HENPeCKS*). Third-generation drugs include cefotaxime, ceftazidime (*Fortum*) and ceftriaxone (*Rocephin*).

Fourth-generation cefalosporins are in development. The first drug of this group, cefepime (*Maxipime*), is active against Gram-negative and Gram-positive organisms, including cefalosporin-resistant staphylococci and *P. aeruginosa*.

Fifth-generation cefalosporins are also in development and appear to be less susceptible to resistance. The first drug of this group, ceftaroline (*Zinforo*) is active against Gram-positive and Gram-negative organisms, including Methicillin-resistant *Staphlococcus aureus* (MRSA) and penicillin resistant *Streptococcus pneumoniae*.

Therapeutic actions and indications

The cefalosporins are both bactericidal and bacteriostatic, depending on the dose used and the specific drug involved. In susceptible species, these agents basically interfere with the cell wall–building ability of bacteria when they divide; that is, they prevent the bacteria from biosynthesising the framework of their cell walls. The bacteria with weakened cell walls swell and burst as a result of the osmotic pressure within the cell (see Figure 9.1).

Cefalosporins are indicated for the treatment of infections caused by susceptible bacteria. See Table 9.3 for usual indications for each of these agents. Selection of an antibiotic from this class depends on the sensitivity of the involved organism, the route of choice and sometimes the cost involved. It is important to reserve cefalosporins for appropriate situations because cefalosporin-resistant bacteria are appearing in increasing numbers. Before therapy begins, perform a culture and sensitivity test to evaluate the causative organism and appropriate sensitivity to the antibiotic being used.

Pharmacokinetics

The following cefalosporins are well absorbed from the GI tract: the first-generation drug cefalexin; the second-generation drugs cefaclor and cefuroxime; the third-generation drug cefotaxime; and the fourth-generation drug cefepime. The others are absorbed well after IM injection or IV administration. (Box 9.4 provides calculation practice using cefaclor.)

The cefalosporins are primarily metabolised in the liver and excreted in the urine. These drugs cross the placenta and enter breast milk (see contraindications and cautions).

BOX 9.4 FOCUS ON Calculations

You are caring for a 20 kg child with a severe case of tonsillitis. An order is written for cefaclor *(Ceclor)* 20 mg/kg/day q 8 hours for 10 days. The drug comes in an oral suspension 125 mg/5 mL. What amount should you administer at each dose?

The order is for 20 mg/kg, so 20 mg/kg × 20 = 400 mg per day.

$$\frac{\text{stock required}}{\text{stock strength}} \times \frac{\text{volume}}{1}$$

$$\frac{400}{125} \times \frac{5}{1} = \frac{2000}{125} = 16 \text{ mL/day}$$

therefore, each dose = 16/3 = 5.3 mL per dose

TABLE 9.3 DRUGS IN FOCUS Cefalosporins

Drug name	Dosage/route	Usual indications
First-generation cefalosporins		
cefalotin *(Keflin)*	Adult: 500 mg–1 g IM or IV q 4–6 hour	Treatment of respiratory tract, skin, GU, biliary tract, bone and joint infections, as well as sepsis
cefazolin *(Cefazolin)*	Adult: 250–500 mg IM or IV q 4–8 hours; reduce dose in renal impairment Paediatric: 25–50 mg/kg/day IM or IV in 3–4 divided doses	Treatment of respiratory tract, skin, GU, biliary tract, bone, joint and myocardial infections, as well as sepsis
cefalexin *(Keflex, Cilex)*	Adult: 250 mg PO q 6 hours Paediatric: 25–50 mg/kg/day PO in divided doses	Treatment of respiratory, skin, bone, and GU infections; used for otitis media in children
Second-generation cefalosporins		
(P) cefaclor *(Ceclor, Keflor)*	Adult: 250 mg PO q 8 hours – do not exceed 4 g/day; must be taken every 8–12 hours around the clock Paediatric: 20 mg/kg/day PO in divided doses q 8 hours; do not exceed 1 g/day	Treatment of respiratory tract infections, skin infections, UTIs, otitis media, typhoid fever, anthrax exposure
cefoxitin (generic)	Adult: 1–2 g IM or IV q 6–8 hours; reduce dose with renal impairment Paediatric: 30–40 mg IM or IV q 6 hours	Treatment of severe infections; preoperative prophylaxis for caesarean section and abdominal, vaginal, biliary or colorectal surgery; more effective in gynaecological and intra-abdominal infections than some other agents
cefuroxime *(Zinnat)*	Adult: 250–500 mg PO bd Paediatric: 125–250 mg PO bd; 50–100 mg/kg/day IM or IV in divided doses q 6–8 hours	Treatment of a wide range of infections, as listed for other second-generation drugs; Lyme disease; preferred treatment in situations involving an anticipated switch from parenteral to oral drug use
Third-generation cefalosporins		
cefotaxime (generic)	Adult: 2–8 g/day IM or IV in divided doses q 6–8 hours; reduce dose with renal impairment Paediatric: 50–180 mg/kg/day IM or IV in divided doses q 4–6 hours	Treatment of moderate to severe skin, urinary tract and respiratory tract infections; pelvic inflammatory disease; intra-abdominal infections; peritonitis; septicaemia; bone infections; CNS infections; preoperative prophylaxis
ceftazidime *(Fortum)*	Adult: 1 g q 8–12 hours IM or IV; reduce dose with renal impairment Paediatric: 25–100 mg/kg/day IV or IM tds or qid	Treatment of moderate to severe skin, urinary tract and respiratory tract infections; intra-abdominal infections; septicaemia; bone infections; CNS infections
ceftriaxone *(Rocephin)*	Adult: 1–2 g/day IM or IV in divided doses bd–qid Paediatric: 50–75 mg/kg/day IV or IM in divided doses q 12 hours	Treatment of moderate to severe skin, urinary tract and respiratory tract infections; pelvic inflammatory disease; intra-abdominal infections; peritonitis; septicaemia; bone infections; CNS infections; preoperative prophylaxis; off-label use for treatment of Lyme disease
Fourth-generation cefalosporins		
cefepime *(Maxipime)*	Adult: 0.5–2 g IM or IV q 12 hours; must be injected for greatest effectiveness q 12 hours for 7–10 days; reduce dose with renal impairment Paediatric: 50 mg/kg per dose q 12 hours IV or IM for 7–10 days	Treatment of moderate to severe skin, urinary tract and respiratory tract infections
Fifth-generation cefalosporins		
ceftaroline *(Zinforo)*	Adult: 600 mg IV q 12 hours	Treatment of complicated skin and soft tissue infectioins or community-acquired pneumonia

Contraindications and cautions

Avoid the use of cefalosporins in people with known allergies to cefalosporins or penicillins *because cross-sensitivity is common.* Use with caution in people with hepatic or renal impairment *because these drugs are toxic to the kidneys and could interfere with the metabolism and excretion of the drug.* In addition, use with caution in pregnant or breastfeeding women *because potential effects on the fetus and infant are not known; use only if the benefits clearly outweigh the potential risk of toxicity to the fetus or infant.*

Reserve cefalosporins for appropriate situations because cefalosporin-resistant bacteria are appearing in increasing numbers. Before therapy begins, perform a culture and sensitivity test to evaluate the causative organism and appropriate sensitivity to the antibiotic being used.

Adverse effects

The most common adverse effects of the cefalosporins involve the GI tract and include nausea, vomiting, diarrhoea, anorexia, abdominal pain and flatulence. Pseudomembranous colitis – a potentially dangerous disorder – has also been reported with some cefalosporins. A particular drug should be discontinued immediately at any sign of violent, bloody diarrhoea or abdominal pain.

CNS symptoms include headache, dizziness, lethargy and paraesthesias. Nephrotoxicity is also associated with the use of cefalosporins, most particularly in people who have a predisposing renal insufficiency. Other adverse effects include superinfections, which occur frequently because of the death of protective bacteria of the normal flora. Monitor people receiving parenteral cefalosporins for the possibility of phlebitis with IV administration or local abscess at the site of an IM injection.

Clinically important drug–drug interactions

Concurrent administration of cefalosporins with aminoglycosides increases the risk for nephrotoxicity. Frequently monitor people receiving this combination, and evaluate serum blood urea nitrogen (BUN) and creatinine levels.

People who receive oral anticoagulants in addition to cefalosporins may experience increased bleeding. Teach these people how to monitor for blood loss (eg, bleeding gums, easy bruising) and to be aware that the dose of the oral anticoagulant may need to be reduced.

Instruct the person receiving cefalosporins to avoid alcohol for up to 72 hours after discontinuation of the drug to prevent a disulfiram-like reaction, which results in unpleasant symptoms such as flushing, throbbing headache, nausea and vomiting, chest pain, palpitations, dyspnoea, syncope, vertigo, blurred vision and, in extreme reactions, cardiovascular collapse, convulsions or even death.

 **Prototype summary: cefaclor**

Indications: treatment of respiratory, dermatological, urinary tract and middle-ear infections caused by susceptible strains of bacteria.

Actions: inhibits the synthesis of bacterial cell walls, causing cell death in susceptible bacteria.

Pharmacokinetics:

Route	Peak	Duration
Oral	30–60 minutes	8–10 hours

$T_{1/2}$: 30–60 minutes; excreted unchanged in the urine.

Adverse effects: nausea, vomiting, diarrhoea, rash, superinfection, bone marrow depression, risk for pseudomembranous colitis.

Care considerations for people receiving cefalosporins

Assessment: history and examination

- Assess for *possible contraindications or cautions*: known allergy to any cefalosporin, penicillin or any other allergens *because cross-sensitivity often occurs* (obtain specific information about the nature and occurrence of the allergic reactions); history of renal disease, *which could exacerbate nephrotoxicity related to the cefalosporin*; and current pregnancy or breastfeeding status.
- Perform physical assessment *to establish baseline data for assessing the effectiveness of the drug and the occurrence of any adverse effects associated with drug therapy.*
- Examine the skin for any rash or lesions, examine injection sites for abscess formation and note respiratory status – including rate, depth and adventitious sounds – *to provide a baseline for determining adverse reactions.*
- Perform culture and sensitivity tests at the site of infection.
- Check renal function test results, including BUN and creatinine clearance, *to assess the status of renal functioning and to detect the possible need to alter dose.*

Implementation with rationale

- Check culture and sensitivity reports *to ensure that this is the drug of choice for this person.*
- Monitor renal function test values before and periodically during therapy *to arrange for appropriate dose reduction as needed.*
- Ensure that person receives the full course of the cefalosporin as prescribed, divided around the clock *to increase effectiveness and to decrease the risk of development of resistant strains.*
- Monitor the infection site and presenting signs and symptoms (eg, fever, lethargy) throughout the course of drug therapy. *Failure of these signs and symptoms to resolve may indicate the need to reculture the site.* Arrange to continue drug therapy for at least 2 days after the resolution of all signs and symptoms *to help prevent the development of resistant strains of bacteria.*
- Provide small, frequent meals as tolerated, frequent mouth care and ice chips or sugarless lollies to suck if stomatitis and sore mouth are problems *to relieve discomfort and provide nutrition.*
- Provide adequate fluids *to replace fluid lost through diarrhoea.*
- Monitor the person for any signs of superinfection *to arrange for treatment if superinfection occurs.*
- Monitor injection sites regularly *to provide warm compresses and gentle massage to injection sites if they are painful or swollen.* If signs of phlebitis occur, remove the IV line and reinsert in a different vein.
- Initiate safety measures, including adequate lighting, side rails on the bed and assistance with ambulation *to protect the person from injury if CNS effects occur.*
- Instruct the person about the appropriate dosage schedule and about possible side effects *to enhance knowledge about drug therapy and to promote compliance.*
- Provide the following teaching:
  - Take safety precautions, including changing position slowly and avoiding driving and hazardous tasks, if CNS effects occur.
  - Try to drink a lot of fluids and to maintain nutrition (very important) even though nausea, vomiting and diarrhoea may occur.
  - Report difficulty breathing, severe headache, severe diarrhoea, dizziness or weakness.
  - Avoid consuming alcoholic beverages while receiving cefalosporins and for at least 72 hours after completing the drug course because serious side effects could occur.

Evaluation

- Monitor person's response to the drug (resolution of bacterial infection).
- Monitor for adverse effects (orientation and affect; renal toxicity; hepatic dysfunction; GI effects; and local irritation, including phlebitis at injection and IV sites).
- Evaluate effectiveness of the teaching plan (person can name drug, dosage, possible adverse effects to expect and specific measures to help avoid adverse effects).
- Monitor effectiveness of comfort and safety measures and the person's compliance with the regimen.

KEY POINTS

- Cefalosporins are a large group of antibiotics, similar to penicillin, that are effective against a wide range of bacteria.
- Monitor for GI upsets and diarrhoea, pseudomembranous colitis, headache, dizziness and superinfections.

MACROLIDES

The macrolides (Table 9.9) are antibiotics that interfere with protein synthesis in susceptible bacteria. Macrolides include erythromycin *(Erythrocin, Eryc and others)*, azithromycin *(Zithromax)*, clarithromycin *(Clarac, Kalixocin, Klacid)* and roxithromycin *(Rulide)*.

Therapeutic actions and indications

The macrolides, which may be bactericidal or bacteriostatic, exert their effect by binding to the bacterial cell membrane and changing protein function (see Figure 9.1). This action can prevent the cell from dividing or cause cell death, depending on the sensitivity of the bacteria and the concentration of the drug.

Macrolides are indicated for treatment of:

- acute infections caused by susceptible strains of *S. pneumoniae*, *M. pneumoniae*, *Listeria monocytogenes* and *Legionella pneumophila*
- infections caused by group A beta-haemolytic streptococci
- pelvic inflammatory disease caused by *N. gonorrhoeae*
- URTIs caused by *H. influenzae* (with sulfonamides)
- infections caused by *Corynebacterium diphtheriae* and *Corynebacterium minutissimum* (with antitoxin)
- intestinal amoebiasis
- infections caused by *C. trachomatis*.

See Table 9.9 for usual indications for each of these agents.

In addition, macrolides may be used as prophylaxis for endocarditis before dental procedures in people with valvular heart disease who are allergic to penicillin. Topical macrolides are indicated for the treatment of ocular infections caused by susceptible organisms and for acne vulgaris, and they may also be used prophylactically against infection in minor skin abrasions and for the treatment of skin infections caused by sensitive organisms.

Pharmacokinetics

The macrolides are widely distributed throughout the body; they cross the placenta and enter the breast milk (see contraindications and cautions). These drugs are absorbed in the GI tract.

Erythromycin is metabolised in the liver, with excretion mainly in the bile to faeces. The half-life of erythromycin is 1.6 hours.

Azithromycin and clarithromycin are mainly excreted unchanged in the urine, making it necessary to monitor renal function when people are taking these drugs. The half-life of azithromycin is 68 hours, making it useful for people who have trouble remembering to take pills because it can be given once a day. The half-life of clarithromycin is 3–7 hours.

Contraindications and cautions

Macrolides are contraindicated in people with known allergy to any macrolide *because cross-sensitivity occurs*. Ocular preparations are contraindicated for viral, fungal or mycobacterial infections of the eye, *which could be exacerbated by loss of bacteria of the normal flora*. Use with caution in people with hepatic dysfunction, *which could alter the metabolism of the drug*, and in those with renal disease, *which could interfere with the excretion of some of the drug*. Also use with caution in breastfeeding women *because macrolides secreted in breast milk can cause diarrhoea and superinfections in the infant* and in pregnant women *because of potential adverse effects on the developing fetus*; use only if the benefit clearly outweighs the risk to the fetus or the infant.

Adverse effects

Relatively few adverse effects are associated with the macrolides. The most frequent ones, which involve the direct effects of the drug on the GI tract, are often uncomfortable enough to limit the use of the drug. These include abdominal cramping, anorexia, diarrhoea, vomiting and pseudomembranous colitis. Other effects include neurological symptoms such as confusion, abnormal thinking and uncontrollable emotions, which could be related to drug effects on the CNS membranes; hypersensitivity reactions ranging from rash to anaphylaxis; and superinfections related to the loss of normal flora.

Clinically important drug–drug interactions

Increased serum levels of digoxin occur when digoxin is taken concurrently with macrolides. People who receive both drugs should have their digoxin levels monitored and dose adjusted during and after treatment with the macrolide.

In addition, when oral anticoagulants, theophyllines, carbamazepine or corticosteroids are administered concurrently with macrolides, the effects of these drugs reportedly increase as a result of metabolic changes in the liver. People who take any of these combinations may require reduced dose of the particular drug and careful monitoring.

Clinically important drug–food interactions

Food in the stomach decreases absorption of oral macrolides. Therefore, the antibiotic should be taken on an empty stomach with a full 150 mL glass of water 1 hour before or at least 2–3 hours after meals.

LINCOSAMIDES

The lincosamides (Table 9.9) are similar to the macrolides but are more toxic. These drugs include clindamycin *(Cleocin)* and lincomycin *(Lincocin)*.

Therapeutic actions and indications

The lincosamides react at almost the same site as macrolide antibiotics in bacterial protein synthesis and are effective against the same strains of bacteria (Figure 9.2). These drugs are used in the treatment of severe infections when a less toxic antibiotic cannot be used.

Pharmacokinetics

The lincosamides are rapidly absorbed from the GI tract or from IM injections and are metabolised in the liver and excreted in the urine and faeces. These drugs cross the placenta and enter breast milk (see contraindications and cautions).

Clindamycin has a half-life of 2–3 hours. It is available in parenteral and oral forms, as well as in topical and vaginal forms for the treatment of local infections.

Lincomycin has a half-life of 5 hours. It can be given orally, IM or IV.

Contraindications and cautions

Use lincosamides with caution in people with hepatic or renal impairment, which could interfere with the metabolism and excretion of the drug. Use during pregnancy and breastfeeding only if the benefit clearly outweighs the risk to the fetus or neonate.

Adverse effects

Severe GI reactions, including fatal pseudomembranous colitis, have occurred, limiting the usefulness of lincosamides. However, for a serious infection caused by a susceptible bacterium, a lincosamide may be the drug of choice. Some other toxic effects that limit usefulness are pain, skin infections and bone marrow depression.

MONOBACTAM ANTIBIOTIC

The only monobactam antibiotic currently available for use is aztreonam *(Azactam)* (Table 9.9).

Therapeutic actions and indications

Among the antibiotics, aztreonam's structure is unique, and little cross-resistance occurs. It is effective against Gram-negative enterobacteria and has no effect on Gram-positive or anaerobic bacteria. Aztreonam disrupts bacterial cell wall synthesis, which promotes leakage of cellular contents and cell death in susceptible bacteria (see Figure 9.2). The drug is indicated for the treatment of urinary tract, skin, intra-abdominal and gynaecological infections, as well as septicaemia caused by susceptible bacteria, including *E. coli and Enterobacter*, *Serratia*, *Proteus*, *Salmonella*, *Providencia*, *Pseudomonas*, *Citrobacter*, *Haemophilus*, *Neisseria* and *Klebsiella* species.

Pharmacokinetics

Aztreonam is available for IV and IM use only and reaches peak effect levels in 1–1.5 hours. Its half-life is 1.5–2 hours. The drug is excreted unchanged in the urine. It crosses the placenta and enters breast milk (see contraindications and cautions).

Contraindications and cautions

Aztreonam is contraindicated with any known allergy to aztreonam. Use with caution in people with a history of acute allergic reaction to penicillins or cefalosporins *because of the possibility of cross-reactivity*; in those with renal or hepatic dysfunction *that could interfere with the clearance and excretion of the drug*; and in pregnant and breastfeeding women *because of potential adverse effects on the fetus or neonate.*

Adverse effects

The adverse effects associated with the use of aztreonam are relatively mild. Local GI effects include nausea, GI upset, vomiting and diarrhoea. Hepatic enzyme elevations related to direct drug effects on the liver may also occur. Other effects include inflammation, phlebitis and discomfort at injection sites, as well as the potential for allergic response, including anaphylaxis.

Care considerations for people receiving macrolides, lincosamides or monobactams

Assessment: history and examination

- Assess for *possible contraindications or precautions*: known allergy to lincosamides, macrolides and monobactams (obtain specific information about the nature and occurrence of allergic reactions); history of liver disease *that could interfere with metabolism of the drug*; and current pregnancy or breastfeeding status *because of potential adverse effects on the fetus or infant.*
- Perform a physical assessment *to establish baseline data for assessing the effectiveness of the drug and the occurrence of any adverse effects associated with drug therapy.*
- Examine the skin for any rash or lesions *to provide a baseline for possible adverse effects.*
- Obtain specimens for culture and sensitivity testing from the site of infection.
- Monitor temperature *to detect infection.*
- Conduct assessment of orientation, affect and reflexes *to establish a baseline for any CNS effects of the drug.*
- Assess liver and renal function test values *to determine the status of renal and liver functioning and to determine any needed alteration in dosage.*
- Obtain baseline electrocardiogram *to rule out conditions that could put the person at risk for serious arrhythmias.*

Implementation with rationale

- Check culture and sensitivity reports *to ensure that this is the drug of choice for this person.*
- Monitor hepatic and renal function test values before therapy begins *to arrange to reduce dose as needed.*
- Ensure that the person receives the full course of the medication as prescribed *to eradicate the infection and to help prevent the emergence of resistant strains.*
- Ensure that the person swallows the tablet whole; it should not be cut, crushed or chewed, *to ensure a therapeutic dose of the drug.*
- Monitor the site of infection and presenting signs and symptoms (eg, fever, lethargy, urinary tract signs and symptoms) throughout the course of drug therapy. *Failure of these signs and symptoms to resolve may indicate the need to reculture the*

site. Arrange to continue drug therapy for at least 2 days after all signs and symptoms resolve, *to help prevent the development of resistant strains*.
- Provide small frequent meals as tolerated *to ensure adequate nutrition with GI upset*; frequent mouth care and ice chips or sugarless lollies to suck *to provide relief of discomfort if dry mouth is a problem*; and adequate fluids *to replace fluid lost through diarrhoea*.
- Ensure ready access to bathroom facilities *to assist people with problems associated with diarrhoea*.
- Institute safety measures *to protect person from injury if CNS effects occur*.
- Arrange for appropriate treatment of superinfections as needed *to decrease the severity of infection and complications*.
- Instruct the person about the appropriate dosage regimen and possible adverse effects *to enhance knowledge about drug therapy and to promote compliance*. For the monobactam agent aztreonam: this drug can be given only IV or IM, so the person will not be responsible for administering the drug.
- For lincosamides, take additional precautions that include careful monitoring of GI activity and fluid balance and stopping the drug at the first sign of severe or bloody diarrhoea.
- Provide the following teaching:
  - Take safety precautions, including changing position slowly and avoiding driving and hazardous tasks, if CNS effects occur.
  - Try to drink a lot of fluids and to maintain nutrition (very important) even though nausea, vomiting and diarrhoea may occur.
  - Report difficulty breathing, severe headache, severe diarrhoea, severe skin rash, and mouth or vaginal sores.

Evaluation

- Monitor person's response to the drug (resolution of bacterial infection).
- Monitor for adverse effects (orientation and affect, GI effects, superinfections).
- Evaluate the effectiveness of the teaching plan (person can name the drug, dosage, possible adverse effects to expect and specific measures to help avoid adverse effects).
- Monitor the effectiveness of comfort and safety measures and compliance with the regimen.

KEY POINTS

- Lincosamides are similar to macrolides but are more toxic. They are used to treat severe infections. Monitor the person for pseudomembranous colitis, bone marrow depression, pain and CNS effects.
- Macrolides are in a class of older antibiotics that can be bactericidal or bacteriostatic. They are used to treat URTIs and urinary tract infections (UTIs) and are often used when people are allergic to penicillin. Monitor the person for nausea, vomiting, diarrhoea, dizziness and other CNS effects.
- The monobactam antibiotic aztreonam is effective against only Gram-negative enterobacteria; it is safely used when people are allergic to penicillin or cefalosporins. Monitor the person taking aztreonam for GI problems, liver toxicity and pain at the injection site.

FLUOROQUINOLONES

The fluoroquinolones (Table 9.4) are a relatively new synthetic class of antibiotics with a broad spectrum

TABLE 9.4 ***DRUGS IN FOCUS*** **Fluoroquinolones**

Drug name	Dosage/route	Usual indications
(P) ciprofloxacin *(Ciproxin, Ciprol)*	Adult: 100–500 mg bd PO for up to 6 weeks; reduce dose in renal failure Paediatric: not recommended because of potential effects on developing cartilage	Treatment of infections caused by a wide spectrum of Gram-negative bacteria
moxifloxacin *(Avelox)*	Adult: 400 mg/day PO or IV for 5–10 days; reduce dose in renal impairment	Treatment of adults with sinusitis, bronchitis, or community-acquired pneumonia
norfloxacin *(Noroxin, Nufloxib)*	Adult: 400 mg PO q 12 hours for up to 28 days; reduce dose in renal impairment	Treatment of various urinary tract infections
ofloxacin *(Ocuflox)*	Adult: 1–2 guttae into affected eye q 30 min–6 hours	Treatment of corneal ulcers, bacterial conjunctivitis

of activity. Fluoroquinolones include ciprofloxacin *(Ciproxin, Ciprol)*, which is the most widely used fluoroquinolone; moxifloxacin *(Avelox)*, norfloxacin *(Noroxin, Nufloxib)* and ofloxacin *(Ocuflox)*.

Therapeutic actions and indications

The fluoroquinolones enter the bacterial cell by passive diffusion through channels in the cell membrane. Once inside, they interfere with the action of DNA enzymes necessary for the growth and reproduction of the bacteria (see Figure 9.1). This leads to cell death because the bacterial DNA is damaged and the cell cannot be maintained. The fluoroquinolones have the advantage of a unique way of disrupting bacterial activity. There is little cross-resistance with other forms of antibiotics. However, misuse of these drugs in the short time the class has been available has led to the existence of resistant strains of bacteria (see contraindications and cautions).

The fluoroquinolones are indicated for treating infections caused by susceptible strains of Gram-negative bacteria, including *E. coli*, *P. mirabilis*, *K. pneumoniae*, *Enterobacter cloacae*, *Proteus vulgaris*, *Proteus rettgeri*, *Morganella morganii*, *Moraxella catarrhalis*, *H. influenzae*, *H. parainfluenzae*, *P. aeruginosa*, *Citrobacter freundii*, *S. aureus*, *Staphylococcus epidermidis*, some *Neisseria gonorrhoeae* and group D streptococci. These infections frequently include urinary tract, respiratory tract and skin infections. Ciprofloxacin is effective against a wide spectrum of Gram-negative bacteria. In 2001, it was approved for prevention of anthrax infection in areas that might be exposed to germ warfare. It is also effective against typhoid fever. See Table 9.4 for usual indications for each of these agents.

Pharmacokinetics

The fluoroquinolones are absorbed from the GI tract, metabolised in the liver and excreted in the urine and faeces. These drugs are widely distributed in the body and cross the placenta and enter breast milk (see contraindications and cautions).

Ciprofloxacin is available in injectable, oral and topical forms. Moxifloxacin is available in oral and IV forms. Norfloxacin is only available in an oral form. Ofloxacin is available as an ophthalmic solution for the treatment of ocular infections caused by susceptible bacteria.

Contraindications and cautions

Fluoroquinolones are contraindicated in people with known allergy to any fluoroquinolone and in pregnant or breastfeeding women *because potential effects on the fetus and infant are not known.* Use with caution in the presence of renal dysfunction, *which could interfere with the metabolism and excretion of the drug*, and seizures, *which could be exacerbated by the drugs' effects on cell membrane channels.*

Because so many resistant strains are emerging, always perform culture and sensitivity tests of infected tissue *to determine the exact bacterial cause and sensitivity.* These drugs have been associated with lesions in developing cartilage and therefore are not recommended for use in children younger than 18 years of age.

Adverse effects

These drugs are associated with relatively mild adverse reactions. The most common are headache, dizziness, insomnia and depression related to possible effects on the CNS membranes. GI effects include nausea, vomiting, diarrhoea and dry mouth, related to direct drug effect on the GI tract and possibly to stimulation of the chemoreceptor trigger zone in the CNS.

Immunological effects include bone marrow depression, which may be related to drug effects on the cells of the bone marrow that rapidly turn over. Other adverse effects include fever, rash and photosensitivity, a potentially serious adverse effect that can cause severe skin reactions. Advise people to avoid sun and ultraviolet light exposure and to use protective clothing and sunscreens.

Clinically important drug–drug interactions

When fluoroquinolones are taken concurrently with iron salts, sucralfate, mineral supplements or antacids, the therapeutic effect of the fluoroquinolone is decreased. If this drug combination is necessary, administration of the two agents should be separated by at least 4 hours.

If fluoroquinolones are taken with drugs that increase the QTc interval or cause *torsades de pointes* (amiodarone, sotalol, erythromycin, pentamidine, tricyclics, phenothiazines), severe-to-fatal cardiac reactions are possible. These combinations should be avoided, but if they must be used, the person should be hospitalised with continual cardiac monitoring.

Combining fluoroquinolones with theophylline leads to increased theophylline levels because the two drugs use similar metabolic pathways. The theophylline dose should be decreased by half and serum theophylline levels monitored carefully. In addition, when fluoroquinolones are combined with non-steroidal anti-inflammatory drugs (NSAIDs), an increased risk of CNS stimulation is possible. If this combination is used, closely monitor the person, especially those who have a history of seizures or CNS problems.

Prototype summary: ciprofloxacin

Indications: treatment of respiratory, dermatological, urinary tract, ear, eye, bone and joint infections; treatment after anthrax exposure, typhoid fever.

Actions: interferes with DNA replication in susceptible Gram-negative bacteria, preventing cell reproduction.

Pharmacokinetics:

Route	Onset	Peak	Duration
Oral	Varies	60–90 minutes	4–5 hours
IV	10 minutes	30 minutes	4–5 hours

$T_{1/2}$: 3.5–4 hours; metabolised in the liver, excreted in bile and urine.

Adverse effects: headache, dizziness, hypotension, nausea, vomiting, diarrhoea, fever, rash.

Care considerations for people receiving fluoroquinolones

Assessment: history and examination

- Assess for *possible contraindications or cautions*: known allergy to any fluoroquinolone (obtain specific information about the nature and occurrence of allergic reactions); history of renal disease, *which could interfere with excretion of the drug*; and current pregnancy or breastfeeding status *because of potential adverse effects on the fetus or infant.*
- Perform physical assessment *to establish baseline data for assessing the effectiveness of the drug and the occurrence of any adverse effects associated with drug therapy.*
- Examine the skin for any rash or lesions *to provide a baseline for possible adverse effects.*
- Perform culture and sensitivity tests at the site of infection.
- Conduct assessment of orientation, affect and reflexes *to establish a baseline for any CNS effects of the drug.*
- Perform renal function tests, including BUN and creatinine clearance, *to evaluate the status of renal functioning and to assess necessary changes in dose.*

Implementation with rationale

- Check culture and sensitivity reports *to ensure that this is the drug of choice for this person.*
- Monitor renal function tests before initiating therapy *to appropriately arrange for dose reduction if necessary.*
- Ensure that the person receives the full course of the fluoroquinolone as prescribed *to eradicate the infection and to help prevent the emergence of resistant strains.*
- Monitor the site of infection and presenting signs and symptoms (eg, fever, lethargy, urinary tract signs and symptoms) throughout the course of drug therapy. *Failure of these signs and symptoms to resolve may indicate the need to reculture the site.* Arrange to continue drug therapy for at least 2 days after resolution of all signs and symptoms *to help decrease the development of resistant strains.*
- Provide small, frequent meals as tolerated, frequent mouth care and ice chips or sugarless lollies to suck if dry mouth is a problem *to relieve discomfort and provide nutrition*, and provide *adequate fluids to replace those lost through diarrhoea.*
- Implement safety measures, including adequate lighting, use of side rails and assistance with ambulation *to protect the person from injury if CNS effects occur.*
- Instruct the person about the appropriate dosage schedule and possible adverse effects *to enhance knowledge about drug therapy and to promote compliance.*
- Provide the following teaching:
  - Take safety precautions, including changing position slowly and avoiding driving and hazardous tasks, if CNS effects occur.
  - Try to drink a lot of fluids and to maintain nutrition (very important), although nausea, vomiting and diarrhoea may occur.
  - Avoid ultraviolet light and sun exposure, using protective clothing and sunscreens.
  - Report difficulty breathing, severe headache, severe diarrhoea, severe skin rash, fainting spells and heart palpitations.

Evaluation

- Monitor person's response to the drug (resolution of bacterial infection).
- Monitor for adverse effects (orientation and affect, GI effects, photosensitivity).
- Evaluate effectiveness of the teaching plan (person can name drug, dosage, possible adverse effects to expect and specific measures to help avoid adverse effects).
- Monitor effectiveness of comfort and safety measures and compliance with the therapeutic regimen.

KEY POINTS

- Fluoroquinolones inhibit the action of DNA enzymes in susceptible Gram-negative bacteria. They are used to treat a wide range of infections.
- Monitor the person for headache, dizziness, GI upsets and bone marrow depression, and caution the person about the risk of photosensitivity reactions.

PENICILLINS AND PENICILLINASE-RESISTANT ANTIBIOTICS

Penicillin (Table 9.5) was the first antibiotic introduced for clinical use. Sir Alexander Fleming used *Penicillium* moulds to produce the original penicillin in the 1920s. Subsequent versions of penicillin were developed to

TABLE 9.5 *DRUGS IN FOCUS* Penicillins and penicillinase-resistant antibiotics

Drug name	Dosage/route	Usual indications
Penicillins		
benzathine penicillin *(Bicillin)*	675 mg–1.8 g IM	Mild to moderate upper respiratory tract infection, streptococcal infections, syphilis, rheumatic fever
benzylpenicillin *(BenPen)*	Adult and paediatric > 10 years: 300 mg IM or IV q 6 hours Paediatric 3–10 years: 150–300 mg IM or IV q 6 hours Paediatric: < 3 years: 60 mg IM or IV q 6 hours	Treatment of infections caused by sensitive organisms; treatment of syphilis, prevention of bacterial endocarditis, wound infection and sepsis
dicloxacillin *(Diclocil, Distaph)*	Adult: 250–500 mg IV or 250 mg PO q 6 hours Paediatric: 25–50 mg/kg/day IV q 6 hours	Severe staphylococcal and other Gram-positive coccal infections; skin and wound infections, pneumonia, osteomyelitis
flucloxacillin *(Flopen, Staphylex)*	Adult: 250 mg PO of IV q 6 hours	Treatment of staphylococcal or other Gram-positive coccal infection; pneumonia, osteomyelitis skin and wound infection
phenoxymethylpenicillin benzathine *(Abbocillin, Cilicaine V)*	Adult: 250–500 mg PO q 4–6 hours Paediatric: 15–50 mg/kg/day in 3–6 divided doses	Treatment of mild to moderate infections due to sensitive organisms
phenoxymethylpenicillin potassium *(Abbocillin VK, Cilicaine VK)*	Adult: 250–500 mg PO q 4–6 hours	Treatment of mild to moderate infections due to sensitive organisms
procaine penicillin *(Cilicaine)*	Adult: 1.5 g/day IM for 2–5 days	Moderately severe infections due to organisms sensitive to penicillin
Broad-spectrum penicillins		
(P) amoxicillin *(Amoxil, Augmentin, Cilamox)*	Adult: 250–500 mg PO q 8 hours Paediatric: 20 mg/kg/day PO in divided doses q 8 hours	Broad spectrum of uses for adults and children
ampicillin *(Amicyn, Ibimicyn)*	Adult: 250–500 mg IM or IV q 6 hours, then 500 mg PO q 6 hours when oral use is feasible Paediatric: 60 mg/kg/day IM or IV in 4–6 divided doses, then 250 mg PO q 6 hours	Broad spectrum of activity; useful form if switch from parenteral to oral is anticipated; monitor for nephritis
piperacillin *(Tazocin, Tazopip)*	Adult and paediatric > 12 years: 4 g IV q 8 hours Paediatric < 12 years: 100 mg/kg IV q 8 hours	Treatment of serious bacterial infections caused by sensitive organisms; lower respiratory tract infection, skin and intra-abdominal infection, bacterial septicaemia, gynaecological infection
ticarcillin *(Timentin)*	Adult: 1 g IM or direct IV q 6 hours; reduce dose with renal impairment Paediatric: 50–100 mg/kg/day IM or direct IV q 6–8 hours	Severe infections caused by susceptible bacteria

decrease the adverse effects of the drug and to modify it to act on resistant bacteria. Penicillins include benzylpenicillin *(BenPen)*, flucloxacillin *(Flopen)*, procaine penicillin *(Cilicaine)*, dicloxacillin *(Diclocil)*, amoxicillin *(Amoxil, Augmentin)*, ampicillin *(Amicyn, Ibimicyn)* and ticarcillin *(Timentin)*.

With the prolonged use of penicillin, more and more bacterial species have synthesised the enzyme penicillinase to counteract the effects of penicillin. Researchers have developed a group of drugs with a resistance to penicillinase, which allows them to remain effective against bacteria that are now resistant to the penicillins. The actual drug chosen depends on the sensitivity of the bacteria causing the infection, the desired and available routes and the personal experience of the clinician with the particular agent.

Therapeutic actions and indications

The penicillins and penicillinase-resistant antibiotics produce bactericidal effects by interfering with the ability of susceptible bacteria to build their cell walls when they are dividing (see Figure 9.2). These drugs prevent the bacteria from biosynthesising the framework of the cell wall, and the bacteria with weakened cell walls swell and then burst from osmotic pressure within the cell. Because human cells do not use the biochemical process that the bacteria use to form the cell wall, this effect is a selective toxicity.

The penicillins are indicated for the treatment of:

- streptococcal infections, including pharyngitis, tonsillitis, scarlet fever and endocarditis
- pneumococcal infections
- staphylococcal infections
- fusospirochetal infections
- rat-bite fever
- diphtheria
- anthrax
- syphilis
- uncomplicated gonococcal infections
- (at high doses) meningococcal meningitis.

See Table 9.5 for usual indications for each agent.

Pharmacokinetics

Most of the penicillins are rapidly absorbed from the GI tract, reaching peak levels in 1 hour. They are sensitive to the gastric acid levels in the stomach and should be taken on an empty stomach to ensure adequate absorption. Penicillins are excreted unchanged in the urine, making renal function an important factor in safe use of the drug. Penicillins enter breast milk and can cause adverse reactions (see contraindications and cautions).

Contraindications and cautions

These drugs are contraindicated in people with allergies to penicillin or cefalosporins or other allergens. Penicillin sensitivity tests are available if the person's history of allergy is unclear and a penicillin is the drug of choice. Use with caution in people with renal disease (lowered doses are necessary *because excretion is reduced*). Although there are no adequate studies of use during pregnancy, use in women who are pregnant and in breastfeeding women should be limited to situations in which the mother clearly would benefit from the drug, *because diarrhoea and superinfections may occur in the infant*.

Perform culture and sensitivity tests *to ensure that the causative organism is sensitive to the penicillin selected for use*. With the emergence of many resistant strains of bacteria, this has become increasingly important.

Adverse effects

The major adverse effects of penicillin therapy involve the GI tract. Common adverse effects include nausea, vomiting, diarrhoea, abdominal pain, glossitis, stomatitis, gastritis, sore mouth and furry tongue. These effects are primarily related to the loss of bacteria from the normal flora and the subsequent opportunistic infections that occur. Superinfections, including yeast infections, are also very common and are again associated with the loss of bacteria from the normal flora. Pain and inflammation at the injection site can occur with injectable forms of the drugs. Hypersensitivity reactions may include rash, fever, wheezing and, with repeated exposure, anaphylaxis that can progress to anaphylactic shock and death.

Clinically important drug–drug interactions

If penicillins and penicillinase-resistant antibiotics are taken concurrently with tetracyclines, a decrease in the effectiveness of the penicillins results. This combination should be avoided if at all possible, or the penicillin doses should be raised, which could increase the occurrence of adverse effects.

In addition, when the parenteral forms of penicillins and penicillinase-resistant drugs are administered in combination with any of the parenteral aminoglycosides, inactivation of the aminoglycosides occurs. These combinations should also be avoided.

Prototype summary: amoxicillin

Indications: treatment of infections caused by susceptible strains of bacteria, postexposure prophylaxis for anthrax, treatment of *Helicobacter* infections as part of combination therapy.

Actions: inhibits synthesis of the cell wall in susceptible bacteria, causing cell death.

Pharmacokinetics:

Route	Onset	Peak	Duration
Oral	Varies	1 hours	6–8 hours

$T_{1/2}$: 1–1.4 hours; excreted unchanged in the urine.

Adverse effects: nausea, vomiting, diarrhoea, glossitis, stomatitis, bone marrow suppression, rash, fever, superinfections, lethargy.

Care considerations for people receiving penicillins and penicillinase-resistant antibiotics

Assessment: history and examination

- Assess for *possible contraindications or cautions*: known allergy to any cefalosporins, penicillins or other allergens *because cross-sensitivity often occurs* (obtain specific information about the nature and occurrence of allergic reactions); history of renal disease *that could interfere with excretion of the drug*; and current pregnancy or breastfeeding status.
- Perform a physical assessment *to establish baseline data for evaluating the effectiveness of the drug and the occurrence of any adverse effects associated with drug therapy.*
- Examine skin and mucous membranes for any rashes or lesions and injection sites for abscess formation *to provide a baseline for possible adverse effects.*
- Perform culture and sensitivity tests at the site of infection *to ensure that this is the drug of choice for this person.*
- Note respiratory status *to provide a baseline for the occurrence of hypersensitivity reactions.*
- Examine the abdomen *to monitor for adverse effects.* Evaluate renal function test findings, including BUN and creatinine clearance, *to assess the status of renal functioning and to determine any needed alteration in dose.*

Implementation with rationale

- Check culture and sensitivity reports *to ensure that this is the drug of choice for this person.*
- Monitor renal function tests before and periodically during therapy *to arrange for dose reduction as needed.*
- Ensure that the person receives the full course of the penicillin as prescribed, in doses around the clock, *to increase effectiveness.*
- Explain storage requirements for suspensions and the importance of completing the prescribed therapeutic course even if signs and symptoms have disappeared, *to increase the effectiveness of the drug and decrease the risk of developing resistant strains.*
- Monitor the site of infection and presenting signs and symptoms (eg, fever, lethargy) throughout the course of drug therapy. *Failure of these signs and symptoms to resolve may indicate the need to reculture the site.* Arrange to continue drug therapy for at least 2 days after the resolution of all signs and symptoms *to reduce the risk of development of resistant strains.*
- Provide small frequent meals as tolerated, ensure frequent mouth care and offer ice chips or sugarless lollies to suck if stomatitis and sore mouth are problems *to relieve discomfort and ensure nutrition.*
- Provide adequate fluids *to replace fluid lost through diarrhoea.*
- Monitor the person for any signs of superinfection *to arrange for treatment if superinfections occur.*
- Monitor injection sites regularly and *provide warm compresses and gentle massage to injection sites if they are painful or swollen.* If signs of phlebitis occur, remove the IV line and reinsert it in a different vein to continue the drug regimen.
- Instruct the person regarding the appropriate dosage regimen and possible adverse effects *to enhance knowledge about drug therapy and promote compliance.*
- Provide the following teaching:
  - Try to drink a lot of fluids and to maintain nutrition (very important) even though nausea, vomiting and diarrhoea may occur.
  - Report difficulty breathing, severe headache, severe diarrhoea, dizziness, weakness, mouth sores and vaginal itching or sores to a health care provider. Box 9.5 contains a teaching checklist for penicillins.

Evaluation

- Monitor person's response to the drug (resolution of bacterial infection).
- Monitor for adverse effects (GI effects; local irritation, phlebitis at injection and IV sites; superinfections).

- Evaluate the effectiveness of the teaching plan (person can name the drug, dosage, possible adverse effects to expect and specific measures to help avoid adverse effects).
- Monitor the effectiveness of comfort and safety measures and compliance with the therapeutic regimen.

KEY POINTS

- The penicillins are one of the oldest classes of antibiotics, and many resistant strains have developed. The penicillinase-resistant antibiotics were created to combat bacteria that produce an enzyme to destroy the penicillin. Penicillins are used to treat a broad spectrum of infections, including respiratory tract infections and UTIs.
- Monitor the person on penicillin for nausea, vomiting, diarrhoea, superinfections and the possibility of hypersensitivity reactions.

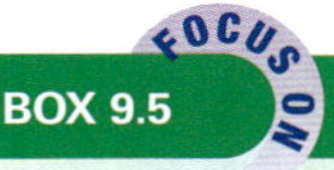

BOX 9.5 Individual and family teaching

Penicillins

- The penicillins are used to help destroy specific bacteria that are causing infections in the body. They are effective against only certain bacteria; they are not effective against viruses (such as cold germs) or other bacteria. To clear up a bacterial infection, the penicillins must act on the bacteria over a period of time, so it is very important to complete the full course to avoid recurrence of the infection.
- The drug should be taken on an empty stomach with a full 150 mL glass of water – 1 hour before meals or 2–3 hours after meals is best. Do not use fruit juice, soft drinks or milk to take your drug, because these foods may interfere with its effectiveness. (This does not apply to amoxicillin or penicillin V.)
- Common effects of these drugs include stomach upset, diarrhoea, changes in taste and change in the colour of the tongue. Small frequent meals may help. It is important to try to maintain good nutrition. These effects should go away when the drug is stopped.
- Report any of the following to your health care provider: hives, rash, fever, difficulty breathing, severe diarrhoea.
- Tell any doctor, nurse, or other health care provider that you are taking this drug.
- Keep this drug and all medications out of the reach of children and pets.
- Do not share this drug with other people and do not use this medication to self-treat other infections.
- It is very important that you complete the full course of your prescription, even if you feel better before you finish it.

SULFONAMIDES

The sulfonamides, or sulpha drugs (Table 9.6), are drugs that inhibit folic acid synthesis. Sulfonamides include sulfasalazine *(Salazopyrin)* and sulfamethoxazole *(Septrin, Bactrim).*

Therapeutic actions and indications

Folic acid is necessary for the synthesis of purines and pyrimidines, which are precursors of RNA and DNA. For cells to grow and reproduce, they require folic acid. Humans cannot synthesise folic acid and depend on the folate in their diet to obtain this essential substance. Bacteria are impermeable to folic acid and must synthesise it inside the cell. The sulfonamides competitively block *para*-aminobenzoic acid (PABA) to prevent the synthesis of folic acid in susceptible bacteria that synthesise their own folates for the production of RNA and DNA (see Figure 9.2). This includes Gram-negative and Gram-positive bacteria such as *Chlamydia trachomatis* and *Nocardia* and some strains of *H. influenzae*, *E. coli* and *P. mirabilis*.

Because of the emergence of resistant bacterial strains and the development of newer antibiotics, the sulpha drugs are no longer commonly used. However, they remain an inexpensive and effective treatment for UTIs and trachoma, especially in developing countries and when cost is an issue. These drugs are used to treat trachoma (a leading cause of blindness), nocardiosis (which causes pneumonias, as well as brain abscesses and inflammation), UTIs and sexually transmitted diseases. See Table 9.6 for usual indications for each of these agents.

Pharmacokinetics

The sulfonamides are teratogenic; they are distributed into breast milk (see contraindications and cautions). These drugs, given orally, are absorbed from the GI tract, metabolised in the liver and excreted in the urine. The time to peak level and the half-life of the individual drug vary.

Sulfasalazine is a sulfapyridine that is carried by aminosalicylic acids (aspirin), which release the aminosalicylic acid in the colon. In a delayed-release form, this sulpha drug is also used to treat rheumatoid arthritis that does not respond to other treatments. It is rapidly absorbed from the GI tract, reaching peak levels in 2–6 hours. After being metabolised in the liver, it is excreted in the urine with a half-life of 5–10 hours.

Sulfamethoxazole is a combination drug with trimethoprim, another antibacterial drug. It is rapidly absorbed from the GI tract, reaching peak levels in 2 hours. After being metabolised in the liver, it is excreted in the urine with a half-life of 7–12 hours.

TABLE 9.6 DRUGS IN FOCUS Sulfonamides

Drug name	Dosage/route	Usual indications
sulfadiazine (generic)	Adult: 2–4 g PO loading dose, then 2–4 g/day PO in 4–6 divided doses Paediatric: 75 mg/kg PO, then 120–150 mg/kg/day PO in 4–6 divided doses	Treatment of a broad spectrum of infections
sulfasalazine *(Salazopyrin)*	Adult: 3–4 g/day PO in evenly divided doses, then 500 mg PO qid; 500 mg PO qid (arthritis) Paediatric: 40–60 mg/kg/day PO in divided doses, then 20–30 mg/kg/day PO in 4 equally divided doses	Treatment of ulcerative colitis and Crohn's disease; rheumatoid arthritis
sulfamethoxazole–trimethoprim (co-trimoxazole) *(Bactrim)*	Adult: 2 tablets PO q 12 hours; reduce dose with renal impairment Paediatric: 8 mg/kg/day trimethoprim plus 40 mg sulfamethoxazole PO q 12 hours	Treatment of otitis media, bronchitis, urinary tract infections, and pneumonitis caused by *Pneumocystis carinii*

Contraindications and cautions

The sulfonamides are contraindicated with any known allergy to any sulfonamide, to sulfonylureas or to thiazide diuretics *because cross-sensitivities occur*; during pregnancy *because the drugs can cause birth defects, as well as kernicterus*; and during breastfeeding *because of a risk of kernicterus, diarrhoea and rash in the infant*. They should be used with caution in people with renal disease or a history of kidney stones *because of the possibility of increased toxic effects of the drugs*.

Adverse effects

Adverse effects associated with sulfonamides include GI effects such as nausea, vomiting, diarrhoea, abdominal pain, anorexia, stomatitis and hepatic injury, which are all related to direct irritation of the GI tract and the death of normal bacteria. Renal effects are related to the filtration of the drug in the glomerulus and include crystalluria, haematuria and proteinuria, which can progress to a nephritic syndrome and possible toxic nephrosis. CNS effects include headache, dizziness, vertigo, ataxia, convulsions and depression (possibly related to drug effects on the nerves). Bone marrow depression may occur and is related to drug effects on the cells that turn over rapidly in the bone marrow.

Dermatological effects include photosensitivity and rash related to direct effects on the dermal cells. A wide range of hypersensitivity reactions may also occur.

Clinically important drug–drug interactions

If sulfonamides are taken with glipizide, glibenclamide or glicazide, the risk of hypoglycaemia increases. If this combination is needed, the person should be monitored and the dose of the antidiabetic agent should be adjusted. An increase in dose will then be needed when sulfonamide therapy stops.

When sulfonamides are taken with ciclosporin, the risk of nephrotoxicity rises. If this combination is essential, the person should be monitored closely and the sulfonamide stopped at any sign of renal dysfunction.

Care considerations for people receiving sulfonamides

Assessment: history and examination

- Assess for *possible contraindications or cautions*: known allergy to any sulfonamide, sulfonylureas or thiazide diuretic *because cross-sensitivity often results* (obtain specific information about the nature and occurrence of allergic reactions); history of renal disease *that could interfere with excretion of the drug and lead to increased toxicity*; and current pregnancy or breastfeeding status.
- Perform a physical assessment *to establish baseline data for assessing the effectiveness of the drug and the occurrence of any adverse effects associated with drug therapy*.
- Examine skin and mucous membranes for any rash or lesions *to provide a baseline for possible adverse effects*.
- Obtain specimens for culture and sensitivity tests at the site of infection *to ensure that this is the appropriate drug for this person*.
- Note respiratory status *to provide a baseline for the occurrence of hypersensitivity reactions*.
- Conduct assessment of orientation, affect and reflexes *to monitor for adverse drug effects* and examination of the abdomen *to monitor for adverse effects*.
- Monitor renal function test findings, including BUN and creatinine clearance, *to evaluate the status of renal functioning and to determine any needed alteration in dosage*. Also perform a full blood count (FBC) *to establish a baseline to monitor for adverse effects*.

Implementation with rationale

- Check culture and sensitivity reports *to ensure that this is the drug of choice for this person and repeat cultures if response is not as anticipated.*
- Monitor renal function tests before and periodically during therapy *to arrange for a dose reduction as necessary.*
- Ensure that the person receives the full course of the sulfonamide as prescribed *to increase therapeutic effects and decrease the risk for development of resistant strains.*
- Administer oral drug on an empty stomach 1 hour before or 2 hours after meals with a full glass of water *to promote adequate absorption of the drug.*
- Discontinue immediately if hypersensitivity reactions occur *to prevent potentially fatal reactions.*
- Provide small, frequent meals and adequate fluids as tolerated, encourage frequent mouth care, and offer ice chips or sugarless lollies to suck if stomatitis and sore mouth are problems *to relieve discomfort, ensure nutrition and replace fluid lost through diarrhoea.*
- Monitor FBC and urinalysis test results before and periodically during therapy *to check for adverse effects.*
- Instruct the person about the appropriate dosage regimen, the proper way to take the drug (on an empty stomach with a full glass of water) and possible adverse effects, *to enhance knowledge about drug therapy and to promote compliance.*
- Provide the following teaching:
  - Avoid driving or operating dangerous machinery because dizziness, lethargy and ataxia may occur.
  - Try to drink a lot of fluids and maintain nutrition (very important), even though nausea, vomiting and diarrhoea may occur.
  - Report difficulty in breathing, rash, ringing in the ears, fever, sore throat or blood in the urine.

Evaluation

- Monitor person's response to the drug (resolution of bacterial infection).
- Monitor for adverse effects (GI effects, CNS effects, rash and crystalluria).
- Evaluate the effectiveness of the teaching plan (person can name the drug, dosage, possible adverse effects to expect and specific measures to help avoid adverse effects).
- Monitor the effectiveness of comfort and safety measures and compliance with the regimen.

KEY POINTS

- Sulfonamides are older drugs; many strains have developed resistance to the sulfonamides, so they are no longer widely used.
- Monitor the person for CNS toxicity, nausea, vomiting, diarrhoea, liver injury, renal toxicity and bone marrow depression.

TETRACYCLINES

The tetracyclines (Table 9.7) were developed as semi-synthetic antibiotics based on the structure of a common soil mould. They are composed of four rings, which is how they got their name. Researchers have developed newer tetracyclines to increase absorption and tissue penetration. Widespread resistance to the tetracyclines has limited their use in recent years. Tetracyclines include doxycycline *(Doryx, Frakas),* tigecycline *(Tygacil)* and minocycline *(Akamin).*

Therapeutic actions and indications

The tetracyclines work by inhibiting protein synthesis in a wide range of bacteria, leading to the inability of the bacteria to multiply (see Figure 9.2). Because the affected protein is similar to a protein found in human cells, these drugs can be toxic to humans at high concentrations.

Tetracyclines are indicated for treatment:

- of infections caused by *Rickettsiae*, *M. pneumoniae*, *Borrelia recurrentis*, *H. influenzae*, *Haemophilus ducreyi*, *Pasteurella pestis*, *Pasteurella tularensis*, *Bartonella bacilliformis*, *Bacteroides* species, *Vibrio comma*, *Vibrio fetus*, *Brucella* species, *E. coli*, *E. aerogenes*, *Shigella* species, *Acinetobacter calcoaceticus*, *Klebsiella* species, *Diplococcus pneumoniae* and *S. aureus*
- against agents that cause psittacosis, ornithosis, lymphogranuloma venereum and granuloma inguinale
- when penicillin is contraindicated in susceptible infections
- for treatment of acne and uncomplicated GU infections caused by *C. trachomatis*.

Some of the tetracyclines are also used as adjuncts in the treatment of certain protozoal infections. See Table 9.7 for usual indications for each agent.

Pharmacokinetics

Tetracyclines are absorbed adequately, but not completely, from the GI tract. Their absorption is affected by food, iron, calcium and other drugs in the stomach. Tetracyclines are concentrated in the liver and excreted unchanged in the urine, with half-lives ranging from

TABLE 9.7 DRUGS IN FOCUS Tetracyclines

Drug name	Dosage/route	Usual indications
(P) doxycycline *(Doryx, Doxsig, Frakas)*	Adult and paediatric > 8 years: initially 200 mg/day PO followed by 100 mg/day PO	Treatment of a wide variety of infections, including traveller's diarrhoea and sexually transmitted diseases; periodontal disease
minocycline *(Akamin, Minomycin)*	Adult: 200 mg PO initially, followed by 100 mg/day PO	Treatment of meningococcal carriers and of various uncomplicated genitourinary and gynaecological infections
tetracycline *(Optycin Eye Ointment)*	Applied to lower conjunctival sac q 2 hours	Ocular infection
tigecycline *(Tygacil)*	Adult: initially, 100 mg IV followed by 50 mg IV q 12 hours	Complicated skin and intra-abdominal infections, including those with MRSA

12 to 25 hours. These drugs cross the placenta and pass into breast milk (see contraindications and cautions).

Tetracycline is available in oral and topical forms, in addition to being available as an ophthalmic agent. Doxycycline and minocycline are available in IV and oral forms.

Contraindications and cautions

Tetracyclines are contraindicated in people with known allergy to tetracyclines or to tartrazine (eg, in specific oral preparations that contain tartrazine) and during pregnancy and breastfeeding *because of effects on developing bones and teeth.* The ophthalmic preparation is contraindicated in people who have fungal, mycobacterial or viral ocular infections *because the drug kills not only the undesired bacteria, but also bacteria of the normal flora, which increases the risk for exacerbation of the ocular infection that is being treated.*

Tetracyclines should be used with caution in children younger than 8 years of age *because they can potentially damage developing bones and teeth*; and in people with hepatic or renal dysfunction *because they are concentrated in the bile and excreted in the urine.*

Adverse effects

The major adverse effects of tetracycline therapy involve direct irritation of the GI tract and include nausea, vomiting, diarrhoea, abdominal pain, glossitis and dysphagia. Fatal hepatotoxicity related to the drug's irritating effect on the liver has also been reported. Skeletal effects involve damage to the teeth and bones. Because tetracyclines have an affinity for teeth and bones, they accumulate there, weakening the structure and causing staining and pitting of teeth and bones. Dermatological effects include photosensitivity and rash. Superinfections, including yeast infections, occur when bacteria of the normal flora are destroyed. Local effects, such as pain and stinging with topical or ocular application, are fairly common. Haematological effects are less frequent, such as haemolytic anaemia and bone marrow depression secondary to the effects on bone marrow cells that turn over rapidly. Hypersensitivity reactions reportedly range from urticaria to anaphylaxis and also include intracranial hypertension.

Clinically important drug–drug interactions

When penicillin G and tetracyclines are taken concurrently, the effectiveness of penicillin G decreases. If this combination is used, the penicillin dose should be increased.

When oral contraceptives are taken with tetracyclines, the effectiveness of the contraceptives decreases, and women who take oral contraceptives should be advised to use an additional form of contraception while receiving the tetracycline. (See Critical thinking scenario.)

When methoxyflurane is combined with tetracycline, the risk of nephrotoxicity increases. If at all possible, this combination should be avoided. In addition, digoxin toxicity rises when tetracyclines are taken concurrently. Digoxin levels should be monitored and dose adjusted appropriately during treatment and after tetracycline therapy is discontinued. Finally, decreased absorption of tetracyclines results from oral combinations with calcium salts, magnesium salts, zinc salts, aluminium salts, bismuth salts, iron, urinary alkalinisers and charcoal.

Clinically important drug–food interactions

Because oral tetracyclines are not absorbed effectively if taken with food or dairy products, they should be administered on an empty stomach 1 hour before or 2–3 hours after any meal or other medication.

CRITICAL THINKING SCENARIO

Antibiotics and oral contraceptives

THE SITUATION

G.S., a 27-year-old married female postgraduate student, is seen in the student health clinic a few weeks into the autumn semester. She has developed a severe sinusitis and complains of head pressure, difficulty sleeping, fever, and muscle aches and pains. A culture is done, and the next day the culture and sensitivity report identifies the infecting organism as a strain of *Klebsiella* that is sensitive to doxycycline. G.S. returns to the clinic to get the prescription for doxycycline.

In talking with you, G.S. tells you that she began university with plans to start a family in 2 years, after completing her program. She is a very organised person and has carefully planned her rigorous course work and her non-academic activities so that almost every hour is scheduled. She states that she has successfully used low-dose oral contraceptives for 4 years and plans to continue this method of birth control.

CRITICAL THINKING

How does doxycycline and some other antibiotics and oral contraceptives interact? What are the possible ramifications of continuing to take doxycycline during a pregnancy?

What care interventions are appropriate for G.S.?

What teaching points should be stressed with G.S.? Think about the nature of her personality and the problems that an unplanned pregnancy might cause. How can you help G.S. to cope with her infection, her drug regimen and her rigorous schedule?

DISCUSSION

Several antibiotics, including tetracycline, are known to lead to the failure of oral contraceptives as evidenced by breakthrough bleeding and unplanned pregnancy. Although the exact way in which these drugs interact is incompletely understood, it is thought that the antibiotics destroy certain bacteria in the normal flora of the GI tract. These bacteria are necessary for the breakdown and eventual absorption of the female hormones contained in the contraceptives. The 5 days of antibiotic treatment together with the time necessary for rebuilding the normal flora can be long enough for the hypothalamus to lose the negative feedback signal provided by the contraceptives that prevents ovulation and preparation of the uterus. Sensing the low hormone levels, the hypothalamus releases gonadotropin-releasing hormone, which leads to the release of follicle-stimulating hormone and luteinising hormone, with subsequent ovulation.

G.S. will need a clear explanation and follow-up in written form about the risks of oral contraceptive failure while she is receiving doxycycline therapy. She should be encouraged to use an additional form of contraception during the course of her antibiotic use and to read all the literature that comes with oral contraceptives, as well as teaching information that should be provided with the antibiotic.

G.S. also may need a great deal of support and encouragement at this time. The sinus infection may increase her stress by interfering with her ability to stick to her rigid schedule. Discussing the possibility of an unplanned pregnancy may cause even more stress. The health clinic visit could be used as an opportunity to allow G.S. to talk, to vent any frustrations and stress, and then to encourage her to make time for herself. The nurse should stress the importance of a good diet, which will ensure that her body has the components she will need to fight this infection, to heal and to ward off other infections, as well as the importance of adequate rest and exercise. The nurse should also make sure that G.S. is receiving annual gynaecological examinations and has been advised not to smoke.

All health care professionals who are involved with G.S. should consider the impact that an unplanned pregnancy could have on this very organised woman and use this as an example of the importance of clear, concise teaching in the administration of drug therapy.

CARE GUIDE FOR G.S.: TETRACYCLINES

Assessment: history and examination

Allergy to any tetracycline

Hepatic or renal dysfunction

Pregnancy or breastfeeding

Concurrent use of oral contraceptives, antacids, iron products, digoxin or penicillins

General: site of infection, culture and sensitivity

Skin: colour, lesions

Respiratory: respiration, adventitious sounds

GI: liver evaluation, bowel sounds, usual output

Laboratory data: liver and renal function tests, urinalysis

Implementation

Perform culture and sensitivity tests before beginning therapy.

Administer drug on an empty stomach, 1 hour before or 2–3 hour after meals. Do not give with antacids, milk or iron products.

Do not use outdated drug because of the risk of nephrotoxicity.

Monitor for and provide hygiene measures and treatment if superinfections occur.
Monitor nutritional status and fluid intake.
Provide ready access to bathroom facilities if diarrhoea is a problem.
Provide support and reassurance for dealing with the drug effects and infection.
Provide teaching regarding drug name, dosage, adverse effects, precautions, warnings to report and drugs that might cause a drug–drug interaction, including the need to use a second form of contraception if using oral contraceptives.

Evaluation

Evaluate drug effects: resolution of bacterial infections.
Monitor for adverse effects: GI effects, superinfections, CNS effects.
Monitor for drug–drug interactions: lack of effectiveness of oral contraceptives, lack of antibacterial effect with antacids or iron.
Evaluate effectiveness of teaching program.
Evaluate effectiveness of comfort and safety measures.

Teaching for G.S.

- Doxycycline is an antibiotic that is specific for your infection. You should take it throughout the day for best results.
- Take this drug on an empty stomach, 1 hour before or 2–3 hours after meals, with a full glass of water.
- Do not take this drug with fooc, dairy products, iron preparations or antacids.
- Take the full course of this antibiotic. Do not stop taking it if you feel better.
- Do not save doxycycline; outdated products can be very toxic to your kidneys.
- Oral contraceptives may become ineffective while you are taking this drug. If you rely on oral contraceptives for birth control, use a second form of contraceptive while on this drug.
- You may experience stomach upset or diarrhoea.
- You may develop other infections in your mouth or vagina. (If this occurs, consult with your health care provider for appropriate treatment.)
- Tell any health care provider who is caring for you that you are taking this drug.
- Keep this, and all medications, out of the reach of children and pets.
- Report any of the following to your health care provider: changes in colour of urine or stool, severe cramps, difficulty breathing, rash or itching, yellowing of the skin or eyes.

Prototype summary: doxycycline

Indications: treatment of various infections caused by susceptible strains of bacteria; acne; when penicillin is contraindicated for eradication of susceptible organisms.

Actions: inhibits protein synthesis in susceptible bacteria, preventing cell replication.

Pharmacokinetics:

Route	Onset	Peak
Oral	Varies	2–4 hours
Topical	Minimal absorption occurs	

$T_{1/2}$: 6–12 hours; excreted unchanged in the urine.

Adverse effects: nausea, vomiting, diarrhoea, glossitis, discolouring and inadequate calcification of primary teeth of fetus when used in pregnant women or of secondary teeth when used in children, bone marrow suppression, photosensitivity, superinfections, rash, local irritation with topical forms.

Care considerations for people receiving tetracyclines

Assessment: history and examination

- Assess for *possible contraindications or cautions*: known allergy to any tetracycline or to tartrazine in certain oral preparations *because cross-sensitivity often occurs* (obtain specific information about the nature and occurrence of allergic reactions); any history of renal or hepatic disease *that could interfere with metabolism and excretion of the drug and lead to increased toxicity*; current pregnancy or breastfeeding status *because of the potential for adverse effects to the fetus or infant*; and age *because of the risk of damage to bones and teeth.*
- Perform a physical examination *to establish baseline data for assessing the effectiveness of the drug and the occurrence of any adverse effects associated with drug therapy.*
- Examine the skin for any rash or lesions *to provide a baseline for possible adverse effects.*
- Perform culture and sensitivity tests at the site of infection *to ensure that this is the appropriate drug for this person.*
- Note respiratory status *to provide a baseline for the occurrence of hypersensitivity reactions.*

- Evaluate renal and liver function test reports, including BUN and creatinine clearance, *to assess the status of renal and liver functioning, which helps to determine any needed changes in dose.*

Implementation with rationale

- Check culture and sensitivity reports *to ensure that this is the drug of choice for this person.* Arrange for repeated cultures if response is not as anticipated.
- Monitor renal and liver function test results before and periodically during therapy *to arrange for a dose reduction as needed.*
- Ensure that the person receives the full course of the tetracycline as prescribed. The oral drug should be taken on an empty stomach 1 hour before or 2 hours after meals with a full 150 mL glass of water. Concomitant use of antacids or salts should be avoided because they interfere with drug absorption. *These precautions will increase drug effectiveness and decrease the development of resistant strains of bacteria.*
- Discontinue the drug immediately if hypersensitivity reactions occur *to avoid the possibility of severe reactions.*
- Provide small frequent meals as tolerated, frequent mouth care and ice chips or sugarless lollies to suck if stomatitis and sore mouth are problems *to relieve discomfort and ensure nutrition.* Also provide adequate fluids *to replace fluid lost through diarrhoea.*
- Monitor for signs of superinfections *to arrange for treatment as appropriate.*
- Encourage the person to apply sunscreen and wear appropriate clothing *to protect exposed skin from skin rashes and sunburn associated with photosensitivity reactions.*
- Instruct the person about the appropriate dosage regimen, how to take the oral drug and possible side effects *to enhance knowledge about drug therapy and to promote compliance.*
- Provide the following teaching:
  - Try to drink a lot of fluids and maintain nutrition (very important) even though nausea, vomiting and diarrhoea may occur.
  - Use a barrier contraceptive method because oral contraceptives may not be effective while a tetracycline is being used.
  - Know that superinfections may occur. Appropriate treatment can be arranged through the health care provider.
  - Use sunscreens and protective clothing if sensitivity to the sun occurs.
  - Know when to report dangerous adverse effects, such as difficulty breathing, rash, itching, watery diarrhoea, cramps or changes in colour of urine or stool.

Evaluation

- Monitor the person's response to the drug (resolution of bacterial infection).
- Monitor for adverse effects (GI effects, rash and superinfections).
- Evaluate the effectiveness of the teaching plan (person can name the drug, dosage, possible adverse effects to expect and specific measures to help avoid adverse effects).
- Monitor the effectiveness of comfort and safety measures and compliance with the regimen.

KEY POINTS

- Tetracyclines inhibit protein synthesis and prevent bacteria from multiplying.
- Tetracyclines can cause damage to developing teeth and bones and should not be used with pregnant women or children.
- Monitor the person for GI effects, bone marrow depression, rash and superinfections. Caution women that tetracyclines may make oral contraceptives ineffective.

ANTIMYCOBACTERIALS

Mycobacteria – the group of bacteria that contain the pathogens that cause tuberculosis and leprosy – are classified on the basis of their ability to hold a stain even in the presence of a 'destaining' agent such as acid. Because of this property, they are called 'acid-fast' bacteria. The mycobacteria have an outer coat of mycolic acid that protects them from many disinfectants and allows them to survive for long periods in the environment. It may be necessary to treat these slow-growing bacteria for several years before they can be eradicated.

Mycobacteria cause serious infectious diseases. The bacterium *Mycobacterium tuberculosis* causes tuberculosis, the leading cause of death from infectious disease in the world. For several years the disease was thought to be under control, but with the increasing number of people with compromised immune systems and the emergence of resistant bacterial strains, tuberculosis is once again on the rise.

Mycobacterium leprae causes leprosy, also known as Hansen disease, which is characterised by disfiguring skin lesions and destructive effects on the respiratory

TABLE 9.8 DRUGS IN FOCUS Antimycobacterials

Drug name	Dosage/route	Usual indications
Antituberculosis drugs		
First-line drugs		
ethambutol *(Myambutol)*	Adult: 15 mg/kg/day PO as a single dose Paediatric: not recommended for children < 13 years	Treatment of *Mycobacterium tuberculosis* infection
(P) isoniazid (INH) (generic)	Adult: 5 mg/kg/day PO Paediatric: 10–12 mg/kg/day PO	Treatment of *M. tuberculosis* infection
rifampicin *(Rifadin, Rimycin)*	Adult: 600 mg PO or IV as a single daily dose Paediatric: 10–20 mg/kg/day PO or IV	Treatment of *M. tuberculosis* infection
Second-line drug		
rifabutin *(Mycobutin)*	Adult: 300 mg PO daily	Second-line treatment of *M. tuberculosis* infection
Leprostatic drugs		
dapsone (generic)	Adult: 50–100 mg/day PO Paediatric: adjust dosage according to body weight	Treatment of leprosy, *Pneumocystis carinii* pneumonia in people with AIDS, and a variety of infections caused by susceptible bacteria and brown recluse spider bites

tract. Leprosy is also a worldwide health problem; it is infectious when the mycobacteria invade the skin or respiratory tract of susceptible individuals. *Mycobacterium avium-intracellulare*, which causes mycobacterium avium complex (MAC), is seen in people with AIDS or in other people who are severely immunocompromised. Rifabutin *(Mycobutin)*, which was developed as an antituberculosis drug, is most effective against *M. avium-intracellulare*.

Antituberculosis drugs

Tuberculosis can lead to serious damage in the lungs, the GU tract, bones and the meninges. Because *M. tuberculosis* is so slow growing, the treatment must be continued for 6 months to 2 years. Using the drugs in combination helps to decrease the emergence of resistant strains and to affect the bacteria at various phases during their long and slow life cycle (Table 9.8).

First-line drugs for treating tuberculosis are used in combinations of two or more agents until bacterial conversion occurs or maximum improvement is seen. The first-line drugs for treating tuberculosis are isoniazid (generic), rifampicin *(Rifadin)*, and ethambutol *(Myambutol)*.

If the person cannot take one or more of the first-line drugs, or if the disease continues to progress because of the emergence of a resistant strain, second-line drugs can be used. The second-line drugs include rifabutin *(Mycobutin)*.

In addition, drugs from other antibiotic classes have been found to be effective in second-line treatment, such as ciprofloxacin *(Ciloxan, Ciprol)* which is a fluoroquinolone.

Leprostatic drugs

The main antibiotic used to treat leprosy is dapsone (generic), which has been the mainstay of leprosy treatment for many years, although resistant strains are emerging (Table 9.8). Like the sulfonamides, dapsone inhibits folate synthesis in susceptible bacteria. In addition to its use in leprosy, dapsone is used to treat *Pneumocystis carinii* pneumonia in people with AIDS and for a variety of infections caused by susceptible bacteria, as well as for bites by the brown recluse spider (rarely found in Australia).

Recently, the hypnotic drug thalidomide *(Thalomid)* has also been used in erythema nodosum leprosum that occurs after treatment for leprosy (Box 9.6).

Therapeutic actions and indications

Most of the antimycobacterial agents act on the DNA and/or RNA of the bacteria, leading to a lack of growth and eventually to bacterial death (see Figure 9.2). Isoniazid specifically affects the mycolic acid coat around the bacterium. Although many of the antimycobacterial agents are effective against other species of susceptible bacteria, their primary indications are in the treatment of tuberculosis or leprosy (as previously indicated). The antituberculosis drugs are always used in combination to affect the bacteria at various stages and to help decrease the emergence of resistant strains. See Table 9.8.

BOX 9.6 New indication for thalidomide

In the 1950s, the drug thalidomide became internationally known because it caused serious abnormalities (eg, lack of limbs, defective limbs) in the fetuses of many women who received the drug during pregnancy to help them sleep and to decrease stress. This tragedy led to the recall of thalidomide in the US and the establishment of more stringent standards for drug testing and labelling. In 2010, the TGA approved the use of this controversial drug for the treatment of erythema nodosum leprosum, which is a painful inflammatory condition related to an immune reaction to dead bacteria that occurs after treatment for leprosy. It is also approved for use in the treatment of multiple myeloma, brain tumours, Crohn's disease, human immunodeficiency virus–wasting syndrome and graft–host reaction in bone marrow transplant.

To take thalidomide, a woman must have a negative pregnancy test, receive instruction in using contraception and sign a release stating that she understands the risks associated with the drug. These limits on the use of a drug were the first such restrictions ever ordered by the TGA.

Thalidomide *(Thalomid)* is given in doses of 100–400 mg/day PO at bedtime for at least 2 weeks, followed by tapered dose in 50-mg increments over the next 2–4 weeks.

Pharmacokinetics

The antimycobacterial agents are generally well absorbed from the GI tract. These drugs, given orally, are metabolised in the liver and excreted in the urine; they cross the placenta and enter breast milk, placing the fetus or child at risk for adverse reactions (see contraindications and cautions).

Contraindications and cautions

Antimycobacterials are contraindicated for people with any known allergy to these agents; in those with severe renal or hepatic failure, *which could interfere with the metabolism or excretion of the drug*; in those with severe CNS dysfunction, *which could be exacerbated by the actions of the drug*; and in pregnancy *because of possible adverse effects on the fetus*. If an antituberculosis regimen is necessary during pregnancy, the combination of isoniazid, ethambutol and rifampicin is considered the safest.

Adverse effects

CNS effects, such as neuritis, dizziness, headache, malaise, drowsiness and hallucinations, are often reported and are related to direct effects of the drugs on neurons. These drugs also are irritating to the GI tract, causing nausea, vomiting, anorexia, stomach upset and abdominal pain. Rifampicin and rifabutin cause discolouration of body fluids from urine to sweat and tears. Alert people that in many instances orange-tinged urine, sweat and tears may stain clothing and permanently stain contact lenses. This can be frightening if the person is not alerted to the possibility that it will happen. As with other antibiotics, there is always a possibility of hypersensitivity reactions. Monitor the person on a regular basis.

Clinically important drug–drug interactions

When rifampicin and isoniazid are used in combination, the possibility of toxic liver reactions increases. People should be monitored closely.

Increased metabolism and decreased drug effectiveness occur as a result of administration of metoprolol, propranolol, corticosteroids, oral contraceptives, oral anticoagulants, oral antidiabetic agents, digoxin, theophylline, methadone, phenytoin, verapamil or ciclosporin in combination with rifampicin or rifabutin. People who are taking these drug combinations should be monitored closely and dose adjustments made as needed.

Prototype summary: isoniazid

Indications: treatment of tuberculosis as part of combination therapy; prophylactic treatment of household members of people recently diagnosed with tuberculosis.

Actions: interferes with lipid and nucleic acid synthesis in actively growing tubercle bacilli.

Pharmacokinetics:

Route	Onset	Peak	Duration
Oral	Varies	1–2 hours	24 hours

$T_{1/2}$: 1–4 hours; metabolised in the liver, excreted in the urine.

Adverse effects: peripheral neuropathies, nausea, vomiting, hepatitis, bone marrow suppression, fever, local irritation at injection sites, gynaecomastia, lupus syndrome.

Care considerations for people receiving antimycobacterials

Assessment: history and examination

- Assess for *possible contraindications or cautions*: known allergy to any antimycobacterial drug (obtain specific information about the nature and occurrence of allergic reactions); history of renal or hepatic disease, *which could interfere with*

metabolism and excretion of the drug and lead to toxicity; history of CNS dysfunction, including seizure disorders and neuritis, *which could be exacerbated by adverse drug effects*; and current pregnancy status *to ensure appropriate drug selection to prevent adverse effects on the fetus*.
- Perform a physical examination *to establish baseline data for assessing the effectiveness of the drug and the occurrence of any adverse effects associated with drug therapy*.
- Examine the skin for any rash or lesions *to provide a baseline for possible adverse effects*.
- Obtain specimens for culture and sensitivity testing *to establish the sensitivity of the organism being treated*.
- Evaluate CNS for orientation, affect and reflexes *to establish a baseline and to monitor for adverse effects*.
- Note respiratory status *to provide a baseline for the occurrence of hypersensitivity reactions*.
- Evaluate renal and liver function tests, including BUN and creatinine clearance, *to assess the status of renal and liver functioning to determine any needed alteration in dose*.

Implementation with rationale

- Check culture and sensitivity reports *to ensure that this is the drug of choice for this person, and arrange repeated cultures if response is not as anticipated*.
- Monitor renal and liver function test results before and periodically during therapy *to arrange for dose reduction as needed*.
- Ensure that the person receives the full course of the drugs *to improve effectiveness and decrease the risk of development of resistant bacterial strains*. These drugs are taken for years and often in combination. Periodic medical evaluation and reteaching are often essential to ensure compliance.
- Discontinue drug immediately if hypersensitivity reactions occur *to avert potentially serious reactions*.
- Encourage the person to eat small frequent meals as tolerated, perform frequent mouth care and drink adequate fluids *to ensure adequate nutrition and hydration*. Monitor nutrition if GI effects become a problem.
- Instruct the person about the appropriate dosage regimen, use of drug combinations and possible adverse effects *to enhance knowledge about drug therapy and to promote compliance*.
- Provide the following teaching:
  - Try to drink a lot of fluids to maintain nutrition (very important) even though nausea, vomiting and diarrhoea may occur.
  - Use barrier contraceptives and understand that oral contraceptives may not be effective if antimycobacterials are being used.
  - Understand that normally some of these drugs impart an orange stain to body fluids. If this occurs, the fluids may stain clothing and tears may stain contact lenses.
  - Report difficulty breathing, hallucinations, numbness and tingling, worsening of condition, fever and chills or changes in colour of urine or stool.

Evaluation

- Monitor person's response to the drug (resolution of mycobacterial infection).
- Monitor for adverse effects (GI effects, CNS changes and hypersensitivity reactions).
- Evaluate the effectiveness of the teaching plan (person can name the drug, dosage, possible adverse effects to expect and specific measures to help avoid adverse effects).
- Monitor the effectiveness of comfort and safety measures and compliance with the regimen.

KEY POINTS

- The mycobacteria have an outer coat of mycolic acid that protects them from many disinfectants and allows them to survive for long periods in the environment. These slow-growing bacteria may need to be treated for several years before they can be eradicated. They cause tuberculosis and leprosy.
- Antituberculosis drugs are used in combination to increase effectiveness and decrease the emergence of resistant strains. These drugs are divided into first-line and second-line drugs. Adverse effects include rashes, an orange tint to body fluids and GI reactions.
- Dapsone is the only antibiotic now used on its own to treat leprosy. Thalidomide was recently reintroduced to treat an unusual reaction many people develop after being on dapsone.

NEW CLASSES OF ANTIBIOTICS AND ADJUNCTS

Research is constantly being done to develop new antibiotics to affect the emerging resistant strains of bacteria. New classes of antibiotics are daptomycin *(Cubicin)*, linezolid *(Zyvox)* and tigecycline *(Tygacil)*.

TABLE 9.9 DRUGS IN FOCUS Other antibiotics

Drug name	Dosage/route	Usual indications
Lincosamides		
(P) clindamycin *(Cleocin)*	Adult: 150–300 mg PO q 6 hours or 600–2700 mg/day in 2–4 equal doses; reduce dose with renal impairment Paediatric: 8–25 mg/kg/day PO or 15–40 mg/kg/day IM or IV in 3–4 divided doses	Severe bacterial infections of the skin and soft tissue, abdomen, respiratory, bone and joint, pelvic infections, sepsis, endocarditis, due to anaerobic organisms, staphylococci, streptococci, pneumococci
lincomycin *(Lincocin)*	Adult: 500 mg PO q 6–8 hours, 600 mg IM q 12–24 hours, or 600 mg–1 g q 8–12 hours; reduce dose with renal impairment Paediatric: 30–60 mg/kg/day PO in 3–4 divided doses, 10 mg/kg IM q 12–24 hours, or 10–20 mg/kg/day IV in divided doses	Treatment of severe infections when penicillin or other less toxic antibiotics cannot be used
Macrolides		
azithromycin *(Azith, Zedd, Zithromax)*	Adult: 500 mg/day IV or 500 mg–1 g/day PO Paediatric: 10 mg/kg PO as a single dose on day 1, then 5 mg/kg PO on day 2–5 or 30 mg/kg PO as a single dose	Treatment of mild to moderate respiratory infections and urethritis in adults and otitis media and pharyngitis/tonsillitis in children
clarithromycin *(Clarac, Kalixocin)*	Adult: 150–450 mg PO q 6 hours Paediatric: 15 mg/kg/day PO given q 12 hours for 10 days	Treatment of various respiratory, skin, sinus, and maxillary infections; effective against mycobacteria
(P) erythromycin *(E-Mycin, EES)*	Adult: 15–20 mg/kg/day IV or PO Paediatric: 30–50 mg/kg/day PO in divided doses	Treatment of infections in people allergic to penicillin; drug of choice for treatment of Legionnaire's disease, infections caused by *Corynebacterium diphtheriae*, *Ureaplasma* species, syphilis, mycoplasma pneumonia, and chlamydial infections
roxithromycin *(Biaxsig, Rulide)*	Adults: 300 mg/day PO Paediatric > 40 kg:150 mg PO bd 24–40 kg: 100 mg PO bd 12–23 kg: 50 mg PO bd 6–11 kg: 25 mg PO bd	Upper and lower respiratory tract infection, skin infection, tonsillitis, impetigo
Monobactam		
(P) aztreonam *(Azactam)*	Adult: 500 mg–1 g q 8–12 hours IM or IV; reduce dose in renal and hepatic impairment Paediatric: 30 mg/kg IM or IV q 6–8 hours	Treatment of Gram-negative enterobacterial infections; safe alternative for treating infections caused by susceptible bacteria in people who may be allergic to penicillins or cefalosporins

See the following for additional information about each of these agents.

Adjuncts to antibiotic therapy include clavulanic acid and thalidomide (see Box 9.6).

Daptomycin was introduced in 2003 as a cyclic lipopeptide antibiotic. This class of drug binds to bacterial cell membranes, causing a rapid depolarisation of membrane potential. The loss of membrane potential leads to the inhibition of protein and DNA and RNA synthesis, which results in bacterial cell death. Daptomycin is approved for treating complicated skin and skin structure infections caused by susceptible Gram-positive bacteria, including MRSA. It must be given IV over 30 minutes, once each day for 7–14 days, which makes its use inconvenient. People should be monitored for pseudomembranous colitis and myopathies.

Linezolid *(Zyvox)* was introduced in 2000. This drug is indicated specifically for treatment of infections caused by vancomycin-resistant and methicillin-resistant strains of bacteria. It is available in IV and oral forms. The usual adult dosage is 600 mg PO, or it may be administered IV q 12 hours for 10–14 days. This drug must also be used cautiously and only when a sensitive bacterial species has been clearly identified. It is the first oral drug approved for the treatment of diabetic foot ulcers. These drugs are part of a wide variety of compounds that are being investigated to deal with the increasing problem of resistant bacteria.

 **Prototype summary: erythromycin**

Indications: treatment of respiratory, dermatological, urinary tract and GI infections caused by susceptible strains of bacteria.

Actions: binds to cell membranes, causing a change in protein function and cell death; can be bacteriostatic or bactericidal.

Pharmacokinetics:

Route	Onset	Peak
Oral	1–2 hours	1–4 hours
IV	Rapid	1 hour

$T_{1/2}$: 3–5 hours; metabolised in the liver, excreted in bile and urine.

Adverse effects: abdominal cramping, vomiting, diarrhoea, rash, superinfection, liver toxicity, risk for pseudomembranous colitis, potential for hearing loss.

 **Prototype summary: clindamycin**

Indications: treatment of serious infections caused by susceptible strains of bacteria, including some anaerobes; useful in septicaemia and chronic bone and joint infections.

Actions: inhibits protein synthesis in susceptible bacteria, causing cell death.

Pharmacokinetics:

Route	Onset	Peak	Duration
Oral	Varies	1–2 hours	8–12 hours
IM	20–30 minutes	1–3 hours	8–12 hours
IV	Immediate	Minutes	8–12 hours
Topical	Minimal absorption		

$T_{1/2}$: 2–3 hours; metabolised in the liver, excreted in the urine and faeces.

Adverse effects: nausea, vomiting, diarrhoea, pseudomembranous colitis, bone marrow suppression, hypotension, cardiac arrest with rapid IV infusion, rash, pain on injection, abscess at injection site.

Tigecycline *(Tygacil)* was the first drug of a new class of antibiotics called glycylcyclines. This antibiotic inhibits protein translation on ribosomes of certain bacteria, leading to their inability to maintain their integrity and culminating in the death of the bacterium. It is used in the treatment of complicated skin and skin structure infections and intra-abdominal infections caused by susceptible bacteria. Caution should be used with a known allergy to tetracycline antibiotics because

 **Prototype summary: aztreonam**

Indications: treatment of lower respiratory, dermatological, urinary tract, intra-abdominal, and gynaecological infections caused by susceptible strains of Gram-negative bacteria.

Actions: interferes with bacterial cell wall synthesis, causing cell death in susceptible Gram-negative bacteria; is not effective against Gram-positive or anaerobic bacteria.

Pharmacokinetics:

Route	Onset	Peak	Duration
IM	Varies	60–90 minutes	6–8 hours
IV	Immediate	30 minutes	6–8 hours

$T_{1/2}$: 1.5–2 hours; excreted unchanged in the urine.

Adverse effects: nausea, vomiting, diarrhoea, rash, superinfection, anaphylaxis, local discomfort at injection sites.

a cross-sensitivity may occur. Women should be advised to use a barrier form of contraceptive when on this drug. People should be monitored for pseudomembranous colitis, rash and superinfections. Tigecycline is given as 100 mg IV followed by 50 mg IV every 12 hours, infused over 30–60 minutes for 5–14 days.

CHAPTER SUMMARY

- Antibiotics work by disrupting protein or enzyme systems within a bacterium, causing cell death (bactericidal) or preventing multiplication (bacteriostatic).
- The proteins or enzyme systems affected by antibiotics are more likely to be found or used in bacteria than in human cells.
- The primary therapeutic use of each antibiotic is determined by the bacterial species that are sensitive to that drug, the clinical condition of the person receiving the drug and the benefit-to-risk ratio for the person.
- The longer an antibiotic has been available, the more likely it is that mutant bacterial strains resistant to the mechanisms of antibiotic activity will have developed.
- The most common adverse effects of antibiotic therapy involve the GI tract (nausea, vomiting, diarrhoea, anorexia, abdominal pain) and superinfections (invasion of the body by normally occurring microorganisms that are usually kept in check by the normal flora).
- To prevent or contain the growing threat of drug-resistant strains of bacteria, it is very important to

use antibiotics cautiously, to complete the full course of an antibiotic prescription and to avoid saving antibiotics for self-medication in the future. A person and family teaching program should address these issues, as well as the proper dosing procedure for the drug (even if the person feels better) and the importance of keeping a record of any reactions to antibiotics.

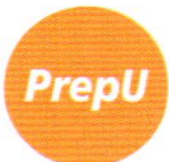

Knowing your strengths and weaknesses helps you to study more effectively. Take a PrepU Practice Quiz to find out how you measure up!

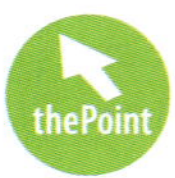

ONLINE RESOURCES

An extensive range of additional resources to enhance teaching and learning and to facilitate understanding of this chapter may be found online at the text's accompanying website, located on thePoint at http://thepoint.lww.com. These include Watch and Learn videos, Concepts in Action animations, journal articles, review questions, case studies, discussion topics and quizzes.

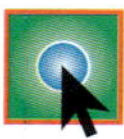

WEB LINKS

Health care providers and students may want to consult the following web resources:

www.health.gov.au/internet/main/publishing.nsf/content/cda-cdi3303e.htm
Australian Government Department of Health. Tuberculosis in Australia.

www.nps.org.au/about-us/what-we-do/campaigns-events/antibiotic-resistance-fighter
National Prescribing Service. Antibiotic Resistance.

www.who.int/mediacentre/factsheets/fs194/en/
World Health Organization. Antimicrobial Resistance.

BIBLIOGRAPHY

Bancroft, E. (2007). Antimicrobial resistance. *Journal of the American Medical Association, 298*, 1803–1804.

Coates, H. (2008). Ear drops and ototoxicity. *Australian Prescriber, 31(2)*, 40–41.

Collignon, P. J. (2002). Antibiotic resistance. *Medical Journal of Australia, 177(6)*, 325–329.

Farrell, M. & Dempsey, J. (2014). *Smeltzer & Bare's Textbook of Medical-Surgical Nursing* (3rd edn). Sydney: Lippincott, Williams & Wilkins.

Ferguson, J. (2004). Antibiotic prescribing: How can emergence of antibiotic resistance be delayed? *Australian Prescriber, 27*, 39–42.

Gillespie, E., Rodrigues, A., Wright, L., Williams, N. & Stuart, R. L. (2013). Improving antibiotic stewardship by involving nurses. *American Journal of Infection Control, 41(4)*, 365–367.

Klevens, R. M., Morrison, M. A., Nadle, J., Petit, S., Gershman, K., Ray, S., et al. (2007). Invasive methicillin-resistant *Staphylococcus aureus* infections in the United States. *Journal of the American Medical Association, 298*, 1763–1771.

Liebert, W. & Rom, W. N. (2004). Principles of tuberculosis management. *Tuberculosis*. Philadelphia: Lippincott Williams & Wilkins.

Looke, D. F. M. & McDougall, D. A. J. (2012). Parenteral antibiotics at home. *Australian Prescriber, 35(6)*, 194–197.

McKenna, L. & Mirkov, S. (2019). *McKenna's Drug Handbook for Nursing and Midwifery* (8th edn). Sydney: Wolters Kluwer Health Australia.

McKenzie, D., Rawlins, M. & Del Mar, C. (2013). Antimicrobial stewardship: What's it all about? *Australian Prescriber, 36(4)*, 116–120.

NHMRC (2010) Australian Guidelines for the Prevention and Control of Infection in Healthcare. Commonwealth of Australia. www.nhmrc.gov.au/_files_nhmrc/publications/attachments/cd33_complete.pdf.

Porth, C. M. (2011). *Essentials of Pathophysiology: Concepts of Altered Health States* (3rd edn). Philadelphia: Lippincott Williams & Wilkins.

Porth, C. M. (2009). *Pathophysiology: Concepts of Altered Health States* (8th edn). Philadelphia: Lippincott Williams & Wilkins.

Rosenstein, N., Phillips, W. R., Gerber, M. A., Marcy, S. M., Schwartz, B. & Dowell, S. F. (1998). The common cold—Principles of judicious use of antimicrobial agents. *Pediatrics, 100*, 181–184.

Turnidge, J. (2010). Multiresistant organisms at the front line. *Australian Prescriber, 33(3)*, 68–71.

CHECK YOUR UNDERSTANDING

Answers to the questions in this chapter can be found in Appendix A at the back of this book.

MULTIPLE CHOICE

Select the best answer to the following.

1. A bacteriostatic substance is one that:
   a. directly kills any bacteria it comes in contact with.
   b. directly kills any bacteria that are sensitive to the substance.
   c. prevents the growth of any bacteria.
   d. prevents the growth of specific bacteria that are sensitive to the substance.
2. Gram-negative bacteria:
   a. are mostly found in the respiratory tract.
   b. are mostly associated with soft tissue infections.
   c. are mostly found in the GI and GU tracts.
   d. accept a positive stain when tested.

3. Antibiotics that are used together to increase their effectiveness and limit the associated adverse effects are said to be:
   a. broad-spectrum.
   b. synergistic.
   c. bactericidal.
   d. anaerobic.

4. An aminoglycoside antibiotic might be the drug of choice in treating:
   a. serious infections caused by susceptible strains of Gram-negative bacteria.
   b. otitis media in an infant.
   c. cystitis in a woman who is 4 months pregnant.
   d. suspected pneumonia before the culture results are available.

5. Which of the following is not a caution for the use of cefalosporins?
   a. allergy to penicillin
   b. renal failure
   c. allergy to aspirin
   d. concurrent treatment with aminoglycosides

6. The fluoroquinolones:
   a. are found freely in nature.
   b. are associated with severe adverse reactions.
   c. are widely used to treat Gram-positive infections.
   d. are broad-spectrum antibiotics with few associated adverse effects.

7. Ciprofloxacin, a widely used antibiotic, is an example of:
   a. a penicillin.
   b. a fluoroquinolone.
   c. an aminoglycoside.
   d. a macrolide antibiotic.

8. A person receiving a fluoroquinolone should be cautioned to anticipate:
   a. increased salivation.
   b. constipation.
   c. photosensitivity.
   d. cough.

9. The goal of antibiotic therapy is:
   a. to eradicate all bacteria from the system.
   b. to suppress resistant strains of bacteria.
   c. to reduce the number of invading bacteria so that the immune system can deal with the infection.
   d. to stop the drug as soon as the person feels better.

10. The penicillins:
    a. are bacteriostatic.
    b. are bactericidal, interfering with bacteria cell walls.
    c. are effective only if given intravenously.
    d. do not produce cross-sensitivity within their class.

MULTIPLE RESPONSE

Select all that apply.

1. A young woman is found to have a soft tissue infection that is most responsive to doxycycline. Your teaching plan for this woman should include which of the following points?
   a. Doxycycline can cause grey baby syndrome.
   b. Do not use this drug if you are pregnant because it can cause tooth and bone defects in the fetus.
   c. Doxycycline can cause severe acne.
   d. You should use a second form of contraception if you are using oral contraceptives because doxycycline can make them ineffective.
   e. This drug should be taken in the middle of a meal to decrease GI upset.
   f. You may experience a vaginal yeast infection as a result of this drug therapy.

2. In general, all people receiving antibiotics should receive teaching that includes which of the following points?
   a. the need to complete the full course of drug therapy
   b. the possibility of oral contraceptive failure
   c. when to take the drug related to food and other drugs
   d. the need for assessment of blood tests
   e. advisability of saving any leftover medication for future use
   f. how to detect superinfections and what to do if they occur

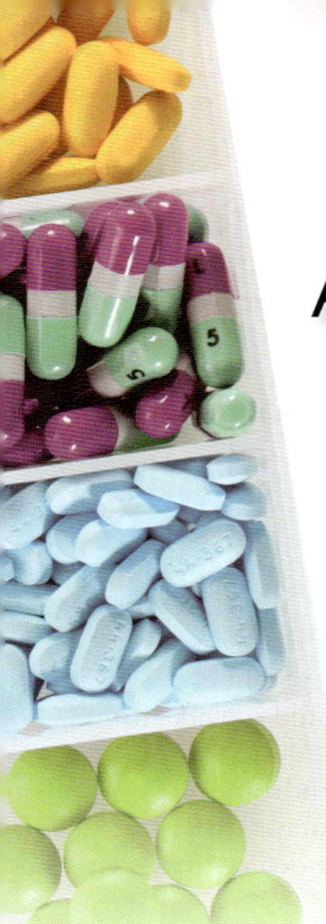

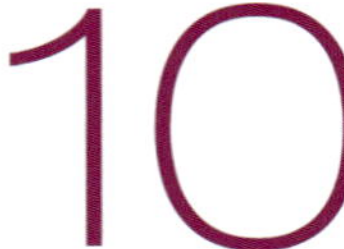

Antiviral agents

Learning objectives

On completing this chapter you should be able to:

1. Discuss problems with treating viral infections in humans and the use of antiviral agents across the lifespan.
2. Describe characteristics of common viruses and the resultant clinical presentations of common viral infections.
3. Describe the therapeutic actions, indications, pharmacokinetics, contraindications, most common adverse reactions and important drug–drug interactions associated with each of the types of antiviral agents discussed in the chapter.
4. Compare and contrast the prototype drugs for each type of antiviral agent with the other drugs within that group.
5. Outline the care considerations for people receiving each class of antiviral agent.

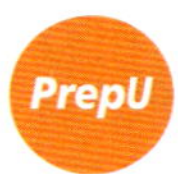

Test your current knowledge of antiviral agents with a PrepU Practice Quiz!

Glossary of key terms

acquired immune deficiency syndrome (AIDS): collection of opportunistic infections and cancers that occurs when the immune system is severely depressed by a decrease in the number of functioning helper T cells; caused by infection with human immunodeficiency virus (HIV)

AIDS-related complex (ARC): collection of less serious opportunistic infections with HIV infection; the decrease in the number of helper T cells is less severe than in fully developed AIDS

CCR5 co-receptor antagonist: a drug that blocks the receptor site the HIV virus needs to interact with in order to enter the cell

cytomegalovirus (CMV): DNA virus that accounts for many respiratory, ophthalmic and liver infections

fusion inhibitor: a drug that prevents the fusion of the HIV-1 virus with the human cellular membrane, preventing it from entering the cell

helper T cell: human lymphocyte that helps to initiate immune reactions in response to tissue invasion

hepatitis B: a serious to potentially fatal viral infection of the liver, transmitted by body fluids

herpes: DNA virus that accounts for many diseases, including shingles, cold sores, genital herpes and encephalitis

human immunodeficiency virus (HIV): retrovirus that attacks helper T cells, leading to a decrease in immune function and AIDS or ARC

influenza A: RNA virus that invades tissues of the respiratory tract, causing the signs and symptoms of the common cold or 'flu'

integrase inhibitor: a drug that inhibits the activity of the virus-specific enzyme integrase, an encoded enzyme needed for viral replication, blocking this enzyme prevents the formation of the HIV-1 provirus

interferon: tissue hormone that is released in response to viral invasion; blocks viral replication

non-nucleoside reverse transcriptase inhibitors: drugs that bind to sites on the reverse transcriptase, preventing RNA and DNA-dependent DNA polymerase activities needed to carry out the viral DNA synthesis; prevents the transfer of information that allows the virus to replicate and survive

nucleoside reverse transcriptase inhibitors: drugs that prevent the growth of the viral DNA chain, preventing it from inserting into the host DNA, so viral replication cannot occur

protease inhibitors: drugs that block the activity of the enzyme protease in HIV; protease is essential for the maturation of infectious virus, and its absence leads to the formation of an immature and non-infective HIV particle

virus: particle of DNA or RNA surrounded by a protein coat that survives by invading a cell to alter its functioning

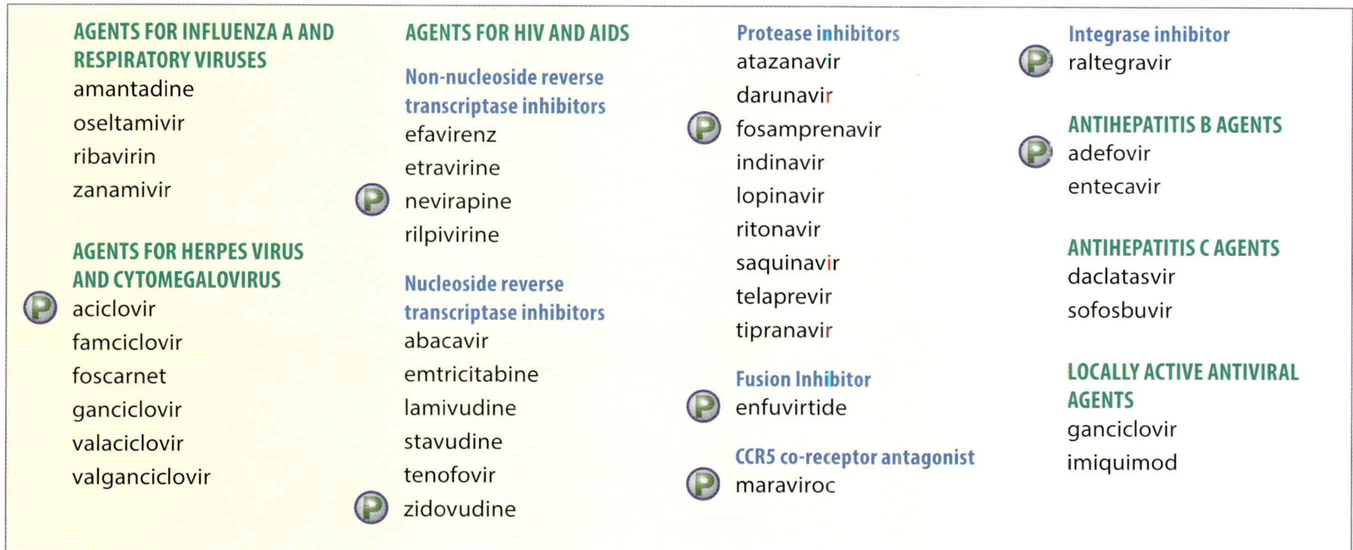

AGENTS FOR INFLUENZA A AND RESPIRATORY VIRUSES
amantadine
oseltamivir
ribavirin
zanamivir

AGENTS FOR HERPES VIRUS AND CYTOMEGALOVIRUS
aciclovir
famciclovir
foscarnet
ganciclovir
valaciclovir
valganciclovir

AGENTS FOR HIV AND AIDS

Non-nucleoside reverse transcriptase inhibitors
efavirenz
etravirine
nevirapine
rilpivirine

Nucleoside reverse transcriptase inhibitors
abacavir
emtricitabine
lamivudine
stavudine
tenofovir
zidovudine

Protease inhibitors
atazanavir
darunavir
fosamprenavir
indinavir
lopinavir
ritonavir
saquinavir
telaprevir
tipranavir

Fusion Inhibitor
enfuvirtide

CCR5 co-receptor antagonist
maraviroc

Integrase inhibitor
raltegravir

ANTIHEPATITIS B AGENTS
adefovir
entecavir

ANTIHEPATITIS C AGENTS
daclatasvir
sofosbuvir

LOCALLY ACTIVE ANTIVIRAL AGENTS
ganciclovir
imiquimod

Viruses cause a variety of conditions, ranging from warts, to the common cold and 'flu', to diseases such as chickenpox and measles. A single virus particle is composed of a piece of DNA or RNA inside a protein coat. To carry on any metabolic processes, including replication, a virus must enter a cell. After a virus has fused with a cell wall and injected its DNA or RNA into the host cell, that cell is altered – that is, it is 'programmed' to control the metabolic processes that the virus needs to survive. The virus, including the protein coat, replicates in the host cell (Figure 10.1). When the host cell can no longer carry out its own metabolic functions because of the viral invader, the host cell dies and releases the new viruses into the body to invade other cells.

Because viruses are contained inside human cells while they are in the body, researchers have difficulty developing effective drugs that destroy a virus without harming the human host. **Interferons** (see Chapter 15) are released by the host in response to viral invasion of a cell and act to prevent the replication of that particular virus. Some interferons that affect particular viruses can now be genetically engineered to treat particular

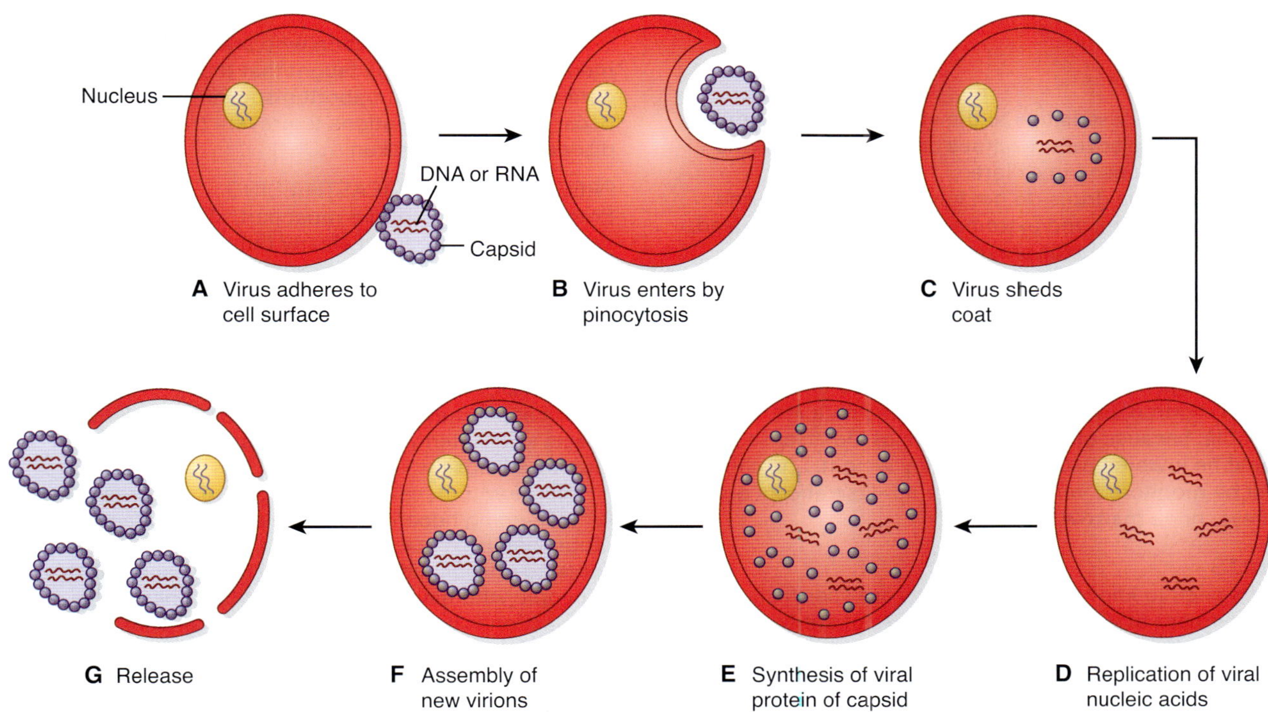

FIGURE 10.1 The stages in the replication cycle of a virus.

viral infections. Other drugs that are used in treating viral infections are not natural substances and have been effective against only a limited number of viruses. Viruses that respond to some antiviral therapy include influenza A and some respiratory viruses, herpes viruses, cytomegalovirus (CMV), the human immunodeficiency virus (HIV) that causes acquired immune deficiency syndrome (AIDS), hepatitis B, and some viruses that cause warts and certain eye infections. People need to be cautioned against using certain complementary and alternative therapies while on antiviral medication (Box 10.1). Box 10.2 discusses the use of antivirals across the lifespan. Figures 10.2 and 10.3 show sites of action for these agents.

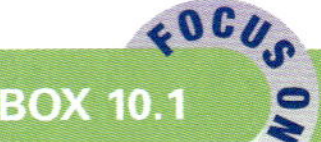

BOX 10.1 Herbal and alternative therapies

Alternative therapies and antiviral drugs

An increasing number of people are using alternative therapies as part of their daily regimen. St John's wort is one of the more popular alternative therapies sold today. This herb has been used as an anti-inflammatory agent, as an antidepressant, as a diuretic, and as a treatment for gastritis and insomnia.

St John's wort is promoted as being able to increase one's sense of wellbeing and to decrease depression. Many people with viral infections just do not feel well. They are tired, have muscle aches and pains, and feel feverish and low on energy. This herbal remedy seems to be aimed at these people.

Unfortunately, St John's wort has been shown to interact with many prescription drugs. When taken with St John's wort, the protease inhibitors used in treating HIV were found to have decreased serum levels, leading to possible treatment failure. Because St John's wort may induce the cytochrome P450 system in the liver, there is a possibility that it could increase the metabolism of many other antiviral drugs that are metabolised by that system and cause treatment failures with those drugs.

People may be reluctant to discuss their use of alternative therapies with the health care provider because they want to maintain control over that aspect of their medical regimen or because they believe that the health care provider would not approve of the use of these therapies. It is important, when a person is prescribed an antiviral agent, to ask specifically about the use of herbal or alternative medicines. Explain to the person that antiviral drugs may interact with some herbal medicines and that it is important to try to avoid any adverse effects or drug failures.

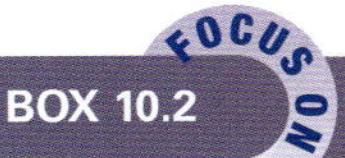

BOX 10.2 Drug therapy across the lifespan

Antivirals

CHILDREN

Children are very sensitive to the effects of most antiviral drugs and more severe reactions can be expected when these drugs are used in children.

Many of these drugs do not have proven safety and efficacy in children, and extreme caution should be used.

Most of the drugs for prevention and treatment of influenza virus infections can be used, in smaller doses, for children.

Aciclovir is the drug of choice for children with herpes virus or cytomegalovirus infections.

The drugs used in the treatment of AIDS are frequently used in children, even when no scientific data are available, because of the seriousness of the disease. Dose should be lowered according to body weight, and children must be monitored very closely for adverse effects on kidneys, bone marrow and liver.

ADULTS

Adults need to know that these drugs are specific for the treatment of viral infections. The use of antibiotics to treat such infections can lead to the development of resistant strains and superinfections that can cause more problems.

People with HIV infection who are taking antiviral medications need to be taught that these drugs do not cure the disease, that opportunistic infections can still occur and that precautions to prevent transmission of the disease need to be taken.

PREGNANCY AND BREASTFEEDING

Pregnant women, for the most part, should not use these drugs unless the benefit clearly outweighs the potential risk to the fetus or neonate. Women of childbearing age should be advised to use barrier contraceptives if they take any of these drugs. Zidovudine has been safely used in pregnant women.

OLDER ADULTS

Older people may be more susceptible to the adverse effects associated with these drugs; they should be monitored closely.

People with hepatic dysfunction are at increased risk for worsening hepatic problems and toxic effects of those drugs that are metabolised in the liver. Drugs that are excreted unchanged in the urine can be especially toxic to people who have renal dysfunction. If hepatic or renal dysfunction is expected (extreme age, alcohol abuse, use of other hepatotoxic or nephrotoxic drugs), the dose may need to be lowered and the person should be monitored more frequently.

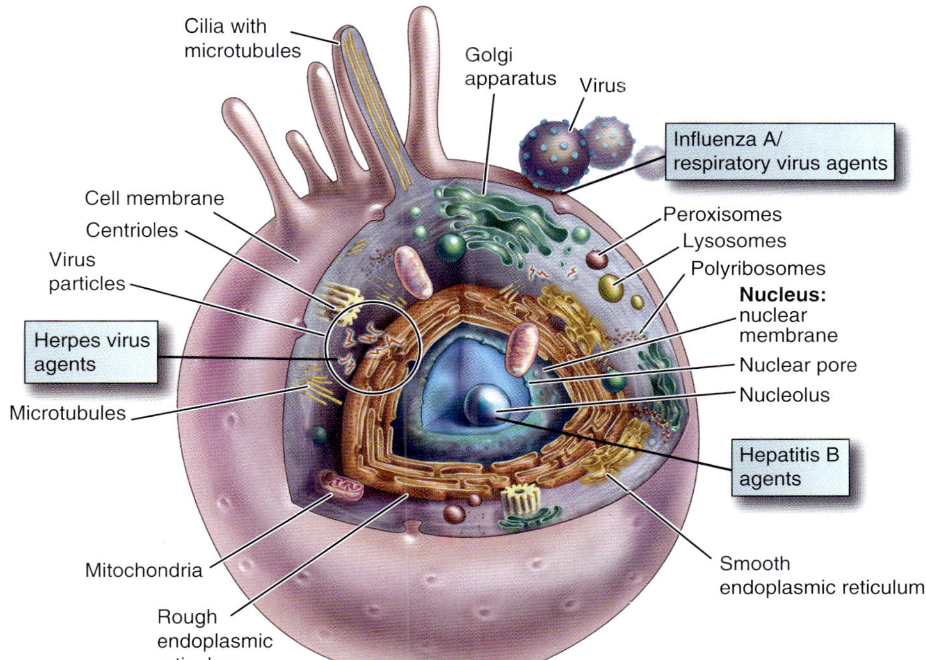

FIGURE 10.2 Agents for treating influenza A and respiratory viruses prevent shedding of the protein coat and entry of virus into the cell. Herpes virus agents alter viral DNA production. Anti–hepatitis B agents block DNA formation, preventing the formation of new viruses.

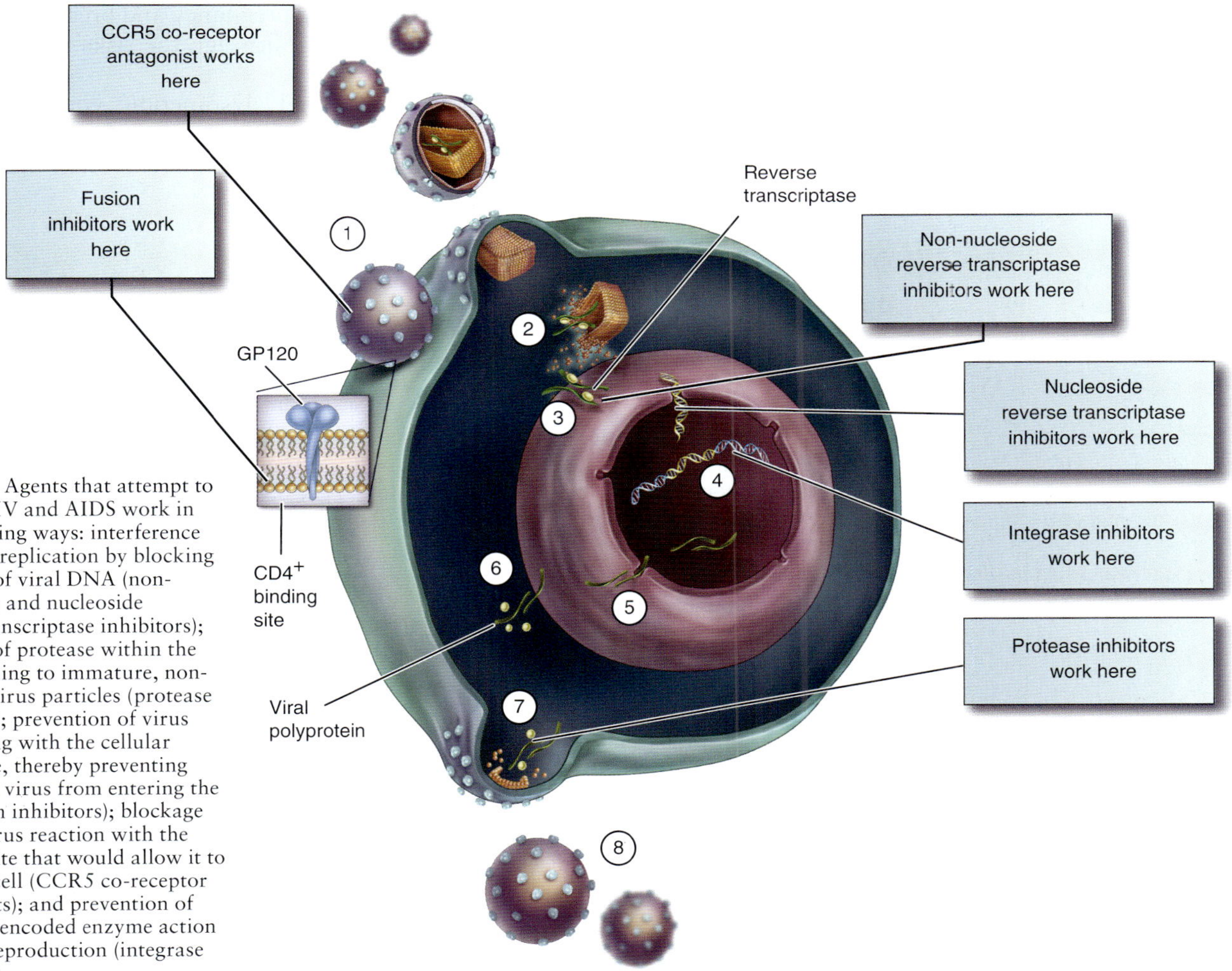

FIGURE 10.3 Agents that attempt to control HIV and AIDS work in the following ways: interference with HIV replication by blocking synthesis of viral DNA (non-nucleoside and nucleoside reverse transcriptase inhibitors); blockage of protease within the virus, leading to immature, non-infective virus particles (protease inhibitors); prevention of virus from fusing with the cellular membrane, thereby preventing the HIV-1 virus from entering the cell (fusion inhibitors); blockage of HIV virus reaction with the receptor site that would allow it to enter the cell (CCR5 co-receptor antagonists); and prevention of necessary encoded enzyme action for viral reproduction (integrase inhibitors).

AGENTS FOR INFLUENZA A AND RESPIRATORY VIRUSES

Influenza A and other respiratory viruses, including influenza B and respiratory syncytial virus (RSV), invade the respiratory tract and cause the signs and symptoms of respiratory 'flu'. Vaccines have been developed (see Chapter 18) to stimulate immunity against influenza A and RSV. Preventing the viral infection is the best option, but if people do develop a viral infection, some drug therapies are available. Agents for influenza A and respiratory viruses include amantadine (*Symmetrel*), oseltamivir (*Tamiflu*), ribavirin (*Virazide*) and zanamivir (*Relenza*). These drugs are described in detail in Table 10.1.

Therapeutic actions and indications

The exact mechanism of action of drugs that combat influenza A and respiratory viruses is not known. The belief is that these agents prevent shedding of the viral protein coat and entry of the virus into the cell (Figure 10.2). This action prevents viral replication, causing viral death. These agents for influenza A and respiratory viruses are especially important for health care workers and other high-risk individuals and for reducing the severity of infection if it occurs. See Table 10.1 for usual indications specific to each antiviral drug. Oseltamivir is the only antiviral agent that has been shown to be effective in treating avian flu.

Pharmacokinetics

Amantadine is slowly absorbed from the gastrointestinal (GI) tract, reaching peak levels in 4 hours. Excretion occurs unchanged through the urine, with a half-life of 15 hours. Oseltamivir is readily absorbed from the GI tract, extensively metabolised in the urine and excreted in the urine with a half-life of 6–10 hours.

Ribavirin, an inhaled drug, is slowly absorbed through the respiratory tract. It is metabolised at the cellular level and is excreted in the faeces and urine with a half-life of 9.5 hours. It is teratogenic and is rated pregnancy category X.

Zanamivir must be delivered by a Diskhaler device, which comes with every prescription. It is absorbed through the respiratory tract and excreted unchanged in the urine with a half-life of 2.5–5.1 hours.

Contraindications and cautions

Because of its renal clearance, amantadine must be used at reduced doses and with caution in people who have any renal impairment *to avoid altered metabolism and excretion of the drug.* Amantadine is embryotoxic in animals and crosses into breast milk. Therefore, it should be used during pregnancy and breastfeeding only if the benefits clearly outweigh the risks to the fetus or neonate.

People with renal dysfunction who are taking oseltamivir require reduced doses and close monitoring *to avoid altered metabolism and excretion of the drug.*

TABLE 10.1 *DRUGS IN FOCUS* Agents for influenza A and respiratory viruses

Drug name	Dosage/route	Usual indications
amantadine (*Symmetrel*)	Adult and paediatric > 10 years: 100 mg PO bd Paediatric 5–9 years: 100 mg PO daily	Treatment of Parkinson's disease; treatment and prevention of respiratory virus infections
oseltamivir (*Tamiflu*)	Adult: 75 mg PO bd for 5 days (treatment); 75 mg/day PO for 7 days (prevention) Paediatric (1–12 years): 30–75 mg bd PO for 5 days (treatment); 30–75 mg/day for 7 days (prevention)	Treatment and prevention of uncomplicated influenza for person who is symptomatic for < 2 days; only antiviral agent effective in treatment of avian flu
ribavirin (*Rebetol, Virazide*)	Adult < 65 kg: 800 mg/day PO; 65–85 kg: 1000 mg/day PO; 86–105 kg 1400 mg/day PO; > 105 kg: 1400 mg/day PO	Used in combination with interferon alfa-2b as an oral drug for the treatment of chronic hepatitis C in children and adults who relapse after interferon-alpha therapy Treatment of influenza A, respiratory syncytial virus (RSV), and herpes virus infections; treatment of children with RSV; has undergone testing for use in several other viral conditions
zanamivir (*Relenza*)	2 inhalations bd for 5 days	Approved in 1999 for treatment and prevention of uncomplicated influenza infections in adults and in children > 7 years of age who have had symptoms for < 2 days

There are no adequate studies in pregnancy and breastfeeding, so oseltamivir should be used during pregnancy and breastfeeding only if the benefits clearly outweigh the risks to the fetus or neonate.

Women of childbearing age should be advised to use barrier contraceptives if they are taking ribavirin. The drug has been associated with serious fetal effects.

Because of the renal excretion, zanamivir must be used cautiously in people with any renal impairment. It should be used during pregnancy and breastfeeding only if the benefits clearly outweigh the risks to the fetus or neonate.

People with renal dysfunction who are taking oseltamivir require reduced doses and close monitoring *to avoid altered metabolism and excretion of the drug.* There are no adequate studies in pregnancy and breastfeeding, so oseltamivir should be used during pregnancy and breastfeeding only if the benefits clearly outweigh the risks to the fetus or neonate.

Women of childbearing age should be advised to use barrier contraceptives if they are taking ribavirin. The drug has been associated with serious fetal effects.

Because of the renal excretion, zanamivir must be used cautiously in people with any renal impairment. It should be used during pregnancy and breastfeeding only if the benefits clearly outweigh the risks to the fetus or neonate.

Adverse events, including bronchospasm and/or decline in respiratory function, some of which have been serious, have been reported in association with the use of *Relenza* during the Northern Hemisphere influenza season. These events have been reported rarely in people with underlying respiratory disease (asthma, chronic obstructive pulmonary disease (COPD)) and have also been reported very rarely in individuals without underlying respiratory disease.

Adverse effects

Use of these antiviral agents is frequently associated with various adverse effects that may be related to possible effects on dopamine levels in the brain. These adverse effects include light-headedness, dizziness and insomnia; nausea; orthostatic hypotension; and urinary retention.

Clinically important drug–drug interactions

People who receive amantadine may experience increased atropine-like effects if this drug is given with an anticholinergic drug. Ribavirin levels may be reduced if given with antacids. The use of ribavirin should be avoided if the person is also receiving a nucleoside reverse transcriptase inhibitor. Rifampicin is known to decrease the effectiveness of many drugs, including antiarrhythmics, digoxin, hormonal contraceptives, corticosteroids, antifungals and central nervous system (CNS) depressants. People should be monitored closely for loss of effectiveness of these drugs if this combination is used. There is an increased incidence of rifampicin-related hepatitis if it is used concurrently with isoniazid. This combination should be avoided.

Care considerations for people receiving agents for influenza A and respiratory viruses

Assessment: history and examination

- Assess for *contraindications or cautions*: known history of allergy to antiviral agents *to avoid hypersensitivity reactions*; history of liver or renal dysfunction *that might interfere with drug metabolism and excretion*; and current status related to pregnancy or breastfeeding.
- Perform a physical assessment to *establish baseline data for evaluating the effectiveness of the drug and the occurrence of any adverse effects associated with drug therapy.*
- Assess for orientation and reflexes *to evaluate any CNS effects of the drug*; vital signs (temperature, respiratory rate, breath sounds for adventitious sounds) *to assess for signs and symptoms of the viral infection;* blood pressure *to monitor for orthostatic hypotension;* urinary output *to monitor genitourinary (GU) effects of the drug;* and renal and liver function tests *to determine baseline function of these organs.*
- Assess for adverse events such as bronchospasm or decline in respiratory function in people using zanamivir and seek medical advice immediately.

Implementation with rationale

- Start the drug regimen as soon after exposure to the virus as possible *to enhance effectiveness and decrease the risk of complications due to viral infection.*
- Administer influenza A vaccine before the flu season begins, if at all possible, *to decrease the risk of contracting the flu and also decrease the risk of complications.*
- Administer the full course of the drug *to obtain the full beneficial effects.*
- Provide safety provisions if CNS effects occur *to protect the person from injury.*
- Instruct the person about the appropriate dosage scheduling regimen; safety precautions, including changing position slowly and avoiding driving and hazardous tasks, that should be taken if CNS effects occur; and the need to report any adverse effects such as difficulty walking or talking *to enhance knowledge about drug therapy and to promote compliance.*

Evaluation

- Monitor person's response to the drug (prevention of respiratory flu-like symptoms; alleviation of flu-like symptoms).
- Monitor for adverse effects (changes in orientation and affect, blood pressure, urinary output).
- Determine the effectiveness of the teaching plan (person can name the drug, dosage, possible adverse effects to watch for and specific measures to help to avoid or minimise adverse effects).
- Monitor the effectiveness of comfort and safety measures and compliance with the regimen.

KEY POINTS

- Viruses are segments of RNA or DNA enclosed in a protein coat.
- A virus must enter a human cell to survive, making it difficult to treat without serious toxic effects for the host.
- Antiviral drugs that prevent the viral replication of respiratory viruses can be used to prevent or treat influenza A or other respiratory viruses.

AGENTS FOR HERPES AND CYTOMEGALOVIRUS

Herpes viruses account for a broad range of conditions, including cold sores, encephalitis, shingles and genital infections. **Cytomegalovirus (CMV)**, although slightly different from the herpes virus, can affect the eye, respiratory tract and liver and reacts to many of the same drugs. Antiviral drugs used to combat these infections include aciclovir (*Zovirax*), famciclovir (*Famvir*), foscarnet (*Foscavir*), ganciclovir (*Cymevene*), valaciclovir (*Shilova*, *Vaclovir*) and valganciclovir (*Valcyte*). See Table 10.2.

Therapeutic actions and indications

Drugs that combat herpes and CMV inhibit viral DNA replication by competing with viral substrates to form shorter, non-effective DNA chains (see Figure 10.2). This action prevents replication of the virus, but it has little effect on the host cells of humans because human cell DNA uses different substrates. These antiviral agents are indicated for treatment of the DNA viruses herpes simplex, herpes zoster and CMV. Research has shown that they are very effective in immunocompromised individuals, such as those with AIDS, those taking immunosuppressants and those with multiple infections. See Table 10.2 for usual indications for each of these agents.

TABLE 10.2 *DRUGS IN FOCUS* Agents for herpes virus and cytomegalovirus (CMV)

Drug name	Dosage/route	Usual indications
(P) aciclovir (*Zovirax, Lovir*)	5–10 mg/kg q 8 hours or 200–800 mg 3–5 times daily for 5–10 days	Treatment of herpes virus infections
famciclovir (*Ezovir, Famvir, Favic*)	Herpes zoster: 250 mg PO q 8 hours for 7 days Genital herpes: 125 mg bd PO for 5 days	Treatment of herpes virus infections such as herpes zoster or shingles and for recurrent episodes of genital herpes
foscarnet (*Foscavir*)	Adult: 40–60 mg/kg q 8–12 hours IV given as a 2 hour infusion Paediatric: safety and efficacy not established	Treatment of CMV and aciclovir-resistant mucocutaneous herpes simplex infections in immunocompromised individuals
ganciclovir (*Cymevene, Vitrasert*)	Adult: 5 m/kg q 12 hours IV given over 1 hour for 14–21 days, then over 1 hour daily 7 days/ week or 6 mg/kg/day for 5 days/week for prophylaxis	Long-term treatment and prevention of CMV infection
valaciclovir (*Shilova, Vaclovir*)	Herpes zoster: 1 g PO tds for 7 days Genital herpes: 500 mg bd PO for 5 days	Treatment of herpes zoster and recurrent genital herpes; cold sores (herpes labialis)
valganciclovir (*Valcyte*)	900 mg PO bd for 21 days, then 900 mg PO once a day for maintenance; reduce dose with renal impairment	Treatment of CMV retinitis in people with AIDS

Pharmacokinetics

Most of the agents for herpes and CMV are readily absorbed in the body and excreted in the urine. Although a former agent in this class, cidofovir (now discontinued) proved to be embryotoxic in animals, no adequate studies have been completed for the other agents.

Aciclovir, which can be given orally and parenterally or applied topically, reaches peak levels within 1 hour and has a half-life of 2.5–5 hours. It is excreted unchanged in the urine. It crosses into breast milk, which exposes the neonate to high levels of the drug.

Famciclovir, an oral drug, is well absorbed from the GI tract, reaching peak levels in 2–3 hours. Famciclovir is metabolised in the liver and excreted in the urine and faeces. It has a half-life of 2 hours and is known to cross the placenta.

Foscarnet is available in IV form only. It reaches peak levels at the end of the infusion and has a half-life of 4 hours. About 90% of foscarnet is excreted unchanged in the urine, making it highly toxic to the kidneys. Use caution and at reduced dose in individuals with renal impairment.

Ganciclovir is available in IV and oral forms. It has a slow onset and reaches peak levels at 1 hour if given IV and 2–4 hours if given orally. This drug is primarily excreted unchanged in the faeces with some urinary excretion, with a half-life of 2–4 hours.

Valaciclovir is an oral agent and is rapidly absorbed from the GI tract and metabolised in the liver to aciclovir. Excretion occurs through the urine, so caution should be used in individuals with renal impairment.

Valganciclovir is the oral prodrug, that is, it is immediately converted to ganciclovir once it is in the body. It is rapidly absorbed and reaches peak levels in 3 hours. It is primarily excreted unchanged in the faeces with some urinary excretion, with a half-life of 2.5–3 hours.

Contraindications and cautions

Drugs indicated for the treatment of herpes and CMV are highly toxic and should not be used during pregnancy or breastfeeding, *to prevent adverse effects on the fetus or infant*; use only if the benefits clearly outweigh the potential risks to the fetus or infant. Avoid use in people with known allergies to antiviral agents *to prevent serious hypersensitivity reactions*; in individuals with renal disease, *which could interfere with excretion of the drug*; or in people with severe CNS disorders *because the drug can affect the CNS, causing headache, neuropathy, paraesthesias, confusion and hallucinations*.

For famciclovir, safety of use in children younger than 18 years of age has not been established.

Foscarnet has been shown to affect bone development and growth. Foscarnet, as well as ganciclovir and valganciclovir, should not be used in children unless the benefit clearly outweighs the risk and the child is monitored very closely.

Adverse effects

The adverse effects most commonly associated with these antiviral agents include nausea and vomiting, headache, depression, paraesthesias, neuropathy, rash and hair loss. Rash, inflammation and burning often occur at sites of IV injection and topical application. Renal dysfunction and renal failure also have been reported. Ganciclovir and valganciclovir have been associated with bone marrow suppression. Foscarnet has been associated with seizures, especially in individuals with electrolyte imbalance.

Clinically important drug–drug interactions

The risk of nephrotoxicity increases when agents indicated for the treatment of herpes and CMV are used in combination with other nephrotoxic drugs, such as the aminoglycoside antibiotics.

The risk of drowsiness also rises when these antiviral agents are taken with zidovudine, an antiretroviral agent.

P Prototype summary: aciclovir

Indications: treatment of herpes simplex virus (HSV) 1 and 2 infections; treatment of severe genital HSV infections; treatment of HSV encephalitis; acute treatment of shingles and chickenpox; ointment for the treatment of genital herpes infections; cream for the treatment of cold sores (herpes labialis).

Actions: inhibits viral DNA replication.

Pharmacokinetics:

Route	Onset	Peak	Duration
Oral	Varies	1.5–2 hours	Not known
IV	Immediate	1 hour	8 hour
Topical	Not generally absorbed systemically		

$T_{1/2}$: 2.5–5 hours; excreted unchanged in the urine.

Adverse effects: headache, vertigo, tremors, nausea, vomiting, rash.

Care considerations for people receiving agents for herpes virus and cytomegalovirus

Assessment: history and examination

- Assess people receiving DNA-active antiviral agents for *contraindications or cautions*: any history of allergy to antiviral agents *to avoid hypersensitivity reactions*; renal dysfunction *that might interfere with the metabolism and excretion of the drug and increase the risk of renal toxicity*; severe CNS disorders *that could be aggravated*; and pregnancy or breastfeeding.
- Perform a physical assessment *to establish baseline data for assessing the effectiveness of the DNA-active antiviral drug and the occurrence of any adverse effects associated with drug therapy.*
- Assess orientation and reflexes *to monitor CNS baseline and adverse effects of the drug.*
- Examine skin (colour, temperature and lesions) *to monitor adverse effects such as rashes.*
- Evaluate renal function tests *to determine baseline function of the kidneys and to assess adverse effects on the kidney and need to adjust the dose of the drug.*

Implementation with rationale

- Administer the drug as soon as possible after the diagnosis has been made *to improve effectiveness of the antiviral activity.*
- Ensure good hydration *to decrease the toxic effects on the kidneys.*
- Ensure that the person takes the complete course of the drug regimen *to improve effectiveness and decrease the risk of the emergence of resistant viruses.*
- Wear protective gloves when applying the drug topically *to decrease the risk of exposure to the drug and inadvertent absorption.*
- Provide safety precautions (eg, use of side rails, appropriate lighting, orientation, assistance) if CNS effects occur *to protect the person from injury.*
- Warn the person that GI upset, nausea and vomiting can occur *to prevent undue anxiety and increase awareness of the importance of nutrition.*
- Monitor renal function tests periodically during treatment *to ensure prompt detection and early intervention if renal toxicity develops.*
- Instruct the person about the drug *to enhance knowledge about drug therapy and to promote compliance.*
- Provide the following teaching:
  - Avoid sexual intercourse if genital herpes is being treated because these drugs do not cure the disease.
  - Wear protective gloves when applying topical agents.
  - Avoid driving and hazardous tasks if dizziness or drowsiness occurs.

Evaluation

- Monitor person's response to the drug (alleviation of signs and symptoms of herpes or CMV infection).
- Monitor for adverse effects (orientation and affect, GI upset and renal function).
- Evaluate the effectiveness of the teaching plan (person can name the drug, dosage, possible adverse effects to watch for and specific measures to help avoid adverse effects).
- Monitor the effectiveness of comfort and safety measures and compliance with the regimen.

KEY POINTS

- Drugs that interfere with viral DNA replication are used to treat herpes infections and CMV infections.
- Antiviral drugs are associated with GI upset and nausea, confusion, insomnia and dizziness.

AGENTS FOR HIV AND AIDS

The **human immunodeficiency virus** (**HIV**) attacks the **helper T cells** (CD4 cells) within the immune system. This virus (an RNA strand) enters the helper T cell, where it uses reverse transcriptase to copy the RNA and produce a double-stranded viral DNA. The virus uses various nucleosides found in the cell to synthesise this DNA strand. The DNA enters the host cell nucleus and slides into the chromosomal DNA to change the cell's processes to ones that produce new viruses. This changes the cell into a virus-producing cell. As a result, the cell loses its ability to perform normal immune functions. The newly produced viruses mature through the action of various proteases and then are released from the cell. On release, they find a new cell to invade, and the process begins again. Eventually, as more and more viruses are released and invade more CD4 cells, the immune system loses an important mechanism responsible for propelling the immune reaction into full force when the body is invaded.

Loss of T cell function causes **acquired immune deficiency syndrome** (**AIDS**) and **AIDS-related complex** (**ARC**), diseases that are characterised by the emergence of a variety of opportunistic infections and cancers that occur when the immune system is depressed and unable to function properly. The HIV mutates over time, presenting a slightly different configuration with each new generation. Treatment of AIDS and ARC has been difficult for two reasons: (1) the length of time the virus can remain dormant within the T cells (i.e. months to years), and (2) the adverse effects of many potent drugs, which may include further depression of the immune system.

A combination of several different antiviral drugs is used to attack the virus at various points in its life cycle to achieve maximum effectiveness with the least amount of toxicity. The types of antiviral agents that are used to treat HIV infections are the non-nucleoside and nucleoside reverse transcriptase inhibitors, the protease inhibitors and three newer classes of drugs – the **fusion inhibitors**, **CCR5 co-receptor antagonists**, and **integrase inhibitors** (Table 10.3). Collectively, these drugs are known as antiretroviral agents. The HIV virus poses a serious health risk. The person and the family of the person diagnosed with HIV infection will need tremendous support and teaching to cope with the disease and its treatment. See Box 10.3 for public education information regarding AIDS.

NON-NUCLEOSIDE REVERSE TRANSCRIPTASE INHIBITORS

The non-nucleoside reverse transcriptase inhibitors have direct effects on the HIV virus activities within the cell. The non-nucleoside reverse transcriptase inhibitors available include efavirenz (*Stocrin*) and nevirapine (*Viramune*).

Therapeutic actions and indications

The **non-nucleoside reverse transcriptase inhibitors** bind directly to HIV reverse transcriptase, blocking both RNA and DNA-dependent DNA polymerase activities. They prevent the transfer of information that would allow the virus to carry on the formation of viral DNA. As a result, the virus is unable to take over the cell and reproduce. These antiviral agents are indicated for the treatment of people with documented AIDS or ARC who have decreased numbers of T cells and evidence of increased opportunistic infections in combination with other antiviral drugs (see Table 10.3).

Pharmacokinetics

Efavirenz is absorbed rapidly from the GI tract, reaching peak levels in 3–5 hours. Efavirenz is metabolised in the liver by the cytochrome P450 system and is excreted in the urine and faeces with a half-life of 52–76 hours.

Nevirapine is recommended for use in adults and children older than 2 months. After rapid GI absorption with a peak effect occurring at 4 hours, nevirapine is metabolised by the cytochrome P450 system in the liver. Excretion is through the urine with a half-life of 45 hours.

Contraindications and cautions

There are no adequate studies of non-nucleoside reverse transcriptase inhibitors in pregnancy, so use should be limited to situations in which the benefits clearly outweigh any risks.

Adverse effects

The adverse effects most commonly experienced with these drugs are GI related – dry mouth, constipation or diarrhoea, nausea, abdominal pain and dyspepsia. Dizziness, blurred vision and headache have also been reported. A flu-like syndrome of fever, muscle aches and pains, fatigue and loss of appetite often occurs with the anti-HIV drugs, but these signs and symptoms may also be related to the underlying disease.

Clinically important drug–drug interactions

There is a risk of serious adverse effects if efavirenz is combined with midazolam, rifabutin, triazolam or ergot derivatives; these combinations should be avoided. There may be a lack of effectiveness if nevirapine is combined with hormonal contraceptives or protease inhibitors. St John's wort should not be used with these drugs; a decrease in antiviral effects can occur.

Prototype summary: nevirapine

Indications: treatment of HIV-1–infected people who have experienced clinical or immunological deterioration, in combination with other antiretrovirals.

Actions: binds to HIV-1 reverse transcriptase and blocks replication of the HIV by changing the structure of the HIV enzyme.

Pharmacokinetics:

Route	Onset	Peak
Oral	Rapid	4 hours

$T_{1/2}$: 45 hours, then 25–30 hours; metabolised in the liver and excreted in the urine.

Adverse effects: headache, nausea, vomiting, diarrhoea, rash, liver dysfunction, chills, fever.

NUCLEOSIDE REVERSE TRANSCRIPTASE INHIBITORS

The **nucleoside reverse transcriptase inhibitors** (Table 10.3) were the first class of drugs developed to

TABLE 10.3 DRUGS IN FOCUS Agents for HIV and AIDS

Drug name	Dosage/route	Usual indications
Non-nucleoside reverse transcriptase inhibitors		
efavirenz (*Stocrin*)	Adult: 600 mg/day PO Paediatric: dose determined by age and weight	Treatment of adults and children with HIV in combination with other antiretroviral agents
etravirine (*Intelence*)	Adult: 200 mg/day PO	Treatment of adults with HIV where viral replication is evident and resistant to other antiretrovirals
(P) nevirapine (*Viramune*)	Adult: 200 mg/day PO for 14 days, then 200 mg PO bd Paediatric: 4 mg/kg PO for 14 days, then 4–7 mg/kg PO bd	Treatment of adults or children with HIV in combination with other antiretroviral agents
rilpivirine (*Edurant*)	Adult: 25 mg/day PO	Treatment of adults with HIV
Nucleoside reverse transcriptase inhibitors		
abacavir (*Ziagen*)	Adult: 300 mg PO bd Paediatric: 8 mg/kg PO bd	Combination therapy for the treatment of adults and children with HIV
emtricitabine (*Emtriva*)	Adult: 200 mg/day PO or 240 mg oral solution/day	Part of combination therapy for treatment of HIV-1 infection
lamivudine (*Combivir, 3TC, Zeffix*)	Adult: 150 mg twice daily or 300 mg once daily PO Paediatric 2–11 years: 3 mg/kg/day PO	With other antiretroviral agents for the treatment of adults and children with HIV; as an oral solution for the treatment of chronic hepatitis B
stavudine (*Zerit*)	Adults > 60 kg: 40 mg PO q 12 hours Adults < 60 kg: 30 mg PO q 12 hours	Treatment of adults with HIV in combination with other antiretroviral agents
tenofovir (*Viread*)	Adult: 300 mg/day PO	Treatment of adults with HIV infection in combination with other antiretroviral drugs
(P) zidovudine [AZT] (*Retrovir*)	Adults ≥ 30 kg: usual dose 500-600 mg/day in 2–5 divided doses	Treatment of symptomatic HIV in adults as part of combination therapy
Protease inhibitors		
atazanavir (*Reyataz*)	Adult: 400 mg/day PO	Treatment of adults with HIV as part of combination therapy
darunavir (*Prezista*)	Adult: 800 mg/day PO Paediatric: no more than 600 mg/day PO with ritonavir 100 mg PO bd	Treatment of adults and children with HIV as part of combination therapy
(P) fosamprenavir (*Telzir*)	Adult: 1400 mg/day PO with 100 mg/day ritonavir PO *or* 700 mg PO bd with ritonavir 100 mg PO bd	Part of combination therapy for the treatment of HIV in adults
indinavir (*Crixivan*)	Adult: 800 mg PO q 8 hours	Treatment of adults with HIV as part of combination therapy
lopinavir (*Kaletra*)	Adult and paediatric > 35 kg: 400 mg PO bd	Treatment of adults and children with HIV in combination with other antiretroviral agents
ritonavir (*Norvir*)	Adult and paediatric (> 2 years): 600 mg PO bd	Part of combination therapy for the treatment of adults and children with HIV
saquinavir (*Invirase*)	1000 mg PO bd with ritonavir 100 mg PO bd	Treatment of adults with HIV as part of combination therapy

TABLE 10.3 DRUGS IN FOCUS Agents for HIV and AIDS *continued*

Drug name	Dosage/route	Usual indications
Protease inhibitors *(continued)*		
tipranavir (*Aptivus*)	Adults: 500 mg PO bd with ritonavir 200 mg PO bd Paediatric > 2 years: 375 mg/m² bd with ritonavir 150 mg/m² bd	Treatment of adults and children with HIV in combination with ritonavir
Fusion inhibitor		
(P) enfuvirtide (*Fuzeon*)	Adult: 90 mg PO bd by SC injection Paediatric 6–16 years: 2 mg/kg bd by SC injection	Part of combination therapy in treatment of people with HIV with evidence of HIV replication despite antiretroviral therapy
CCR5 co-receptor antagonist		
(P) maraviroc (*Celsentri*)	Adult: 150 mg PO bd	Part of combination therapy for treatment of HIV-1 infections
Integrase inhibitor		
(P) raltegravir (*Isentress*)	Adult: 400 mg PO bd	Part of combination therapy for treatment of HIV-1 infections

treat HIV infections. These are drugs that compete with the naturally occurring nucleosides within a human cell that the virus would need to develop. The nucleoside reverse transcriptase inhibitors include the following agents: abacavir (*Ziagen*), emtricitabine (*Emtriva*), lamivudine (*Combivir, 3TC, Zeffix*), stavudine (*Zerit*), tenofovir (*Viread*) and zidovudine (*Retrovir*).

Therapeutic actions and indications

Nucleoside reverse transcriptase inhibitors compete with the naturally occurring nucleosides within the cell that the virus would use to build the DNA chain. These nucleosides, however, lack a substance needed to extend the DNA chain. As a result, the DNA chain cannot lengthen and cannot insert itself into the host DNA. Thus the virus cannot reproduce. They are used as part of combination therapy for the treatment of HIV infection. See Table 10.3 for usual indications for each of these agents.

Pharmacokinetics

Abacavir is an oral drug that is rapidly absorbed from the GI tract. It is metabolised in the liver and excreted in faeces and urine with a half-life of 1–2 hours.

Emtricitabine has the advantage of being a one-capsule-a-day therapy. Emtricitabine has a rapid onset and peaks in 1–2 hours. It has a half-life of 10 hours, and after being metabolised in the liver is excreted in the urine and faeces. Dose needs to be reduced in individuals with renal impairment. It has been associated with severe and even fatal hepatomegaly with steatosis, a fatty degeneration of the liver.

Lamivudine is rapidly absorbed from the GI tract and is excreted primarily unchanged in the urine. It peaks within 4 hours and has a half-life of 5–7 hours. Because excretion depends on renal function, dose reduction is recommended in the presence of renal impairment.

Stavudine is rapidly absorbed from the GI tract, reaching peak levels in 1 hour. Most of the drug is excreted unchanged in the urine, making it important to reduce dose and monitor people carefully in the presence of renal dysfunction. It can be used for adults and children and is only available in an extended-release form, allowing for once-a-day dosing.

Tenofovir is a newer drug that affects the virus at a slightly different point in replication – a nucleotide that becomes a nucleoside. It is used only in combination with other antiretroviral agents. It is rapidly absorbed from the GI tract, reaching peak levels in 45–75 minutes. Its metabolism is not known, but it is excreted in the urine.

Zidovudine was one of the first drugs found to be effective in the treatment of AIDS. It is rapidly absorbed from the GI tract, with peak levels occurring within 30–75 minutes. Zidovudine is metabolised in the liver and excreted in the urine, with a half-life of 1 hour.

Contraindications and cautions

Of the nucleosides, zidovudine is the only agent that has been proven to be safe when used during pregnancy. Of the other agents, there have been no adequate studies in pregnancy, so use should be limited to situations in which the benefits clearly outweigh any risks. Women infected with HIV are urged not to breastfeed. Tenofovir, zidovudine and emtricitabine should be used with caution in the presence of hepatic dysfunction or severe renal impairment. Zidovudine should also be used with caution with any bone marrow suppression.

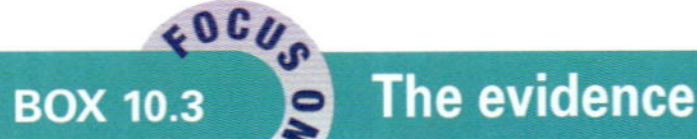

BOX 10.3 The evidence

Public education about AIDS

When AIDS was first diagnosed in the early 1980s, it was found in a certain population in New York City. The people in this group tended to be homosexual, intravenous drug users, and debilitated persons with poor hygiene and nutrition habits.

Originally, a number of health care practitioners thought that the disease was a syndrome of opportunistic infections that occurred in a population with repeated exposures to infections that naturally deplete the immune system. It was not until several years later that the human immunodeficiency virus (HIV) was identified.

Since then, it has been discovered that HIV infection is rampant in many African countries. The infection has also spread throughout Australia and New Zealand in populations that are not homosexual or intravenous drug users and who have good nutrition and hygiene habits. As health care practitioners have learned, HIV is not particular about the body it invades. Once introduced into a body, it infects T cells and causes HIV infection.

The evidence shows that when a person is diagnosed with HIV infection, the health professional faces a tremendous challenge in providing education and support. The person and any significant others should be counselled about the risks of transmission and reassured about ways in which the virus is not transmitted. They will need to learn about drug protocols, T-cell levels, adverse drug effects and anticipated progress of the disease. They also will need consistent support. Many communities have AIDS support groups and other resources that can be very helpful; the health professional can direct the person to these resources as appropriate.

The combinations of drugs that are being used today and the constant development of more drugs make the disease less of a death sentence than it was in the past. The result, however, is that many people must take a large number of pills each day, at tremendous cost and inconvenience. Many people today do live for long periods with HIV infection. An AIDS vaccine is currently being studied and offers hope for preventing this disease in the future.

Public education is key for promoting the acceptance and care of people with HIV infection or AIDS, who need a great deal of support and assistance. Health professionals can be role models for dealing with people with HIV and can provide informal public education whenever the opportunity presents.

Adverse effects

Serious-to-fatal hypersensitivity reactions have occurred with abacavir, and it must be stopped immediately at any sign of a hypersensitivity reaction (fever, chills, rash, fatigue, GI upset, flu-like symptoms).

Emtricitabine has been associated with severe and even fatal hepatomegaly with steatosis.

Severe hepatomegaly with steatosis has been reported with tenofovir, so it must be used with extreme caution in any individual with hepatic impairment or lactic acidosis. People also need to be alerted that the drug may cause changes in body fat distribution, with loss of fat from arms, legs and face and deposition of fat on the trunk, neck and breasts.

Severe bone marrow suppression has occurred with zidovudine.

Clinically significant drug–drug interactions

Clarithromycin tablets reduce the absorption of zidovudine. This can be avoided by separating the administration of zidovudine and clarithromycin by at least two hours. Serum phenytoin levels can be affected by concomitant administration of zidovudine, and close monitoring of phenytoin serum levels is required. The nucleoside analogue ribavirin antagonises the antiviral activity of zidovudine and so concomitant use of this active substance should be avoided. Aspirin, codeine, morphine, methadone, indomethacin, ketoprofen, naproxen, oxazepam, lorazepam, cimetidine, dapsone may alter the metabolism of zidovudine by competitively inhibiting glucuronidation or directly inhibiting hepatic microsomal metabolism. Concomitant treatment with potentially nephrotoxic or myelosuppressive medicinal products (eg, systemic pentamidine, dapsone, pyrimethamine, co-trimoxazole, amphotericin, flucytosine, ganciclovir, interferon, vincristine, vinblastine and doxorubicin) may also increase the risk of adverse reactions to zidovudine. If concomitant therapy is necessary monitor renal function and haematological

Prototype summary: zidovudine

Indications: management of adults with symptomatic HIV infection in combination with other antiretrovirals; prevention of maternal–fetal HIV transmission.

Actions: a thymidine analogue that is activated to a triphosphate form, which inhibits the replication of various retroviruses, including HIV.

Pharmacokinetics:

Route	Onset	Peak
Oral	Varies	30–90 minutes
IV	Rapid	End of infusion

$T_{1/2}$: 30–60 minutes; metabolised in the liver and excreted in the urine.

Adverse effects: headache, insomnia, dizziness, nausea, diarrhoea, fever, rash, bone marrow suppression.

parameters, the dosage of one or more agents should be reduced. There have been reports of severe drowsiness and lethargy if zidovudine is combined with ciclosporin; warn the person to take appropriate safety precautions.

PROTEASE INHIBITORS

The **protease inhibitors** block protease activity within the HIV virus. The protease inhibitors that are available for use include atazanavir (*Reyataz*), darunavir (*Prezista*), fosamprenavir (*Telzir*), indinavir (*Crixivan*), lopinavir (*Kaletra*), ritonavir (*Norvir*), saquinavir (*Invirase*) and tipranavir (*Aptivus*).

Therapeutic actions and indications

Protease is essential for the maturation of an infectious virus; without it, an HIV particle is immature and non-infective, unable to fuse with and inject itself into a cell. All these drugs are used as part of combination therapy for the treatment of HIV infection (see Table 10.3).

Pharmacokinetics

Atazanavir is rapidly absorbed from the GI tract and can be taken with food. After metabolism in the liver, it is excreted in the urine and faeces with a half-life of 6.5–7.9 hours. It is not recommended for people with severe hepatic impairment; for those with moderate hepatic impairment, the dose should be reduced.

Fosamprenavir is rapidly absorbed after oral administration, reaching peak levels in 1.5–4 hours. It is metabolised in the liver and excreted in urine and faeces.

Indinavir is rapidly absorbed from the GI tract, reaching peak levels in 0.8 of an hour. Indinavir is metabolised in the liver by the cytochrome P450 system. It is excreted in the urine with a half-life of 1.8 hours. People with hepatic or renal impairment are at risk for increased toxic effects, necessitating a reduction in dose.

Lopinavir is used as a fixed combination drug that combines lopinavir and ritonavir. The ritonavir inhibits the metabolism of lopinavir, leading to increased lopinavir serum levels and effectiveness. It is readily absorbed from the GI tract, reaching peak levels in 3–4 hours, and undergoes extensive hepatic metabolism by the cytochrome P450 system. Lopinavir is excreted in urine and faeces.

Tipranavir is used for the treatment of HIV infection in adults in combination with 200 mg of ritonavir. It is taken orally with food, two 250 mg capsules each day with the ritonavir. It is slowly absorbed, reaching peak levels in 2.9 hours. It is metabolised in the liver with a half-life of 4.8–6 hours; excretion is through urine and faeces.

Ritonavir is rapidly absorbed from the GI tract, reaching peak levels in 2–4 hours. Ritonavir undergoes extensive metabolism in the liver and is excreted in faeces and urine.

BOX 10.4 Fixed combination drugs for treatment of HIV infection

People who are taking combination drug therapy for HIV infection may have to take a very large number of pills each day. Keeping track of these pills and swallowing such a large number each day can be an overwhelming task. In an effort to improve compliance and make it easier for some of these people, some anti-HIV agents are now available in combination products.

Combivir is a combination of 150 mg lamivudine and 300 mg zidovudine. The person takes one tablet twice a day. Because this is a fixed combination drug, it is not the drug of choice for people who require a dose reduction because of renal impairment or adverse effects that limit dose tolerance.

In 2005, a new combination product was approved to make compliance with an HIV drug regimen easier. *Truvada* (200 mg emtricitabine with 300 mg tenofovir) is a once-a-day tablet. People should be stabilised on each antiviral individually before being switched to the combination form.

The year 2009 saw another combination product, Atripla – 600 mg efavirenz, 200 mg emtricitabine and 300 mg tenofovir – which is recommended for people 18 years of age and older who have already been stabilised on each antiviral individually.

The following combination antivirals are now available:

- atazanavir with cobicistat (Evotaz)
- bictegravir with emtricitabine and tenofovir (Biktarvy)
- darunavir with cobicistat (Prezcobix)
- elbasvir with grazoprevir (Zepatier)
- elvitegravir with cobicistat, emtricitabine and tenofovir (Genvoya)
- emtricitabine with efavirenz and tenofovir (Atripla)
- glecaprevir with pibrentasvir (Maviret)
- lamivudine with zidovudine (Combivir)
- ledipasvir with sofosbuvir (Harvoni)
- sofosbuvir with velpatasvir (Epclusa)
- sofosbuvir with velpatasvir and voxilaprevir (Vosevi)
- tenofovir with emtricitabine (Truvada)
- tenofovir with emtricitabine, cobicistat and elvitegravir (Stribild)
- tenofovir with emtricitabine and rilpivirine (Eviplera)

Saquinavir is slowly absorbed from the GI tract and is metabolised in the liver by the cytochrome P450 mediator, so it must be used cautiously in the presence of hepatic dysfunction. It is primarily excreted in the faeces with a short half-life.

Because therapy for HIV infection involves the use of several different antiviral drugs, many are now available as combination drugs, which reduces the number of tablets a person has to take each day. Box 10.4 discusses combination drugs.

Contraindications and cautions

Of the protease inhibitors listed, saquinavir is the only agent that has not been shown to be teratogenic; however, its use during pregnancy should be limited. Saquinavir crosses into breast milk, and women are advised not to breastfeed while taking this drug. For the other agents, there are no adequate studies in pregnancy, so use should be limited to situations in which the benefits clearly outweigh any risks. It is suggested that women not breastfeed if they are infected with HIV.

People with mild to moderate hepatic dysfunction should receive a lower dose of fosamprenavir, and people with severe hepatic dysfunction should not receive this drug because of its toxic effects on the liver. People receiving tipranavir must have liver function monitored regularly because of the possibility of potentially fatal liver dysfunction. Saquinavir must also be used cautiously in the presence of hepatic dysfunction.

The safety of indinavir for use in children younger than 12 years has not been established.

Adverse effects

As with the other antiviral agents, people taking these drugs often experience GI effects, including nausea, vomiting, diarrhoea, anorexia and changes in liver function. Elevated cholesterol and triglyceride levels may occur. There is often a redistribution of fat to a buffalo hump with thinning of arms and legs. Rashes, pruritus and the potentially fatal Steven–Johnson syndrome have also occurred.

Clinical significant drug–drug interactions

Fosamprenavir should not be used in people who are receiving ritonavir if they have used protease inhibitors to treat their disease, because of a risk of serious adverse effects.

Tipranavir and fosamprenavir have been shown to interact with many other drugs. Before administering these drugs, it is important to check a drug guide to assess for potential interactions with other drugs being given.

Many potentially serious toxic effects can occur when ritonavir is taken with non-sedating antihistamines, sedative/hypnotics or antiarrhythmics because of the activity of ritonavir in the liver. Individuals with hepatic dysfunction are at increased risk for serious effects when taking ritonavir and require a reduced dose and close monitoring.

FUSION INHIBITOR

A new class of drug called a fusion inhibitor (Table 10.3) was introduced in 2003. This agent acts at a different site than do other HIV antiviral agents. The fusion inhibitor prevents the fusion of the virus with the human cellular membrane, which prevents the HIV-1 virus from entering the cell. Enfuvirtide (*Fuzeon*) is used in combination with other antiretroviral agents to treat adults and children older than 6 years who have evidence of HIV-1 replication despite ongoing antiretroviral therapy.

Enfuvirtide is given by subcutaneous injection and peaks in effect in 4–8 hours. After metabolism in the liver, it is recycled in the tissues and not excreted. The half-life of enfuvirtide is 3.2–4.4 hours. Enfuvirtide is contraindicated with hypersensitivity to any component of the drug and in breastfeeding women. It should be used with caution in the presence of lung disease or pregnancy. The drug has been associated with insomnia,

Prototype summary: fosamprenavir

Indications: management of adults with symptomatic HIV infection in combination with other antiretrovirals.

Actions: inhibits protease activity, leading to the formation of immature, non-infectious virus particles.

Pharmacokinetics:

Route	Onset	Peak
Oral	Varies	1.5–4 minutes

$T_{1/2}$: 7.7 hours; metabolised in the liver and excreted in the faeces and urine.

Adverse effects: headache, mood changes, nausea, diarrhoea, fatigue, rash, Stevens–Johnson syndrome, redistribution of body fat (buffalo hump, thin arms and legs).

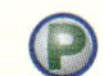

Prototype summary: enfuvirtide

Indications: treatment of HIV-1–infected individuals who have experienced clinical or immunological deterioration after treatment with other agents, in combination with other antiretrovirals.

Actions: prevents the entry of the HIV-1 virus into cells by inhibiting the fusion of the virus membrane with the cellular membrane.

Pharmacokinetics:

Route	Onset	Peak
Subcutaneous	Slow	4–8 hours

$T_{1/2}$: 3.2–4.4 hours; metabolised in the liver, tissues recycle the amino acids, not excreted.

Adverse effects: headache, nausea, vomiting, diarrhoea, rash, anorexia, pneumonia, chills, injection-site reactions.

depression, peripheral neuropathy, nausea, diarrhoea, pneumonia and injection-site reactions. There are no reported drug interactions, but caution should be used when it is combined with any other drug.

CCR5 CO-RECEPTOR ANTAGONIST

In 2007, another new class of drugs was introduced for the treatment of HIV. Maraviroc (*Celsentri*) is a CCR5 co-receptor antagonist. It blocks the receptor site to which the HIV virus needs to interact to enter the cell. It is indicated for the treatment of HIV in adults as part of combination therapy with other antiviral agents. Maraviroc is rapidly absorbed from the GI tract, metabolised in the liver and excreted primarily through the faeces. It has a half-life of 14–18 hours. Maraviroc should not be used with known hypersensitivity to any component of the drug or by breastfeeding women. Caution should be used in the presence of liver disease or co-infection with hepatitis B because of the risk of serious hepatic toxicity. People at increased risk for cardiovascular events or with hypotension should be monitored very closely if this is the drug of choice for them. As with other antiviral agents, it should be used in pregnancy only if the benefit outweighs the potential risk to the fetus.

Severe hepatotoxicity has been reported with this drug, often preceded by a systemic allergic reaction with eosinophilia and rash. Regular monitoring of liver function should be routine when using this drug. CNS effects including dizziness and changes in consciousness have been reported; people experiencing these should be cautioned to take measures to assure safety. People may also be at increased risk of infections because of the way the drug affects the cell membrane of the CD4 cells. Appropriate precautions are necessary.

There is a risk of increased serum levels and toxicity when combined with cytochrome P450 CYP3A inhibitors (ketoconazole, lopinavir/ritonavir, ritonavir, saquinavir, atazanavir), and the maraviroc dose should be adjusted accordingly. Decreased serum levels and loss of effectiveness may occur if maraviroc is combined with CYP3A inducers (rifampicin, efavirenz), and the maraviroc dose should be adjusted accordingly. Individuals should not use St John's wort while on this drug because there is a loss of antiviral effects when the two are combined.

INTEGRASE INHIBITOR

In late 2007, another class of drugs – integrase inhibitors – was introduced to treat HIV infection. The drug raltegravir (*Isentress*) belongs to this class. Raltegravir inhibits the activity of the virus-specific enzyme integrase, an encoded enzyme needed for viral replication. Blocking this enzyme prevents the formation of the HIV-1 provirus and leads to a decrease in viral load and increase in active CD4 cells. It is reserved for use in people who have been treated with other antiviral agents and have evidence of a return to viral replication.

Raltegravir is rapidly absorbed from the GI tract and metabolised in the liver. It has a half-life of 3 hours and is excreted primarily in the faeces.

P Prototype summary: maraviroc

Indications: combination antiretroviral treatment of adults infected with CCR5-tropic HIV-1 who have evidence of viral replication and HIV-1 strains resistant to multiple antiretroviral agents.

Actions: selectively binds to the human chemokine receptor CCR5 on the cell membrane, preventing interaction of HIV-1 and CCR5, which is necessary for the HIV to enter the cell; HIV cannot enter the cell and cannot multiply.

Pharmacokinetics:

Route	Onset	Peak
Oral	Slow	0.5–4 hours

$T_{1/2}$: 14–28 hours; metabolised in the liver, excreted in the faeces and urine.

Adverse effects: dizziness, paraesthesias, nausea, vomiting, diarrhoea, cough, URTI, fever, musculoskeletal symptoms, hepatotoxicity.

Prototype summary: raltegravir

Indications: in combination with other antiviral agents for the treatment of HIV-1 infection in treatment-experienced adults who have evidence of viral replication and HIV-1 strains resistant to multiple antiretroviral agents.

Actions: inhibits the activity of the virus-specific enzyme integrase, an encoded enzyme needed for viral replication. Blocking this enzyme prevents the formation of the HIV-1 provirus and leads to a decrease in viral load and an increase in active CD4 cells.

Pharmacokinetics:

Route	Onset	Peak
Oral	Rapid	3 hours

$T_{1/2}$: 9 hours; metabolised in the liver, excreted in the faeces and urine.

Adverse effects: headache, dizziness, nausea, vomiting, diarrhoea, fever, rhabdomyolysis.

Raltegravir is contraindicated with known hypersensitivity to any component of the drug, as initial treatment in adults, for use in children and for breastfeeding women. Caution should be used if the person is at risk for rhabdomyolysis or myopathy and during pregnancy. People taking this drug must be very careful to continue the drug regimen to help decrease the development of resistant strains of the virus.

Common adverse effects include headache, dizziness and an increase risk for the development of rhabdomyolysis and myopathy. There is a risk of decreased serum levels of raltegravir if it is combined with rifampicin; monitor the person and adjust the dose if this combination must be used. People should avoid the use of St Johns wort, which can interfere with the drug's effectiveness.

Care considerations for people receiving agents for HIV and AIDS

Assessment: history and examination

- Assess for *contraindications and cautions to the use of these drugs*: any history of allergy to antiviral agents *to avoid hypersensitivity reactions*; renal or hepatic dysfunction *that might interfere with the metabolism and excretion of the drug*; and pregnancy or breastfeeding *because of possible adverse effects on the fetus or infant*.
- Perform a physical assessment *to establish baseline data for assessing the effectiveness of the drug and the occurrence of any adverse effects associated with drug therapy*.
- Assess level of orientation and reflexes *to evaluate any CNS effects of the drug*.
- Examine the skin (colour, temperature and lesions) *to monitor for adverse effects of the drug*.
- Check temperature *to monitor for infections*.
- Evaluate hepatic and renal function tests *to determine baseline function of the kidneys and liver*. Check results of a full blood count (FBC) with differential *to monitor bone marrow activity* and T cell number *to determine the severity of the disease and indicate the effectiveness of the drugs*.

Implementation with rationale

- Monitor renal and hepatic function before and periodically during therapy *to detect changes requiring dose adjustments or additional treatment as needed*.
- Ensure that the person takes the complete course of the drug regimen and takes all drugs included in a particular combination *to improve the effectiveness of the drug and decrease the risk of emergence of resistant viral strains*.
- Administer the drug throughout the 24-hour period, if indicated, *to provide the critical concentration needed for the drug to be effective*.
- Monitor nutritional status if GI effects are severe, and take appropriate action *to maintain nutrition, including small frequent meals and balanced nutrition to provide protein and other nutrients*.
- Stop drug if severe rash occurs, especially if accompanied by blisters, fever and other signs, *to avert potentially serious reactions*.
- Provide safety precautions (eg, the use of side rails, appropriate lighting, orientation, assistance) if CNS effects occur, *to protect person from injury*.
- Teach the person about the drugs prescribed *to enhance knowledge about drug therapy and to promote compliance*. Include as a teaching point that these drugs do not cure the disease, so appropriate precautions should still be taken *to prevent transmission*.
- Provide the following teaching:
  - Have regular medical care.
  - Set up a regular schedule for taking all your drugs at the correct time during the day.
  - Have periodic blood tests, which are necessary to monitor the effectiveness and toxicity of the drug.
  - Realise that GI upset, nausea and vomiting may occur but that efforts must be taken to maintain adequate nutrition.
  - Avoid driving and hazardous tasks if dizziness or drowsiness occurs.
  - Report extreme fatigue, severe headache, difficulty breathing or severe rash to a health care provider.

See the Critical thinking scenario for a case study and focused follow-up for the antiviral agents used for HIV and AIDS.

Evaluation

- Monitor the person's response to the drug (alleviation or reduction of signs and symptoms of AIDS or ARC and maintenance of T cell levels).
- Monitor for adverse effects (level of orientation and affect, GI upset, renal and hepatic function, skin, levels of blood components).
- Evaluate the effectiveness of the teaching plan (the person can name the drug, dosage, possible adverse effects to watch for and specific measures to help avoid adverse effects).
- Monitor the effectiveness of comfort and safety measures and compliance with the regimen.

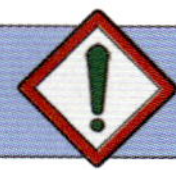

CRITICAL THINKING SCENARIO

Antiviral agents for HIV and AIDS

THE SITUATION

H.P. is a 34-year-old attorney who was diagnosed with AIDS, having had a positive HIV test 3 years ago. Although his T cell count had been stabilised with treatment with zidovudine and efavirenz, it recently dropped remarkably. He presents with numerous opportunistic infections and Kaposi sarcoma. H.P. admits that he has been under tremendous stress at work and at home in the last few weeks. He begins a combination regimen of lamivudine, zidovudine and ritonavir.

CRITICAL THINKING

What are the important care implications in this case?
What role would stress play in the progress of this disease?
What specific issues should be discussed?
What other clinical implications should be considered?

DISCUSSION

Combination therapy with antivirals has been found to be effective in decreasing some of the morbidity and mortality associated with HIV and AIDS. However, this treatment does not cure the disease. H.P. needs to understand that opportunistic infections can still occur and that regular medical help should be sought. He also needs to understand that these drugs do not decrease the risk of transmitting HIV by sexual contact or through blood contamination and he should be encouraged to take appropriate precautions.

It is important to make a dosing schedule for H.P., or even to prepare a weekly medication dispenser, to ensure that all medications are taken as indicated. H.P. should also receive interventions to help him decrease his stress because activation of the sympathetic nervous system during periods of stress depresses the immune system. Further depression of his immune system could accelerate the development of opportunistic infections and decrease the effectiveness of his antiviral drugs. Measures that could be used to decrease stress should be discussed and tried with H.P.

Discussing the adverse effects that H.P. may experience is important because GI upset and discomfort may occur while he is taking all these anti-HIV/AIDS medications. Small frequent meals may help alleviate the discomfort. It is important that every effort be made to maintain H.P.'s nutritional state, and a nutritional consultation may be necessary if GI effects are severe. H.P. also may experience dizziness, fatigue and confusion, which could cause more problems for him at work and may necessitate changes in his workload.

Because some of the prescribed drugs must be taken around the clock, provisions may be needed to allow H.P. to take his drugs on time throughout the day. For example, he may need to wear an alarm wristwatch, establish planned breaks in his schedule at dosing times, or devise other ways to follow his drug regimen without interfering with his work schedule. The adverse effects and inconvenience of taking this many drugs may add to his stress. It is important that a health care provider work consistently with him to help him to manage his disease and treatment as effectively as possible.

CARE GUIDE FOR H.P.: ANTIVIRAL AGENTS FOR HIV AND AIDS

Assessment: history and examination

Allergies to any of these drugs
Bone marrow depression
Renal or liver dysfunction
Skin: colour, lesions, texture
CNS: affect, reflexes, orientation
GI: abdominal and liver evaluation
Haematological: FBC and differential; viral load; T-cell levels; renal and liver function tests

Implementation

Monitor FBC and differential before and every 2 weeks during therapy.
Provide comfort and implement safety measures: assistance, temperature control, lighting control, mouth care, back rubs.
Provide small, frequent meals and monitor nutritional status.
Monitor for opportunistic infections and arrange treatment as indicated.
Provide support and reassurance for dealing with drug effects and discomfort.
Provide teaching regarding drug name, dosage, adverse effects, warnings, precautions, use of OTC or herbal remedies, and signs to report.

Evaluation

Evaluate drug effects: relief of signs and symptoms of AIDS and AIDS-related complex (ARC) and stabilisation of T-cell levels.
Monitor for adverse effects: GI alterations, dizziness, confusion, headache, fever.
Monitor for drug–drug interactions as indicated for each drug.
Evaluate effectiveness of teaching plan.
Evaluate effectiveness of comfort and safety measures.

Teaching for H.P.

A combination of antiviral drugs has been prescribed to treat your HIV infection. These drugs work in combination to stop the replication of HIV, to control AIDS and to maintain the functioning of your immune system. A schedule will be plotted out to show exactly when to take each of the drugs. It is very important that you take all the drugs and that you adhere to this schedule to ensure that the drugs can be effective and reduce the development of resistant strains of the virus.

These drugs are not a cure for HIV, AIDS or ARC. Opportunistic infections may occur and regular medical follow-up should be sought to deal with the disease.

These drugs do not reduce the risk of transmission of HIV to others by sexual contact or by blood contamination; use appropriate precautions.

Common effects of these drugs include:

- *Dizziness, weakness and loss of feeling:* change positions slowly. If you feel drowsy, avoid driving and dangerous activities.
- *Headache, fever, muscle aches:* analgesics may be ordered to alleviate this discomfort. Consult with your health care provider.
- *Nausea, loss of appetite, change in taste:* small, frequent meals may help. It is important to try to maintain good nutrition. Consult your health care provider if this becomes a severe problem.
- Report any of the following to your health care provider: excessive fatigue, lethargy, severe headache, difficulty breathing or skin rash.
- Avoid over-the-counter medications and herbal therapies; many of them interact with your drugs and may make them ineffective. If you feel that you need one of these, check with your health care provider first.
- Schedule regular medical evaluations, including blood tests, which are needed to monitor the effects of these drugs on your body and to adjust doses as needed.
- Tell any doctor, nurse, or other health care provider that you are taking these drugs.
- Keep these drugs and all medications out of the reach of children. Do not share these drugs with other people.

KEY POINTS

- The HIV virus infects helper T cells, leading to a loss of immune function and the development of opportunistic infections.
- Drugs used to treat HIV are usually given in combination to affect the virus at various points in the body: non-nucleoside and nucleoside reverse transcriptase inhibitors block RNA and DNA activity in the cell; protease inhibitors prevent maturation of the virus; fusion inhibitors prevent the entry of the virus into the cell; CCR5 co-receptor antagonists prevent the virus from reacting with the receptor on the cell membrane, preventing its entry into the cell; and integrase inhibitors block an enzyme essential for formation of the provirus within the cell, leading to decrease in the number of viruses.
- People taking drugs to treat HIV need to take all their medications continuously as prescribed and take precautions to prevent the spread of the disease to others.

ANTI-HEPATITIS B AND C AGENTS

Hepatitis B and C are serious-to-potentially fatal viral infections of the liver. The hepatitis B and C virus can be spread by blood or blood products, sexual contact or contaminated needles or instruments. Health care workers are at especially high risk for contracting hepatitis infection due to needlestick injuries. Hepatitis B has a higher mortality than other types of hepatitis. Individuals infected may also develop a chronic condition or become a carrier. In the past, hepatitis B and C were treated with interferons (see Chapter 17). In 2004 and 2005, adefovir (*Hepsera*) and entecavir (*Baraclude*) were approved specifically for treating chronic hepatitis B. More recently, daclatasvir and sofosbuvir have become available specifically for hepatitis C.

Therapeutic actions and indications

Adefovir and entecavir are indicated for the treatment of adults with chronic hepatitis B who have evidence of active viral replication and either evidence of persistent elevations in serum aminotransferases or histologically active disease. The drugs inhibit reverse transcriptase in the hepatitis B virus and cause DNA chain termination, leading to blocked viral replication and decreased viral load (see Table 10.4). Boceprevir and telaprevir block the HCV NS3 serine protease essential for replication of the hepatitis C virus.

Pharmacokinetics

These drugs are rapidly absorbed from the GI tract, with peak effects occurring in 0.5–1.5 hours (entecavir) and 0.5–4 hours (adefovir). Entecavir and adefovir are metabolised in the liver and excreted in the urine. Adefovir has a half-life of 7.5 hours, and entecavir 128–149 hours. It is not known whether any of these drugs crosses the placenta or enters breast milk. Peak effects of boceprevir occur in 2 hours and for telaprevir in 4–5 hours. Telaprevir has a half-life of 4.0–4.7 hours and boceprevir has a half-life of 3.4 hours.

Contraindications and cautions

These drugs are contraindicated with any known allergy to the drugs and with breastfeeding because of potential toxicity to the infant. Use caution when administering these drugs to individuals with renal impairment and severe liver disease and women who are pregnant.

Adverse effects

The adverse effects most frequently seen with these drugs are headache, dizziness, nausea, diarrhoea and elevated liver enzyme levels. Severe hepatomegaly with steatosis, sometimes fatal, has been reported with use of adefovir. Lactic acidosis and renal impairment have been reported with entecavir and adefovir. A potential risk for hepatitis B exacerbation could occur when the drugs are stopped. Therefore, teach people the importance of not running out of their drugs and use extreme caution when discontinuing these drugs.

Clinically important drug–drug interactions

There is an increased risk of renal toxicity if these drugs are taken with other nephrotoxic drugs. If such a combination is used, monitor the person closely. An evaluation of risks versus benefits may be necessary if renal function begins to deteriorate.

Ⓟ Prototype summary: adefovir

Indications: treatment of chronic hepatitis B in adults with evidence of active viral replication and either evidence of persistent elevations in alanine aminotransferase (ALT) and aspartate aminotransferase (AST) or histologically active disease.

Actions: inhibits hepatitis B virus reverse transcriptase, causes DNA chain termination and blocks viral replication.

Pharmacokinetics:

Route	Onset	Peak	Duration
Oral	Rapid	0.6–4 hours	Unknown

$T_{1/2}$: 7.5 hours; excreted in the urine.

Adverse effects: headache, asthenia, nausea, severe-to-fatal hepatomegaly with steatosis, nephrotoxicity, lactic acidosis, exacerbation of hepatitis B when discontinued.

TABLE 10.4 *DRUGS IN FOCUS* Anti-hepatitis B and C agents

Drug name	Dosage/route	Usual indications
Hepatitis B		
Ⓟ adefovir (*Hepsera*)	Adult: 10 mg/day PO Renal impairment: CrCl 30–49 mL/min: 10 mg PO q 48 hours CrCl 10–29 mL/min: 10 mg PO q 72 hours	Treatment of hepatitis B with evidence of active viral replication and persistent elevations in liver enzymes
entecavir (*Baraclude*)	Adults and children (≥ 16 years): 0.5 mg/day; also receiving lamivudine: 1 mg/day Reduce dose with renal impairment	Treatment of chronic hepatitis B in adults with evidence of active viral replication and persistent liver enzyme elevations
Hepatitis C		
daclatasvir	Adult: 60 mg PO once daily for 12–24 weeks 30 mg PO once daily if with concomitant use of potent CYP450 inhibitors 90 mg once daily; with concomitant use of moderate CYP3A4 inducers	Treatment of chronic hepatitis C infection in combination with other antiviral treatment
sofosbuvir	Adult: 400 mg PO once daily	Treatment of chronic hepatitis C infection in combination with other antiviral treatment

CrCl, creatinine clearance.

Care considerations for people receiving anti-hepatitis B or C agents

Assessment: history and examination

- Assess for *contraindications or cautions*: any history of allergy to any of the agents *to avoid hypersensitivity reactions*; renal dysfunction, *which could be exacerbated by the nephrotoxic effects of these drugs*; severe liver impairment, *which could affect the metabolism and exacerbate the liver toxicity of these drugs*; and pregnancy and breastfeeding *because the potential effects of these drugs on the fetus or baby are not known.*
- Perform a physical assessment *to establish baseline data for assessing the effectiveness of these drugs and the occurrence of any adverse effects associated with drug toxicity.*
- Assess body temperature *to monitor underlying disease.*
- Assess level of orientation and reflexes *to assess for CNS changes.*
- Evaluate renal and liver function tests *to monitor for developing toxicity and to determine drug effectiveness.*

Implementation with rationale

- Monitor renal and hepatic function before and periodically during therapy *to detect renal or hepatic function changes and determine the need for possible dose reduction or institute treatment as needed.*
- Withdraw the drug and monitor the person if they develop signs of lactic acidosis or hepatotoxicity *because these adverse effects can be life threatening.*
- Caution person to not stop the medication and to take it continually *because acute exacerbation of hepatitis B or C can occur when the drug is stopped.*
- Advise women of childbearing age to use barrier contraceptives *because the potential adverse effects of this drug on the fetus are not known.*
- Advise women who are breastfeeding to find another method of feeding the baby while using the drug *because the potential toxic effects on the baby are not known.*
- Advise people that these drugs do not cure the disease and there is still a risk of transferring the disease, *so the person should continue to take appropriate steps to prevent transmission of hepatitis B or C.*
- Instruct the person about the drug prescribed *to enhance knowledge about drug therapy and to promote compliance.*
- Provide the following teaching:
  - Have regular blood tests and medical follow-up.
  - Take precautions to maintain a constant supply of the drug, because it must be taken continually, and avoid missing doses.
  - Realise that GI upset, with nausea and diarrhoea, is common with these drugs.
  - Report severe weakness, muscle pain, palpitations, yellowing of the eyes or skin and trouble breathing.

Evaluation

- Monitor response to the drug (decreased viral load of hepatitis B or C).
- Monitor for adverse effects (liver or renal dysfunction, headache, nausea, diarrhoea).
- Evaluate the effectiveness of the teaching plan (person can name the drug, dosage, possible adverse effects to watch for and specific measures to avoid adverse effects).
- Monitor the effectiveness of comfort and safety measures and compliance with the drug regimen.

KEY POINTS

- Hepatitis B and C are serious-to-potentially fatal viral infections of the liver spread by blood or blood products, sexual contact, or contaminated needles or instruments. Hepatitis B has a higher mortality than other types of hepatitis.
- Prevention of infection through use of hepatitis B vaccines and avoiding exposure is essential in stopping the spread of this disease.
- Hepatitis B and C used to be treated only with interferons and rest. Entecavir and adefovir are antivirals now available for the treatment of hepatitis B. Boceprevir and telaprevir are used for the treatment of hepatitis C.

LOCALLY ACTIVE ANTIVIRAL AGENTS

Some antiviral agents are given locally to treat local viral infections. These agents include ganciclovir (*Cymevene*) and imiquimod (*Aldara*).

Therapeutic actions and indications

These antiviral agents act on viruses by interfering with normal viral replication and metabolic processes. They are indicated for specific, local viral infections (see Table 10.5).

TABLE 10.5 DRUGS IN FOCUS Locally active antiviral agents

Drug name	Usual indications
ganciclovir (*Cymevene*)	Implanted for treatment of CMV in people with AIDS
imiquimod (*Aldara*)	Local treatment of genital and perianal warts

Contraindications and cautions

Locally active antiviral drugs are not absorbed systemically, but caution must be used in people with known allergic reactions to any topical drugs.

Adverse effects

Because these drugs are not absorbed systemically, the adverse effects most commonly reported are local burning, stinging and discomfort. These effects usually occur at the time of administration and reduce and disappear over time.

Care considerations for people receiving locally active antiviral agents

Assessment: history and examination

- Assess for history of allergy to antiviral agents *to avoid allergic response to these drugs.*
- Perform a physical assessment *to establish baseline data for evaluating the effectiveness of the drug and the occurrence of any adverse effects associated with drug therapy.*
- Assess the infected area, including location, size and character of lesions.
- Evaluate for signs of inflammation at the site of infection.

Implementation with rationale

- Ensure proper administration of the drug *to improve effectiveness and decrease risk of adverse effects.*
- Stop the drug if severe local reaction occurs or if open lesions occur near the site of administration *to prevent systemic absorption and adverse effects.*
- Instruct the person about the drug being used *to enhance knowledge about drug therapy and to promote compliance.* Include as a teaching point that these drugs do not cure the disease but should alleviate discomfort and prevent damage to healthy tissues.
- Encourage the person to report severe local reaction or discomfort.

Evaluation

- Monitor person's response to the drug (alleviation of signs and symptoms of viral infection).
- Monitor for adverse effects (local irritation and discomfort).
- Evaluate the effectiveness of the teaching plan (the person can name the drug, the dosage, proper administration technique, and adverse effects to watch for and report to a health care provider).
- Monitor the effectiveness of comfort and safety measures and compliance with the regimen.

KEY POINTS

- Some antiviral agents are available only for the local treatment of viral infections, including warts and eye infections.
- Topical antiviral agents should not be applied to open wounds; local reactions can occur with administration.

CHAPTER SUMMARY

- Viruses are particles of DNA or RNA surrounded by a protein coat that survive by injecting their own DNA or RNA into a healthy cell and taking over its functioning.
- Because viruses are contained within human cells, it has been difficult to develop drugs that are effective antiviral agents and yet do not destroy human cells. Antiviral agents are available that are effective against only a few types of viruses.
- Influenza A and respiratory viruses cause the signs and symptoms of the common cold or 'flu'. The drugs that are available to prevent the replication of these viruses are used for prophylaxis against these diseases during peak seasons and to treat disease when it occurs.
- Herpes viruses and CMV are DNA viruses that cause a multitude of problems, including cold sores,

encephalitis, infections of the eye and liver, and genital herpes.

- Helper T cells are essential for maintaining a vigilant, effective immune system. When these cells are decreased in number or effectiveness, opportunistic infections occur. AIDS and ARC are syndromes of opportunistic infections that occur when the immune system is depressed.
- HIV, which specifically attacks helper T cells, may remain dormant in T cells for long periods and has been known to mutate easily.
- Antiviral agents that are effective against HIV and AIDS include non-nucleoside and nucleoside reverse transcriptase inhibitors, protease inhibitors, fusion inhibitors, CCR5 co-receptor antagonists and integrase inhibitors, all of which affect the way the virus communicates, replicates or matures within the cell. These drugs are known as antiretroviral agents. They are given in combination to most effectively destroy the HIV virus and prevent mutation.
- Two drugs are used to treat hepatitis B infection: adefovir and entecavir.

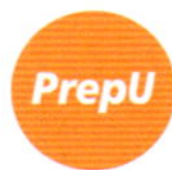

Knowing your strengths and weaknesses helps you to study more effectively. Take a PrepU Practice Quiz to find out how you measure up!

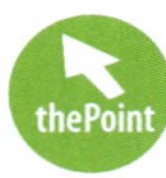

ONLINE RESOURCES

An extensive range of additional resources to enhance teaching and learning and to facilitate understanding of this chapter may be found online at the text's accompanying website, located on thePoint at http://thepoint.lww.com. These include Watch and Learn videos, Concepts in Action animations, journal articles, review questions, case studies, discussion topics and quizzes.

BIBLIOGRAPHY

Australasian Society for HIV Medicine. (2009). *HIV Management in Australasia: A Guide for Clinical Care*. Sydney: Australasian Society for HIV Medicine. www.ashm.org.au/images/Publications/Monographs/HIV_Management_Australasia/HIV-Management-Australia-2009.pdf.

Batey, R. (2006). Managing hepatitis C in the community. *Australian Prescriber, 29*, 36–39.

Bell, S. J. & Nguyen, T. (2009). The management of hepatitis B. *Australian Prescriber, 32*, 99–104.

Boyd, M. & Pett, S. (2008). HIV fusion inhibitors: A review. *Australian Prescriber, 31*, 66–69.

Coery, L., Wald, A., Patel, R., Sacks, S. L., Tyring, S. K., Warren, T., et al. (2004). Once-daily valacyclovir to reduce the risk of transmission of genital herpes. *New England Journal of Medicine 350*, 11–20. Farrell, M. & Dempsey, J. (2014). *Smeltzer & Bare's Textbook of Medical-Surgical Nursing* (3rd edn). Sydney: Lippincott, Williams & Wilkins.

Gilman, A., Hardman, J. G. & Limbird, L. E. (Eds.). (2006). *Goodman and Gilman's the Pharmacological Basis of Therapeutics* (11th edn). New York: McGraw-Hill.

Idemyor, V. (2003). Twenty years since human immunodeficiency virus discovery: Considerations for the next decade. *Pharmacotherapy, 23*, 384–387.

Kaiser, L., Wat, C., Mills, T., Mahoney, P., Ward, P. & Hayden, F. (2003). Impact of oseltamivir treatment on influenza-related lower respiratory tract complications and hospitalizations. *Archives of Internal Medicine, 163*, 1667–1672.

McKenna, L. & Mirkov, S. (2019). *McKenna's Drug Handbook for Nursing and Midwifery* (8th edn). Sydney: Wolters Kluwer Health Australia.

Porth, C. M. (2011). *Essentials of Pathophysiology: Concepts of Altered Health States* (3rd edn). Philadelphia: Lippincott Williams & Wilkins.

Porth, C. M. (2009). *Pathophysiology: Concepts of Altered Health States* (8th edn). Philadelphia: Lippincott Williams & Wilkins.

Wehrhahn, M. C. & Dwyer, D. E. (2012). Herpes zoster: epidemiology, clinical features, treatment and prevention. *Australian Prescriber, 35*, 143–147.

CHECK YOUR UNDERSTANDING

Answers to the questions in this chapter can be found in Appendix A at the back of this book.

MULTIPLE CHOICE

Select the best answer to the following.

1. In assessing a person, a viral cause might be suspected if the person was diagnosed with:
   a. tuberculosis.
   b. leprosy.
   c. the common cold.
   d. gonorrhoea.
2. Virus infections have proved difficult to treat because they:
   a. have a protein coat.
   b. inject themselves into human cells to survive and to reproduce.
   c. are bits of RNA or DNA.
   d. easily resist drug therapy.
3. Naturally occurring substances that are released in the body in response to viral invasion are called:
   a. antibodies.
   b. immunoglobulins.
   c. interferons.
   d. interleukins.

4. Herpes viruses cause a broad range of conditions but have not been identified as the causative agent in:
   a. cold sores.
   b. shingles.
   c. genital infections.
   d. leprosy.

5. Which of the following would be an important teaching point for the person receiving an agent to treat herpes virus or CMV?
   a. Stop taking the drug as soon as the lesions have disappeared.
   b. Sexual intercourse is fine – as long as you are taking the drug, you are not contagious.
   c. Drink plenty of fluids to decrease the drug's toxic effects on the kidneys.
   d. There are few if any associated GI adverse effects.

6. HIV selectively enters which of the following cells:
   a. B clones.
   b. helper T cells.
   c. suppressor T cells.
   d. cytotoxic T cells.

7. Care interventions for the person receiving antiviral drugs for the treatment of HIV probably would include:
   a. monitoring renal and hepatic function periodically during therapy.
   b. administering the drugs just once a day to increase drug effectiveness.
   c. encouraging the person to avoid eating if GI upset is severe.
   d. stopping the drugs and notifying the prescriber if severe rash occurs.

8. Locally active antiviral agents can be used to treat:
   a. HIV infection.
   b. warts.
   c. RSV.
   d. CMV systemic infections.

MULTIPLE RESPONSE

Select all that apply.

1. When explaining to a person the reasoning behind using combination therapy in the treatment of HIV, the nurse or midwife would include which of the following points?
   a. The virus can remain dormant within the T cell for a very long time; they can mutate while in the T cell.
   b. Adverse effects of many of the drugs used to treat this virus include immunosuppression, so the disease could become worse.
   c. The drugs are cheaper if used in combination.
   d. The virus slowly mutates with each generation.
   e. Attacking the virus at many points in its life cycle has been shown to be most effective.
   f. Research has shown that using only one type of drug that targeted only one point in the virus life cycle led to more mutations and more difficulty in controlling the disease.

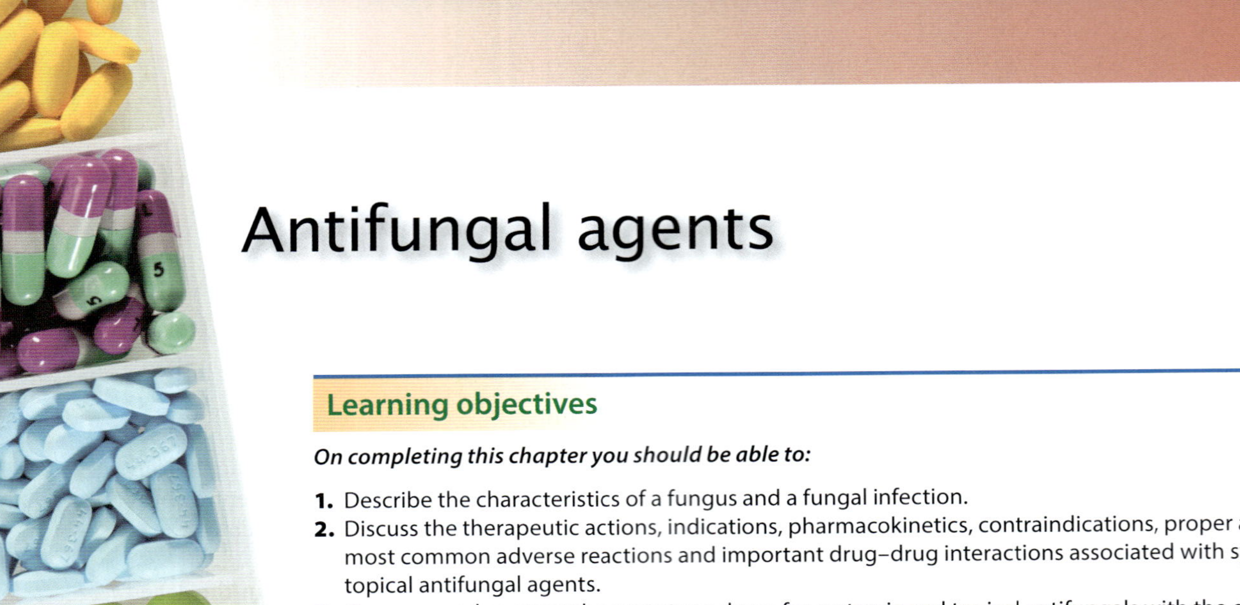

11 Antifungal agents

Learning objectives

On completing this chapter you should be able to:

1. Describe the characteristics of a fungus and a fungal infection.
2. Discuss the therapeutic actions, indications, pharmacokinetics, contraindications, proper administration, most common adverse reactions and important drug–drug interactions associated with systemic and topical antifungal agents.
3. Compare and contrast the prototype drugs for systemic and topical antifungals with the other drugs in each class.
4. Discuss the impact of using antifungal agents across the lifespan.
5. Outline the care considerations for people receiving a systemic or topical antifungal.

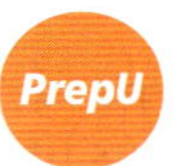

Test your current knowledge of antifungal agents with a PrepU Practice Quiz!

Glossary of key terms

azoles: a group of drugs used to treat fungal infections
***Candida*:** fungus that is normally found on mucous membranes; can cause yeast infections or thrush of the GI tract and vagina in immunosuppressed individuals
ergosterol: steroid-type protein found in the cell membrane of fungi; similar in configuration to adrenal hormones and testosterone
fungus: a cellular organism with a hard cell wall that contains chitin and many polysaccharides, as well as a cell membrane that contains ergosterols
mycosis: disease caused by a fungus
tinea: fungus called ringworm that causes such infections as athlete's foot, jock itch and others

SYSTEMIC ANTIFUNGALS

Azole antifungals
(P) fluconazole
itraconazole
posaconazole
voriconazole

Echinocandin antifungals
anidulafungin
caspofungin

Other antifungals
amphotericin B
flucytosine
griseofulvin
nystatin
terbinafine

TOPICAL ANTIFUNGALS

Azole topical antifungals
(P) clotrimazole
econazole
ketoconazole
miconazole
terbinafine

Other topical antifungals
ciclopirox
tolnaftate
undecenoic acid

Fungal infections in humans range from conditions such as the annoying "athlete's foot" to potentially fatal systemic infections. An infection caused by a **fungus** is called a **mycosis**. Fungi differ from bacteria in that the fungus has a rigid cell wall that is made up of chitin and various polysaccharides and a cell membrane that contains **ergosterol**. The composition of the protective layers of the fungal cell makes the organism resistant to antibiotics. Conversely, because of their cellular makeup, bacteria are resistant to antifungal drugs.

The incidence of fungal infections has increased with the rising number of immunocompromised individuals – people with acquired immune deficiency syndrome (AIDS) and AIDS-related complex (ARC), those taking immunosuppressant drugs, those who have undergone transplantation surgery or cancer treatment and members of the increasingly large elderly population, whose body is no longer able to protect itself from the many fungi that are found throughout the environment (Box 11.1). For example, ***Candida***, a fungus that is normally found on mucous membranes, can cause yeast infections or 'thrush' in the gastrointestinal (GI) tract and yeast infections or 'vaginitis' in the vagina.

SYSTEMIC ANTIFUNGALS

The drugs used to treat systemic fungal infections (Table 11.1) can be toxic to the host and are not used indiscriminately. It is important to get a culture of the fungus causing the infection to ensure that the right drug is being used so that the person is not put at additional risk from the toxic adverse effects associated with these drugs.

AZOLE ANTIFUNGALS

The **azoles** are a large group of antifungals used to treat systemic and topical fungal infections (Table 11.1). The azoles include fluconazole (*Canesoral*, *Diflucan*, *Dizole*), itraconazole (*Sporanox*), ketoconazole (*Nizoral*), posaconazole (*Noxafil*), terbinafine (*Lamisil*, *Tamsil*) and voriconazole (*Vfend*). Although azoles are considered less toxic than some other antifungal agents, such as amphotericin B, they may also be less effective in very severe and progressive infections.

Therapeutic actions and indications

These drugs bind to sterols and can cause cell death (a fungicidal effect) or interfere with cell replication (a fungistatic effect), depending on the type of fungus being affected and the concentration of the drug. (See Figure 11.1.)

Ketoconazole, fluconazole and itraconazole work by blocking the activity of a sterol in the fungal wall. In addition, they may block the activity of human steroids, including testosterone and cortisol (see usual indications in Table 11.1).

BOX 11.1 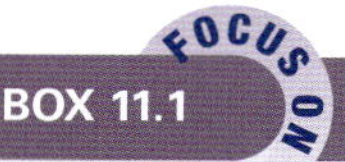 Drug therapy across the lifespan

Antifungal agents

CHILDREN

Children are very sensitive to the effects of most antifungal drugs and more severe reactions can be expected when these drugs are used in children.

Many of these drugs do not have proven safety and efficacy in children and extreme caution should be exercised when using them. Fluconazole, ketoconazole, terbinafine and griseofulvin have established paediatric doses and would be drugs of choice if appropriate for a particular infection.

Topical agents should not be used over open or draining areas that would increase the risk of systemic absorption and toxicity. Occlusive dressings, including tight nappies, should be avoided over the affected areas.

ADULTS

These drugs can be very toxic to the body, and their use should be reserved for situations in which the causative organism has been identified. Over-the-counter topical preparations are widely used, and people should be cautioned to follow the instructions and to report continued problems to their health care provider.

PREGNANCY AND BREASTFEEDING

Pregnant and breastfeeding women should not use these drugs unless the benefit clearly outweighs the potential risk to the fetus or neonate. Women of childbearing age should be advised to use barrier contraceptives if any of these drugs are used. A severe fungal infection may threaten the life of the mother and/or fetus; in these situations, the potential risk of treatment should be carefully explained.

Topical agents should not be used over open or draining areas, which would increase the risk of systemic absorption.

OLDER ADULTS

Older people may be more susceptible to the adverse effects associated with these drugs and should be monitored closely.

People with hepatic dysfunction are at increased risk for worsening hepatic problems and toxic effects of many of these drugs (ketoconazole, itraconazole, griseofulvin). If hepatic dysfunct on is expected (extreme age, alcohol abuse, use of other hepatotoxic drugs), the dose may need to be lowered and the person monitored more frequently.

Other agents are associated with renal toxicity (flucytosine, fluconazole, griseofulvin) and should be used cautiously in the presence of renal impairment. People at risk for renal toxicity should be monitored carefully.

TABLE 11.1 DRUGS IN FOCUS Systemic antifungals

Drug name	Dosage/route	Usual indications
Azole antifungals		
(P) fluconazole (*Canesoral, Diflucan, Dizole*)	Adult (serious infections): 400mg on day 1, then 200–400 mg PO for 4 weeks; IV route can be used, but do not exceed 200 mg/hour Paediatric: 3–6 mg/kg/day PO; maximum 12 mg/kg/day	Treatment of candidiasis, cryptococcal meningitis, other systemic fungal infections; prophylaxis for reducing the incidence of candidiasis in bone marrow transplant recipients
itraconazole (*Sporanox*)	Adult: 100–400 mg/day PO Paediatric: safety and efficacy not established	Treatment of blastomycosis, histoplasmosis and aspergillosis
ketoconazole (*Nizoral*)	Topical: as a shampoo and topical	Topical treatment of mycoses (cream) and to reduce the scaling of dandruff (shampoo)
posaconazole (*Noxafil*)	Adults and children ≥ 13 years: 200 mg PO tds with food	Prophylaxis of invasive *Aspergillus* and *Candida* infections in adults and children > 13 years who are immunosuppressed secondary to antineoplastic, chemotherapy, graft-versus-host disease following transplants or haematological malignancies
terbinafine (*Lamisil, Tamsil*)	250 mg/d PO for 6 weeks (fingernail) or 12 weeks (toenail)	Treatment of onychomycosis of the fingernail or toenail caused by dermatophytes; the drug was approved in late 2007 for treatment of tinea capitis (ringworm of the scalp) in children ≥ 4 years
voriconazole (*Vfend*)	Adult: 6 mg/kg IV q 12 hours for two doses, then 4 mg/kg IV q 12 hours; switch to oral dose as soon as possible > 40 kg: 200 mg PO q 12 hours < 40 kg: 100 mg PO q 12 hours	Treatment of invasive aspergillosis; treatment of serious fungal infections caused by *Scedosporium apiospermum* or *Fusarium* species when the person is intolerant to or not responding to other therapy
Echinocandin antifungals		
anidulafungin (*Eraxis*)	Single 200 mg loading dose administered on day 1, followed by 100 mg daily thereafter for at least 14 days after the last positive culture Duration of treatment should not exceed 1 month	Treatment of candidaemia (infection of the blood stream) and other forms of *Candida* infection, intra-abdominal infections and oesophageal candidiasis
caspofungin acetate (*Cancidas*)	Adult: 70 mg/day IV loading dose, then 50 mg/day IV infusion; dose should be reduced to 35 mg/day IV infusion with hepatic impairment	Treatment of invasive aspergillosis in people who do not respond or are intolerant to other therapies
Other antifungals		
amphotericin B (*Abelcet, AmBisome, Fungilin*)	Abelcet dose: 5 mg/kg/day as single IV infusion at 2.5 mg/kg/hour; administer initial test dose (1 mg IV infusion over 15 minutes) AmBisome: for systemic mycoses, initially 1 mg/kg/day of body weight, and increased stepwise to 5 mg/kg/day Fungilin lozenge dose: 10 mg PO qid	Treatment of aspergillosis, leishmaniasis, cryptococcosis, blastomycosis, moniliasis, coccidioidomycosis, histoplasmosis and mucormycosis; use is reserved for progressive, potential fatal infections due to many associated adverse effects
flucytosine (*Ancotil*)	Adult: 37.5–50 mg/kg IV over 20–40 min q 6 hours	Treatment of systemic infections caused by *Candida* or *Cryptococcus*

TABLE 11.1 DRUGS IN FOCUS Systemic antifungals *continued*

Drug name	Dosage/route	Usual indications
griseofulvin (*Grisovin*)	Tinea corporis, tinea cruris and tinea capitis: Adult: 500 mg/day Tinea pedis and tinea unguium: Adult: 500 mg/day Paediatric: 10 mg/kg/day in divided doses	Treatment of variety of ringworm or tinea infections caused by susceptible *Trichophyton* species, including tinea corporis, tinea pedis, tinea cruris, tinea barbae, tinea capitis and tinea unguium
nystatin (*Kenacomb, Mycostatin, Nilstat*)	500,000–1,000,000 units tds PO; continue for 48 hours after resolution to prevent relapse; also used topically	Treatment of candidiasis (oral form); treatment of local candidiasis, vaginal candidiasis, and cutaneous and mucocutaneous infections caused by *Candida* species

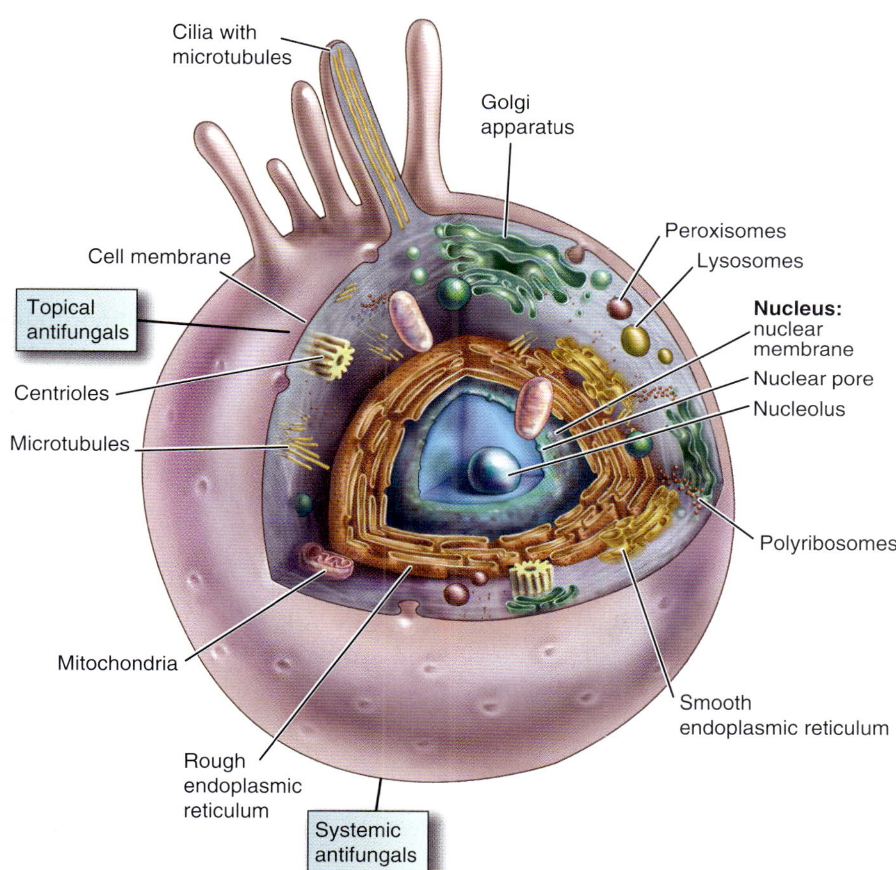

FIGURE 11.1 Sites of action of antifungal agents. Both systemic and topical antifungals alter fungal cell permeability, leading to prevention of replication and cell death.

Posaconazole is one of the newest antifungals (see Table 11.1 for uses). This drug and voriconazole inhibit the synthesis of ergosterol, which leads to the inability of the fungus to form a cell wall, which results in cell death. Terbinafine is a similar drug that blocks the formation of ergosterol. It inhibits a cytochrome P450 2D6 (CYP2D6) enzyme system, so it may be a better choice for people who need to take drugs metabolised by the cytochrome P450 (CYP450) system. It is available in a sprinkle formulation for children.

Pharmacokinetics

Itraconazole, posaconazole and terbinafine are administered orally. Ketoconazole is available as a shampoo and a cream.

Fluconazole and voriconazole are available in oral and intravenous (IV) preparations, making it possible to start the drug intravenously for a serious infection and then switch to an oral form when the person's condition improves and they are able to take oral medications.

Fluconazole reaches peak levels within 1–2 hours after administration. Most of the drug is excreted unchanged in the urine, so extreme caution should be used in the presence of renal dysfunction. Itraconazole is slowly absorbed from the GI tract and is metabolised in the liver by the CYP450 system. It is excreted in the urine and faeces. Posaconazole is given orally, has a rapid onset of action and peaks within 3–5 hours. It is metabolised in the liver and excreted in the faeces. Terbinafine is rapidly absorbed from the GI tract, extensively metabolised in the liver and excreted in the urine with a half-life of 36 hours.

Voriconazole reaches peak levels in 1–2 hours if given orally, and at the onset of the infusion if given IV. It is metabolised in the liver with a half-life of 24 hours and is excreted in the urine.

Contraindications and cautions

Itraconazole has been associated with hepatic failure, should not be used in people with hepatic failure and so should be used with caution in those with hepatic impairment. It is not known whether posaconazole crosses the placenta or enters breast milk, so it should not be used during pregnancy or breastfeeding unless the benefits clearly outweigh the potential risks. Caution should be used if posaconazole is used in the presence of liver impairment. Carefully monitor people for bone marrow suppression and GI and liver toxicity if using this drug. Terbinafine has been associated with severe liver toxicity and is contraindicated with liver failure. It may cross the placenta and may enter breast milk, so it should not be used in pregnant or breastfeeding women because of the potential toxic effects on the fetus or baby.

Voriconazole should not be used with any other drugs that prolong the QTc interval and can cause ergotism if taken with ergot alkaloids.

Adverse effects

Many of the azoles are associated with liver toxicity and can cause severe effects on a fetus or breastfeeding infant.

Clinically important drug–drug interactions

Azole antifungals inhibit the CYP450 enzyme system in the liver and are associated with many drug–drug interactions, such as increased serum levels of the following agents: ciclosporin, digoxin, oral hypoglycaemics, warfarin, oral anticoagulants and phenytoin. If these combinations cannot be avoided, closely monitor individuals and anticipate the need for dose adjustments. A drug guide should be consulted whenever one of these drugs is added to or removed from a drug regimen. Itraconazole has a black box warning regarding the potential for serious cardiovascular effects if it is given with simvastatin, triazolam or midazolam. These combinations should be avoided. Voriconazole and posaconazole should not be used with any other drugs that prolong the QTc interval and can cause ergotism if taken with ergot alkaloids. Box 11.2 highlights important information about hazardous interactions between voriconazole and posaconazole and the herb ergot.

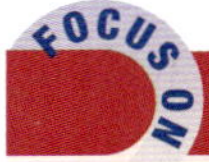

Safe medication administration

Name confusion has occurred between Lamisil *(terbinafine) and* Lamictal *(lamotrigine), an antiepileptic agent. Use extreme caution if a person is receiving either of these drugs to make sure that the correct drug is being used.*

ECHINOCANDIN ANTIFUNGALS

The echinocandin antifungals are another group of antifungals. Drugs in this class include anidulafungin and caspofungin.

Therapeutic actions and indications

The echinocandins work by inhibiting glucan synthesis. Glucan is an enzyme that is present in the fungal cell wall but not in human cell walls. If this enzyme is inhibited, the fungal cell wall cannot form, leading to death of the cell wall. See Table 11.1 for usual indications for each of these agents.

Pharmacokinetics

Anidulafungin is given as a daily IV infusion for at least 14 days. It has a rapid onset of action, is metabolised by degradation and has a half-life of 40–50 hours. This drug is excreted in the faeces.

Caspofungin is available for IV use. This drug is slowly metabolised in the liver, with half-lives of 9–11 hours, then 6–48 hours and then 40–50 hours. It is bound to protein and widely distributed throughout the body. It is excreted through the urine.

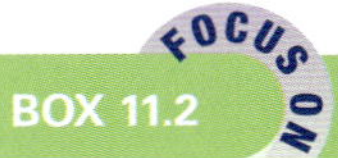

BOX 11.2 Herbal and alternative therapies

People being treated with voriconazole or posaconazole should be cautioned about the risk of ergotism if they combine this drug with ergot, a herb frequently used to treat migraine headache and menstrual problems. If the person is using voriconazole, it should be suggested that ergot not be used until the antifungal therapy is finished.

Concomitant administration of St John's wort with voriconazole and posaconazole is contraindicated. St John's wort is an inducer of CYP450 and P-glycoprotein and decreases serum concentration of voriconazole and posaconazole, leading to treatment failure.

Contraindications and cautions

Anidulafungin may cross the placenta and enter breast milk and should not be used by pregnant or breastfeeding women. Caution must be used in the presence of hepatic impairment because it can be toxic to the liver. Caspofungin can be toxic to the liver; therefore, reduced doses must be used if a person has known hepatic impairment. Caspofungin is embryotoxic in animal studies and is known to enter breast milk; therefore, it should be used with great caution during pregnancy and breastfeeding.

Adverse effects

Anidulafungin and caspofungin are associated with hepatic toxicity, and liver function should be monitored closely when using these drugs.

Clinically important drug–drug interactions

Concurrent use of ciclosporin with caspofungin is contraindicated unless the benefit clearly outweighs the risk of hepatic injury.

OTHER ANTIFUNGAL AGENTS

Other antifungal drugs that are available do not fit into either of these classes. These include amphotericin B (*Abelcet, AmBisome, Fungilin*), flucytosine (*Ancotil*), griseofulvin (*Grisovin*) and nystatin (*Kenacomb, Mycostatin, Nilstat*).

Therapeutic actions and indications

Other antifungal agents work to cause fungal cell death or to prevent fungal cell reproduction. Amphotericin B is a very potent drug with many unpleasant adverse effects (see Adverse effects). The drug binds to the sterols in the fungus cell wall, changing cell wall permeability. This change can lead to cell death (fungicidal effect) or prevent the fungal cells from reproducing (fungistatic effect). (See Table 11.1 for usual indications.) Because of the many adverse effects associated with this agent, its use is reserved for progressive, potentially fatal infections.

Flucytosine is a less toxic drug that alters the cell membrane of susceptible fungi, causing cell death (see Table 11.1 for usual indications).

Griseofulvin is an older antifungal that acts in much the same way, changing cell membrane permeability and causing cell death.

Nystatin binds to sterols in the cell wall, changing membrane permeability and allowing leaking of the cellular components, which will result in cell death.

Pharmacokinetics

Amphotericin B and flucytosine are available in IV form. They are excreted in the urine. Amphotericin liposomal (AmBisone) has an elimination half-life of 26–38 hours, depending on the dosing regimen. Amphotericin phospholipid complex (Abelcet) has a much longer half-life 90–173 hours. Different amphotericin B preparations are not interchangeable and dosages will vary. Their metabolism is not fully understood. Flucytosine is excreted unchanged in the urine and a small amount in the faeces, with a half-life of 3–6 hours in adults with normal kidney function, and 6–7 hours in premature infants. Impaired renal function results in prolongation of the half-life. Griseofulvin is administered orally and reaches peak levels in around 4 hours. It is metabolised in the liver and excreted in the urine with a half-life of 24 hours. Nystatin is not absorbed from the GI tract and passes unchanged in the stool.

Contraindications and cautions

Amphotericin B has been used successfully during pregnancy, but it should be used cautiously. It crosses into breast milk and should not be used during breastfeeding because of the potential risk to the neonate. Because flucytosine is excreted primarily in the urine, extreme caution is needed in the presence of renal impairment because drug accumulation and toxicity can occur. Toxicity is associated with serum levels higher than 100 mcg/mL. Because of the potential for adverse reactions in the fetus or neonate, flucytosine should be used during pregnancy and breastfeeding only if the benefits clearly outweigh the risks. Nystatin is a Category A pregnancy rated drug as referred above it is poorly absorbed from the GI tract.

All drugs taken during pregnancy should always only be taken when benefits outweigh potential risks.

Adverse effects

Adverse effects of these drugs are related to their toxic effects on the liver and kidneys. People should be monitored closely for any changes in liver or kidney functions. Bone marrow suppression has also been reported with the use of these drugs as well as rash and dermatological changes. Amphotericin B is associated with severe renal impairment, bone marrow suppression, GI irritation with nausea, vomiting and potentially severe diarrhoea, anorexia and weight loss, and pain at the injection site with the possibility of phlebitis or thrombophlebitis. Adverse effects of griseofulvin are relatively mild, with headache and central nervous system (CNS) changes occurring most frequently.

Clinically important drug–drug interactions

People who receive amphotericin B should not take other nephrotoxic drugs such as nephrotoxic antibiotics or antineoplastics, ciclosporin or corticosteroids unless absolutely necessary *because of the increased risk of severe renal toxicity.*

Prototype summary: fluconazole

Indications: treatment of oropharyngeal, oesophageal and vaginal candidiasis; cryptococcal meningitis; systemic fungal infections; prophylaxis to decrease the incidence of candidiasis in bone marrow transplants.

Actions: binds to sterols in the fungal cell membrane, changing membrane permeability; fungicidal or fungistatic, depending on the concentration of drug and the organism.

Pharmacokinetics:

Route	Onset	Peak	Duration
Oral	Slow	1–2 hours	2–4 days
IV	Rapid	1 hour	2–4 days

$T_{1/2}$: 30 hours; metabolised in the liver and excreted in the urine.

Adverse effects: headache, nausea, vomiting, diarrhoea, abdominal pain, rash.

Care considerations for people receiving systemic antifungals

Assessment: history and examination

- Assess the person for *contraindications or cautions*: history of allergy to antifungals *to prevent potential hypersensitivity reactions*; history of liver or renal dysfunction *that might interfere with metabolism and excretion of the drug*; and pregnancy or breastfeeding *because of potential adverse effects to the fetus or infant*.
- Perform a physical assessment *to establish baseline data for assessing the effectiveness of the drug and the occurrence of any adverse effects associated with drug therapy*; test orientation and reflexes *to evaluate any CNS effects*; and examine skin for colour changes and lesions *to monitor for any dermatological effects*.
- Obtain a culture of the infected area *to make an accurate determination of the type and responsiveness of the fungus*.
- Evaluate renal and liver function tests and full blood count *to determine baseline function of these organs and to assess possible toxicity during drug therapy*.

Implementation with rationale

- Arrange for appropriate culture and sensitivity tests before beginning therapy *to ensure that the appropriate drug is being used*. However, in some cases, treatment can begin before test results are known because of the seriousness of the systemic infections.
- Administer the entire course of the drug *to get the full beneficial effects*; this may take as long as 6 months for some chronic infections.
- Monitor IV sites *to ensure that phlebitis or infiltration does not occur*. Treat appropriately and restart IV at another site if phlebitis occurs.
- Monitor renal and hepatic function before and periodically during treatment to assess for possibly dysfunction *and arrange to stop the drug if signs of organ failure occur*.
- Provide comfort and safety provisions if CNS effects occur (eg, side rails and assistance with ambulation for dizziness and weakness, analgesics for headache, antipyretics for fever and chills, temperature regulation for fever) *to protect the person from injury*.
- Provide small, frequent, nutritious meals if GI upset is severe. Monitor nutritional status and arrange a dietary consultation as needed *to ensure nutritional status*. GI upset may be decreased by taking an oral drug with food.
- Instruct the person *to enhance knowledge about drug therapy and to promote compliance*.
- Provide the following teaching:
  - Follow the appropriate dosage regimen.
  - Take safety precautions, including changing position slowly and avoiding driving and hazardous tasks, if CNS effects occur.
  - Take an oral drug with meals and try small, frequent meals if GI upset is a problem.
  - Report to a health care provider any of the following: sore throat, unusual bruising and bleeding or yellowing of the eyes or skin, all of which could indicate hepatic toxicity; or severe nausea and vomiting, which could interfere with nutritional state and slow recovery.

Evaluation

- Monitor person's response to the drug (resolution of fungal infection).
- Monitor for adverse effects (orientation and affect, nutritional state, skin colour and lesions, renal and hepatic function).
- Evaluate the effectiveness of the teaching plan (person can name the drug, dosage, possible adverse effects to watch for and specific measures to help avoid adverse effects).
- Monitor the effectiveness of comfort and safety measures and compliance with the regimen.

KEY POINTS

- Fungi can cause many different infections in humans.
- Fungi differ from bacteria in that a fungus has a rigid cell wall that is made up of chitin and various polysaccharides and a cell membrane that contains ergosterol.
- Systemic antifungal drugs can be very toxic; extreme care should be taken to ensure that the right drug is used to treat an infection and that the person is monitored closely to prevent severe toxicity.
- Systemic antifungals are associated with many drug–drug interactions because of their effects on the liver. Monitor a person closely when adding or removing a drug from a drug regimen if the person is receiving a systemic antifungal.

TOPICAL ANTIFUNGALS

Some antifungal drugs are available only in topical forms for treating a variety of mycoses of the skin and mucous membranes. Some of the systemic antifungals are also available in topical forms. Fungi that cause these mycoses are called *dermatophytes*. These diseases include a variety of **tinea** infections, which are often referred to as ringworm, although the causal organism is a fungus, not a worm. These mycoses include tinea infections such as athlete's foot (tinea pedis), jock itch (tinea cruris) and yeast infections of the mouth and vagina often caused by *Candida*. Because the antifungal drugs reserved for use as topical agents are often too toxic for systemic administration, care is necessary when using them near open or draining wounds that might permit systemic absorption. Topical antifungals include the azole-type antifungals clotrimazole (*Canesten*, *Clonea*), econazole (*Pevaryl*), ketoconazole (*Nizoral*), miconazole (*Daktarin*, *Resolve*) and terbinafine (*Lamisil*), and other antifungals – ciclopirox (*Rejuvenail*), gentian violet (generic), tolnaftate (*Mycil*, *Tinaderm*, *Tineafax*) and undecenoic acid (*Gordochom*). (See Table 11.2.)

Therapeutic actions and indications

The topical antifungal drugs work to alter the cell permeability of the fungus, causing prevention of replication and fungal death (see Figure 11.1). They are indicated only for local treatment of mycoses, including tinea infections. See Table 11.2 for usual indications. (See also Critical thinking scenario related to drug therapy.)

Pharmacokinetics

These drugs are not absorbed systemically and do not undergo metabolism or excretion in the body.

Contraindications and cautions

Because these drugs are not absorbed systemically, contraindications are limited to a known allergy to any of these drugs and open lesions. Econazole can cause

TABLE 11.2 DRUGS IN FOCUS Topical antifungals

Drug name	Dosage/route	Usual indications
Azole topical antifungals		
(P) clotrimazole (*Canesten, Clonea*)	Available OTC as a cream, lotion, or solution; applied as a thin layer twice a day for 2–4 weeks	Available OTC for treatment of oral and vaginal *Candida* infections; tinea infections
econazole (*Pevaryl*)	Applied to affected wet body on three consecutive evenings	Treatment of tinea, candidiasis of skin or external genitalia
ketoconazole (*DaktaGOLD Nizoral, Sebizole*)	Shampoo: applied twice weekly for 2–4 weeks	Treatment of seborrhoeic dermatitis, tinea corporis, tinea cruris, tinea pedis
miconazole (*Daktarin, Resolve*)	Available as an OTC product in several topical forms (cream, powder, solution, ointment, gel and spray); applied twice daily for 2–4 weeks	Treatment of local, topical mycoses, including bladder and vaginal infections and athlete's foot
terbinafine (*Lamisil*)	Available as a cream or gel; used for 1–4 weeks; applied twice daily	Short-term (1–4 weeks) treatment of topical mycosis; treatment of tinea infections
Other topical antifungals		
ciclopirox (*Rejuvenail*)	Available as a liquid for use as a shampoo	Treatment of dandruff, seborrhoeic dermatitis
tolnaftate (*Mycil, Tinaderm, Tineafax*)	Available as a cream, powder, and spray; applied twice a day for 2–4 weeks	Available OTC for treatment of athlete's foot, topical fungal infections, tinea
undecenoic acid (*Gordochom*)	Available as a solution	Treatment of onychomycosis, cutaneous fungal infections

intense, local burning and irritation and should be discontinued if these conditions become severe. Terbinafine should not be used for longer than 4 weeks. This drug should be stopped when the fungal condition appears to be improved or if local irritation and pain become too great to avoid toxic effects.

Adverse effects

When these drugs are applied locally as a cream, lotion or spray, local effects include irritation, burning, rash and swelling. When they are taken as a suppository or troche (lozenge), adverse effects include nausea, vomiting and hepatic dysfunction (related to absorption of some of the drug by the GI tract) or urinary frequency, burning and change in sexual activity (related to local absorption in the vagina).

Prototype summary: clotrimazole

Indications: treatment of oropharyngeal candidiasis (troche); prevention of oropharyngeal candidiasis in people receiving radiation or chemotherapy; local treatment of vulvovaginal candidiasis (vaginal preparations); topical treatment of tinea pedis tinea cruris and tinea corporis.

Actions: binds to sterols in the fungal cell membrane, changing membrane permeability and allowing leakage of intracellular components, causing cell death.

Pharmacokinetics: not absorbed systemically; pharmacokinetics is unknown.

Adverse effects: troche: nausea, vomiting, abnormal liver function tests. Topical: stinging, redness, urticaria, oedema. Vaginal: lower abdominal pain, urinary frequency, burning or irritation in the sexual partner.

CRITICAL THINKING SCENARIO

Poor nutrition and opportunistic infections

THE SITUATION

P.P., a 19-year-old woman and aspiring model, complains of abdominal pain, difficulty swallowing and a very sore throat. The strict diets she has followed for long periods have sometimes amounted to a starvation regimen. In the last 18 months, she has received treatment for a variety of bacterial infections (eg, pneumonia, cystitis) with a series of antibiotics.

P.P. appears to be a very thin, extremely pale young woman who looks older than her stated age. Her mouth is moist, and small, white colonies that extend down the pharynx cover the mucosa. A vaginal examination reveals similar colonies. Cultures are performed, and it is determined that she has mucocutaneous candidiasis. Fluconazole (Diflucan) is prescribed and P.P. is asked to return in 14 days for follow-up.

CRITICAL THINKING

What are the effects of taking a variety of antibiotics on the normal flora? *Think about the possible cause of the mycosis.*

What happens to the immune system and to the skin and mucous membranes when a person's nutritional status becomes insufficient?

How is P.P.'s chosen profession affecting her health? What are the possible ramifications of suggesting that P.P. change her profession or her lifestyle?

What are the important nursing implications for P.P.? *Think about how the nurse can work with P.P. to ensure some compliance with therapy and a return to a healthy state.*

DISCUSSION

Because of P.P.'s appearance, a complete physical examination should be performed before drug therapy is initiated. It is necessary to know baseline functioning to evaluate any underlying problems that may exist. Poor nutrition and total starvation result in characteristic deficiencies that predispose individuals to opportunistic infections and prevent their bodies from protecting themselves adequately through inflammatory and immune responses. In this case, the fact that liver changes often occur with poor nutrition is particularly important; such hepatic dysfunction may cause deficient drug metabolism and lead to toxicity.

An intensive program of teaching and support should be started for P.P., who should have an opportunity to vent her feelings and fears. She needs help accepting her diagnosis and adapting to the drug therapy and nutritional changes that are necessary for the effective treatment of this infection. She should understand the possible causes of her infection (poor nutrition and the loss of normal flora secondary to antibiotic therapy); the specifics of her drug therapy, including timing and administration; and adverse effects and warning signs that should be reported. P.P. should be monitored closely for adverse effects and should return for follow-ups regularly while taking the ketoconazole. Nutritional counselling or referral to a dietician for thorough nutritional teaching may prove beneficial.

The actual resolution of the fungal infection may occur only after a combination of prolonged drug and nutritional therapy. Because the required therapy will affect P.P.'s lifestyle tremendously, she will need a great deal of support and encouragement to make the necessary changes and to maintain compliance. A health care provider, such as a nurse who P.P. trusts and with whom she can regularly discuss her concerns, may be an essential element in helping to eradicate the fungal infection.

Fluconazole is a potent inhibitor of CYP2C9, CYP2C19 and moderate inhibitor of CYP3A4. Caution should be exercised when fluconazole is coadministered with other compounds metabolised by these isoenzymes, and these individuals should be carefully monitored.

CARE GUIDE FOR P.P.: ANTIFUNGAL AGENTS

Assessment: history and examination

Assess history of allergy to any antifungal drug. Also check history of renal or hepatic dysfunction and pregnancy or breastfeeding status.

Focus the physical examination on the following:

Local: culture of infected site

Skin: colour, lesions, texture

GU: urinary output

GI: abdominal, liver evaluation

Haematological: renal and liver function tests

Implementation

Culture infection before beginning therapy.

Provide comfort and implement safety measures (eg, provide assistance and raise side rails).

Ensure temperature control, lighting control, mouth care and skin care.

Provide small, frequent meals and monitor nutritional status.

Provide support and reassurance for dealing with drug effects and discomfort.

Provide teaching regarding drug name, dosage, adverse effects, precautions and warning signs to report.

Evaluation

Evaluate drug effects: relief of signs and symptoms of fungal infection.

Monitor for adverse effects: GI alterations, dizziness, confusion, headache, fever, renal or hepatic dysfunction, local pain, discomfort.

Monitor for drug–drug interactions as indicated for each drug.

Evaluate effectiveness of teaching program and of comfort and safety measures.

TEACHING FOR P.P.

- Fluconazole is an azole antifungal drug that works to destroy the fungi that have invaded the body. Because of the way that antifungal drugs work, they may need to be taken over a long period of time.
- It is very important to take all of the prescribed medication.
- Common adverse effects of this drug include the following:
  - *Headache and weakness* – change positions slowly; an analgesic may be ordered to help alleviate the headache; if you feel drowsy, avoid driving or dangerous activities.
  - *Stomach upset, nausea and vomiting* – small, frequent meals may help; take the drug with food if appropriate because this may decrease the gastrointestinal upset associated with these drugs; maintain adequate nutrition.
- Report any of the following to your health care provider: severe vomiting, abdominal pain, fever or chills, yellowing of the skin or eyes, dark urine or pale stools, or skin rash.
- Avoid over-the-counter medications. If you feel that you need one of these, check with your health care provider first.
- Take the full course of your prescription. Never use this drug to self-treat any other infection and never give this drug to any other person.
- Tell any doctor, nurse or other health care provider involved in your care that you are taking this drug.
- Keep this drug and all medications out of the reach of children.

Care considerations for people receiving topical antifungals

Assessment: history and examination

- Assess for known allergy to any topical antifungal agent.
- Perform a physical assessment *to establish baseline data for evaluation of the effectiveness of the drug and the occurrence of any adverse effects associated with drug therapy.*
- Perform culture and sensitivity testing of the affected area *to determine the causative fungus and appropriate medication.*
- Inspect the area of application for colour, temperature and evidence of lesions to establish a baseline *to monitor the effectiveness of the drug and to monitor for local adverse effects of the drug.*

Implementation with rationale

- Culture the affected area before beginning therapy *to identify the causative fungus.*

- Ensure that the person takes the complete course of the drug regimen *to achieve maximal results.*
- Instruct the person in the correct method of administration, depending on the route, *to improve effectiveness and decrease the risk of adverse effects*:
  - Troches should be dissolved slowly in the mouth.
  - Vaginal suppositories, creams and tablets should be inserted high into the vagina with the woman remaining recumbent for at least 10–15 minutes after insertion.
  - Topical creams and lotions should be gently rubbed into the affected area after it has been cleansed with soap and water and patted dry. Occlusive bandages should be avoided.
- Advise the person to stop the drug if a severe rash occurs, especially if it is accompanied by blisters or if local irritation and pain are very severe. *This development may indicate a sensitivity to the drug or worsening of the condition being treated.*
- Provide instruction *to enhance the person's knowledge about drug therapy and to promote compliance.*
- Provide the following teaching:
  - The correct method of drug administration; demonstrate proper application.
  - The length of time necessary to treat the infection adequately.
  - Use of clean, dry socks when treating athlete's foot, to help eradicate the infection.
  - The need to keep the infected area clean, washing with mild soap and water and patting dry; keeping area dry.
  - The need to avoid scratching the infected area; use of cool compresses to decrease itching can be advised.
  - The need to avoid occlusive dressings because of the risk of increasing systemic absorption.
  - The importance of not placing drugs near open wounds or active lesions because these agents are not intended to be absorbed systemically.
  - The need to report severe local irritation, burning or worsening of the infection to a health care provider.

Evaluation

- Monitor response to the drug (alleviation of signs and symptoms of the fungal infection).
- Monitor for adverse effects: rash, local irritation and burning.
- Evaluate the effectiveness of the teaching plan (person can name the drug, dosage, possible adverse effects to watch for and specific measures to help avoid adverse effects).
- Monitor the effectiveness of comfort and safety measures and compliance with the regimen.

KEY POINTS

- Local fungal infections include vaginal and oral yeast infections (*Candida*) and a variety of tinea infections, including athlete's foot and jock itch.
- Topical antifungals are agents that are too toxic to be used systemically but are effective in the treatment of local fungal infections.
- Proper administration of topical antifungals improves their effectiveness. They should not be used near open wounds or lesions.
- Topical antifungals can cause serious local irritation, burning and pain. The drug should be stopped if these conditions occur.

CHAPTER SUMMARY

- A fungus is a cellular organism with a hard cell wall that contains chitin and polysaccharides and a cell membrane that contains ergosterols.
- Any infection with a fungus is called a mycosis. Systemic fungal infections, which can be life threatening, are increasing with the rise in the number of immunocompromised individuals.
- Systemic antifungals alter the cell permeability, leading to leakage of cellular components. This causes prevention of cell replication and cell death.
- Because systemic antifungals can be very toxic, individuals should be monitored closely while receiving them.
- Adverse effects may include hepatic and renal failure.
- Local fungal infections include vaginal and oral yeast infections (*Candida*) and a variety of tinea infections, including athlete's foot and jock itch.
- Topical antifungals are agents that are too toxic to be used systemically but are effective in the treatment of local fungal infections.
- Proper administration of topical antifungals improves their effectiveness. They should not be used near open wounds or lesions.
- Topical antifungals can cause serious local irritation, burning and pain. The drug should be stopped if these conditions occur.

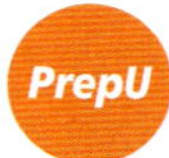

Knowing your strengths and weaknesses helps you to study more effectively. Take a PrepU Practice Quiz to find out how you measure up!

ONLINE RESOURCES

An extensive range of additional resources to enhance teaching and learning and to facilitate understanding of this chapter may be found online at the text's accompanying website, located on thePoint at http://thepoint.lww.com. These include Watch and Learn videos, Concepts in Action animations, journal articles, review questions, case studies, discussion topics and quizzes.

BIBLIOGRAPHY

Brouwer, A. E., Rajanuwong, A., Chierakul, W., Griffin, G. E., Larsen, R. A., White, N. J., et al. (2004). Combination antifungal therapies for HIV associated cryptococcal meningitis: A randomised trial. *Lancet, 363*, 1764–1767.

Chen, S. C. A. & Sorrell, T. C. (2007). Antifungal agents. *Medical Journal of Australia*, 187, 404–409.

Dempsey, J., Hillege, S. & Hill, R. (2014). *Fundamentals of Nursing and Midwifery: A Person-centred Approach to Care* (2nd Australian and New Zealand edn). Sydney: Lippincott Williams & Wilkins.

Farrell, M. & Dempsey, J. (2014). *Smeltzer & Bare's Textbook of Medical-Surgical Nursing* (3rd edn). Sydney: Lippincott, Williams & Wilkins.

Jen, L., Piacenti, F. J. & Lyakhovetskiy, A. G. (2003). Voriconazole. *Clinical Therapeutics, 25*, 1321–1381.

Johnson, M. D. & Perfect, J. R. (2003). Caspofungin: First approved agent in a new class of antifungals. *Expert Opinion on Pharmacotherapy, 4*, 807–823.

Kontoyiannis, D. P., Mantadaki, E. & Samonis, G. (2003). Systemic mycoses in immune-compromised host: An update in antifungal therapy. *Journal of Hospital Infection, 53*, 243–258.

McKenna, L. & Mirkov, S. (2019). *McKenna's Drug Handbook for Nursing and Midwifery* (8th edn). Sydney: Wolters Kluwer Health Australia.

Pfaller, M. A. (2012). Antifungal drug resistance: Mechanisms, epidemiology, and consequences for treatment. *American Journal of Medicine, 125*, S3–S13.

Porth, C. M. (2011). *Essentials of Pathophysiology: Concepts of Altered Health States* (3rd edn). Philadelphia: Lippincott Williams & Wilkins.

Porth, C. M. (2009). *Pathophysiology: Concepts of Altered Health States* (8th edn). Philadelphia: Lippincott Williams & Wilkins.

Van Onselen, J. (2012). Prescribing for superficial fungal skin and nail infections. *Nurse Prescribing, 10*, 229–234.

CHECK YOUR UNDERSTANDING

Answers to the questions in this chapter can be found in Appendix A at the back of this book.

MULTIPLE CHOICE

Select the best answer to the following.

1. A person with a fungal infection asks the health professional why she cannot take antibiotics. The health professional explains that the reason for this is that a fungus is resistant to antibiotics because:
- **a.** a fungal cell wall has fewer but more selective protective layers.
- **b.** the composition of the fungal cell wall is highly rigid and protective.
- **c.** a fungus does not reproduce by the usual methods of cell division.
- **d.** antibiotics are developed to affect only bacterial cell walls.

2. When administering a systemic antifungal agent, the nurse or midwife incorporates understanding that all systemic antifungal drugs function to:
- **a.** break apart the fungus nucleus.
- **b.** interfere with fungus DNA production.
- **c.** alter cell permeability of the fungus, leading to cell death.
- **d.** prevent the fungus from absorbing needed nutrients.

3. After assessing a person, the nurse or midwife would question an order for amphotericin B to prevent the possibility of serious nephrotoxicity if the person was also receiving which of the following?
- **a.** digoxin
- **b.** oral anticoagulants
- **c.** phenytoin
- **d.** corticosteroids

4. The health professional is describing fungi that cause infections of the skin and mucous membranes, appropriately calling these which of the following?
- **a.** mycoses
- **b.** meningeal fungi
- **c.** dermatophytes
- **d.** worms

5. After teaching a group of students about topical fungal infections, the instructor determines that the students need additional instruction when they identify which of the following as an example?
- **a.** athlete's foot
- **b.** Rocky Mountain spotted fever
- **c.** jock itch
- **d.** vaginal yeast infections

6. Which of the following would the nurse or midwife recommend that a woman with repeated vaginal yeast infections keep on hand?
- **a.** undecenoic acid
- **b.** terbinafine
- **c.** clotrimazole
- **d.** ciclopirox

7. The nurse or midwife instructs a person to use care when applying topical antifungal agents to prevent systemic absorption because:
   a. the fungus is only on the surface.
   b. these drugs are too toxic to be given systemically.
   c. absorption would prevent drug effectiveness.
   d. these drugs can cause serious local burning and pain.

8. A person with a severe case of athlete's foot is seen with lesions between the toes, which are oozing blood and serum. After teaching the person, the health professional determines that the instruction was effective if the person states which of the following?
   a. 'I have to wear black socks and must be careful not to change them very often because it could pull more skin off my feet.'
   b. 'I need to apply a thick layer of the antifungal cream between my toes, making sure that all of the lesions are full of cream.'
   c. 'I should wear white socks and keep my feet clean and dry. I shouldn't use the antifungal cream in areas where I have open lesions.'
   d. 'After I apply the cream to my feet, I should cover my feet in plastic wrap for several hours to make sure the drug is absorbed.'

MULTIPLE RESPONSE

Select all that apply.

1. When administering a systemic antifungal, the health professional would include which of the following in the person's plan of care?
   a. ensuring that a culture of the affected area had been done
   b. having the person swallow the troche used for oral Candida infections
   c. ensuring that the person stays flat for at least 1 hour if receiving a vaginal suppository
   d. monitoring the IV site to prevent phlebitis
   e. keeping the person NBM (nothing by mouth) if GI upset occurs to prevent vomiting
   f. providing antipyretics if fever occurs with IV antifungals

2. The nurse or midwife would include which of the following in a teaching plan for a person who is receiving an oral antifungal drug?
   a. It is important that you complete the full course of your drug therapy.
   b. You can share this drug with other family members if they develop the same symptoms.
   c. If you feel drowsy or dizzy, you should avoid driving or operating dangerous machinery.
   d. If GI upset occurs, avoid eating and drinking so you don't vomit and lose the drug.
   e. Use over-the-counter drugs to counteract any adverse effects like headache, fever or rash.
   f. Notify your health care provider if you experience yellowing of the skin or eyes, dark urine or light-coloured stools, or fever and chills.

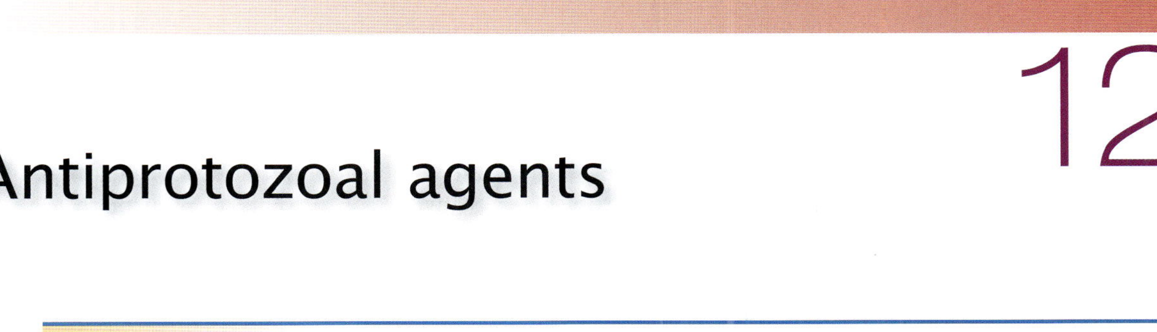

12

Antiprotozoal agents

Learning objectives

On completing this chapter you should be able to:

1. Outline the life cycle of the protozoan that causes malaria.
2. Describe the therapeutic actions, indications, pharmacokinetics, contraindications, proper administration, most common adverse reactions and important drug–drug interactions associated with drugs used to treat malaria.
3. Describe other common protozoal infections, including cause and clinical presentation.
4. Compare and contrast the antimalarials with other drugs used to treat protozoal infections.
5. Outline the care considerations for individuals receiving an antiprotozoal agent across the lifespan.

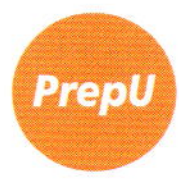

Test your current knowledge of antiprotozoal agents with a PrepU Practice Quiz!

Glossary of key terms

amoebiasis: amoebic dysentery, which is caused by intestinal invasion by the trophozoite stage of the protozoan *Entamoeba histolytica*

***Anopheles* mosquito:** type of mosquito that is essential to the life cycle of *Plasmodium*; injects the protozoa into humans for further maturation

cinchonism: syndrome of quinine toxicity characterised by nausea, vomiting, tinnitus and vertigo

giardiasis: protozoal intestinal infection that causes severe diarrhoea and epigastric distress; may lead to serious malnutrition

leishmaniasis: skin, mucous membrane or visceral infection caused by a protozoan passed to humans by the bites of sand flies

malaria: protozoal infection with *Plasmodium*, characterised by cyclic fever and chills as the parasite is released from ruptured red blood cells; causes serious liver, CNS, heart and lung damage

***Plasmodium*:** a protozoan that causes malaria in humans; its life cycle includes the *Anopheles* mosquito, which injects protozoa into humans

***Pneumocystis carinii* pneumonia (PCP):** opportunistic infection that occurs when the immune system is depressed; a frequent cause of pneumonia in people with AIDS and in those who are receiving immunosuppressive therapy

protozoa: single-celled organisms that pass through several stages in their life cycle, including at least one phase as a human parasite; found in areas of poor sanitation and hygiene and crowded living conditions

trichomoniasis: infestation with a protozoan that causes vaginitis in women but no signs or symptoms in men

trophozoite: a developing stage of a parasite, which uses the host for essential nutrients needed for growth

trypanosomiasis: African sleeping sickness, which is caused by a protozoan that inflames the CNS and is spread to humans by the bite of the tsetse fly; also, Chagas disease, which causes a serious cardiomyopathy after the bite of the house fly

ANTIMALARIALS
- artemether with lumefantrine
- doxycycline
- (P) hydroxychloroquine
- mefloquine
- primaquine
- quinine
- tafenoquine

OTHER ANTIPROTOZOALS
- atovaquone
- (P) metronidazole
- pentamidine
- pyrimethamine
- tinidazole

Infections caused by **protozoa** – single-celled organisms that pass through several stages in their life cycles, including at least one phase as a human parasite – are very common in several parts of the world. In tropical areas, where protozoal infections are most prevalent, many people suffer multiple infestations at the same time. These illnesses are relatively rare in Australia and New Zealand, but with people travelling throughout the world in increasing numbers, it is not unusual to find an individual who returns home from a trip to Africa, Asia or South America with fully developed protozoal infections. Protozoa thrive in tropical climates, but they may also survive and reproduce in any area where people live in very crowded and unsanitary conditions. This chapter focuses on agents used for protozoal infections that are caused by insect bites (malaria, trypanosomiasis and leishmaniasis) and those that result from ingestion or contact with the causal organism (amoebiasis, giardiasis and trichomoniasis). Box 12.1 discusses the use of antiprotozoals across the lifespan. Figure 12.1 shows sites of action for these agents.

MALARIA

Malaria is a parasitic disease that has killed hundreds of millions of people and even changed the course of history. The progress of several African battles and the building of the Panama Canal were altered by outbreaks of malaria. Even with the introduction of drugs for the treatment of this disease, it remains endemic in many parts of the world. In our local region, malaria remains a significant cause of mortality in countries such as Papua New Guinea and Indonesia. The only known method of transmission of malaria is through the bite of a female ***Anopheles* mosquito**, an insect that harbours the protozoal parasite and carries it to humans.

Four protozoal parasites, all in the genus ***Plasmodium***, have been identified as causes of malaria:

- *Plasmodium falciparum* is considered to be the most dangerous type of protozoan. Infection with this protozoan results in an acute, rapidly fulminating disease with high fever, severe hypotension, swelling and reddening of the limbs, loss of red blood cells and even death.
- *Plasmodium vivax* causes a milder form of the disease, which seldom results in death.
- *Plasmodium malariae* is endemic in many tropical countries and causes very mild signs and symptoms in the local population. It can cause more acute disease in travellers to endemic areas.
- *Plasmodium ovale*, which is rarely seen, seems to be in the process of being eradicated.

A major problem with controlling malaria involves the mosquito that is responsible for transmitting the disease, which has developed a resistance to the insecticides designed to eradicate it. Over the years, widespread efforts at mosquito control were successful, with fewer cases of malaria being seen each year. However, the rise of insecticide-resistant mosquitoes has allowed malaria to continue to flourish, increasing the incidence of the

BOX 12.1 FOCUS ON Drug therapy across the lifespan

Antiprotozoal agents

CHILDREN

Children are very sensitive to the effects of most antiprotozoal drugs, and more severe reactions can be expected when these drugs are used in children.

Many of these drugs do not have proven safety and efficacy in children, and extreme caution should be used. The dangers of infection resulting from travel to areas endemic with many of these diseases are often much more severe than the potential risks associated with cautious use of these drugs.

If a child needs to travel to an area with endemic protozoal infections, the CDC or local health department should be consulted about the safest possible preventive measures.

ADULTS

Adults should be well advised about the need for prophylaxis against various protozoal infections and the need for immediate treatment if the disease is contracted. It is very helpful to mark calendars as reminders of the days before, during and after exposure on which the drugs should be taken.

PREGNANCY AND BREASTFEEDING

Pregnant and breastfeeding women should not use these drugs unless the benefit clearly outweighs the potential risk to the fetus or neonate. Women of childbearing age should be advised to use barrier contraceptives if any of these drugs are used. A pregnant woman travelling to an area endemic with protozoal infections should be advised of the serious risks to the fetus associated with both preventive therapy and treatment of acute attacks, as well as the risks associated with contracting the disease.

OLDER ADULTS

Older people may be more susceptible to the adverse effects associated with these drugs. They should be monitored closely.

People with hepatic dysfunction are at increased risk for worsening hepatic problems and toxic effects of many of these drugs. If hepatic dysfunction is expected (extreme age, alcohol abuse, use of other hepatotoxic drugs), the dose may need to be lowered and the person monitored more frequently.

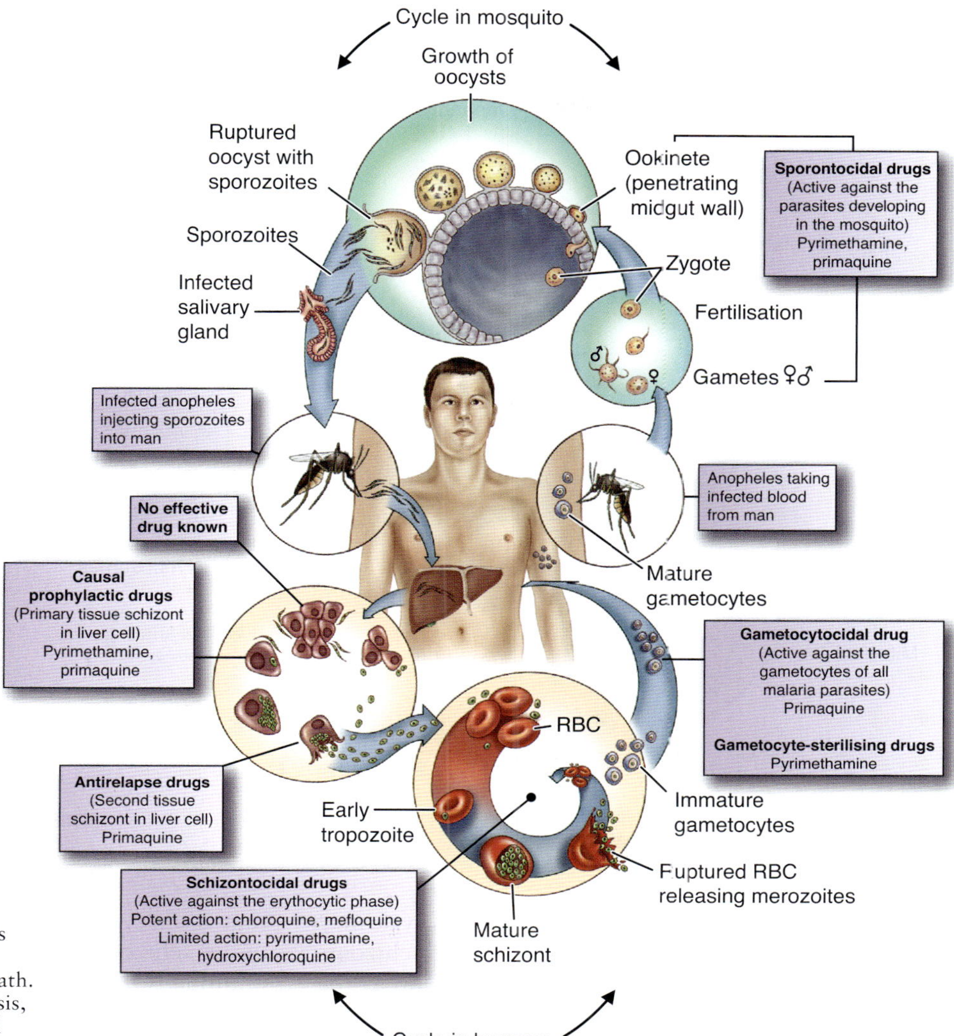

FIGURE 12.1 Sites of action of antimalarials and other antiprotozoals. Antimalarials block protein synthesis and cause cell death. Other antiprotozoals block DNA synthesis, prevent cell reproduction and lead to cell death. RBC, red blood cell.

disease. In addition, the protozoa that cause malaria have developed strains resistant to the usual antimalarial drugs. This combination of factors has led to a worldwide public health challenge.

Life cycle of plasmodium

The parasites that cause human malaria spend part of their life in the *Anopheles* mosquito and part in the human host (see Figure 12.1). When a mosquito bites a human who is infected with malaria, it sucks blood infested with gametocytes, which are male and female forms of the *Plasmodium*. These gametocytes mate in the stomach of the mosquito and produce a zygote that goes through several phases before forming sporozoites (spore animals) that make their way to the mosquito's salivary glands. The next person who is bitten by that mosquito is injected with thousands of sporozoites. These organisms travel through the bloodstream, where they quickly become lodged in the human liver and other tissues, and invade the cells.

Inside human cells, the organisms undergo asexual cell division and reproduction. Over the next 7–10 days, these primary tissue organisms called schizonts grow and multiply within their invaded cells, using the cell for needed nutrients (as **trophozoites**). Merozoites are then formed from the primary schizonts and burst from invaded cells when they rupture because of overexpansion. These merozoites enter the circulation and invade red blood cells. Here they continue to divide until the blood cells also burst, sending more merozoites into the circulation to invade yet more red blood cells.

Eventually, there are a large number of merozoites in the body, as well as many ruptured and invaded red blood cells. At this point, the acute malarial attack occurs. The rupture of the red blood cells causes chills and fever related to the pyrogenic effects of the protozoa and the toxic effects of the red blood cell components on the system. This cycle of chills and fever usually occurs about every 72 hours.

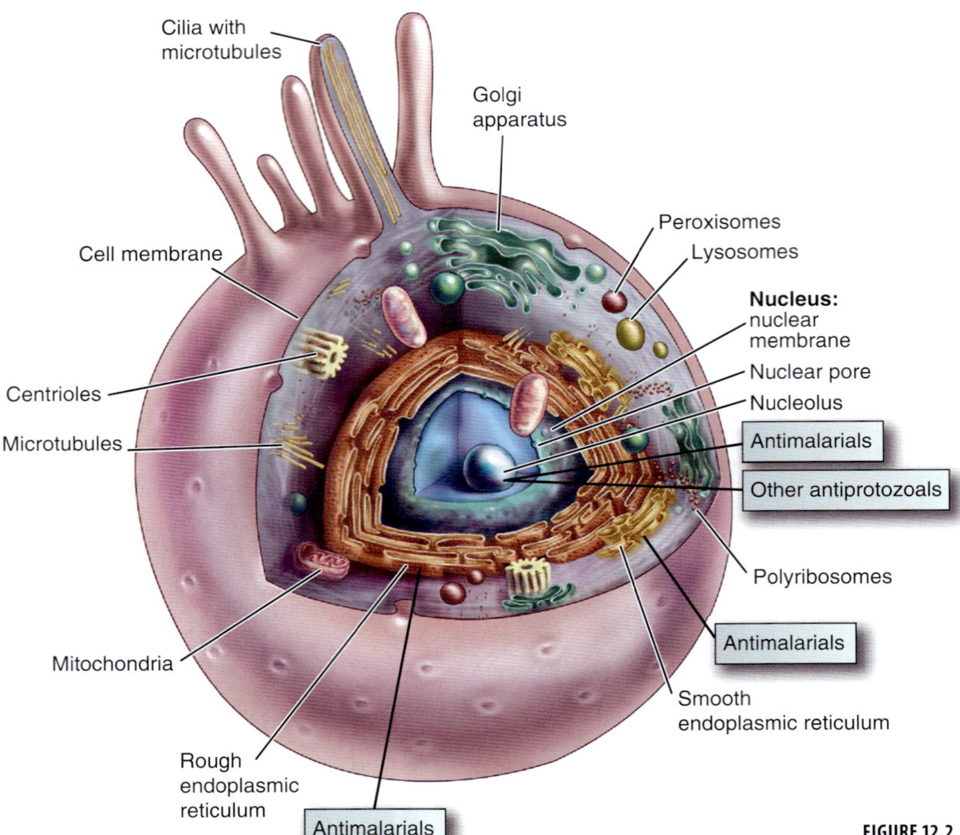

FIGURE 12.2 Types of antimalarial drugs in relation to the stages in the life cycle of *Plasmodium*.

With *P. vivax* and *P. malariae* malaria, this cycle may continue for a long period. Many of the tissue schizonts lay dormant until they eventually find their way to the liver, where they multiply and then invade more red blood cells, again causing the acute cycle. This cycle of emerging from dormancy to cause a resurgence of the acute cycle may occur for years in an untreated individual.

With *P. falciparum* malaria, there are no extra-hepatic sites for the schizonts. If the person survives an acute attack, no prolonged periods of relapse occur. The first attack of this type of malaria can destroy so many red blood cells that the person's capillaries become clogged and the circulation to vital organs is interrupted, leading to death.

ANTIMALARIALS

Antimalarial drugs (see Table 12.1) are usually given in combination form to attack the *Plasmodium* at various stages of its life cycle. Using this approach, it is possible to prevent the acute malarial reaction in individuals who have been infected by the parasite. These drugs can be schizonticidal (acting against the red blood–cell phase of the life cycle), gametocytocidal (acting against the gametocytes), sporontocidal (acting against the parasites that are developing in the mosquito) or work against tissue schizonts as prophylactic or anti-relapse agents. Quinine (*Quinate, Quinbisul*) was the first drug found to be effective in the treatment of malaria. Antimalarials used today include doxycycline (*Doryx*, *Frakas*), hydroxychloroquine (*Plaquenil*), mefloquine (*Lariam*) and primaquine (*Primacin*). Tafenoquine (*Kodatef*) is a new drug for treatment of relapsing malaria. It has activity against all stages of the *P. vivax* life cycle. Fixed-dose combination drugs for malaria prevention and treatment are discussed in Box 12.2.

Therapeutic actions and indications

Chloroquine has previously been the mainstay of antimalarial therapy. However, due to resistance to this drug, it is no longer readily accessible in Australia, and is only available through the Special Access Scheme. This drug enters human red blood cells and changes the metabolic pathways necessary for the reproduction of the *Plasmodium* (see Figure 12.2). In addition, this agent is directly toxic to parasites that absorb it; it is acidic and it decreases the ability of the parasite to synthesise DNA, leading to a blockage of reproduction. Because many strains of the parasite are developing resistance to chloroquine, the U.S. Centers for Disease Control and Prevention often recommends the use of

TABLE 12.1 DRUGS IN FOCUS Antimalarials

Drug name	Dosage/route	Usual indications
artemether with lumefantrine (*Riamet*)	Adults, adolescents and children over 35 kg or 12 years of age: 6 doses of 4 tablets over 60 hours 25 to < 35 kg: 18 tablets over 60 hours 15 to < 25 kg: 12 tablets over 60 hours 5 to < 15 kg: 6 tablets over 60 hours	Treatment of acute, uncomplicated malaria due to *Plasmodium falciparum*
doxycycline (*Doryx, Frakas*)	Suppression: Adult and paediatric (> 8 years and 50 kg): 100 mg PO daily, beginning 2 days before entering malaria area, continued throughout stay in the area, then for 2 weeks after leaving	Prevention of *Plasmodium falciparum* malaria Prevention of *Plasmodium vivax* malaria in combination
(P) hydroxychloroquine (*Plaquenil*)	Suppression: Adult: 310 mg PO every week, starting 2 weeks before exposure and continuing for 8 weeks after exposure Paediatric: 5 mg/kg/week, following adult schedule Acute attack: Adult: 800 mg (620 mg) base PO, followed by 400 mg (310 mg) PO in 6–8 hours on 2 consecutive days	Treatment of *Plasmodium* malaria in combination with other drugs, particularly primaquine
mefloquine (*Lariam*)	Adults and children of > 45 kg body weight Treatment: A loading dose of 3 tablets (750 mg), followed 6–8 hours later by 2 tablets (500 mg) Prevention: 250 mg PO once weekly, starting 1 week before travel and continuing for 2 weeks after leaving endemic area	Prevention and treatment of *Plasmodium* malaria in combination with other drugs
primaquine (*Primacin*)	Radical cure. 15 mg/day for 14 days, 21 days in Southeast Asia, Pacific regions; up to 30 mg/day for 14 days if unresponsive or resistant malaria	Prevention of relapses of *P. vivax* and *P. malariae* infections; radical cure of *P. vivax* malaria
quinine (*Quinbisul*)	For chloroquine-resistant *Plasmodium falciparum* malaria: 600 mg PO every eight hours for at least 3 days in most areas of the world (7 days in Southeast Asia) with concurrent or consecutive administration of 1.5 g of sulfadoxine and 75 mg of pyrimethamine combination as a single dose; or concurrent or consecutive administration of 900 mg of clindamycin tid for 3 days	Treatment of malaria due to strains of *P. falciparum* resistance to 4-aminoquinolones

certain antibiotics as part of combination therapy for treatment of malaria caused by these resistant strains. Box 12.3 lists the antibiotics used to treat malaria. See Table 12.1 for usual indications. Mechanisms of action are as follows:

- Hydroxychloroquine inhibits parasite reproduction, and by blocking the synthesis of protein production, it can cause the death of the *Plasmodium*. This drug is used in combination therapy, usually with primaquine, for greatest effectiveness.
- Mefloquine increases the acidity of plasmodial food vacuoles, causing cell rupture and death. In combination therapy, mefloquine is used in malarial prevention, as well as treatment.
- Primaquine, another very old drug for treating malaria, similar to quinine, disrupts the mitochondria of the *Plasmodium*. It also causes death of gametocytes and exoerythrocytic (outside of the red blood cell) forms and prevents other forms from reproducing.
- Tafenoquine is an 8-aminoquinoline derivative with activity against all stages of the *Plasmodium vivax*

BOX 12.2 Combination drugs used for malaria prevention and treatment

Two fixed-dose combination drugs are available for use in the prevention and treatment of malaria. Combining two different preparations in one drug may increase compliance by reducing the number of pills a person has to take, and it conforms to the treatment protocol of taking drugs that affect the protozoa at different stages of their life cycle.

Riamet is a combination of artemether and lumefantrine. It is indicated for treatment of *P. falciparum* malaria. *Riamet* is contraindicated in the first trimester of pregnancy and women should be advised to use barrier contraceptives while taking it. Breastfeeding should not begin for at least 4 weeks after the last dose, as few data exist on effects on the infant.

Usual dosage, acute attack:

Adult and paediatric (> 35 kg or > 12 years): 6 doses of 4 tablets PO over 60 hours

Paediatric (5–35 kg and > 3 months–12 years): 6 doses of 1–3 tablets PO over 60 hours

Malarone and *Malarone Junior* combine atovaquone and proguanil. They are indicated for the prevention of *P. falciparum* malaria when chloroquine resistance has been reported. They are used for the treatment of uncomplicated *P. falciparum* malaria when mefloquine has not proved successful, most likely because of resistance. This combination should be used in pregnancy and breastfeeding only if the benefit clearly outweighs the potential risk to the fetus or neonate.

Usual dosage, acute attack:

Adult: 4 tablets PO as a single daily dose for 3 consecutive days

Paediatric (11–20 kg): 1 adult tablet PO daily for 3 consecutive days

Paediatric (21–30 kg): 2 adult tablets PO daily as a single daily dose for 3 consecutive days

Paediatric (31–40 kg): 3 adult tablets PO daily as a single daily dose for 3 consecutive days

Paediatric (> 40 kg): 4 adult tablets PO daily as a single daily dose for 3 consecutive days

Prevention:

Adult: 1 tablet PO daily

Paediatric (11–20 kg): 1 junior tablet PO daily

Paediatric (21–30 kg): 2 junior tablets PO daily

Paediatric (31–40 kg): 3 junior tablets PO daily

Paediatric (> 40 kg): 1 adult tablet PO daily

Prevention should start 1–2 days before exposure and continue throughout plus 7 days after leaving the area.

lifecycle: pre-erythrocytic (liver) forms, erythrocytic (asexual) forms and gametocytes.

Pharmacokinetics

Chloroquine is readily absorbed from the gastrointestinal (GI) tract, with peak serum levels occurring in 1–6 hours. It is concentrated in the liver, spleen, kidney and brain and is excreted very slowly in the urine, primarily as an unchanged drug.

BOX 12.3 Antibiotics used to treat malaria

With the emergence of chloroquine-resistant strains of *Plasmodium*, doxycycline, quinine with concurrent sulfadoxine and pyrimethamine or quinine with concurrent clindamycin are recommended for the prophylaxis of malaria caused by strains with unknown resistance.

Doxycycline: adult and paediatric (> 8 years): 100 mg/day PO for 2 days before entering malaria region, continuing during stay and for 4 weeks after leaving.

Hydroxychloroquine is readily absorbed from the GI tract, with peak serum levels occurring in 1–6 hours. It is excreted slowly in the urine, primarily as an unchanged drug.

Mefloquine is a mixture of molecules that are absorbed, metabolised and excreted at different rates. The terminal half-life is 13–24 days. Metabolism occurs in the liver; caution should be used in individuals with hepatic dysfunction.

Primaquine is readily absorbed and metabolised in the liver. Excretion occurs primarily in the urine. Safety for use during pregnancy has not been established.

Contraindications and cautions

Antimalarials are contraindicated in the presence of known allergy to any of these drugs; liver disease or alcoholism, *both because of the parasitic invasion of the liver and because of the need for the hepatic metabolism to prevent toxicity*; and breastfeeding *because the drugs can enter breast milk and could be toxic to the infant.* Another method of feeding the baby should be used if treatment is necessary. These drugs should be avoided during pregnancy *because they are associated with birth defects.* With mefloquine, which is teratogenic in preclinical studies, pregnancy should be avoided during, and for 2 months after completing, therapy. Use caution in people with retinal disease or damage *because many of these drugs can affect vision and the retina, and the likelihood of problems increases if the retina is already damaged*; with psoriasis or porphyria *because of skin damage*; or with damage to mucous membranes, *which can occur as a result of the effects of the drug on proteins and protein synthesis.* There have been some genetic enzyme differences identified in various groups that predispose them to adverse effects associated with these drugs. See Box 12.4 for cultural considerations and the use of some antimalarials.

Oesophageal ulceration has been associated with the use of doxycycline. Therefore, it is important that doxycycline should be administered with adequate amounts of fluid or food and the person should remain sitting

BOX 12.4 FOCUS ON Cultural considerations

Potential for haemolytic crisis

People with glucose-6-phosphate dehydrogenase (G6PD) deficiency – which is more likely to occur in Greeks, Italians and other people of Mediterranean descent – may experience a haemolytic crisis if they are taking the antimalarial agent chloroquine or primaquine. People of Greek, Italian or other Mediterranean ancestry should be questioned about any history of potential G6PD deficiency. If no history is known, the person should be tested before any of these drugs are prescribed. If testing is not possible and the drugs are needed, the person should be monitored very closely and informed about the potential need for hospitalisation and emergency services.

or standing for up to 2 hours afterwards to prevent the possible development of oesophageal irritation.

Adverse effects

A number of adverse effects may be encountered with the use of these antimalarial agents. Central nervous system (CNS) effects include headache and dizziness. Immune reaction effects related to the release of merozoites include fever, shaking, chills and malaise. Nausea, vomiting, dyspepsia and anorexia are associated with direct effects of the drug on the GI tract and the effects on CNS control of vomiting caused by the products of cell death and protein changes. Hepatic dysfunction is associated with the toxic effects of the drug on the liver and the effects of the disease on the liver. Dermatological effects include rash, pruritus and loss of hair associated with changes in protein synthesis of the hair follicles. Visual changes, including possible blindness related to

Prototype summary: hydroxychloroquine

Indications: treatment and prophylaxis of acute attacks of malaria caused by susceptible strains of *Plasmodium*; treatment of extraintestinal amoebiasis.

Actions: inhibits protozoal reproduction and protein synthesis.

Pharmacokinetics:

Route	Onset	Peak	Duration
Oral	Varies	1–2 hours	1 week

$T_{1/2}$: 70–120 hours; metabolised in the liver and excreted in the urine.

Adverse effects: visual disturbances, retinal changes, abdominal pain, nausea, vomiting, diarrhoea, skin rashes.

Care considerations for people receiving antimalarial agents

Assessment: history and examination

- Assess for contraindications or cautions: history of allergy to any of the antimalarials *to prevent hypersensitivity reactions*; liver dysfunction or alcoholism *that might interfere with the metabolism and excretion of the drug*; porphyria or psoriasis, *which could be exacerbated by the drug effects*; retinal disease *that could increase the visual disturbances associated with these drugs*; and pregnancy and breastfeeding *because these drugs could affect the fetus and could enter the breast milk and be toxic to the infant.*
- Perform a physical assessment *to establish baseline data for assessment of the effectiveness of the drug and the occurrence of any adverse effects associated with drug therapy.* Assess CNS (reflexes and muscle strength).
- Perform ophthalmic and retinal examinations and auditory screening *to determine the need for cautious administration and to evaluate changes that occur as a result of drug therapy.*
- Assess the person's liver function, including liver function tests *to determine appropriateness of therapy and to monitor for toxicity.*
- Obtain blood culture to *identify the causative* Plasmodium *species.*
- Inspect the skin closely for colour, temperature, texture and evidence of lesions *to monitor for adverse effects.*

Implementation with rationale

- Arrange for appropriate culture and sensitivity tests before beginning therapy *to ensure proper drug for susceptible* Plasmodium *species.* Treatment may begin before test results are known.
- Administer the complete course of the drug *to get the full beneficial effects.* Mark a calendar for prophylactic doses. Use combination therapy as indicated.
- Monitor hepatic function and perform ophthalmological examination before and periodically during treatment *to ensure early detection and prompt intervention with cessation of drug if signs of failure or deteriorating vision occur.*
- Provide comfort and safety measures if CNS effects occur (eg, side rails and assistance with ambulation if dizziness and weakness are present) *to prevent injury.* Provide oral hygiene and ready access to bathroom facilities as needed *to cope with GI effects.*

- Provide small, frequent, nutritious meals if GI upset is severe *to ensure adequate nutrition.* Monitor nutritional status and arrange a dietary consultation as needed. Taking the drug with food may also decrease GI upset.
- Instruct the person concerning the appropriate dosage regimen and the importance of adhering to the drug schedule *to enhance knowledge about drug therapy and to promote compliance.*
- Provide the following teaching:
  - Take safety precautions, including changing position slowly and avoiding driving and hazardous tasks, if CNS effects occur.
  - Take the drug with meals and try small, frequent meals if GI upset is a problem.
  - Report blurring of vision, which could indicate retinal damage; loss of hearing or ringing in the ears, which could indicate CNS toxicity; and fever or worsening of condition, which could indicate a resistant strain or non-effective therapy.

Evaluation

- Monitor response to the drug (resolution of malaria or prevention of malaria).
- Monitor for adverse effects (orientation and affect, nutritional state, skin colour and lesions, hepatic function, and visual and auditory changes).
- Evaluate the effectiveness of the teaching plan (person can name the drug, dosage, possible adverse effects to watch for and specific measures to help avoid adverse effects).
- Monitor the effectiveness of comfort and safety measures and compliance with the regimen.

retinal damage from the drug, and ototoxicity related to other nerve damage may occur. **Cinchonism** (nausea, vomiting, tinnitus and vertigo) may occur with high levels of hydroxychloroquine or primaquine.

Clinically important drug–drug interactions

The person who is receiving combinations of the quinine derivatives and quinine is at increased risk for cardiac toxicity and convulsions. Therefore, monitor the person closely, checking drug levels and anticipating dose adjustments as needed.

KEY POINTS

- A protozoan is a parasitic single-celled organism. Its life cycle includes a parasitic phase inside human tissues or cells.
- Malaria is the most common protozoal infection and is spread to humans by the bite of an *Anopheles* mosquito. The signs and symptoms of malaria are related to the destruction of red blood cells and toxicity to the liver.
- Antimalarial agents attack the parasite at the various stages of its development inside and outside the human body.

OTHER PROTOZOAL INFECTIONS

Other protozoal infections that are encountered in clinical practice include amoebiasis, leishmaniasis, trypanosomiasis, trichomoniasis and giardiasis. These infections, which are caused by single-celled protozoa, are usually associated with unsanitary, crowded conditions and use of poor hygienic practices. People travelling to other countries may encounter these infections, which are also now appearing increasingly in Australia and

BOX 12.5 FOCUS ON The evidence

World travel and the spread of pathogens

Nowadays, people are travelling to more exotic areas of the world than ever before. Because of this, people are being exposed to more pathogens than ever before, and they are also potentially spreading pathogens to different areas of the world. Pathogens that are endemic in one area of the world and cause mild disease to the local population there can be quite devastating in a population that has not previously been exposed to that pathogen.

World health agencies and governments have established guidelines for prophylaxis and treatment of such diseases for travellers. People who are planning to travel out of the country should contact their local Health Department, the Australian Government Department of Foreign Affairs and Trade, or SmartTraveller (http://smartraveller.gov.au/index.html) for the latest information on what prophylactic measures are required in the area they plan to visit and to learn about potential health hazards in that area. The information is updated frequently; treatment and prophylaxis suggestions are based on current clinical experience in the area and should be consulted regularly. Nurses should access this information when working with people who are travelling to provide pertinent teaching points and to ensure that appropriate prophylactic measures are taken. Nurses and midwives caring for people with tropical diseases should access this information regularly for best treatment practices.

People who have been travelling to other areas of the world and who present with any illness should be questioned about where they travelled, what precautions (including prophylactic measures) they took, and when they first experienced any signs or symptoms of illness. The SmartTraveller website can be consulted about diagnosis and treatment guidelines for any tropical disease that is unfamiliar to a health care provider, as well as about what precautions should be used in caring for such people.

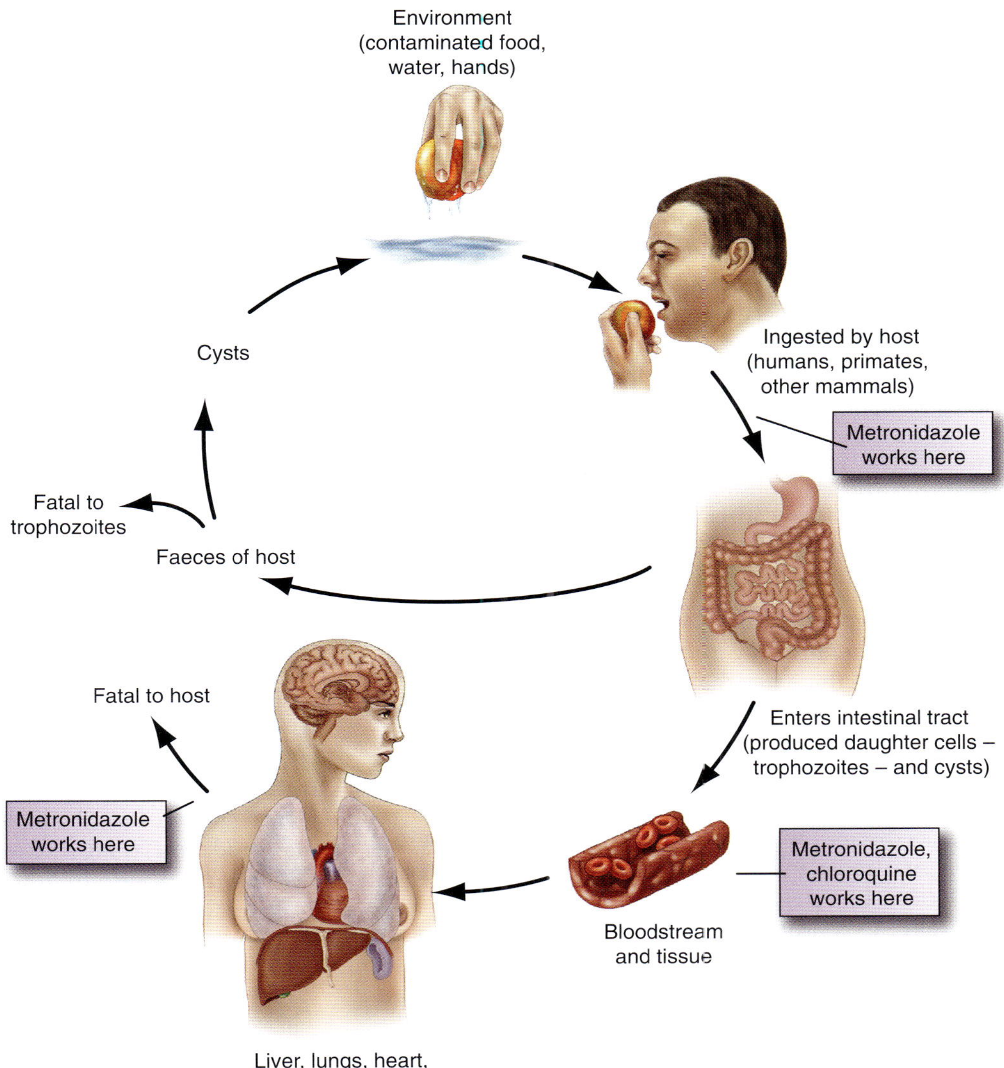

FIGURE 12.3 Life cycle of *Entamoeba histolytica* and the sites of action of metronidazole and chloroquine, which are used to treat amoebiasis. Cysts ingested by the host enter the intestinal tract and produce trophozoites. Trophozoites enter the bloodstream to reach tissue. Trophozoites enter the liver, lungs, heart, brain and spleen, which can be fatal to the host. Trophozoites are excreted in the stool and die. Cysts excreted in the stool contaminate water and can be ingested by the host.

New Zealand. Box 12.5 discusses the impact of travel and tourism on the spread of pathogens.

Amoebiasis

Amoebiasis, an intestinal infection caused by *Entamoeba histolytica*, is often known as amoebic dysentery. *E. histolytica* has a two-stage life cycle (see Figure 12.3). The organism exists in two stages: (1) a cystic, dormant stage, in which the protozoan can live for long periods outside the body or in the human intestine, and (2) a trophozoite stage in the ideal environment – the human large intestine.

The disease is transmitted while the protozoan is in the cystic stage in faecal matter, from which it can enter water and the ground. It can be passed to other humans who drink this water or eat food that has been grown in this ground. The cysts are swallowed and pass, unaffected by gastric acid, into the intestine. Some of these cysts are passed in faecal matter, and some of them become trophozoites that grow and reproduce. The trophozoites migrate into the mucosa of the colon, where they penetrate into the intestinal wall, forming erosions. These forms of *Entamoeba* release a chemical that dissolves mucosal cells, and eventually they eat away tissue until they reach the vascular system, which carries them throughout the body. The trophozoites lodge in the liver, lungs, heart, brain, and so on.

Early signs of amoebiasis include mild to fulminate diarrhoea. In the worst cases, if the protozoan is able to invade extraintestinal tissue, it can dissolve the tissue and eventually cause the death of the host. Some individuals can become carriers of the disease without having any overt signs or symptoms. These people seem to be resistant to the intestinal invasion but pass the cysts on in the stool.

Leishmaniasis

Leishmaniasis is a disease caused by a protozoan that is passed from sand flies to humans. The sand fly injects an asexual form of this flagellated protozoan, called a promastigote, into the body of a human, where it is rapidly attacked and digested by human macrophages. Inside the macrophages, the promastigote divides, developing many new forms called amastigotes, which keep dividing and eventually kill the macrophage, releasing the amastigotes into the system to be devoured by more macrophages. Thus, a cyclic pattern of infection is established. These amastigotes can cause serious lesions in the skin, the viscera or the mucous membranes of the host.

Trypanosomiasis

Trypanosomiasis is caused by infection with *Trypanosoma*. Two parasitic protozoal species cause very serious and often fatal diseases in humans:

- African sleeping sickness, which is caused by *Trypanosoma brucei gambiense,* is transmitted by the tsetse fly. After the pathogenic organism has lived and grown in human blood, it eventually invades the CNS, leading to an acute inflammation that results in lethargy, prolonged sleep and even death.
- Chagas disease, which is caused by *Trypanosoma cruzi,* is almost endemic in many South American countries. It is passed to humans by the common housefly. This protozoan results in a severe cardiomyopathy that accounts for numerous deaths and disabilities in certain regions.

Trichomoniasis

Trichomoniasis, which is caused by another flagellated protozoan, *Trichomonas vaginalis*, is a common cause of vaginitis. This infection is usually spread during sexual intercourse by men who have no signs and symptoms of infection. In women, this protozoan causes reddened, inflamed vaginal mucosa, itching, burning and a yellowish-green discharge. Trichomoniasis is particularly prevalent among the Aboriginal and Torres Strait Islander population in Australia.

Giardiasis

Giardiasis, which is caused by *Giardia lamblia*, is a very commonly diagnosed intestinal parasite in Australia. This protozoan forms cysts, which survive outside the body and allow transmission through contaminated water or food, and trophozoites, which break out of the cysts in the upper small intestine and eventually cause signs and symptoms of disease. Diarrhoea, rotten egg–smelling stool, and pale and mucus-filled stool are commonly seen. Some individuals experience epigastric distress, weight loss and malnutrition as a result of the invasion of the mucosa.

Pneumocystis carinii pneumonia

Pneumocystis carinii is an endemic protozoan that does not usually cause illness in humans. When an individual's immune system becomes suppressed because of acquired immune deficiency syndrome (AIDS) or AIDS-related complex (ARC), the use of immunosuppressant drugs or advanced age, this parasite is able to invade the lungs, leading to severe inflammation and the condition known as ***Pneumocystis carinii* pneumonia (PCP)**. This disease is the most common opportunistic infection in people with AIDS.

OTHER ANTIPROTOZOAL AGENTS

Drugs that are available specifically for the treatment of these various protozoan infections include many of the malarial drugs; chloroquine is effective against extraintestinal amoebiasis, and pyrimethamine is effective in treating toxoplasmosis. Other drugs, including some tetracyclines and aminoglycosides, are used for treating these conditions at various stages of the disease. Other antiprotozoals include atovaquone (*Wellvone*), metronidazole (*Flagyl, Metronide*), pentamidine (*DBL Pentamidine Isethionate*), pyrimethamine (*Daraprim*) and tinidazole (*Fasigyn, Simplotan*). (See Table 12.2.)

Therapeutic actions and indications

These antiprotozoal agents act to inhibit DNA synthesis in susceptible protozoa, interfering with the cell's ability to reproduce, subsequently leading to cell death (see Figure 12.1). These drugs are indicated for the treatment of infections caused by susceptible protozoa. See Table 12.2 for usual indications for each of these agents.

Pharmacokinetics

Atovaquone is slowly absorbed and is highly protein bound in circulation. It is excreted slowly through the faeces, with a half-life of 2.2–3.2 days.

Metronidazole is well absorbed orally, reaching peak levels in 1–2 hours. It is metabolised in the liver with a half-life of 6–12 hours. Excretion occurs primarily through the urine.

Pentamidine is readily absorbed through the lungs. Excretion occurs in the urine, with traces found in the urine for up to 6 weeks.

Pyrimethamine is readily absorbed from the GI tract, with peak levels occurring within 2–6 hours. It is metabolised in the liver and has a half-life of 4 days. It usually maintains suppressive concentrations in the body for about 2 weeks.

TABLE 12.2 DRUGS IN FOCUS Other antiprotozoals

Drug name	Dosage/route	Usual indications
atovaquone with proguanil (*Malarone, Malarone Junior, Promozio*)	Prevention: 1–2 days before entering a malaria-endemic area, continued daily until 7 days after leaving Adult: 1 Malarone tablet (atoaquone 250mg with proguanil 100mg) per day Paediatric: depending on the body weight, 1–3 tablets of Malarone Junior (atoaquone 62.5mg with proguanil 25mg per tablet) Treatment: Adult: 4 Malarone tablets (adult strength), total daily dose 1 g atovaquone / 400 mg proguanil as a single dose for 3 consecutive days Paediatric: depending on body weight, 1–4 tablets of Malarone (adult strength)	Prevention and treatment of *Pneumocystis carinii* pneumonia; used in combination with proguanil for treatment of chloroquine-resistant malaria
(P) metronidazole (*Flagyl, Metronide*)	Amoebiasis: Adults, children > 12 years: 400–800 mg tid for 5–10 days Paediatric: 35–50 mg/kg/day PO in 3 divided doses for 10 days Trichomoniasis: Adults, children > 12 years: 200 mg tid for 7 days; or 2 g single dose Paediatric: 40 mg/kg orally as a single dose or 15–30 mg/kg/day divided in 2–3 doses; not to exceed 2000 mg/dose	Treatment of amoebiasis, trichomoniasis, giardiasis
pentamidine (*DBL Pentamidine, Isethionate* for Injection)	Injection: 4 mg/kg/day IM or slow IV infusion for 14 days Inhalation: 300 mg once a month by inhalation using a suitable nebuliser fitted with either a portable compressor or piped oxygen	As nhalation treatment of *P. carinii* pneumonia; as a systemic agent in the treatment of trypanosomiasis and leishmaniasis
pyrimethamine (*Daraprim*)	Adult: 50–75 mg/day PO with 1–4 g of a sulfonamide for 4–5 weeks Paediatric (> 6 years): same as adult Paediatric: 1 mg/kg/day PO, divided into two equal doses, for 2–4 days; then cut dose in half and continue for 1 month	Treatment of toxoplasmosis
tinidazole (*Fasigyn, Simplotan*)	Trichomoniasis, giardiasis: Adult: 2 g PO as a single dose with food Paediatric (≥3 years): 50 mg/kg PO as a single dose with food Amoebiasis: Adult: 2 g/day PO with food for 3 days Paediatric (≥3 years): 50 mg/kg/day PO with food. Maximum dose 2g/day for 5 days	Treatment of trichomoniasis, giardiasis, amoebiasis

Tinidazole is rapidly absorbed after oral administration, reaching peak levels within 60–90 minutes. It is excreted in the urine with a half-life of 12–14 hours.

Contraindications and cautions

Contraindications include the presence of any known allergy or hypersensitivity to any of these drugs and pregnancy *because drug effects on developing fetal DNA and proteins can cause fetal abnormalities and even death*. Use caution when administering these drugs to people with CNS disease *because of possible disease exacerbation due to drug effects on the CNS*; hepatic disease *because of possible exacerbation when hepatic drug effects occur*; candidiasis *because of the risk of superinfections*; and women who are breast-feeding *because these drugs may pass into breast milk and could have severe adverse effects on the infant.* The safety and efficacy of pentamidine in children have not been established. Tinidazole and metronidazole should never be combined with alcohol and should be used with caution in people with renal dysfunction, *which could interfere with excretion of the drug.*

Adverse effects

Adverse effects that can be seen with these antiprotozoal agents include CNS effects such as headache, dizziness, ataxia, loss of coordination and peripheral neuropathy related to drug effects on the neurons. GI effects include nausea, vomiting, diarrhoea, unpleasant taste, cramps and changes in liver function. Superinfections can also occur when the normal flora are disrupted.

Clinically important drug–drug interactions

Tinidazole and metronidazole should not be combined with alcohol, which could cause severe adverse effects; individuals are advised to avoid alcohol for at least 3 days after treatment has ended. Metronidazole and tinidazole combined with oral anticoagulants can lead to increased bleeding; people should be monitored closely and dose adjustments made to the anticoagulant during therapy and for up to 8 days after stopping therapy. Psychotic reactions have been reported when tinidazole or metronidazole is combined with disulfiram; this combination should be avoided, and 2 weeks should elapse between tinidazole therapy and the starting of disulfiram.

Increased bone marrow suppression may occur if antifolate drugs (methotrexate, sulfonamides, etc.) are combined with pyrimethamine; discontinue pyrimethamine if signs of folate deficiency develop (diarrhoea, fatigue, weight loss, anaemia).

Prototype summary: metronidazole

Indications: acute intestinal amoebiasis, amoebic liver abscess, trichomoniasis, acute infections caused by susceptible strains of anaerobic bacteria, and preoperative and postoperative prophylaxis for people undergoing colorectal surgery.

Actions: inhibits DNA synthesis of specific anaerobes, causing cell death; mechanism of action as an antiprotozoal and amoebicidal is not known.

Pharmacokinetics:

Route	Onset	Peak
Oral	Varies	1–2 hours
IV	Rapid	1–2 hours

$T_{1/2}$: 6–8 hours; metabolised in the liver and excreted in the urine and faeces.

Adverse effects: headache, dizziness, ataxia, nausea, vomiting, metallic taste, diarrhoea, darkening of the urine.

Care considerations for people receiving antiprotozoal agents

Assessment: history and examination

- Assess for contraindications and cautions: history of allergy to any of the antiprotozoals *to prevent hypersensitivity reactions*; liver dysfunction *that might interfere with metabolism and excretion of the drug or be exacerbated by the drug*; pregnancy, *which is a contraindication*, and breastfeeding *because these drugs could enter the breast milk and be toxic to the infant*; CNS disease *that could be exacerbated by the drug*; and candidiasis *that could become severe as a result of the effects of these drugs on the normal flora.*
- Perform a physical assessment *to establish baseline data for determining the effectiveness of the drug and the occurrence of any adverse effects associated with drug therapy.*
- Evaluate the CNS *to check reflexes and muscle strength to identify the need for cautious drug use and to evaluate changes that occur as a result of drug therapy.*
- Examine the skin and mucous membranes to check for lesions, colour, temperature and texture *to monitor for adverse effects and superinfections.*
- Evaluate liver function, including liver function tests, *to determine the appropriateness of therapy and to monitor for toxicity.*
- Obtain cultures *to determine the exact protozoal species causing the disease.*

Implementation with rationale

- Arrange for appropriate culture and sensitivity tests before beginning therapy *to ensure proper drug for susceptible organisms.* Treatment may begin before test results are known.
- Administer a complete course of the drug *to get the full beneficial effects.* Use combination therapy as indicated.
- Monitor hepatic function before and periodically during treatment *to arrange to effectively stop the drug if signs of failure or worsening liver function occur.*
- Provide comfort and safety measures if CNS effects occur, such as side rails and assistance with ambulation if dizziness and weakness are present, *to prevent injury to the person.*
- Provide oral hygiene and ready access to bathroom facilities as needed *to cope with GI effects.*
- Arrange for the treatment of superinfections as appropriate *to prevent severe infections.*
- Provide small, frequent, nutritious meals if GI upset is severe *to ensure proper nutrition.* Monitor nutritional status and arrange a dietary consultation as needed. Taking the drug with food may also decrease GI upset.
- Instruct the person about the appropriate dosage regimen *to enhance knowledge about drug therapy and to promote compliance.*
- Provide the following teaching:
  - Take safety precautions, including changing position slowly and avoiding driving and hazardous tasks, if CNS effects occur.
  - Take the drug with meals and try small, frequent meals if GI upset is a problem.
  - Follow drug dosing guidelines carefully.

– Report severe GI problems and interference with nutrition; fever and chills, which may indicate the presence of a superinfection; and dizziness, unusual fatigue or weakness, which may indicate CNS effects.

Evaluation

- Monitor response to the drug (resolution of infection and negative cultures for parasite).
- Monitor for adverse effects (orientation and affect, nutritional state, skin colour and lesions, hepatic function and occurrence of superinfections).
- Evaluate the effectiveness of the teaching plan (person can name the drug, dosage, possible adverse effects to watch for and specific measures to help avoid adverse effects).
- Monitor the effectiveness of comfort and safety measures and compliance with the regimen.

See Critical thinking scenario for additional information related to coping with amoebiasis and the use of metronidazole.

KEY POINTS

- Other protozoal infections include amoebiasis, leishmaniasis, trypanosomiasis, trichomoniasis, giardiasis and *Pneumocystis carinii* infection.
- People receiving antiprotozoal agents should be monitored regularly to detect any serious adverse effects, including loss of vision, liver toxicity and so on.

CHAPTER SUMMARY

- A protozoan is a parasitic single-celled organism. Its life cycle includes a parasitic phase inside human tissues or cells.
- Malaria is caused by *Plasmodium* protozoa, which must go through a cycle in the *Anopheles* mosquito before being passed to humans by the mosquito bite. Once inside a human, the protozoa invade red blood cells.
- The characteristic cyclic chills and fever of malaria occur when red blood cells burst, releasing more protozoa into the bloodstream.
- Malaria is treated with a combination of drugs that attack the protozoan at various stages in its life cycle.
- Amoebiasis is caused by the protozoan *Entamoeba histolytica*, which invades human intestinal tissue after being passed to humans through unsanitary food or water. It is best treated with metronidazole or tinidazole.
- Leishmaniasis, a protozoan-caused disease, can result in serious lesions in the mucosa, viscera and skin. It is treated with systemic pentamidine.
- Trypanosomiasis, which is caused by infection with a *Trypanosoma* parasite, may assume two

CRITICAL THINKING SCENARIO

Coping with amoebiasis

THE SITUATION

J.C., a 20-year-old male university student, reported to the university health centre complaining of severe diarrhoea, abdominal pain and, most recently, blood in his stool. He had a mild fever and appeared to be dehydrated and very tired. The young man, who denied he had travelled outside the country, reported eating most of his meals at the local café, where he worked in the kitchen each night making pizza.

A stool sample for ova and parasites (O&P) was obtained, and a diagnosis of amoebiasis was made. Metronidazole was prescribed. A public health referral was sent to find the source of the infection, which was the kitchen of the café where J.C. worked. The kitchen was shut down until all the food, utensils and environment passed state health inspection. Although a potential epidemic was averted (only three other cases of amoebiasis were reported), the action of the public health officials added new stress to this student's life because he was unemployed for several months.

CRITICAL THINKING

What are the important care implications for J.C.? *Think about the usual nutritional state of a university student who eats most of his meals in a pizza place.*

What are the implications for recovery when a person is malnourished and then has a disease that causes severe diarrhoea, dehydration and potential malnourishment? *Consider how difficult it will be for J.C. to be a full-time student while trying to cope with the signs and symptoms of his disease, as well as the adverse effects associated with his drug therapy and the need to maintain adequate nutrition to allow some healing and recovery.*

What potential problems could the added stress of being out of work have for J.C.? *Consider the physiological impact of stress, as well as the psychological problems of trying to cope with one more stressor.*

DISCUSSION

J.C. needed a great deal of reassurance and an explanation of his disease. He learned that oral hygiene and small, frequent meals would help alleviate some of his discomfort until the metronidazole could control the amoebiasis and that good hygiene and strict hand washing when the disease is active would help to prevent transmission. He was advised to watch for the occurrence of specific adverse drug effects, such as a possible severe reaction to alcohol (he was advised to avoid alcoholic beverages while taking this drug); gastrointestinal upset and a strange metallic taste (the importance of good nutrition to promote healing of the gastrointestinal tract was stressed); dizziness or light-headedness; and superinfections.

J.C. was scheduled for a follow-up examination for stool O&P and nutritional status. Metronidazole was continued until the stool sample came back negative. He needed and received a great deal of support and encouragement because he was far from home and the disease and the drug effects were sometimes difficult to cope with. The effects of stress – decreasing blood flow to the gastrointestinal tract, for example – can make it more difficult for people such as J.C. to recover from this disease. Support and encouragement can be major factors in their eventual recovery. J.C. was given a telephone number to call if he needed information or support and a complete set of written instructions regarding the disease and the drug therapy.

CARE GUIDE FOR J.C.: METRONIDAZOLE

Assessment: history and examination

Allergies to metronidazole, renal or liver dysfunction
Concurrent use of barbiturates, oral anticoagulants, alcohol
Local: culture of stool for accurate diagnosis of infection
CNS: orientation, affect, vision, reflexes
Skin: colour, lesions, texture
GI: abdominal, liver evaluation
Haematological: full blood count, liver function tests

Implementation

Culture infection before beginning therapy.
Provide comfort and safety measures: oral hygiene, safety precautions, treatment of superinfections, maintenance of nutrition.
Provide small, frequent meals and monitor nutritional status.
Provide support and reassurance for dealing with drug effects and discomfort.
Provide teaching regarding drug name, dosage, adverse effects, precautions and warning signs to report and hygiene measures to observe.

Evaluation

Evaluate drug effects: resolution of protozoal infection.
Monitor for adverse effects: GI alterations, dizziness, confusion, central nervous system changes, vision loss, hepatic function, superinfections.
Monitor for drug–drug interactions with oral anticoagulants, alcohol or barbiturates.
Evaluate effectiveness of teaching program.
Evaluate effectiveness of comfort and safety measures.

TEACHING FOR J.C.

You have been prescribed metronidazole to treat your amoebic infection. This antiprotozoal drug acts to destroy certain protozoa that have invaded your body. Because it affects specific phases of the protozoal life cycle, it must be taken over a period of time to be effective. It is very important to take all the drug that has been ordered for you.

- This drug frequently causes stomach upset. If it causes you to have nausea, heartburn or vomiting, take the drug with meals or a light snack.
- Common effects of this drug include the following:
  - *Nausea, vomiting and loss of appetite:* take the drug with food and have small, frequent meals.
  - *Superinfections of the mouth, skin:* these go away when the course of the drug has been completed. If they become uncomfortable, notify your health care provider for an appropriate solution.
  - *Dry mouth, strange metallic taste:* frequent mouth care and sucking sugarless lozenges may help. This effect will also go away when the course of the drug is finished.
  - *Intolerance to alcohol (nausea, vomiting, flushing, headache and stomach pain):* avoid alcoholic beverages or products containing alcohol while taking this drug.
- Report any of the following to your health care provider: sore throat, fever or chills; skin rash or redness; severe GI upset; and unusual fatigue, clumsiness or weakness.
- Take the full course of your prescription. Never use this drug to self-treat any other infection or give it to any other person.
- Tell any doctor, nurse or other health care provider that you are taking this drug.
- Keep this drug and all medications out of the reach of children.

forms: African sleeping sickness which leads to inflammation of the CNS, and Chagas disease which results in serious cardiomyopathy. These diseases can be treated with systemic pentamidine.

- Trichomoniasis is caused by *Trichomonas vaginalis*. This common cause of vaginitis results in no signs or symptoms in men but serious vaginal inflammation in women. It is treated with metronidazole and tinidazole.
- Giardiasis, which is caused by *Giardia lamblia*, is a very commonly diagnosed intestinal parasititic infection in Australia. This disease may lead to

serious malnutrition when the pathogen invades intestinal mucosa. It is treated with metronidazole and tinidazole.
- *Pneumocystis carinii* is an endemic protozoan that does not usually cause illness in humans unless they become immunosuppressed. *P. carinii* pneumonia (PCP) is the most common opportunistic infection seen in people with AIDS. It is treated with inhaled pentamidine and oral atovaquone.
- Individuals receiving antiprotozoal agents should be monitored regularly to detect any serious adverse effects, including loss of vision and liver toxicity.

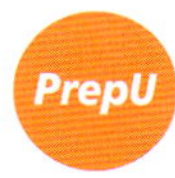

Knowing your strengths and weaknesses helps you to study more effectively. Take a PrepU Practice Quiz to find out how you measure up!

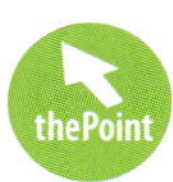

ONLINE RESOURCES

An extensive range of additional resources to enhance teaching and learning and to facilitate understanding of this chapter may be found online at the text's accompanying website, located on thePoint at http://thepoint.lww.com. These include Watch and Learn videos, Concepts in Action animations, journal articles, review questions, case studies, discussion topics and quizzes.

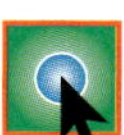

WEB LINKS

Health care providers and students may want to consult the following web resources:

https://trove.nla.gov.au/work/8306835?q&versionId=9572356
Northern Territory Government Malaria Guidelines for Health Professionals in the Northern Territory.

www.medsafe.govt.nz/profs/PUarticles/doxyou.htm
Medsafe information about oesophageal ulcer and doxycycline.

http://smartraveller.gov.au
Australian Government Department of Foreign Affairs and Trade, Smart Traveller.

www.who.int/malaria/en
World Health Organization resources and guidelines for managing malaria.

www.who.int/countries/png/en
World Health Organization country profile: Papua New Guinea.

www.who.int/malaria/publications/country-profiles/profile_idn_en.pdf
World Health Organization country profile: Indonesia.

BIBLIOGRAPHY

Dempsey, J., Hillege, S. & Hill, R. (2014). *Fundamentals of Nursing and Midwifery: A Person-centred Approach to Care* (2nd Australian and New Zealand edn). Sydney: Lippincott Williams & Wilkins.

Farrell, M. & Dempsey, J. (2014). *Smeltzer & Bare's Textbook of Medical-Surgical Nursing* (3rd edn). Sydney: Lippincott Williams & Wilkins.

Gawthrop, M., Stillwell, A., Wong, C. S. & Simons, H. (2012). Preventing malaria in travellers: An overview. *Nursing Times, 108*, 23–25.

Gherardin, A. (2012). Assessing fever in the returned traveller. *Australian Prescriber, 35*, 10–14.

McKenna, L. & Mirkov, S. (2019). *McKenna's Drug Handbook for Nursing and Midwifery* (8th edn). Sydney: Wolters Kluwer Health Australia.

O'Brien, D. & Biggs, B. (2002). Malaria prevention in the expatriate and long-term traveller. *Australian Prescriber, 25*, 66–69.

Panaretto, K. S., Lee, H. M., Mitchell, M. R., Larkins, S. L., Manessis, V., Buettner, P. G. & Watson, D. (2006). Prevalence of sexually transmitted infections in pregnant urban Aboriginal and Torres Strait Islander women in Northern Australia. *Australian and New Zealand Journal of Obstetrics and Gynaecology, 46*, 217–224.

Porth, C. M. (2011). *Essentials of Pathophysiology: Concepts of Altered Health States* (3rd edn). Philadelphia: Lippincott Williams & Wilkins.

Porth, C. M. (2009). *Pathophysiology: Concepts of Altered Health States* (8th edn). Philadelphia: Lippincott Williams & Wilkins.

Stanley, S. (2003). Amebiasis. *Lancet, 362*, 1025–1034.

Thomas, C. F. & Limper, A. H. (2004). *Pneumocystis* pneumonia. *New England Journal of Medicine, 350*, 2487–2498.

Turner, C. & Zuckerman, J. (2011). Advice for travellers on avoiding malaria. *Practice Nursing, 22*, 134–139.

Umeed, M. (2010). Prescribing in travel health: Malaria. *Nurse Prescribing, 8*, 215–220.

CHECK YOUR UNDERSTANDING

Answers to the questions in this chapter can be found in the Appendix A at the back of this book.

MULTIPLE CHOICE

Select the best answer to the following.

1. After a group of students is taught about protozoal infections, which infection, if stated by the group as caused by an insect bite, would indicate the need for additional teaching?
   a. malaria
   b. trypanosomiasis
   c. leishmaniasis
   d. giardiasis

2. When describing the development of malaria caused by the *Plasmodium* protozoan, the instructor would explain that the organism depends on:
   a. a snail to act as intermediary in the life cycle of the protozoan.
   b. a mosquito and a red blood cell for maturation.
   c. a human liver cell for cell division and reproduction.
   d. stagnant water for maturation.

3. A person who is receiving a combination drug to treat malaria asks the nurse why. The nurse responds to the person based on the understanding that combination drugs are:
   a. associated with a much lower degree of toxicity when used in combination.
   b. absorbed more completely when administered and taken together.
   c. more effective in preventing mosquitoes from biting the individual.
   d. effective at various stages in the life cycle of the protozoan.

4. A person travelling to an area of the world where malaria is known to be endemic should be taught to:
   a. avoid drinking the water.
   b. begin prophylactic antimalarial therapy before travelling and continue it through the visit and for 2–3 weeks after the visit.
   c. take a supply of antimalarial drugs in case they get a mosquito bite.
   d. begin prophylactic antimalarial therapy 2 weeks before travelling and stop the drugs on arriving at the destination.

5. Amoebiasis or amoebic dysentery:
   a. is seen only in Third World countries.
   b. is caused by a protozoan that enters the body through an insect bite.
   c. is caused by a protozoan that can enter the body in the cyst stage in water or food.
   d. usually has no signs and symptoms.

6. Giardiasis is a very common intestinal parasite seen in Australia, and it:
   a. does not respond to drug therapy.
   b. can invade the liver and cause death.
   c. is seen only in areas with no sanitation.
   d. is associated with rotten egg–smelling stool, diarrhoea and mucus-filled stool.

7. PCP (*Pneumocystis carinii* pneumonia) is:
   a. an endemic protozoan found in the human respiratory system.
   b. responsive to inhaled pentamidine.
   c. an opportunistic bacterial infection.
   d. frequently associated with children in day care settings.

8. Trypanosomiasis may assume two different forms:
   a. African sleeping sickness and Chagas disease.
   b. elephantiasis and malaria.
   c. dysentery and African sleeping sickness.
   d. malaria and Chagas disease.

9. It would be noted that a person had a good understanding of his antimalarial drug regimen if the person reported:
   a. 'I keep these pills with me at all times while I'm away and take them only when I have been bitten by a mosquito.'
   b. 'I will need to start these pills now and then continue to take them every day for the rest of my life.'
   c. 'I'll start the pills before my trip, keep taking them during the trip and for a period of time after I'm home.'
   d. 'I start taking these pills as soon as I arrive at my destination, but before I get off the plane.'

MULTIPLE RESPONSE

Select all that apply.

1. A mother calls in concerned that her son, a university student, has been diagnosed with giardiasis. The nurse would respond to the mother's concerns by telling her which of the following?
   a. You should have your son come home immediately so that he can be treated appropriately.
   b. This is a very rare disorder; it is not usually seen in this country.
   c. This is the most common protozoal infection seen in this country and is usually transmitted through food or water.
   d. This infection can be treated with oral drugs, and he should be able to get the drugs where his infection was diagnosed.
   e. This is an infection that has to be treated quickly with IV medications.
   f. Encourage your son to get the medicine and to try very hard to eat nutritious food.

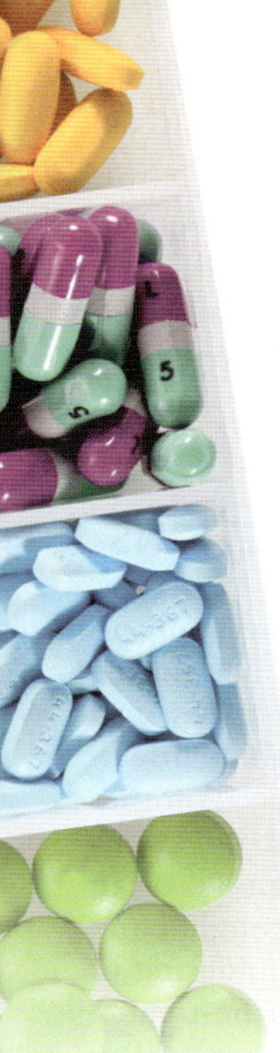

13

Anthelmintic agents

Learning objectives

On completing this chapter you should be able to:

1. List the common worms that cause disease in humans.
2. Describe the therapeutic actions, indications, pharmacokinetics, contraindications, most common adverse reactions and important drug–drug interactions associated with the anthelmintics.
3. Discuss the use of anthelmintics across the lifespan.
4. Compare and contrast the prototype drug mebendazole with other anthelmintics.
5. Outline the care considerations, including important teaching points to stress, for people receiving an anthelmintic.

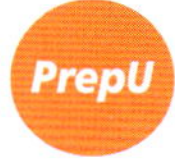

Test your current knowledge of anthelmintic agents with a PrepU Practice Quiz!

Glossary of key terms

***Ascaris*:** the most prevalent helminthic infection; fertilised roundworm eggs are ingested, which hatch in the small intestine and then make their way to the lungs, where they may cause cough, fever and other signs of a pulmonary infiltrate

cestode: tapeworm with a head and segmented body parts that is capable of growing to several metres n the human intestine

filariasis: infection of the blood and tissues of healthy individuals by worm embryos or filariae

helminth: worm that can cause disease by invading the human body

hookworms: worms that attach themselves to the small intestine of infected individuals, where they suck blood from the walls of the intestine, damaging the intestinal wall and leading to severe anaemia with lethargy, weakness and fatigue

nematode: roundworms such as the commonly encountered pinworm, whipworm, threadworm, *Ascaris* or hookworm that cause a common helminthic infection in humans; can cause intestinal obstruction as the adult worms clog the intestinal lumen, or severe pneumonia when the larvae migrate to the lungs and form a pulmonary infiltrate

pinworm: nematode that causes a common helminthic infection in humans; lives in the intestine and causes anal and possible vaginal irritation and itching

platyhelminth: flatworms, including the cestodes or tapeworms; a worm that can live in the human intestine or can invade other human tissues (flukes)

schistosomiasis: infection with a blood fluke that is carried by a snail; it poses a common problem in tropical countries, where the snail is the intermediary in the life cycle of the worm; larvae burrow into the skin in fresh water and migrate throughout the human body, causing a rash and then symptoms of diarrhoea, and liver and brain inflammation

threadworm: pervasive nematode that can send larvae into the lungs, liver and CNS; can cause severe pneumonia or liver abscess

trichinosis: disease that results from ingestion of encysted roundworm larvae in undercooked pork; larvae migrate throughout the body to invade muscles, nerves and other tissues; can cause pneumonia, heart failure and encephalitis

whipworm: worm that attaches itself to the intestinal mucosa and sucks blood; may cause severe anaemia and disintegration of the intestinal mucosa

ANTHELMINTICS
albendazole
ivermectin

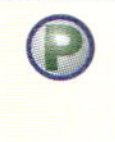 mebendazole
praziquantel
pyrantel

Helminthic infections, or infections in the gastrointestinal (GI) tract or other tissues due to worm infection, affect about one billion people, making these types of infections among the most common of all diseases. These infestations are very common in tropical areas, but they are also often found in other regions, including countries such as Australia and New Zealand. With so many people travelling to many parts of the world, it is not uncommon for a traveller to contract a helminthic infection in one country and inadvertently bring it home, where the worms can then infect other individuals (see Box 13.1). The **helminths** that most commonly infect humans are of two types: the nematodes (or roundworms) and the platyhelminths (or flatworms) that cause intestine-invading worm infections; and tissue-invading worms.

Being diagnosed with a worm infestation may be personally confronting. Nurses and midwives need to take care to avoid forming preconceptions or judgements. It is very important for the nurse or midwife to understand the disease process and to explain the disease and treatment carefully to help the person to cope with both the diagnosis and the treatment.

BOX 13.1 FOCUS ON **Cultural considerations**

Travellers and helminths

People who come from or travel to areas of the world where schistosomiasis is endemic should always be assessed for the possibility of infection with such a disease when seen for health care. Areas of the world in which this disease is endemic are mainly tropical settings, such as Puerto Rico, islands of the West Indies, Africa, parts of South America, the Philippines, China, Japan and Southeast Asia. People travelling to these areas should be warned about wading, swimming or bathing in freshwater streams, ponds or lakes. For example, swimming in the Nile River is a popular attraction on Egyptian vacation tours; however, this activity may result in a lasting (unhappy) memory when the traveller returns home and is diagnosed with schistosomiasis. The nurse or midwife can suggest to people who are planning a visit to one of these areas that they contact the SmartTraveller website for health and safety guidelines, as well as what signs and symptoms to watch for after returning home. SmartTraveller information can be reached online at www.smartraveller.gov.au/.

INTESTINE-INVADING WORM INFECTIONS

Many of the worms that infect humans live only in the intestinal tract. Proper diagnosis of a helminthic infection requires a stool examination for ova (eggs) and parasites. Treatment of a helminthic infection entails the use of an anthelmintic drug. Another important part of therapy for helminthic infections involves the prevention of re-infection or spread of an existing infection. Measures such as thorough hand washing after use of the toilet; frequent laundering of bed linens and underwear in very hot, chlorine-treated water; disinfection of toilets and bathroom areas after each use; and good personal hygiene to wash away ova are important to prevent the spread of the disease. See Table 13.1 for a summary of worms that cause intestinal infections.

Infections by nematodes

Nematodes, or roundworms, include the commonly encountered pinworms, whipworms, threadworms, *Ascaris* and hookworms. These worms cause diseases that range from mild to potentially fatal.

Pinworm infections

Pinworms are usually transmitted when the worm eggs are ingested, either by transfer by touching the eggs when they are shed to clothing, toys or bedding; or by the inhalation of eggs that become airborne and are then swallowed. Pinworms, which remain in the intestine, cause little discomfort except for perianal itching or occasionally vaginal itching. Infection with pinworms is the most common helminthic infection among school-aged children.

TABLE 13.1 Helminthic infections

Intestine-invading worm	Mechanism of disease	Manifestations
Pinworms	Remain in intestine	Perianal itching Occasionally, vaginal itching
Whipworms	Attach to wall of colon	Colic Bloody diarrhoea (with large numbers of worms)
Threadworms	Burrow into intestine; can enter lungs, liver and other tissue	Pneumonia, liver abscess
Ascaris	Burrow into intestine; enter the blood and infect lungs	Cough, fever, pulmonary infiltrates; abdominal distension and pain
Hookworms	Attach to the wall of the intestine	Anaemia, fatigue, malabsorption
Cestodes	Live in the intestine, ingesting nutrients from the host	Weight loss, abdominal distension

Whipworm infections

Whipworms are transmitted when eggs found in the soil are ingested. Whipworms attach to the wall of the colon. In large numbers, they cause colic and bloody diarrhoea. In severe cases, whipworm infestation may result in prolapse of the intestinal wall and anaemia related to blood loss.

Threadworm infestation

Threadworms can cause more damage to humans than most of the other helminths. Threadworms are transmitted as larvae found in the soil and inadvertently ingested. The larvae mature into worms, and, after burrowing into the wall of the small intestine, female worms lay eggs. These eggs hatch into larvae that invade many body tissues, including the lungs, liver and heart. In very severe cases, death may occur from pneumonia or from lung or liver abscesses that result from larval invasion.

Ascaris

Worldwide, ***Ascaris*** infection is the most prevalent helminthic infection. It may occur wherever sanitation is poor. Eggs in the soil are ingested with vegetables or other improperly washed foods. Many individuals are unaware that they have this infestation unless they see a worm in their stool. However, others become quite ill.

Initially, the individual ingests fertilised roundworm eggs, which hatch in the small intestine and then make their way to the lungs, where they may cause cough, fever and other signs of a pulmonary infiltrate. The larvae then migrate back to the intestine, where they grow to adult size (i.e. about as long and as big around as an earthworm), causing abdominal distension and pain. In the most severe cases, intestinal obstruction by masses of worms can occur.

Hookworm infections

Hookworm eggs are found in the soil, where they hatch into larvae that moult and become infective to humans. The larvae penetrate the skin and then enter the blood and within about a week reach the intestine. Hookworms attach to the small intestine of infected individuals. The worms suck blood from the walls of the intestine, damaging the intestinal wall and leading to severe anaemia with lethargy, weakness and fatigue. Malabsorption problems may occur as the small intestinal mucosa is altered. Treatment for anaemia and fluid and electrolyte disturbances is an important part of the therapy for this infection.

Infections caused by platyhelminths

The **platyhelminths** (flatworms) include the cestodes (tapeworms) that live in the human intestine and the flukes (schistosomes) that live in the intestine and that also invade other tissues as part of their life cycle. Because schistosomes invade tissues, they are discussed in the following section on tissue-invading worm infections.

Cestodes

Cestodes are segmented flatworms with a head, or scolex, and a variable number of segments that grow from the head. Cestodes enter the body as larvae that are found in undercooked meat or fish; they sometimes form worms that are several metres long. Persons with a tapeworm may experience some abdominal discomfort and distension, as well as weight loss because the worm eats ingested nutrients. Many infected people require a great deal of psychological support when they excrete parts of the tapeworm or when the worm occasionally exits through the mouth or nose.

TISSUE-INVADING WORM INFECTIONS

Some of the worms that invade the body exist outside of the intestinal tract and can seriously damage the tissues they invade. Because of their location within healthy tissue, they can also be more difficult to treat.

Trichinosis

Trichinosis is the disease caused by ingestion of the encysted larvae of the roundworm, *Trichinella spiralis*, in undercooked pork. Once ingested, the larvae are deposited in the intestinal mucosa, pass into the bloodstream and are carried throughout the body. They can penetrate skeletal muscle and can cause an inflammatory reaction in cardiac muscle and in the brain. Fatal pneumonia, heart failure and encephalitis may occur.

The best treatment for trichinosis is prevention. Because the larvae are ingested by humans in undercooked pork, freezing pork meat, monitoring the food eaten by pigs and instructing individuals about properly cooking pork can be most beneficial.

Filariasis

Filariasis refers to infection of the blood and tissues of healthy individuals by worm embryos, which enter the body via insect bites. These thread-like embryos, or filariae, can overwhelm the lymphatic system and cause massive inflammatory reactions. This may lead to severe swelling of the hands, feet, legs, arms, scrotum or breast – a condition called elephantiasis.

Schistosomiasis

Schistosomiasis (see Figure 13.1) is a platyhelminthic infection by a fluke that is carried by a snail. This disease is a common problem in parts of Africa, Asia

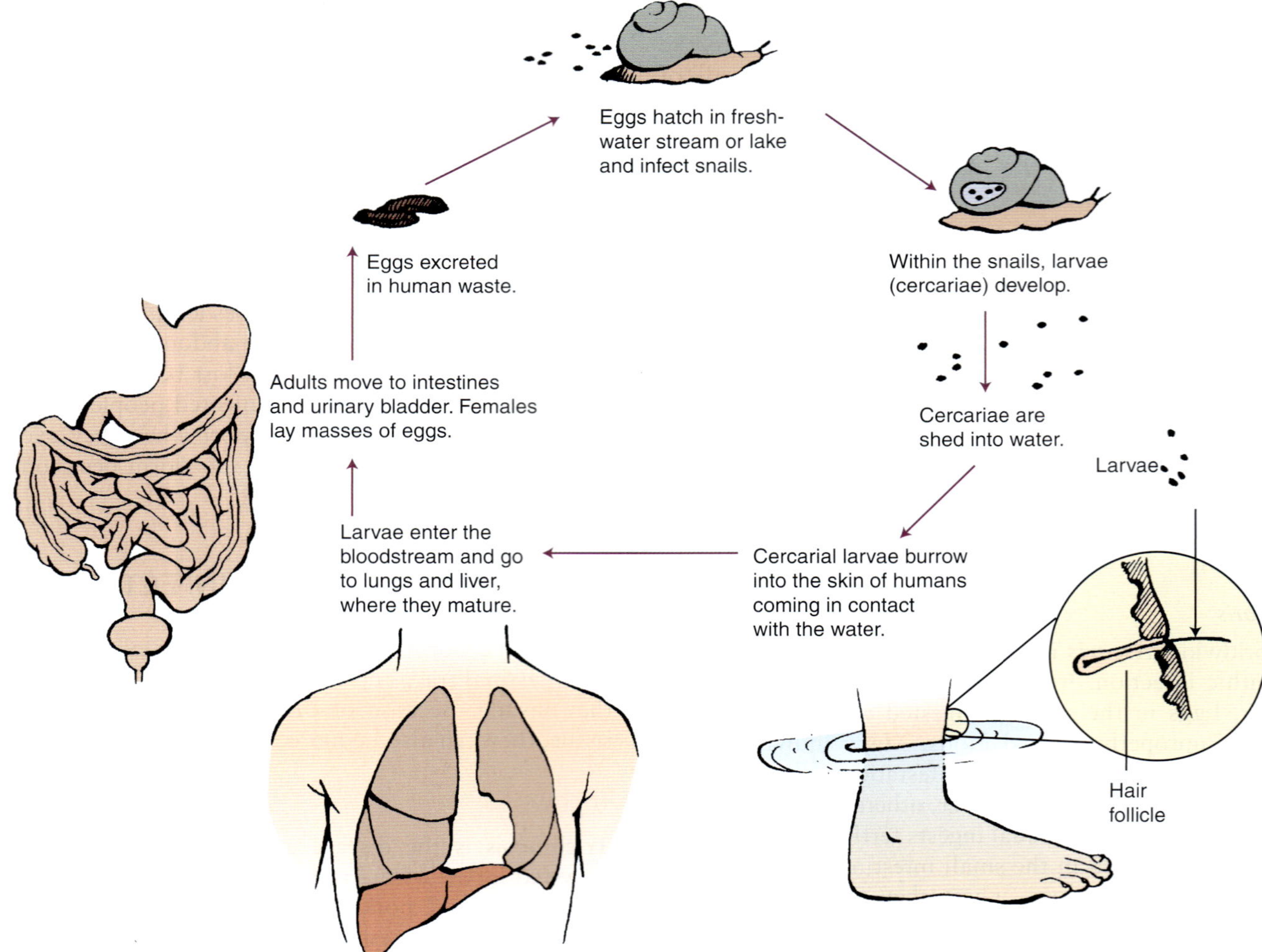

FIGURE 13.1 Life cycle of schistosomes.

and certain South American and Caribbean countries that have climates and snails conducive to the life cycle of schistosomes.

Eggs that are excreted in the urine and faeces of infected individuals hatch in fresh water into a form that infects a certain snail. In the snail, larvae known as cercariae develop. The snail sheds the cercariae back into the freshwater pond or lake. People become infected when they come in contact with the infested water. The larvae attach to the skin and quickly burrow into the bloodstream and lymphatics. Then they move into the lungs, and later to the liver, where they mature into adult worms that mate and migrate to the intestines and urinary bladder. The female worms then lay large numbers of eggs, which are expelled in the faeces and urine, and the cycle begins again.

Signs and symptoms may include a pruritic rash, often called swimmer's itch, where the larva attaches to the skin. About 1 or 2 months later, affected individuals may experience several weeks of fever, chills, headache and other symptoms. Chronic or severe infestation may lead to abdominal pain and diarrhoea, as well as blockage of blood flow to areas of the liver, lungs and central nervous system (CNS). These blockages can lead to liver and spleen enlargement, as well as signs of CNS and cardiac ischaemia. (See Critical thinking scenario for a case study of a person diagnosed with chronic schistosomiasis.)

KEY POINTS

- Helminths are worms that cause disease by invading the human body. Some helminths invade body tissues and can seriously damage lymphatic tissue, lungs, CNS, heart or liver.
- Pinworms are the most frequent cause of helminth infection in Australia and New Zealand, and roundworms called *Ascaris* are the most frequent cause of helminth infections throughout the world.
- Education is important for decreasing the stress and anxiety that may occur when individuals are diagnosed with a worm infestation.

ANTHELMINTICS

The anthelmintic drugs (see Table 13.2) act on metabolic pathways that are present in the invading worm but are absent or significantly different in the human host. Anthelmintic drugs include albendazole (*Eskazole, Zentel*), ivermectin (*Stromectol*), mebendazole (*Ridworm, Vermox*), praziquantel (*Biltricide*) and pyrantel (*Anthel, Combantrin*). Box 13.2 includes information about use of these drugs across the lifespan. See the Critical thinking scenario for a case study of a person receiving anthelmintics.

TABLE 13.2 *DRUGS IN FOCUS* Anthelmintics

Drug name	Dosage/route	Usual indications
albendazole (*Eskazole, Zentel*)	Hydatid disease: ≥ 60 kg: 400 mg bd PO < 60 kg: 15 mg/kg/day PO in divided doses, bd, on a 28-day cycle, followed by 14 days of rest, for a total of three cycles Neurocysticercosis: ≥ 60 kg: 400 mg bd PO < 60 kg: 15/mg/kg/day PO in divided doses, bd, for 3–7 days of treatment	Treatment of active lesions caused by pork tapeworm and cystic disease of the liver, lungs and peritoneum caused by dog tapeworm
ivermectin (*Stromectol*)	150–200 micrograms/kg PO as a single dose	Treatment of threadworm disease or strongyloidiasis; onchocerciasis or river blindness, which is found in tropical areas of Africa, Mexico and South America
(P) mebendazole (*Ridworm, Vermox*)	100 mg PO morning and evening on three consecutive days Enterobiasis: 100 mg PO as a single dose	Treatment of diseases caused by pinworms, roundworms, whipworms and hookworms
praziquantel (*Biltricide*)	Three doses of 20–25 mg/kg PO as a 1-day treatment	Treatment of a wide number of schistosomes or flukes
pyrantel (*Anthel, Combantrin*)	10 mg/kg PO as a single dose; maximum dose, 1 g	Treatment of diseases caused by pinworms and roundworms; because administered in single dose, may be preferred for people who could have trouble remembering to take medication or following drug regimens

BOX 13.2 FOCUS ON Drug therapy across the lifespan

Anthelmintic agents

CHILDREN

Culture of the suspected worm is important before beginning any drug therapy.

The more toxic drugs – albendazole, ivermectin and praziquantel – should be avoided in children.

The most commonly used anthelmintic, mebendazole, comes in a chewable tablet that is convenient for use in children.

Nutritional status and hydration are major concerns with children taking these drugs who develop serious gastrointestinal effects.

ADULTS

Adults may be somewhat repulsed by the idea that they have a worm infestation, and they may be reluctant to discuss the needed lifestyle adjustments and treatment plans.

PREGNANCY AND BREASTFEEDING

Pregnant and breastfeeding women should not use these drugs unless the benefit clearly outweighs the potential risk to the fetus or neonate. If a severe helminth infestation threatens the mother, some of the drugs can be used as long as the mother is informed of the potential risk.

OLDER ADULTS

Older people may be more susceptible to the central nervous system and gastrointestinal effects of some of these drugs. Dose adjustment is needed for these agents.

Monitor hydration and nutritional status carefully.

CRITICAL THINKING SCENARIO

Anthelmintics

THE SITUATION

V.Y., a 33-year-old man from Sudan, underwent a complete physical examination in preparation for a training job in custodial work at a local hospital. He was a refugee who had come to Australia 6 months ago as part of a sponsored resettlement program. In the course of the examination, it was found that he had a history of chronic diarrhoea, hepatomegaly, pulmonary rales and splenomegaly. Further tests indicated that he had chronic schistosomiasis. Because of V.Y.'s limited use of the English language, he was hospitalised so that his disease, which was unfamiliar to most of the associated health care providers, could be monitored. He was treated with praziquantel.

CRITICAL THINKING

What are the important care implications for V.Y.? *Think about the serious limitations that are placed on medical care, particularly teaching, when the person and the health care workers do not speak the same language.*

What innovative techniques could be used to teach this person about the disease, the drugs and the hygiene measures that are important for him to follow?

Are the other people or workers in the hospital exposed to any health risks? What sort of educational program should be developed to teach them about this disease and to allay any fears or anxieties they may have?

What special interventions are needed to explain the drug therapy and any adverse effects or warning signs that V.Y. should be watching for?

DISCUSSION

A language barrier can be a real handicap in the health care system. In many cases, pictures can assist communication. For example, the need for nutritious food is conveyed by using appropriate pictures of foods that should be eaten. Frequent reinforcement is necessary because the person has no way of letting you know that they really understand the message that you are trying to convey. The person is prepared for discharge through careful teaching that may involve pictures, calendars and clocks so that they are given every opportunity to comply with their medical regimen.

In addition, the staff should contact the local health department to determine whether the local sewer system can properly handle contaminated wastes. In this case, the staff learned from the local health department that the snail's intermediate host does not live in this country, so the hazards posed by this waste are small, and normal disposal of the wastes should be appropriate.

V.Y. should also be observed for signs of adverse effects, although praziquantel is a relatively mild drug. Drug fever, abdominal pain or dizziness may occur. If dizziness occurs, safety precautions, such as assistance with ambulation, use of side rails and adequate lighting, need to be taken without alarming the person.

CARE GUIDE FOR V.Y.: ANTHELMINTIC AGENTS

Assessment: history and examination

Allergies to this drug, renal or liver dysfunction
Drug history: use of albendazole
Local: culture of infection
CNS: orientation, affect
Skin: colour, lesions, texture
GI: abdominal and liver evaluation, including liver function tests
GU: renal function tests

Implementation

Culture for ova and parasites before beginning therapy.
Provide comfort and safety measures: small, frequent meals; safety precautions; hygiene measures; maintenance of nutrition.
Monitor nutritional status as needed.
Provide support and reassurance to deal with drug effects, discomfort and diagnosis.
Provide teaching regarding drug name, dosage regimen, adverse effects and precautions to report, and hygiene measures to observe.

Evaluation

Evaluate drug effects: resolution of helminth infection.
Monitor for adverse effects: GI alterations, CNS changes, dizziness and confusion, renal and hepatic function.
Monitor for drug–drug interactions: concurrent use of albendazole.
Evaluate effectiveness of teaching program.
Evaluate effectiveness of comfort and safety measures.

TEACHING FOR V.Y.

- This drug is called an anthelmintic. It works to destroy certain helminths, or worms, that have invaded your body.
- It is important that you take the full course of the drug – three doses the first day, then retesting to repeat this course if needed to ensure that all of the worms, in all phases of their life cycle, have disappeared from your body.
- You may take this drug with meals or with a light snack to help decrease any stomach upset that you may

experience. Swallow the tablets whole and avoid holding them in your mouth for any length of time because a very unpleasant taste may occur.
- Common effects of this drug include
  - *Nausea, vomiting and loss of appetite:* take the drug with food, and eat small, frequent meals.
  - *Dizziness and drowsiness:* if this occurs, avoid driving a car or operating dangerous machinery. Change positions slowly to avoid falling or injury.
- Report any of the following conditions to your health care provider: fever, chills, rash, headache, weakness or tremors.
- Take all of the drug that has been prescribed. Never use this drug to self-treat any other infection or give it to any other person.
- Tell any doctor, nurse or other health care provider that you are taking this drug.
- Keep this drug and all medications out of the reach of children.

Therapeutic actions and indications

Anthelmintic agents are indicated for the treatment of infections by certain susceptible worms and are very specific in the worms that they affect; they are not interchangeable for treating various worm infections. See Table 13.2 for usual indications for each of these agents. Anthelmintics interfere with metabolic processes in particular worms, as described previously. Figure 13.2 shows sites of actions for these drugs.

Pharmacokinetics

Mebendazole is available in the form of a chewable tablet, and a typical 3-day course can be repeated in 3 weeks if needed. Very little of the mebendazole is absorbed systemically, so adverse effects are few. The drug is not metabolised in the body, and most of it is excreted unchanged in the faeces. A small amount may be excreted in the urine.

Albendazole is poorly absorbed from the GI tract, reaching peak plasma levels in about 5 hours. It is metabolised in the liver and primarily excreted in urine.

Ivermectin is readily absorbed from the GI tract and reaches peak plasma levels in 4 hours. It is completely metabolised in the liver with a half-life of 16 hours; excretion is through the faeces.

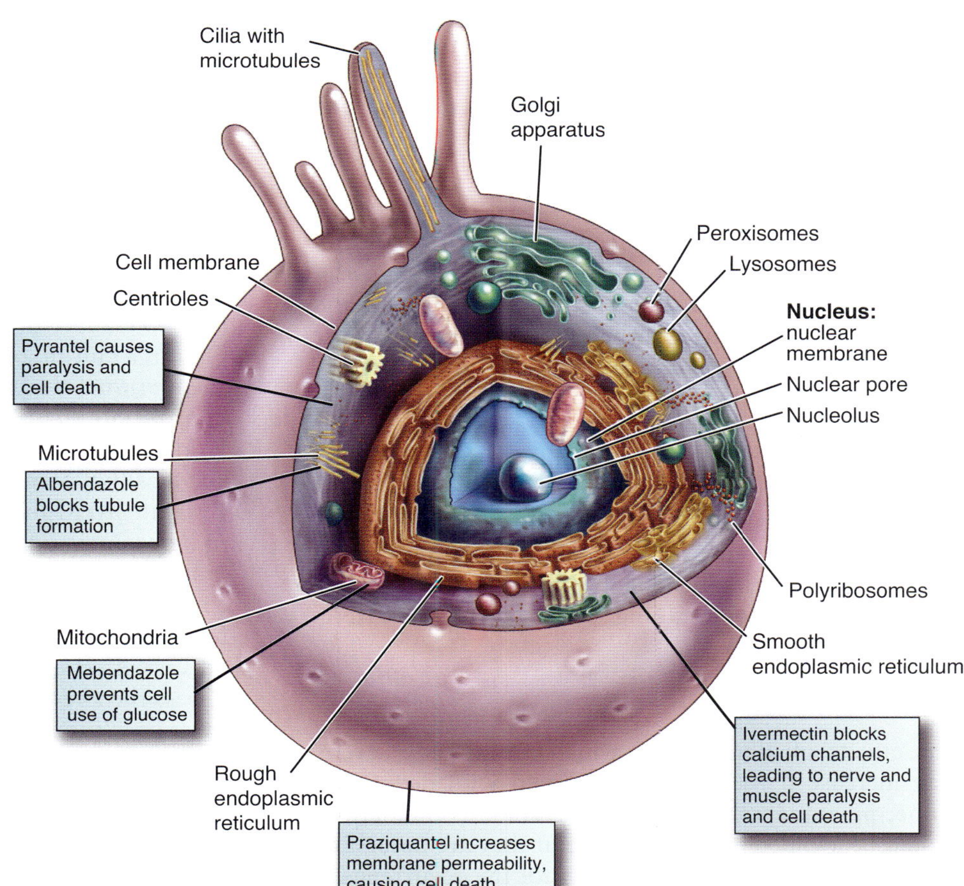

FIGURE 13.2 General structure of a cell, showing the sites of action of the anthelmintic agents. Mebendazole interferes with the ability to use glucose, leading to an inability to reproduce and cell death. Albendazole blocks tubule formation, resulting in cell death. Ivermectin blocks calcium channels, leading to nerve and muscle paralysis and cell death. Pyrantel is a neuromuscular polarising agent that causes paralysis and cell death. Praziquantel increases membrane permeability, leading to a loss of intracellular calcium and muscular paralysis; it may also result in disintegration of the integument.

Praziquantel is taken in a series of three oral doses at 4–6-hour intervals. It is rapidly absorbed from the GI tract and reaches peak plasma levels within 1–3 hours. It is metabolised in the liver with a half-life of 0.8–1.5 hours. Excretion of praziquantel occurs primarily through the urine.

Pyrantel is poorly absorbed, and most of the drug is excreted unchanged in the faeces, although a small amount may be found in the urine.

Contraindications and cautions

Overall contraindications to the use of anthelmintic drugs include the presence of known allergy to any of these drugs; breastfeeding *because the drugs can enter breast milk and could be toxic to the infant* – women are advised to refrain from breastfeeding when using these drugs; and pregnancy (in most cases) *because of reported associated fetal abnormalities or death.* Women of childbearing age should be advised to use barrier contraceptives while taking these drugs. Pyrantel has not been established as safe for use in children younger than 2 years. Albendazole should be used only after the causative worm has been identified *because it can cause adverse effects on the liver, which could be problematic if the person has liver involvement.*

Use caution in the presence of renal or hepatic disease *that interferes with the metabolism or excretion of drugs that are absorbed systemically* and in cases of severe diarrhoea and malnourishment, *which could alter the effects of the drug on the intestine and any pre-existing helminths.*

Adverse effects

Adverse effects frequently encountered with the use of these anthelmintic agents are related to their absorption or direct action in the intestine. Mebendazole and pyrantel, which are not absorbed systemically, may cause abdominal discomfort, diarrhoea or pain but have very few other effects and are well tolerated. Anthelmintics that are absorbed systemically may cause the following effects: headache and dizziness; fever, shaking, chills and malaise associated with an immune reaction to the death of the worms; rash; pruritus; and loss of hair.

Renal failure and severe bone marrow depression are associated with albendazole, which is toxic to some human tissues. People taking this drug require careful monitoring.

Clinically important drug–drug interactions

The effects of albendazole, which are already severe, may increase if the drug is combined with dexamethasone, praziquantel or cimetidine. These combinations should be avoided if at all possible; if they are necessary, people should be monitored closely for the occurrence of adverse effects.

Prototype summary: mebendazole

Indications: treatment of whipworm, pinworm, roundworm and hookworm infections.

Actions: irreversibly blocks glucose uptake by susceptible helminths, depleting glycogen stores needed for survival and reproduction, causing the death of the helminth.

Pharmacokinetics:

Route	Onset	Peak
Oral	Slow	2–4 hours

$T_{1/2}$: 2.5–9 hours; metabolised in the liver and excreted in the faeces.

Adverse effects: transient abdominal pain, diarrhoea, fever.

Care considerations for people receiving anthelmintics

Assessment: history and examination

- Assess for possible contraindications or cautions: history of allergy to any of the anthelmintics *to avoid hypersensitivity reactions*; history of hepatic or renal dysfunction *that might interfere with drug metabolism and excretion of the drug*; and current status related to pregnancy and breastfeeding, *which are contraindications to the use of these drugs.*
- Perform a physical assessment *to establish baseline data for determining the effectiveness of the drug and the occurrence of any adverse effects associated with drug therapy.*
- Obtain a culture of stool for ova and parasites *to determine the infecting worm and establish appropriate treatment.*
- Examine reflexes and muscle strength *to evaluate changes that occur as a result of drug therapy.*
- Evaluate liver function and renal function tests *to determine appropriateness of therapy and to monitor for toxicity.*
- Examine skin, including colour, temperature and texture, and note any lesions to assess for possible adverse effects.
- Assess the abdomen *to evaluate for any changes from baseline related to the infection, identify possible adverse effects and monitor for improvement.*

Implementation with rationale

- Arrange for appropriate culture and sensitivity tests before beginning therapy *to ensure identification of the correct cause and use of the appropriate drug.*
- Administer the complete course of the drug *to obtain the full beneficial effects.* Ensure that chewable tablets are chewed. Give the drug with food if necessary, but avoid giving the drug with high-fat meals, which might interfere with drug effectiveness.
- Monitor hepatic and renal function before and periodically during treatment *to allow for early identification and prompt intervention if signs of failure due to albendazole administration occur.*
- Provide comfort and safety measures if CNS effects occur (eg, side rails and assistance with ambulation in the presence of dizziness and weakness) *to protect the person from injury.* Provide oral hygiene and ready access to bathroom facilities as needed *to cope with GI effects.*
- Provide small, frequent, nutritious meals if GI upset is severe *to ensure adequate nutrition.* Monitor nutritional status and arrange a dietary consultation as needed. Taking the drug with food may also decrease GI upset.
- Instruct the person about the appropriate dosage regimen and other measures *to enhance knowledge about drug therapy and to promote compliance.*
- Provide the following teaching:
  - Take safety precautions, including changing position slowly and avoiding driving and hazardous tasks, if CNS effects occur.
  - Take the drug with meals and try small, frequent meals if GI upset is a problem.
  - Identify the importance of strict hand washing and hygiene measures, including daily laundering of underwear and bed linens, daily disinfection of toilet facilities and periodic disinfection of bathroom floors (see Box 13.3).
  - Report fever, severe diarrhoea or aggravation of condition, which could indicate a resistant strain or non-effective therapy, to a health care provider.

Evaluation

- Monitor response to the drug (resolution of helminth infestation and improvement in signs and symptoms).
- Monitor for adverse effects (changes in orientation and affect, nutritional state, skin colour and evidence of lesions, hepatic and renal function and reports of abdominal discomfort and pain).
- Evaluate the effectiveness of the teaching plan (person can name the drug, dosage, possible adverse effects to watch for and specific measures to help avoid adverse effects).
- Monitor the effectiveness of comfort and safety measures and compliance with the regimen.

BOX 13.3 FOCUS ON **Individual and family teaching**

Managing pinworm infections

Infestation with worms can be a frightening and traumatic experience for most people. Seeing the worm can be an especially difficult experience. Some worm infestations are not that uncommon in Australia and New Zealand, especially infestation with pinworms.

Pinworms can spread very rapidly among children in schools, summer camps and other institutions. Once the infestation starts, careful hygiene measures and drug therapy are required to eradicate the disease. After the diagnosis has been made and appropriate drug therapy started, proper hygiene measures are essential. Some suggested hygiene measures that might help to control the infection include the following:

- Keep the child's nails cut short and hands well scrubbed because reinfection results from the worm's eggs being carried back to the mouth after becoming lodged under the fingernails when the child scratches the pruritic perianal area.
- Give the child a shower in the morning to wash away any ova deposited in the anal area during the night.
- Change and launder undergarments, bed linen and pyjamas every day.
- Disinfect toilet seats daily and the floors of bathrooms and bedrooms periodically.
- Encourage the child to wash hands vigorously after using the toilet.
- It is important to reassure individuals and families that these types of infections do not necessarily reflect negatively on their hygiene or lifestyle. It takes a coordinated effort among health personnel, families and individuals to control a pinworm infestation.

KEY POINTS

- Anthelmintic drugs affect metabolic processes that are either different in worms than in human hosts or are not found in humans. These agents all cause death of the worm by interfering with normal functioning.
- Proper hygiene and sanitation processes are an important part in preventing the spread of helminths, including good hand hygiene, and preparation and storage of food.

CHAPTER SUMMARY

- Helminths are worms that cause disease by invading the human body. Helminths that affect humans include nematodes (round-shaped worms) such as pinworms, hookworms, threadworms, whipworms and roundworms; and platyhelminths (flatworms), which include tapeworms and flukes.
- Pinworms are the most frequent cause of helminth infection in Australia and New Zealand, and roundworms called *Ascaris* are the most frequent cause of helminth infections throughout the world.
- Some helminths invade body tissues and can seriously damage lymphatic tissue, lungs, CNS, heart, liver and so on. These include trichinosis-causing tapeworms, which are found in undercooked pork; filariae, which occur when thread-like worm embryos clog up vascular spaces; and schistosomiasis-causing flukes. Schistosomiasis is a common problem in many tropical areas where the snail, that is necessary in the life cycle of the fluke, lives.
- Anthelmintic drugs affect metabolic processes that are either different in worms than in human hosts or are not found in humans. These agents all cause death of the worm by interfering with normal functioning.
- Prevention is a very important part of the treatment of helminths. Thorough hand washing; laundering of bed linen, pyjamas and underwear to destroy ova that are shed during the night; and disinfection of toilet facilities at least daily and of bathroom floors periodically, help to stop the spread of these diseases. In addition, proper sanitation and hygiene in food preparation and storage is essential for reducing the incidence of these infestations.
- Education is important for decreasing the stress and anxiety that may occur when individuals are diagnosed with a worm infestation.

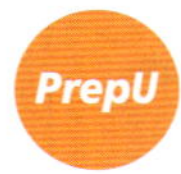

Knowing your strengths and weaknesses helps you to study more effectively. Take a PrepU Practice Quiz to find out how you measure up!

ONLINE RESOURCES

An extensive range of additional resources to enhance teaching and learning and to facilitate understanding of this chapter may be found online at the text's accompanying website, located on thePoint at http://thepoint.lww.com. These include Watch and Learn videos, Concepts in Action animations, journal articles, review questions, case studies, discussion topics and quizzes.

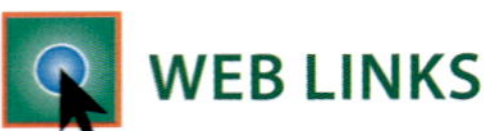

WEB LINKS

Health care providers and students may want to consult the following web resources:

www.betterhealth.vic.gov.au/bhcv2/bhcarticles.nsf/pages/Pinworms
Victorian Government information on pinworms.

http://smartraveller.gov.au
Australian Government Department of Foreign Affairs and Trade Smart Traveller.

www.who.int/topics/helminthiasis/en/
World Health Organization Information on helminth infections.

BIBLIOGRAPHY

Abbas, A. & Newsholme, W. (2011). Diagnosis and recommended treatment of helminth infections. *Prescriber, 22*, 56–64.

Dempsey, J., Hillege, S. & Hill, R. (2014). *Fundamentals of Nursing and Midwifery: A Person-centred Approach to Care* (2nd Australian and New Zealand edn). Sydney: Lippincott Williams & Wilkins.

Drudge-Coates, L. & Turner, B. (2013). Schistosomiasis: An endemic parasitic waterborne disease. *British Journal of Nursing, 22*, S12–S14.

Falcone, F. & Pritchard, D. (2005). Parasite reversal: Worms on trial. *Trends in Parasitology, 21*, 157–160.

Farrell, M. & Dempsey, J. (2014). *Smeltzer & Bare's Textbook of Medical-Surgical Nursing* (3rd edn). Sydney: Lippincott Williams & Wilkins.

Gherardin, A. (2012). Assessing fever in the returned traveller. *Australian Prescriber, 35*, 10–14.

Hamilton, S. (2005). Alleviating the distress of threadworms. *Practice Nursing, 16*, 430–432.

Horton, J. (2003). Global anthelmintic chemotherapy programs: Learning from history. *Trends in Parasitology, 19*, 405–409.

Hotez, P. J., Brooker, S., Bethony, J., Bottazzi, M. E., Loukas, A. & Xiao, S. (2004). Hookworm infection. *New England Journal of Medicine, 351*, 799–807.

Keiser, J. & Utzinger, J. (2008). Efficacy of current drugs against soil transmitted helminth infections: Systematic review. *JAMA, 299*, 1937–1948.

McKenna, L. & Mirkov, S. (2019). *McKenna's Drug Handbook for Nursing and Midwifery* (8th edn). Sydney: Wolters Kluwer Health Australia.

Porth, C. M. (2011). *Essentials of Pathophysiology: Concepts of Altered Health States* (3rd edn). Philadelphia: Lippincott Williams & Wilkins.

Porth, C. M. (2009). *Pathophysiology: Concepts of Altered Health States* (8th edn). Philadelphia: Lippincott Williams & Wilkins.

CHECK YOUR UNDERSTANDING

Answers to the questions in this chapter can be found in Appendix A at the back of this book.

MULTIPLE CHOICE

Select the best answer to the following.

1. To ensure effective treatment of pinworm infections, which instruction would be most important to emphasise to the individual and family?
   a. Keep nails long so cutting will not introduce more infection.
   b. Launder undergarments, bed linen and pyjamas every day.
   c. Boil all drinking water.
   d. Maintain a clear liquid diet for at least 7–10 days.
2. Which of the following would you expect to assess in a person who is suspected of having an *Ascaris* infection?
   a. cough and signs of pulmonary infestation
   b. cardiac arrhythmias and low blood pressure
   c. seizures and disorientation
   d. bloody diarrhoea and excessive vomiting
3. The nurse describes schistosomiasis to a group of students as an infection caused by:
   a. a protozoan carried by a mosquito.
   b. improperly cooked pork.
   c. a fluke carried by a snail.
   d. eating food contaminated by faecal material.
4. A person has travelled to Egypt and come home with schistosomiasis. The family is very concerned about spreading the disease. Which of the following would be most helpful to teach the family?
   a. Strict hand washing will stop the spread of the disease.
   b. Isolating the person will be necessary to stop the spread of the disease.
   c. Carefully cooking all of the person's food will help to stop the spread of the disease.
   d. The snail needed for the life cycle of this worm does not live in this climate.
5. A person is prescribed mebendazole. The nurse knows that this is the most commonly used anthelmintic, being the drug of choice for treating:
   a. pinworms, roundworms, whipworms and hookworms.
   b. trichinosis, flukes, cestodes and hookworms.
   c. pork tapeworm, threadworms, cestodes and whipworms.
   d. all stages of schistosomal infections.
6. Teaching regarding the use of anthelmintics should include counselling about:
   a. the use of oral contraceptives.
   b. maintenance of nutrition during therapy.
   c. the use of oral anticoagulants.
   d. cardiac drug effects.
7. People may experience anxiety about the diagnosis and treatment of helminthic infections. Teaching may help to alleviate this anxiety and should include:
   a. what they may experience if the worms are passed from the body.
   b. focus on the cleanliness of the home.
   c. measures to isolate the organism in the home.
   d. criticism of their personal hygiene practices.

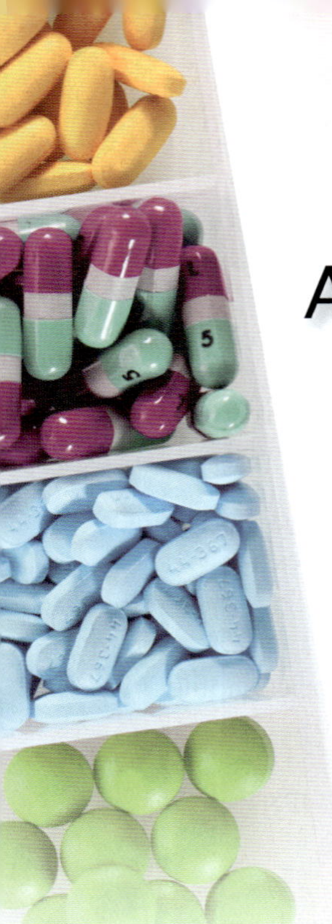

14 Antineoplastic agents

Learning objectives

On completing this chapter you should be able to:

1. Describe the nature of cancer and the changes the body undergoes when cancer occurs.
2. Describe the therapeutic actions, indications, pharmacokinetics, contraindications, most common adverse reactions and important drug–drug interactions associated with each class of antineoplastic agents and with adjunctive therapy used with these drugs.
3. Discuss the use of antineoplastic drugs across the lifespan.
4. Compare and contrast the prototype drugs for each class of antineoplastic agents with the other drugs in that class.
5. Outline the care considerations and teaching needs for people receiving each class of antineoplastic agents.

Test your current knowledge of antineoplastic agents with a PrepU Practice Quiz!

Glossary of key terms

alopecia: hair loss; a common adverse effect of many antineoplastic drugs, which are more effective against rapidly multiplying cells such as those of hair follicles

anaplasia: loss of organisation and structure; property of cancer cells

angiogenesis: the generation of new blood vessels; cancer cells release an enzyme that will cause angiogenesis or the growth of new blood vessels to feed the cancer cells

antineoplastic agent: drug used to combat cancer or the growth of neoplasms

autonomy: loss of the normal controls and reactions that inhibit growth and spreading; property of cancer cells

bone marrow suppression: inhibition of the blood-forming components of the bone marrow; a common adverse effect of many antineoplastic drugs, which are more effective against rapidly multiplying cells, such as those in bone marrow; also seen in anaemia, thrombocytopenia and leucopenia

carcinoma: tumour that originates in epithelial cells

metastasis: ability to enter the circulatory or lymphatic system and travel to other areas of the body that are conducive to growth and survival; property of cancer cells

neoplasm: new or cancerous growth; occurs when abnormal cells have the opportunity to multiply and grow

sarcoma: tumour that originates in the mesenchyme and is made up of embryonic connective tissue cells

ALKYLATING AGENTS

busulfan
carboplatin
carmustine
(P) chlorambucil
cisplatin
cyclophosphamide
dacarbazine
fotemustine
ifosfamide
lomustine
melphalan
oxaliplatin
procarbazine
temozolomide
thiotepa

ANTIMETABOLITES

asparaginase (colaspase)
azacitidine
capecitabine
cladribine
clofarabine
cytarabine
fludarabine
fluorouracil
gemcitabine
mercaptopurine
(P) methotrexate
pemetrexed
raltitrexed
thioguanine

ANTINEOPLASTIC ANTIBIOTICS

bleomycin
dactinomycin
daunorubicin
(P) doxorubicin
epirubicin
idarubicin

mitomycin
mitozantrone

MITOTIC INHIBITORS
docetaxel
etoposide
paclitaxel
vinblastine
(P) vincristine
vinorelbine

HORMONES AND HORMONE MODULATORS
abiraterone
anastrozole
bicalutamide
cabazitaxel
degarelix
exemestane
flutamide
fulvestrant
goserelin
letrozole
megestrol
nilutamide
(P) tamoxifen
toremifene
triptorelin

CANCER CELL–SPECIFIC AGENTS
bortezomib
erlotinib
everolimus
gefitinib
(P) imatinib
lapatinib
nilotinib
sorafenib
sunitinib
temsirolimus

MISCELLANEOUS ANTINEOPLASTICS
arsenic trioxide
hydroxycarbamide (hydroxyurea)
irinotecan
topotecan
tretinoin

ANTINEOPLASTIC ADJUNCTIVE THERAPY
amifostine
leucovorin
mesna
rasburicase

The use of the term chemotherapy implies cancer treatment to most people. However, only one branch of chemotherapy involves drugs developed to act on and kill or alter human cells – the **antineoplastic agents**, which are designed to fight **neoplasms**, or cancers.

Antineoplastic drugs alter human cells in a variety of ways. Their action is intended to target the abnormal cells that compose the neoplasm or cancer, having a greater impact on them than on normal cells. Unfortunately, normal cells also are affected by antineoplastic agents.

This area of pharmacology, which has grown tremendously in recent years, now includes many drugs that act on, or are part of, the immune system. These substances fight the cancerous cells using components of the immune system instead of destroying cells directly (see Chapter 15). This chapter discusses the classic antineoplastic agents and includes those drugs that are used in cancer chemotherapy.

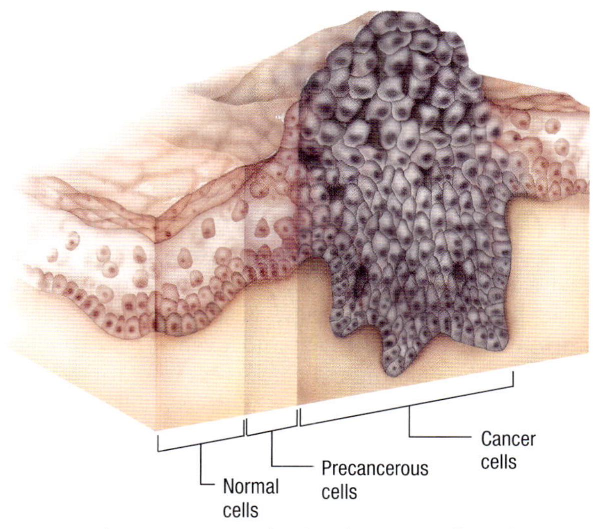

FIGURE 14.1 Malignant tumours develop from one cell, with somatic mutations occurring during cell division as the tumour grows.

CANCER

Cancer is a disease that can strike a person at any age and is one of the leading causes of death in Australia and New Zealand. Treatment of cancer can be prolonged and often debilitating. The person can experience numerous and wide-ranging complications and effects.

All cancers start with a single cell that is genetically different from the other cells in the surrounding tissue. This cell divides, passing along its abnormalities to daughter cells, eventually producing a tumour or neoplasm that has characteristics quite different from those of the original tissue (see Figure 14.1). As the abnormal cells continue to divide, they lose more and more of their original cell characteristics. The cancerous cells exhibit **anaplasia** – a loss of cellular differentiation and organisation, which leads to a loss of their ability to function normally. They also exhibit **autonomy**, growing without the usual homeostatic restrictions that regulate cell growth and control. This loss of control allows the cells to form a tumour.

Over time, these neoplastic cells grow uncontrollably, invading and damaging healthy tissue in the area and even undergoing **metastasis**, or travelling from the place of origin to develop new tumours in other areas of the body where conditions are favourable for cell growth (see Figure 14.2). The abnormal cells release enzymes that generate blood vessels (**angiogenesis**) in the area to supply both oxygen and nutrients to the cells, thus contributing to their growth. Overall, the cancerous cells rob the host cells of energy and nutrients and block normal lymph and vascular vessels as the result of pressure and intrusion on normal cells, leading to a loss of normal cellular function.

The body's immune system can damage or destroy some neoplastic cells. T cells, which recognise the abnormal cells and destroy them; antibodies, which form in response to parts of the abnormal cell protein;

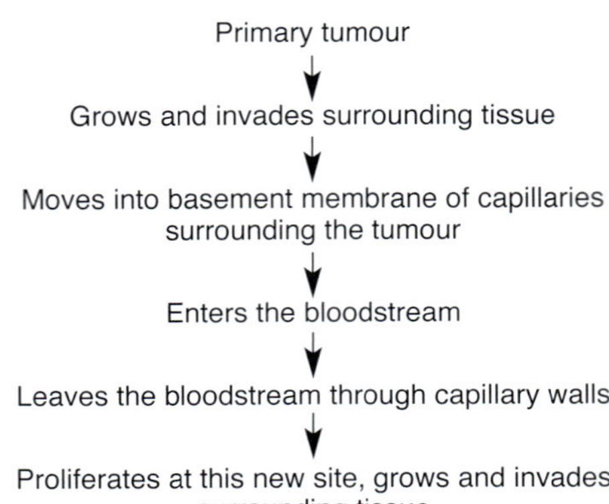

FIGURE 14.2 Metastasis of cancer cells.

interferons; and tissue necrosis factor (TNF) all play a role in the body's attempt to eliminate the abnormal cells before they become uncontrollable and threaten the life of the host. Once the neoplasm has grown and enlarged, it may overwhelm the immune system, which is no longer able to manage the problem.

Causes of cancer

What causes the cells to mutate and become genetically different is not clearly understood. In some cases, a genetic predisposition to such a mutation can be found. Breast cancer, for example, seems to have a definite genetic link. In other cases, viral infection, constant irritation and cell turnover and even stress have been blamed for the ensuing cancer. Stress reactions suppress the activities of the immune system (see Chapter 29), so if a cell is mutating while a person is under prolonged stress, research suggests that the cell has a better chance of growing into a neoplasm than when the person's immune system is fully active. Pipe smokers are at increased risk for development of tongue and mouth cancers because the heat of the pipe and chemicals in the pipe tobaccos and smoke continuously destroy normal cells, which must be replaced rapidly, increasing the chances for development of a mutant cell. People living in areas with carcinogenic or cancer-causing chemicals in the air, water or even the ground are at increased risk of developing mutant cells in response to exposure to these toxic chemicals. Cancer clusters are often identified in such high-risk areas. Not everyone exposed to carcinogens or undergoing stress or having a genetic predisposition to develop cancer actually develops cancer. Researchers have not discovered what the actual trigger for cancer development is or what protective abilities some people have that other people lack. Most likely, a mosaic of factors coming together in one person leads to development of the neoplasm.

The estimated total number of new cancers diagnosed in Australia in 2019 was 144,713. Of these new cancers diagnosed, 78,081 were diagnosed in males and 66,632 in females. The most common cancers in Australia (excluding non-melanoma skin cancer) are prostate, breast, colorectal (bowel), melanoma and lung cancer. These five cancers account for around 60% of all cancers diagnosed in Australia. Cancer control is one of the Australian government's nine National Health Priority Areas. For more information on cancer-associated indicators and risk factors, see www.aihw.gov.au/reports/cancer/cancer-data-in-australia/contents/summary and https://canceraustralia.gov.au/affected-cancer/what-cancer/cancer-australia-statistics.

Types of cancer

Cancers can be divided into two groups: (1) solid tumours; and (2) haematological malignancies such as the leukaemias and lymphomas, which occur in the blood-forming organs. Solid tumours may originate in any body organ and may be further divided into **carcinomas**, or tumours that originate in epithelial cells, and **sarcomas**, or tumours that originate in the mesenchyme and are made up of embryonic connective tissue cells. Examples of carcinomas include granular cell tumours of the breast, bronchogenic tumours arising in cells that line the bronchial tubes and squamous and basal tumours of the skin. Sarcomas include osteogenic tumours, which form in the primitive cells of the bone, and rhabdomyosarcomas, which occur in striated muscles. Haematological malignancies involve the blood-forming organs of the body, the bone marrow and the lymphatic system. These malignancies alter the body's ability to produce and regulate the cells found in the blood.

KEY POINTS

- Cancers arise from a single abnormal cell that multiplies and grows.
- Cancer cells lose their normal function (anaplasia), develop characteristics that allow them to grow in an uninhibited way (autonomy) and have the ability to travel to other sites in the body that are conducive to their growth (metastasis). They also have the ability to grow new blood vessels to feed the tumour (angiogenesis).
- The goal of cancer chemotherapy is to decrease the size of the neoplasm so that the human immune system can deal with it.

ANTINEOPLASTIC DRUGS

Antineoplastic drugs can work by affecting cell survival or by boosting the immune system in its efforts to combat the abnormal cells (see Figure 14.3). Chapter 17 discusses the immune agents that are used to combat cancer. This chapter focuses on those drugs that affect cell survival. The antineoplastic drugs that are commonly

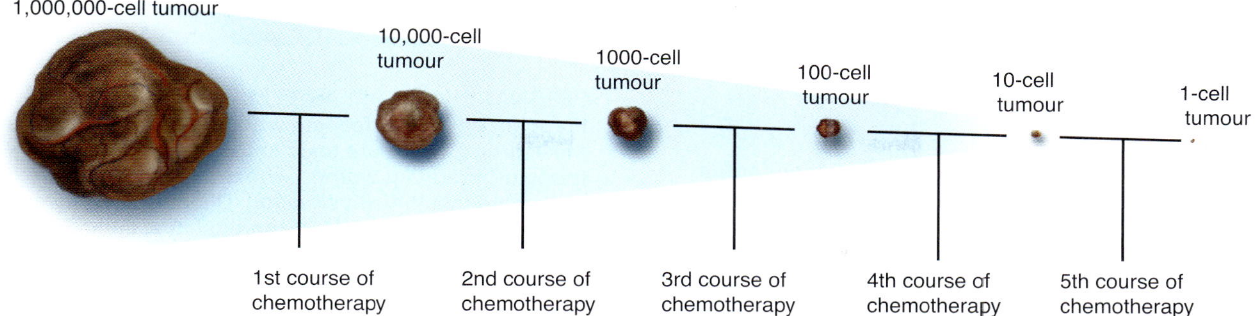

FIGURE 14.3 Cell kill theory. A set percentage of cells is killed after each dose of chemotherapy. The percentage killed is dependent upon the drug therapy. In this example, each course of chemotherapy kills 90% of cells in a cancerous tumour. After the fifth course of chemotherapy in this example, a 1-cell tumour remains; the person's immune system would destroy this malignant cell.

used today include alkylating agents, antimetabolites, antineoplastic antibiotics, mitotic inhibitors, hormones and hormone modulators, cancer cell–specific agents, protein tyrosine kinase inhibitors (which target enzymes specific to the cancer cells) and a group of antineoplastic agents that cannot be classified elsewhere. Other drugs are used to combat the serious adverse effects that can be associated with the antineoplastic drugs. These drugs are used as adjunctive therapy. Figure 14.4 shows sites of action of these drugs. Box 14.1 discusses use of these drugs across the lifespan.

As discussed in Chapter 7, all cells progress through a cell cycle. Different types of cells progress at different rates (see Figure 7.6). Rapidly multiplying cells, or cells that replace themselves quickly, include those lining the gastrointestinal (GI) tract and those in hair follicles, skin and bone marrow. These cells complete the cell cycle every few days. Cells that proceed very slowly through

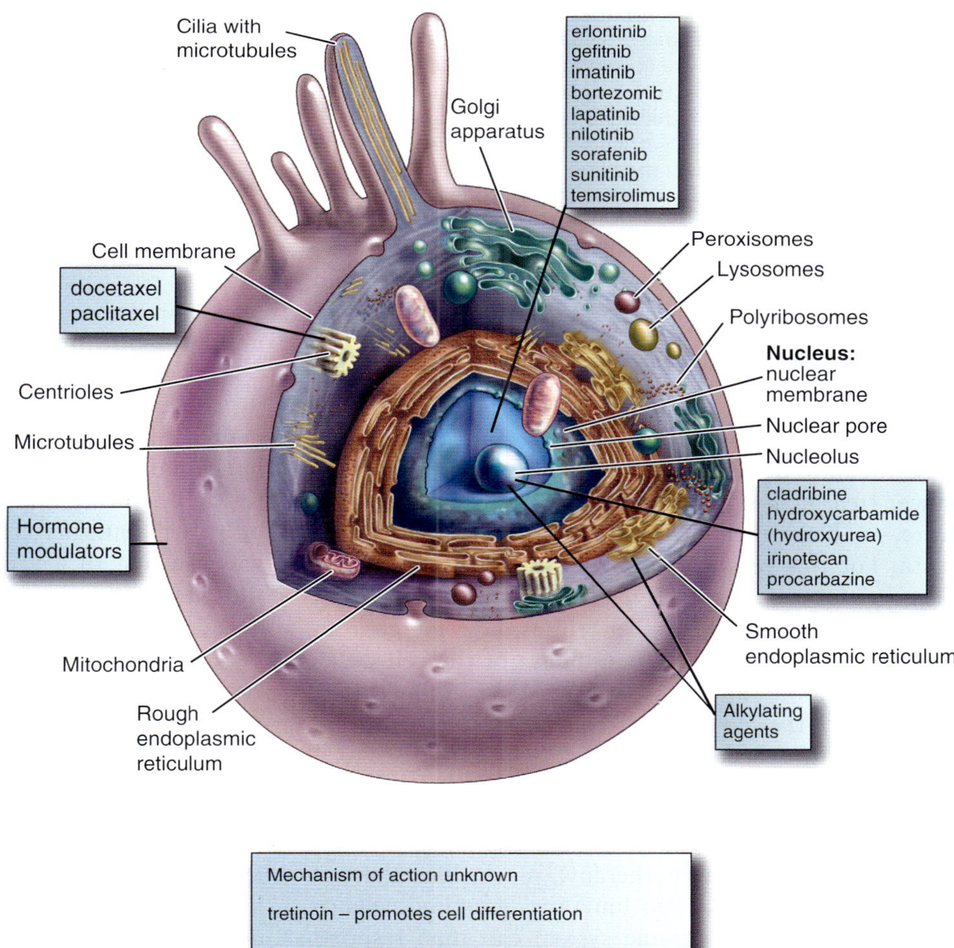

FIGURE 14.4 Sites of action of non–cell cycle-specific antineoplastic agents. Alkylating agents interfere with RNA, DNA or other cellular proteins. For example, procarbazine blocks DNA, RNA and protein synthesis. Hormone modulators react with specific receptor sites to block cell growth and activity. Mitotic inhibitors such as docetaxel and paclitaxel inhibit microtubular reorganisation. The antimetabolite cladribine and miscellaneous agent hydroxycarbamide (hydroxyurea) block DNA synthesis. The miscellaneous agent irinotecan disrupts DNA strands. Cell-specific agents such as gefitinib, erlotinib, lapatinib, nilotinib, sorafenib, sunitinib, temsirolimus and imatinib inhibit protein tyrosine kinases. Bortezomib is a proteasome inhibitor.

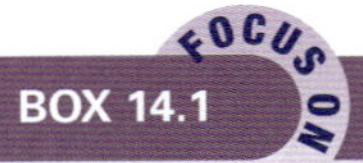

BOX 14.1 Drug therapy across the lifespan

Antineoplastic agents

CHILDREN

Antineoplastic protocols have been developed for the treatment of most paediatric cancers. Combination therapy is stressed to eliminate as many of the mutant cells as possible. Dose and timing of these combinations is crucial.

Independent checking of dose, including recalculating desired dose and verifying the drug amount with another nurse, is good practice when giving these toxic drugs to children.

Children need to be monitored closely for hydration and nutritional status. The nutritional needs of a child are greater than those of an adult, and this needs to be considered when formulating a care plan.

These children need support and comfort. They also need to be allowed to explore and learn like any other children. Body image problems, lack of energy and the need to protect the child from exposure to infection can isolate a child receiving antineoplastic agents. The total care plan of the child needs to include social, emotional and intellectual stimulation.

Monitor bone marrow activity very carefully and adjust the dose accordingly.

ADULTS

The adult receiving antineoplastic drugs is confronted with many dilemmas that the care provider needs to address. Changes in body image are common, with loss of hair, skin changes, gastrointestinal (GI) complaints and weight loss. Fear of the diagnosis and the treatment is also common with these individuals. Networking support systems and providing teaching, reassurance and comfort can have a tremendous impact on the success of the drug therapy.

PREGNANCY AND BREASTFEEDING

Pregnant and breastfeeding women should not receive these drugs, which are toxic to the developing cells of the fetus. Pregnant women who are diagnosed with cancer are in a difficult situation. The drug therapy can have serious adverse effects on the fetus, and not using the drug therapy can be detrimental to the mother. Education, support and referrals to appropriate specialists are important. Breastfeeding women should find another method of feeding the baby to prevent the adverse effects to the fetus that occur when these drugs cross into breast milk. Use of barrier contraceptives is urged when these drugs are being used by women of childbearing age.

OLDER ADULTS

Older adults may be more susceptible to the central nervous system (CNS) and GI effects of some of these drugs. Older people should be monitored for hydration and nutritional status regularly. Safety precautions should be instituted if CNS effects occur, including increased lighting, assistance with ambulation and use of supports.

Many older people have decreased renal and/or hepatic function. Many of these drugs depend on the liver and kidney for metabolism and excretion. Renal and liver function tests should be done before (baseline) and periodically during the use of these drugs, and dose should be adjusted accordingly.

Protecting these people from exposure to infection and injury is a very important aspect of their care. Older people are naturally somewhat immunosuppressed because of age, and giving drugs that further depress the immune system can lead to infections that are serious and difficult to treat. Monitor blood counts carefully, and arrange for rest or reduced dose as indicated.

the cell cycle include those in the breasts, testicles and ovaries. Some cells take weeks, months or even years to complete the cycle.

Cancer cells tend to move through the cell cycle at about the same rate as their cells of origin. Malignant cells that remain in a dormant phase for long periods are difficult to destroy. These cells can emerge long after cancer treatment has finished – after weeks, months or years – to begin their division and growth cycle all over again. For this reason, antineoplastic agents are often given in sequence over periods of time, in the hope that the drugs will affect the cancer cells as they emerge from dormancy or move into a new phase of the cell cycle. A combination of antineoplastic agents targeting different phases of the cell cycle is frequently most effective in treating many cancers.

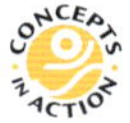

Oncology: Cell cycle

The goal of cancer therapy, much like that of anti-infective therapy, is to limit the offending cells to the degree that the immune system can then respond without causing too much toxicity to the host. However, this is a particularly difficult task when using antineoplastic drugs because, for the most part, these agents are not specific to mutant cells, and affect normal human cells as well. In most cases, antineoplastic drugs primarily affect human cells that are rapidly multiplying with many cells in many phases of the cell cycle (eg, those in the hair follicles, GI tract and bone marrow). Much research is being done to develop drugs that will affect only the abnormal cells. *Imatinib*, released in 2001, was the first of a growing number of drugs to target the enzymes used by very specific abnormal cells. Other agents that affect only the mechanisms of cancer cells have been marketed. It is anticipated that many more such drugs will be released in the near future.

Antineoplastic drugs are associated with many adverse effects, with specific adverse effects occurring with particular drugs. These effects are often unpleasant and debilitating. Some antineoplastic drugs exert toxic effects on ova and sperm production, affecting the person's fertility. These agents are also usually selective for rapidly growing cells, posing a danger to the developing fetus during pregnancy. Consequently, pregnancy is a contraindication to the use of antineoplastic

BOX 14.2 FOCUS ON The evidence

New drugs for the battle against cancer

Arsenic trioxide (*Phenasen*), known as a poison in forensic medicine, has been approved for the induction and remission of promyelocytic leukaemia (PML) in people whose disease is refractory to conventional therapy and whose leukaemia is characterised by t(15;17) translocation of *PML/RAR-alpha* gene expression. It is given intravenously (IV) at a rate of 0.15 mg/kg/day until bone marrow remission occurs and then 0.15 mg/kg/day starting 3–6 weeks after induction. The person needs to be screened carefully for toxic reactions.

Other drugs are under development that target specific areas of the human genome. In the future, antineoplastic drugs may be able to target abnormal cells and not affect the healthy cells. This could relieve the suffering of many people undergoing cancer chemotherapy.

Several familiar drugs are being studied for their ability to block angiogenesis. By blocking the development of new blood vessels to feed the tumour, the growing cells in the tumour will lack nutrition and oxygen and will not be able to survive. Celecoxib (Celebrex), an anti-inflammatory drug, is being studied in various cancer combination-drug trials for this effect. Some low-molecular-weight heparins, such as dalteparin (*Fragmin*), are also being studied for this effect.

drugs. These agents also jeopardise the immune system by causing **bone marrow suppression**, inhibiting the blood-forming components of the bone marrow and interfering with the body's normal protective actions against abnormal cells. The person's haematological profile must always be assessed for toxic effects. People also need to understand the importance of returning every few weeks to go through the chemotherapy, with its adverse effects, over and over again.

Many antineoplastic drugs often result in another adverse effect: cancer itself. Cell death due to these agents increases the need for cellular growth, placing the person at increased risk for mutant cell development.

Most people with cancer are not considered to be 'cured' until they have been cancer-free for a period of 5 years because of the possibility that cancer cells will emerge from dormancy to cause new tumours or problems. No cells have yet been identified that can remain dormant for longer than 5 years, so the chance of the emergence of one after that time is very slim.

A cancerous mass may be so large that no therapy can arrest its growth without killing the host. In such cases, antineoplastic agents are used as palliative therapy to shrink the size of the tumour and alleviate some of the signs and symptoms of the cancer, decreasing pain and increasing function. Here the goal of drug therapy is not to cure the disease but to try to improve the person's quality of life in a situation in which there is no cure. Some emerging antineoplastic agents are discussed in Box 14.2.

ALKYLATING AGENTS

Because alkylating agents can affect cells even in the resting phase, these drugs are said to be non-cell-cycle specific (see Figure 14.4). They are most useful in the treatment of slow growing cancers, which have many cells in the resting phase. Alkylating agents (see Table 14.1) include the following drugs: busulfan (*Busulfex*, *Myleran*), carboplatin (*Carbaccord*), carmustine (*BiCNU*, *Gliadel*), chlorambucil (*Leukeran*), cisplatin (generic), cyclophosphamide (*Endoxan*), dacarbazine (generic), fotemustine (*Muphoran*), ifosfamide (*Holoxan*), lomustine (*CeeNU*), melphalan (*Alkeran*), oxaliplatin (*Oxalatin*, *Xalox*), procarbazine (*Natulan*), temozolomide (*Astromide*, *Temizole*, *Temodal*) and thiotepa (generic).

Therapeutic actions and indications

Alkylating agents produce their cytotoxic effects by reacting chemically with portions of the RNA, DNA or other cellular proteins, being most potent when they bind with cellular DNA. The oldest drugs in this class are the nitrogen mustards, and modifications of the structure of these drugs have led to the development of the nitrosoureas.

These drugs are most useful in the treatment of slow growing cancers such as various lymphomas, leukaemias, myelomas, some ovarian, testicular and breast cancers, and some pancreatic cancers. See Table 14.1 for usual indications for each of the alkylating agents. These agents are not used interchangeably.

Pharmacokinetics

The alkylating agents vary in their degree of absorption, and little is known about their distribution in the tissues. They are metabolised and sometimes activated in the liver, with many of these agents using the cytochrome P450 systems. They are excreted in the urine.

Contraindications and cautions

Alkylating agents are contraindicated during pregnancy and breastfeeding because of their potential for severe effects on the fetus and neonate. Caution is necessary when giving alkylating agents to any individual with a known allergy to any of them; with bone marrow suppression, *which is often the index for redosing and dosing levels*; or with suppressed renal or hepatic function, *which may interfere with metabolism or*

TABLE 14.1 **DRUGS IN FOCUS** **Alkylating agents**

Drug name	Dosage/route	Usual indications
busulfan (*Busulfex, Myleran*)	Dosing complex*	Treatment of chronic myelogenous leukaemia; not effective in blastic phase or without the Philadelphia chromosome **Special considerations:** dosing monitored by effects on bone marrow; always push fluids to decrease toxic renal effects; alopecia is common
carboplatin (*Carbaccord*)	Dosing complex*	Palliative or initial treatment of recurring ovarian cancer after prior chemotherapy; initial treatment of ovarian cancer with other chemotherapy; may be useful in several other cancers **Special considerations:** dose and timing determined by bone marrow response; alopecia is common
carmustine (*BiCNU, Gliadel*)	Dosing complex*	Treatment of brain tumours, Hodgkin disease and multiple myelomas; available in implantable wafer form for treatment of glioblastoma **Special considerations:** dose determined by bone marrow toxicity; do not repeat for 6 weeks because of delayed toxicity; often used in combination therapy
(P) chlorambucil (*Leukeran*)	Dosing complex*	Palliative treatment of lymphomas and leukaemias, including Hodgkin disease; being considered for the treatment of rheumatoid arthritis and other conditions **Special considerations:** toxic to liver and bone marrow; dosing based on bone marrow response
cisplatin (generic)	Dosing complex*	Combination therapy for metastatic testicular or ovarian tumours, advanced bladder cancers **Special considerations:** neurotoxic, nephrotoxic, and can cause serious hypersensitivity reactions
cyclophosphamide (*Endoxan*)	Dosing complex*	Treatment of lymphoma, myelomas, leukaemias and other cancers in combination with other drugs **Special considerations:** haemorrhagic cystitis is a potentially fatal side effect; alopecia is common
dacarbazine (generic)	Dosing complex*	Treatment of metastatic malignant melanoma and as second-line therapy with other drugs for the treatment of Hodgkin disease **Special considerations:** bone marrow depression, GI toxicity, severe photosensitivity are common; extravasation can cause tissue necrosis or cellulitis – use extreme care, and monitor injection sites regularly
fotemustine (*Muphoran*)	Dosing complex*	Management of disseminated malignant melanoma, including cerebral metastases **Special considerations:** monitor liver function, blood counts before each administration

TABLE 14.1 DRUGS IN FOCUS Alkylating agents *(continued)*

Drug name	Dosage/route	Usual indications
ifosfamide (*Holoxan*)	Dosing complex*	Combination therapy as a third-line agent in treating germ cell testicular cancers; being tested for treatment of other cancers **Special considerations:** alopecia is common
lomustine (*CeeNU*)	Dosing complex*	Palliative combination therapy for Hodgkin disease and primary and metastatic brain tumours **Special considerations:** immune suppression and gastrointestinal (GI) effects are common
melphalan (*Alkeran*)	Dosing complex*	Nitrogen mustard; treatment for multiple myeloma, ovarian cancers **Special considerations:** oral route is preferred; pulmonary fibrosis, bone marrow suppression and alopecia are common
oxaliplatin (*Oxalatin, Xalox*)	Dosing complex*	Treatment of metastatic carcinoma of the colon or rectum when disease progresses after standard therapy; used in combination therapy **Special considerations:** premedicate with antiemetics and dexamethasone; monitor for potentially dangerous anaphylactic reactions
procarbazine (*Natulan*)	Dosing complex*	Used in combination therapy for treatment of stages III and IV of Hodgkin disease **Special considerations:** bone marrow toxicity; GI toxicity and skin lesions also limit use in some people; severity of adverse effects regulates the dose of the drug
temozolomide (*Astromide, Temizole, Temodal*)	Dosing complex*	Treatment of refractory astrocytoma or glioblastoma in people refractory to other treatments **Special considerations:** monitor bone marrow closely; especially toxic in women and the elderly
thiotepa (generic)	Dosing complex*	Treatment of adenocarcinoma of the breast and uterus and papillary carcinoma of the bladder; available intrathecally to treat effusion **Special considerations:** infertility, rash, GI toxicity, dizziness, headache and bone marrow suppression are common

*Chemotherapy regimens and doses are complex and a part of fixed treatment protocols. eviQ (www.eviq.org.au) is a freely available, Australian Government online resource of cancer treatment protocols developed by multidisciplinary teams of cancer specialists. The website offers evidence-based, consensus-driven cancer treatment protocols and information for use at the point of care. eviQ is developed for the Australian context and supports health professionals in the delivery of cancer treatments.

excretion of these drugs and often indicates a need to change the dose.

Adverse effects

Adverse effects frequently encountered with the use of these alkylating agents are listed here; see Table 14.1 for a list of adverse effects specific to each agent. Amifostine (*Ethyol*) and mesna (*Uromitexan*) are cytoprotective (cell-protecting) drugs that may be given to limit certain effects of cisplatin and ifosfamide, respectively (see Box 14.3).

Haematological effects include bone marrow suppression, with leucopenia, thrombocytopenia, anaemia and pancytopenia, secondary to the effects of the drugs on the rapidly multiplying cells of the bone marrow.

GI effects include nausea, vomiting, anorexia, diarrhoea and mucous membrane deterioration, all of which are related to the drugs' effects on the rapidly multiplying cells of the GI tract. Hepatic toxicity and renal toxicity may occur, depending on the exact mechanism of action. **Alopecia**, or hair loss, related to effects on the hair follicles, may also occur. All drugs that cause cell death can cause a potentially toxic increase in uric acid levels. In 2006, rasburicase, was introduced to manage uric acid levels in children (see Box 14.4).

BOX 14.3 Drugs that protect cells from alkylating agents

Amifostine (*Ethyol*) is a cytoprotective (cell-protecting) drug that preserves healthy cells from the toxic effects of cisplatin. It is thought to react to the specific acidity and vascularity of non-tumour cells to protect them, and it may also act as a scavenger of free radicals released by cells that have been exposed to cisplatin. Amifostine is given at a dose of 910 mg/m^2 four times a day as a 15-minute IV infusion starting within 30 minutes after starting cisplatin therapy; timing is very important to its effectiveness. Now approved for use to prevent the renal toxicity associated with the use of cisplatin in individuals with advanced ovarian cancer, amifostine is under investigation as an agent for protecting lung fibroblasts from the effects of paclitaxel. Because amifostine is associated with severe nausea and vomiting, concurrent administration of an antiemetic is recommended. It also can cause hypotension and individuals should be monitored closely for this condition.

Mesna (*Uromitexan*) is a cytoprotective agent that is used to reduce the incidence of haemorrhagic cystitis caused by ifosfamide or cyclophosphamide. Mesna, which is known to react chemically with urotoxic metabolites of ifosfamide, is given IV at the time of the ifosfamide injection at a dose that is 20% of the ifosfamide dose and is repeated 4 and 8 hours afterwards. Because mesna has been associated with nausea and vomiting, an antiemetic may be useful.

BOX 14.4 Drug to manage rising uric acid levels associated with tumour lysis

Rasburicase (*Fasturtec*) was approved in 2006 for the management of plasma uric acid levels in children with leukaemia, lymphoma and solid tumour malignancies who are receiving antineoplastic therapy associated with tumour lysis and subsequent elevated serum uric acid levels. It is administered as a single daily IV infusion of 0.15–0.2 mg/kg over 30 minutes for 5 days. Chemotherapy should be started 4–24 hours after the first dose of rasburicase. Uric acid levels should be monitored frequently, using prechilled, heparinised vials that are kept in an ice-water bath. This analysis should be done within 4 hours of each rasburicase dose.

Clinically important drug–drug interactions

Alkylating agents that are known to cause hepatic or renal toxicity should be used cautiously with any other drugs that have similar effects. In addition, drugs that are toxic to the liver may adversely affect drugs that are metabolised in the liver or that act in the liver (eg, oral anticoagulants). Always check for specific drug–drug interactions for each agent in a drug guide.

Prototype summary: chlorambucil

Indications: palliative treatment of chronic lymphocytic leukaemia, malignant lymphomas and Hodgkin disease.

Actions: alkylates cellular DNA, interfering with the replication of susceptible cells.

Pharmacokinetics:

Route	Onset	Peak	Duration
Oral	Varies	1 hour	15–20 hours

$T_{1/2}$: 60–90 minutes, metabolised in the liver and excreted in the urine.

Adverse effects: tremors, muscle twitching, confusion, nausea, hepatotoxicity, bone marrow suppression, sterility, cancer.

Care considerations for people receiving alkylating agents

Assessment: history and examination

- Assess for contraindications or cautions: history of allergy to any of the alkylating agents *to avoid hypersensitivity reactions*; bone marrow suppression *to prevent further suppression*; renal or hepatic dysfunction *that might interfere with drug metabolism and excretion*; and current status related to pregnancy or breastfeeding *to prevent potentially serious adverse effects on the fetus or breastfeeding baby.*
- Perform a physical assessment *to establish baseline data for determining the effectiveness of the drug and the occurrence of any adverse effects associated with drug therapy.*
- Assess orientation and reflexes *to evaluate any central nervous system effects*; respiratory rate and adventitious sounds *to monitor the disease and to evaluate for respiratory or hypersensitivity effects*; pulse, rhythm and auscultation to monitor for systemic or cardiovascular effects; and bowel sounds and mucous membrane status *to monitor for gastrointestinal (GI) effects.*

- Monitor the results of laboratory tests such as full blood count (FBC) with differential *to identify possible bone marrow suppression and toxic drug effects*; and renal and liver function tests to determine need for *possible dose adjustment and identify toxic drug effects.*

Implementation with rationale

- Arrange for blood tests before, periodically during, and for at least 3 weeks after therapy *to monitor bone marrow function to aid in determining the need for a change in dose or discontinuation of the drug.*
- Administer medication according to scheduled protocol and in combination with other drugs as indicated *to improve effectiveness.*
- Ensure that the person is well hydrated *to decrease risk of renal toxicity.*
- Protect the person from exposure to infection; limit invasive procedures *when bone marrow suppression limits the person's immune* or *inflammatory responses.*
- Provide small, frequent meals, frequent mouth care and dietary consultation as appropriate *to maintain nutrition when GI effects are severe.* Anticipate the need for antiemetics if necessary. (See Box 14.5.)
- Arrange for proper head covering at extremes of temperature if alopecia occurs; a wig, scarf or hat *is important for maintaining body temperature.* If alopecia is an anticipated effect of drug therapy, advise the person to obtain a wig or head covering before the condition occurs *to promote self-esteem and a positive body image.*
- Provide teaching about the following:
  - Follow the appropriate dosage regimen, including dates to return for further doses.
  - Cover the head at extremes of temperature.
  - Maintain nutrition if GI effects are severe.
  - Avoid exposure to infection.
  - Plan for appropriate rest periods because fatigue and weakness are common effects of the drugs.
  - Consult with a health care provider, if appropriate, due to the possibility of impaired fertility.
  - Use barrier contraceptives *to reduce the risk of pregnancy during therapy.*

Evaluation

- Monitor response to the drug (alleviation of cancer being treated, palliation of signs and symptoms of cancer).
- Monitor for adverse effects (bone marrow suppression, GI toxicity, neurotoxicity, alopecia, renal or hepatic dysfunction).
- Evaluate the effectiveness of the teaching plan (person can name the drug, dosage, possible adverse effects to watch for and specific measures to help avoid adverse effects).

KEY POINTS

- Alkylating agents affect cellular RNA, DNA or other cellular proteins, are cell-cycle-non-specific, and are most effective against slow-growing tumours.
- People receiving alkylating agents may experience alopecia, nausea and vomiting and need to be monitored for bone marrow suppression and CNS toxicity.

BOX 14.5 Antiemetics and cancer chemotherapy

Antineoplastic drugs can directly stimulate the chemoreceptor trigger zone (CTZ) in the medulla to induce nausea and vomiting. These drugs also cause cell death, which releases many toxins into the system, which in turn stimulate the CTZ. Because people expect nausea and vomiting with the administration of antineoplastic agents, the higher cortical centres of the brain can stimulate the CTZ to induce vomiting just at the thought of the chemotherapy.

A variety of antiemetic agents have been used in the course of antineoplastic therapy. Sometimes a combination of drugs is most helpful. It should also be remembered that an accepting environment, plenty of comfort measures (eg, environmental control, mouth care, ice chips), and support for the person can help to decrease the discomfort associated with the emetic effects of these drugs. Antihistamines to decrease secretions and corticosteroids to relieve inflammation are useful as adjunctive therapies.

Drugs that are known to help in treating antineoplastic chemotherapy–induced nausea and vomiting include the following:

- Ondansetron (*Zofran*), granisetron (*Kytril*) and palonosetron (*Aloxi*) block serotonin receptors in the CTZ and are among the most effective antiemetics, especially if combined with a corticosteroid such as dexamethasone. The usual dosage is three 0.15 mg/kg doses IV or 8 mg PO three times a day starting 30 minutes before chemotherapy (ondansetron) or 10 mg/kg IV or 1 mg PO twice a day (granisetron), or 0.25 mg IV over 30 seconds, starting 30 minutes before chemotherapy (palonosetron).
- Aprepitant (*Emend*) blocks human substance P/neurokinin 1 receptors in the CNS, blocking the nausea and vomiting caused by severely emetogenic antineoplastic drugs without effects on dopamine or serotonin. The usual dosage is 125 mg PO 1 hour before chemotherapy (day 1) and 80 mg PO once daily in the morning on days 2 and 3; given in combination with 12 mg dexamethasone PO on day 1

■ BOX 14.5 Antiemetics and cancer chemotherapy *(continued)*

and 8 mg dexamethasone PO on days 2–4, and 32 mg ondansetron IV on day 1 only.

- Two benzodiazepines – alprazolam (*Xanax*), 0.5 mg PO four times a day, and lorazepam (*Ativan*), 2–6 mg/day PO – seem to be effective in directly blocking the CTZ to relieve nausea and vomiting caused by cancer chemotherapy; they are especially effective when combined with a corticosteroid.
- Haloperidol (*Haldol*), 0.5–2.0 mg PO four times a day, or 2–25 mg intramuscularly (IM) or IV, is a dopaminergic blocker that also is believed to have direct CTZ effects.
- Metoclopramide (*Maxolon*), 2 mg/kg IV over at least 30 minutes, calms the activity of the GI tract; it is especially effective if combined with a corticosteroid, an antihistamine, and a centrally acting blocker such as haloperidol or lorazepam.
- Prochlorperazine (*Stemetil*), 5–10 mg PO three to four times a day, or 5–10 mg IM, is a phenothiazine that has been found to have strong antiemetic action in the CNS; it can be given by a variety of routes.

Nausea and vomiting are unavoidable aspects of many chemotherapeutic regimens. However, treating the person as the chemotherapy begins, using combination regimens, and providing plenty of supportive and comforting care can help to alleviate some of the distress associated with these adverse effects.

ANTIMETABOLITES

Antimetabolites (see Table 14.2) are drugs that have chemical structures similar to those of various natural metabolites that are necessary for the growth and division of rapidly growing neoplastic cells and normal cells. Antimetabolites include azacitidine (*Vidaza*), capecitabine (*Xeloda*), cladribine (*Leustatin, Litak*), clofarabine (*Evoltra*), asparaginase (colaspase) (*Leunase*), cytarabine (generic), fludarabine (*Farine, Fludara*), fluorouracil (*Efudix*), gemcitabine (*Gemcite, Gemzar*), mercaptopurine (*Puri-Nethol*), methotrexate (*Methoblastin*), pemetrexed (*Alimta*), raltitrexed (*Tomudex*) and thioguanine (*Lanvis*).

Therapeutic actions and indications

Antimetabolites inhibit DNA production in cells that depend on certain natural metabolites to produce their DNA. They replace these needed metabolites and thereby prevent normal cellular function. Many of these agents inhibit thymidylate synthetase, DNA polymerase or folic acid reductase, all of which are needed for DNA synthesis. They are considered to be S phase specific in the cell cycle. They are most effective in rapidly dividing cells, preventing cell replication and leading to cell death (see Figure 14.5). The antimetabolites are indicated for the treatment of various leukaemias and some GI and basal cell cancers (see Table 14.2 for usual indications for each agent). Use of these drugs has been somewhat limited because neoplastic cells rapidly develop resistance to these agents. For this reason, these drugs are usually administered as part of a combination therapy.

TABLE 14.2 *DRUGS IN FOCUS* Antimetabolites

Drug name	Dosage/route	Usual indications
azacitidine (*Vidaza*)	Dosage: 75 mg/m²/day SC for 7 days q 4 weeks	Treatment of myelodysplastic syndrome **Special considerations:** premedicate for nausea; monitor for bone marrow suppression; avoid pregnancy or fathering children while on drug
capecitabine (*Xeloda*)	2500 mg/m²/day PO in 2 divided doses for 2 weeks, then 1 week of rest, for 3 cycles Dukes C colon cancer: 1250 mg/m² PO bd for 2 weeks, then 1 week of rest for a total of eight 3-week cycles	Treatment of metastatic breast cancer with resistance to paclitaxel or anthracyclines; treatment of metastatic colorectal cancer as first-line therapy treatment of breast cancer with docetaxel in people with metastatic disease; postsurgery Dukes C colon cancer **Special considerations:** severe diarrhoea can occur – monitor hydration and nutrition; monitor for bone marrow suppression
cladribine (*Leustatin, Litak*)	0.09 mg/kg/day IV for 7 consecutive days	Treatment of active hairy cell leukaemia **Special considerations:** severe bone marrow depression can occur – monitor person closely and reduce dose as needed; fever is common, especially early in treatment

TABLE 14.2 DRUGS IN FOCUS Antimetabolites *(continued)*

Drug name	Dosage/route	Usual indications
clofarabine (*Evoltra*)	52 mg/m² by IV infusion over 2 hours daily for 5 days; repeat every 2–6 weeks, based on baseline function	Treatment of people 1–21 years of age with acute lymphocytic leukaemia (ALL) after at least two relapses on other regimens **Special considerations:** GI toxicity, bone marrow suppression and infection are common
asparaginase (colaspase) (*Leunase*)	50–200 KU/kg IV daily or every alternate day	Treatment of acute lymphoblastic leukaemia, myeloid leukaemia and malignant lymphoma **Special considerations:** test dose usually administered to check for hypersensitivity. Use with caution in people with renal or hepatic impairment
cytarabine (generic)	200 mg/m² per day by continuous IV infusion for 5 days, repeat every 2 weeks; intrathecal use, 30 mg/m² every 4 days	Treatment of meningeal and myelocytic leukaemias; used in combination with other agents; lymphomatous meningitis; non-Hodgkin lymphoma in children **Special considerations:** GI toxicity and cytarabine syndrome (fever, myalgia, bone pain, chest pain, rash, conjunctivitis, and malaise) are common – this syndrome sometimes responds to corticosteroids; alopecia may occur
fludarabine (*Fludara*)	25 mg/m² per day IV for 5 days; repeat every 28 days; or 40 mg/m²/day PO for 5 days every 28 days	Treatment of chronic lymphocytic leukaemia (CLL); unresponsive B cell CLL with no progress with at least one other treatment **Special considerations:** CNS toxicity can be severe; GI toxicity, respiratory complications, renal failure and a tumour lysis syndrome are common
fluorouracil (*Efudix*)	12 mg/kg/day IV on days 1–3, then 6 mg/kg IV on days 5, 7, 9; Maintenance: 5–10 mg/kg once weekly	Palliative treatment of various GI cancers; topical treatment of basal cell carcinoma and actinic and solar keratoses **Special considerations:** GI toxicity, bone marrow suppression, alopecia and skin rash are common; avoid occlusive dressings with topical forms; wash hands thoroughly after coming in contact with drug
gemcitabine (*Gemzar*)	1000–1250 mg/m² IV over 30 minutes once a week; timing based on other therapies and response	Treatment of locally advanced or metastatic adenocarcinoma of the pancreas; given with cisplatin for the treatment of inoperable non-small-cell lung cancer; metastatic breast cancer, ovarian cancer after failure of a platinum-based therapy **Special considerations:** can cause severe bone marrow depression, GI toxicity, pain, alopecia, interstitial pneumonitis
mercaptopurine (*Puri-Nethol*)	Usual dose is 2.5 mg/kg/day, but dose and duration of administration depend on nature and dosage of other cytotoxic agents given in conjunction with Puri-Nethol. Dosage should be carefully adjusted to suit the individual patient	Remission induction and maintenance therapy in acute leukaemias **Special considerations:** bone marrow toxicity and GI toxicity are common; hyperuricaemia is a true concern – ensure that the person is well hydrated during therapy

Continued on following page

TABLE 14.2 DRUGS IN FOCUS Antimetabolites *(continued)*

Drug name	Dosage/route	Usual indications
(P) methotrexate (*Methoblastin*)	Dose varies with route and disease being treated; for trophoblastic neoplasms, 15–30 mg/day PO or IM for 5 days and repeated after 1–2 weeks for 3–5 cycles For rheumatoid arthritis dose is usually once weekly starting at 7.5 mg/week to a maximum of 20 mg/week	Treatment of leukaemias, psoriasis, rheumatoid arthritis and choriocarcinomas **Special considerations:** hypersensitivity reactions can be severe; liver toxicity and GI complications are common; monitor for bone marrow suppression and increased susceptibility to infections; dose pack available for the oral treatment of psoriasis and rheumatoid arthritis
pemetrexed (*Alimta*)	500 mg/m² IV over 10 minutes on day one with 75 mg/m² cisplatin IV over 2 hours; repeat cycle every 21 days	Treatment of malignant mesothelioma in people whose disease is unresectable or who are not candidates for surgery; locally advanced or metastatic non–small cell lung cancer as a single agent after other chemotherapy **Special considerations:** pretreat with corticosteroids, folic acid and vitamin B12; monitor for bone marrow suppression and GI effects
raltitrexed (*Tomudex*)	Dosage: 3 mg/m² IV over 15 minutes; repeated q 3 weeks	Palliative treatment for advanced colorectal cancer **Special considerations:** GI and haematologic toxicity; full blood count before each treatment
thioguanine (*Lanvis*)	2–2.5 mg/kg/day PO for 4 weeks; then dose may be increased if tolerated well	Remission induction and maintenance of acute leukaemias alone or as part of combination therapy **Special considerations:** bone marrow suppression, GI toxicity, miscarriage and birth defects have been reported; monitor bone marrow status to determine dose and redosing; ensure that the person is well hydrated during therapy to minimise hyperuricaemia – person may respond to allopurinol and urine alkalinisation

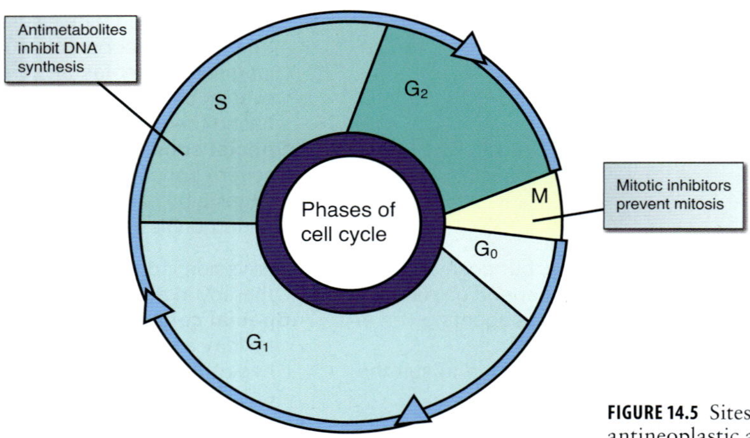

FIGURE 14.5 Sites of action of cell cycle–specific antineoplastic agents.

Pharmacokinetics

Methotrexate is absorbed well from the GI tract and is excreted unchanged in the urine. People with renal impairment may require reduced dose and increased monitoring when taking methotrexate. Methotrexate readily crosses the blood–brain barrier. Cytarabine, clofarabine, asparaginase (colaspase), fluorouracil, gemcitabine and pemetrexed are not absorbed well from the GI tract and need to be administered parenterally. They are metabolised in the liver and excreted in the urine, necessitating close monitoring of individuals with hepatic or renal impairment who are receiving these drugs. Mercaptopurine and thioguanine are absorbed slowly from the GI tract and are metabolised in the liver and excreted in the urine.

Contraindications and cautions

Antimetabolites are contraindicated for use during pregnancy and breastfeeding *because of the potential for severe effects on the fetus and neonate.* Caution is necessary when administering antimetabolites to any individual with a known allergy to any of them; with bone marrow suppression, *which is often the index for redosing and dosing levels*; with renal or hepatic dysfunction, *which might interfere with the metabolism or excretion of these drugs and often indicates a need to change the dose*; and with known GI ulcerations or ulcerative diseases *that might be exacerbated by the effects of these drugs.*

Adverse effects

Adverse effects frequently encountered with the use of the antimetabolites are listed here. To counteract the effects of treatment with one antimetabolite – methotrexate – the drug Leucovorin is sometimes given (see Box 14.6).

BOX 14.6 A drug that protects against an antimetabolite

Leucovorin (calcium folinate) is an active form of folic acid that is used to 'rescue' normal cells from the adverse effects of methotrexate therapy in the treatment of osteosarcoma. This drug is also used to treat folic acid deficiency conditions such as sprue, nutritional deficiency, pregnancy and breastfeeding. Leucovorin is given orally or IV at the time of methotrexate therapy and for the next 72 hours at a dose of 12–15 g/m^2 PO or IV followed by 10 mg/m^2 PO q 6 hours for 72 hours. Use of this drug has been associated with pain at the injection site.

Haematological effects include bone marrow suppression, with leucopenia, thrombocytopenia, anaemia and pancytopenia, secondary to the effects of the drugs on the rapidly multiplying cells of the bone marrow. Toxic GI effects include nausea, vomiting, anorexia, diarrhoea and mucous membrane deterioration, all of which are related to drug effects on the rapidly multiplying cells of the GI tract. CNS effects include headache, drowsiness, aphasia, fatigue, malaise and dizziness. People should be advised to take precautions if these conditions occur. There is a risk of pulmonary toxicity, including interstitial pneumonitis with these drugs. As with alkylating agents, effects of the antimetabolites may include possible hepatic or renal toxicity, depending on the exact mechanism of action. Alopecia may also occur.

Clinically important drug–drug interactions

Antimetabolites that are known to cause hepatic or renal toxicity should be used with care with any other drugs known to have the same effect. In addition, drugs that are toxic to the liver may adversely affect drugs that are metabolised in the liver or that act in the liver (eg, oral anticoagulants). Check for specific drug–drug interactions for each agent in a drug guide.

Prototype summary: methotrexate

Indications: treatment of gestational choriocarcinoma, chorioadenoma destruens, hydatidiform, meningeal leukaemia; symptomatic control of severe psoriasis; rheumatoid arthritis; juvenile rheumatoid arthritis.

Actions: inhibits folic acid reductase, leading to inhibition of DNA synthesis and inhibition of cellular replication; affects the most rapidly dividing cells.

Pharmacokinetics:

Route	Onset	Peak
Oral	Varies	1–4 hours
IV	Rapid	0.5–2 hours

$T_{1/2}$: 2–4 hours, excreted unchanged in the urine.

Adverse effects: fatigue, malaise, rashes, alopecia, ulcerative stomatitis, hepatic toxicity, severe bone marrow suppression, interstitial pneumonitis, chills, fever, anaphylaxis.

Care considerations for people receiving antimetabolites

Assessment: history and examination

- Assess for contraindications and cautions: history of allergy to the specific antimetabolite *to avoid hypersensitivity reactions*; bone marrow suppression *to prevent further suppression*; renal or hepatic dysfunction *that might interfere with drug metabolism and excretion*; current status related to pregnancy or breastfeeding *to prevent potentially serious effects to the fetus or breastfeeding baby*; and a history of GI ulcerative disease, *which could be exacerbated with the use of these drugs.*
- Perform a physical assessment *to establish baseline data for determining the effectiveness of the drug and the occurrence of any adverse effects associated with drug therapy.*
- Assess orientation and reflexes *to evaluate any CNS effects*; respiratory rate and adventitious sounds *to monitor the disease and to evaluate for respiratory or hypersensitivity effects*; pulse, rhythm and cardiac auscultation *to monitor for systemic or cardiovascular effects*; and bowel sounds and mucous membrane status *to monitor for GI effects.*
- Monitor the results of laboratory tests such as full blood count (FBC) with differential to identify possible bone marrow suppression and toxic drug effects; and renal and liver function tests *to determine the need for possible dose adjustment and toxic drug effects.*

Implementation with rationale

- Arrange for blood tests to monitor bone marrow function before, periodically during, and for at least 3 weeks after therapy *to arrange to discontinue the drug or reduce the dose as needed.*
- Administer medication according to the scheduled protocol and in combination with other drugs as indicated *to improve the effectiveness of drug therapy.*
- Ensure the person is well hydrated *to decrease the risk of renal toxicity.*
- Provide small, frequent meals, frequent mouth care and dietary consultation as appropriate *to maintain nutrition when GI effects are severe.* Anticipate the use of antiemetics as necessary. (See Box 14.5.)
- Arrange for proper head covering at extremes of temperature if alopecia occurs; a wig, scarf or hat *is important for maintaining body temperature.* If alopecia is an anticipated effect of drug therapy, advise the person to obtain a wig or head covering before the condition occurs *to promote self-esteem and a positive body image.*
- Protect the individual from exposure to infections *because bone marrow suppression will limit immune/inflammatory responses.*
- Provide support and encouragement to help the person cope with the diagnosis and the effects of drug therapy.
- Provide the following teaching:
  - Follow the appropriate dosage regimen, including dates to return for further doses. People need to be reminded to report all other drugs and alternative therapies that they might be using. Box 14.7 discusses alternative therapies often used by cancer sufferers that could interact with their drug regimen.
  - Maintain nutrition if GI effects are severe.
  - Cover the head at extremes of temperature if alopecia is anticipated.
  - Plan for appropriate rest periods because fatigue and weakness are common effects of the drugs.
  - Avoid situations that might lead to infection, including crowded places, sick people and working in the soil.
  - Use safety measures such as not driving or using dangerous equipment, because of possible dizziness, headache and drowsiness.
  - Think about consulting with a health care provider, if appropriate, due to the possibility of impaired fertility.
  - Use barrier contraceptives to reduce the risk of pregnancy during therapy.

Evaluation

- Monitor response to the drug (alleviation of cancer being treated, palliation of signs and symptoms of cancer, palliation of rheumatoid arthritis or psoriasis).
- Monitor for adverse effects (bone marrow suppression, GI toxicity, neurotoxicity, alopecia, renal or hepatic dysfunction).
- Evaluate the effectiveness of the teaching plan (person can name the drug, dosage, possible adverse effects to watch for and specific measures to help avoid adverse effects).
- Monitor the effectiveness of comfort and safety measures and compliance with the regimen.

KEY POINTS

- Antimetabolites inhibit DNA production by inhibiting metabolites needed for the synthesis of DNA in susceptible cells.
- Antimetabolites are S phase cell cycle–specific and are used for some leukaemias, as well as some GI and basal cell cancers.
- Bone marrow suppression, alopecia and toxic GI effects are common adverse effects of antimetabolites.

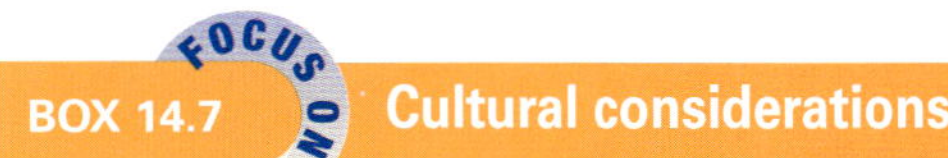

BOX 14.7 Cultural considerations

Alternative therapies and cancer

The diagnosis of cancer and the sometimes devastating effects of cancer treatment often drive people to seek out alternative therapies, either as adjuncts to traditional cancer therapy or sometimes instead of traditional therapy. Because people of Asian and Pacific Islander descent often see drug therapy and other cancer therapies as part of a 'yin/yang' belief system, they may turn to a variety of herbal therapies to 'balance' their systems.

Nurses and midwives should be aware of some potential interactions that may occur when alternative therapies are used:

- Echinacea – may be hepatotoxic; increases the risk of hepatotoxicity when taken with antineoplastics that are hepatotoxic
- Ginkgo – inhibits blood clotting, which can cause problems after surgery or with bleeding neoplasms
- Saw palmetto – may increase the effects of various oestrogen hormones and hormone modulators; advise people taking such drugs to avoid this herb
- St John's wort – can greatly increase photosensitivity, which can cause problems with people who have received radiation therapy or are taking drugs that cause other dermatological effects; has been shown to interfere with the effectiveness of some antineoplastic agents

If a person has an unexpected reaction to a drug, ask about whether they are using alternative therapies. Many of these agents are untested, and interactions and adverse effects are not well documented.

ANTINEOPLASTIC ANTIBIOTICS

Antineoplastic antibiotics (Table 14.3), although selective for bacterial cells, are also toxic to human cells. Because these drugs tend to be more toxic to cells that are multiplying rapidly, they are more useful in the treatment of certain cancers. Antineoplastic antibiotics include bleomycin (*Blenamax*), dactinomycin (*Cosmegen*), daunorubicin (generic), doxorubicin (*Adriamycin*, *Caelyx*), epirubicin (generic), idarubicin (*Zavedos*), mitomycin (*Mitomycin C*) and mitoxantrone (generic).

Therapeutic actions and indications

Some antineoplastic antibiotics break up DNA links, and others prevent DNA synthesis.

The antineoplastic antibiotics are cytotoxic and interfere with cellular DNA synthesis by inserting themselves between base pairs in the DNA chain. This, in turn, causes a mutant DNA molecule, leading to cell death (see Figure 14.4). See Table 14.3 for usual indications for each antineoplastic antibiotic. Like other antineoplastics, the main adverse effects of these drugs are seen in cells that multiply rapidly, such as those in the bone marrow, GI tract and skin. Their potentially serious adverse effects may limit their usefulness in people with pre-existing diseases and in those who are debilitated and, therefore, more susceptible to these effects.

TABLE 14.3 *DRUGS IN FOCUS* **Antineoplastic antibiotics**

Drug name	Dosage/route	Usual indications
bleomycin (*Blenamax*)	10,000–20,000 IU/m^2 IM, IV, or SC once or twice weekly	Palliative treatment of squamous cell carcinomas, testicular cancers and lymphomas; used to treat malignant pleural effusion **Special considerations:** GI toxicity, severe skin reactions and hypersensitivity reactions may occur; pulmonary fibrosis can be a serious problem – baseline and periodic chest radiographs and pulmonary function tests are necessary
dactinomycin (*Cosmegen*)	Adult: 0.5 mg/day IV for up to 5 days Paediatric: 0.015 mg/kg/day IV for up to 5 days or a total dose of 2.5 mg/m^2/week	Part of combination drug regimen in the treatment of a variety of sarcomas and carcinomas; potentiates the effects of radiation therapy **Special considerations:** bone marrow suppression and GI toxicity, which may be severe, limit the dose; effects may not appear for 1–2 weeks; local extravasation can cause necrosis and should be treated with injectable corticosteroids, ice to the area and restarting of the IV line in a different vein

Continued on following page

TABLE 14.3 DRUGS IN FOCUS Antineoplastic antibiotics *(continued)*

Drug name	Dosage/route	Usual indications
daunorubicin (generic)	0.5–1 mg/kg/day IV or 2 mg/kg q 4 days IV, or 2.5–3 mg/kg q 7–14 days. Maximum lifetime adult dose 550 mg/m² or 20 mg/kg	First-line treatment of advanced HIV infection and associated Kaposi sarcoma **Special considerations:** complete alopecia is common, and GI toxicity and bone marrow suppression may also occur; severe necrosis may occur at sites of local extravasation – immediate treatment with corticosteroids, normal saline and ice may help; if ulcerations occur, a plastic surgeon should be called
(P) doxorubicin (*Adriamycin*)	60–75 mg/m² as a single IV dose; repeat every 21 days Lifetime cumulative dose limit 550 mg/m² (adults)	Treatment of a number of leukaemias and cancers; used to induce regression; available in a liposomal form for treatment of AIDS-associated Kaposi sarcoma **Special considerations:** complete alopecia is common; GI toxicity and bone suppression may occur; severe necrosis may occur at sites of local extravasation – immediate treatment with corticosteroids, normal saline and ice may help; if ulcerations occur, a plastic surgeon should be called; toxicity is dose related – an accurate record of each dose received is important in determining dose; severe pulmonary toxicity, alopecia, and injection-site and GI toxicity occur
epirubicin (generic)	75–135 mg/m² IV given in repeated 3–4-week cycles all on day 1 or divided on days 1 and 8. Maximum lifetime cumulative dose 900 mg/m²	Adjunctive therapy in people with evidence of axillary node tumour involvement after resection of primary breast cancer **Special considerations:** may cause cardiotoxicity and delayed cardiomyopathy; monitor for myelosuppression and hyperuricaemia; severe local cellulitis and tissue necrosis can occur with extravasation
idarubicin (*Zavedos*)	12 mg/m²/day IV for 3 days with cytarabine or 30 mg/m²/day × 3 days PO	Combination therapy for treatment of acute myeloid leukaemia in adults **Special considerations:** may cause severe bone marrow suppression, which regulates dose; associated with cardiac toxicity, which can be severe; GI toxicity and local necrosis with extravasation are also common; severe necrosis may occur at sites of local extravasation – immediate treatment with corticosteroids, normal saline and ice may help; if ulcerations occur, a plastic surgeon should be called; it is essential to monitor heart and bone marrow function to protect the person from potentially fatal adverse effects
mitomycin (generic)	20 mg/m² IV as a single dose at 6–8-week intervals	Treatment of disseminated adenocarcinoma of the stomach and pancreas **Special considerations:** severe pulmonary toxicity, alopecia, and injection-site and GI toxicity occur

TABLE 14.3 DRUGS IN FOCUS Antineoplastic antibiotics *(continued)*

Drug name	Dosage/route	Usual indications
mitozantrone (generic)	14 mg/m²/day IV every 21 days	Part of combination therapy in the treatment of adult leukaemias; treatment of bone pain in advanced prostatic cancer **Special considerations:** severe bone marrow suppression may occur and limits dose; alopecia, GI toxicity and congestive heart failure often occur; avoid direct skin contact with the drug – use gloves and goggles; monitor bone marrow activity and cardiac activity to adjust dose or discontinue drug as needed

Pharmacokinetics

The antineoplastic antibiotics are not absorbed well from the GI tract. They are given IV or injected into specific sites. They are metabolised in the liver and excreted in the urine at various rates. Many of them have very long half-lives (eg, 45 hours for idarubicin; more than 5 days for mitozantrone). Daunorubicin and doxorubicin do not cross the blood–brain barrier, but they are widely distributed in the body and are taken up by the heart, lungs, kidneys and spleen. This can lead to toxic effects in these organs.

Contraindications and cautions

All of these agents are contraindicated for use during pregnancy and breastfeeding *because of the potential risk to the fetus and neonate.* Use caution when giving antineoplastic antibiotics to an individual with a known allergy to the antibiotic or related antibiotics. Care is necessary when administering these agents to individuals with the following conditions: bone marrow suppression, *which is often the index for re-dosing and dosing levels*; suppressed renal or hepatic function, *which might interfere with the metabolism or excretion of these drugs and often indicates a need to change the dose*; known GI ulcerations or ulcerative diseases, *which may be exacerbated by the effects of these drugs*; pulmonary problems with bleomycin or mitomycin, or cardiac problems with idarubicin or mitozantrone, *which are specifically toxic to these organ systems.*

Adverse effects

Adverse effects frequently encountered with the use of these antibiotics include bone marrow suppression, with leucopenia, thrombocytopenia, anaemia and pancytopenia, secondary to the effects of the drugs on the rapidly multiplying cells of the bone marrow. Toxic GI effects include nausea, vomiting, anorexia, diarrhoea and mucous membrane deterioration, all of which are related to drug effects on the rapidly multiplying cells of the GI tract. As with the alkylating agents and antimetabolites, effects of antineoplastic antibiotics may include renal or hepatic toxicity, depending on the exact mechanism of action. Alopecia may also occur. Specific antineoplastic antibiotics are toxic to the heart and lungs.

Clinically important drug–drug interactions

Antimetabolites that are known to cause hepatic or renal toxicity should be used with care with any other drugs known to have the same effect. Drugs that result in toxicity to the heart or lungs should be used with caution with any other drugs that produce that particular toxicity. Check for specific drug–drug interactions for each agent in a nursing drug guide.

Prototype summary: doxorubicin

Indications: to produce regression in acute lymphoblastic lymphoma, acute myeloblastic leukaemia, Wilms tumour, neuroblastoma, soft tissue and bone sarcoma, breast carcinoma, ovarian carcinoma, thyroid carcinoma, Hodgkin and non-Hodgkin lymphomas, bronchogenic carcinoma; also to treat AIDS-related Kaposi sarcoma.

Actions: binds to DNA and inhibits DNA synthesis in susceptible cells, causing cell death.

Pharmacokinetics:

Route	Onset	Peak	Duration
IV	Rapid	2 hours	24–36 hours

$T_{1/2}$: 12 minutes, then 3.3 hours, then 29.6 hours; metabolised in the liver and excreted in the bile, faeces and urine.

Adverse effects: cardiac toxicity, complete but reversible alopecia, nausea, vomiting, mucositis, red urine, myelosuppression, fever, chills, rash.

Care considerations for people receiving antineoplastic antibiotics

Assessment: history and examination

- Assess for contraindications and cautions: history of allergy to the antibiotic in use *to avoid hypersensitivity reactions*; bone marrow suppression *to prevent further suppression*; renal or hepatic dysfunction *that might interfere with drug metabolism and excretion*; respiratory or cardiac disease; current status related to pregnancy or breastfeeding *to prevent potentially serious adverse effects to the fetus or breastfeeding baby*; and GI ulcerative disease, *which could be exacerbated by these drugs.*
- Perform a physical assessment *to establish baseline data for determining the effectiveness of the drug and the occurrence of any adverse effects associated with drug therapy.*
- Assess orientation and reflexes *to evaluate any CNS effects*; respiratory rate and adventitious sounds *to monitor the disease and evaluate for respiratory or hypersensitivity effects*; pulse, rhythm, cardiac auscultation and baseline electrocardiogram *to monitor for systemic or cardiovascular effects*; and bowel sounds and mucous membrane status *to monitor for GI effects.*
- Monitor the results of laboratory tests such as FBC with differential to identify possible bone marrow suppression and toxic drug effects, as well as renal and liver function tests, *to determine the need for possible dose adjustment.*

Implementation with rationale

- Arrange for blood tests to monitor bone marrow function before, periodically during, and for at least 3 weeks after therapy *to arrange to discontinue the drug or reduce the dose as needed.*
- Monitor cardiac and respiratory function, as well as clotting times as appropriate for the drug being used, *to arrange to discontinue the drug or reduce the dose as needed.*
- Protect the person from exposure to infection *because bone marrow suppression will decrease immune/inflammatory reactions.*
- Administer medication according to scheduled protocol and in combination with other drugs as indicated *to improve the effectiveness of drug therapy.*
- Ensure that the person is well hydrated *to decrease the risk of renal toxicity.*
- Provide small, frequent meals, frequent mouth care and dietary consultation as appropriate *to maintain nutrition when GI effects are severe.* Anticipate the need for antiemetics as necessary. (See Box 14.5.)
- Arrange for proper head covering at extremes of temperature if alopecia occurs; a wig, scarf or hat *is important for maintaining body temperature.* If alopecia is an anticipated effect of drug therapy, advise the person to obtain a wig or head covering before the condition occurs *to promote self-esteem and a positive body image.*
- Provide the following teaching:
  - Follow the appropriate dosage regimen, including dates to return for further doses.
  - Maintain nutrition if GI effects are severe.
  - Cover the head at extremes of temperature if alopecia is anticipated.
  - Plan for appropriate rest periods because fatigue and weakness are common effects of the drugs.
  - Avoid exposure to possible infection, including avoiding crowded places, sick people and working in soil.
  - Use safety measures such as avoiding driving or using dangerous equipment to prevent injury due to possible dizziness, headache and drowsiness.
  - Consult with a health care provider, if appropriate, due to the possibility of impaired fertility.
  - Use barrier contraceptives to reduce the risk of pregnancy during therapy.

Evaluation

- Monitor response to the drug (alleviation of cancer being treated and palliation of signs and symptoms of cancer).
- Monitor for adverse effects (bone marrow suppression, GI toxicity, neurotoxicity, alopecia, renal or hepatic dysfunction, and cardiac or respiratory dysfunction).
- Evaluate the effectiveness of the teaching plan (person can name the drug, dosage, possible adverse effects to watch for and specific measures to help avoid adverse effects).

KEY POINTS

- Antineoplastic antibiotics are toxic to rapidly dividing cells.
- These drugs are cell cycle–specific, affecting the S phase.
- Bone marrow suppression, alopecia and toxic GI effects are common adverse effects of the antineoplastic antibiotics.

MITOTIC INHIBITORS

Mitotic inhibitors (Table 14.4) are drugs that kill cells as the process of mitosis begins (see Figure 14.5). These cell cycle–specific agents inhibit DNA synthesis. Like other antineoplastics, the main adverse effects of the mitotic inhibitors occur with cells that rapidly multiply: those in the bone marrow, GI tract and skin. Mitotic inhibitors include docetaxel (generic), etoposide (*Etopophos*, *Vepesid*), paclitaxel (*Abraxane*), teniposide (*Vumon*), vinblastine (generic), vincristine (generic) and vinorelbine (*Navelbine*).

TABLE 14.4 ***DRUGS IN FOCUS*** **Mitotic inhibitors**

Drug name	Dosage/route	Usual indications
docetaxel (generic)	75–100 mg/m² IV over 1 hour every 3 weeks	Treatment of breast cancer and non-small-cell lung cancer; androgen-dependent prostate cancer; gastric adenocarcinoma **Special considerations:** monitor person closely – deaths have occurred during use; severe fluid retention can occur – premedicate with corticosteroids and monitor for weight gain; skin rash and nail disorders are usually reversible; monitor people closely during use
etoposide (*Etopophos*, *Vepesid*)	Usually 50–100 mg/m²/day IV for 4–5 days or 100–200 mg/m² PO per day	Treatment of testicular cancers refractory to other agents; non-small-cell lung carcinomas **Special considerations:** fatigue, GI toxicity, bone marrow depression and alopecia are common side effects; avoid direct skin contact with the drug; use protective clothing and goggles; monitor bone marrow function to adjust dose; rapid fall in blood pressure can occur during IV infusion – monitor person carefully
paclitaxel (*Abraxane*)	260 mg/m² IV over 30 minutes every 3 weeks	Treatment of advanced ovarian cancer, breast cancer, non-small-cell lung cancer and AIDS-related Kaposi sarcoma **Special considerations:** anaphylaxis and severe hypersensitivity reactions have occurred – monitor very closely during administration; also monitor for bone marrow suppression; cardiovascular toxicity and neuropathies have occurred
vinblastine (generic)	Adult: 3.7 mg/m² IV once weekly Dose may then be increased based on leucocyte count and response	Palliative treatment of various lymphomas and sarcomas; advanced Hodgkin disease; alone or as part of combination therapy for the treatment of advanced testicular germ cell cancers **Special considerations:** GI toxicity, CNS effects and total loss of hair are common; antiemetics may help; avoid contact with drug; monitor injection sites for reactions
(P) vincristine (generic)	Adult: usually 0.4–1.4 mg/m² IV at weekly intervals	Treatment of acute leukaemia, various lymphomas and sarcomas **Special considerations:** extensive CNS effects are common; GI toxicity, local irritation at injection IV site and hair loss commonly occur; syndrome of inappropriate secretion of antidiuretic hormone (SIADH) has been reported – monitor urine output and arrange for fluid restriction and diuretics as needed

Continued on following page

TABLE 14.4 DRUGS IN FOCUS Mitotic inhibitors *(continued)*

Drug name	Dosage/route	Usual indications
vinorelbine (*Navelbine*)	Usually 25–30 mg/m^2 IV once weekly, based on granulocyte count	First-line treatment of unresectable advanced non-small-cell lung cancer; stage IV non-small-cell once weekly lung cancer and stage III non-small-cell lung cancer with cisplatin **Special considerations:** GI and CNS toxicity are common; total loss of hair, local reaction at injection site and bone marrow depression also occur; prepare a calendar with return dates for the series of injections; avoid extravasation but arrange for hyaluronidase infusion if it occurs; antiemetics may be helpful if reaction is severe

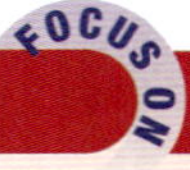

Safe medication administration

Special care needs to be taken when administering these drugs. The care provider should avoid any skin, eye or mucous membrane contact with the drug. This type of contact can cause serious reactions and toxicity.

Therapeutic actions and indications

The mitotic inhibitors interfere with the ability of a cell to divide; they block or alter DNA synthesis, thus causing cell death. They work in the M phase of the cell cycle. These drugs are used for the treatment of a variety of tumours and leukaemias. See Table 14.4 for usual indications for each of these agents.

Pharmacokinetics

Generally, these drugs are given IV because they are not well absorbed from the GI tract. They are metabolised in the liver and excreted primarily in the faeces, making them safer for use in people with renal impairment than the antineoplastics that are cleared through the kidney.

Contraindications and cautions

These drugs should not be used during pregnancy or breastfeeding *because of the potential risk to the fetus or neonate*. Use caution when giving these drugs to anyone with a known allergy to the drug or related drugs. Care is necessary for individuals with the following conditions: bone marrow suppression, *which is often the index for redosing and dosing levels*; renal or hepatic dysfunction, *which could interfere with the metabolism or excretion of these drugs and often indicates a need to change the dose*; and known GI ulcerations or ulcerative diseases, *which may be exacerbated by the effects of these drugs*.

Adverse effects

Adverse effects frequently encountered with the use of mitotic inhibitors include bone marrow suppression, with leucopenia, thrombocytopenia, anaemia and pancytopenia, secondary to the effects of the drugs on the rapidly multiplying cells of the bone marrow. GI effects include nausea, vomiting, anorexia, diarrhoea and mucous membrane deterioration. As with the other antineoplastic agents, effects of the mitotic inhibitors may include possible hepatic or renal toxicity, depending on the exact mechanism of action. Alopecia may also occur. These drugs also cause necrosis and cellulitis if extravasation occurs, so it is necessary to regularly monitor injection sites and take appropriate action as needed.

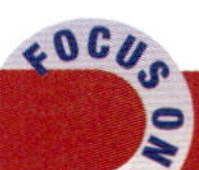

Safe medication administration

Preventing and treating extravasation

When an IV antineoplastic drug extravasates or infiltrates into the surrounding tissue, serious tissue damage can occur. These drugs are toxic to cells, and the resulting tissue injury can result in severe pain, scarring, nerve and muscle damage, infection and, in very severe cases, even amputation of the limb.

Prevention is the best way to deal with extravasation. Interventions that can help to prevent extravasation include the following: use a distal vein, and avoid small veins on the wrist or digits; never use an existing line unless it is clearly open and running well; start the infusion with plain 5% dextrose in water (D5W) and monitor for any sign of extravasation; check the site frequently and ask the person to report any discomfort in the area; and, if at all possible, do not use an infusion pump to administer one of these drugs because it will continue to deliver the drug under pressure and can cause severe extravasation.

Clinically important drug–drug interactions

Mitotic inhibitors that are known to be toxic to the liver or the CNS should be used with care with any other drugs known to have the same adverse effect. Check specific drug–drug interactions for each agent in a drug guide.

Prototype summary: vincristine

Indications: acute leukaemia, Hodgkin disease, non-Hodgkin lymphoma, rhabdomyosarcoma, neuroblastoma, Wilms tumour.

Actions: arrests mitotic division at the stage of metaphase; the exact mechanism of action is not understood.

Pharmacokinetics:

Route	Onset	Peak
IV	Varies	15–30 min

$T_{1/2}$: 5 minutes, then 2.3 hours, then 85 hours; metabolised in the liver and excreted in the faeces and urine.

Adverse effects: ataxia, cranial nerve manifestations, neuritic pain, muscle wasting, constipation, leucopenia, weight loss, loss of hair, death.

Care considerations for people receiving mitotic inhibitors

Assessment: history and examination

- Assess for contraindications or cautions: history of allergy to the drug used (or related drugs) *to avoid hypersensitivity reactions*; bone marrow suppression *to prevent further suppression*; renal or hepatic dysfunction *that might interfere with drug metabolism and excretion*; current status of pregnancy or breastfeeding *to prevent potentially serious adverse effects on the fetus or breastfeeding baby*; and GI ulcerative disease, *which could be exacerbated by these drugs.*
- Perform a physical assessment *to establish baseline data for determining the effectiveness of the drug and the occurrence of any adverse effects associated with drug therapy.*
- Assess orientation and reflexes *to evaluate any CNS effects*; skin *to evaluate for lesions*; hair and hair distribution *to monitor for adverse effects*; respiratory rate and adventitious sounds *to monitor the disease and to evaluate for respiratory or hypersensitivity effects*; and bowel sounds and mucous membrane status *to monitor for GI effects.*
- Monitor the results of laboratory tests such as FBC with differential *to identify possible bone marrow suppression and toxic drug effects*; and renal and liver function tests *to determine the need for possible dose adjustment as needed and to evaluate toxic drug effects.*
- Regularly inspect IV insertion sites *for signs of extravasation or inflammation, which need to be treated quickly.*

Implementation with rationale

- Arrange for blood tests to monitor bone marrow function before, periodically during, and for at least 3 weeks after therapy *to arrange to discontinue the drug or reduce the dose as needed.*
- Avoid direct skin or eye contact with the drug. Wear protective clothing and goggles while preparing and administering the drug *to prevent toxic reaction to the drug.*
- Administer medication according to scheduled protocol and in combination with other drugs as indicated *to improve the effectiveness of drug therapy.*
- Ensure that the person is well hydrated *to decrease the risk of renal toxicity.*
- Monitor injection sites *to arrange appropriate treatment for extravasation, local inflammation or cellulitis.*
- Protect the person from exposure to infection *because bone marrow suppression will decrease immune/inflammatory responses.*
- Provide small, frequent meals, frequent mouth care and dietary consultation as appropriate *to maintain nutrition if GI effects are severe.* Anticipate the need for antiemetics as necessary. (See Box 14.5.)
- Arrange for proper head covering at extremes of temperature if alopecia or epilation occurs; a wig, scarf or hat *is important for maintaining body temperature.* If alopecia is an anticipated effect of drug therapy, advise the person to obtain a wig or head covering before the condition occurs *to promote self-esteem and positive body image.*
- Provide the following teaching:
  - Follow the appropriate dosage regimen, including dates to return for further doses.
  - Maintain nutrition if GI effects are severe.
  - Cover the head at extremes of temperature if alopecia is anticipated.
  - Plan for appropriate rest periods because fatigue and weakness are common effects of the drugs.

- Avoid situations that might lead to infection, including crowded areas, sick people and working in the soil.
- Use safety measures such as avoiding driving or using dangerous equipment, due to possible dizziness, headache and drowsiness.
- Consult with a health care provider, as appropriate, due to the possibility of impaired fertility.
- Use barrier contraceptives to reduce the risk of pregnancy during therapy.

Evaluation

- Monitor response to the drug (alleviation of cancer being treated and palliation of signs and symptoms of cancer).
- Monitor for adverse effects (bone marrow suppression, GI toxicity, neurotoxicity, alopecia, renal or hepatic dysfunction, and local reactions at the injection site).
- Evaluate the effectiveness of the teaching plan (person can name the drug, dosage, possible adverse effects to watch for and specific measures to help avoid adverse effects).

KEY POINTS

- Mitotic inhibitors kill cells during the M phase and are used to treat a variety of cancers.
- These drugs are usually given IV. Extravasation could be a serious problem.
- Bone marrow suppression, alopecia and toxic GI effects are common adverse effects of the mitotic inhibitors.

HORMONES AND HORMONE MODULATORS

Some cancers, particularly those involving the breast tissue, ovaries, uterus, prostate and testes, are sensitive to oestrogen stimulation. Oestrogen-receptor sites on the tumour react with circulating oestrogen, and this reaction stimulates the tumour cells to grow and divide. Several antineoplastic agents are used to block or interfere with these receptor sites to prevent growth of the cancer and in some situations to actually cause cell death. Some hormones are used to block the release of gonadotropic hormones in breast or prostate cancer if the tumours are responsive to gonadotropic hormones. Others may block androgen-receptor sites directly and are useful in the treatment of advanced prostate cancers. Hormones and hormone modulators include abiraterone (*Zytiga*), anastrozole (*Arianna, Arimidex*), bicalutamide (*Calutex, Cosudex*), cabazitaxel (*Jevtana*), degarelix (*Firmagon*), exemestane (*Aromasin*), flutamide (*Flutamin*), fulvestrant (*Faslodex*), goserelin (*Zoladex*), letrozole (*Femara*), megestrol (*Megace*), nilutamide (*Anandron*), tamoxifen (*Nolvadex, Tamosin*), toremifene (*Fareston*) and triptorelin (*Diphereline*) (see Table 14.5).

Therapeutic actions and indications

The hormones and hormone modulators used as antineoplastics are receptor-site specific or hormone specific to block the stimulation of growing cancer cells that are sensitive to the presence of that hormone (see Figure 14.4). These drugs are indicated for the treatment of breast cancer in postmenopausal women or in other women without ovarian function. Some drugs are indicated for the treatment of prostatic cancers that are sensitive to hormone manipulation. Table 14.5 shows usual indications for each of the hormones and hormone modulators.

Pharmacokinetics

These drugs are readily absorbed from the GI tract, metabolised in the liver and excreted in the urine. Caution must be used with any individual who has hepatic or renal impairment. These drugs cross the placenta and enter into breast milk.

Contraindications and cautions

These drugs are contraindicated during pregnancy and breastfeeding *because of toxic effects on the fetus and neonate*. Hypercalcaemia is a contraindication to the use of toremifene, *which is known to increase calcium levels*. Use caution when giving hormones and hormone modulators to anyone with a known allergy to any of these drugs. Care is necessary in people with bone marrow suppression, *which is often the index for redosing and dosing levels*, and in those with renal or hepatic dysfunction, *which could interfere with the metabolism or excretion of these drugs and often indicates a need to change the dose*.

Adverse effects

Adverse effects frequently encountered with the use of these drugs involve the effects that are seen when oestrogen is blocked or inhibited. Menopause-associated effects include hot flushes, vaginal spotting, vaginal dryness, moodiness and depression. Other effects include bone marrow suppression and GI toxicity, including hepatic dysfunction. Hypercalcaemia is also encountered as the calcium is pulled out of the bones without oestrogen activity to promote calcium deposition. Many of these drugs increase the risk for cardiovascular disease because of their effects on the body.

TABLE 14.5 **DRUGS IN FOCUS** **Hormones and hormone modulators**

Drug name	Dosage/route	Usual indications
abiraterone (*Zytiga*)	1 g PO once daily	Treatment of metastatic advanced prostate cancer **Actions:** reduces androgen levels **Special considerations:** administered with prednisone or prednisolone. Monitor cardiovascular and hepatic function
anastrazole (*Arianna, Arimidex*)	1 mg/day PO	Treatment of advanced breast cancer in postmenopausal women after tamoxifen therapy; first-line and adjunctive treatment of postmenopausal women with locally advanced breast cancer **Actions:** antioestrogen drug; blocks oestradiol production without effects on adrenal hormones **Special considerations:** GI effects, signs and symptoms of menopause – hot flushes, mood swings, oedema, vaginal dryness and itching – as well as bone pain and back pain, treatable with analgesics, may occur; monitor lipid concentrations in people at risk for high cholesterol level
bicalutamide (*Calutex, Cosamide, Cosudex*)	50 mg/day PO	In combination with a luteinising hormone for the treatment of advanced prostate cancer **Actions:** antiandrogen drug that competitively binds androgen-receptor sites **Special considerations:** gynaecomastia and breast tenderness occur in 33% of people; GI complaints are common; pregnancy category X
cabazitaxel (*Jevtana*)	Adults: 20 mg/m^2 (25 mg/m^2 for selected patients) by IV infusion over 1 hour every 3 weeks	Treatment of hormone refractory metastatic prostate cancer **Actions:** inhibits mitotic and interphase cellular functions **Special considerations:** administered with prednisone or prednisolone. Weekly blood counts during cycle 1 and before each subsequent treatment. Closely monitor hydration status
degarelix (*Firmagon*)	240 mg by subcutaneous injection given in two 120 mg injections, then 80 mg SC every 28 days for maintenance	Treatment of people with advanced prostate cancer **Actions:** gonadotropin-releasing hormone–receptor-site antagonist, leads to decreased follicle-stimulating hormone and luteinising hormone and decreased testosterone levels **Special considerations:** pregnancy category X; risk of prolonged QT interval; injection-site reactions, hot flushes, increased weight are common
exemestane (*Aromasin*)	25 mg/day PO with food	Treatment of advanced, metastatic breast cancer in postmenopausal women whose disease has progressed after tamoxifen therapy **Actions:** inactivates steroid aromatase, lowering circulating oestrogen levels and preventing the conversion of androgens to oestrogen **Special considerations:** avoid use in premenopausal women or in people with liver or renal dysfunction; hot flushes, headache, GI upset, anxiety and depression are common

Continued on following page

TABLE 14.5 DRUGS IN FOCUS Hormones and hormone modulators *(continued)*

Drug name	Dosage/route	Usual indications
flutamide (*Flutamin*)	250 mg PO tds. given 8 hours apart	With a luteinising hormone for treatment of locally confined and metastatic prostate cancer **Actions:** antioestrogenic drug, inhibits androgen uptake and binding on target cells **Special considerations:** may cause liver toxicity, so liver function should be monitored regularly; associated with impaired fertility and cancer development; urine may become greenish; protect person from exposure to the sun – photosensitivity is common
fulvestrant (*Faslodex*)	250 mg IM injection into each buttock (total dose 500 mg), then a further 500 mg after 2 weeks and at 1 month intervals	Treatment of hormone receptor–positive metastatic breast cancer in postmenopausal women with disease progression after antioestrogen therapy **Actions:** competitively binds to oestrogen receptors, downregulating the oestrogen receptor protein in breast cancer cells **Special considerations:** pregnancy category X; hot flushes, depression, headache and GI upset are common; mark calendar with monthly injection dates; injection-site reactions may occur
goserelin (*Zoladex*)	3.6–10.8 mg implant, SC, every 28 days to 12 weeks, varies with diagnosis	Treatment of advanced prostatic and breast cancers; management of endometriosis **Actions:** synthetic luteinising hormone that inhibits pituitary release of gonadotropic hormones **Special considerations:** a 3.6 mg dose is effective in decreasing the signs and symptoms of endometriosis; associated with hypercalcaemia and bone density loss – monitor serum calcium levels regularly; impairs fertility and is carcinogenic; monitor males for possible ureteral obstruction, especially during the first month
letrozole (*Femara*)	2.5 mg/day PO	Treatment of advanced breast cancer in postmenopausal women with disease after antioestrogen therapy; postsurgery adjunct for postmenopausal women with early hormone receptor–positive breast cancer **Actions:** prevents the conversion of precursors to oestrogens in all tissues **Special considerations:** GI toxicity, bone marrow depression, alopecia, hot flushes and CNS depression are common effects; discontinue drug at any sign that the cancer is progressing

TABLE 14.5 DRUGS IN FOCUS **Hormones and hormone modulators *(continued)***

Drug name	Dosage/route	Usual indications
megestrol (*Megace*)	160 mg/day PO	Palliative treatment of advanced breast or endometrial cancer; appetite stimulant for people with HIV infection **Actions:** blocks luteinising-hormone release; efficacy not understood **Special considerations:** monitor for thromboembolic events and weight gain; not for use during pregnancy
nilutamide (*Anandron*)	300 mg/day PO for 30 days, then 150 mg/day PO	With surgical castration for treatment of metastatic prostate cancer **Actions:** antioestrogenic drug, inhibits androgen uptake and binding on target cells **Special considerations:** may cause liver toxicity, and liver function test results should be monitored regularly; associated with interstitial pneumonitis – baseline and periodic chest radiographs should be obtained and drug discontinued at first sign of dyspnoea
(P) tamoxifen (*Nolvadex, Tamosin*)	20–40 mg/day PO	In combination therapy with surgery to treat breast cancer; treatment of advanced breast cancer in men and women; first drug approved for the prevention of breast cancer in women at high risk **Actions:** antioestrogen, competes with oestrogen for receptor sites in target tissues **Special considerations:** signs and symptoms of menopause are common effects; CNS depression, bone marrow depression and GI toxicity are also common; can change visual acuity and cause corneal opacities and retinopathy – pretherapy and periodic ophthalmic examinations are indicated
toremifene (*Fareston*)	60 mg/day PO	Treatment of advanced breast cancer in women with oestrogen receptor–positive disease **Actions:** binds to oestrogen receptors and prevents growth of breast cancer cells **Special considerations:** signs and symptoms of menopause are common effects; CNS depression and GI toxicity are also common
triptorelin (*Diphereline*)	3.75 mg IM depot monthly or 11.25 mg IM depot every 3 months or 22.5 mg IM depot every 6 months	Treatment of advanced prostatic cancer **Actions:** analogue of luteinising hormone–releasing hormone; causes a decrease in follicle-stimulating hormone and luteinising hormone levels, leading to a suppression of testosterone production **Special considerations:** monitor prostate-specific antigen and testosterone levels regularly; sexual dysfunction, urinary tract symptoms, bone pain and hot flushes are common; schedule depot injections and mark calendar for person

Clinically important drug–drug interactions

If hormones and hormone modulators are taken with oral anticoagulants, there is often an increased risk of bleeding. Care is also necessary when administering these agents with any drugs that might increase serum lipid levels.

 **Prototype summary: tamoxifen**

Indications: treatment of metastatic breast cancer, reduction of risk of invasive breast cancer in women with ductal carcinoma in situ, reduction in occurrence of contralateral breast cancer in people receiving adjuvant tamoxifen therapy, reduction in incidence of breast cancer in women at high risk for breast cancer, treatment of McCune–Albright syndrome, and treatment of precocious puberty in females 2–10 years of age.

Actions: competes with oestrogen for binding sites in target tissues, such as the breast; a potent antioestrogenic agent.

Pharmacokinetics:

Route	Onset	Peak
Oral	Varies	4–7 hours

$T_{1/2}$: 7–14 days; metabolised in the liver and excreted in the faeces.

Adverse effects: hot flushes, rash, nausea, vomiting, vaginal bleeding, menstrual irregularities, oedema, pain, cerebrovascular accident, pulmonary emboli.

Care considerations for people receiving hormones and hormone modulators

Assessment: history and examination

- Assess for contraindications or cautions: history of allergy to the drug in use or any related drugs *to avoid hypersensitivity reactions*; bone marrow suppression *to prevent further suppression*; renal or hepatic dysfunction *that might interfere with drug metabolism and excretion*; current status of pregnancy or breastfeeding *to prevent potentially serious adverse effects on the fetus or breastfeeding baby*; history of hypercalcaemia and hypercholesterolaemia *to avoid further increases in levels.*
- Perform a physical assessment *to establish baseline data for determining the effectiveness of the drug and the occurrence of any adverse effects associated with drug therapy.*
- Assess orientation and reflexes *to evaluate any CNS effects*; skin *to evaluate for lesions*; hair and hair distribution *to monitor for adverse drug effects*; blood pressure, pulse and perfusion *to evaluate the status of the cardiovascular system and monitor for adverse drug effects*; and bowel sounds and mucous membrane status *to monitor for GI effects.*
- Monitor the results of laboratory tests such as FBC with differential to identify bone marrow suppression and toxic drug effects, serum calcium levels to evaluate for hypercalcaemia, and renal and liver function tests *to determine the need for possible dose adjustment to evaluate toxic drug effects.*
- *See the Critical thinking scenario for a full discussion of assessing and evaluating antineoplastic therapy for a woman with breast cancer.*

Implementation with rationale

- Arrange for blood tests to monitor bone marrow function before and periodically during therapy *to discontinue the drug or reduce the dose as needed.*
- Provide small, frequent meals, frequent mouth care and dietary consultation as appropriate *to maintain nutrition when GI effects are severe.*
- Provide comfort measures *to help the person cope with menopausal signs and symptoms* such as hygiene measures, temperature control and stress reduction. Expect to reduce the dose if these effects become severe or intolerable.
- Advise the individual of the need to use barrier contraceptive measures while taking these drugs *to avert serious fetal harm.*
- Provide the following teaching:
  - Follow the appropriate dosage regimen, including dates to return for further doses.
  - Maintain nutrition even if GI effects are severe.
  - Use barrier contraceptives to prevent pregnancy during therapy.
  - Try using comfort measures such as staying in a cool environment.
  - Perform hygiene and skin care and use measures to reduce stress to help cope with menopausal effects.
  - You may need to have periodic blood tests to monitor the effects of this drug on your body.

Evaluation

- Monitor response to the drug (alleviation of cancer being treated and palliation of signs and symptoms of cancer being treated).
- Monitor for adverse effects (bone marrow suppression, GI toxicity, menopausal signs and symptoms, hypercalcaemia and cardiovascular effects).

- Evaluate the effectiveness of the teaching plan (person can name the drug, dosage, possible adverse effects to watch for and specific measures to help avoid adverse effects).

KEY POINTS

- Hormones and hormonal agents are used to treat specific cancers that respond to hormone stimulation such as breast cancer or prostate cancer.
- The adverse effects of hormones and hormonal agents used to treat cancers are increased or decreased effects of the hormones on the body: virilisation, increased risk of cardiovascular disease, increased calcium levels.

CANCER CELL–SPECIFIC AGENTS

The goal of much of the current antineoplastic drug research is directed at finding drugs that are cancer cell specific. These drugs would not have the devastating effects on healthy cells in the body and would be more effective against particular cancer cells. Four groups of drugs are available for cancer cell–specific actions: monoclonal antibodies, protein tyrosine kinase inhibitors, an epidermal growth factor inhibitor and a proteasome inhibitor (see Table 14.6).

MONOCLONAL ANTIBODIES

Monoclonal antibodies (mAbs) are genetically engineered, protein antibody molecules used to treat cancer as well as other immunological conditions. They are made using identical clones of a unique parent immune cell. The mAbs bind to specific cancer cells, leading to an immune response against the cells. There are many examples, with varying indications, dosage and routes of administration. Table 14.6 lists some of the more commonly used ones.

PROTEIN TYROSINE KINASE INHIBITORS

The protein kinase inhibitors (Table 14.6) act on specific enzymes that are needed for protein building by specific tumour cells. Blocking of these enzymes inhibits tumour cell growth and division.

Each drug that has been developed inhibits a very specific protein kinase and acts on very specific tumours. They do not affect healthy human cells, so the person does not experience the numerous adverse effects associated with antineoplastic chemotherapy. Imatinib (*Glivec*), the first drug approved in this class, is

CRITICAL THINKING SCENARIO

Antineoplastic therapy and breast cancer

THE SITUATION

B.P., a 34-year-old woman, is a schoolteacher with two young daughters. She noticed a slightly painful lump under her arm when showering. About 2 weeks later, she found a mass in her right breast. Initial assessment found that she had no other underlying medical problems, had no allergies and took no medications. Her family history was most indicative: many of the women in her family – her mother, two grandmothers, three aunts, two older sisters and one younger sister – died of breast cancer when they were in their early 30s. All data from the initial examination, including an evaluation of the lump in the upper outer quadrant of her breast and the presence of a fixed axillary node, were recorded as baseline data for further drug therapy and treatment. B.P. underwent a radical mastectomy with biopsy report for grade IV infiltrating ductal carcinoma (28 of 35 lymph nodes were positive for tumour) and then radiation therapy. Then she began a 1-year course of doxorubicin, cyclophosphamide and paclitaxel (AC/paclitaxel/sequential).

CRITICAL THINKING

What are the important implications for B.P.? *Think about the outlook for B.P., based on her biopsy results and her family history.*

What are the effects of high levels of stress on the immune system and the body's ability to fight cancer?

What impact will this disease have on B.P.'s job and her family? *Think about the adverse drug effects that can be anticipated.*

How can good teaching help B.P. to anticipate and cope with these many changes and unpleasant effects?

What future concerns should be addressed or at least approached at this point in the treatment of B.P.'s disease? What are the implications for her two daughters? How may a coordinated health team work to help the daughters cope with their mother's disease, as well as the prospects for their future?

DISCUSSION

The extent of B.P.'s disease, as evidenced by the biopsy results, does not signify a very hopeful prognosis. In this case, the overall care plan should take into account not only the acute needs related to surgery and drug therapy, but also future needs related to potential debilitation and even the prospect of death. Immediate needs include comfort and teaching measures to help B.P. deal with the mastectomy and recovery from the surgery. She should be given an opportunity to vent her feelings and thoughts in a protected environment. Effort should be made to help her to organise her life and plans around her radiation therapy and chemotherapy.

The adverse effects associated with the antineoplastic agents she will be given should be explained and possible ways to cope should be discussed. These effects include the following:

Alopecia. B.P. should be reassured that her hair will grow back, but she will need to cover her head in extremes of temperature. Purchasing a wig before the hair loss begins may be a good alternative to trying to remember later what her hair was like.

Nausea and vomiting. These effects will most often occur immediately after the drugs are given. Antiemetics may be ordered, but they are frequently not very effective.

Bone marrow suppression. This will make B.P. more susceptible to disease, which could be a problem for a teacher and a mother with young children. Ways to avoid contact and infection, as well as warning signs to report immediately, should be discussed.

Mouth sores. Stomatitis and mucositis are common problems. Frequent mouth care is important. The person should be encouraged to maintain fluid intake and nutrition.

Because the antineoplastic therapy will be a long-term regimen, it might help to prepare a calendar of drug dates for use in planning other activities and events. All of B.P.'s treatment should be incorporated into a team approach that helps B.P. and her family deal with the impact of this disease and its therapy, as well as with the potential risk to her daughters. B.P.'s daughters are in a very high–risk group for this disease, so the importance of frequent examinations as they grow up needs to be stressed. In some areas of the country, health care providers are encouraging prophylactic mastectomies for women in this very high–risk group.

CARE GUIDE FOR B.P.: ANTINEOPLASTIC AGENTS

Assessment: history and examination

Allergies to any of these drugs, renal or hepatic dysfunction, pregnancy or breastfeeding, bone marrow suppression, or GI ulceration

Concurrent use of diazepam, verapamil, dexamethasone, cisplatin, ciclosporin, etoposide, vincristine, testosterone or digoxin, which could interact with these drugs

Local: evaluation of injection site

CNS: orientation, affect, reflexes

Skin: colour, lesions, texture

GI: abdominal, liver evaluation

Laboratory tests: FBC with differential; renal and liver function tests

Implementation

Ensure safe administration of the drug.

Provide comfort and safety measures: mouth and skin care, rest periods, safety precautions, antiemetics as needed, maintenance of nutrition and head covering.

Provide support and reassurance to deal with drug effects, body image changes, discomfort and diagnosis.

Provide teaching regarding drug name, dosage, adverse effects, precautions to take, signs and symptoms to report and comfort measures to observe.

Evaluation

Evaluate drug effects: resolution of cancer.

Monitor for adverse effects: GI toxicity, bone marrow suppression, CNS changes, renal and hepatic damage, alopecia, extravasation of drug.

Monitor for drug–drug interactions as listed.

Evaluate effectiveness of teaching program.

Evaluate effectiveness of comfort and safety measures.

TEACHING FOR B.P.

Antineoplastic agents work to destroy cells at various phases of their life cycle. The drugs are given in combination to affect the cells at these various stages. These drugs are prescribed to kill cancer cells that are growing in the body. Because these drugs also affect normal cells, they sometimes cause many adverse effects. Your drug combination includes doxorubicin, cyclophosphamide and paclitaxel.

- These drugs are given in a 21-day cycle, followed by a rest period. You will need to mark your calendar with the treatment days and rest days. You will need to have regular blood tests to follow the effects of these drugs on your blood cells.

- Common adverse effects of these drugs include the following:
  - *Nausea and vomiting.* Antiemetic drugs and sedatives may help. Your health care provider will be with you to help if these effects occur.
  - *Loss of appetite.* It is very important to keep up your strength. Tell people if there is something that you would be interested in eating – anything that appeals to you. Alert someone if you feel hungry, regardless of the time of day.
  - *Loss of hair.* Your hair will grow back, although its colour or consistency may be different from what it was originally. It may help to purchase a wig before you lose your hair so that you can match appearance if you would like to. Hats and scarves may also be worn. It is very important to keep your head covered in extremes of temperature and to protect yourself from sun, heat and cold. Because much of the body's heat can be lost through the head, not protecting yourself could cause serious problems.
  - *Mouth sores.* Frequent mouth care is very helpful. Try to avoid very hot or spicy foods.
  - *Fatigue, malaise.* Frequent rest periods and careful planning of your day's activities can be very helpful.
  - *Bleeding.* You may bruise more easily than you normally do and your gums may bleed while you are brushing your teeth. Special care should be taken when shaving or brushing your teeth. Avoid activities that might cause an injury and avoid medications that contain aspirin.
  - *Susceptibility to infection.* Avoid people with infections or colds, and avoid crowded, public places. In some cases, the people who are caring for you may wear gowns and masks to protect you from their germs. Avoid working in your garden because soil can be full of bacteria.
- Report any of the following to your health care provider: bruising and bleeding, fever, chills, sore throat, difficulty breathing, flank pain, and swelling in your ankles or fingers.
- Take the full course of your prescription. It is very important to take the complete regimen that has been ordered for you. Cancer cells grow at different rates, and they go through rest periods during which they are not susceptible to the drugs. The disease must be attacked over time to eradicate the problem.
- Tell any doctor, nurse or other health care provider that you are taking this drug.
- Try to maintain a balanced diet while you are taking this drug. Drink 10–12 glasses of water each day during the drug therapy.
- Use a barrier contraceptive while you are taking this drug. These drugs can cause serious effects to a developing fetus, and precautions must be taken to avoid pregnancy. If you think that you are pregnant, consult your health care provider immediately.
- You need to have periodic blood tests and examinations while you are taking this drug. These tests help to guard against serious adverse effects and may be needed to determine the next dose of your drug.

TABLE 14.6 DRUGS IN FOCUS Cancer cell–specific agents

Drug name	Dosage/route	Usual indications
Protein tyrosine kinase inhibitors		
everolimus (*Afinitor, Certican*)	10 mg/day PO with food	Treatment of people with advanced renal cell carcinoma after failure of treatment with sunitinib or sorafenib **Special considerations:** pneumonitis, serious-to-fatal infections, oral ulcerations, and elevations in blood glucose, lipid and creatinine levels may occur, monitor person very closely; do not use in pregnancy
gefitinib (*Iressa*)	250 mg/day PO	Monotherapy for treatment of people with locally advanced or metastatic non-small-cell lung cancer after failure with platinum-based or docetaxel chemotherapies; use limited to people doing well on therapy – not for new use **Special considerations:** interstitial lung disease may occur; monitor pulmonary function closely; eye changes may require stopping the drug for a while; do not use during pregnancy; numerous drug–drug interactions are possible

Continued on following page

TABLE 14.6 DRUGS IN FOCUS Cancer cell–specific agents *(continued)*

Drug name	Dosage/route	Usual indications
Protein tyrosine kinase inhibitors *(continued)*		
(P) imatinib (*Glivec*)	Chronic-phase chronic myelocytic leukaemia (CML): 400 mg/day PO, may be increased to 600 mg/day if needed, then may consider 800 mg/day after 4 weeks Blast-crisis CML: 600 mg/day PO, may be increased to 400 mg PO bd First-line CML treatment: 400 mg/day PO GI stromal tumours: 400–600 mg/day PO	Treatment of CML people in blast crisis or in chronic phase after interferon-alpha therapy; treatment of people with Kit-positive malignant GIST; first-line treatment of CML **Special considerations:** administer with a meal and a full glass of water; arrange for small, frequent meals if GI upset is a problem; provide analgesics for headache and muscle pain; monitor full blood count and for oedema to arrange for dose reduction if needed; person should receive consultation to deal with high cost of drug
lapatinib (*Tykerb*)	1250 mg (5 tablets) orally once daily on days 1–21 in combination with capecitabine 2000 mg/m^2/day PO in 2 doses approximately 12 hours apart on days 1–14; give in a repeating 21-day cycle; reduce dose to 750 mg/day PO with severe hepatic dysfunction	In combination with capecitabine for the treatment of people with advanced or metastatic breast cancer whose tumours overexpress HER2 and who have received prior treatment including an anthracycline, taxane and trastuzumab **Special considerations:** monitor heart function closely and decrease dose as needed; monitor for rash, GI toxicity; avoid grapefruit juice; many drug–drug interactions are possible
nilotinib (*Tasigna*)	300–400 mg PO bd, approximately 12 hours apart without food	Treatment of chronic-phase and accelerated-phase Philadelphia chromosome–positive chronic myelogenous leukaemia in adults resistant to, or intolerant of, prior therapy that included imatinib **Special considerations:** monitor for prolonged QT interval, bone marrow suppression and possible liver toxicity
sorafenib (*Nexavar*)	400 mg PO bd on an empty stomach	Treatment of people with advanced renal cell carcinoma and unresectable hepatocellular carcinoma **Special considerations:** monitor for skin reactions, hand–foot syndrome, hypertension
sunitinib (*Sutent*)	50 mg/day PO for 4 weeks, followed by 2 weeks of rest; repeat cycle	Treatment of GI stromal tumour if person is intolerant of, or tumour progresses after, imatinib therapy **Special considerations:** monitor for GI disturbances, bone marrow suppression; adjust dose as needed
temsirolimus (*Torisel*)	25 mg IV, infused over 30–60 minutes once per week	Treatment of advanced renal cell carcinoma **Special considerations:** monitor lung function, blood glucose, renal function; may experience slowed healing; avoid grapefruit juice, St John's wort
Epidermal growth factor inhibitor		
erlotinib (*Tarceva*)	150 mg/day PO 1 hour before or 2 hours after meal; may increase to 300 mg daily or 450 mg daily	Treatment of locally advanced or metastatic non-small-cell lung cancer after failure of at least one other drug regimen; first-line treatment of pancreatic cancer when used in combination with gemcitabine **Special considerations:** serious-to-fatal interstitial lung disease – monitor with hepatic impairment; do not use during pregnancy

TABLE 14.6 DRUGS IN FOCUS Cancer cell–specific agents *(continued)*

Drug name	Dosage/route	Usual indications
Proteasome inhibitor		
bortezomib (*Velcade*)	1.3 mg/m² by bolus IV injection on days 1, 4, 8 and 11, followed by 10 days of rest, then repeat Administer 2 additional cycles beyond confirmed complete response, or a total 8 cycles in responding patients without complete remission	Treatment of multiple myeloma in people with disease progression after two other therapies **Special considerations:** may cause peripheral neuropathies, hypotension and bone marrow suppression; do not use during pregnancy
Monoclonal antibodies		
bevacizumab (*Avastin*), denosumab (*Prolia, Xgeva*), pembrolizumab (*Keytruda*), rituximab (*Mabthera*)	Various. See McKenna's *Drug Handbook for Nursing and Midwifery*, 2019.	Various. See McKenna's *Drug Handbook for Nursing and Midwifery*, 2019.

given orally and is approved to treat chronic myelocytic leukaemia (CML). Individuals who have CML and who have been switched to imatinib after traditional chemotherapy have been amazed at how good they feel and how much they have recovered from the numerous adverse effects of the traditional chemotherapy. Examples of protein tyrosine kinase inhibitors include bortezomib (*Velcade*), erlotinib (*Tarceva*), everolimus (*Afinitor, Certican*), gefitinib (*Iressa*), imatinib (*Glivec*), lapatinib (*Tykerb*), nilotinib (*Tasigna*), sorafenib (*Nexavar*), sunitinib (*Sutent*) and temsirolimus (*Torisel*).

Epidermal growth factor inhibitor

In 2006, the Australian Therapeutic Goods Administration (TGA) approved erlotinib (*Tarceva*), a drug that inhibits cell epidermal growth factor receptors. This growth factor is found on normal and cancerous cells but is more abundant on rapidly growing cells.

Proteasome inhibitor

The TGA has approved bortezomib (*Velcade*) for the treatment of multiple myeloma in people whose disease has progressed after one other standard therapy. This drug inhibits proteasome in human cells, a large protein complex that works to maintain cell homeostasis and protein production. Without it, the cell loses homeostasis and dies. This drug was shown to delay growth in selected tumours.

Therapeutic actions and indications

Imatinib, an oral antineoplastic drug, is a protein tyrosine kinase inhibitor that selectively inhibits the Bcr-Abl tyrosine kinase created by the Philadelphia chromosome abnormality in CML. Blocking this enzyme inhibits proliferation and induces cell division in Bcr-Abl–positive cell lines, as well as in new leukaemic cells, thereby inhibiting tumour growth in people with CML in blast crisis. It also inhibits a specific receptor site in individuals with gastrointestinal stromal tumour (GIST). Because of its specific effects on these tumour cells, it is not associated with adverse effects on normal human cells.

Gefitinib, lapatinib, nilotinib, sorafenib, sunitinib and temsirolimus work by inhibiting various kinases in the cancer cell. Table 14.6 shows usual indications for all protein tyrosine kinase inhibitors.

Gefitinib inhibits tyrosine kinases, including ones associated with epidermal growth factor receptors. It is usually indicated for localised, advanced or metastatic non-small-cell lung cancer (NSCLC).

Erlotinib is an oral drug that inhibits enzymes associated with epidermal growth factor. It is approved for the treatment of non-small-cell lung cancer and for first-line treatment of pancreatic cancer when used in combination with gemcitabine.

Bortezomib blocks a large protein complex that is necessary for maintaining cell homeostasis, leading to cell death. It must be given IV and is approved for the treatment of mantle cell lymphoma and multiple myeloma.

Pharmacokinetics

Imatinib is slowly absorbed from the GI tract, reaching peak levels in 2–4 hours. It is extensively metabolised in the liver, with a half-life of 18 and then 40 hours. Gefitinib is slowly absorbed from the GI tract, reaching peak levels in 3–7 hours. It is metabolised in the liver with a half-life of 48 hours. Lapatinib, given orally, is absorbed from the GI tract, reaching peak levels in 1–1.5 hours. Lapatinib is metabolised in the liver, with a half-life of 24 hours. Nilotinib, given orally, reaches peak levels 3 hours after GI absorption. Most of the drug is excreted unchanged in the stool with a half-life of 17 hours. Sorafenib is well absorbed from the GI tract after oral administration, reaching peak levels in 1–2 hours. Most of the drug is excreted unchanged in the stool with a half-life of 24–48 hours. Sunitinib, given orally, is slowly absorbed from the GI tract, reaching peak levels in 6–12 hours. After metabolism in the liver, it has a half-life of 40–60 hours and then 80–110 hours for its active metabolite. Temsirolimus, only available for IV use, reaches peak levels at the end of the infusion. It is metabolised in the liver and primarily excreted in the faeces with a half-life of 17 hours and then 55 hours for its active metabolite. Erlotinib is well absorbed orally from the GI tract, reaching peak levels in 4 hours. It is metabolised in the liver with a half-life of 36 hours. Bortezomib, given IV, reaches peak effects at the end of the infusion. It is metabolised in the liver and has a half-life of 40–193 hours.

Contraindications and cautions

All of these drugs are in either pregnancy category C or pregnancy category D (see Chapter 1). Women of childbearing age should be advised to use barrier contraceptives while taking these drugs. They can enter breast milk, and should be used during breastfeeding only if the benefits to the mother clearly outweigh the risks to the baby. With imatinib, caution should be used in people with known hepatic dysfunction. Nilotinib is contraindicated with individuals who have, or are at risk for, prolonged QT intervals (hypokalaemia, hypomagnesaemia or taking another drug that prolongs the QT interval) because it prolongs the QT interval, and sudden deaths could occur. These drugs should not be given to anyone who has a history of hypersensitivity to any component of the drug being given.

Adverse effects

The adverse effects associated with imatinib include GI upset, muscle cramps, heart failure, fluid retention and skin rash. The severe bone marrow suppression, alopecia and severe GI effects associated with more traditional antineoplastic therapy do not occur. Gefitinib has been associated with potentially severe interstitial lung disease and various eye symptoms. Nilotinib causes prolonged QT intervals and can impair liver and kidney function. Lapatinib causes diarrhoea and can cause liver impairment and alter heart function. Erlotinib and bortezomib are associated with cardiovascular events and pulmonary toxicity. Bortezomib has also been associated with peripheral neuropathy and liver and kidney impairment.

Clinically important drug–drug interactions

Use caution when administering imatinib with other drugs affected by the cytochrome P450 enzyme system. In addition, St John's wort decreases the effectiveness of many of these drugs and should be avoided. When using nilotinib avoid any other drugs that are known to prolong the QT interval.

Prototype summary: imatinib

Indications: treatment of adults with CML who are in blast crisis, accelerated phase, or chronic phase after failure with interferon-alpha therapy. It has since also been approved for use in the treatment of people with CD117-positive unresectable or metastatic GIST.

Actions: tyrosine kinase inhibitor that selectively inhibits the Bcr-Abl tyrosine kinase created by the Philadelphia chromosome abnormality in CML and certain tumour cells present in GIST; blocking this enzyme inhibits proliferation and induces cell division.

Pharmacokinetics:

Route	Onset	Peak
Oral	Slow	2–4 hours

$T_{1/2}$: 18–40 hours; metabolised in the liver and excreted in the faeces.

Adverse effects: nausea, vomiting, bone marrow suppression, heart failure, headache, dizziness, oedema, rash.

Care considerations for people receiving cancer cell–specific agents

These are similar to care considerations for people receiving alkylating agents.

KEY POINTS

- Cancer cell–specific drugs have been developed to target processes that occur in cancer cells but not in healthy cells. This specificity results in fewer toxic effects than with traditional antineoplastic therapy.
- Protein tyrosine kinase inhibitors, epidermal growth factor inhibitors and proteasome inhibitors have been developed to target cancer cells specifically.

MISCELLANEOUS ANTINEOPLASTICS

Many other agents that do not fit into one of the previously discussed groups are used as antineoplastics to cause cell death. These drugs are used for treating a wide variety of cancers. Table 14.7 lists the unclassified antineoplastic drugs, their indications and any special

TABLE 14.7 **DRUGS IN FOCUS** **Miscellaneous antineoplastics**

Drug name	Dosage/route	Usual indications
arsenic trioxide (*Phenasen*)	Complex dosing. Newly diagnosed promyelocytic leukaemia (APL) Induction (cycle 1): 0.15 mg/kg/day from day 9 for 28 days, last dose on day 36 Consolidation (cycle 2): start 3–4 weeks after cycle 1, 0.15 mg/kg/day from day 1–28 Consolidation (cycle 3): start 3–4 weeks after cycle 2, 0.15 mg/kg/day for 5 days/week (5 days on, 2 days off) for a total of 5 weeks	Induction and consolidation in people with acute promyelocytic leukaemia (APL) who are refractory to, or relapsed from, standard therapy **Actions:** causes damage to fusion proteins and DNA failure, leading to cell death **Special considerations:** monitor for cardiac toxicity; do not use during pregnancy
hydroxycarbamide (hydroxyurea) (*Hydrea*)	80 mg/kg PO every third day; 20–30 mg/kg PO daily for continual therapy	Inhibits enzymes essential for the synthesis of DNA, causing cell death **Actions:** treatment of melanoma, ovarian cancer, chronic myelocytic leukaemia; in combination therapy for primary squamous cell cancers of the head and neck; also used in the treatment of sickle cell anaemia **Special considerations:** can cause bone marrow depression, headache, rash, GI toxicity and renal dysfunction; encourage person to drink 10–12 glasses of water each day while taking this drug
irinotecan (*Camptosar*)	125 mg/m² IV over 90 minutes, once a week for 4 weeks, followed by 2 weeks of rest; repeat every 6 weeks	Treatment of metastatic colon or rectal cancer after treatment with fluorouracil (5-FU) or given with 5-FU **Actions:** disrupts DNA strands during DNA synthesis, causing cell death **Special considerations:** can cause severe bone marrow depression, which regulates dose of the drug; causes GI toxicity, dyspnoea, and alopecia
topotecan (*Hycamtin*)	1.5 mg/m²/day IV for 5 days; as part of a 21-day course; minimum of four courses	Treatment of people with metastatic ovarian cancer after failure of other agents **Actions:** damages DNA strand, causing cell death during cell division **Special considerations:** can cause severe bone marrow depression, which regulates the dose of the drug; total alopecia, GI toxicity and CNS effects may also limit the use of the drug; analgesics may be helpful
Drug name	**Dosage/route**	**Usual indications**
tretinoin (*Vesanoid*)	45 mg/m² per day in 2 divided doses PO for 30–120 days	Used to induce remission in APL; can cause severe respiratory and cardiac toxicity, including myocardial infarction and cardiac arrest **Actions:** promotes cell differentiation and the repopulation of the bone marrow with normal cells in people with APL **Special considerations:** GI toxicity, pseudotumour cerebri (papilloedema, headache, nausea, vomiting, visual changes), skin rash and fragility may limit use in some people; discontinue drug at first sign of toxic effects; use for induction of remission only – then other chemotherapeutic agents should be used

considerations associated with the drug. Specific information about each drug may be obtained in a nursing drug guide. (See Figure 14.4 for sites of action of the miscellaneous antineoplastic agents.)

CHAPTER SUMMARY

- Cancers arise from a single abnormal cell that multiplies and grows.
- Cancers can manifest as diseases of the blood and lymph tissue or as growth of tumours arising from epithelial cells (carcinomas) or from mesenchymal cells and connective tissue (sarcomas).
- Cancer cells lose their normal function (anaplasia), develop characteristics that allow them to grow in an uninhibited way (autonomy), have the ability to travel to other sites in the body that are conducive to their growth (metastasis) and can stimulate the production of blood vessels to bring nutrients to the growing tumour (angiogenesis).
- Antineoplastic drugs affect both normal cells and cancer cells by disrupting cell function and division at various points in the cell cycle; new drugs are being developed, such as protein kinase inhibitors, to target cancer cell–specific functions.
- Cancer drugs are usually most effective against cells that multiply rapidly (i.e. proceed through the cell cycle quickly). These cells include most neoplasms, bone marrow cells, cells in the GI tract and cells in the skin or hair follicles.
- The goal of cancer chemotherapy is to decrease the size of the neoplasm so that the human immune system can deal with it.
- Antineoplastic drugs are often given in combination so that they can affect cells in various stages of the cell cycle, including cells that are emerging from rest or moving to a phase of the cycle that is disrupted by these drugs.
- Adverse effects associated with antineoplastic therapy include effects caused by damage to the rapidly multiplying cells, such as bone marrow suppression, which may limit the drug use; GI toxicity, with nausea, vomiting, mouth sores and diarrhoea; and alopecia (hair loss).
- Chemotherapeutic agents should not be used during pregnancy or breastfeeding because they may result in potentially serious adverse effects on the rapidly multiplying cells of the fetus and neonate.
- The newest drugs developed as antineoplastic agents target very specific enzyme systems or processes used by the cancer cells but not by healthy human cells. These drugs are not as toxic to the person as traditional antineoplastic drugs.

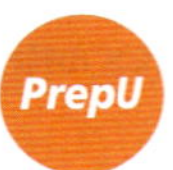

Knowing your strengths and weaknesses helps you to study more effectively. Take a PrepU Practice Quiz to find out how you measure up!

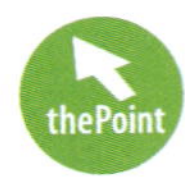

ONLINE RESOURCES

An extensive range of additional resources to enhance teaching and learning and to facilitate understanding of this chapter may be found online at the text's accompanying website, located on thePoint at http://thepoint.lww.com. These include Watch and Learn videos, Concepts in Action animations, journal articles, review questions, case studies, discussion topics and quizzes.

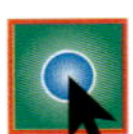

WEB LINKS

Health care providers and students may want to consult the following web resources:

www.eviq.org.au
Australian Government online resource of evidence-based, consensus-driven cancer treatment protocols developed by multidisciplinary teams of cancer specialists.

www.cancer.org.au
The Cancer Council Australia. Information on cancer including research, protocols and new information.

http://canceraustralia.gov.au
Cancer Australia, Australian Government.

www.cancernz.org.nz
The Cancer Society of New Zealand. Information on cancer including research, protocols and new information.

www.cnsa.org.au
The Cancer Nurses Society of Australia

www.ons.org
Information about the Oncology Nursing Society.

BIBLIOGRAPHY

Carrington, C. (2013). Safe use of oral cytotoxic medicines. *Australian Prescriber*, *36*, 9–12.

Chabner, B. A. & Roberts, T. G. (2005). Timeline: Chemotherapy and the war on cancer. *Nature Reviews. Cancer*, *5*, 65–72.

De Vita, V. T., Laurence, T. S. & Rosenberg, S. A. (2011). *Cancer: Principles and Practice of Oncology*. Philadelphia: Lippincott, Williams & Wilkins.

Dempsey, J., Hillege, S. & Hill, R. (2014). *Fundamentals of Nursing and Midwifery: A Person-centred Approach to Care* (2nd Australian and New Zealand edn). Sydney: Lippincott Williams & Wilkins.

Krishnasamy, M., Kwok-Wei, W., Yates, P., de Calvo, L.E.A., Annab, R., Wisniewski, T. & Aranda, S. (2013). The nurse's role in managing chemotherapy-induced nausea and vomiting: An international survey. *Cancer Nursing*, DOI: 10.1097/NCC.0b013e3182a3534a.

Liauw, W. S. (2013). Molecular mechanisms and clinical use of targeted anticancer drugs. *Australian Prescriber*, *36*, 126–131.

McKenna, L. & Mirkov, S. (2019). *McKenna's Drug Handbook for Nursing and Midwifery* (8th edn). Sydney: Wolters Kluwer Health Australia.

Middleton, J. & Lennan, E. (2011). Effectively managing chemotherapy-induced nausea and vomiting. *British Journal of Nursing*, *20*, *(sup10)*, S7–15.

Porth, C. M. (2011). *Essentials of Pathophysiology: Concepts of Altered Health States* (3rd edn). Philadelphia: Lippincott Williams & Wilkins.

Porth, C. M. (2009). *Pathophysiology: Concepts of Altered Health States* (8th edn). Philadelphia: Lippincott Williams & Wilkins.

Priestman, T. (2012). *Cancer Chemotherapy in Clinical Practice*. London: Springer-Verlag.

Roe, H. (2011). Chemotherapy-induced alopecia: Advice and support for hair loss. *British Journal of Nursing*, *20 (sup5)*, 4–11.

Schlumeister, L. (2007). Extravasation management. *Seminars in Oncology Nursing*, *23*, 184–190.

Vardy, J. (2008). Neurocognitive effects of chemotherapy in adults. *Australian Prescriber*, *31*, 22–24.

CHECK YOUR UNDERSTANDING

Answers to the questions in this chapter can be found in Appendix A at the back of this book.

MULTIPLE CHOICE

Select the best answer to the following.

1. Some properties of neoplastic cells are the same as the properties of normal cells, including:
   a. anaplasia.
   b. metastasis.
   c. mitosis.
   d. autonomy.
2. Carcinomas are tumours that originate in:
   a. mesenchyme.
   b. bone marrow.
   c. striated muscle.
   d. epithelial cells.
3. The goal of traditional antineoplastic drug therapy is to:
   a. reduce the size of abnormal cell mass for immune system destruction.
   b. eradicate all of the abnormal cells that have developed.
   c. destroy all cells of the originating type.
   d. stimulate the immune system to destroy the neoplastic cells.
4. Cancer can be a difficult disease to treat because:
   a. cells no longer progress through the normal cell cycle.
   b. cells can develop resistance to drug therapy.
   c. cells remain dormant, emerging months to years later.
   d. the exact cause of cancer is not known.
5. Antineoplastic drugs destroy human cells. They are most likely to cause cell death among healthy cells that:
   a. have poor cell membranes.
   b. are rapidly turning over.
   c. are in dormant tissues.
   d. cross the blood–brain barrier.
6. Cancer treatment usually occurs in several different treatment phases. In assessing the appropriateness of another round of chemotherapy for a particular person, which of the following would be evaluated as the most important?
   a. hair loss
   b. bone marrow function
   c. anorexia
   d. heart rate
7. It is important to explain to women that chemotherapeutic agents should not be used during pregnancy because:
   a. the tendency to cause nausea and vomiting will be increased.
   b. of potential serious adverse effects on the rapidly multiplying cells of the fetus.
   c. bone marrow toxicity could alter hormone levels.
   d. people may be weakened by the drug regimen.
8. Cancer drugs are given in combination and over a period of time because it is difficult to affect:
   a. slowly growing cells.
   b. cells in the dormant phase of the cell cycle.
   c. cells that multiply rapidly and go through the cell cycle quickly.
   d. cells that have moved from their normal site in the body.

MULTIPLE RESPONSE

Select all that apply.

1. Which of the following points would be most important to stress when developing a teaching plan for a person receiving antineoplastic therapy?
   a. the importance of keeping the head covered at extremes of temperature
   b. the need to use barrier contraceptives because of the risk of serious fetal effects
   c. the importance of avoiding exposure to infection because the ability to heal or to fight infection is impaired
   d. the importance of avoiding food if nausea or vomiting is a problem
   e. the importance of avoiding digging in the dirt without protective coverings because of the many pathogens that live in the dirt that could cause infection
   f. the importance of taking periodic rest periods during the day because you will feel tired when your red blood cell count falls

2. Hair loss, or alopecia, is an adverse effect of many antineoplastic agents. If a person is receiving a drug that usually causes alopecia, it is important that the care provider do which of the following?
   a. Warn the person that alopecia will occur.
   b. Encourage the person to arrange for an appropriate head covering at extremes of temperature.
   c. Advise the person to lie with the legs elevated and head low to promote circulation and prevent hair loss.
   d. Encourage the person to arrange for a wig or other head covering before the hair loss occurs.
   e. Advise the person that people will stare and can be rude when hair loss occurs.
   f. Make arrangements for the person to attend a support group before hair loss happens.

PART 3

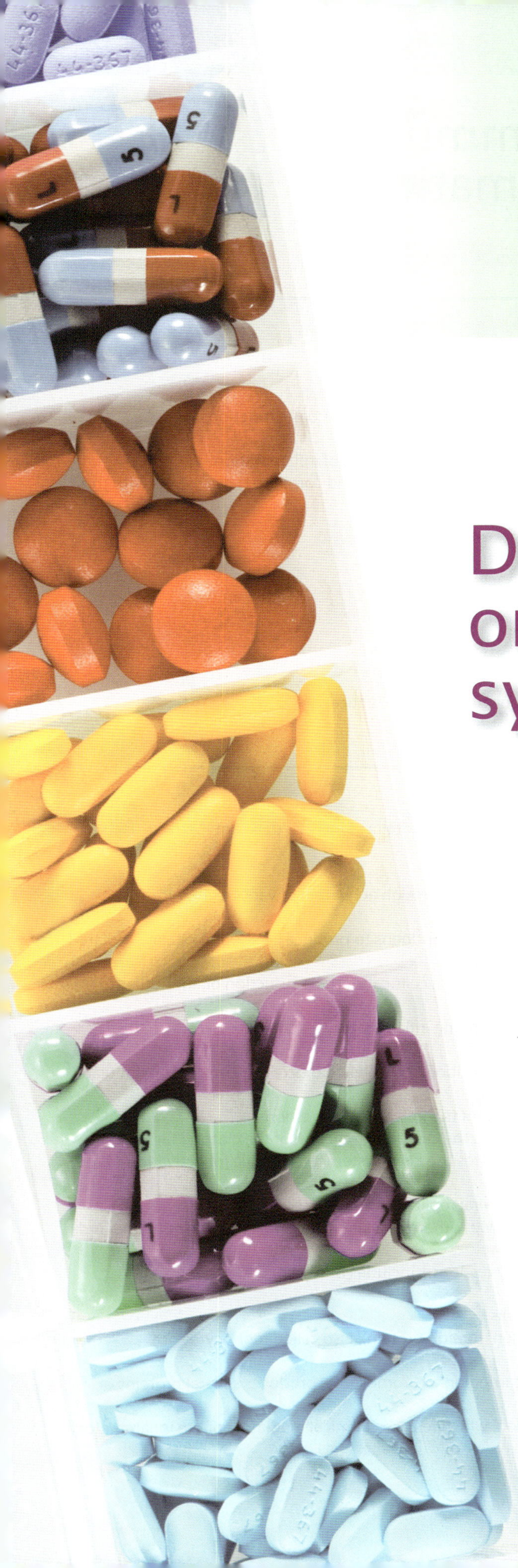

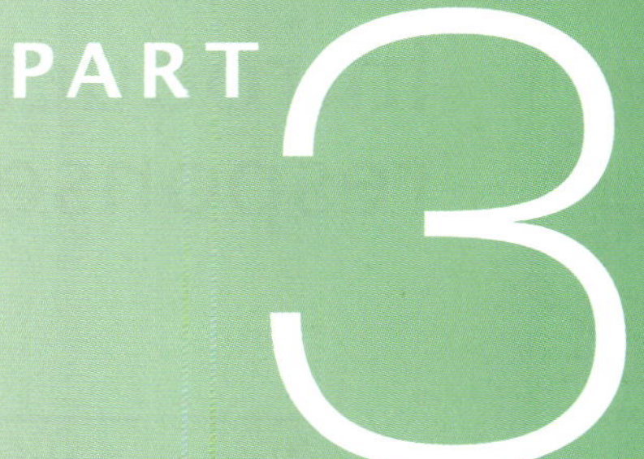

Drugs acting on the immune system

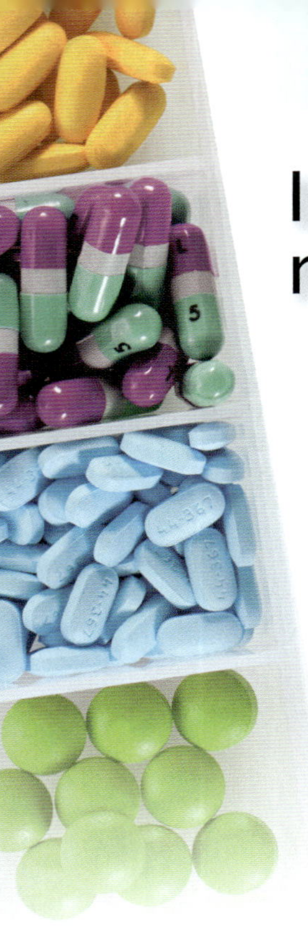

Introduction to the immune response and inflammation

15

Learning objectives

On completing this chapter you should be able to:

1. List four natural body defences against infection.
2. Describe the cells associated with the body's fight against infection and their basic functions.
3. Outline the sequence of events in the inflammatory response.
4. Correlate the events in the inflammatory response with the clinical picture of inflammation.
5. Outline the sequence of events in an antibody-related immune reaction and correlate these events with the clinical presentation of such a reaction.

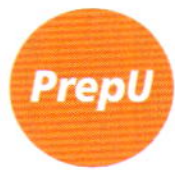

Test your current knowledge of immune response and inflammation with a PrepU Practice Quiz!

Glossary of key terms

antibodies: immunoglobulins; produced by B cell plasma cells in response to a specific protein; react with that protein to cause its destruction directly or through activation of the inflammatory response

antigen: foreign protein that induces specific immune responses

arachidonic acid: released from injured cells to stimulate the inflammatory response through activation of various chemical substances

autoimmune disease: a disorder that occurs when the body responds to specific self-antigens to produce antibodies or cell-mediated responses against its own cells

B cells: lymphocytes programmed to recognise specific proteins; when activated, these cells cause the production of antibodies to react with that protein

calour: heat, one of the four cardinal signs of inflammation; caused by activation of the inflammatory response

chemotaxis: property of drawing neutrophils to an area

complement proteins: series of cascading proteins that react with the antigen–antibody complex to destroy the protein or stimulate an inflammatory reaction

dolour: pain, one of the four cardinal signs of inflammation; caused by activation of the inflammatory response

Hageman factor: first factor activated when a blood vessel or cell is injured; starts the cascading reaction of the clotting factors, activates the conversion of plasminogen to plasmin to dissolve clots and activates the kinin system responsible for activation of the inflammatory response

interferon: tissue hormone that is released in response to viral invasion; blocks viral replication

interleukins: chemicals released by white blood cells (WBCs) to communicate with other WBCs and to support the inflammatory and immune reactions

kinin system: system activated by Hageman factor as part of the inflammatory response; includes bradykinin

leucocytes: white blood cells; can be neutrophils, basophils or eosinophils

lymphocytes: white blood cells with large, varied nuclei; can be T cells or B cells

macrophages: mature leucocytes that are capable of phagocytising an antigen (foreign protein); also called monocytes or mononuclear phagocytes

major histocompatibility complex (MHC): the genetic identification code carried on a chromosome; produces several proteins or antigens that allow the body to recognise cells as being self cells

mast cells: fixed basophils found in the respiratory and GI tracts and in the skin, which release chemical mediators of the inflammatory and immune responses when they are stimulated by local irritation

myelocytes: leucocyte-producing cells in the bone marrow that can develop into neutrophils, basophils, eosinophils, monocytes or macrophages
non-self cells: cells that are foreign; not identified as part of the organism itself
phagocytes: neutrophils that are able to engulf and digest foreign material
phagocytosis: the process of engulfing and digesting foreign pyrogens
pyrogen: fever-causing substance
rubor: redness, one of the four cardinal signs of inflammation; caused by activation of the inflammatory response
T cells: lymphocytes programmed in the thymus gland to recognise self cells; may be effector T cells, helper T cells, or suppressor T cells
tumour: swelling, one of the four cardinal signs of inflammation; caused by activation of the inflammatory response

The body has many defence systems in place to keep it intact and to protect it from external stressors. These stressors can include bacteria, viruses, other foreign pathogens or **non-self cells**, trauma and exposure to extremes of environmental conditions. The same defence systems that protect the body also help to repair it after cellular trauma or damage. Understanding the basic mechanisms involved in these defence systems is important in order to be able to explain the actions of the drugs that affect the immune system and inflammation.

BODY DEFENCES

The human body can mount two types of immune defences. The innate or natural (or non-specific) immunity and the specific or acquired immunity. The innate or natural immunity defences are factors that are present in the body before exposure to a particular infectious organism. The specific or acquired immune defences occur only after exposure to substances called antigens.

The body's defences include barrier defences, cellular defences, the inflammatory response and the immune response. Each of these defences plays a major role in maintaining homeostasis and preventing disease.

Barrier defences

Certain anatomical barriers exist to prevent the entry of foreign pathogens and to serve as important lines of defence in protecting the body. These barriers include the skin and mucous membranes, gastric acid and the major histocompatibility complex.

Skin

The skin is the first line of defence. The skin acts as a physical barrier to protect the internal tissues and organs of the body. Glands in the skin secrete chemicals that destroy or repel many pathogens. The top layer of the skin sheds daily, which makes it difficult for any pathogen to colonise on the skin. In addition, normal bacterial flora of the skin help to destroy many disease-causing pathogens.

Mucous membranes

Mucous membranes line the areas of the body that are exposed to external influences but do not have the benefit of skin protection. These body areas include the respiratory tract, which is exposed to air; the gastrointestinal (GI) tract, which is exposed to anything ingested by mouth; and the genitourinary (GU) tract, which is exposed to many pathogens from the perineal and rectal area. Like the skin, the mucous membrane acts as a physical barrier to invasion. It also secretes a sticky mucous capable of trapping invaders and inactivating them for later destruction and removal by the body.

In the conducting airways of the respiratory tract, the mucous membrane is lined with tiny, hair-like processes called cilia. The cilia sweep any captured pathogens or foreign materials upwards towards the mouth, where they will be swallowed. The cilia can also move the captured material to an area causing irritation, which leads to removal by coughing or sneezing.

In the GI tract, the mucous membrane serves as a protective coating, preventing erosion of GI cells by the acidic environment of the stomach, the digestive enzymes of the small intestine and the waste products that accumulate in the large intestine. The mucous membrane also secretes mucus, which serves as a lubricant throughout the GI tract to facilitate movement of the food bolus and of waste products. The mucous membrane acts as a thick barrier to prevent foreign pathogens from penetrating the GI tract and entering the body.

In the GU tract, the mucous membrane provides direct protection against injury and trauma and traps any pathogens in the area for destruction by the body.

Gastric acid

The stomach secretes acid in response to many stimuli. The acidity of the stomach not only aids digestion, but also destroys many would-be pathogens that are either ingested or swallowed after removal from the respiratory tract.

Major histocompatibility complex

The body's last barrier of defence is the ability to distinguish between self cells and foreign cells. All of the cells and tissues of each person are marked for identification as part of that individual's genetic code. No two people have exactly the same code. In humans, the genetic identification code is carried on a chromosome and is called the **major histocompatibility complex** (MHC). The MHC produces several proteins called histocompatibility antigens, or human leucocyte antigens (HLAs). These **antigens** (proteins) are located on the cell membrane and allow the body to recognise cells as being self cells. Cells that do not have these proteins are identified as foreign and are targeted for destruction by the body.

Cellular defences

Any foreign pathogen that manages to get past the barrier defences will encounter the human inflammatory and immune systems, or mononuclear phagocyte system (MPS). Previously called the reticuloendothelial system, the MPS is composed primarily of leucocytes, lymphocytes, lymphoid tissues and numerous chemical mediators.

Stem cells in the bone marrow produce two types of white blood cells, or **leucocytes**: the lymphocytes and the myelocytes. The **lymphocytes** are the key components of the immune system and consist of T cells, B cells and natural killer cells (see later discussion of the immune response). The **myelocytes** develop into a number of different cell types that are important in both the basic inflammatory response and the immune response. Myelocytes include neutrophils, basophils, eosinophils and monocytes, or macrophages (Figure 15.1).

Neutrophils

Neutrophils are polymorphonuclear leucocytes that are capable of moving outside of the blood stream (diapedesis) and engulfing and digesting foreign material (**phagocytosis**). When the body is injured or invaded by a pathogen, neutrophils are rapidly produced and move to the site of the insult to attack the foreign substance. Because neutrophils are able to engulf and digest foreign material, they are called **phagocytes**. Phagocytes are able to identify non-self cells by use of the MHC, and they can engulf these cells or mark them for destruction by cytotoxic T lymphocytes.

Basophils

Basophils are myelocytic leucocytes that are not capable of phagocytosis. They contain chemical substances or mediators that are important for initiating and maintaining an immune or inflammatory response. These substances include histamine, heparin and other chemicals used in the inflammatory response.

Basophils that are fixed and do not circulate are called **mast cells**. They are found in the respiratory and GI tracts and in the skin. They release many of the chemical mediators of the inflammatory and immune responses when they are stimulated by local irritation.

Eosinophils

Eosinophils are circulating myelocytic leucocytes whose exact function is not understood. They are often found at the site of allergic reactions and may be responsible for removing the proteins and active components of the immune reaction from the site of an allergic response.

Monocytes/Macrophages

Monocytes or mononuclear phagocytes are also called **macrophages**. They are mature leucocytes that are capable of phagocytising an antigen. Macrophages help to remove foreign material from the body, including pathogens, debris from dead cells and necrotic tissue from injury sites, so that the body can heal. They can

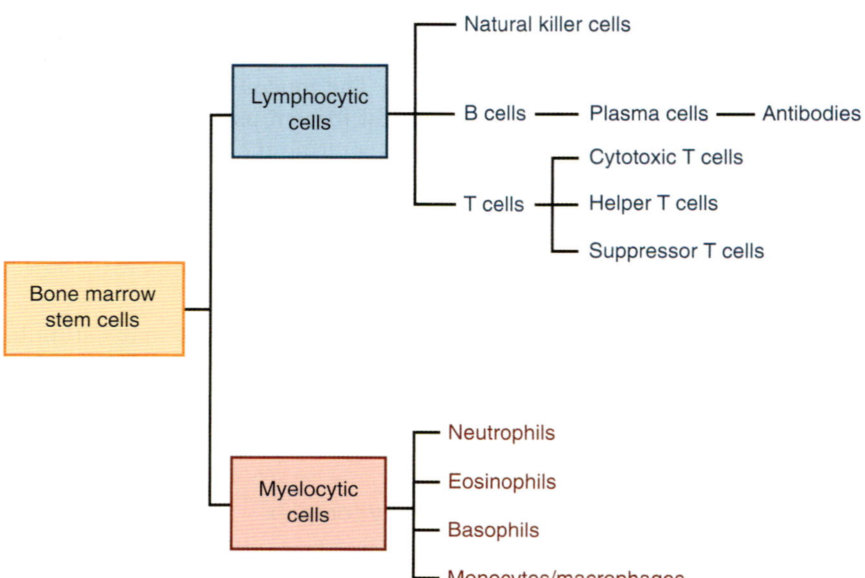

FIGURE 15.1 Types of white blood cells, or leucocytes, produced by the body.

also process antigens and present them to active lymphocytes for destruction.

Macrophages can circulate in the blood stream or they can be fixed in specific tissues, such as the Kupffer cells in the liver, the cells in the alveoli of the respiratory tract, and the microglia in the central nervous system (CNS), GI, circulatory and lymph tissues. As active phagocytes, macrophages release chemicals that are necessary to elicit a strong inflammatory reaction. These cells also respond to chemical mediators released by other cells that are active in the inflammatory and immune responses to increase the intensity of a response and to facilitate the body's reaction.

Lymphoid tissues

Lymphoid tissues that play an important part in the cellular defence system include the lymph nodes, spleen, thymus gland (a bipolar gland located in the middle of the chest, which becomes smaller with age), bone marrow and lymphoid tissue throughout the respiratory and GI tracts. The bone marrow and the thymus gland are important for creation of the cellular components of the MPS. The bone marrow has a role in the differentiation of these cellular components. The thymus gland is responsible for the final differentiation of the T cells and for regulating the actions of the immune system. The lymph nodes and lymphoid tissue store concentrated populations of neutrophils, basophils, eosinophils and lymphocytes in areas of the body that facilitate their surveillance for, and destruction of, foreign proteins. Other cells travel through the cardiovascular and lymph systems to search for foreign proteins or to reach the sites of injury or pathogen invasion.

KEY POINTS

- The body has several defence mechanisms in place to protect it from injury or foreign invasion.
- Barrier defences include the skin, mucous membranes, normal flora and gastric acid.
- Cellular defences include blood cells such as the lymphocytes (T and B cells) and the myelocytes (neutrophils, eosinophils, basophils and macrophages).

The inflammatory response

The inflammatory response is the local reaction of the body to invasion or injury. Any insult to the body that injures cells or tissues sets off a series of events and chemical reactions.

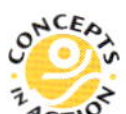

Nutritional: Immune: acute inflammation

Cell injury causes the activation of a chemical in the plasma called factor XII, or **Hageman factor.** Hageman factor is responsible for activating at least three systems in the body: the **kinin system**, which is discussed here; the clotting cascade, which initiates blood clotting; and the plasminogen system, which initiates the dissolution of blood clots. The last two systems are discussed in Part 8, Drugs acting on the cardiovascular system.

Kinin system

Hageman factor activates kallikrein, a substance found in the local tissues, which causes the precursor substance kininogen to be converted to bradykinin and other kinins. Bradykinin was the first kinin identified and remains the one that is best understood.

Bradykinin causes local vasodilation, which brings more blood to the injured area and allows white blood cells to escape into the tissues. It also stimulates nerve endings to cause pain, which alerts the body to the injury.

Bradykinin also causes the release of **arachidonic acid** from the cell membrane. Arachidonic acid causes the release of other substances called autacoids. These substances act like local hormones – they are released from cells, cause an effect in the immediate area and are then broken down. These autacoids include the following:

- Prostaglandins, some of which augment the inflammatory reaction and some of which block it.
- Leukotrienes, some of which can cause vasodilation and increased capillary permeability, and some of which can block the reactions.
- Thromboxanes, which cause local vasoconstriction and facilitate platelet aggregation and blood coagulation.

Histamine release

While this series of Hageman factor-initiated events is proceeding, another locally mediated response is occurring. Injury to a cell membrane causes the local release of histamine. Histamine causes vasodilation, which brings more blood and blood components to the area. It also alters capillary permeability, making it easier for neutrophils and blood chemicals to leave the bloodstream and enter the injured area. In addition, histamine stimulates pain perception. The vasodilation and changes in capillary permeability bring neutrophils to the area to engulf and get rid of the invader or to remove the cell that has been injured.

Chemotaxis

Some leukotrienes activated by arachidonic acid have a property called **chemotaxis,** which is the ability to attract neutrophils and to stimulate them and other macrophages in the area to be very aggressive. Activation of the neutrophils and release of other chemicals into the area can lead to cell injury and destruction. When destroyed, the cell releases various lysosomal enzymes that dissolve or destroy cell membranes and cellular proteins. The lysosomal enzymes are an important part of biological recycling and the breakdown of once-living tissues after death. In the case of an inflammatory reaction, they can cause local cellular breakdown and further inflammation, which can develop into a vicious cycle leading to cell death.

Many inflammatory diseases, such as rheumatoid arthritis and systemic lupus erythematosus, are examples of these uncontrolled cycles. The prostaglandins and leukotrienes are important to the inflammatory response because they act to moderate the reaction, thus preventing this destructive cycle from happening on a regular basis. Many of the drugs used to affect the inflammatory and immune systems modify or interfere with these inflammatory reactions.

Clinical presentation

Activation of the inflammatory response produces a characteristic clinical presentation. The Latin words calour, tumour, rubor and dolour describe a typical inflammatory reaction. **Calour**, or heat, occurs because of the increased blood flow to the area. **Tumour**, or swelling, occurs because of the fluid that leaks into the tissues as a result of the change in capillary permeability. **Rubor**, or redness, is related again to the increase in blood flow caused by the vasodilation. **Dolour**, or pain, comes from the activation of pain fibres by histamine and the kinin system. These signs and symptoms occur whenever a cell is injured (Figure 15.2). For example, if you scratch the top of your hand and wait for about a minute, the direct line of the scratch will be red (rubor) and raised (tumour). If you feel it gently, it will be warmer than the surrounding area (calour). You should also experience a burning sensation or discomfort at the site of the scratch (dolour). Invasion of the lungs by bacteria can produce pneumonia. If the lungs could be examined closely, they would also show the signs and symptoms of inflammation. They would be red from increased blood flow; fluid

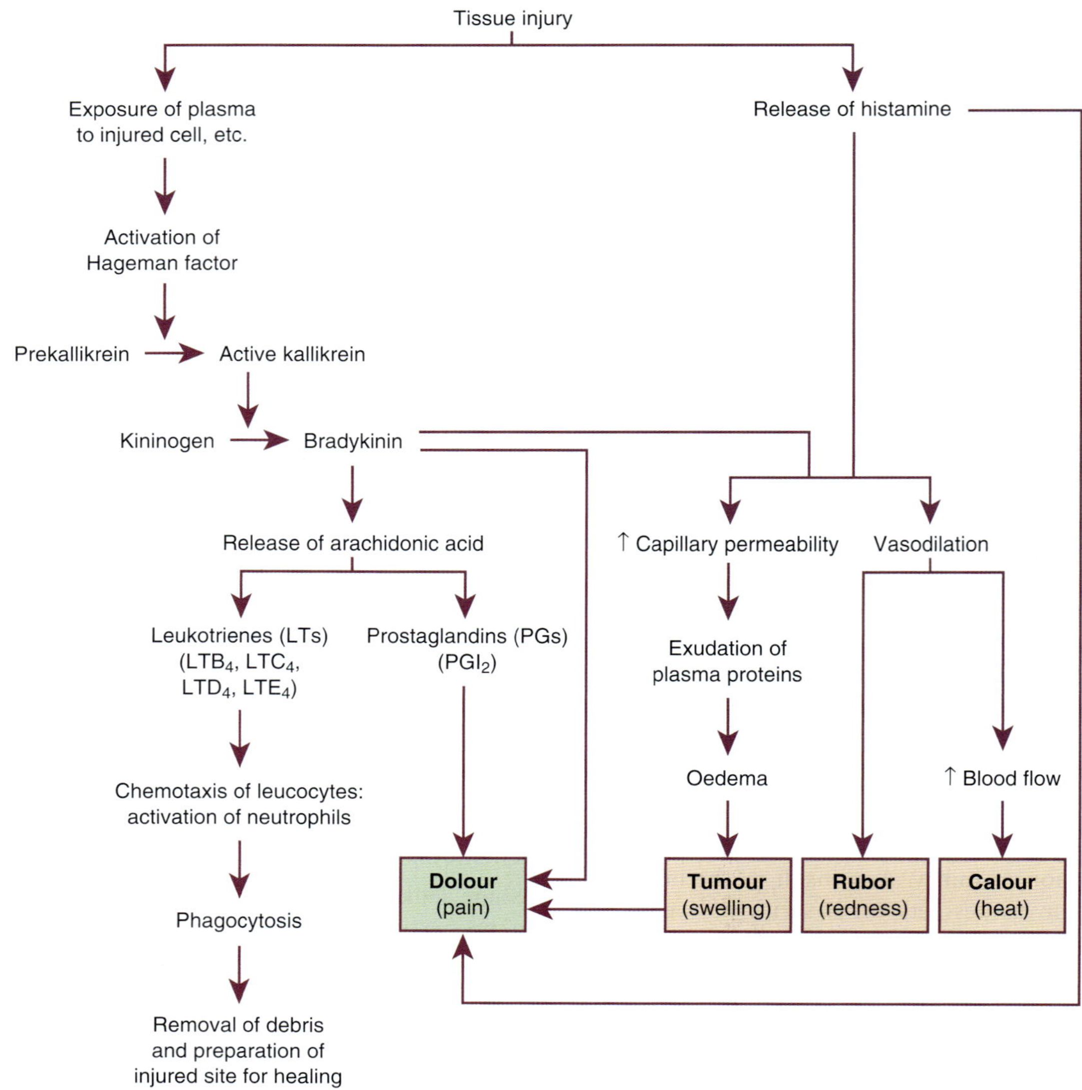

FIGURE 15.2 The inflammatory response in relation to the four cardinal signs of inflammation.

would start to leak out of the capillaries (often this can be heard as rales); the person would complain of chest discomfort; and the increased blood flow to the area of infection would make it appear hot or very active on a scan. No matter what the cause of the insult, the body's local response is the same.

Once the inflammatory response is under way and neutrophils become active, engulfing and digesting injured cells or the invader, they release a chemical that is a natural **pyrogen**, or fever-causing substance. This pyrogen resets specific neurons in the hypothalamus to maintain a higher body temperature, seen clinically as a fever. The higher temperature acts as a catalyst to many of the body's chemical reactions, making the inflammatory and immune responses more effective. Treating fevers remains a controversial subject because lowering a fever decreases the efficiency of the immune and inflammatory responses.

The leukotrienes (autocoids activated through the kinin system) affect the brain to induce slow-wave sleep, which is believed to be an important energy conservation measure for fighting the invader. They also cause myalgia and arthralgia (muscle and joint pain) – common signs and symptoms of various inflammatory diseases – which also cause reduced activity and save energy. All of these chemical responses make up the total clinical picture of an inflammatory reaction.

The immune response

More specific invasion can stimulate a more specific response through the immune system. As mentioned previously, stem cells in the bone marrow produce lymphocytes that can develop into T lymphocytes (so named because they migrate from the bone marrow to the thymus gland for activation and maturation) or B lymphocytes (so named because they are activated in the bursa of Fabricius in chickens, although the specific point of activation in humans has not been identified). Other identified lymphocytes include natural killer cells and lymphokine-activated killer cells. Both of these cells are aggressive against neoplastic or cancer cells and promote rapid cellular death. They do not seem to be programmed for specific identification of cells.

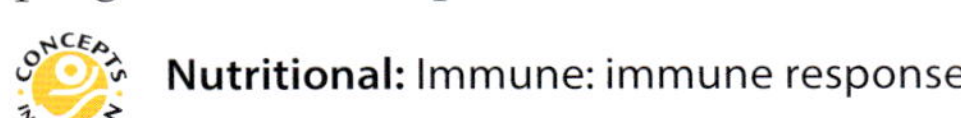

Research in the area of lymphocyte identification is relatively new and continues to grow. There may be other lymphocytes with particular roles in the immune response that have not yet been identified.

T cells

T cells are programmed in the thymus gland and provide what is called cell-mediated immunity (Figure 15.3). T cells develop into at least three different cell types.

1. *Effector or cytotoxic T cells* are found throughout the body. These T cells are aggressive against non-self cells, releasing cytokines, or chemicals, that can either directly destroy a foreign cell or mark it for aggressive destruction by phagocytes in the area via an inflammatory response. These non-self cells have membrane-identifying antigens that are different from those established by the person's MHC. They may be the body's own cells that have been invaded by a virus, which changes the cell membrane; neoplastic cancer cells; or transplanted foreign cells.
2. *Helper T cells* respond to the chemical indicators of immune activity and stimulate other lymphocytes, including B cells, to be more aggressive and responsive.
3. *Suppressor T cells* respond to rising levels of chemicals associated with an immune response to suppress or slow the reaction. The balance of the helper and suppressor T cells allows for a rapid response to body injury or invasion by pathogens, which may destroy foreign antigens immediately and then be followed by a slowing reaction if the invasion continues. This slowing allows the body to conserve energy and the components of the immune and inflammatory reaction necessary for basic protection and to prevent cellular destruction from a continued inflammatory reaction.

B cells

B cells are found throughout the MPS in groups called clones. B cells are programmed to identify specific proteins or antigens. They provide what is called humoral immunity (Figure 15.4). When a B cell reacts with its specific antigen, it changes to become a plasma cell. Plasma cells produce **antibodies**, or immunoglobulins, which circulate in the body and react with this specific antigen when it is encountered. This is a direct chemical reaction. When the antigen and antibody react, they

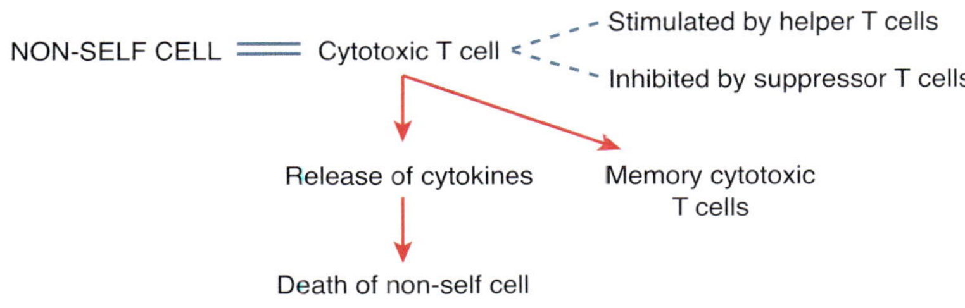

FIGURE 15.3 Cell-mediated immune response. Cytotoxic T cells are activated when recognising a non-self cell. Memory T cells are formed. Cytokines are released to destroy the non-self cell.

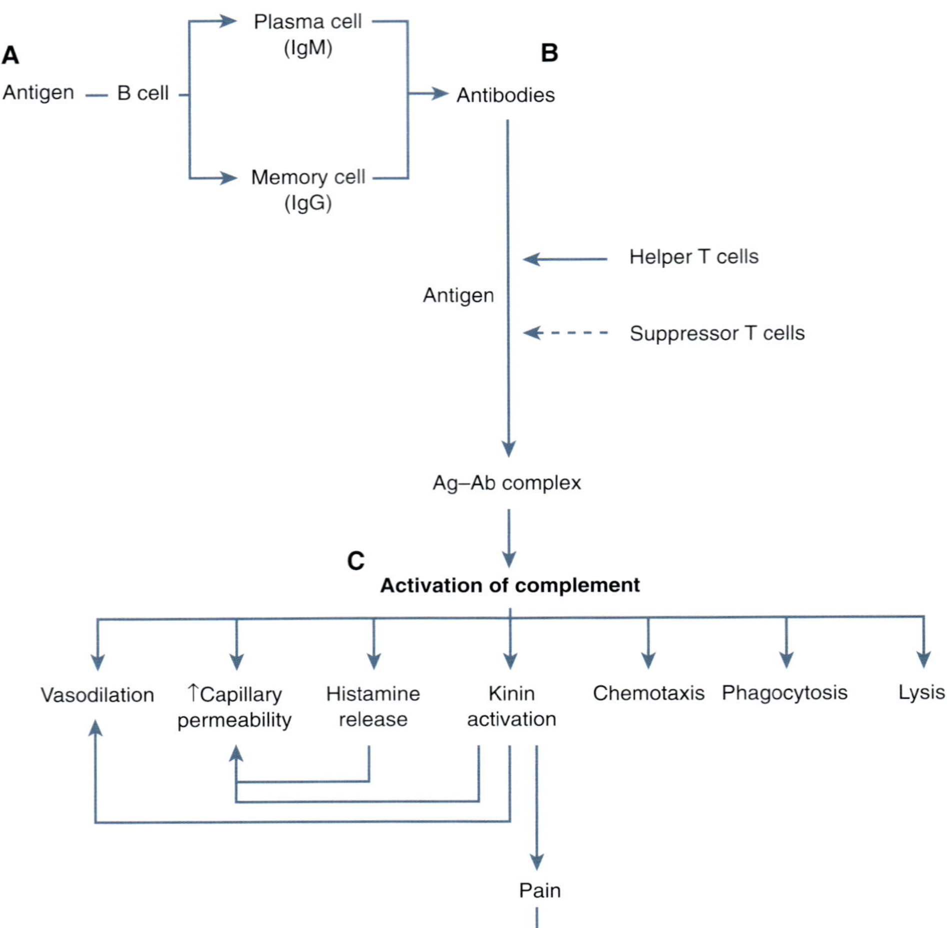

FIGURE 15.4 The humoral immune response. **A.** A B cell reacts with a specific antigen to form plasma cells and memory cells, which produce antibodies. **B.** Circulating antibodies react with the antigen to form an antigen–antibody (Ag–Ab) complex. This process is facilitated by helper T cells and suppressed by suppressor T cells. **C.** The antigen–antibody complex activates circulating complement, which facilitates aggressive inflammatory reactions. **D.** This process destroys the antigen.

form an antigen–antibody complex. This new structure reveals a new receptor site on the antibody that activates a series of plasma proteins in the body called complement proteins.

Complement proteins

Complement proteins react in a cascade fashion to form a ring around the antigen–antibody complex. The complement can destroy the antigen by puncturing its membrane, allowing an osmotic inflow of fluid that causes the cell to burst. They also induce chemotaxis (attraction of phagocytic cells to the area), increase the activity of phagocytes and release histamine. Histamine release causes vasodilation, which increases blood flow to the area and brings in all of the components of the inflammatory reaction to destroy the antigen. The antigen–antibody–complement complex precipitates out of the circulatory system and deposits in various sites, including end arteries in joints, the eyes, the kidneys and the skin. The signs and symptoms of the inflammatory response can be seen where the antigen–antibody complexes are deposited. Chickenpox eruptions are an example of an antigen–antibody–complement complex that deposits in the skin and causes a local inflammatory reaction.

Antibody formation

The initial formation of antibodies, or primary response, takes several days. Once activated, the B cells form memory cells that will produce antibodies for immediate release in the future if the antigen is encountered. The antibodies are released in the form of immunoglobulins. Five different types of immunoglobulins have been identified:

- The first immunoglobulin released is M (IgM), which contains the antibodies produced at the first exposure to the antigen.
- IgG, another form of immunoglobulin, contains antibodies made by the memory cells that circulate and enter the tissue; most of the immunoglobulin found in the serum is IgG.
- IgA is found in tears, saliva, sweat, mucus and bile. It is secreted by plasma cells in the GI and respiratory tracts and in epithelial cells. These antibodies react with specific pathogens that are encountered in exposed areas of the body.

- IgE is present in small amounts and seems to be related to allergic responses and to the activation of mast cells.
- IgD is another identified immunoglobulin whose role has not been determined.

This process of antibody formation, called acquired or active immunity, is a lifelong reaction. For example, a person exposed to chickenpox will have a mild respiratory reaction when the virus (varicella) first enters the respiratory tract. There will then be a 2–3-week incubation period as the body is forming IgM antibodies and preparing to attack any chickenpox virus that appears. The chickenpox virus enters a cell and multiplies. The cell eventually ruptures and ejects more viruses into the system. When this happens, the body responds with the immediate release of antibodies, and a full scale antigen–antibody response is seen throughout the body. Fever, myalgia, arthralgia and skin lesions are all part of the immune response to the virus. Once all of the invading chickenpox viruses have been destroyed or have entered the CNS to safely hibernate away from the antibodies, the clinical signs and symptoms resolve. (Varicella can enter the CNS and stay dormant for many years. The antibodies are not able to cross into the CNS, and the virus remains unaffected while it stays there.)

The B memory cells will continue to make a supply of immunoglobulin, IgG, for use on future exposure to the chickenpox virus. That exposure does not usually evolve into a clinical case because the viruses are destroyed immediately on entering the body and do not have a chance to multiply. Older people with weakened immune systems, people who are immunosuppressed and individuals who have depleted their immune system fighting an infection are at risk for development of shingles if they had chickenpox earlier in their lives. The dormant virus, which has aged and changed somewhat, is able to leave the CNS along a nerve root because the immunosuppressed body is slow to respond. The antibodies do eventually respond to the varicella, and the signs and symptoms of shingles occur as the virus is attacked along the nerve root. Figure 15.5 outlines this entire process.

B clones cluster in areas where they are most likely to encounter the specific antigen that they have been programmed to recognise. For example, pathogens or antigens that are introduced into the body via the respiratory tract will meet up with the B cells in the tonsils and upper respiratory tract; antigens that enter the body through the GI tract will meet their B cells situated in the oesophagus and GI tract. Theorists believe that the B cells are programmed genetically and are formed by the time of birth. Clones of B cells contain similar cells. The introduction of an antigen to which there are no preprogrammed B cells could result in widespread disease because the body would have no way of responding. A major concern about space travel has always been the introduction of a completely new antigen to Earth; for this reason, long periods of decontamination have been used after rocks or debris are brought back to Earth. Germ warfare research is ongoing in some countries to develop an antigen that has not been seen before and to which people would have no response.

Other mediators

Several other factors also play an important role in the immune reaction. **Interferons** are chemicals that are secreted by cells that have been invaded by viruses and possibly by other stimuli. The interferons prevent viral replication and also suppress malignant cell replication and tumour growth.

Interleukins are chemicals secreted by active leucocytes to influence other leucocytes. Interleukin 1 (IL-1) stimulates T and B cells to initiate an immune response. IL-2 is released from active T cells to stimulate the production of more T cells and to increase the activity of B cells, cytotoxic cells and natural killer cells. Interleukins also cause fever, arthralgia, myalgia and slow-wave sleep induction – all things that help the body to conserve energy for use in fighting off the invader. Several other factors released by lymphocytes and basophils have been identified. These include interleukins such as B-cell growth factor, macrophage-activating factor, macrophage inhibiting factor, platelet-activating factor, eosinophil chemotactic factor and neutrophil chemotactic factor.

The thymus gland also releases a number of hormones that aid in the maturation of T cells and that circulate in the body to stimulate and communicate with T cells. Thymosin, a thymus hormone that has been replicated, is important in the maturation of T cells and cell-mediated immunity. Research is ongoing on the use of thymosin in certain leukaemias and melanomas to stimulate the immune response.

Tumour necrosis factor (TNF), a cytokine, is a chemical released by macrophages that inhibits tumour growth and can actually cause tumour regression. It also works with other chemicals to make the inflammatory and immune responses more aggressive and efficient. Research is ongoing to determine the therapeutic effectiveness of TNF. TNF receptor sites are now available for injection into people with acute rheumatoid arthritis. These receptor sites react with TNF released by the macrophages in this inflammatory disease. All of these chemicals act as communication factors within the immune system, allowing the coordination of the immune response.

Interrelationship of the immune and inflammatory responses

The immune and inflammatory responses work together to protect the body and to maintain a level of homeostasis. Helper T cells stimulate the activity of B cells and

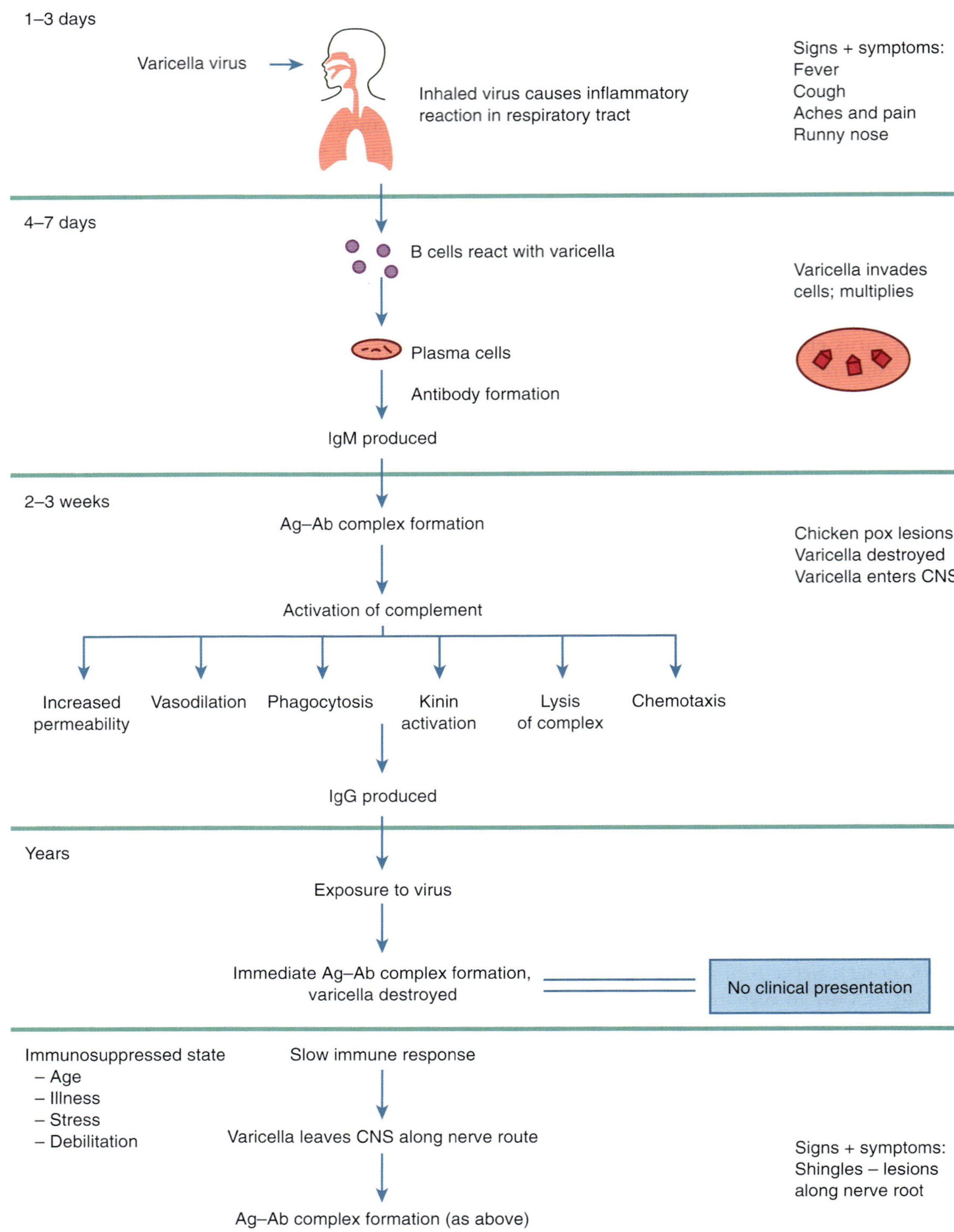

FIGURE 15.5 Process of response to varicella exposure in humans. Ag–Ab, antigen–antibody complex; Ig, immunoglobulin.

effector T cells. Suppressor T cells monitor the chemical activity in the body and act to suppress B-cell and T-cell activity when the foreign antigen is under control. Both B cells and T cells ultimately depend on an effective inflammatory reaction to achieve the end goal of destruction of the foreign protein or cell (Figure 15.6).

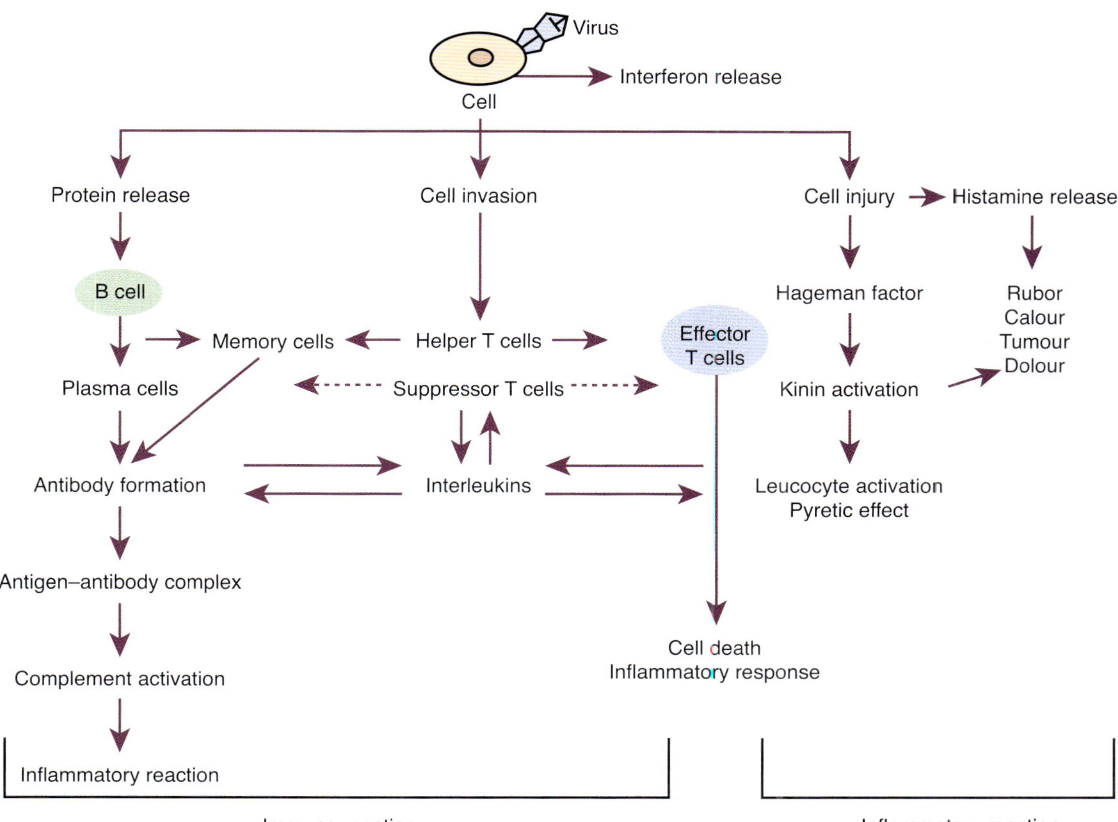

FIGURE 15.6 Interrelationship of immune and inflammatory reactions.

KEY POINTS

- The response to the inflammatory stimuli involves local vasodilation, increased capillary permeability and the stimulation of pain fibres. These reactions alert the person to the injury and bring an increased blood flow to the area.
- The immune response provides a specific reaction to foreign cells or proteins.
- T cells can be cytotoxic, destroying non-self cells; helper, augmenting an immune reaction; or suppressor, damping the immune response to save energy and prevent cell damage.
- B cells produce antibodies in response to exposure to specific antigens or proteins. Antibodies react with this antigen to produce an antigen–antibody complex that activates complement and will result in destruction of the antigen.
- Other mediators that affect the immune and inflammatory responses include interferons, tissue necrosis factor and interleukins.
- The immune and inflammatory responses work together to protect the body from injury or foreign pathogens.

PATHOPHYSIOLOGY INVOLVING THE IMMUNE SYSTEM

Several conditions can arise that cause problems involving the immune system. These conditions, many of which are treated by drugs that stimulate or suppress the immune system, include neoplasm, viral invasion, autoimmune disease and transplant rejection.

Neoplasms

Neoplasms occur when mutant cells escape the normal surveillance of the immune system and begin to grow and multiply. This can happen in many ways. For example, ageing causes a decreased efficiency of the immune system, allowing some cells to escape detection. Location of the mutant cells can make it difficult for lymphocytes to get to an area to respond. Mutant cells in breast tissue, for example, are not well perfused with blood and may escape detection until they are quite abundant. Sometimes cells are able to avoid detection by the T cells until the growing mass of cells is so large that the immune system cannot deal with it. Tumours can also produce blocking antibodies that cover the antigen-receptor sites on the tumour and prevent recognition by cytotoxic T cells. In addition, a weakly antigenic tumour may develop; such a tumour elicits a mild response from the immune system and somehow tricks the T cells into allowing it to survive.

Viral invasion of cells

Viruses are genetic parasites that can survive only by invading a host cell that provides the nourishment necessary for viral replication. Invasion of a cell alters the cell membrane and the antigenic presentation of the cell (the MHC). This change can activate cellular immunity, or it can be so subtle that the immune system's response to the cell is mild or absent. In some cases, the response activates a cellular immune reaction to normal cells similar to the one that was invaded. This is one theory for the development of autoimmune disease.

Autoimmune disease

Autoimmune disease occurs when the body responds to specific self-antigens to produce antibodies or cell-mediated immune responses against its own cells. The cause of autoimmune disease is not known, but theories speculate that (1) it could be a result of response to a cell that was invaded by a virus, leading to antibody production to similar cells; (2) production of autoantibodies is a normal process that goes on all the time, but in a state of immunosuppression the suppressor T cells do not suppress autoantibody production; or (3) there is a genetic predisposition to develop autoantibodies.

Transplant rejection

With the growing field of organ transplantation, more is being learned about the reaction to foreign cells that are introduced into the body. Typically, self-transplantation, or autotransplantation, results in no immune response. All other transplants produce an immune reaction. Therefore, matching a donor's HLA markers as closely as possible to those of the recipient for histocompatibility is essential. The more closely the foreign cells can be matched, the less aggressive the immune reaction to the donated tissue will be.

CHAPTER SUMMARY

- The body has several defence mechanisms in place to protect it from injury or foreign invasion: the skin, mucous membranes, normal flora, gastric acid, and the inflammatory and immune responses.
- The inflammatory response is a general response to any cell injury and involves activation of Hageman factor to stimulate the kinin system and release of histamine from injured cells to generate local inflammatory responses.
- The clinical presentation of an inflammatory reaction is heat (calour), redness (rubor), swelling (tumour) and pain (dolour).
- The inflammatory response is a non-specific reaction to any cellular injury and involves the activation of various chemicals and neutrophil activity. The immune response is specific to an antigen or protein that has entered the body and involves B cells, antibodies and T cells.
- Several types of T cells exist: effector or cytotoxic T cells, helper T cells and suppressor T cells. Effector or cytotoxic T cells immediately destroy foreign cells. Helper T cells stimulate the immune and inflammatory reactions. Suppressor T cells damp the immune and inflammatory responses to conserve energy and prevent cellular damage.
- B cells are programmed to recognise specific proteins or foreign antigens. Once in contact with that protein, the B cell produces antibodies (immunoglobulins) that react directly with the protein.
- Reaction of an antibody with the specific receptor site on the protein activates the complement cascade of proteins and lyses the associated protein or precipitates an aggressive inflammatory reaction around it.
- Other chemicals are involved in communication among parts of the immune system and in local response to invasion. Any of these chemicals has the potential to alter the immune response.
- The T cells, B cells and inflammatory reaction work together to protect the body from invasion, limit the response to that invasion and return the body to a state of homeostasis.
- Problems that occur within the immune system include the development of neoplasms, viral invasions of cells that trigger immune responses, autoimmune diseases and rejection of transplanted organs.

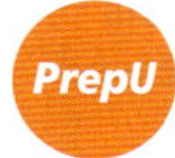

Knowing your strengths and weaknesses helps you to study more effectively. Take a PrepU Practice Quiz to find out how you measure up!

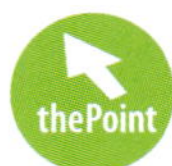

ONLINE RESOURCES

An extensive range of additional resources to enhance teaching and learning and to facilitate understanding of this chapter may be found online at the text's accompanying website, located on thePoint at http://thepoint.lww.com. These include Watch and Learn videos, Concepts in Action animations, journal articles, review questions, case studies, discussion topics and quizzes.

BIBLIOGRAPHY

Abbas, A., Lichtman, A. H. & Pillai, S. (2014). *Basic Immunology: Functions and Disorders of the Immune System* (4th edn). Philadelphia: Elsevier Saunders.

Barrett, K. E. & Ganong, W. F. (2012). *Ganong's Review of Medical Physiology* (24th edn). New York: McGraw-Hill.

Doan, T. (2013). *Lippincott's Illustrated Reviews: Immunology* (2nd edn). Philadelphia: Lippincott Williams & Wilkins.

Hall, J. (2011). *Guyton and Hall Textbook of Medical Physiology* (12th edn). Philadelphia: Saunders.

McKenna, L. & Mirkov, S. (2019). *McKenna's Drug Handbook for Nursing and Midwifery* (8th edn). Sydney: Wolters Kluwer Health Australia.

Peakman, M. & Vergani, D. (2009). *Basic and Clinical Immunology* (2nd edn). London: Churchill-Livingstone.

Porth, C. M. (2011). *Essentials of Pathophysiology: Concepts of Altered Health States* (3rd edn). Philadelphia: Lippincott Williams & Wilkins.

Porth, C. M. (2009). *Pathophysiology: Concepts of Altered Health States* (8th edn). Philadelphia: Lippincott Williams & Wilkins.

Sompayrac, L. (2012). *How the Immune System Works* (4th edn). Hoboken, NJ; Wiley-Blackwell.

CHECK YOUR UNDERSTANDING

Answers to the questions in this chapter can be found in Appendix A at the back of this book.

MULTIPLE CHOICE

Select the best answer to the following.

1. Antibodies:
   a. are carbohydrates.
   b. are secreted by activated T cells.
   c. are not found in circulating gamma globulins.
   d. are effective only against specific antigens.
2. B and T cells are similar in that they both:
   a. secrete antibodies.
   b. play important roles in the immune response.
   c. are activated in the thymus gland.
   d. release cytotoxins to destroy cells.
3. Which of the following is not a cytokine?
   a. interleukin 2
   b. antibody
   c. tumour necrosis factor
   d. interferon
4. As part of the non-specific defence against infection,
   a. blood flow and vascular permeability to proteins increase throughout the circulatory system.
   b. particles in the respiratory tract are engulfed by phagocytes.
   c. B cells are released from the bone marrow.
   d. neutrophils release lysosomes, heparin and kininogen into the extracellular fluid.
5. B cells respond to an initial antigen challenge by:
   a. reducing in size.
   b. immediately producing antigen-specific antibodies.
   c. producing a large number of cells that are unlike the original B cell.
   d. producing new cells that become plasma cells and memory cells.
6. Interleukins are:
   a. chemicals released when a virus enters a cell.
   b. chemicals secreted by activated leucocytes.
   c. part of the kinin system.
   d. activated by arachidonic acid.
7. Treating fevers remains a controversial subject because:
   a. fevers make people feel ill.
   b. higher temperatures act as catalysts to many of the body's chemical reactions.
   c. higher temperatures can suppress the body's normal metabolism.
   d. higher temperatures can alter the body's hormone levels, particularly that of progesterone.
8. After describing the function of T cells, the nurse or midwife would identify the need for additional teaching if the person stated that T cells become which of the following?
   a. cytotoxic T cells
   b. helper T cells
   c. suppressor T cells
   d. antibody-secreting T cells

MULTIPLE RESPONSE

Select all that apply.

1. Which of the following statements could be used to describe a neutrophil?
   a. They possess the property of phagocytosis.
   b. When activated, they release a pyrogen that causes fever.
   c. When the body is injured, they are produced rapidly and in large numbers.
   d. They are not capable of movement outside the circulatory system.
   e. They are most often seen in response to an allergic reaction.
   f. They float around in the blood and release chemicals in response to injury.
2. The inflammatory response is activated whenever cell injury occurs. An inflammatory response would involve which of the following activities?
   a. activation of Hageman factor
   b. vasodilation in the area of the injury
   c. generalised oedema and tumour development
   d. changes in capillary permeability to allow proteins to leak out of the capillaries
   e. activation of complement
   f. production of interferon

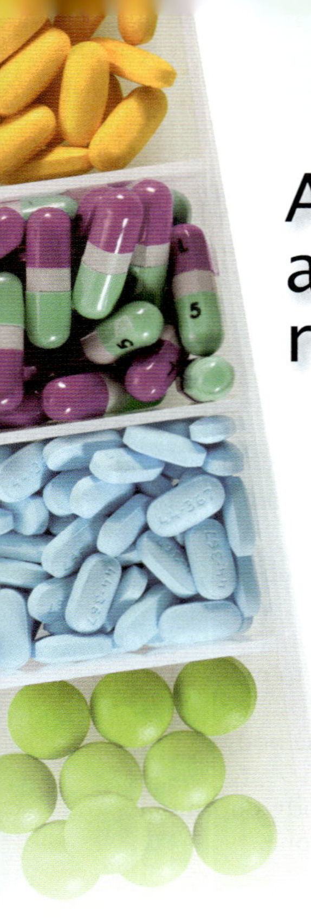

Anti-inflammatory, antiarthritis and related agents

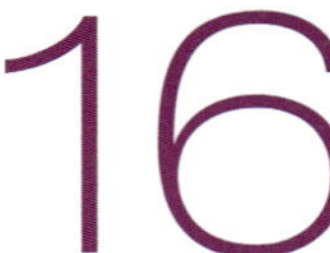

Learning objectives

On completing this chapter you should be able to:

1. Describe the sites of action of the various anti-inflammatory agents.
2. Describe the therapeutic actions, indications, pharmacokinetics, contraindications, most common adverse reactions and important drug–drug interactions associated with each class of anti-inflammatory agents.
3. Discuss the use of anti-inflammatory drugs across the lifespan.
4. Compare and contrast the prototype drugs for each class of anti-inflammatory drugs with the other drugs in that class.
5. Outline the care considerations and teaching needs for people receiving each class of anti-inflammatory agents.

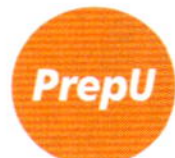

Test your current knowledge of anti-inflammatory, antiarthritis and related agents with a PrepU Practice Quiz!

Glossary of key terms

analgesic: compounds with pain-blocking properties, capable of producing analgesia

anti-inflammatory agents: drugs that block the effects of the inflammatory response

antipyretic: blocking fever, often by direct effects on the thermoregulatory centre in the hypothalamus or by blockade of prostaglandin mediators

chrysotherapy: treatment with gold salts; gold is taken up by macrophages, which then exhibit inhibited phagocytosis; it is reserved for use in people who are unresponsive to conventional therapy, and can be very toxic

inflammatory response: the body's non-specific response to cell injury, resulting in pain, swelling, heat and redness in the affected area

non-steroidal anti-inflammatory drugs (NSAIDs): drugs that block prostaglandin synthesis and act as anti-inflammatory, antipyretic and analgesic agents

salicylates: salicylic acid compounds, used as anti-inflammatory, antipyretic and analgesic agents; they block the prostaglandin system

salicylism: syndrome associated with high levels of salicylates – dizziness, ringing in the ears, difficulty hearing, nausea, vomiting, diarrhoea, mental confusion and lassitude

stool guaiac: a test to detect occult blood in the stool

SALICYLATES

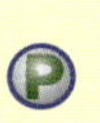 aspirin
balsalazide
mesalazine
olsalazine

NON-STEROIDAL ANTI-INFLAMMATORY DRUGS AND RELATED AGENTS

Non-steroidal anti-inflammatory drugs (NSAIDs)

Propionic acids

flurbiprofen
ibuprofen
ketoprofen
naproxen

Acetic acids

diclofenac
indometacin
ketorolac
sulindac

Fenamates

mefenamic acid

Oxicam derivatives

meloxicam
piroxicam

Cyclo-oxygenase-2 inhibitor

celecoxib
etoricoxib
parecoxib

Related agent

paracetamol

ANTIARTHRITIS AGENTS

Gold compounds

auranofin
sodium aurothiomalate

Other antiarthritis drugs

anakinra
etanercept
hydroxychloroquine
leflunomide
penicillamine
sodium hyaluronate

The **inflammatory response** is designed to protect the body from injury and pathogens. It employs a variety of potent chemical mediators to produce the reaction that helps to destroy pathogens and promote healing. As the body reacts to these chemicals, it produces signs and symptoms of disease, such as swelling, fever, aches and pains. Occasionally, the inflammatory response becomes a chronic condition and can result in damage to the body, leading to increased inflammatory reactions. **Anti-inflammatory agents** generally block or alter the chemical reactions associated with the inflammatory response to stop one or more of the signs and symptoms of inflammation.

ANTI-INFLAMMATORY, ANTIARTHRITIS AND RELATED AGENTS

Several different types of drugs are used as anti-inflammatory agents. Corticosteroids (discussed in Chapter 36) are used systemically to block the inflammatory and immune systems. Blocking these important protective processes may produce many adverse effects, including decreased resistance to infection and neoplasms. Corticosteroids also are used topically to produce a local anti-inflammatory effect without as many adverse effects. Antihistamines (discussed in Chapter 54) are used to block the release of histamine in the initiation of the inflammatory response. In this chapter, discussion of anti-inflammatory agents focuses on drugs that have a direct effect on the inflammatory response, including salicylates, non-steroidal anti-inflammatory drugs (NSAIDs) and related agents, and antiarthritis drugs.

Because many anti-inflammatory drugs are available over the counter (OTC), there is a potential for abuse and overdosing. In addition, individuals may take these drugs and block the signs and symptoms of a present illness, thus potentially causing the misdiagnosis of a problem. In some situations, individuals may combine these drugs and unknowingly induce toxicity. All of these drugs have adverse effects that can be dangerous if toxic levels of the drug circulate in the body. See Box 16.1 for information on using these drugs with various age groups.

SALICYLATES

Salicylates (Table 16.1) are popular anti-inflammatory agents not only because of their ability to block the inflammatory response, but also because of their **antipyretic** (fever-blocking) and **analgesic** (pain-blocking) properties.

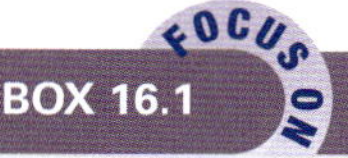

BOX 16.1 Drug therapy across the lifespan

Anti-inflammatory agents

CHILDREN

Children are more susceptible to the gastrointestinal (GI) and central nervous system (CNS) effects of these drugs. Care must be taken to make sure that the child receives the correct dose of any anti-inflammatory agent. This can be a problem because many of these drugs are available in OTC pain, cold, flu and combination products. Parents need to be taught to read the label to find out the ingredients and the dose they are giving the child.

Aspirin is not recommended for children < 12 years of age. The drug should not be used when any risk of Reye syndrome exists.

Ibuprofen, naproxen, meloxicam and, in some cases, indometacin are the NSAIDs approved for use in children.

Paracetamol is the most used anti-inflammatory drug for children. Care must be taken to avoid overdose, which can cause severe hepatotoxicity.

Children with arthritis may receive treatment with gold salts or etanercept; they must be monitored very closely for toxic effects.

ADULTS

Adults need to be cautioned about the presence of these drugs in many OTC products and taught to be aware of exactly what they are taking to avoid serious toxic effects. They should also be cautioned to report OTC drug use to their health care provider when they are receiving any other prescription drug to avoid possible drug–drug interactions and the masking of signs and symptoms of disease.

PREGNANCY AND BREASTFEEDING

Pregnant and breastfeeding women should not use these drugs unless the benefit clearly outweighs the potential risk to the fetus or neonate. The salicylates, NSAIDs and gold products have potentially severe adverse effects on the neonate and possibly the mother. Paracetamol can be used cautiously if a pain preparation or antipyretic is needed. Non-drug measures should be taken when at all possible to decrease the potential risk. These women also need to be urged to avoid OTC drugs unless they are suggested by their health care providers.

OLDER ADULTS

Older people may be more susceptible to the CNS and GI effects of some of these drugs. Dose adjustment is not needed for many of these agents.

Geriatric warnings have been associated with naproxen, ketorolac and ketoprofen because of reports of increased toxicity when they are used by older people. These NSAIDs should be avoided if possible.

Gold salts, used to treat arthritis, which is more common in older people, are particularly toxic for people in this age group. Accumulations in tissues can lead to increased renal, GI and even liver problems. If gold is used in this group, the dose should be reduced and the person monitored very closely for toxic effects.

TABLE 16.1 DRUGS IN FOCUS Salicylates

Drug name	Dosage/route	Usual indications
aspirin (*Aspro* and others)	Adult: 325–650 mg PO or PR q 4 hours Myocardial infarction (MI): 75–100 mg PO Paediatric ≥ 12 years: 325–650 mg PO every 4–6 hours as needed; maximum 4 g in 24 hours	Treatment of fever, pain, inflammatory conditions; at low dose to prevent the risk of death and MI in people with history of MI, prevention of transient ischaemic attacks
balsalazide (*Colazide*)	Three 750 mg capsules PO tds until remission or maximum of 12 weeks	Treatment of mildly to moderately acute ulcerative colitis in adults
mesalazine (*Pentasa, Mesasal*)	500 mg PO tds up to 1.5–4 g in divided doses; one enema at bedtime, or one suppository once daily	Treatment of ulcerative colitis and other inflammatory bowel diseases in adults
olsalazine (*Dipentum*)	250 mg–2 g/day PO in 2 divided doses Maintenance of remission: 1 g/day PO in 2 divided doses	Treatment of ulcerative colitis and other inflammatory bowel diseases in adults
sulfasalazine (*Pyralin EN, Salazopyrin*)	Adult: initially, 1–2 g PO qid, then 2 g PO daily in divided doses as maintenance Paediatric > 2 years: initially, 40–60 mg/kg PO daily, divided into 3–6 doses; then 40 mg/kg daily in 4 doses; may be started at lower dosage if GI intolerance occurs	Mild to moderate ulcerative colitis; adjunctive therapy in severe ulcerative colitis and Crohn's disease

Salicylates are some of the oldest anti-inflammatory drugs used. They were extracted from willow bark, poplar trees and other plants by ancient peoples to treat fever, pain and what we now call inflammation. They are generally available without prescription and are relatively non-toxic when used as directed. Aspirin (*Aspro* and others), which is available OTC, is one of the most widely used drugs for treating inflammatory conditions.

BOX 16.2 FOCUS ON Cultural considerations

Sensitivity to anti-inflammatory drugs

African Americans have a documented decreased sensitivity to the pain-relieving effects of many of the anti-inflammatory drugs. They do, however, have an increased risk of developing GI adverse effects to these drugs, including paracetamol. This should be taken into consideration when using these drugs as analgesics. Increased doses may be needed to achieve a pain-blocking effect, but the increased dose will put these people at an even greater risk for development of the adverse GI effects associated with these drugs. Monitor these people closely, and use non-drug measures to decrease pain, such as positioning, environmental control, physiotherapy, warm soaks and so on. If African American people are prescribed anti-inflammatory drugs, provide teaching about the signs and symptoms of GI bleeding and what to report, and monitor regularly for any adverse reactions to these drugs. Sensitivity to anti-inflammatory drugs has been reported in other ethnic groups such as Japanese, Koreans and Chinese. However, evidence is still inconclusive and more multicentre research in the future is needed to establish pharmacogenetic considerations in prescribing NSAIDs in some ethnic populations.

Additional synthetic salicylates include balsalazide (*Colazide*), mesalazine (*Pentasa, Mesasal*), olsalazine (*Dipentum*) and sulfasalazine (*Pyralin EN, Salazopyrin*), which are mostly used to reduce inflammation in ulcerative colitis and other inflammatory bowel diseases. A person who does not respond to one salicylate may respond to a different one.

Therapeutic actions and indications

Salicylates inhibit the synthesis of prostaglandins, important mediators of the inflammatory reaction (Figure 16.1). The antipyretic effect of salicylates may be related to blocking of a prostaglandin mediator of pyrogens (chemicals that cause an increase in body temperature and that are released by active white blood cells) at the thermoregulatory centre of the hypothalamus. At low levels, aspirin also affects platelet aggregation by inhibiting the synthesis of thromboxane A_2, a potent vasoconstrictor that normally increases platelet aggregation and blood clot formation. At higher levels, aspirin inhibits the synthesis of prostacyclin, a vasodilator that inhibits platelet aggregation.

Salicylates are indicated for the treatment of mild to moderate pain, fever and numerous inflammatory conditions, including rheumatoid arthritis and osteoarthritis. (See Box 16.3 and the Critical thinking scenario for more on rheumatoid arthritis.) See Table 16.1 for usual indications for each type of salicylate.

Pharmacokinetics

Salicylates are readily absorbed directly from the stomach, reaching peak levels within 5–30 minutes. They are metabolised in the liver to salicylic acid, an

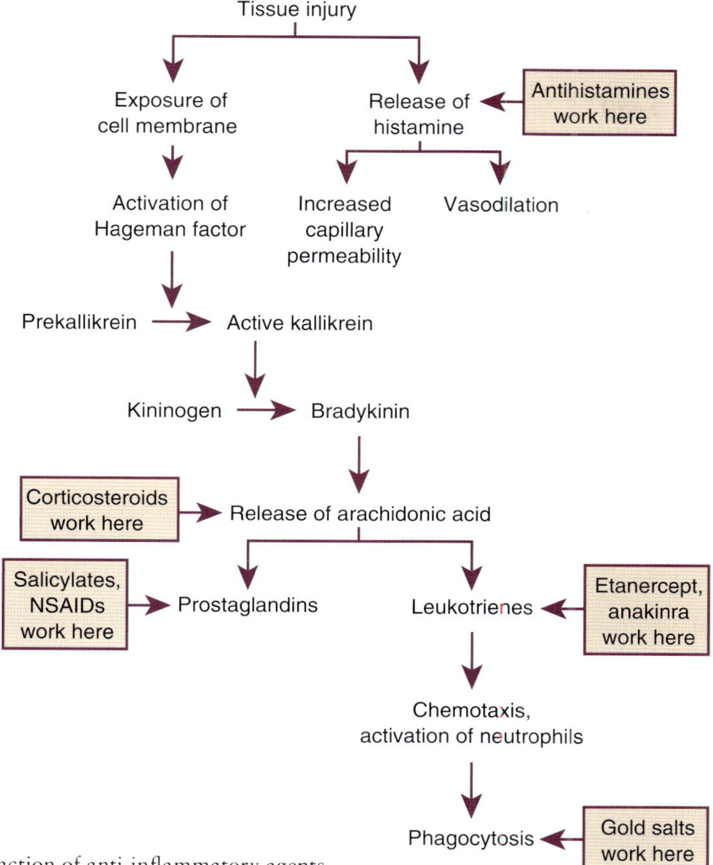

FIGURE 16.1 Sites of action of anti-inflammatory agents.

BOX 16.3 Pathophysiology of rheumatoid arthritis

Rheumatoid arthritis is a chronic, systemic disease that affects people of all ages. It is considered to be an autoimmune disease. People with rheumatoid arthritis have high levels of rheumatoid factor (RF), an antibody to immunoglobulin G (IgG). RF interacts with circulating IgG to form immune complexes, which tend to deposit in the synovial fluid of joints, as well as in the eye and other small vessels. The formation of the immune complex activates complement and precipitates an inflammatory reaction. During the immune reaction, lysosomal enzymes are released that destroy the tissues surrounding the joint. This destruction of normal tissue causes a further inflammatory reaction, and a cycle of destruction and inflammation ensues. Over time, the joint becomes severely damaged and the synovial space fills with scar tissue.

active metabolite, and excreted in the urine, with a half-life of 15 minutes to 12 hours, depending on the salicylate. Salicylates cross the placenta and enter breast milk; they are not indicated for use during pregnancy or breastfeeding because of the potential adverse effects on the neonate and associated bleeding risks for the mother.

Contraindications and cautions

Salicylates are contraindicated in the presence of known allergy to salicylates, other NSAIDs (more common with a history of nasal polyps, asthma or chronic urticaria) or tartrazine (a dye that has a cross-sensitivity with aspirin) *because of the risk of allergic reaction*; allergic reaction to aspirin can induce bronchospasm and, in rare cases, this reaction can lead to death in aspirin-sensitive people with asthma; bleeding abnormalities *because of the changes in platelet aggregation associated with these drugs*; impaired renal function *because the drug is excreted in the urine*; chickenpox or influenza *because of the risk of Reye syndrome in children and teenagers*; surgery or other invasive procedures scheduled within 1 week *because of the risk of increased bleeding*; and pregnancy or breastfeeding *because of the potential adverse effects on the neonate or mother.*

Adverse effects

The adverse effects associated with salicylates may be the result of direct drug effects on the stomach (nausea, dyspepsia, heartburn, epigastric discomfort) and on clotting systems (blood loss, bleeding abnormalities). **Salicylism** can occur with high levels

CRITICAL THINKING SCENARIO

Aspirin and rheumatoid arthritis

THE SITUATION

G.T. is an 82-year-old man on a fixed income with a 14-year history of rheumatoid arthritis. He is seen in the clinic for evaluation of his arthritis and to address his complaint that his medicines are not helping him. On examination, it is found that G.T.'s range of motion (ROM), physical examination of joints and overall presentation have not changed since his last visit. G.T. states that he had been taking aspirin, as prescribed, for his arthritis. But the aspirin prescribed by his doctor is more expensive than he could handle on his income, so he started taking it only once every 3 days.

CRITICAL THINKING

Think about the pathophysiology of rheumatoid arthritis and how the drugs ordered act on the inflammatory process.

How can the nurse best explain the disease and the drug regimen to G.T.?

What could be contributing to G.T.'s perception that his condition has worsened?

What interventions would be appropriate to help G.T. cope with his disease and his need for medication?

DISCUSSION

G.T. should be offered encouragement and support to deal with his progressive disease and the drug regimen required. The fact that his physical status has not changed but he perceives that the disease is worse may reflect other underlying problems that are making it more difficult for him to cope with chronic pain and limitations. The nurse should explore his social situation, any changes in his living situation, and support services. An examination should be done to determine whether other physical problems have emerged that could be adding to his sense that things are getting worse. The actions of aspirin on the arthritic process should be reviewed in basic terms, with emphasis on the importance of preventing further damage and maintaining high enough levels of aspirin to control the arthritis signs and symptoms. Pictures of the process involved in rheumatoid arthritis may help – the simpler the better in most cases.

G.T. should also be taught that all aspirin is the same, so it is acceptable to buy the cheapest generic aspirin. He can check the expiration date to make sure that the drug is fresh and still therapeutic and check that it does not smell like vinegar. Tell G.T. that the expensive combination product that G.T. has been using has not been proven to be any more effective at helping arthritis or at decreasing adverse effects than generic aspirin.

If G.T. has been having GI complaints with the aspirin, he can be encouraged to take the drug with food and to have small, frequent meals to keep stomach acid levels at a more steady state. If G.T. has not been having any GI complaints, he should be asked to report any immediately. The importance of the placebo effect cannot be overlooked with this person. Many people actually state that they feel better when they are using well-recognised, brand-name products. With support and encouragement, G.T. can be helped to follow his prescribed drug regimen and delay further damage from his arthritis.

CARE GUIDE FOR G.T.: ASPIRIN AND RHEUMATOID ARTHRITIS

Assessment: *history and examination*

Allergies to aspirin; renal or hepatic impairment; ulcerative GI disease; peptic ulcer; hearing impairment; blood dyscrasias

Concurrent use of anticoagulants, steroids, ascorbic acid, alcohol, frusemide, acetazolamide, antacids, methotrexate, sodium valproate, sulfonylureas, insulin, captopril, beta-adrenergic blockers, probenecid, spironolactone, glyceryl trinitrate

Neurological: orientation, reflexes, affect

Musculoskeletal system: ROM, joint assessment

Skin: colour, lesions

CV: pulse, cardiac auscultation, blood pressure, perfusion

GI: liver evaluation, bowel sounds

Lab tests: FBC, liver and renal function tests

Implementation

Ensure proper administration of the drug.

Administer with food if GI upset occurs.

Provide support and comfort measures to deal with adverse effects: small, frequent meals; safety measures if CNS effects occur; measures for headache; bowel training as needed.

Provide teaching regarding drug name, dosage, side effects, precautions and warnings to report; supplementary measures to help decrease arthritis pain.

Evaluation

Evaluate drug effects: decrease in signs and symptoms of inflammation.

Monitor for adverse effects: CNS changes, rash, GI upset, GI bleeding.

Monitor for drug–drug interactions as listed.

Evaluate effectiveness of teaching program.

Evaluate effectiveness of comfort/safety measures.

TEACHING FOR G.T.

- Your doctor has prescribed aspirin to help relieve the signs and symptoms of your rheumatoid arthritis. Aspirin works as an anti-inflammatory drug. It works in the body to decrease inflammation and to relieve the signs and symptoms of inflammation, such as pain, swelling, heat, tenderness and redness. It does not cure your arthritis, but will help you to live with it more comfortably.
- Take your aspirin exactly as prescribed, every day. It is important to take the drug every day so that the blood levels of the aspirin are high enough to be effective. Do not use any aspirin that has a vinegar odour.
- Some of the following adverse effects may occur:
  - *Nausea, vomiting, abdominal discomfort:* taking the drug with food or eating small, frequent meals may help. If these effects persist, consult with your health care provider.
  - *Diarrhoea, constipation:* these effects may decrease over time; ensure ready access to bathroom facilities and consult with your health care provider for possible treatment.
  - *Drowsiness, dizziness, blurred vision:* avoid driving or performing tasks that require alertness if you experience any of these problems.
  - *Headache:* if this becomes a problem, consult with your health care provider. Do not self-treat with more aspirin or other analgesics.
- Tell any health care provider who is taking care of you that you are taking this drug.
- Avoid using other over-the-counter preparations while you are taking this drug. If you feel that you need one of these drugs, consult with your health care provider for the most appropriate choice. Many of these drugs may also contain aspirin and could cause an overdose.
- Report any of the following to your health care provider: fever, rash, GI pain, nausea, itching, black or tarry stools, or difficulty with breathing.
- Keep this drug and all medications out of the reach of children.

of aspirin; dizziness, ringing in the ears, difficulty hearing, nausea, vomiting, diarrhoea, mental confusion and lassitude can occur. Acute salicylate toxicity may occur at doses of 20–25 g in adults or 4 g in children. Signs of salicylate toxicity include hyperpnoea, tachypnoea, haemorrhage, excitement, confusion, pulmonary oedema, convulsions, tetany, metabolic acidosis, fever, coma and cardiovascular (CV), renal and respiratory collapse.

Prototype summary: aspirin

Indications: treatment of mild to moderate pain, fever, inflammatory conditions; reduction of risk of transient ischaemic attack (TIA) or stroke; reduction of risk of MI.

Actions: inhibits the synthesis of prostaglandins; blocks the effects of pyrogens at the hypothalamus; inhibits platelet aggregation by blocking thromboxane A_2.

Pharmacokinetics:

Route	Onset	Peak	Duration
Oral	5–30 min	0.25–2 hours	3–6 hours

$T_{1/2}$: 15 minutes to 12 hours; metabolised in the liver and excreted in the urine.

Adverse effects: nausea, vomiting, heartburn, epigastric discomfort, occult blood loss, dizziness, tinnitus, acidosis.

Clinically important drug–drug interactions

The salicylates interact with many other drugs, primarily because of alterations in absorption, effects on the liver or extension of the therapeutic effects of the salicylate or the interacting drug (or both). Drugs such as anticoagulants, coumarin, heparin or thrombolytic agents may lead to increased anticoagulation and risk of bleeding, as salicylates may displace these medicines from protein-binding sites and may cause hypoprothrombinaemia. A list of interacting drugs in each drug monograph in a nursing drug guide should be consulted and the prescriber consulted before adding or removing a salicylate from any drug regimen.

Care considerations for people receiving salicylates

Assessment: history and examination

- Assess for contraindications or cautions: history of allergy to any salicylate or tartrazine *to avoid hypersensitivity reactions*; renal disease *because these drugs are excreted through the urine;* bleeding disorders *because of the drug effects on blood clotting*; chickenpox or influenza in children *to avoid the risk of Reye syndrome*; and pregnancy or breastfeeding *to avoid adverse effects on the fetus or baby and risk of bleeding in the mother.*

- Perform physical assessment to establish baseline status before beginning therapy and *to monitor for any potential adverse effects.*
- Assess for the presence of any skin lesions *to monitor for dermatological effects.*
- Monitor temperature *to evaluate the drug's effectiveness in lowering temperature.*
- Evaluate CNS status – orientation, reflexes, eighth cranial nerve function and affect – *to assess CNS effects of the drug.*
- Monitor pulse, blood pressure and perfusion *to assess for bleeding effects of CV effects of the drug.*
- Evaluate respirations and adventitious sounds *to detect hypersensitivity reactions.*
- Perform a liver evaluation and monitor bowel sounds *to detect hypersensitivity reactions, bleeding and gastrointestinal (GI) effects of the drug.*
- Monitor laboratory tests for full blood count (FBC), liver and renal function tests, urinalysis, **stool guaiac** and clotting times *to detect bleeding or other adverse effects of the drug and changes in function that could interfere with drug metabolism and excretion.*

Implementation with rationale

- Administer with food if GI upset is severe; provide small, frequent meals *to alleviate GI effects.*
- Administer drug as indicated; check all drugs being taken for possible salicylate ingredients; monitor dose *to avoid toxic levels.*
- Monitor for severe reactions *to avoid problems and provide emergency procedures* (gastric lavage, induction of vomiting, administration of charcoal) if they occur.
- Arrange for supportive care and comfort measures (rest, environmental control) *to decrease body temperature or to alleviate inflammation.*
- Ensure that the person is well hydrated during therapy *to decrease the risk of toxicity.*
- Provide thorough teaching, including measures to avoid adverse effects and warning signs of problems, as well as proper administration, *to increase knowledge about drug therapy and to increase compliance with the drug regimen.*
- Offer support and encouragement *to deal with the drug regimen.*

Evaluation

- Monitor response to the drug (improvement in condition being treated, relief of signs and symptoms of inflammation).
- Monitor for adverse effects (GI upset, CNS changes, bleeding).
- Evaluate the effectiveness of the teaching plan (person can name drug, dosage, adverse effects to watch for, specific measures to avoid adverse effects).
- Monitor the effectiveness of comfort measures and compliance with the drug regimen.

KEY POINTS

- Salicylates block prostaglandin activity, which decreases the inflammatory response and relieves the signs and symptoms of inflammation.
- Salicylates can cause GI irritation, eighth cranial nerve stimulation, and salicylism – ringing in the ears, acidosis, nausea, vomiting, diarrhoea, mental confusion and lassitude.

NON-STEROIDAL ANTI-INFLAMMATORY DRUGS AND RELATED AGENTS

Non-steroidal anti-inflammatory drugs (NSAIDs) provide strong anti-inflammatory and analgesic effects without the adverse effects associated with the corticosteroids (Table 16.2). Paracetamol (*Dymadon, Panadol*) is a related drug and a widely used agent. It has antipyretic and analgesic properties but does not have the anti-inflammatory effects of the salicylates or the NSAIDs. It is discussed in this chapter because it is used for many of the same reasons that NSAIDs are used, and nurses and midwives need to understand the similarities and differences of these drugs.

NON-STEROIDAL ANTI-INFLAMMATORY DRUGS

The NSAIDs are a drug class that has become one of the most commonly used drug types in Australia and New Zealand. Following unanticipated study results linking drugs in this class to an increased risk of CV events and death as well as increased bleeding in the GI tract, a black box warning was added to all of these drugs pointing out the CV and GI risks associated with taking them.

This group of drugs includes propionic acids, acetic acids, fenamates, oxicam derivatives and cyclooxygenase-2 inhibitors. The classes are defined by chemical structural differences, but, clinically, the NSAIDs are all-inclusive. See Table 16.2 for a list of these drugs by group, as well as their specific indications. The choice of NSAID depends on personal experience and the person's response to the drug. A person may have little response to one NSAID and a huge response to another. It may take several trials to determine the drug of choice for any particular person (Box 16.4).

TABLE 16.2 DRUGS IN FOCUS Non-steroidal anti-inflammatory drugs (NSAIDs) and related agents

Drug name	Dosage/route	Usual indications
NSAIDs		
Propionic acids		
(P) ibuprofen (*Advil, Brufen*, others)	Adult: 400–800 mg PO tds to qid up to a maximum of 2400 mg/day Paediatric: 30–40 mg/kg/day PO in 3–4 divided doses for arthritis; 5–10 mg/kg PO q 6–8 hours for fever	Treatment of pain, arthritis, dysmenorrhoea, juvenile arthritis
ketoprofen (*Orudis*)	Adult: 100–200 mg PO/day or one suppository rectally at night	Short-term management of pain; long-term management of arthritis (SR form); ophthalmic form to relieve ocular itching
naproxen (*Naprosyn*)	Adult: 250–500 mg PO bd; do not give > 250 mg q 12 hours for older people Paediatric: 10 mg/kg/day PO in 2 divided doses for juvenile arthritis; do not give OTC versions to children < 12 years without consulting health care provider	Treatment of pain, arthritis, dysmenorrhoea, juvenile arthritis
Acetic acids		
diclofenac (*Voltaren, Clonac, Dinac*)	75–150 mg/day PO or PR	Treatment of acute and chronic pain associated with inflammatory conditions in adults
indometacin (*Arthrexin, Indocid*)	50–200 mg/day PO or PR. Patent ductus arteriosus (PDA) in premature neonate: 0.1–0.25 mg/kg q 12–24 hours × 3 doses	Relief of moderate to severe pain in PO, topical and PR forms; closure of PDA in premature infants (given IV)
ketorolac (*Toradol*)	Adults < 65 years: initially 10–30 mg followed by 10–30 mg q 4–6 hours up to a maximum of 90 mg/day Elderly > 65 years: initially 10–15 mg followed by 10–15 mg q 4–6 hours up to a maximum of 60 mg/day Ophthalmic: 1 drop to affected eye qid; reduce dose with renal impairment and in people > 65 years	Short-term management of pain in adults; topically to relieve ocular itching
sulindac (*Aclin*)	150–200 mg PO bd	Treatment of various inflammatory conditions in adults
Fenamates		
mefenamic acid (*Ponstan*)	500 mg PO, then 250 mg PO tid q 6 hours as needed for a maximum of 7 days	Short-term treatment of pain in adults and children > 14 years; primary dysmenorrhoea
Oxicam derivative		
meloxicam (*Mobic*)	Adult: 7.5 mg/day PO to a maximum of 15 mg/day Paediatric: contraindicated in children and adolescents < 18 years	Treatment of osteoarthritis, rheumatoid arthritis and juvenile arthritis
piroxicam (*Feldene*)	10–20 mg/day PO as a single dose	Treatment of acute and chronic arthritis in adults
Cyclo-oxygenase-2 inhibitors		
celecoxib (*Celebrex*)	Initially 100–200 mg PO bd (acute pain: 400 mg) PO then 200 mg PO bd for familial adenomatous polyposis (FAP)	Treatment of acute and chronic arthritis in adults; acute pain; primary dysmenorrhoea; reduction of the number of colorectal polyps in FAP; ankylosing spondylitis

Continued on following page

TABLE 16.2 DRUGS IN FOCUS Non-steroidal anti-inflammatory drugs (NSAIDs) and related agents *(continued)*

Drug name	Dosage/route	Usual indications
etoricoxib (*Arcoxia*)	60–90mg PO daily as a single dose	Treatment of osteoarthritis, chronic musculoskeletal pain, rheumatoid arthritis, ankylosing spondylitis, acute gouty arthritis and acute pain in adults
paracoxib (*Dynastat*)	40 mg IV or IM as a single perioperative dose	Postoperative pain in adults
Related agent		
paracetamol (*Panadol, Panamax, Febridol* and others)	Adults and children > 12 years: 1–2 tablets (500–1000 mg) every 4–6 hours with water Maximum of 8 tablets in 24 hours; maximum daily dose: 4 g; do not use for more than a few days at a time, except on medical advice Paediatric 7–12 years: half to 1 (250–500 mg) tablet every 4–6 hours with water Maximum of 2 g in 24 hours For adults: do not use for more than a few days at a time, except on medical advice Paediatric 7–17 years: do not use for more than 48 hours, except on medical advice	Relief of pain and fever in a variety of situations

BOX 16.4 FOCUS ON **The evidence**

Cyclo-oxygenase-2 inhibitors

In late 2004, Merck voluntarily withdrew their cyclo-oxygenase-2 (COX-2) inhibitor, rofecoxib (Vioxx), from the market following release of a midstudy finding that the use of the drug over an 18-month period led to a significant increase in CV mortality in those taking the drug compared with a placebo group. The study, called the APPROVe study (Adenomatous Polyp Prevention on *Vioxx*), was targeted at testing whether the blocking of such growth factors as angiogenesis could decrease cancer risk in a specific population. The study participants took 25 mg of *Vioxx* each day for 18 months (the halfway point in the study), when the finding of increased CV events was announced and the study was stopped. The CV outcomes were not noted earlier than 18 months. Interestingly, other studies, including a 4-year study of the effects on Alzheimer disease, did not show a significant difference in CV events between the placebo and drug groups. Yet, in the VIGOR (Vioxx Gastrointestinal Outcomes Research) study, in which rofecoxib was compared with naproxen (another NSAID) for 12 months, increased CV events were noted in the rofecoxib group after only 2 months.

The U.S. Food and Drug Administration (FDA) formed a committee to study the COX-2 inhibitors and then all of the NSAIDs on the market to see if there were any problems in oversight of drug safety and to make recommendations about the future use of these drugs.

Valdecoxib (*Bextra*) was withdrawn from the market at FDA request after the committee reviewed data. A small study did show an increase in CV events, including death, when Bextra was used immediately in postoperative people recovering from coronary artery bypass graft (CABG) surgery. The drug was not proven to be especially more effective than other NSAIDs for relieving pain, and already had a black-box warning about the increased possibility of severe skin reactions, including Stevens–Johnson syndrome. With those facts in mind and the possibility of a COX-2 link to increased CV events, the FDA believed that the benefits of marketing the drug did not outweigh the potential risks for using the drug.

Celecoxib (*Celebrex*) remains on the market. The APC study (Adenoma Prevention with Celecoxib) did show a two- to threefold increase in CV events among people using the drug compared with a placebo over 33 months. There did seem to be a dose correlation, with more events in the group using a higher dose. A nearly identical study, the PreSAP trial (Prevention of Spontaneous Adenomatous Polyps), showed no increase in CV events in the group using celecoxib. A small study, the ADAPT (Alzheimer's Disease Anti-inflammatory Prevention Trial), did not appear to show an increase in CV events in the people in that study.

The FDA has recommended that the packaging information of all NSAIDs include warnings that there is potential risk for increased CV events as well as the risk of GI bleeding, and that health care providers use caution in recommending these drugs to anyone with an established CV risk; that all prescription NSAIDs be contraindicated in people immediately after CABG surgery; and that the prescribing information for celecoxib include a black-box warning referencing the available data about increased CV risk. All NSAIDs should be used at the lowest effective dose for the shortest possible duration to reduce the risk of serious adverse effects.

Therapeutic actions and indications

The anti-inflammatory, analgesic and antipyretic effects of the NSAIDs are largely related to inhibition of prostaglandin synthesis (see Figure 16.1). The NSAIDs block two enzymes, known as cyclo-oxygenase-1 (COX-1) and cyclo-oxygenase-2 (COX-2). COX-1 is present in all tissues and seems to be involved in many body functions, including blood clotting, protecting the stomach lining, and maintaining sodium and water balance in the kidney. COX-1 turns arachidonic acid into prostaglandins, as needed, in a variety of tissues. COX-2 is active at sites of trauma or injury when more prostaglandins are needed, but it does not seem to be involved in the other tissue functions. By interfering with this part of the inflammatory reaction, NSAIDs block inflammation before all of the signs and symptoms can develop. Most NSAIDs also block various other functions of the prostaglandins, including protection of the stomach lining, regulation of blood clotting and water and salt balance in the kidney. The COX-2 inhibitors are thought to act only at sites of trauma and injury to more specifically block the inflammatory reaction.

The adverse effects associated with most NSAIDs are related to blocking of both of these enzymes and changes in the functions that they influence – GI integrity, blood clotting and sodium and water balance. The COX-2 inhibitors are designed to affect only the activity of COX-2, the enzyme that becomes active in response to trauma and injury. They do not interfere with COX-1, which is needed for normal functioning of these systems. Consequently, these drugs should not have the associated adverse effects seen when both COX-1 and COX-2 are inhibited. Experience has shown that the COX-2 inhibitors still have some effect on these other functions, and people should still be evaluated for GI effects, changes in bleeding time and water retention. Recent studies suggest that they may block some protective responses in the body, such as vasodilation and inhibited platelet clumping, which is protective if vessel narrowing or blockage occurs; blocking this effect could lead to CV problems. Box 16.5 summarises the actions and adverse effects of the COX-1 and COX-2 receptors.

The NSAIDs are indicated for relief of the signs and symptoms of rheumatoid arthritis and osteoarthritis, for relief of mild to moderate pain, for treatment of primary dysmenorrhoea and for fever reduction.

Pharmacokinetics

The NSAIDs are rapidly absorbed from the GI tract, reaching peak levels in 1–3 hours. They are metabolised in the liver and excreted in the urine. NSAIDs cross the placenta and enter into breast milk. Therefore, they are not recommended during pregnancy and breastfeeding because of the potential adverse effects on the fetus or neonate.

Contraindications and cautions

- The NSAIDs are contraindicated in the presence of allergy to any NSAID or salicylate, and celecoxib is also contraindicated in the presence of allergy to sulfonamides. Additional contraindications are CV dysfunction or hypertension *because of the varying effects of the prostaglandins*; peptic ulcer or known GI bleeding *because of the potential to exacerbate the GI bleeding*; and pregnancy or breastfeeding *because of potential adverse effects on the neonate or mother*. The risk for CV dysfunction is increased with high doses, increasing duration of use and in people

BOX 16.5 Comparison of cyclo-oxygenase (COX) receptors

COX-1

Site of action
Found in many tissues, important for homeostasis

Effects
- Converts arachidonic acid to inflammatory prostaglandins
- Maintains renal function
- Provides for gastric mucosa integrity
- Promotes vascular haemostasis, increases bleeding
- Autocrine effects causing fever

Effects of blocking
- Decreases swelling, pain, inflammation
- Sodium retention, oedema, increased blood pressure
- Gastrointestinal erosion, bleeding
- Decreases fever

COX-2

Site of action
Induced by inflammatory stimuli at the site of inflammation

Effects
- Increases pain, inflammation
- Vasodilates
- Blocks platelet clumping

Effects of blocking
- Decreases pain, inflammation
- Prevents protective vasodilation, allows platelet clumping, which can lead to MI and cerebrovascular accident
- Myriad of skin reactions, including Stevens–Johnson syndrome

with other CV risk factors. The lowest effective NSAID dose should be used for the shortest possible duration; caution should be used with renal or hepatic dysfunction, *which could alter the metabolism and excretion of these drugs*, and with any other known allergies, *which indicate increased sensitivity.*
- All NSAIDs (including COX-2 inhibitors) have been associated with the development of acute kidney injury. Acute kidney injury is more likely to occur in individuals with other risk factors – particularly hypovolaemic states. Renal function should be monitored in at-risk individuals. If acute kidney injury occurs, the NSAID should be stopped. NSAIDs should be avoided in people who develop or have a history of interstitial nephritis.
- Colonic ulceration, perforation and haemorrhage have been associated with NSAIDs. NSAID-induced diaphragm strictures are usually found in the ascending colon. Symptoms suggestive of ulceration and diaphragm strictures in the large intestine are chronic diarrhoea, iron deficiency anaemia and weight loss, rather than pain and subacute obstruction.

Adverse effects

People receiving NSAIDs often experience nausea, dyspepsia, GI pain, constipation, diarrhoea or flatulence caused by direct GI effects of the drug. The potential for GI bleeding is often a cause of discontinuation of the drug. Headache, dizziness, somnolence and fatigue also occur frequently and could be related to prostaglandin activity in the CNS. Bleeding, platelet inhibition and even bone marrow depression have been reported with chronic use and probably are related to the blocking of prostaglandin activity. Rash and mouth sores may occur, and anaphylactoid reactions ranging up to fatal anaphylactic shock have been reported in cases of severe hypersensitivity.

Severe cutaneous adverse reactions (SCARs) have been reported with NSAIDs. These include bullous eruptions, erythema multiforme, epidermal necrolysis, toxic epidermal necrolysis and Stevens–Johnson syndrome. SCARs may cause permanent sequelae such as disfigurement, blindness and death. Importantly, these reactions may occur without warning.

Clinically important drug–drug interactions

There is often a decreased diuretic effect when these drugs are taken with loop diuretics; there is a potential for decreased antihypertensive effect of beta-blockers if these drugs are combined; and there have been reports of lithium toxicity, especially when combined with ibuprofen. People who receive these combinations should be monitored closely, and appropriate dose adjustments should be made by the prescriber. Avoid the concomitant use of more than one NSAID, or an NSAID with a COX-2 inhibitor and/or an anticoagulant where possible. If such a combination is necessary, a gastroprotective agent such as a proton pump inhibitor should be considered.

 **Prototype summary: ibuprofen**

Indications: relief of the signs and symptoms of rheumatoid arthritis and osteoarthritis; relief of mild to moderate pain; treatment of primary dysmenorrhoea; fever reduction.

Actions: inhibits prostaglandin synthesis by blocking cyclo-oxygenase-1 and -2 receptor sites, leading to an anti-inflammatory effect, analgesia and antipyretic effects.

Pharmacokinetics:

Route	Onset	Peak	Duration
Oral	30 min	1–2 hours	4–6 hours

$T_{1/2}$: 1.8–2.5 hours; metabolised in the liver and excreted in the urine.

Adverse effects: headache, dizziness, somnolence, fatigue, rash, nausea, dyspepsia, bleeding, constipation.

PARACETAMOL

Paracetamol (*Dymadon, Panadol*) is used to treat moderate to mild pain and fever and is often used in place of the NSAIDs or salicylates. It is the most frequently used drug for managing pain and fever in children. It is widely available over the counter and is found in many combination products. It can be extremely toxic. It causes severe liver toxicity that can lead to death when taken in high doses. Every year people die from inadvertent paracetamol overdose when they take more than one OTC drug containing paracetamol or accidentally administer a high dose of paracetamol. The US FDA and drug manufacturers have joined forces to produce mass media ads warning parents about this possibility.

Therapeutic actions and indications

Paracetamol acts directly on the thermoregulatory cells in the hypothalamus to cause sweating and vasodilation; this in turn causes the release of heat and lowers fever. The mechanism of action related to the analgesic effects of paracetamol has not been identified.

Paracetamol is indicated for the treatment of pain and fever associated with a variety of conditions, including influenza; as prophylaxis in children receiving diphtheria–pertussis–tetanus (DPT) immunisations (aspirin may mask Reye syndrome in children); and for the relief of musculoskeletal pain associated with arthritis (see Table 16.2).

Pharmacokinetics

Paracetamol is rapidly absorbed from the GI tract, reaching peak levels in 30 minutes to 2 hours. It is extensively metabolised in the liver and excreted in the urine, with a half-life of about 2 hours. Caution should be used in people with hepatic or renal impairment, which could interfere with metabolism and excretion of the drug, leading to toxic levels. Paracetamol crosses the placenta and enters breast milk; it should be used cautiously during pregnancy or breastfeeding because of the potential adverse effects on the fetus or neonate.

Contraindications and cautions

Paracetamol is contraindicated in the presence of allergy to paracetamol. It should be used cautiously in pregnancy or breastfeeding and in hepatic dysfunction or chronic alcoholism *because of associated toxic effects on the liver.*

Adverse effects

Adverse effects associated with paracetamol use include headache, haemolytic anaemia, renal dysfunction, skin rash and fever. Hepatotoxicity is a potentially fatal adverse effect that is usually associated with chronic use and overdose, and is related to direct toxic effects on the liver. The dose that could prove toxic varies with the age of the person, other drugs that the person might be taking and the underlying hepatic function of that person. When overdose occurs, acetylcysteine can be used as an antidote. Life support measures may also be necessary.

Clinically important drug–drug interactions

There is an increased risk of bleeding with oral anticoagulants *because of effects on the liver;* of toxicity with chronic ethanol ingestion *because of toxic effects on the liver;* and of hepatotoxicity with barbiturates, carbamazepine, hydantoins, rifampicin or sulfinpyrazone. These combinations should be avoided, but if they must be used, appropriate dose adjustment should be made and the person should be monitored closely.

Prototype summary: paracetamol

Indications: treatment of mild to moderate pain, fever, or signs and symptoms of the common cold or flu; musculoskeletal pain associated with arthritis and rheumatic disorders.

Actions: acts directly on the hypothalamus to cause vasodilation and sweating, which will reduce fever; mechanism of action as an analgesic is not understood.

Pharmacokinetics:

Route	Onset	Peak	Duration
Oral	Varies	0.5–2 hours	3–6 hours

$T_{1/2}$: 1–3 hours; metabolised in the liver and excreted in the urine.

Adverse effects: rash, fever, chest pain, liver toxicity and failure, bone marrow suppression.

BOX 16.6 Withdrawal of dextropropoxyphene with paracetamol fixed-dose combination (*Paradex, Capadex*)

In December 2009 the New Zealand Medicines Adverse Reactions Committee (MARC) reviewed the benefits and risk of dextropropoxyphene-containing medicines.[1] The MARC assessed the published literature; adverse reactions reported in New Zealand (NZ) and internationally; and NZ Poisons Centre data, the results of a Paradex utilisation study conducted in New Zealand in 2007. The MARC also considered reviews conducted by other medicine regulators.

After analysis and discussion of the available data the MARC concluded there is evidence that:

- These medicines are no more effective than maximum recommended doses of paracetamol alone.
- These medicines have the potential to cause more adverse reactions than paracetamol used at recommended doses.
- These medicines are more dangerous than other simple analgesics in overdose, particularly when combined with alcohol. Deaths have occurred in association with dextropropoxyphene use in NZ.
- Deaths related to dextropropoxyphene overdose have occurred within 1 hour of ingestion and before medical intervention could be obtained.

Prescribing restrictions introduced in 2006 have failed to ensure that these medicines were only used in people for whom the benefits are likely to outweigh the risks. Overall the risks of these medicines exceed their benefits. Therefore, in the interests of public safety, the MARC recommended that Capadex and Paradex be withdrawn from sale in New Zealand. Dextropropoyxphene was discontinued in Australia in August 2018.

[1] www.medsafe.govt.nz/profs/PUArticles/Dextropropoxyphene%20-%20review%20concludes%20risk-benefit%20balance%20unfavourable.htm

Source: MEDSAFE – NZ Medicines and Medical Devices Safety Authority (2010)

Care considerations for people receiving NSAIDs and related agents

Assessment: history and examination

(Refer to the section on salicylates for implementation with rationale and evaluation.)

- Assess for *contraindications or cautions*: known allergies to any salicylates, NSAIDs or tartrazine; pregnancy or breastfeeding; hepatic or renal disease; CV dysfunction; hypertension; and GI bleeding or peptic ulcer.
- Assess for *baseline status before beginning therapy and for any potential adverse effects*: presence of any skin lesions; temperature; orientation, reflexes and affect; pulse, blood pressure and perfusion; respirations and adventitious sounds; liver evaluation; bowel sounds; and FBC, liver and renal function tests, urinalysis, stool guaiac and serum electrolytes.

KEY POINTS

- NSAIDs block prostaglandin synthesis at COX-1 and COX-2 sites. This blocks inflammation but also blocks protection of the stomach lining, as well as the kidneys' regulation of water.
- There are many different NSAIDs. If one does not work for a particular person, another one might.
- Paracetamol causes vasodilation and heat release, lowering fever and working to relieve pain.
- Paracetamol can cause liver failure. It is found in many OTC products. Teach people to avoid toxic doses of paracetamol.

ANTIARTHRITIS AGENTS

Other drugs that are used to block the inflammatory process include the antiarthritis drugs. Arthritis is a potentially debilitating inflammatory process in the joints that causes pain and bone deformities. Antiarthritis drugs include the gold compounds, which are used to prevent and suppress arthritis in selected people with rheumatoid arthritis. The other antiarthritis drugs are specifically used to block the inflammation and tissue damage of rheumatoid arthritis (see Table 16.3).

GOLD COMPOUNDS

Some individuals with rheumatic inflammatory conditions do not respond to the usual anti-inflammatory therapies, and their conditions worsen despite weeks or months of standard pharmacological treatment. Some of these individuals respond to treatment with gold salts, also known as **chrysotherapy**, in which gold is taken up by macrophages, which then exhibit inhibited phagocytosis; it is reserved for use in people who are unresponsive to conventional therapy, and can be very toxic. The gold salts available for use include auranofin (*Ridaura*) and sodium aurothiomalate (*Myocrisin*).

Therapeutic actions and indications

Chrysotherapy results in inhibition of phagocytosis (see Figure 16.1). Because phagocytosis is blocked, the release of lysosomal enzymes is inhibited and tissue destruction is decreased. This action allows gold salts to suppress and prevent some arthritis and synovitis. Gold salts are indicated to treat selected cases of rheumatoid and juvenile rheumatoid arthritis in people whose disease has been unresponsive to standard therapy (see Table 16.3 for usual indications). These drugs do not repair damage; they prevent further damage and so are most effective if used early in the disease.

Pharmacokinetics

The gold salts are absorbed at varying rates, depending on their route of administration. They are widely distributed throughout the body but seem to concentrate in the hypothalamic–pituitary–adrenocortical (HPA) system and in the adrenal and renal cortices. The gold salts are excreted in urine and faeces. These drugs cross the placenta and enter into breast milk. They have been shown to be teratogenic in animal studies and should not be used during pregnancy or breastfeeding. Barrier contraceptives should be recommended to women of childbearing age, and another method of feeding the baby should be used if gold therapy is needed in a breastfeeding woman.

Contraindications and cautions

Gold salts can be quite toxic and are contraindicated in the presence of any known allergy to gold, uncontrolled diabetes, congestive heart failure, severe debilitation, renal or hepatic impairment, hypertension, blood dyscrasias, recent radiation treatment, history of toxic levels of heavy metals, and pregnancy or breastfeeding.

Adverse effects

A variety of adverse effects is common with the use of gold salts, which are probably related to their deposition in the tissues and effects at that local level: stomatitis, glossitis, gingivitis, pharyngitis, laryngitis, colitis, diarrhoea and other GI inflammation; gold bronchitis and interstitial pneumonitis; bone marrow depression; vaginitis and nephrotic syndrome; dermatitis, pruritus and exfoliative dermatitis; and allergic reactions ranging from flushing, fainting and dizziness to anaphylactic shock.

TABLE 16.3 **DRUGS IN FOCUS** **Antiarthritis agents**

Drug name	Dosage/route	Usual indications
Gold compounds		
(P) auranofin (*Ridaura*)	Adult: 6 mg/day PO; monitor elderly people carefully Paediatric: not recommended in children < 16 years	Oral agent for long-term therapy of rheumatic disorders
sodium aurothiomalate (*Myocrisin*)	Adult: initially test dose of 1 mg 1st week, 5 mg in 2nd week, 10 mg in 3rd week then 50 mg at weekly intervals to a total of 1 g. Maintenance: 50 mg/month to total 3 g or for ≥ 2 years after remission, or indefinitely Paediatric: not recommended	Injected drug for early treatment of rheumatic disorders
Other antiarthritis drugs		
anakinra (*Kineret*)	Adult: 100 mg/day SC	Reduction of signs and symptoms of rheumatoid arthritis in people ≥ 18 years if one or more other arthritis agents have failed
etanercept (*Enbrel*)	Adult: 25 mg SC twice a week or 50 mg SC once a week Paediatric (2–17 years): 0.8 mg/kg (maximum of 50 mg per dose) SC once weekly	Reduction of signs and symptoms of severe rheumatoid arthritis in people whose disease is unresponsive to other therapy; prevention of damage early in the disease; ankylosing spondylosis; psoriatic arthritis
hyaluronidase (*Hyalase*)	2 mL once a week for 3 weeks injected into the affected knee	Relief of pain in the knees of people with arthritis whose disease is unresponsive to conventional treatment
leflunomide (*Arava*)	100 mg PO daily for 3 days, then 20 mg PO daily. If doses are not tolerated, reduce to 10 mg PO daily	Treatment of active rheumatoid arthritis, to relieve signs and symptoms and to slow the progression of disease in adults
penicillamine (*D-Penamine*)	250 mg/day PO for 1 month, increasing to 1500 mg/day PO	Treatment of severe, active rheumatoid arthritis in adults whose disease is unresponsive to conventional therapy
sodium hyaluronate (*Fermathron*)	20 mg once a week for 5 weeks injected into affected knee	Relief of pain in the knees of people with arthritis whose disease is unresponsive to conventional treatment

Clinically important drug–drug interactions

These drugs should not be combined with penicillamine, antimalarials, cytotoxic drugs or immunosuppressive agents other than low-dose corticosteroids because of the potential for severe toxicity.

DISEASE-MODIFYING ANTIRHEUMATIC DRUGS

Other antiarthritis drugs, called disease-modifying antirheumatic drugs (DMARDs), are available for treating arthritis and aggressively affect the process of inflammation. Because they alter the course of the inflammatory process, many rheumatologists are selecting to use DMARDs early in the diagnosis, before damage to the joints has occurred. Adverse effects associated with these drugs (see Adverse effects) can be severe to life-threatening because they alter the ability of the body to initiate or carry on an inflammatory reaction.

DMARDs discussed in this chapter include drugs used when people do not respond to conventional therapy – anakinra (*Kineret*), etanercept (*Enbrel*), leflunomide (*Arava*) and penicillamine (*D-Penamine*) – and drugs used to directly decrease pain in joints affected by arthritis, including hyaluronidase derivative (*Hyalase*) and sodium hyaluronate (*Fermathron*).

Additional drugs also used to modify the disease process in rheumatoid arthritis include the antineoplastic drug methotrexate (see Chapter 14), the monoclonal antibodies infliximab (*Remicade*), golimumab (*Simponi*) and adalimumab (*Humira*) (see Chapter 17), the T-cell suppressor abatacept (*Orencia*) (see Chapter 17), certain antimalarial drugs (see Chapter 12), some additional antineoplastic drugs such as cyclophosphamide (see Chapter 14) and the immune modulators ciclosporin A and azathioprine (see Chapter 17).

Prototype summary: auranofin

Indications: treatment of selected cases of adult and juvenile rheumatoid arthritis, most effective early in disease.

Actions: although the mechanism of action has not been fully elucidated, auranofin exhibits a variety of anti-inflammatory, antiarthritic and immunoregulatory activities. These properties include: stimulation of cell-mediated immunity, suppression of immunoglobulin synthesis and antibody-dependent cytotoxicity, suppression of the respiratory burst/superoxide radicals, inhibition of neutrophil release of lysosomal enzymes and secretion of inflammatory eicosanoids, inhibition of platelet aggregation, serotonin production and protein kinase C activity.

Pharmacokinetics:

Route	Onset	Peak
Oral	Rapid	2 hours

$T_{1/2}$: 10–30 days; excreted mainly in faeces and some in urine.

Adverse effects: dermatitis, nausea, diarrhoea, anaemia, membranous glomerulonephritis and nephrotic syndrome.

Therapeutic actions and indications

Anakinra is indicated for treatment of arthritis. This drug is an interleukin-1 receptor antagonist. It blocks the increased interleukin-1, which is responsible for the degradation of cartilage in rheumatoid arthritis. This drug must be given each day by subcutaneous (SC) injection and is often used in combination with other antiarthritis drugs.

Etanercept contains genetically engineered tumour necrosis factor (TNF) receptors derived from Chinese hamster ovary cells. These receptors react with free-floating TNF released by active leucocytes in autoimmune inflammatory disease to prevent the damage caused by TNF. See Table 16.3 for usual indications.

Hyaluronidase derivatives, such as hylan G-F 20 and sodium hyaluronate, have elastic and viscous properties. These drugs are injected directly into the joints of people with severe rheumatoid arthritis of the knee. They seem to cushion and lubricate the joint and relieve the pain associated with degenerative arthritis. They are given weekly for 3–5 weeks.

Leflunomide directly inhibits an enzyme, dihydroorotate dehydrogenase (DHODH), which is active in the autoimmune process that leads to rheumatoid arthritis, relieving signs and symptoms of inflammation and blocking the structural damage this inflammation can cause, slowing disease progression.

Penicillamine lowers the immunoglobulin M (IgM) rheumatoid factor levels in people with acute rheumatoid arthritis, relieving the signs and symptoms of inflammation. It may take 2–3 months of therapy before a response is noted.

Pharmacokinetics

Anakinra is slowly absorbed from the subcutaneous tissue, reaching peak levels in 3–7 hours. It is metabolised in the tissues and excreted in the urine. It has a half-life of 4–6 hours. Etanercept is very slowly absorbed after SC injection, reaching peak levels in 72 hours. It is metabolised and destroyed in the tissues with a half-life of 115 hours. The hyaluronidase derivatives are not absorbed systemically. Leflunomide is slowly absorbed from the GI tract, reaching peak levels in 6–12 hours. It undergoes hepatic metabolism and excretion in the urine. The half-life of leflunomide is 14–18 days. Penicillamine is an oral drug that reaches peak levels 1–3 hours after administration. It is extensively metabolised in the liver and excreted in the urine with a half-life of 2–3 hours.

Contraindications and cautions

These drugs are contraindicated in the presence of allergy to the drugs or to the animal products from which they were derived (Chinese hamster products in etanercept; chicken products in hylan G-F 20 and sodium hyaluronate); pregnancy or breastfeeding *because of the potential for adverse effects on the fetus or neonate*; acute infection *because of the blocking of normal inflammatory pathways*; and liver or renal impairment, *which could be exacerbated by these drugs.*

Adverse effects

A variety of adverse effects are common with the use of these drugs, including local irritation at injection sites (anakinra, etanercept, hyaluronidase derivatives and sodium hyaluronate), pain with injection and increased risk of infection. Leflunomide is associated with potentially fatal hepatic toxicity and rashes. Penicillamine is associated with a potentially fatal myasthenic syndrome, bone marrow depression and assorted hypersensitivity reactions. Etanercept is associated with severe bone marrow suppression, and a warning has been issued stating that the drug has been associated with the development of serious CNS problems, including multiple sclerosis. It can also cause severe myelosuppression and increased risk of infections and cancer development. People who use this drug need to be monitored very closely. Leflunomide has been associated with severe hepatic toxicity, and the person's liver function needs to be monitored closely.

Clinically important drug–drug interactions

Hyaluronidase derivatives such as sodium hyaluronate should not be injected at the same time as local anaesthetics.

Because leflunomide can cause severe liver dysfunction if it is combined with other hepatotoxic drugs, this combination should be avoided.

The absorption of penicillamine is decreased if it is taken with iron salts or antacids; if these are both being given, they should be separated by at least 2 hours.

Anakinra and etanercept should not be used together because of an increased risk of serious infections.

Care considerations for people receiving antiarthritis agents

Care considerations for people receiving the drugs listed in this section are similar to those for people receiving NSAIDs and related agents. Details related to each individual drug can be found in the specific drug monograph in your drug guide.

KEY POINTS

- Gold salts prevent macrophage phagocytosis, lysosomal release and tissue damage because the gold salts are taken up by phagocytes, which then are not able to function in a normal way.
- Gold salts are deposited in the tissues and cause an assortment of inflammatory reactions, including stomatitis, glossitis, gingivitis, pharyngitis, laryngitis, colitis, diarrhoea and other GI inflammation; gold bronchitis and interstitial pneumonitis; bone marrow depression; vaginitis and nephrotic syndrome; dermatitis, pruritus and exfoliative dermatitis; and allergic reactions ranging from flushing, fainting and dizziness to anaphylactic shock.
- Drugs used to alter the inflammatory process involved in arthritis are called disease-modifying antirheumatic drugs (DMARDs) and can be associated with serious to potentially fatal infections. If used early in the disease, they can prevent or slow down the damage caused to the joints.
- The DMARDs can cause local irritation at the injection site, liver impairment and a variety of CNS problems, including demyelinating disorders.

CHAPTER SUMMARY

- The inflammatory response, which is important for protecting the body from injury and invasion, produces many of the signs and symptoms associated with disease, including fever, aches and pains and lethargy.
- Chronic or excessive activity by the inflammatory response can lead to the release of lysosomal enzymes and tissue destruction.
- Anti-inflammatory drugs block various chemicals associated with the inflammatory reaction. Anti-inflammatory drugs may also have antipyretic (fever-blocking) and analgesic (pain-blocking) activities.
- Salicylates block prostaglandin activity. NSAIDs block prostaglandin synthesis. Paracetamol causes vasodilation and heat release, lowering fever and working to relieve pain. Gold salts prevent macrophage phagocytosis, lysosomal release and tissue damage. DMARDs alter the course of the inflammatory process and treat arthritis by aggressively affecting the process of inflammation.
- Salicylates can cause acidosis and eighth cranial nerve damage. NSAIDs are mostly associated with GI irritation and bleeding. Paracetamol can cause serious liver toxicity. The gold salts cause many systemic inflammatory reactions. Other antiarthritis drugs are associated with local injection-site irritation and increased susceptibility to infection; leflunomide is associated with severe hepatic toxicity.
- Many anti-inflammatory drugs are available OTC, and care must be taken to prevent abuse or overuse of these drugs.

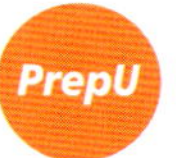

Knowing your strengths and weaknesses helps you to study more effectively. Take a PrepU Practice Quiz to find out how you measure up!

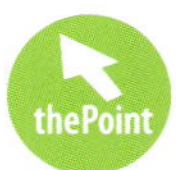

ONLINE RESOURCES

An extensive range of additional resources to enhance teaching and learning and to facilitate understanding of this chapter may be found online at the text's accompanying website, located on thePoint at http://thepoint.lww.com. These include Watch and Learn videos, Concepts in Action animations, journal articles, review questions, case studies, discussion topics and quizzes.

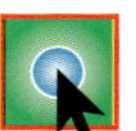

WEB LINKS

Health care providers and students may want to consult the following web resources:

www.arthritisaustralia.com.au
Arthritis Australia. Information about arthritis and support services.

www.arthritis.org.nz
Arthritis New Zealand. Information about arthritis and support services.

BIBLIOGRAPHY

Cavagna, L., Caporali, R., Trifiro, G., Arcoraci, V., Rossi, S. & Montecucco, C. (2013). Overuse of prescription and OTC non-steroidal anti-inflammatory drugs in patients with rheumatoid arthritis and osteoarthritis. *International Journal of Immunopathology & Pharmacology, 26*, 279–281.

Corke, P. (2013). Postoperative pain management. *Australian Prescriber, 36*, 202–205.

D'Arcy, Y. (2011). Prescribing nonsteroidal anti-inflammatory drugs. *Nurse Practitioner, 36*, 8–11.

Dempsey, J., Hillege, S. & Hill, R. (2014). *Fundamentals of Nursing and Midwifery: A Person-centred Approach to Care* (2nd Australian and New Zealand edn). Sydney: Lippincott Williams & Wilkins.

Firth, J. (2011). Rheumatoid arthritis: Treating to target with disease-modifying drugs. *British Journal of Nursing, 20*, 1240–1245.

Firth, J. & Critchley, S. (2011). Treating to target in rheumatoid arthritis: Biologic therapies. *British Journal of Nursing, 20*, 1284–1291.

Fitzgerald, G. A. (2004). Coxibs and cardiovascular disease. *New England Journal of Medicine, 351*, 1709–1711.

Kennedy, D. (2011). Analgesics and pain relief in pregnancy and breastfeeding. *Australian Prescriber, 34*, 8–10.

Lu, T.Y-T. & Hill, C. (2006). Managing patients taking tumour necrosis factor inhibitors. *Australian Prescriber, 29*, 67–70.

McKenna, L. & Mirkov, S. (2019). *McKenna's Drug Handbook for Nursing and Midwifery* (8th edn). Sydney: Wolters Kluwer Health Australia.

O'Dell, J. R. (2004). Therapeutic strategies for rheumatoid arthritis. *New England Journal of Medicine, 350*, 2591–2602.

Paul, S. P. & Whibley, J. (2010). Paracetamol prophylaxis: What the evidence says. *Practice Nursing, 21*, 530–532.

Porth, C. M. (2011). *Essentials of Pathophysiology: Concepts of Altered Health States* (3rd edn). Philadelphia: Lippincott Williams & Wilkins.

Porth, C. M. (2009). *Pathophysiology: Concepts of Altered Health States* (8th edn). Philadelphia: Lippincott Williams & Wilkins.

Swaminathan, S. & Riminton, S. (2006). Monoclonal antibody therapy for non-malignant disease. *Australian Prescriber, 29*, 130–133.

Swanson, K. I. & Pfenning, S. (2011). The nurse practitioner's role in the management of rheumatoid arthritis. *Journal for Nurse Practitioners, 7*, 858–870.

Varghese, M. & Lockey, R. F. (2008). Aspirin-induced asthma. *Allergy, Asthma, and Clinical Immunology, 4(2)*, 75–83.

CHECK YOUR UNDERSTANDING

Answers to the questions in this chapter can be found in Appendix A at the back of this book.

MULTIPLE CHOICE

Select the best answer to the following.

1. A drug could be classified as an analgesic if it:
   a. reduces fever.
   b. reduces swelling.
   c. reduces redness.
   d. reduces pain.
2. An antipyretic is a drug that can:
   a. block pain.
   b. block swelling.
   c. block fever.
   d. block inflammation.
3. A nurse or midwife might not see a salicylate used as an anti-inflammatory if a drug was needed for its:
   a. antipyretic properties.
   b. analgesic properties.
   c. OTC availability.
   d. parenteral availability.
4. The NSAIDs affect the COX-1 and COX-2 enzymes. By blocking COX-2 enzymes, the NSAIDs block inflammation and the signs and symptoms of inflammation at the site of injury or trauma. By blocking COX-1 enzymes, these drugs block:
   a. fever regulation.
   b. prostaglandins that protect the stomach lining.
   c. swelling in the periphery.
   d. liver function.
5. A person has been receiving ibuprofen for many years to relieve the pain of osteoarthritis. Assessment of the person should include:
   a. an electrocardiogram.
   b. FBC with differential.
   c. respiratory auscultation.
   d. renal evaluation.

6. People taking NSAIDs should be taught to avoid the use of OTC medications without checking with their prescriber because:
   a. many of the OTC preparations contain NSAIDs and inadvertent toxicity could occur.
   b. no one should take more than one type of pain reliever at a time.
   c. increased GI upset could occur.
   d. there is a risk of Reye syndrome.

7. Chronic or excessive activity by the inflammatory response can lead to:
   a. loss of white blood cells.
   b. coagulation problems.
   c. release of lysosomal enzymes and tissue destruction.
   d. adrenal suppression.

8. A person with rheumatoid arthritis who is on a fixed income and who is being treated with aspirin should be advised:
   a. to use only brand-name aspirin.
   b. to use only enteric-coated aspirin.
   c. to use generic aspirin.
   d. to switch to one of the NSAIDs.

MULTIPLE RESPONSE

Select all that apply.

1. A person is being treated for severe rheumatoid arthritis. The health professional could anticipate treatment with which of the following?
   a. etanercept (TNF inhibitor)
   b. gold therapy
   c. anakinra
   d. ketoprofen
   e. interferon beta-2a
   f. methotrexate

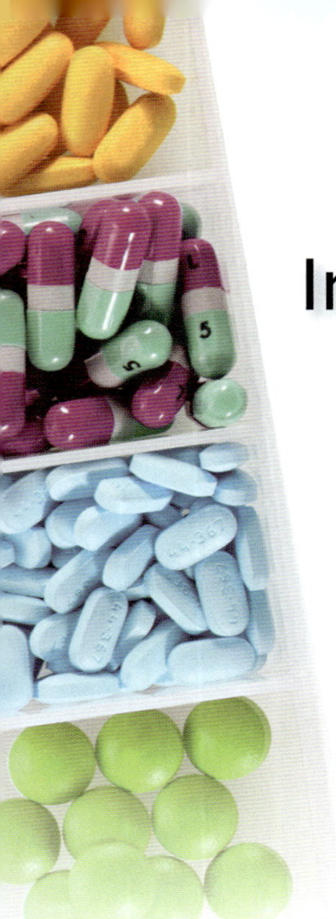

17

Immune modulators

Learning objectives

On completing this chapter you should be able to:

1. Describe the sites of actions of the various immune modulators.
2. Describe the therapeutic actions, indications, pharmacokinetics, contraindications, most common adverse effects and important drug–drug interactions associated with each class of immune stimulants and immune suppressants.
3. Discuss the use of immune modulators across the lifespan.
4. Compare and contrast the prototype drugs for each class of immune modulators with the other drugs in that class and with drugs in other classes.
5. Outline the care considerations and teaching needs for people receiving each class of immune modulator.

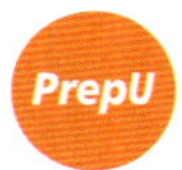

Test your current knowledge of immune modulators with a PrepU Practice Quiz!

Glossary of key terms

immune stimulant: drug used to energise the immune system when it is exhausted from fighting prolonged invasion or needs help fighting a specific pathogen or cancer cell

immune suppressant: drug used to block or suppress the actions of the T cells and antibody production; used to prevent transplant rejection and to treat autoimmune diseases

monoclonal antibodies: specific antibodies produced by a single clone of B cells to react with a very specific antigen

recombinant DNA technology: use of bacteria to produce chemicals normally produced by human cells

IMMUNE STIMULANTS

Interferons
- interferon alfa-2a
- interferon alfa-2b
- interferon beta-1a
- interferon beta-1b
- interferon gamma-1b
- peginterferon alfa-2a
- peginterferon beta-1a

Interleukins

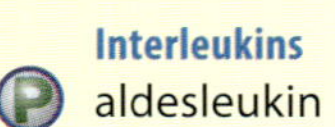

- aldesleukin

IMMUNE SUPPRESSANTS

T- and B-cell suppressors
- abatacept
- azathioprine
- ciclosporin
- glatiramer acetate
- mycophenolate
- pimecrolimus
- sirolimus
- tacrolimus

Interleukin-receptor antagonist
- anakinra

Monoclonal antibodies
- adalimumab
- basiliximab
- bevacizumab
- certolizumab pegol
- cetuximab
- erlotinib
- golimumab
- infliximab
- natalizumab
- nivolumab
- omalizumab
- palivizumab
- panitumumab
- rituximab
- tocilizumab
- trastuzumab
- ustekinumab

As the name implies, immune modulators are used to modify the actions of the immune system. **Immune stimulants** are used to energise the immune system when it is exhausted from fighting prolonged invasion or when it needs help fighting a specific pathogen or cancer cell. **Immune suppressants** are used to block the normal effects of the immune system in cases of organ transplantation (in which non-self cells are transplanted into the body and destroyed by the immune reaction) and in autoimmune disorders (in which the body's defences recognise self-cells as foreign and work to destroy them) in some cancers. Each group acts at various sites within the immune response (Figure 17.1).

The knowledge base about the actions and components of the immune system is continually growing and changing. As new discoveries are made and the actions and interactions of the various components of the system become better understood, new applications will be found for modulating the immune system in a variety of disorders. Box 17.1 discusses the use of immune modulators across the lifespan. Box 17.2 discusses use of these agents during pregnancy.

IMMUNE STIMULANTS

Immune stimulants (Table 17.1) include the interferons, which are naturally released from human cells in response to viral invasion; and interleukins, which are chemicals produced by T cells to communicate between leucocytes.

INTERFERONS

Interferons are substances naturally produced and released by human cells that have been invaded by viruses. They may also be released from cells in response to other stimuli, such as cytotoxic T cell activity. A number of interferons are available for use. Several are produced by **recombinant DNA technology**, including interferon alfa-2a (*Roferon-A*), interferon alfa-2b (*Intron A*), peginterferon alfa-2a (*Pegasys*), peginterferon alfa-2b (*Peg-Intron*) and interferon beta-1b (*Betaferon*). Interferon beta-1a (*Avonex*) is produced from Chinese hamster ovary cells. Interferon gamma-1b (*Imukin*) is produced by *Escherichia coli* bacteria. The interferon of choice depends on the condition being treated (see Table 17.1).

Therapeutic actions and indications

Interferons act to prevent virus particles from replicating inside cells. They also stimulate interferon-receptor sites on non-invaded cells to produce antiviral proteins, which prevent viruses from entering the cell. In addition, interferons have been found to inhibit tumour growth and replication, to stimulate cytotoxic T-cell activity and to enhance the inflammatory response. Of interest, interferon gamma-1b also acts like an interleukin,

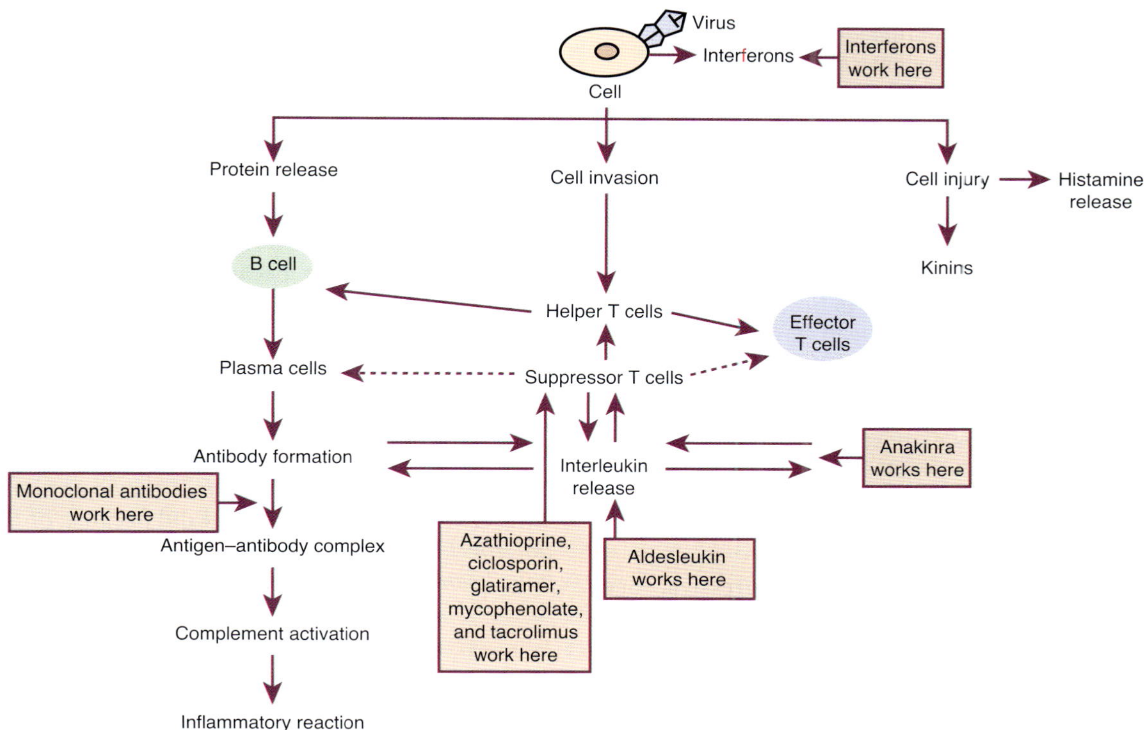

FIGURE 17.1 Sites of action of the immune modulators.

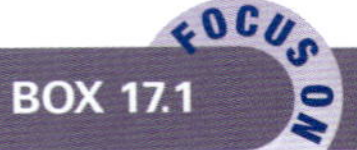

BOX 17.1 Drug therapy across the lifespan

Immune modulators

CHILDREN

Most of the drugs that affect the immune system are not recommended for use in children or have not been tested in children. The exceptions – interferon alfa-2b, azathioprine, ciclosporin, tacrolimus and palivizumab – should be used cautiously, monitoring the child frequently for infection, gastrointestinal (GI), renal, haematological or central nervous system (CNS) effects.

The immune suppressants (azathioprine, ciclosporin, and tacrolimus) are usually needed in higher doses for children than for adults to achieve the same therapeutic effect.

Protecting the child from infection and injury is a very important part of the care of a child taking an immune modulator. This can be a great challenge with an active child.

ADULTS

Both the adult who is receiving a parenteral immune modulator and a significant other should learn the proper technique for injection, disposal of needles and special storage precautions for the drug. It is important to stress ways to avoid exposure to infection and injury to prevent further complications. The person should be encouraged to seek regular follow-up and medical care.

PREGNANCY AND BREASTFEEDING

Immune modulators are contraindicated during pregnancy and breastfeeding because of the potential for adverse effects on the fetus or neonate and complications for the mother. Women of childbearing age should be advised to use barrier contraceptives while taking these drugs and, if breastfeeding, should be counselled to find another method of feeding the baby. Some of these drugs impair fertility, and the person should be advised of this fact before taking the drug.

OLDER ADULTS

Older people may be more susceptible to the effects of the immune modulators, partly because the ageing immune system is less efficient and less responsive.

These people need to be monitored closely for infection, GI, renal, hepatic and CNS effects. Baseline renal and liver function tests can help to determine whether a decreased dosage will be needed before beginning therapy.

Because these people are more susceptible to infection, they need to receive extensive teaching about ways to avoid infection and injury.

BOX 17.2 FOCUS ON Gender considerations

Immune modulators and pregnancy

Generally, immune modulators are contraindicated for use during pregnancy and breastfeeding, largely because these drugs have been associated with fetal abnormalities, increased maternal and fetal infections, and suppressed immune responses in breastfeeding babies. Women should be informed of the risk of using these drugs during pregnancy and receive counselling in the use of barrier contraceptives. (The use of barrier contraceptives is advised because the effects of oral contraceptives may be altered by liver changes or by changes in the body's immune response, potentially resulting in unexpected pregnancy.)

If a woman taking immune modulators becomes pregnant or decides that she wants to become pregnant, she should discuss this with her health care provider and review the risks associated with use of the drug or drugs being taken. The monoclonal antibodies should be used with caution during pregnancy and breastfeeding. Because long-term studies of most of these drugs are not yet available, it may be prudent to advise women taking these drugs to avoid pregnancy if possible.

stimulating phagocytes to be more aggressive. See Table 17.1 for usual indications for each interferon.

Pharmacokinetics

The interferons are generally well absorbed after subcutaneous (SC) or intramuscular injection. They have a rapid onset of action and peak within 3–8 hours, with a half-life ranging from 3–8 hours, with the exception of interferon beta-1a, which has an onset of action of 12 hours and reaches peak levels in 48 hours, with a half-life of 10 hours. They are broken down in the liver and kidneys and seem to be excreted primarily through the kidneys.

Contraindications and cautions

The use of interferons is contraindicated in the presence of known allergy to any interferon or product components. Many of the interferons are teratogenic in animals and therefore should not be used during pregnancy. Use of barrier contraceptives is advised for women of childbearing age. It is not known whether these drugs cross into breast milk, but because of the potential adverse effects on the baby, it is advised that the drugs not be used during breastfeeding unless the benefits to the mother clearly outweigh any risks to the baby. Caution should be used in the presence of known cardiac disease *because hypertension and arrhythmias have been reported with the use of these drugs*; with myelosuppression *because these drugs may further suppress the bone marrow*; and with CNS dysfunction of any kind *because of the potential for CNS depression and personality changes that have been reported.*

Adverse effects

The adverse effects associated with the use of interferons are related to the immune or inflammatory reaction that is being stimulated (stimulating the immune and

TABLE 17.1 DRUGS IN FOCUS Immune stimulants

Drug name	Dosage/route	Usual indications
Interferons		
interferon alfa-2a (*Roferon-A*)	Individualised; dose varies widely	Treatment of leukaemias, Kaposi sarcoma, non-Hodgkin lymphoma, chronic hepatitis C
(P) interferon alfa-2b (*Intron-A*)	Adult: dose varies widely based on indication	Treatment of leukaemias, Kaposi sarcoma, warts, hepatitis B, malignant melanoma
interferon beta-1a (*Avonex*)	30 micrograms IM once a week	Treatment of multiple sclerosis in adults
interferon beta-1b (*Betaferon*)	Individualised; dose varies widely	Treatment of multiple sclerosis in adults
interferon gamma-1b (*Imukin*)	Individualised; dose varies widely	Treatment of serious, chronic granulomatous disease in adults; delaying time to disease progression in severe, malignant osteopetrosis
peginterferon alfa-2a (*Pegasys*)	180 micrograms SC once weekly	Treatment of chronic hepatitis B, C
peginterferon beta-1a (*Plegridy*)	125 micrograms SC q 2 weeks	Treatment of relapsing forms of multiple sclerosis
Interleukins		
(P) aldesleukin (*Proleukin*)	Two 5-day cycles of 600,000 IU/kg IV q 8 hours given over 15 minutes 18 million IU/m^2 per 24 hours as a continuous IV infusion for 5 days, followed by 2–6 days without Proleukin therapy, an additional 5 days of IV Proleukin as a continuous infusion, then 3 weeks without Proleukin therapy This constitutes one induction cycle	The treatment of metastatic melanoma and metastatic renal cell carcinoma

inflammatory response causes a flu-like syndrome with lethargy, myalgia, arthralgia, anorexia, nausea). Other commonly seen adverse effects include headache, dizziness, bone marrow depression, depression and suicidal ideation, photosensitivity and liver impairment.

(P) Prototype summary: interferon alfa-2b

Indications: hairy cell leukaemia, malignant melanoma, AIDS-related Kaposi sarcoma, chronic hepatitis B and C, intralesional treatment of condylomata acuminata in individuals 18 years of age or older.

Actions: inhibits the growth of tumour cells and enhances the immune response.

Pharmacokinetics:

Route	Onset	Peak
IM, SC	Rapid	3–12 hours
IV	Rapid	End of infusion

$T_{1/2}$: 2–3 hours; metabolised in the kidney, excretion is unknown.

Adverse effects: dizziness, confusion, rash, dry skin, anorexia, nausea, bone marrow suppression, flu-like syndrome.

Clinically important drug–drug interactions

There are no reported clinically important drug–drug interactions with the interferons.

INTERLEUKINS

Interleukins are synthetic compounds much like endogenous interleukins; they communicate between lymphocytes, which stimulate cellular immunity and inhibit tumour growth. Interleukin-2 stimulates cellular immunity by increasing the activity of natural killer cells, platelets and cytokines. Aldesleukin (*Proleukin*) (available in New Zealand but not Australia) is a human interleukin produced by recombinant DNA technology using *E. coli* bacteria (see Table 17.1).

Therapeutic actions and indications

Natural interleukin-2 is produced by various lymphocytes to activate cellular immunity and inhibit tumour growth by increasing lymphocyte numbers and their activity. When synthetic interleukins are administered, there are increases in the numbers of natural killer cells and lymphocytes, in cytokine activity and in the number of circulating platelets. See Table 17.1 for usual indications.

Pharmacokinetics

The interleukins are rapidly distributed after injection. Aldesleukin, given IV, reaches peak levels in 13 minutes and has a half-life of 85 minutes. This drug is primarily cleared from the body by the kidneys.

Contraindications and cautions

Interleukins are contraindicated in the presence of any allergy to an interleukin or *E. coli*–produced product. They were shown to be embryocidal and teratogenic in animal studies and should not be used during pregnancy. Use of barrier contraceptives is recommended for women of childbearing age who require one of these drugs. It is not clear whether the drugs cross into breast milk, but it is recommended that they not be used during breastfeeding; if they must be used, another method of feeding the baby must be chosen because of the potential for adverse effects in the baby. Caution should be used with renal, liver or cardiovascular impairment *because of the adverse effects of the drugs*. Interleukins are also contraindicated in individuals with evidence of active infection requiring antibiotic therapy.

Adverse effects

The adverse effects associated with the interleukins can be attributed to their effect on the body during inflammation (flu-like effects: lethargy, myalgia, arthralgia, fatigue, fever). Respiratory difficulties, CNS changes and cardiac arrhythmias have also been reported, and the person should be monitored for these effects and the drug stopped if they do occur.

Prototype summary: aldesleukin (not available in Australia)

Indications: metastatic renal cell carcinoma in adults; treatment of metastatic melanomas (orphan drug use).

Actions: activates human cellular immunity and inhibits tumour growth through increases in lymphocytes, platelets and cytokines.

Pharmacokinetics:

Route	Onset	Peak	Duration
IV	5 min	13 min	3–4 hours

$T_{1/2}$: 85 minutes; metabolised in the kidney and excreted in the urine.

Adverse effects: mental status changes, dizziness, hypotension, sinus tachycardia, arrhythmias, pruritus, nausea, vomiting, diarrhoea, anorexia, GI bleed, bone marrow suppression, respiratory difficulties, fever, chills, pain.

Clinical Important drug–drug interactions

There are no reported drug–drug interactions with interleukins.

Care considerations for people receiving immune stimulants

Assessment: history and examination

- Assess for contraindications and cautions: known allergies to any of these drugs or their components *to prevent hypersensitivity reactions*; current status related to pregnancy or breastfeeding *to avoid serious adverse effects on the fetus or baby*; history of hepatic, renal or cardiac disease, bone marrow depression and CNS disorders, including seizures, *all of which could be exacerbated by the effects of these drugs.*
- Perform a physical assessment *to determine baseline status before beginning therapy and for any potential adverse effects*; inspect for the presence of any skin lesions *to detect early dermatological effects*; obtain weight *to monitor for fluid retention*; monitor temperature *to detect any infection*; check heart rate and rhythm and blood pressure *to monitor for any cardiac effects of the drug*; assess level of orientation and reflexes *to evaluate CNS effects of the drug.*
- Obtain a baseline electrocardiogram (ECG) *to evaluate cardiac function and monitor adverse effects of the drugs.*
- Assess the person's renal and liver function, including renal and liver function tests, *to determine the appropriateness of therapy* and *to determine the need for possible dose adjustment and toxic drug effects.*
- Monitor the results of laboratory tests such as full blood count (FBC) *to identify changes in bone marrow function.*

Implementation with rationale

- Arrange for laboratory tests before and periodically during therapy, including FBC and differential, *to monitor for drug effects and adverse effects.*
- Administer drug as indicated; instruct the person and a significant other if injections are required *to ensure that the drug will be given even if the person is not able to administer it.*
- Monitor for severe reactions, such as severe hypersensitivity reactions, and *arrange to discontinue the drug immediately if they occur.*
- Arrange for supportive care and comfort measures for flu-like symptoms (eg, rest, environmental control, paracetamol) *to help the person cope with*

the drug effects. Ensure that the person is well hydrated during therapy *to prevent severe adverse effects*.

- Instruct women in the use of barrier contraceptives *to avoid pregnancy during therapy because of the potential for adverse effects on the fetus*.
- Offer support and encouragement *to deal with the diagnosis and the drug regimen*.
- Provide teaching about measures to avoid adverse effects; warning signs of problems; and proper administration technique.

Evaluation

- Monitor response to the drug (improvement in condition being treated).
- Monitor for adverse effects (flu-like symptoms, GI upset, CNS changes, bone marrow depression).
- Evaluate the effectiveness of the teaching plan (person can name drug, dosage, adverse effects to watch for, specific measures to avoid adverse effects).
- Monitor the effectiveness of comfort measures and compliance with the regimen.

KEY POINTS

- Immune stimulants assist the immune system to fight specific pathogens or cancer cells; in doing so they cause flu-like symptoms (lethargy, muscle and joint aches and pains, anorexia, nausea).
- Interferons are used to treat various cancers and warts.
- Interleukins stimulate cellular immunity and inhibit tumour growth.

IMMUNE SUPPRESSANTS

Immune suppressants (Table 17.2) often are used in conjunction with corticosteroids, which block the inflammatory reaction and decrease initial damage to cells. They are especially beneficial in cases of organ transplantation and in the treatment of autoimmune diseases. The immune suppressants include T- and B-cell suppressors, an interleukin-receptor antagonist and **monoclonal antibodies** – antibodies produced by a single clone of B cells that react with specific antigens.

T- AND B-CELL SUPPRESSORS

Several T- and B-cell immune suppressors are available for use. Of the numerous agents available, ciclosporin (*Sandimmun*, *Neoral*) is the most commonly used immune suppressant. Additional agents include abatacept (*Orencia*), azathioprine (*Imuran*), glatiramer (*Copaxone*), mycophenolate (*CellCept*), pimecrolimus (*Elidel*), sirolimus (*Rapamune*) and tacrolimus (*Prograf*).

Therapeutic actions and indications

The exact mechanism of action of the T- and B-cell suppressors is not clearly understood. It has been shown that they block antibody production by B cells, inhibit suppressor and helper T cells, and modify the release of interleukins and of T-cell growth factor (see Figure 17.1).

The T- and B-cell suppressors are indicated for the prevention and treatment of specific transplant rejections. See Table 17.2 for usual indications of each agent.

Pharmacokinetics

Ciclosporin is well absorbed from the GI tract, reaching peak levels in 1–2 hours. It is extensively metabolised in the liver by the cytochrome P450 system and is primarily excreted in the bile. The half-life of the drug is about 19 hours for *Sandimmun* and 8.4 hours for *Neoral*. It is available as an oral solution that can be mixed with milk, chocolate milk or orange juice for ease of administration. Abatacept must be given as a 30-minute infusion every 2–4 weeks, depending on the person's response. Peak levels are reached at the end of the infusion. Abatacept has a half-life of 12–23 days and usually reaches a steady state by 60 days of treatment. The drug is cleared from the body by the kidneys.

Azathioprine is rapidly absorbed from the GI tract, reaching peak levels in 1–2 hours. This drug is catabolised in the liver and red blood cells.

Little is known about the pharmacokinetics of glatiramer. Some of it is immediately hydrolysed on injection, some enters the lymph system and some may actually reach the systemic circulation.

Mycophenolate is readily absorbed and immediately metabolised to its active metabolite. Most of the metabolised drug is then excreted in the urine.

Sirolimus is rapidly absorbed from the GI tract, reaching peak levels in 1 hour. It is extensively metabolised in the liver, partly by the cytochrome P450 system. The drug is then excreted primarily in the faeces.

Tacrolimus is rapidly absorbed from the GI tract, reaching peak levels in 1.5–3.5 hours. It is extensively metabolised in the liver by the cytochrome P450 system and is excreted in the urine.

Contraindications and cautions

The use of T- and B-cell suppressors is contraindicated in the presence of any known allergy to the drug or its components and during pregnancy and breastfeeding

TABLE 17.2 DRUGS IN FOCUS **Immunosuppressants**

Drug name	Dosage/route	Usual indications
T- and B-cell suppressors		
abatacept (*Orencia*)	< 60 kg: 500 mg IV repeated at 2 and 4 weeks, then every 4 weeks 60–100 kg: 750 mg IV, repeated at 2 and 4 weeks, then every 4 weeks > 100 kg: 1 g IV, repeated at 2 and 4 weeks, then every 4 weeks	Reduction of the signs and symptoms and slowing structural damage in adults with rheumatoid arthritis who have inadequate response to other drugs
azathioprine (*Imuran*)	Adult: 3–5 mg/kg day PO for prevention of rejection; maintenance: 1–4 mg/kg/day PO Rheumatoid arthritis: 1–2.5 mg/kg/day PO; reduce dose with renal impairment Paediatric: 3–5 mg/kg/day IV or PO to prevent rejection; maintenance: 1–4 mg/kg/day PO	Prevention of rejection in renal homotransplants; treatment of rheumatoid arthritis
(P) ciclosporin (*Sandimmun*)	Solid organ transplantation in combination with other immunosuppressants: 3–6 mg/kg/day in 2 divided doses starting 4–12 hours before transplantation; the dose is adjusted according to serum levels Paediatric: larger doses may be needed to achieve therapeutic levels	Suppression of rejection in a variety of transplant situations
ciclosporin (*Neoral*)	Rheumatoid arthritis: 3 mg/kg/day PO in 2 divided doses Psoriasis: 2.5 mg/kg PO bd	Treatment of rheumatoid arthritis, psoriasis
glatiramer acetate (*Copaxone*)	20 mg SC once daily or 40 mg SC three times weekly	Reduction of the number of relapses in multiple sclerosis in adults
mycophenolate (*CellCept*)	1–1.5 g PO bd; may be started IV during transplantation, with switch to oral route as soon as possible	Prevention of rejection after renal, hepatic, or heart transplantation in adults; not for use in pregnancy
pimecrolimus (*Elidel*)	Applied to affected site bd	Treatment of atopic dermatitis
sirolimus (*Rapamune*)	6 mg PO as soon after transplant as possible; then 2 mg/day PO	Prevention of rejection after renal transplantation in adults
tacrolimus (*Prograf*)	Initial dose of 0.15–0.30 mg/kg/day PO in 2 divided doses. Dose is adjusted according to serum levels	Primary immunosuppression in liver, kidney, pancreas, lung or heart allograft recipients Prevention of allograft rejection
Interleukin-receptor antagonist		
anakinra (*Kineret*)	100 mg/day SC	Prevention of rejection after renal or liver transplantation; reduction of the signs and symptoms and slowing structural damage in adults with rheumatoid arthritis who have inadequate response to other drugs
Monoclonal antibodies		
adalimumab (*Humira*)	40 mg SC every other week; if also taking methotrexate, may require 40 mg SC once a week	Reduction of signs and symptoms and inhibition of structural damage in adults who have moderate to severe rheumatoid arthritis and who have not responded to other drugs
(P) basiliximab (*Simulect*)	20 mg IV twice – first dose within 24 hours of transplantation, then at 4 days	Prevention of renal transplant rejection
certolizumab pegol (*Cimzia*)	400 mg SC, repeated at weeks 2 and 4, then every 4 weeks	Reduction of the signs and symptoms of Crohn disease in adults with moderate to severe disease not controlled by standard therapy

TABLE 17.2 DRUGS IN FOCUS Immunosuppressants (continued)

Drug name	Dosage/route	Usual indications
Monoclonal antibodies *(continued)*		
golimumab (*Simponi*)	Rheumatoid arthritis, psoriatic arthritis, ankylosing spondylitis: 50 mg SC once monthly Ulcerative colitis: 200 mg SC at week 0, then 100 mg at week 2, then 100 mg q 4 weeks thereafter	Management of moderate to severe active rheumatoid arthritis, progressive psoriatic arthritis, active ankylosing spondylitis
infliximab (*Remicade*)	3–5 mg/kg increasing to 10 mg/kg if needed IV over 2 hours; may be repeated at 2 and 6 weeks	Decreases signs and symptoms of Crohn disease in individuals who do not respond to other therapy; treatment of fistulating Crohn disease; also approved for use with methotrexate in the treatment of progressing moderate to severe rheumatoid arthritis
omalizumab (*Xolair*)	Adults and children > 6 years: 75–600 mg, according to patient's body weight and baseline serum IgE, SC in 1–4 injections every 4 weeks	Treatment of asthma with a very strong allergic component and seasonal allergic rhinitis not well controlled with traditional medications
palivizumab (*Synagis*)	15 mg/kg IM one a month during respiratory syncytial virus (RSV) season	Prevention of serious RSV infection in high-risk children
panitumumab (*Vectibix*)	6 mg/kg IV every 2 weeks	Treatment of wild type KRAS metastatic colorectal cancer
rituximab (*Mabthera*)	375 mg/m^2 IV once weekly for 4 doses	Treatment of relapsed follicular B-cell non-Hodgkin lymphoma
tocilizumab (*Actemra*)	8 mg/kg IV every 4 weeks, with methotrexate	Relief of signs and symptoms of moderate to severe rheumatoid arthritis in adults
trastuzumab (*Herceptin, Kadcyla*)	Herceptin IV: initial loading dose 4 mg/kg IV over 90 minutes. Maintenance dosage 2 mg/kg IV weekly as 30-minute IV infusion if initial loading dose is well tolerated Herceptin SC: 600 mg SC q 3 weeks. Kadcyla: 3.6 mg/kg q 3 weeks until disease progression or unacceptable toxicity; then reduce to 3 mg/kg, then to 2.4 mg/kg	Treatment of metastatic breast cancer with tumours that overexpress human epidermal growth factor receptor 2 (HER2) Alert: check the vial labels to ensure the medicine being prepared and administered is Herceptin (trastuzumab) and not Kadcyla (trastuzumab emtansine) Alert: it is important to check the labels to ensure the correct formulation (IV or SC) is being administered to the patient as prescribed
ustekinumab (*Stelara*)	45–90 mg by SC injection once a month, then once q 8–12 weeks as determined by individual condition and response	Treatment of recalcitrant plaque psoriasis in adults not responsive to traditional therapy

because of the potential serious adverse effects on the fetus or neonate. Caution should be used with renal or hepatic impairment, *which could interfere with the metabolism or excretion of the drug*, and in the presence of known neoplasms, *which potentially could spread with immune system suppression.*

Adverse effects

People receiving these drugs are at increased risk for infection and for the development of neoplasms due to their blocking effect on the immune system. Other potentially dangerous adverse effects include hepatotoxicity, renal toxicity, renal dysfunction and pulmonary oedema. Individuals may experience headache, tremors and secondary infections such as acne, GI upset, diarrhoea and hypertension.

Clinically important drug–drug interactions

There is an increased risk of toxicity if these drugs are combined with other drugs that are hepatotoxic or nephrotoxic. Extreme care should be used if such combinations are necessary. Other reported drug–drug interactions are drug specific; consult a drug guide or drug handbook.

 **Prototype summary: ciclosporin**

Indications: prophylaxis for organ rejection in kidney, liver and heart transplants (used with corticosteroids); treatment of chronic rejection in people previously treated with other immunosuppressants; treatment of rheumatoid arthritis and recalcitrant psoriasis.

Actions: reversibly inhibits immunocompetent lymphocytes; inhibits T helper cells and T suppressor cells, lymphokine production, and release of interleukin-2 and T-cell growth factor.

Pharmacokinetics:

Route	Onset	Peak
PO	Varies	3.5 hours
IV	Rapid	1–2 hours

$T_{1/2}$: 19–27 hours; metabolised in the liver and excreted in the bile and urine.

Adverse effects: tremor, hypertension, gum hyperplasia, renal dysfunction, diarrhoea, hirsutism, acne, bone marrow suppression.

Interleukin-receptor antagonist

An interleukin-receptor antagonist works to block the activity of the interleukins that are released in an inflammatory or immune response. The only available interleukin receptor antagonist is anakinra (*Kineret*). See Table 17.2 for additional information about this drug.

Therapeutic actions and indications

Anakinra specifically antagonises human interleukin-1 receptors, blocking the activity of interleukin-1. Interleukin-1 levels are elevated in response to inflammation or immune reactions and are thought to be responsible for the degradation of cartilage that occurs in rheumatoid arthritis. Anakinra is used to reduce the signs and symptoms of moderately to severely active rheumatoid arthritis and active systemic juvenile idiopathic arthritis (SJIA) in patients 2 years and older who are unresponsive to non-biological DMARDs.

As one of the most common chronic conditions in Australia, arthritis is one of the Australian government's nine National Health Priority Areas. Data from the 2014–15 National Health Survey suggest that 407,900 Australians are affected by rheumatoid arthritis (2% prevalence). For more information on arthritis, see www.aihw.gov.au/reports/chronic-musculoskeletal-conditions/rheumatoid-arthritis/contents/who-gets-rheumatoid-arthritis.

Pharmacokinetics

The recommended dosage is 100 mg/day by SC injection. After injection anakinra is absorbed slowly, reaching peak effects in 3–7 hours. It is metabolised in the tissues with a 4- to 6-hour half-life and is excreted in the urine.

Contraindications and cautions

Anakinra is contraindicated with any known allergy to *E. coli*–produced products or to anakinra itself. It should be used with caution during pregnancy and breastfeeding *because the drug may cross the placenta and enter breast milk*. It is also used cautiously in people with renal impairment, immunosuppression or any active infection *because these could be exacerbated by the effects of the drug*. There is an increased risk of infection whenever this drug is used, and the person needs to be protected from exposure to infections and monitored closely after any invasive procedures. Immunisations cannot be given while the person is on this drug.

Adverse effects

Headache, sinusitis, nausea, diarrhoea, upper respiratory and other infections and injection-site reactions are among the most common adverse effects.

Clinically important drug–drug interactions

People who are also receiving etanercept (*Enbrel*) must be monitored very closely because severe and even life-threatening infections have occurred. Anakinra should not be combined with abatacept because of the potential for serious infections.

Monoclonal antibodies

Antibodies that attach to specific receptor sites are being developed to respond to very specific situations. Every year, several new monoclonal antibodies are marketed, showing the rapid pace with which these agents are being developed and approved for clinical use. Monoclonal antibodies include adalimumab (*Humira*), basiliximab (*Simulect*), bevacizumab (*Avastin*), certolizumab pegol (*Cimzia*), cetuximab (*Erbitux*), erlotinib (*Tarceva*), golimumab (*Simponi*), infliximab (*Remicade*), natalizumab (*Tysabri*), nivolumab (*Opdivo*), omalizumab (*Xolair*), palivizumab (*Synagis*), panitumumab (*Vectibix*), rituximab (*Mabthera*), tocilizumab (*Actemra*), trastuzumab (*Herceptin, Kadcyla*) and ustekinumab (*Stelara*).

Therapeutic actions and indications

Adalimumab, certolizumab pegol, golimumab and infliximab are antibodies specific for human tumour necrosis factor. They keep the inflammatory reaction in check by reacting with and deactivating the free-floating tumour necrosis factor released by active leucocytes.

Basiliximab is specific to interleukin-2 receptor sites on activated T lymphocytes; it reacts with those sites and blocks cellular response to allograft transplants.

Cetuximab is an antibody specific to epidermal growth factor receptor sites. Trastuzumab also reacts with human epidermal growth factor receptor 2 (HER2), a genetic defect that is seen in certain metastatic breast cancers. It is used in the treatment of metastatic breast cancer in tumours that over-express HER2.

Erlotinib, bevacizumab and panitumumab are effective against specific malignant receptor sites.

Rituximab is antibodies specific to sites on activated B lymphocytes.

Natalizumab is an antibody specific to surface receptors on all leucocytes except neutrophils.

Nivolumab is an anti-PD-1 immune checkpoint inhibitor antibody. It binds to programmed death-1 (PD-1) receptor on T cells, preventing the binding of PD-1 to its ligands PD-L1 and PD-L2 on tumour cells. This activates T cells by releasing the PD-1 pathway–mediated immune responses against tumour cells.

Omalizumab is an antibody to immunoglobulin E, an important factor in allergic reactions. It has not had a great deal of success because of related respiratory adverse effects.

Palivizumab is specific to the antigenic site on RSV; it inactivates that virus. It is used to prevent RSV disease in high-risk children.

Ustekinumab comprises antibodies specific to interleukins.

Pharmacokinetics

With the exception of erlotinib (an oral agent), all of the monoclonal antibodies have to be injected. They can be given IV, IM or SC. Because antibodies are proteins, they are rapidly broken down in the GI tract. They are processed by the body like naturally occurring antibodies.

Contraindications and cautions

Monoclonal antibodies are contraindicated in the presence of any known allergy to the drug or to murine products and in the presence of fluid overload. They should be used cautiously with fever (treat the fever before beginning therapy) and in individuals who have had previous administration of the monoclonal antibody (*serious hypersensitivity reactions can occur with repeat administration*). Because of the potential for adverse effects, they should not be used during pregnancy or breastfeeding unless the benefit clearly outweighs the potential risk to the fetus or neonate.

Adverse effects

The most serious adverse effects associated with the use of monoclonal antibodies are acute pulmonary oedema (dyspnoea, chest pain, wheezing), which is associated with severe fluid retention, and cytokine release syndrome (flu-like symptoms that can progress to third-spacing of fluids, and shock). Other adverse effects that can be anticipated include fever, chills, malaise, myalgia, nausea, diarrhoea, vomiting and increased susceptibility to infection.

Erlotinib is reserved for individuals whose disease has progressed after other therapies.

The manufacturer of natalizumab stopped marketing the drug weeks after its release because of reports of CNS complications. It was returned to the market in June 2006 with warnings about the potential for CNS complications.

Clinically important drug–drug interactions

Use caution and arrange to reduce the dose if a monoclonal antibody is combined with any other immunosuppressant drug because severe immune suppression with increased infections and neoplasms can occur.

Prototype summary: basiliximab

Indications: treatment of acute organ rejection in individuals who have undergone renal transplantation.

Actions: monoclonal antibody to the antigen of human T cells; functions as an immunosuppressant by enabling T cells.

Pharmacokinetics:

Route	Onset	Peak	Duration
IV	Minutes	2–7 days	7 days

$T_{1/2}$: 47–100 hours; metabolised in the tissues.

Adverse effects: headache, insomnia, vomiting, nausea, diarrhoea, general oedema, upper respiratory tract infection, fever, chills, increased susceptibility to infection.

Care considerations for people receiving immune suppressants

Assessment: history and examination

- Assess for contraindications and cautions: any known allergies to any of these drugs or their components *to prevent hypersensitivity reactions*; current status related to pregnancy or breastfeeding *because of the potential risk to the fetus or baby*; history of renal or hepatic impairment *that might interfere with drug metabolism and excretion*; and history of neoplasm, *which could be exacerbated with the use of these drugs*.

- Perform a physical assessment *to determine baseline status before beginning therapy and for any potential adverse effects*; inspect the skin *to detect the presence of any lesions*; obtain weight *to monitor for fluid retention*; monitor temperature *to monitor for potential infection*; monitor pulse and blood pressure *to assess the cardiac effects of these drugs*; assess level of orientation and reflexes *to monitor for any CNS changes associated with drug use*.
- Obtain a baseline ECG *to evaluate cardiac function*.
- Assess the person's renal and liver function, including renal and liver function tests, *to determine the appropriateness of therapy and determine the need for possible dose adjustment and toxic drug effects*.
- Monitor the results of laboratory tests such as FBC *to identify changes in bone marrow function*.

Implementation with rationale

- Arrange for laboratory tests before and periodically during therapy, including FBC, differential and liver and renal function tests, *to monitor for drug effects and adverse effects*.
- Administer the drug as indicated; instruct the person and a significant other if injections are required *to ensure proper administration of the drug*.
- Protect the person from exposure to infections and maintain strict aseptic technique for any invasive procedures *to prevent infections during immunosuppression*.
- Arrange for supportive care and comfort measures for flu-like symptoms (rest, environmental control, paracetamol) *to decrease discomfort and increase therapeutic compliance*.
- Monitor nutritional status during therapy; provide small frequent meals, mouth care and nutritional consultation as necessary *to ensure adequate nutrition*.
- Instruct women in the use of barrier contraceptives *to avoid pregnancy during therapy because of the risk of adverse effects to the fetus*.
- Offer support and encouragement *to help the person deal with the diagnosis and the drug regimen*.
- Provide thorough teaching, including measures to avoid adverse effects, warning signs of problems and proper administration, *to increase knowledge about drug therapy and to increase compliance with the drug regimen*.

Evaluation

- Monitor response to the drug (prevention of transplant rejection; improvement in autoimmune disease or cancer; prevention of RSV disease; improvement in signs and symptoms of Crohn disease or rheumatoid arthritis).
- Monitor for adverse effects (flu-like symptoms, GI upset, increased infections, neoplasms, fluid overload).
- Evaluate the effectiveness of the teaching plan (person can name drug, dosage, adverse effects to watch for, specific measures to avoid adverse effects, proper administration technique).
- Monitor the effectiveness of comfort measures and compliance to the regimen (see Critical thinking scenario).

KEY POINTS

- Immune suppressants are used to depress the immune system when needed to prevent transplant rejection or severe tissue damage associated with autoimmune disease. Research is ongoing to extend the use of various immune suppressants to other situations, including various autoimmune disorders.
- Increased susceptibility to infection and increased risk of neoplasm are potentially dangerous effects associated with the use of immune suppressants. People need to be protected from infection, injury and invasive procedures.

CRITICAL THINKING SCENARIO

Holistic care for a person with a transplant

THE SITUATION

After waiting on a transplant list for 4 years, T.B. received a human heart transplant to replace his heart, which had been severely damaged by cardiomyopathy. Before getting the transplant, T.B. was bedridden, on oxygen, and near death. The transplant has given T.B. a 'new lease on life', and he is determined to do everything possible to stay healthy and improve his activity and lifestyle. Currently, he is being maintained on ciclosporin, mycophenolate and corticosteroids.

CRITICAL THINKING

What important teaching facts would help T.B. to achieve his goal? *Think about the psychological impact of the heart transplant and the 'new lease on life'.*

What activity, dietary and supportive guidelines should be outlined for T.B.?

What impact will T.B.'s drug regimen have on his plans?

How can all of the aspects of his condition and medical care be coordinated to give T.B. the best possible advantages for the future?

DISCUSSION

T.B.'s medical regimen will include a very complicated combination of rehabilitation, nutrition, drug therapy and prevention. T.B. should know the risks of transplant rejection and the measures that will be used to prevent it. He also should know the names of his medications and when to take them, the signs and symptoms of rejection to watch for, and what to do if they occur. T.B. must understand the need to prevent exposure to infections and the precautions required, such as avoiding crowded areas and people with known diseases, avoiding injury, and taking steps to maintain cleanliness and avoid infection if an injury occurs.

The medications that T.B. is taking may cause him to experience flu-like symptoms, which can be quite unpleasant. A restful, quiet environment may help to decrease his stress. Paracetamol may be ordered to help alleviate the fever, aches and pains.

T.B. also may experience GI upset, nausea and vomiting related to drug effects. A nutritional consultation may be requested to help T.B. maintain a good nutritional state. Frequent mouth care and small, frequent meals may help. Proper nutrition will help T.B. to recover, heal and maintain his health.

T.B.'s primary health care provider will need to work with the transplantation surgeon, rehabilitation team, dietitian and cardiologist to coordinate a total program that will help T.B. to avoid problems and make the most of his transplanted heart.

CARE GUIDE FOR T.B.: CICLOSPORIN, MYCOPHENOLATE AND CORTICOSTEROIDS

Assessment: history and examination

- Assess for history of allergies to any immune suppressant, renal or hepatic impairment, history of neoplasm, concurrent use of colestyramine, theophylline, phenytoin, other nephrotoxic drugs, digoxin, statins, diltiazem, metoclopramide, amiodarone, androgens, azole antifungals, macrolides; grapefruit juice
- Review physical examination findings, including orientation, reflexes, affect (neurological); temperature and weight (general); pulse, cardiac auscultation, blood pressure, oedema, electrocardiogram (cardiovascular); liver evaluation (GI); and laboratory test results (FBC, liver and renal function tests, condition being treated)

Implementation

Arrange for laboratory tests before and periodically during therapy.

Administer drug as indicated.

Protect person from exposure to infection.

Provide supportive and comfort measures to deal with adverse effects.

Monitor nutritional status and intervene as needed.

Provide teaching regarding the drugs and their dosage, adverse effects, precautions and warning signs to report to care provider.

Evaluation

Evaluate drug effects: prevention of transplant rejection, improvement of autoimmune disease.

Monitor for adverse effects: infection, flu-like symptoms, GI upset, fluid overload, neoplasm.

Monitor for drug–drug interactions and drug–food interactions.

Evaluate effectiveness of teaching program and of comfort and safety measures.

TEACHING FOR T.B.: CICLOSPORIN, MYCOPHENOLATE AND CORTICOSTEROIDS

- You will need to take a combination of drugs to prevent your body from rejecting your new organ. These drugs include ciclosporin, mycophenolate and corticosteroids. They suppress the activity of your immune system and prevent your body from rejecting any transplanted tissue.
- You should never stop taking your drugs without consulting your health care provider. If your prescription is low or you are unable to take the medication for *any* reason, notify your health care provider.
- You should not take your ciclosporin with grapefruit juice.
- Some of the following adverse effects may occur:
  - *Nausea, vomiting:* taking the drug with food and eating small frequent meals may help. It is very important that you maintain good nutrition. A consultation with a dietitian may be needed to help you if these GI problems are severe.
  - *Diarrhoea:* this may not decrease; ensure ready access to bathroom facilities.
  - *Flu-like symptoms:* rest and a cool, peaceful environment may help; paracetamol may be ordered to help relieve discomfort.

- *Rash, mouth sores:* frequent skin and mouth care may ease these effects.
- You will be more susceptible to infection because your body's normal defences will be decreased. You should avoid crowded places, people with known infections and working in soil. If you notice any signs of illness or infection, notify your health care provider immediately.
- Tell any doctor, nurse or other health care provider involved in your care that you are taking these drugs.
- You will need to schedule periodic blood tests and perhaps biopsies while you are being treated with these drugs.
- Report any of the following to your health care provider: unusual bleeding or bruising, fever, sore throat, mouth sores, fatigue, and any other signs of infection or injury.
- Keep your medications safely out of the reach of children and pets and do not share medications with anyone else.

CHAPTER SUMMARY

- Immune stimulants boost the immune system when it is exhausted from fighting off prolonged invasion or needs help to fight a specific pathogen or cancer cell. They include interferons and interleukins.
- Interferons are naturally released from cells in response to viral invasion; they are used to treat various cancers and warts.
- Interleukins stimulate cellular immunity and inhibit tumour growth; they are used to treat very specific cancers.
- Adverse effects seen with immune stimulants are related to the immune response (flu-like symptoms, including fever, myalgia, lethargy, arthralgia and fatigue).
- Immune suppressants are used to depress the immune system when needed to prevent transplant rejection or severe tissue damage associated with autoimmune disease. Research is ongoing to extend the use of various immune suppressants to other situations, including various autoimmune disorders.
- Increased susceptibility to infection and increased risk of neoplasm are potentially dangerous effects associated with the use of immune suppressants. People need to be protected from infection, injury and invasive procedures.

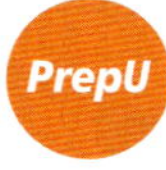

Knowing your strengths and weaknesses helps you to study more effectively. Take a PrepU Practice Quiz to find out how you measure up!

ONLINE RESOURCES

An extensive range of additional resources to enhance teaching and learning and to facilitate understanding of this chapter may be found online at the text's accompanying website, located on thePoint at http://thepoint.lww.com. These include Watch and Learn videos, Concepts in Action animations, journal articles, review questions, case studies, discussion topics and quizzes.

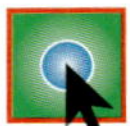

WEB LINKS

Health care providers and students may want to consult the following web resources:

www.arthritisaustralia.com.au
Arthritis Australia. Information, support and research about rheumatoid arthritis.

www.leukaemia.org.au/web/index.php
Leukaemia Foundation. Information, support and research on leukaemia.

www.msaustralia.org.au
MS Australia. Information, support and research about multiple sclerosis.

www.oncolink.org
Information on cancers (including leukaemias and Kaposi sarcoma) and treatments.

BIBLIOGRAPHY

Barrett, K. E. & Ganong, W. F. (2010). *Ganong's Review of Medical Physiology* (23rd edn). New York: McGraw-Hill.

Beatty, K., Winkelman, C., Bokar, J. A., Mazanec, P. & Lystrup, A. (2011). Advances in oncology care: Targeted therapies. *AACN Advanced Critical Care, 22(4)*, 323–336.

Eisenberg, S. (2012). Biologic therapy. *Journal of Infusion Nursing, 35(5)*, 301–313.

Farrell, M. & Dempsey, J. (2014). *Smeltzer & Bare's Textbook of Medical-Surgical Nursing* (3rd edn). Sydney: Lippincott Williams & Wilkins.

Gensicke, H., Leppert, D., Yaldizli, O., Lindberg, R. L., Mehling, M., Kappos, L. & Kuhle, J. (2012). Monoclonal antibodies and recombinant immunoglobulins for the treatment of multiple sclerosis. *CNS Drugs, 26(1)*, 11–37.

Goodman, L. S., Brunton, L. L., Chabner, B. & Knollmann, B. C. (2011). *Goodman and Gilman's Pharmacological Basis of Therapeutics* (12th edn). New York: McGraw-Hill.

Liauw, W. S. (2013). Molecular mechanisms and clinical use of targeted anticancer drugs. *Australian Prescriber, 36(4)*, 126–131.

McKenna, L. & Mirkov, S. (2019). *McKenna's Drug Handbook for Nursing and Midwifery* (8th edn). Sydney: Wolters Kluwer Health Australia.

Porth, C. M. (2011). *Essentials of Pathophysiology: Concepts of Altered Health States* (3rd edn). Philadelphia: Lippincott Williams & Wilkins.

Porth, C. M. (2009). *Pathophysiology: Concepts of Altered Health States* (8th edn). Philadelphia: Lippincott Williams & Wilkins.

Swaminathan, S. & Riminton, S. (2006). Monoclonal antibody therapy for non-malignant disease. *Australian Prescriber, 29*, 130–133.

Vickers, E., Uzzell, M. & Burnet, K. (2012). Understanding how targeted therapies work. *Cancer Nursing Practice, 11(7)*, 14–22.

CHECK YOUR UNDERSTANDING

Answers to the questions in this chapter can be found in Appendix A at the back of this book.

MULTIPLE CHOICE

Select the best answer to the following.

1. In which situation would the health professional be least likely to expect to administer an immune suppressant?
   a. treatment of transplant rejection
   b. treatment of autoimmune disease
   c. reduction of number of relapses in multiple sclerosis
   d. treatment of aggressive cancers
2. Teaching for an individual receiving an interferon would include:
   a. proper use of oral contraceptives.
   b. use of aspirin to control adverse effects.
   c. importance of cardiovascular workouts.
   d. proper methods of injecting the drug.
3. People who are receiving an immune stimulant may experience any of the clinical signs of immune response activity, including:
   a. flu-like symptoms.
   b. diarrhoea.
   c. constipation.
   d. headache.
4. Organ transplants are often rejected by the body because the T cells recognise the transplanted cells as foreign and try to destroy them. Treatment with an immune suppressant would:
   a. activate antibody production.
   b. stimulate interleukin release.
   c. stimulate thymus secretions.
   d. block the initial damage to the transplanted cells.
5. You might use a monoclonal antibody in treating:
   a. warts.
   b. herpes zoster.
   c. tumours that overexpress HER2.
   d. Kaposi sarcoma.

MULTIPLE RESPONSE

Select all that apply.

1. The nurse is assigned to care for a person who is receiving immune suppressants. The nurse would continually assess the person for which of the following anticipated adverse effects?
   a. development of cancers
   b. increased risk of infection
   c. development of secondary infections
   d. increased bleeding tendencies
   e. hepatomegaly
2. Teaching points that the nurse would incorporate into the care of a person receiving ciclosporin would include which of the following?
   a. Use barrier contraceptives to avoid pregnancy.
   b. If mouth sores occur, try to restrict eating as much as possible.
   c. Dilute the solution with milk, chocolate milk, or orange juice and drink immediately.
   d. Avoid drinking grapefruit juice when on this drug.
   e. Stop taking the drug if GI upset or fever occurs.
   f. Refrigerate the oral solution.

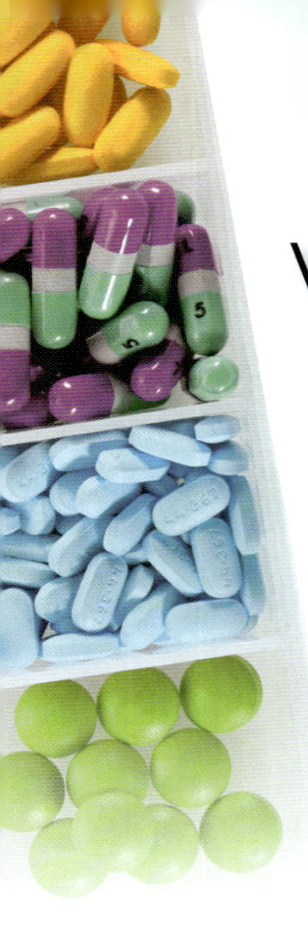

18

Vaccines and sera

Learning objectives

On completing this chapter you should be able to:

1. Define the terms active immunity and passive immunity.
2. Describe the therapeutic actions, indications, pharmacokinetics, contraindications, most common adverse effects and important drug–drug interactions associated with each vaccine, immune serum, antitoxin and antivenin.
3. Discuss the use of vaccines and sera across the lifespan, including recommended immunisation schedules.
4. Compare and contrast the prototype drugs for each class of vaccine and immune serum with others in that class.
5. Outline the care considerations and teaching needs for people receiving a vaccine or immune serum.

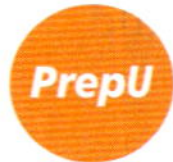

PrepU Test your current knowledge of vaccines and sera with a PrepU Practice Quiz!

Glossary of key terms

active immunity: the formation of antibodies secondary to exposure to a specific antigen; leads to the formation of plasma cells, antibodies and memory cells to immediately produce antibodies if exposed to that antigen in the future; imparts lifelong immunity

antitoxins: immune sera that contain antibodies to specific toxins produced by invaders; may prevent the toxin from adhering to body tissues and causing disease

antivenins: immune sera that contain antibodies to specific venins produced by poisonous snakes or spiders; may prevent the venom from causing cell death

biologicals: vaccines, immune sera and antitoxins that are used to stimulate the production of antibodies, to provide preformed antibodies to facilitate an immune reaction or to react specifically with the toxins produced by an invading pathogen

immune sera: preformed antibodies found in immune globulin from animals or humans who have had a specific disease and developed antibodies to it

immunisation: the process of stimulating active immunity by exposing the body to weakened or less toxic proteins associated with specific disease-causing organisms; the goal is to stimulate immunity without causing the full course of a disease

passive immunity: the injection of preformed antibodies into a host at high risk for exposure to a specific disease; immunity is limited by the amount of circulating antibody

serum sickness: reaction of a host to injected antibodies or foreign sera; host cells make antibodies to the foreign proteins, and a massive immune reaction can occur

toxoid: inactivated toxin used to prepare toxoid vaccines. A toxoid is no longer toxic but is immunogenic and used to stimulate formation of antibodies

vaccine: immunisation containing weakened or altered protein antigens to stimulate a specific antibody formation against a specific disease; refers to a product used to stimulate active immunity

VACCINES

Bacterial vaccines

BCG (tuberculosis) vaccine

Coxiella burnetii (Q fever) vaccine

Haemophilus B conjugate vaccine

Neisseria meningitidis (meningococcal) vaccine

pneumococcal vaccine

Salmonella typhi (typhoid) vaccine

Toxoids

diphtheria and tetanus toxoid

diphtheria and tetanus toxoid and pertussis vaccine

diphtheria and tetanus toxoid, and pertussis and poliomyelitis vaccine

diphtheria and tetanus toxoid, and hepatitis B, pertussis, poliomyelitis and *Haemophilus influenzae* vaccine

Viral vaccines

H1N1 pandemic influenza vaccine

hepatitis A vaccine, inactivated

hepatitis A vaccine, inactivated, with hepatitis B recombinant vaccine

hepatitis B vaccine

human papillomavirus recombinant vaccine

influenza virus vaccine

Japanese encephalitis vaccine

 measles, mumps, rubella vaccine

poliomyelitis vaccine

rabies vaccine

rotavirus vaccine, live, oral

varicella–zoster vaccine, live attenuated

vibrio cholerae vaccine-cholera toxin B

yellow fever vaccine

IMMUNE SERA

antithymocyte globulin

cytomegalovirus immunoglobulin

hepatitis B immunoglobulin

Ⓟ immunoglobulin, normal (human)

rabies immunoglobulin

tetanus immunoglobulin

zoster immunoglobulin

ANTITOXINS AND ANTIVENINS

black snake antivenom

box jellyfish antivenom

brown snake antivenom

death adder antivenom

funnel web spider antivenom

polyvalent snake antivenom

red back spider antivenom

sea snake antivenom

stonefish antivenom

taipan antivenom

tiger snake antivenom

Vaccines and immune sera, including antivenins and antitoxins, are usually referred to as **biologicals**. They are used to stimulate the production of antibodies, to provide preformed antibodies to facilitate an immune reaction, or to react specifically with the toxins produced by an invading pathogen or venins injected by poisonous snakes or spiders. Stimulating the production of antibodies to specific antigens with vaccines provides the person with immunity to that antigen. Vaccines are frequently called immunisations because they stimulate immunity. Many diseases that were once devastating or fatal can now be prevented by stimulating an immune response and the development of antibodies without the need for the person to actually contract the disease. Prudent, prophylactic medical care requires the routine administration of certain vaccines to prevent diseases. The immune sera provide treatments for specific antigens, toxins or venins. They are used after exposure to antigens or toxins or after bites from poisonous snakes or spiders to make diseases less invasive and aggressive or to prevent clinical problems from developing at all. Box 18.1 discusses the use of biologicals among various age groups.

IMMUNITY

Immunity is a state of relative resistance to a disease that develops after exposure to the specific disease-causing agent. People are not born with immunity to diseases, so they must acquire immunity by stimulating B-cell clones to form plasma cells and then antibodies.

Active immunity occurs when the body recognises a foreign protein and begins producing antibodies to react with that specific protein or antigen. After plasma cells are formed to produce antibodies, specific memory cells that produce the same antibodies are created. If the specific foreign protein is introduced into the body again, these memory cells react immediately to release antibodies. This type of immunity is thought to be lifelong.

Passive immunity occurs when preformed antibodies are injected into the system and react with a specific antigen. These antibodies come from animals that have been infected with the disease or from humans who have had the disease and have developed antibodies. The circulating antibodies act in the same manner as those produced from plasma cells, recognising the foreign protein and attaching to it, rendering it harmless. Unlike active immunity, passive immunity is limited. It lasts only as long as the circulating antibodies last because the body does not produce its own antibodies.

In some cases, the host human responds to the circulating injected antibodies, which are foreign proteins to the host's body, by producing its own antibodies to the injected antibodies. This results in **serum sickness**, a massive immune reaction manifested by fever, arthritis, flank pain, myalgia and arthralgia.

IMMUNISATION

Immunisation is the process of artificially stimulating active immunity by exposing the body to weakened

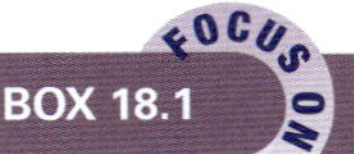

BOX 18.1 Drug therapy across the lifespan

Biologicals

CHILDREN

Routine immunisation for children has become a standard of care in Australia and New Zealand. Parents should receive written records of immunisations given to their children to assure continuity of care. The parent should be asked to report adverse reactions to any immunisation. Sensitive children may receive divided doses of their immunisations to help prevent adverse reactions.

Simple comfort measures – warm soaks at the injection site, paracetamol to reduce fever or aches and pains, comfort from parents or carers – will help the child to deal with the immunisation experience.

Parent education is a very important aspect of the immunisation procedure. Parents may need reassurance and educational materials when concerns about the safety of immunisations arise.

Immune sera are used for specific exposures.

ADULTS

There are a number of reasons why adults should receive certain immunisations. For example, adults who are travelling to areas with high risk for particular diseases – and who may not have previously been exposed to those diseases – are advised to be immunised.

In addition, adults with chronic diseases are advised to be immunised yearly with an influenza vaccine and once with a pneumococcal pneumonia vaccine. These vaccines provide some protection against diseases that can prove dangerous for people with chronic lung, cardiovascular or endocrine disorders. The influenza vaccine changes yearly, depending on predictions of which flu strain might be emergent in that year. The pneumonia vaccine contains 23 strains and is believed to offer lifetime protection.

Tetanus shots also are recommended for adults every 10 years or with any injury that potentially could precipitate a tetanus infection.

Immune sera are used for specific exposures.

OLDER ADULTS

Older people are at greater risk for severe illness from influenza and pneumococcal infections. The yearly flu injection, routine varicella–zoster vaccine, and the pneumococcal vaccine every 5 years should be stressed for this group.

A tetanus booster every 10 years will also help to protect older adults from exposure to that illness. Ask the person about any adverse reaction to previous tetanus boosters and weigh the risk against the possible exposure to tetanus.

Immune sera are used for specific exposures. Older adults are at increased risk for severe reactions and should be monitored closely.

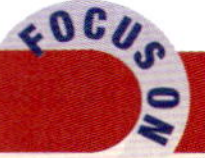

Safe medication administration

Use of allergenic extracts

Many people receive 'allergy shots' or injections of allergenic extracts. These extracts contain various antigens based on specific standardisations. The exact action of these extracts is not completely understood, but it has been shown that, after injection, specific immunoglobulin G (IgG) antibodies appear in the serum. These antibodies compete with IgE for the receptor site on a specific antigen that is the cause of the allergy (IgE is the immune globulin that is associated with allergic reactions; these antibodies react with mast cells, causing the release of histamine and other inflammatory chemicals when they have combined with the antigen). After repeated exposure to the antigens, the levels of IgG antibodies increase and the circulating levels of IgE seem to decrease, leading to less allergic response. It may take 4–6 months of subcutaneous (SC) injections of the allergenic extract every 3–4 days to achieve relief from the symptoms of the allergic reaction. The IgG levels remain high for weeks or sometimes months, but the individual response varies widely. Many people are maintained with a weekly injection once the desired response has been achieved.

or less toxic proteins associated with specific disease-causing organisms. The proteins could be a weakened bacterial cell membrane, the protein coat of a virus or a virus (protein coat with the genetic fragment that makes up the virus) that has been chemically weakened so that it cannot cause disease. The goal is to cause an immune response without having the individual suffer the full course of a disease. Adults may require immunisations in certain situations: exposure, travel to an area endemic for a disease they have not had and have not been immunised against, and occupations that are considered high risk. Children are routinely immunised against many infections that were once quite devastating. For example, smallpox was one of the first diseases against which children were immunised. Today, smallpox is considered to be eradicated worldwide. Concerns over biological terrorism have renewed interest in this disease, and smallpox vaccine is now available for people who might be at high risk for exposure to a potential attack by terrorists.

Diphtheria, pertussis, tetanus, *Haemophilus influenzae* B, hepatitis B, hepatitis A, chickenpox, poliovirus, meningitis, measles, mumps and rubella are all standard childhood immunisations today (see Figures 18.1 and 18.2). The bacille Calmette-Guérin (BCG) vaccine for tuberculosis is widely used throughout the world in countries with a high incidence of tuberculosis to limit the spread of the disease. However, it is not routinely used in Australia because the incidence of tuberculosis is relatively low and it can induce false-positive tuberculin skin test results. The human papillomavirus (HPV) vaccine is now recommended for girls to protect against several of the viruses that cause many cervical cancers.

The use of vaccines is not without controversy. Severe reactions, although rare, have occurred, resulting in concerns about the safety of vaccines and their administration, especially in children (Boxes 18.2 and 18.3). The central reporting of adverse effects or suspected adverse effects may help to clarify concerns about reactions to immunisations.

Antigens are also processed and injected to help some people who have severe allergic reactions. People who receive allergy shots to help them cope with the signs and symptoms of allergic reactions receive antigenic proteins that stimulate antibody production to

National Immunisation Program Schedule
From 1 April 2019

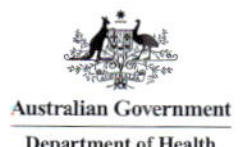

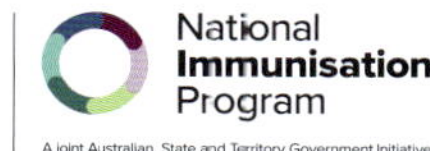

Age	Disease	Vaccine Brand
Childhood vaccination (also see influenza vaccine)		
Birth	• Hepatitis B (usually offered in hospital)[a]	H-B-Vax® II Paediatric or Engerix B® Paediatric
2 months Can be given from 6 weeks of age	• Diphtheria, tetanus, pertussis (whooping cough), hepatitis B, polio, *Haemophilus influenzae* type b (Hib) • Pneumococcal • Rotavirus[b]	Infanrix® hexa Prevenar 13® Rotarix®
4 months	• Diphtheria, tetanus, pertussis (whooping cough), hepatitis B, polio, *Haemophilus influenzae* type b (Hib) • Pneumococcal • Rotavirus[b]	Infanrix® hexa Prevenar 13® Rotarix®
6 months	• Diphtheria, tetanus, pertussis (whooping cough), hepatitis B, polio, *Haemophilus influenzae* type b (Hib)	Infanrix® hexa
Additional vaccines for Aboriginal and Torres Strait Islander children (QLD, NT, WA and SA) and medically at-risk children[c]	• Pneumococcal	Prevenar 13®
12 months	• Meningococcal ACWY • Measles, mumps, rubella • Pneumococcal	Nimenrix® M-M-R® II or Priorix® Prevenar 13®
Additional vaccines for Aboriginal and Torres Strait Islander children (QLD, NT, WA and SA)	• Hepatitis A	Vaqta® Paediatric
18 months	• *Haemophilus influenzae* type b (Hib) • Measles, mumps, rubella, varicella (chickenpox) • Diphtheria, tetanus, pertussis (whooping cough)	ActHIB® Priorix-Tetra® or ProQuad® Infanrix® or Tripacel®
Additional vaccines for Aboriginal and Torres Strait Islander children (QLD, NT, WA and SA)	• Hepatitis A	Vaqta® Paediatric
4 years	• Diphtheria, tetanus, pertussis (whooping cough), polio	Infanrix® IPV or Quadracel®
Additional vaccines for medically at-risk children[c]	• Pneumococcal	Pneumovax 23®

FIGURE 18.1 Australian Government Department of Health, National Immunisation Program Schedule.

Department of Health. (2019). *National immunisation program schedule.* (Used with permission of the Australian Government.) Retrieved September 2019 from https://www.health.gov.au/health-topics/immunisation/immunisation-throughout-life/national-immunisation-program-schedule

Continued on following page

National Immunisation Program Schedule

From 1 April 2019

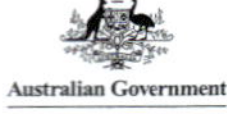

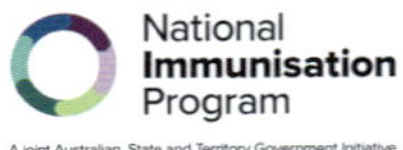

Age	Disease	Vaccine brand
Adolescent vaccination (also see influenza vaccine)		
12–<13 years (School programs[d])	• Human papillomavirus (HPV)[e] • Diphtheria, tetanus, pertussis (whooping cough)	Gardasil®9 Boostrix®
14–<16 years (School programs[d])	• Meningococcal ACWY	Nimenrix®
Adult vaccination (also see influenza vaccine)		
15–49 years Aboriginal and Torres Strait Islander people with medical risk factors[c]	• Pneumococcal	Pneumovax 23®
50 years and over Aboriginal and Torres Strait Islander people	• Pneumococcal	Pneumovax 23®
65 years and over	• Pneumococcal	Pneumovax 23®
70–79 years[f]	• Shingles (herpes zoster)	Zostavax®
Pregnant women	• Pertussis (whooping cough)[g] • Influenza[h]	Boostrix® or Adacel®

Funded annual influenza vaccination[h]
6 months and over with certain medical risk factors[c]
All Aboriginal and Torres Strait Islander people 6 months and over
65 years and over
Pregnant women

a Hepatitis B vaccine: should be given to all infants as soon as practicable after birth. The greatest benefit is if given within 24 hours, and must be given within 7 days.
b Rotavirus vaccine: first dose must be given by 14 weeks of age, the second dose by 24 weeks of age.
c Refer to the current edition of *The Australian Immunisation Handbook* for all medical risk factors.
d Contact your state or territory health service for school grades eligible for vaccination.
e Observe Gardasil®9 dosing schedules by age and at-risk conditions. 2 doses: 9 to < 15 years – 6 months mininimum interval. 3 doses: ≥ 15 years and/or have certain medical conditions – 0, 2 and 6 month schedule. Only 2 doses funded on the NIP unless 12–13 year old has certain medical risk factors.
f All people aged 70 years old, with a five year catch-up program for people aged 71–79 years old until 31 October 2021.
g Single dose recommended each pregnancy, ideally between 20–32 weeks, but may be given up until delivery.
h Refer to annual influenza information for recommended vaccine brand for age.

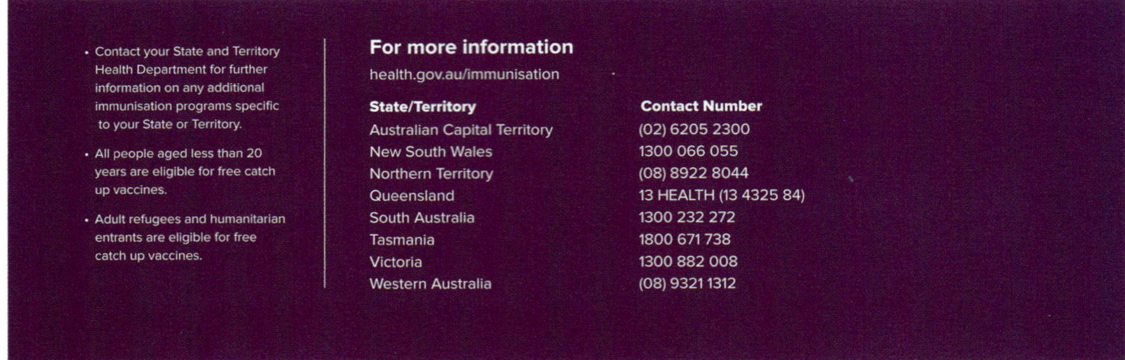

FIGURE 18.1 Australian Government Department of Health, National Immunisation Program Schedule *(continued)*.

National Immunisation Schedule

Antigen(s)	DTaP-IPV-HepB/Hib	PCV10	RV1	MMR	Hib	VV	DTaP-IPV	Tdap	HPV9	Td	Influenza	HZV
Brand name	**Infanrix-hexa**	**Synflorix**	**Rotarix**	**Priorix**	**Hiberix**	**Varilrix**	**Infanrix-IPV**	**Boostrix**	**Gardasil 9**	**ADT Booster**	**Influvac Tetra**	**Zostavax**
Pregnancy								Tdap			Influenza	
6 weeks	DTaP-IPV-HepB/Hib	PCV10	RV1									
3 months	DTaP-IPV-HepB/Hib	PCV10	RV1									
5 months	DTaP-IPV-HepB/Hib	PCV10										
15 months		PCV10		MMR	Hib	VV						
4 years				MMR			DTaP-IPV					
11 or 12 years								Tdap	HPV9 (2 doses)			
45 years										Td		
65 years										Td	Influenza (annually)	HZV

Key:

D = diphtheria; T = tetanus; aP = acellular pertussis; IPV = inactivated polio vaccine; HepB = hepatitis B; Hib = *Haemophilus influenzae* type b; PCV10 = 10-valent pneumococcal conjugate vaccine; RV1 = rotavirus vaccine (monovalent); MMR = measles, mumps and rubella; VV = varicella vaccine; d = adult diphtheria; ap = adult acellular pertussis; HPV9 = human papillomavirus (9 serotypes); HZV = herpes zoster vaccine.

FIGURE 18.2 National Schedule of Immunisation for New Zealand.

New Zealand Ministry of Health. (2018). National Immunisation Schedule. Page 696 in New Zealand Ministry of Health. (2018). *Immunisation Handbook* (2nd ed.). Retrieved August 2019 from https://www.health.govt.nz/system/files/documents/publications/immunisation-handbook-2017-2nd-edition-mar18-v4.pdf

BOX 18.2 FOCUS ON **Individual teaching**

Paediatric immunisation

It is well-documented that by preventing potentially devastating diseases, society prevents unneeded suffering and death, and saves valuable citizens for the future. Paediatric immunisation has helped to greatly decrease the incidence of most childhood diseases and has prevented associated complications. In Australia and New Zealand, routine immunisation is considered standard medical practice.

Ensuring that every child has the opportunity to receive the recommended immunisations has become a political as well as a social issue. The cost of preventing a disease that most people have never even seen may be difficult to justify to families who have trouble putting food on the table. Widespread campaigns to provide free immunisations and health screening to all children have addressed this problem but have not been totally successful.

In addition, periodic reports of severe or even fatal reactions to standard immunisations alarm many parents about the risks of immunisations. These parents need facts as well as reassurance about modern efforts to prevent and screen for these reactions.

Public education efforts should be directed at providing parents with information about paediatric immunisation and encouraging them to act on that information. Nurses and midwives are often in the ideal position to provide this information, during prenatal visits, while screening for other problems, or even standing in line at the supermarket. It is important for nurses and midwives to be well versed on the need for standard immunisations and screening to prevent severe reactions. The Australian Department of Health (www.immunise.health.gov.au) and New Zealand Ministry of Health (www.health.govt.nz/our-work/preventative-health-wellness/immunisation/new-zealand-immunisation-schedule) offer current information and updates for health care providers, as well as teaching materials that can be printed for easy reference.

prevent the allergic response by stimulating production of another antibody in the body.

VACCINES

The word **vaccine** comes from the Latin word for smallpox, *vaccinia*. Vaccines are immunisations containing weakened or altered protein antigens that stimulate the formation of antibodies against a specific disease (Figure 18.3). They are used to promote active immunity (see Table 18.1).

Vaccines can be made from chemically inactivated microorganisms or from live, weakened viruses or bacteria. Toxoids are vaccines that are made from the toxins produced by the microorganism. The toxins are altered so that they are no longer poisonous but still

BOX 18.3 FOCUS ON The evidence

Studies find no link between measles–mumps–rubella (MMR) vaccine and autism

There have been theories circulated in the mass media that MMR vaccine has been linked to the development of autism. This has influenced many parents to choose not to immunise their children, with detrimental outcomes. The Australian Government Department of Health suggests that this has resulted from one study that has since been retracted due to questionable data. From time to time, there have been other myths surrounding different vaccines and these have the potential to lead to unnecessary harm.

Nurses and midwives have a responsibility to be informed about vaccine safety and to be able to educate parents on factors associated with vaccinations.

Source: Australian Government Department of Health and Ageing. (2013). *Myths and Realities: Responding to Arguments against Vaccination – A Guide for Providers* (5th edn). Canberra: Author.

See also https://www.hccc.nsw.gov.au/Publications/Media-releases/2018/Public-Warning—Misleading-and-Unsafe-Practices-by-Anti-Vaccination-Campaigners

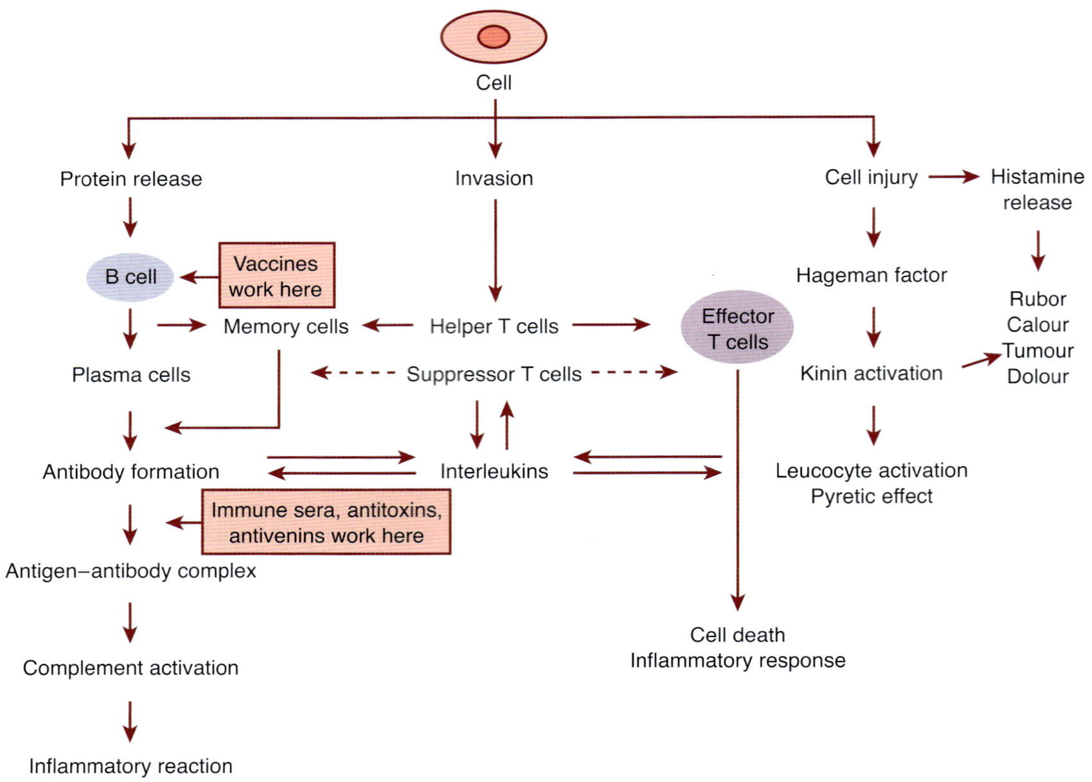

FIGURE 18.3 Sites of action of biologicals.

TABLE 18.1 DRUGS IN FOCUS Vaccines

Drug name	Dosage/route	Usual indications
Bacterial vaccines		
BCG vaccine (OncoTICE [NZ only])	Vaccine: 0.1 mL intradermally Urothelial cell carcinoma of the bladder: OncoTICE for intravesical administration 1 vial once weekly for 6 weeks	Prevention of tuberculosis Urothelial cell carcinoma of the bladder
Coxiella burnetii vaccine (*Q-vax*)	0.5 mL SC	Prevention of Q fever
Haemophilus B conjugate vaccine (*Hiberix*)	0.5 mL IM at 2, 4, 6 and 12 months	Active immunisation against *Haemophilus influenzae* type b

TABLE 18.1 DRUGS IN FOCUS Vaccines *(continued)*

Drug name	Dosage/route	Usual indications
Bacterial vaccines *(continued)*		
Neisseria meningitidis vaccine (*Bexsero, Menactra, Menitorix, Menveo, NeisVacC, Nimenrix, Trumenba*)	Adult and paediatric > 2 years: 0.5 mL SC	Active immunisation against meningococcal meningitis groups A, C, W_{135}, Y
pneumococcal vaccine (*Pneumovax 23, Prevenar*)	*Pneumovax 23*: adult and paediatric > 2 years: 0.5 mL SC or IM *Prevenar*: paediatric 6 weeks–6 months: 0.5 mL IM at 2, 4, 6 months and 12–15 months	Active immunisation against *Streptococcus pneumoniae* disease
Salmonella typhi vaccine (*Typhim Vi, Vivaxim, Vivotif*)	*Typherix, Typhim Vi*: adult and paediatric > 2 years: 0.5 mL slow IM into deltoid at least 14 days before exposure *Vivotif*: adult and paediatric > 6 years: 1 capsule swallowed on days 1, 3 and 5. Booster every 3 years	Active immunisation against typhoid fever
Toxoids		
diphtheria and tetanus toxoid (*ADT Booster*)	0.5 mL intramuscular injection (IMI)	Reimmunisation in adults and children > 5 years
diphtheria and tetanus toxoid and pertussis vaccine (*Adacel, Boostrix*)	0.5 mL deep IMI	Immunisation in adults and children > 10 years
diphtheria and tetanus toxoid and pertussis vaccine (*Tripacel*)	0.5 mL IMI at 2, 4, 6, 18 months and booster 4–6 years	Primary immunisation children 6 weeks or older
diphtheria and tetanus toxoid, pertussis and poliomyelitis vaccine (*Adacel Polio, Boostrix-IPV, Quadracel*)	0.5 mL deep IMI	Booster immunisation in adults or children > 4 years
diphtheria and tetanus toxoid, pertussis and poliomyelitis vaccine (*Infanrix IPV*)	0.5 mL by deep IMI	Primary immunisation in children 6 weeks or older
diphtheria and tetanus toxoid, and hepatitis B, pertussis, poliomyelitis and *Haemophilus influenzae* vaccine (*Infanrix Hexa*)	0.5 mL IM at 2, 4, 6 months	Primary immunisation in children 6 weeks or older
Viral vaccines		
H1N1 pandemic influenza vaccine (*Vapacel*)	Adult: 0.5 mL IM, repeated after 3 weeks	Active immunisation against H1N1 influenza
hepatitis A vaccine, inactivated (*Avaxim, Havrix, VAQTA*)	Adult: 1 mL IM with a booster dose in 6–12 months Paediatric: 0.5 mL IM with a repeat dose in 6–12 months	Immunisation of adults and children against hepatitis A infection
hepatitis A vaccine, inactivated, with hepatitis B recombinant vaccine (*Twinrix*)	1 mL IM followed by booster doses at 1 and 6 months	Immunisation against hepatitis A and hepatitis B infections in people ≥ 18 years of age
hepatitis B vaccine (*Energix-B, H-B-Vax II*)	0.5–1 mL IM, followed by 0.5–1 mL IM at 1 and 6 months	Immunisation against hepatitis B infections in susceptible people and in infants born to mothers with hepatitis B
human papillomavirus, recombinant, quadrivalent (*Cervarix, Gardasil, Gardasil 9*)	Cervarix: females 10–45 years: 0.5 mL IM given at 0, 1, 6 months (total of 3 doses) Gardasil and Gardasil 9: females 9–26 years: 0.5 mL IM at 0, 2, 6 months (total of 3 doses)	Active immunisation against human papillomavirus responsible for causing genital warts and many cervical cancers

Continued on following page

TABLE 18.1 DRUGS IN FOCUS Vaccines *(continued)*

Drug name	Dosage/route	Usual indications
Viral vaccines *(continued)*		
influenza virus vaccine (*Afluria, Fluarix, FluQuadri, Fluvax, Influvac*)	Adult: 0.5 mL IM or deep SC Paediatric: *Afluria,* children from 5–9 years: 0.5 mL IM or deep SC, repeated in 4 weeks *Fluarix,* children from 6 months–9 years 0.25–0.5 mL IM or deep SC, repeated in 4 weeks *FluQuadri:* children aged 6 months–35 months, 0.25 mL dose; children and adults 3 years of age and older, 0.5 mL dose, IM, repeated in 4 weeks *Infuvac:* children > 3 years, 0.5 mL IM or deep SC; children < 9 years who have not previously been vaccinated, a second dose of 0.5 mL in 4 weeks	Prophylaxis in adults and children at high risk for complications of influenza infections
Japanese encephalitis vaccine (*Imojev, Jespect*)	*Jespect,* adults: 0.5 mL IM, repeated at 28 days *Imojev,* 1 mL SC on days 0, 7 and 30 1–3 years: 0.5 mL SC on days 0, 7 and 30 in children 9 months and over: 0.5 mL IM, repeated after 12 months in children 9–17 years, and after 5 years in adults	Immunisation of persons > 1 year of age who reside in, or will travel to, endemic areas
(P) measles, mumps, rubella vaccine (*Priorix*)	0.5 mL SC or IM Adult: single dose Paediatric: dose at 1 year with booster 4–6 years	Immunisation against measles, mumps and rubella in adults and children > 15 months of age
poliomyelitis vaccine, inactivated (*Ipol*)	0.5 mL SC × 3 doses 8 weeks apart, and 4th dose 12 months after the 3rd	Immunisation against polio infections in adults and children
rabies vaccine (*Merieux, Rabipur*)	*Rabipur,* pre-exposure: 1 mL IM on days 0, 7, 21 or and 28; postexposure: 1 mL IM on days 0, 3, 7, 14, 28 *Merieux,* pre-exposure: 1 mL IM or deep SC on days 0, 7, 28; postexposure: 1 mL IM or deep SC on days 0, 3, 7, and 14, 30, 90	Pre-exposure immunisation against rabies for high-risk people; postexposure antirabies regimen with rabies immune globulin
rotavirus vaccine, live, oral pentavalent (*RotaTeq, Rotarix*)	Three doses of 2 mL PO starting at age 6–12 weeks, with subsequent doses at 4–10-week intervals (third dose should be given at 32 weeks)	Prevention of rotavirus gastroenteritis in infants and children
varicella–zoster vaccine (*Zostavax Varilrix*)	*Zostavax*: adult > 60 years: 0.65 mL SC injection *Varilrix*: adult and paediatric > 9 months: 0.5 mL SC with another 0.5 mL SC 6 weeks later	Prevention of herpes zoster (shingles and chicken pox) infection
vibrio cholerae vaccine–cholera toxin B (*Dukoral*)	Dissolve the effervescent granules in approximately 150 mL of cool water to make the buffer solution. Shake the vaccine vial gently and add the contents to the buffer solution. Adult and paediatric > 6 years: 1 dose PO × 2 doses at least 1 week apart Paediatric 2–6 years: pour half the amount of buffer solution away and mix the remaining part (approx. 75 mL) with the entire contents of the vaccine vial, then give 3 doses PO at least 1 week apart	Active immunisation against cholera
yellow fever vaccine (*Stamaril*)	Adult and paediatric > 9 months: 0.5 mL SC or IM. Booster every 10 years	Immunisation of travellers to areas where yellow fever is endemic H1N1 pandemic influenza vaccine is available in New Zealand (as *Vapacel*), but not Australia

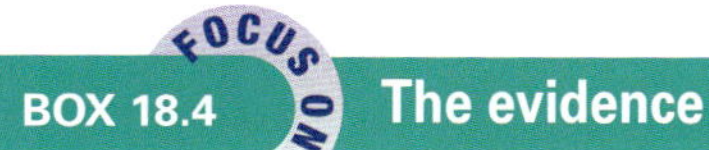

BOX 18.4 The evidence

Vaccine to protect against cervical cancer

In 2006, the Australian Therapeutic Goods Administration (TGA) approved the first vaccine to protect against cancer caused by a virus. The human papillomavirus (HPV) is one of the most common sexually transmitted infections in Australia and New Zealand. Most of the time, the body's defence system will clear the virus, but some types of HPV can be more virulent. There are many types of HPV; some cause genital warts, and others are known to cause abnormal cells on the lining of the cervix, which can lead to cervical cancer years later.

The vaccine Gardasil is effective against HPV types 16 and 18 (which account for 70% of cervical cancers) and against types 6 and 11 (which are responsible for 90% of genital warts). Gardasil 9 protects against 9 HPV types. The vaccine is recommended for girls and women aged 9–26 years. Studies have shown that it is only effective if it is given before HPV infection occurs, so it is best given before the girl or woman becomes sexually active. The vaccine is given as a series of three injections. The second injection given about 2 months after the first, and the last injection given about 6 months later. Tests are being done to evaluate the effectiveness of the vaccine in males and to monitor the long-term effectiveness of the vaccine. It is not yet known whether a booster injection will be needed later and what would be its effects if given inadvertently to a pregnant woman. Side effects that have been reported include the usual flu-like symptoms seen with immunisation and pain at the injection site. In Australia, from February 2013, both males and females aged 12–13 years will receive the HPV vaccine, while a catch-up program for males aged 14–15 years is to be completed by the end of 2014.

This is the first vaccine to protect against cancer, and it is hoped that more such vaccines will be developed in the future. The willingness of parents to listen to the pros and cons and accept the need for this vaccine will have a big impact on the success of this and other such vaccines.

have the recognisable protein antigen that will stimulate antibody production.

The particular vaccine that is used depends on the possible exposure a person will have to a particular disease and the age of the person. Some vaccines are used only in children and some cannot be used in infants. Some vaccines require booster doses – doses that are given a few months after the initial dose to further stimulate antibody production. For example, Box 18.4 discusses the human papillomavirus (HPV) vaccine, which protects young women from many cervical cancers. This vaccine is given in a series of three injections to achieve full protection. In many cases, antibody titres (levels of the antibody in the serum) can be used to evaluate a person's response to an immunisation and determine the need for a booster dose.

Due to recent events and the fear of terrorist activities, concern has risen about the use of various diseases as biological weapons. Box 18.5 discusses vaccines and the use of biological weapons.

Therapeutic actions and indications

Vaccines stimulate active immunity in people who are at high risk for development of a particular disease. The vaccine needed for a person depends on the exposure that person will have to the pathogen. Exposure is usually determined by where the person lives and their travel plans, and work or family environment exposures. Vaccines are thought to provide lifelong immunity to the disease against which the individual is being immunised. Table 18.1 lists the various vaccines available along with usual indications.

Pharmacokinetics

There is no pharmacokinetic information on these biologicals, which are treated like endogenous antibodies in the body.

Contraindications and cautions

The use of vaccines is contraindicated in the presence of immune deficiency *because the vaccine could cause disease, and the body would not be able to respond as anticipated if it is in an immunodeficient state*; during pregnancy *because of potential effects on the fetus and on the success of the pregnancy*; in individuals with known allergies to any of the components of the vaccine (refer to each individual vaccine for specifics, sometimes including eggs, where some pathogens are cultured); or in people who are receiving immune globulin or have received blood or blood products within the last 3 months *because a serious immune reaction could occur.*

Caution should be used whenever a vaccine is given to a child with a history of febrile convulsions or cerebral injury, or in any condition in which a potential fever would be dangerous. Caution also should be used in the presence of any acute infection.

Adverse effects

Adverse effects of vaccines are associated with the immune or inflammatory reaction that is being stimulated: moderate fever, rash, malaise, chills, fretfulness, drowsiness, anorexia, vomiting and irritability. Pain, redness, swelling and even nodule formation at the injection site are also common. In rare instances, severe hypersensitivity reactions have been reported.

Clinically important drug–drug interactions

Vaccines should not be given with any immunosuppressant drugs, including corticosteroids, which could alter the body's response to the vaccine.

BOX 18.5 Vaccines and biological weapons

The events of September 11 2001 and the subsequent war on terrorism have heightened awareness of several diseases that might be in development as biological weapons. Anthrax, plague, tularaemia, smallpox, botulism and a variety of viral haemorrhagic fevers are all considered to be likely biological warfare weapons.

Anthrax

An imported vaccine is available in Australia made from inactivated cell-free filtrate of a virulent strain of the anthrax bacillus. It is available only for military use. Active production stopped in 1998, but production and supply issues were made high priorities. Ciprofloxacin and, in sensitive cases, doxycycline and penicillins are effective in treating postexposure cases. The vaccine is given and repeated in 2 and 4 weeks, along with the appropriate antibiotic, to people who have been exposed.

Plague

Plague is easily spread from person to person, and without treatment can progress rapidly to respiratory failure and death. There is currently no vaccine for plague; a whole-cell vaccine that was used for many years is no longer available. Research is ongoing using a pneumonic plague vaccine that has successfully protected animals. Several drugs have been found to be life-saving with plague – streptomycin, doxycycline, ciprofloxacin and chloramphenicol.

Smallpox

Smallpox was considered eradicated since no new cases had been seen in 20 years. Smallpox is highly transmissible and has a 30% mortality rate in unvaccinated people. Immunisation against smallpox ended in the 1970s. There is now a commercially available vaccine, but use is somewhat limited because of questions raised during studies of the vaccine. It is given to military personnel and people thought to be at high risk. It is currently thought that the vaccine is no longer effective after 20 years, although there is no definite evidence that previously vaccinated people have no protection. The smallpox vaccine uses live virus, placed in punctures made in the skin. After exposure, vaccination given within the first 3–4 days can prevent the disease. If it has been 7 days or longer since exposure, the vaccine and a vaccinia immune globulin should be used, if any are available. So far no drugs are thought to be effective in treating smallpox. Early studies have, however, shown cidofovir (*Vistide*) to be effective in vitro.

Tularaemia

Tularaemia in an aerosolised form can cause systemic and respiratory illness with a 35% mortality rate. It is not passed from person to person. There is no vaccine available, but doxycycline and ciprofloxacin can be used after exposure, and gentamicin has been effective after symptoms appear.

Botulism

Botulism, produced by *Clostridium botulinum*, can be aerosolised or used to contaminate food. The toxin it produces causes cranial nerve palsies that can result in muscle paralysis and respiratory failure. Antitoxin is also available for people with specific exposures, and research is ongoing with an equine antitoxin effective against all seven serotypes of botulism that is thought to cause fewer hypersensitivity reactions than what is currently available.

Viral haemorrhagic fever

Lassa, Marburg, Junin and Ebola viruses cause haemorrhagic fevers with mortality rates as high as 90%. No vaccines are currently available for these agents, although the United States Army has had success with a vaccine for Junin. Ribavirin has been effective in some cases of Lassa fever and has been effective orally for postexposure prophylaxis. It is being studied for effectiveness with these other viruses. Currently there is no established treatment and this area is one of the highest priorities for combating possible biological warfare.

Care considerations for people receiving vaccines

Assessment: history and examination

- Assess for contraindications or cautions: known allergies to any vaccines or to the components of the one being used *to prevent hypersensitivity reactions*; current status related to pregnancy, *which is a contraindication to the use of vaccines*; recent administration of immune globulin or blood products, *which could alter the response to the vaccine*; history of immune deficiency, *which could alter immune reactions*; and evidence of acute infection, *which could be exacerbated by the introduction of other antigens*.
- Perform a physical assessment *to determine baseline status before beginning therapy and for any potential adverse effects*: inspect for the presence of any skin lesions *to monitor for hypersensitivity reactions*; check temperature *to monitor for possible infection*; monitor pulse, respirations and blood pressure; auscultate lungs for adventitious sounds; and assess level of orientation and affect *to monitor for hypersensitivity reactions to the vaccine*.

- Evaluate the range of motion of the extremity to be used for vaccine administration *to assure adequate blood flow to deal with the antigen and inflammatory reaction.*
- Assess tissue perfusion to establish a baseline *to monitor for potential hypersensitivity reactions.*

Implementation with rationale

- Do not use to treat acute infection; *a vaccine is used to prevent infection with future exposures.*
- Do not administer if the person exhibits signs of acute infection or immune deficiency *because the vaccine can cause a mild infection and can exacerbate acute infections.*
- Do not administer if the individual has received blood, blood products or immune globulin within the last 3 months *because a severe immune reaction could occur.*
- Arrange for proper preparation and administration of the vaccine; check on the timing and dose of each injection *because dose, preparation and timing vary with individual vaccines.*
- Maintain emergency equipment on standby, including adrenaline (epinephrine), *in case of severe hypersensitivity reaction.*
- Arrange for supportive care and comfort measures for flu-like symptoms (rest, environmental control, paracetamol) and for injection discomfort (local heat application, anti-inflammatories, resting arm) *to promote comfort.*
- Do not administer aspirin to children to treat discomforts associated with immunisation. *Aspirin can mask warning signs of Reye syndrome, a potentially serious disease.*
- Provide thorough teaching, including measures to avoid adverse effects, warning signs of problems and the need to keep a written record of immunisations, *to increase knowledge about drug therapy and to increase compliance with the drug regimen.*
- Provide a written record of the immunisation, including the need to return for booster immunisations and timing of the boosters, if necessary, *to increase compliance with medical regimens.*

Evaluation

- Monitor response to the drug (prevention of disease, appropriate antibody titre levels).
- Monitor for adverse effects (flu-like symptoms; GI upset; local pain, swelling, nodule formation at the injection site).
- Evaluate the effectiveness of the teaching plan (person can name drug, dosage, adverse effects to watch for; has written record of immunisations; can state when to return for the next immunisation or booster if needed).
- Monitor the effectiveness of comfort measures and adherence to the regimen.

See Critical thinking scenario for additional information on educating a parent about vaccines.

KEY POINTS

- Immunity is a state of relative resistance to a disease that develops only after exposure to the specific disease-causing agent.
- Vaccines provide active immunity by stimulating the production of antibodies to a specific protein, which may produce the signs and symptoms of a mild immune reaction but protects the person from the more devastating effects of disease.

Prototype summary: measles, mumps and rubella vaccine

Indications: active immunisation against measles, mumps, and rubella in children older than 15 months and adults.

Actions: attenuated measles, mumps and rubella viruses produce a modified infection and stimulate an active immune reaction with the production of antibodies to these viruses.

Pharmacokinetics:

Route	Onset	Peak
IM	Rapid	3–12 hours

$T_{1/2}$: unknown; metabolised in the tissues, excretion is unknown.

Adverse effects: moderate fever, rash, or burning or stinging wheal or flare at the site of injection; rarely, febrile convulsions and high fever; Guillain–Barré syndrome, ocular palsies.

IMMUNE SERA

As explained earlier, passive immunity can be achieved by providing preformed antibodies to a specific antigen. These antibodies are found in immune sera, which may contain antibodies to toxins, venins, bacteria, viruses or even red blood cell antigenic factors. The term **immune sera**, or immunoglobulin, is usually used to refer to sera that contain antibodies to specific bacteria or viruses. The term **antitoxin** refers to immune sera that have antibodies to very specific toxins that might be released by invading pathogens. The term **antivenin** is used to refer to immune sera that have antibodies to venom that might

CRITICAL THINKING SCENARIO

Educating a parent about vaccines

THE SITUATION

S.D. is a 25-year-old, first-time mother who has brought her 2-month-old daughter to the maternal and child health centre for a routine evaluation. The baby is found to be healthy, growing well and within normal parameters for her age. At the end of the visit, the nurse prepares to give the baby the first of her routine immunisations. S.D. becomes concerned and expresses fears about paralysis and infant deaths associated with immunisations.

CRITICAL THINKING

What information should S.D. be given about immunisations?

What care interventions would be appropriate at this time?

Think of ways to explain the importance of immunisations to S.D. while supporting her concerns for the welfare of her baby.

How can this experience be incorporated into a teaching plan for S.D. and her baby?

DISCUSSION

S.D. should be reassured before the baby is immunised. The nurse can tell her that in the past, paralysis and infant deaths were reported, but that efforts continue to make the vaccines pure. Careful monitoring of the child and the child's response to each immunisation can help avoid such problems. Reassure S.D. that the immunisations will prevent her daughter from contracting many, sometimes deadly, diseases. Praise S.D.'s efforts for researching information that might affect her baby and for asking questions that could have an impact on her child and her understanding of her care.

The recommended schedule of immunisations should be given to S.D. so that she is aware of what is planned and how the various vaccines are spaced and combined. She should be encouraged to monitor the baby after each injection for fever, chills and flu-like reactions. When she gets home, she can medicate the baby with paracetamol to avert many of these symptoms before they happen. (S.D. should be advised not to give the baby aspirin, which could cover up Reye syndrome, a potentially serious disorder.) S.D. also should be told that the injection site might be sore, swollen and red, but that this will pass in a couple of days. S.D. can ease the baby's discomfort by applying warm soaks to the area for about 10–15 minutes every 2 hours.

S.D. should be encouraged to write down all of the immunisations that the baby has had and to keep this information handy for easy reference. She should also be encouraged to record any adverse effects that occur after each immunisation. If reactions are uncomfortable, it is possible to split doses of future immunisations.

The nurse should give S.D. a chance to vent her concerns and fears. First-time parents may be more anxious than experienced ones when dealing with issues involving a new baby. To alleviate S.D.'s anxiety, the nurse should provide a telephone number that S.D. can call if the baby seems to be having a severe reaction or if S.D. wants to discuss any questions or concerns. She should feel that support is available for any concern that she may have. Because this interaction is likely to form the basis for future interactions with S.D., it is important to establish a sense of respect and trust.

CARE GUIDE FOR S.D.'S BABY: VACCINES

Assessment: history and examination

Allergies to the serum base, acute infection, immunosuppression

General: temperature

CV: pulse, cardiac auscultation, blood pressure, oedema, perfusion

Respiratory: respirations, adventitious sounds

Skin: lesions

Joints: range of motion

Implementation

Ensure proper preparation and administration of vaccine within appropriate time frame.

Provide supportive and comfort measures to deal with adverse effects: anti-inflammatory/antipyretic, local heat application, small meals, rest and a quiet environment.

Provide parent teaching regarding drug name, adverse effects and precautions, and warning signs to report.

Provide emergency life support if needed for acute reaction.

Evaluation

Evaluate drug effects: serum titres reflecting immunisation (if appropriate).

Monitor for adverse effects: pain, flu-like symptoms, local discomfort.

Evaluate effectiveness of parent teaching program.

Evaluate effectiveness of comfort and safety measures.

Evaluate effectiveness of emergency measures if needed.

TEACHING FOR S.D.

- This immunisation will help your baby to develop antibodies to protect her against diphtheria, tetanus and pertussis. The baby will develop antibodies to these diseases, and this will prevent the baby from contracting one of these potentially deadly diseases in the future.
- The injection site might be sore and painful. Heat applied to the area may help this discomfort and speed the baby's recovery.

- Adverse effects that the baby might experience include fever, muscle aches, joint aches, fatigue, malaise, crying and fretfulness. Paracetamol may help these discomforts; check with your health care provider for the correct dose to use for the baby. Rest, small meals and a quiet environment may also help the baby to feel better.
- The adverse effects should pass within 2–3 days. If they seem to be causing undue discomfort or persist longer than a few days, notify your health care provider.
- Booster immunisations are required for this immunisation. Your baby should receive a booster immunisation at your next scheduled checkup. Keep a written record of this immunisation.
- Please contact your health care provider if you have any questions or concerns.

TABLE 18.2 DRUGS IN FOCUS Immune sera

Drug name	Dosage/route	Usual indications
Immune sera		
antithymocyte globulin (*Atgam*)	10–15 mg/kg/day × 14 days, then alternate days for 14 days to total 21 doses in 28 days	Treatment of renal transplant acute rejection in conjunction with immunosuppression
cytomegalovirus immunoglobulin (*CMV Immuno-globulin-VF*)	Prophylaxis: 25,000 U/kg IV 4 days before, 2 days before and the day of surgery Treatment: 50,000 U/kg IV repeated in 4–5 days, then every 10–14 days as needed	Attenuation of primary cytomegalovirus disease after renal transplantation
hepatitis B immunoglobulin (*Hepatitis B Immunoglobulin-VF*)	400 IU deep IM. Babies born to hepatitis B–positive mothers: 100 IU IM at birth	Postexposure prophylaxis against hepatitis B
(P) immunoglobulin, normal (*Intragam P, Octagam* and others)	Dose varies with indication and preparation; always check manufacturer's instructions	Prophylaxis after exposure to hepatitis A, measles, varicella or rubella; bone marrow and other transplants; Kawasaki disease; chronic lymphocytic leukaemia; treatment of people with immunoglobulin deficiency
rabies immunoglobulin (*Imogam Rabies*)	20 IU/kg IM	Protection against rabies in non-immunised people exposed to rabies
tetanus immunoglobulin (generic)	IM preparation: 250–500 IU deep IMI IV preparation: 4000 IU by slow IV infusion	Passive immunisation against tetanus at time of injury
zoster immunoglobulin (*Zoster Immunoglobulin-VF*)	< 10 kg: 125 IU, 10.1–20 kg: 250 IU, 20.1–30 kg: 375 IU, 30.1–40 kg: 500 IU, > 40 kg: 600 IU by deep IMI within 96 hours of exposure	Passive immunisation against varicella–zoster in immunosuppressed people exposed to disease
Antitoxins and antivenins		
black snake antivenom (generic)	18,000 U by slow IV infusion diluted in Hartmann solution or normal saline	Systemic envenoming following bite from king brown or mulga snake
box jellyfish antivenom (generic)	20,000 U by slow IV infusion diluted with Hartmann solution or normal saline	Systemic envenoming or extreme pain following box jellyfish sting, not responding to routine analgesia
brown snake antivenom (generic)	1000 U by slow IV infusion diluted in Hartmann solution or normal saline	Systemic envenoming following bite from snake of genus *Pseudonaja*
death adder antivenom (generic)	6000 U by slow IV infusion diluted in Hartmann solution or normal saline	Systemic envenoming following bite from death adder
Katipo spider (New Zealand)	Use redback spider antivenom 500 units IM (IV for severe or life-threatening envenomation). Up to 3 vials can be administered at 2-hourly intervals	Systemic envenoming after bite from Katipo spider
funnel-web spider antivenom (generic)	2 vials diluted by slow IV injection, simultaneously given with adrenaline (epinephrine). Dose repeated in 15 minutes if required	Systemic envenoming following bite from funnel-web spider

Continued on following page

TABLE 18.2 DRUGS IN FOCUS Immune sera *(continued)*

Drug name	Dosage/route	Usual indications
Antitoxins and antivenins *(continued)*		
polyvalent snake antivenom (generic)	40,000 U by slow IV infusion diluted in Hartmann solution or normal saline	Systemic envenoming following snakebite, where the snake has not been identified. Contains antibodies to king brown, tiger, brown snakes, death adder and taipan. Not used in Victoria or Tasmania
redback spider antivenom (generic)	1 vial (500 IU) IM, or IV diluted in Hartmann solution or normal saline. May be repeated in 2 hours	Systemic envenoming following bite from redback spider
sea snake antivenom (generic)	1000 U by slow IV infusion diluted with Hartmann solution or normal saline	Systemic envenoming following bite from a sea snake
stonefish antivenom (generic)	2000–6000 U IM or IV (diluted in Hartmann solution or normal saline), depending on number of punctures	Systemic envenoming following bite from stonefish, with severe oedema and pain not responsive to first aid
taipan antivenom (generic)	12,000 U by slow IV diluted in Hartmann solution or normal saline	Systemic envenoming following bite from taipan
tiger snake antivenom (generic)	3000 U by slow IV diluted in Hartmann solution or normal saline	Systemic envenoming following bite from tiger, copper head or black snake

be injected through spider or snake bites. These drugs are used to provide early treatment following exposure to known antigens. They are very specific for antigens to which they can respond (see Table 18.2).

Therapeutic actions and indications

Immune sera are used to provide passive immunity to a specific antigen, which could be a pathogen, venom or toxin. They may also be used as prophylaxis against specific diseases after exposure in individuals who are immunosuppressed. In addition, immune sera may be used to lessen the severity of a disease after known or suspected exposure (see Figure 18.3 for sites of action of immune sera and antitoxins). Table 18.2 lists the various available immune sera, antitoxins and antivenins, as well as usual indications.

Pharmacokinetics

No pharmacokinetic data are available for these biologicals.

Contraindications and cautions

Immune sera are contraindicated in individuals with a history of severe reaction to any immune sera or to products similar to the components of the sera *to prevent potential serious hypersensitivity reactions*. They should be used with caution during pregnancy *because of potential risk to the fetus*; with coagulation defects or thrombocytopenia; or in individuals with a known history of previous exposure to the immune sera *because increased risk of hypersensitivity reaction occurs with each use*.

Adverse effects

Adverse effects can be attributed either to the effect of immune sera on the immune system (rash, nausea, vomiting, chills, fever) or to allergic reactions (chest tightness, falling blood pressure, difficulty breathing). Local reactions, such as swelling, tenderness, pain or muscle stiffness at the injection site, are very common.

Clinically important drug–drug interactions

Caution should be used if these drugs are combined with any immune suppressant drugs, including corticosteroids. These can alter the body's response to the biologicals.

Prototype summary: immunoglobulin, normal (human)

Indications: prophylaxis against hepatitis A, measles, varicella, rubella; prophylaxis for people with immunoglobulin deficiency.

Actions: provides preformed antibodies to hepatitis A, measles, varicella, rubella and perhaps other antigens, providing a passive, short-term immunity.

Pharmacokinetics:

Route	Onset	Peak
IM	Slow	2–5 days

$T_{1/2}$: unknown; metabolised in the tissues, excretion is unknown.

Adverse effects: tenderness, muscle stiffness at site of the injection; urticaria, angioedema, nausea, vomiting, chills, fever, chest tightness.

Care considerations for people receiving immune sera

Assessment: history and examination

- Assess for contraindications or cautions: any known allergies to any of these drugs or their components *to prevent hypersensitivity reactions*; current status related to pregnancy, *which would be a contraindication for immune sera*; previous exposure to the serum being used *because hypersensitivity reactions become worse with repeated exposure*; evidence of thrombocytopenia or coagulation disorders, *which could be exacerbated by the effects of immune sera*; and immunisation history *to determine the potential for hypersensitivity reactions*.
- Perform a physical assessment *to determine baseline status before beginning therapy and for any potential adverse effects*: inspect for the presence of any skin lesions *to monitor for hypersensitivity reactions*; check temperature *to monitor for possible infection*; monitor pulse, respirations and blood pressure; auscultate lungs for adventitious sounds; and assess level of orientation and affect *to monitor for hypersensitivity reactions to the vaccine*.

Implementation with rationale

- Do not administer to any individual with a history of severe reaction to immune globulins or to the components of the drug being used *because severe immune reactions can occur*.
- Administer the drug as indicated. *Preparation varies with each product; always check the manufacturer's guidelines*.
- Monitor for severe reactions and have emergency equipment ready *to allow prompt intervention should a severe reaction occur*.
- Arrange for supportive care and comfort measures for flu-like symptoms (rest, environmental control, paracetamol) and for the local reaction (heat to injection site, anti-inflammatories) *to promote comfort*.
- Provide thorough teaching, including measures to avoid adverse effects and warning signs of problems, *to improve compliance*.
- Provide a written record of immune sera use, and encourage the individual or family to keep that information *to ensure proper medical treatment and to avert future reactions*.

Evaluation

- Monitor the person's response to the drug (improvement in disease signs and symptoms, prevention of severe disease).
- Monitor for adverse effects (flu-like symptoms, GI upset, local inflammation and pain).
- Evaluate the effectiveness of the teaching plan (person can name drug, dosage, adverse effects to watch for and specific measures to avoid adverse effects and to promote comfort, and acknowledge the need to retain a written record of injection).
- Monitor the effectiveness of comfort measures and compliance with the regimen.

KEY POINTS

- Immune sera provide preformed antibodies to specific proteins for people who have been exposed to them or are at high risk for exposure.
- The term immune sera typically refers to sera that contain antibodies to specific bacteria or viruses.

CHAPTER SUMMARY

- Immunity (relative resistance to a disease) may be active or passive. Active immunity results from the body making antibodies against specific proteins for immediate release if that protein re-enters the body. Passive immunity results from preformed antibodies to a specific protein, which offers protection against the protein only for the life of the circulating antibodies.
- Immunisations are given to stimulate active immunity in a person who is at high risk for exposure to specific diseases. Immunisations are a standard part of preventive medicine.
- Vaccines can be made from chemically inactivated microorganisms or from live, weakened viruses or bacteria. Toxoids are vaccines that are made from the toxins produced by the microorganism that are altered so that they are no longer poisonous but still have the recognisable protein antigen that will stimulate antibody production.
- Immune sera provide preformed antibodies to specific proteins for people who have been exposed to them or are at high risk for exposure.
- The term immune sera typically refers to sera that contain antibodies to specific bacteria or viruses. Antitoxins are immune sera that have antibodies to very specific toxins that might be released by invading pathogens. Antivenins are immune sera that have antibodies to venom that might be injected through spider or snake bites.
- Serum sickness – a massive immune reaction – occurs more frequently with immune sera than with vaccines. Individuals need to be monitored for any history of hypersensitivity reactions and emergency equipment should be available.

- People should be advised to keep a written record of all immunisations or immune sera used. Booster doses for various vaccines may be needed to further stimulate antibody production.

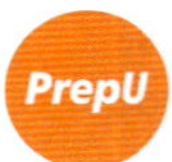

Knowing your strengths and weaknesses helps you to study more effectively. Take a PrepU Practice Quiz to find out how you measure up!

ONLINE RESOURCES

An extensive range of additional resources to enhance teaching and learning and to facilitate understanding of this chapter may be found online at the text's accompanying website, located on thePoint at http://thepoint.lww.com. These include Watch and Learn videos, Concepts in Action animations, journal articles, review questions, case studies, discussion topics and quizzes.

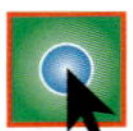

WEB LINKS

Health care providers and students may want to consult the following web resources:

www.anaesthesia.med.usyd.edu.au/resources/venom/snakebite.html
Information on Australian snakes and management of snakebite.

https://immunisationhandbook.health.gov.au
Australian Government Department of Health, *Immunisation Handbook* (10th edition).

https://beta.health.gov.au/file/1161/download?token=_enZ6KjN
Australian Government, Department of Health publication: *Myths and Realities: Responding to arguments against vaccination – a guide for providers.*

www.health.gov.au/health-topics/immunisation
Australian Government Department of Health immunisation guidelines.

www.health.govt.nz/immunisation
New Zealand Ministry of Health Immunisation schedules.

www.smartraveller.gov.au
Information for overseas travellers on vaccines that are needed, and food and travel precautions.

BIBLIOGRAPHY

Australian Government Department of Health and Ageing. (2013). *The Australian Immunisation Handbook* (10th edn). Canberra: Author.

Australian Government Department of Health and Ageing. (2013). *Myths and Realities: Responding to arguments against vaccination – a guide for providers* (5th edn). Canberra: Author.

Braitberg, G. & Segal, L. (2009). Spider bites – Assessment and management. *Australian Family Physician, 38(11)*, 862–867.

Charo, R. (2007). Politics, parents and prophylaxis: Mandating HPV vaccinations. *New England Journal of Medicine, 356*, 1905–1908.

Chiu, C. & McIntyre, P. (2013). Pneumoccocal vaccines – past, present and future. *Australian Prescriber, 36*, 88–93.

Dempsey, J., Hillege, S. & Hill, R. (2014). *Fundamentals of Nursing and Midwifery: A Person-centred Approach to Care* (2nd Australian and New Zealand edn). Sydney: Lippincott Williams & Wilkins.

Dugdale, P. (2007). Influenza vaccination for healthy adults. *Australian Prescriber, 30*, 35–37.

Farrell, M. & Dempsey, J. (2014). *Smeltzer & Bare's Textbook of Medical-Surgical Nursing* (3rd edn). Sydney: Lippincott, Williams & Wilkins.

Goodman, L. S., Brunton, L .L., Chabner, B. & Knollmann, B. C. (2011). *Goodman and Gilman's Pharmacological Basis of Therapeutics* (12th edn). New York: McGraw-Hill.

Isbister, G. (2007). Managing injuries by venomous sea creatures in Australia. *Australian Prescriber, 30*, 117–121.

Isbister, G. (2006). Snake bite: A current approach to management. *Australian Prescriber, 29*, 125–129.

Isbister, G. (2006). Spider bite: A current approach to management. *Australian Prescriber, 29*, 156–158.

McKenna, L. & Mirkov, S. (2019). *McKenna's Drug Handbook for Nursing and Midwifery* (8th edn). Sydney: Wolters Kluwer Health Australia.

O'Malley, P. (2011). Just say no to shingles! The zoster vaccine: Update for the clinical nurse specialist. *Clinical Nurse Specialist, 25(6)*, 281–283.

Porth, C. M. (2011). *Essentials of Pathophysiology: Concepts of Altered Health States* (3rd edn). Philadelphia: Lippincott Williams & Wilkins.

Porth, C. M. (2009). *Pathophysiology: Concepts of Altered Health States* (8th edn). Philadelphia: Lippincott Williams & Wilkins.

Robertus, L. M., Konstantinos, A., Hayman, N. E. & Paterson, D. L. (2011). Tuberculosis in the Australian indigenous population: History, current situation and future challenges. *Australian and New Zealand Journal of Public Health, 35(1)*, 6–9.

Ruff, T. A. & Taylor, K. (2012). Australia's contribution to global immunisation. *Australian and New Zealand Journal of Public Health, 36(5)*, 564–569.

Uahwatanasakul, W. & Carapetis, J. R. (2005). Frequently asked questions about varicella vaccine. *Australian Prescriber, 28*, 2–5.

Whyte, I. & Buckley, N. (2012). Antivenom update. *Australian Prescriber, 35*, 152–155.

Zimet, G. D. (2005). Improving adolescent health. Focus on HPV vaccine acceptance. *Journal of Adolescent Health, 37*, S17–S23.

CHECK YOUR UNDERSTANDING

Answers to the questions in this chapter can be found in Appendix A at the back of this book.

MULTIPLE CHOICE

Select the best answer to the following.

1. When preparing a presentation for a local parent group about vaccines, the nurse or midwife would describe vaccines as being used to stimulate:
   a. passive immunity to a foreign protein.
   b. active immunity to a foreign protein.
   c. serum sickness.
   d. a mild disease in healthy people.
2. After teaching a parent about common adverse effects associated with routine immunisations, which of the following, if stated by the parent, would indicate the need for additional teaching?
   a. difficulty breathing and fainting
   b. fever and rash
   c. drowsiness and fretfulness
   d. swelling and nodule formation at the site of injection
3. Which vaccine would the nurse or midwife be least likely to recommend for a 6-month-old child?
   a. diphtheria, tetanus, pertussis (DTPa) vaccine
   b. Haemophilus influenzae b vaccine
   c. poliovirus vaccine
   d. chickenpox vaccine
4. The health professional recommends that older adults and people who are at high risk of complications of influenza should receive a flu vaccine every autumn based on the understanding that the vaccine is repeated because:
   a. the immunity wears off after a year.
   b. the strains of virus predicted to cause the flu change every year.
   c. a booster shot will activate the immune system.
   d. older people do not produce good antibodies.
5. The care provider reviews a person's record to make sure that tetanus booster shots have been given:
   a. only with exposure to anaerobic bacteria.
   b. every 2 years.
   c. every 5 years.
   d. every 10 years.
6. A health professional suffers a needle-stick injury after injecting a person with suspected hepatitis B. The health professional should:
   a. have repeated titres to determine whether she was exposed to hepatitis B and, if she was, have hepatitis immunoglobulin.
   b. immediately receive hepatitis immunoglobulin and begin hepatitis B vaccines if she has not already received them.
   c. start antibiotic therapy immediately.
   d. go on sick leave until all screening tests are negative.
7. A person is to receive immunoglobulin after exposure to hepatitis A. The person has a previous history of allergies to various drugs. Before giving the immunoglobulin, the nurse or midwife should:
   a. have emergency equipment readily available.
   b. premedicate the person with aspirin.
   c. make sure all of the person's vaccinations are up to date.
   d. make sure the person has a ride home.

MULTIPLE RESPONSE

Select all that apply.

1. A public education campaign to stress the importance of childhood immunisations should include which of the following points?
   a. Prevention of potentially devastating diseases outweighs the discomfort and risks of immunisation.
   b. Routine immunisation is standard practice in Australia and New Zealand.
   c. The practice of routine immunisations has virtually wiped out many previously deadly or debilitating diseases.
   d. The risk of severe adverse reactions is on the rise and is not being addressed.
   e. If there is a family history of autism, that person should avoid immunisations.
   f. The temporary discomfort associated with the immunisation can be treated with over-the-counter drugs.

2. A mother brings her child to his 18-month maternal and child health centre visit. The health professional would not give the child his routine immunisations in which of the following situations?
   a. He cried at his last immunisation.
   b. He developed a fever or rash after his last immunisation.
   c. He currently has a fever and symptoms of a cold.
   d. He is allergic to aspirin.
   e. He is currently taking oral corticosteroids.
   f. His siblings are all currently being treated for a viral infection.

3. When assessing the medical record of an older adult to evaluate the status of his immunisations, the nurse would be looking for evidence of which of the following?
   a. yearly pneumococcal vaccination
   b. yearly flu vaccination
   c. tetanus booster every 10 years
   d. tetanus booster every 5 years
   e. measles, mumps, rubella (MMR) vaccine if the person was born after 1957
   f. varicella vaccine only if there is evidence that the person had chickenpox as a child

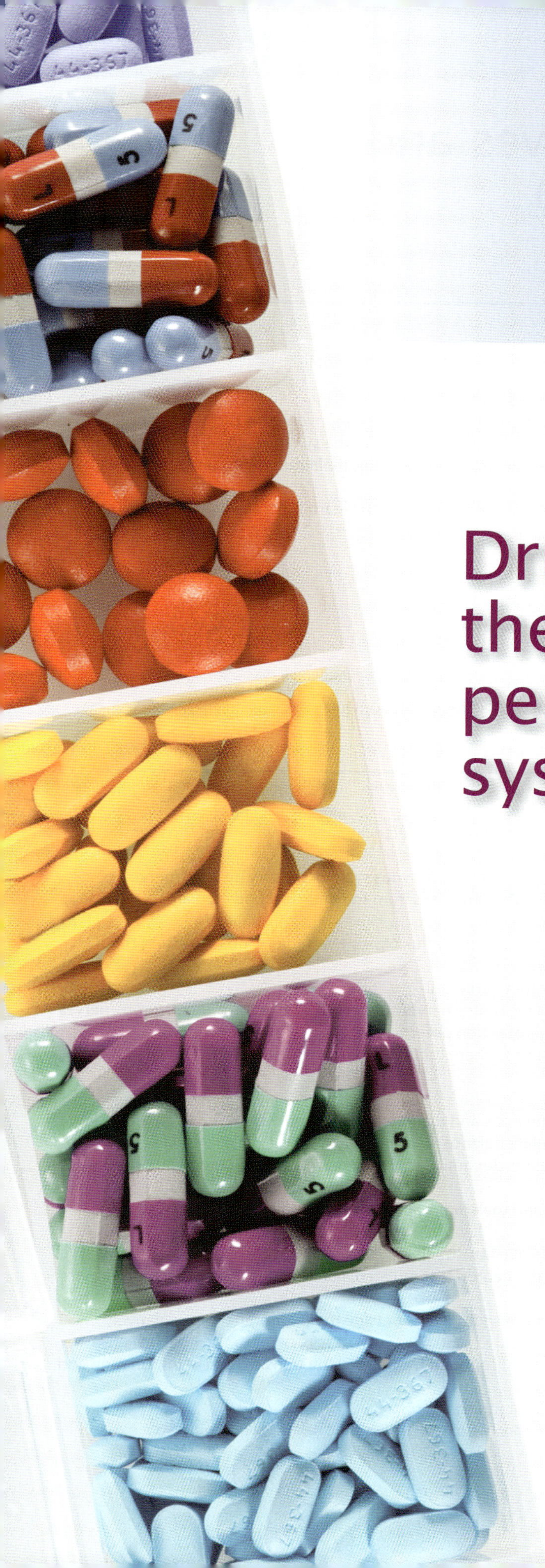

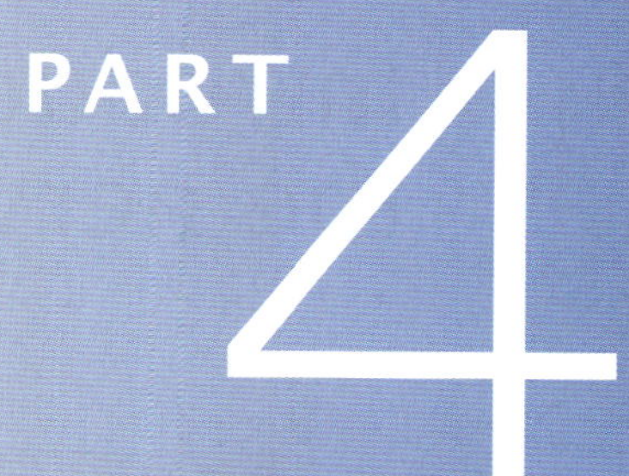

PART 4

Drugs acting on the central and peripheral nervous systems

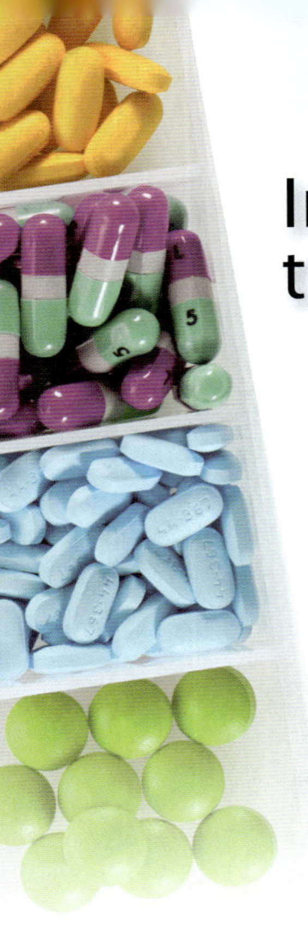

Introduction to nerves and the nervous system

19

Learning objectives

On completing this chapter you should be able to:

1. Label the parts of a neuron and describe the functions of each part.
2. Describe an action potential, including the roles of the various electrolytes involved in the action potential.
3. Explain what a neurotransmitter is, including its origins and functions at the synapse.
4. Describe the function of the cerebral cortex, cerebellum, hypothalamus, thalamus, midbrain, pituitary gland, medulla, spinal cord and reticular activating system.
5. Discuss what is known about learning and the impact of emotion on the learning process.

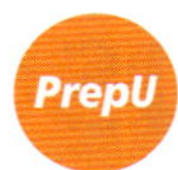

PrepU Test your current knowledge of nerves and the nervous system with a PrepU Practice Quiz!

Glossary of key terms

action potential: sudden change in electrical charge of a neuronal cell membrane; the electrical signal by which neurons send information

afferent: neurons or groups of neurons (nerves) that bring information to the central nervous system; sensory neurons/nerves

axon: nerve fibre; a long projection from a neuronal body that carries electrical impulses from the neuronal body towards a synapse

dendrite: short projection from a neuronal body that transmits information

depolarisation: opening of the sodium channels in a nerve membrane to allow the influx of positive sodium ions, reversing the membrane charge from negative to positive

effector cell: cell stimulated by a nerve; may be a muscle, a gland or another nerve cell

efferent: neurons or groups of neurons (nerves) that carry information from the central nervous system to an effector; motor neurons/nerves

engram: short-term memory made up of a reverberating electrical circuit of action potentials

forebrain: upper level of the brain; consists of the two cerebral hemispheres, where thinking and coordination of sensory and motor activity occur

ganglia: a group of nerve bodies

hindbrain: most primitive area of the brain, the brainstem; consists of the pons and medulla, which control basic, vital functions and arousal, and the cerebellum, which controls motor functions that regulate balance

limbic system: area in the midbrain that is rich in adrenaline, noradrenaline, dopamine and serotonin; involved in motivation, emotion, learning and memory

midbrain: the middle area of the brain; it consists of the hypothalamus and thalamus and includes the limbic system

neuron: structural unit of the nervous system

nerve: the axons of many neurons packed closely together to form cable-like fibre tracts

neurotransmitter: chemical produced by a neuron and released when the neuron is stimulated; reacts with a specific receptor site to cause a reaction

repolarisation: return of a neuronal membrane to a resting state, with more sodium ions outside the membrane and a relatively negative charge inside the membrane

Schwann cell: insulating cell found on nerve axons; allows 'leaping' electrical conduction to speed the transmission of information and prevent tiring of the neuron

soma: cell body of a neuron; contains the nucleus, cytoplasm and various granules

synapse: junction between a neuron and another neuron or an effector; consists of the presynaptic neuronal ending, a space called the synaptic cleft and the postsynaptic cell

The nervous system is responsible for controlling the functions of the human body, analysing incoming stimuli and integrating internal and external responses. The nervous system is composed of the central nervous system (CNS; the brain and spinal cord) and the peripheral nervous system (PNS). The PNS is composed of sensory receptors that bring information into the CNS and motor nerves that carry information away from the CNS to facilitate response to stimuli. The autonomic nervous system, which is discussed in Chapter 29, uses components of the CNS and PNS to regulate automatic or unconscious responses to stimuli.

The structural unit of the nervous system is the nerve cell, or **neuron**. The billions of nerve cells that make up the nervous system are organised to allow movement realisation of various sensations; response to internal and external stimuli; and learning, thinking and emotion. The mechanisms that are involved in all of these processes are not clearly understood. The actions of drugs that are used to affect the functioning of the nerves and the responses that these drugs cause throughout the nervous system provide some of the current theories about the workings of the nervous system.

PHYSIOLOGY OF THE NERVOUS SYSTEM

The nervous system operates through the use of electrical impulses and chemical messengers to transmit information throughout the body and to respond to internal and external stimuli. The properties and functions of the neuron provide the basis for all nervous system function.

Neurons

As noted previously, the neuron is the structural unit of the nervous system. The human body contains about 14 billion neurons. About 10 billion of these are located in the brain, and the remainder make up the spinal cord and PNS.

Neurons have several distinctive cellular features (Figure 19.1). Each neuron is made up of a cell body, or **soma**, which contains the cell nucleus, cytoplasm, and various granules and other particles. Short, branch-like projections that cover most of the surface of a neuron are known as **dendrites**. These structures, which provide increased surface area for the neuron, bring information into the neuron from other neurons.

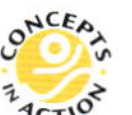

Neurological: Simple neuronal cells

One end of the neuronal body extends into a long process that does not branch out until the very end of the process. This elongated process is called the neuronal **axon** and it emerges from the soma at the axon hillock, a slightly enlarged area of the soma from which the axon emerges. The axon of a neuron can be extremely tiny, or it can extend a lengthy distance. The axon carries information from a neuron to be transmitted to **effector cells** – cells stimulated by a neuron, which may include muscle or gland cells or another neuron. This transmission occurs at the end of the axon, where the axon branches out in what is called the axon terminal.

The axons of many neurons are packed closely together into nerves that look like cable or fibre tracts. **Afferent** fibres are nerve axons that run from peripheral receptors into the CNS. In contrast, **efferent** fibres are nerve axons that carry nerve impulses from the CNS to the periphery to stimulate muscles or glands. (An easy way to remember the difference between afferent and efferent is to recall that efferent fibres exit from the CNS.)

It is currently thought that neurons are unable to reproduce; so, if nerves are destroyed, they are lost. If dendrites and axons are lost, nerves regenerate those structures; however, for this regeneration to occur, the soma and the axon hillock must remain intact. For a clinical example, consider a person who has closed a car door on their finger. Sensation and movement may be lost or limited for a certain period, but because the nerve bodies for most of the nerves in the hand are located in **ganglia** (groups of nerve bodies) in the wrist, they are able to regenerate the damaged axon or dendrites. Over time, sensation and full movement should return.

Research on possible ways to stimulate the reproduction of nerves is under way. Although scientists have used nerve growth factor with fetal cell implants to stimulate some nerve growth, it is currently assumed that nerves are unable to reproduce.

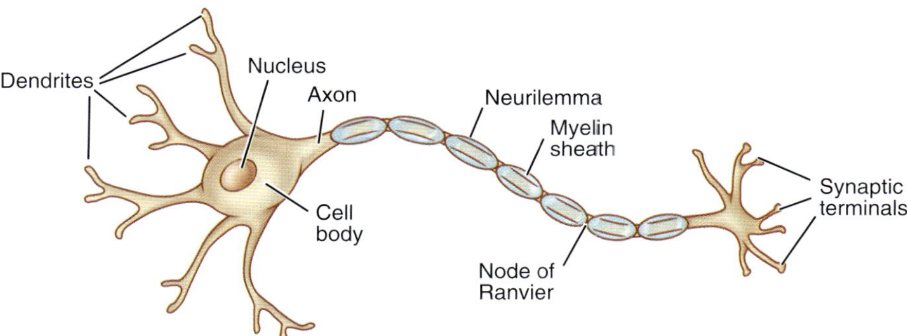

FIGURE 19.1 The neuron, functional unit of the nervous system.

Action potential

Nerves send messages by conducting electrical impulses called **action potentials**.

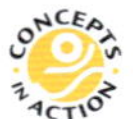

Neurological: Action potential

Nerve membranes, which are capable of conducting action potentials along the entire membrane, send messages to nearby neurons or to effector cells that may be located close or far away via this electrical communication system. Like all cell membranes, nerve membranes have various channels or pores that control the movement of substances into and out of the cell. Some of these channels allow the movement of sodium, potassium and calcium. When cells are at rest, their membranes are impermeable to sodium. However, the membranes are permeable to potassium ions.

The sodium–potassium pump that is active in the membranes of neurons is responsible for this property of the membrane. This system pumps sodium ions out of the cell and potassium ions into the cell. At rest, more sodium ions are outside the cell membrane, and more potassium ions are inside. Electrically, the inside of the cell is relatively negative compared with the outside of the membrane, which establishes an electrical potential along the nerve membrane. When nerves are at rest, this is referred to as the resting membrane potential of the nerve.

Stimulation of a neuron causes **depolarisation** of the nerve, which means that the sodium channels open in response to the stimulus, and sodium ions rush into the cell, following the established concentration gradient. If an electrical monitoring device is attached to the nerve at this point, a positive rush of ions is recorded. The electrical charge on the inside of the membrane changes from relatively negative to relatively positive. This sudden reversal of membrane potential, called the action potential (Figure 19.2), lasts less than a microsecond. Using the sodium–potassium pump, the cell then returns that section of membrane to the resting membrane potential, a process called **repolarisation**. The action potential generated at one point along a nerve membrane stimulates the generation of an action potential in adjacent portions of the cell membrane, and the stimulus travels the length of the cell membrane.

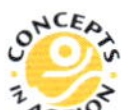

Neurological: Flipping the membrane potential

Nerves can respond to stimuli several hundred times per second, but for a given stimulus to cause an action potential, it must have sufficient strength and must occur when the nerve membrane is able to respond – that is, when it has repolarised. A nerve cannot be stimulated again while it is depolarised. The balance of sodium and potassium across the cell membrane must be re-established.

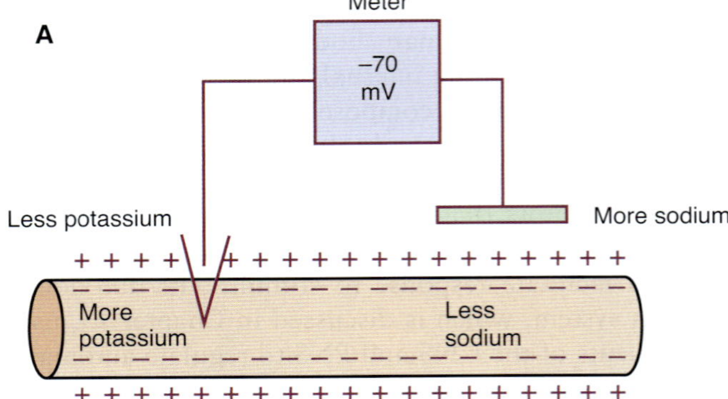

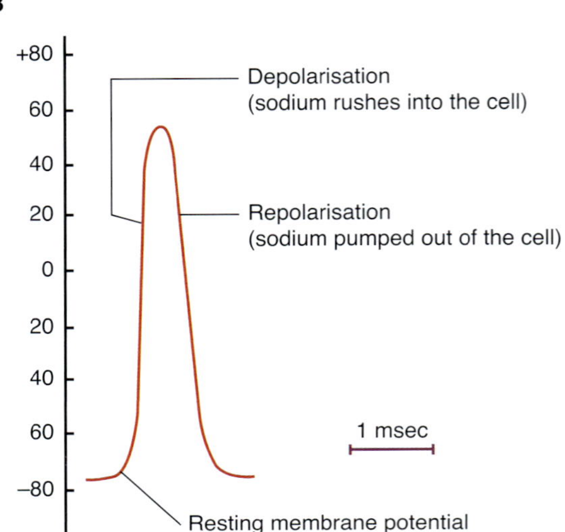

FIGURE 19.2 The action potential. **A.** A segment of an axon showing that, at rest, the inside of the membrane is relatively negatively charged and the outside is positively charged. A pair of electrodes placed as shown would record a potential difference of about –70 mV; this is the resting membrane potential. **B.** An action potential of about 1 msec that would be recorded if the axon shown in panel A were brought to threshold. At the peak of the action potential, the charge on the membrane reverses polarity.

Nerves require energy (i.e. oxygen and glucose) and the correct balance of the electrolytes sodium and potassium to maintain normal action potentials and transmit information into and out of the nervous system. If an individual has anoxia or hypoglycaemia, the nerves might not be able to maintain the sodium–potassium pump, and that individual may become severely irritable or too stable (not responsive to stimuli).

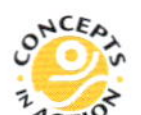

Neurological: Equilibrium potential

Long nerves are myelinated: they have a myelin sheath that speeds electrical conduction and protects the nerves from the fatigue that results from frequent formation of action potentials. Even though many of the tightly packed nerves in the brain do not need to travel far to stimulate another nerve, they are myelinated. The effect of this myelination is not understood.

Myelinated nerves have **Schwann cells,** which are located at specific intervals along nerve axons and are very resistant to electrical stimulation (Figure 19.1). The Schwann cells wrap themselves around the axon in Swiss-roll fashion (Figure 19.3). Between the Schwann cells are areas of uncovered nerve membrane called the nodes of Ranvier. So-called 'leaping' nerve conduction occurs along these exposed nerve fibres. An action potential excites one section of nerve membrane, and the electrical impulse then 'skips' from one node to the next, generating an action potential. Because the membrane is forming fewer action potentials, the speed of conduction is much faster and the nerve is protected from being exhausted or using up energy to form multiple action potentials. This node-to-node mode of conduction is termed *saltatory* or leaping *conduction* (Figure 19.1).

Neurological: Saltatory conduction

If the Schwann cells become enlarged or swollen and block the nodes of Ranvier, which is what occurs in the neuromuscular disease multiple sclerosis, conduction does not occur because the electrical impulse has a limited firing range. A stimulus may simply be 'lost' along the nerve. Believed to be an autoimmune disorder that attacks Schwann cells and leads to swelling and scarring of these cells, multiple sclerosis is characterised by a progressive loss of nerve response and muscle function.

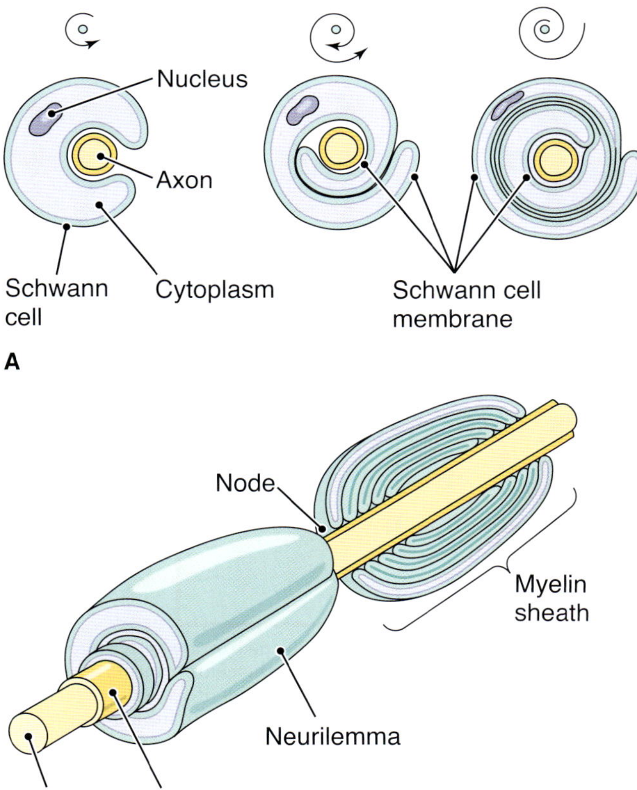

FIGURE 19.3 Formation of a myelin sheath. **A.** Schwann cells wrap around the axon, creating a myelin coating. **B.** The outermost layer of the Schwann cell forms the neurilemma. Spaces between the cells are the nodes of Ranvier.

Nerve synapse

When the electrical action potential reaches the end of an axon, the electrical impulse comes to a halt. At this point the stimulus no longer travels at the speed of electricity. The transmission of information between two nerves or between a nerve and a gland or muscle is chemical. Nerves communicate with other nerves or effectors at the nerve **synapse** (Figure 19.4). The synapse is made up of a presynaptic nerve, the synaptic cleft and the postsynaptic effector cell. The nerve axon, called the presynaptic nerve, releases a chemical called a **neurotransmitter** into the synaptic cleft and the neurotransmitter reacts with a very specific receptor site on the postsynaptic cell to cause a reaction.

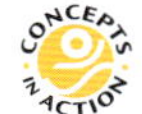

Neurological: Nerve synapse

Neurotransmitters

Neurotransmitters stimulate postsynaptic cells either by exciting or by inhibiting them. The reaction that occurs when a neurotransmitter stimulates a receptor site depends on the specific neurotransmitter that it releases and the receptor site it activates. A nerve may produce only one type of neurotransmitter, using building blocks such as tyrosine or choline from the extracellular fluid, often absorbed from dietary sources. The neurotransmitter, packaged into vesicles, moves to the terminal membrane of the axon, and when the nerve is stimulated, the vesicles contract and push the neurotransmitter into the synaptic cleft. The calcium channels in the nerve membrane are open during the action potential, and the presence of calcium causes the contraction. When the cell repolarises, calcium leaves the cell, and the contraction stops. Once released into the synaptic cleft, the neurotransmitter reacts with very specific receptor sites to cause a reaction.

To return the effector cell to a resting state so that it can be stimulated again, if needed, neurotransmitters must be inactivated. Neurotransmitters may be either reabsorbed by the presynaptic nerve in a process called reuptake (a recycling effort by the nerve to reuse the materials and save resources) or broken down by enzymes in the area (eg, monoamine oxidase breaks down the neurotransmitter noradrenaline; the enzyme acetylcholinesterase breaks down the neurotransmitter acetylcholine). Several neurotransmitters have been identified. As research continues, other neurotransmitters

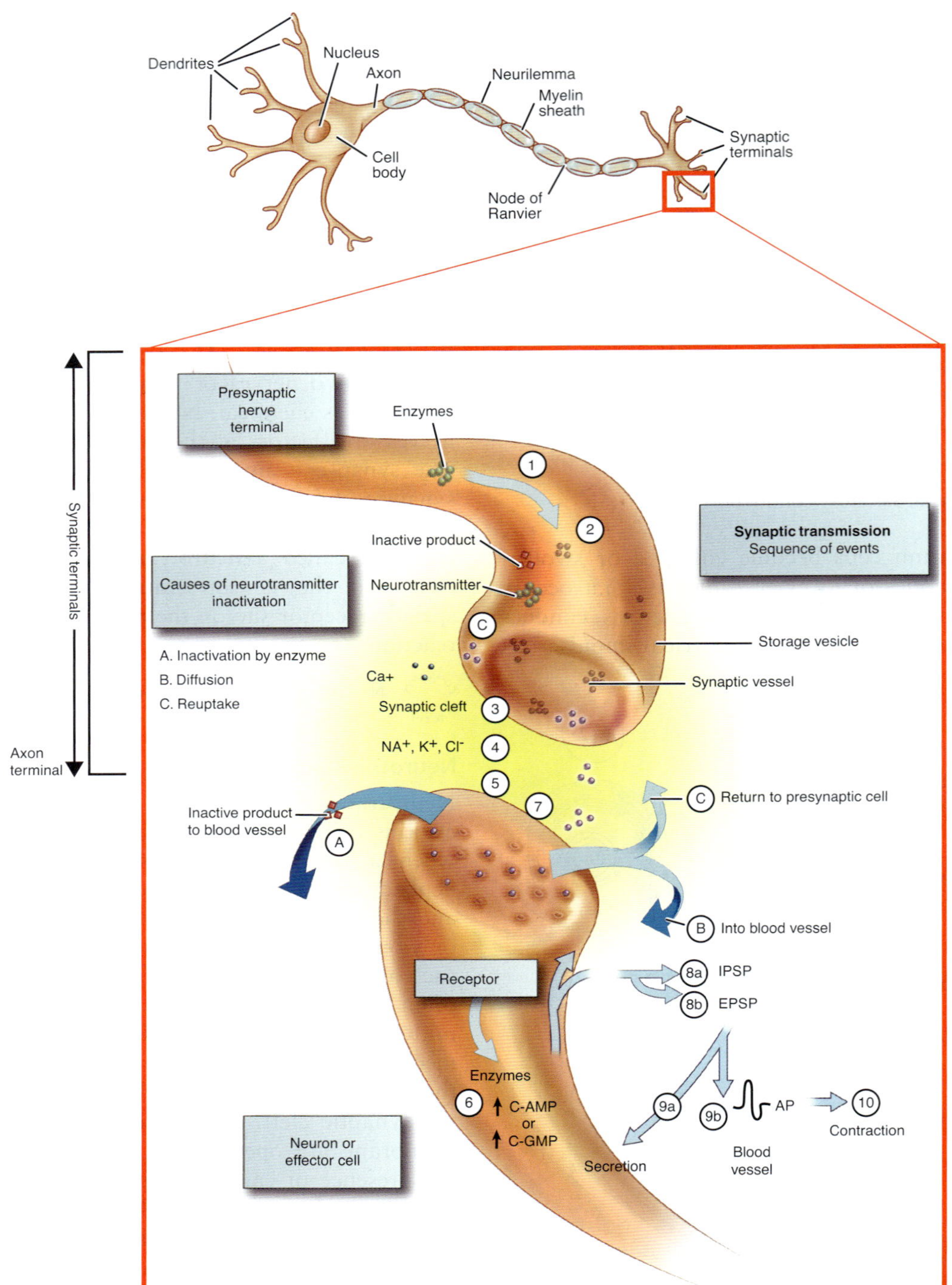

FIGURE 19.4 The sequence of events in synaptic transmission: (**1**) Synthesis of the neurotransmitter; (**2**) uptake of the neurotransmitter into storage vesicles; (**3**) release of the neurotransmitter by an action potential in the presynaptic nerve; (**4**) diffusion of the neurotransmitter across the synaptic cleft; (**5**) combination of the neurotransmitter with a receptor; (**6**) a sequence of events leading to activation of second messengers within the postsynaptic nerve; (**7**) change in permeability of the postsynaptic membrane to one or more ions, causing (**8a**) an inhibitory postsynaptic potential or (**8b**) an excitatory postsynaptic potential. Characteristic responses of the postsynaptic cell are as follows: (**9a**) The gland secretes hormones; (**9b**) the muscle cells have an action potential; and (10) the muscle contracts. The action of the neurotransmitter is terminated by one or more of the following processes. (**A**) inactivation by an enzyme; (**B**) diffusion out of the synaptic cleft and removal by the vascular system; and (**C**) reuptake into the presynaptic nerve followed by storage in a synaptic vesicle or deactivation by an enzyme.

may be discovered, and the actions of known neurotransmitters will be better understood.

The following are selected neurotransmitters:

- *Acetylcholine*, which communicates between nerves and muscles, is also important as the preganglionic neurotransmitter throughout the autonomic nervous system and as the postganglionic neurotransmitter in the parasympathetic nervous system and in several pathways in the brain.
- *Noradrenaline* and *adrenaline* are catecholamines, which are released by nerves in the sympathetic branch of the autonomic nervous system and are classified as hormones when they are released from cells in the adrenal medulla. These neurotransmitters also occur in high levels in particular areas of the brain, such as the limbic system.
- *Dopamine*, which is found in high concentrations in certain areas of the brain, is involved in the coordination of impulses and responses, both motor and intellectual.
- *Gamma-aminobutyric acid (GABA)*, which is found in the brain, inhibits nerve activity and is important in preventing overexcitability or stimulation such as seizure activity.
- *Serotonin*, which is also found in the limbic system, is important in arousal and sleep, as well as in preventing depression and promoting motivation.

Many of the drugs that affect the nervous system involve altering the activity of the nerve synapse. These drugs have several functions, including blocking the reuptake of neurotransmitters so that they are present in the synapse in greater quantities and cause more stimulation of receptor sites; blocking receptor sites so that the neurotransmitter cannot stimulate the receptor site; blocking the enzymes that break down neurotransmitters to cause an increase in neurotransmitter concentration in the synapse; stimulating specific receptor sites when the neurotransmitter is not available; and causing the presynaptic nerve to release greater amounts of the neurotransmitter.

KEY POINTS

- The nervous system controls the body, analyses external stimuli and integrates internal and external responses to stimuli.
- The neuron, comprising a cell body, dendrites and an axon, is the functional unit of the nervous system. Dendrites route information to the cell body and axons take the information away.
- Neurons and nerves (bundled neurons) transmit information by way of action potentials. An action potential is a sudden change in membrane charge from negative to positive that is triggered when stimulation of a nerve opens sodium channels and allows positive sodium ions to flow into the neuronal cells.
- When sodium ions flow into a neuron, the neuronal membrane depolarises. Mechanically, this is recorded as a flow of positive electrical charges. Repolarisation immediately follows, with the sodium–potassium pump in the cell membrane pumping sodium and potassium ions out of the cell, leaving the inside of the membrane relatively negative to the outside.
- At the end of the axon, neurons communicate with chemicals called neurotransmitters, which are produced by the neurons. Neurotransmitters are released into the synapse when the nerve is stimulated; they react with a very specific receptor site to cause a reaction and are immediately broken down or removed from the synapse.

CENTRAL NERVOUS SYSTEM

The CNS consists of the brain and the spinal cord, the two parts of the body that contain the vast majority of nerves. The bones of the vertebrae protect the spinal cord; and the bones of the skull, which are corrugated much like an egg carton and serve to absorb impact, protect the brain (Figure 19.5). In addition, the meninges, which are membranes that cover the nerves in the brain and spine, furnish further protection.

The blood–brain barrier, a functioning boundary, also plays a defensive role. It keeps toxins, proteins and other large structures out of the brain and prevents their contact with the sensitive and fragile neurons. The

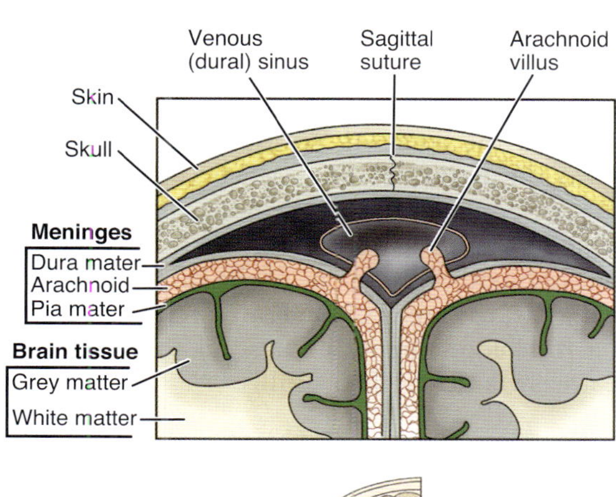

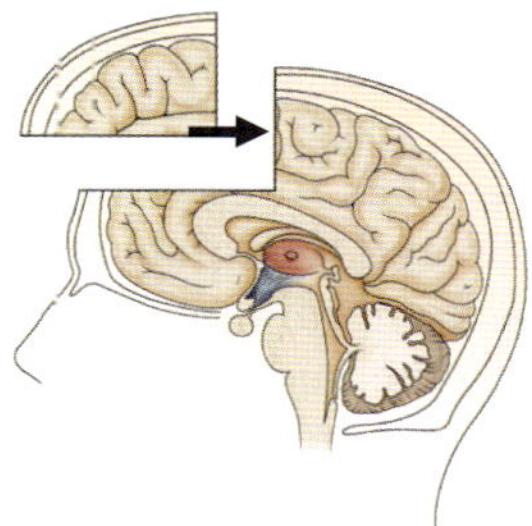

FIGURE 19.5 Bony and membranous protection of the brain.

FIGURE 19.6 The protective blood supply of the brain: the carotid, vertebral and basilar arteries join to form the circle of Willis.

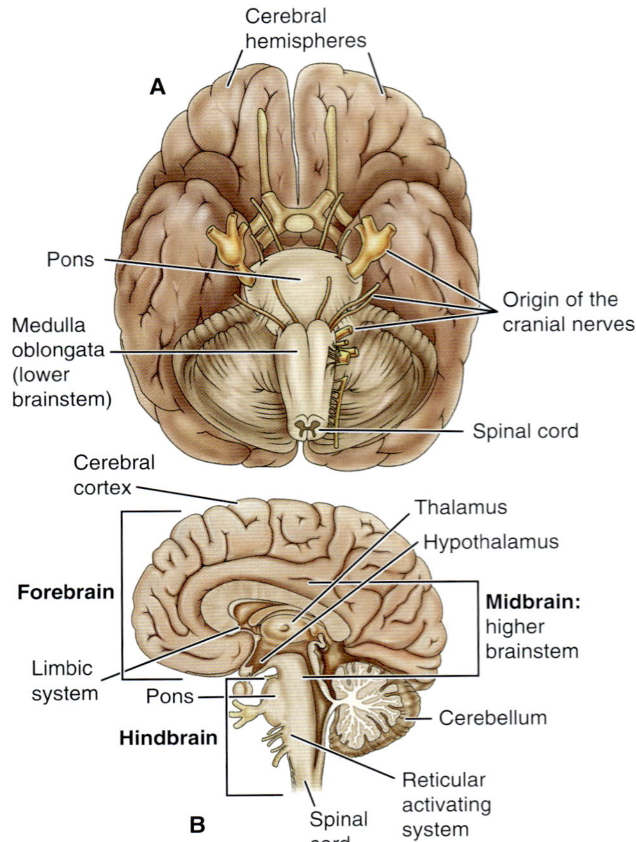

FIGURE 19.7 Anatomy of the brain. **A.** A view of the underside of the brain. **B.** The medial or midsagittal view of the brain.

blood–brain barrier represents a therapeutic challenge to drug treatment of brain-related disorders because a large percentage of drugs are carried bound to plasma proteins and are unable to cross into the brain. When a person is suffering from a brain infection, antibiotics cannot cross into the brain until the infection is so severe that the blood–brain barrier can no longer function.

The brain has a unique blood supply to protect the neurons from lack of oxygen and glucose. Two arteries – the carotids – branch off the aortic arch and go up into each side of the brain at the front of the head, and two other arteries – the vertebrals – enter the back of the brain to become the basilar arteries. These arteries all deliver blood to a common vessel at the bottom of the brain called the circle of Willis, which distributes the blood to the brain as it is needed (Figure 19.6). The role of the circle of Willis becomes apparent when an individual has an occluded carotid artery. Although the passage of blood through one of the carotid arteries may be negligible, the areas of the brain on that side will still have a full blood supply because of the blood sent to those areas via the circle of Willis.

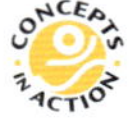
Neurological: Basilar membrane

Anatomy of the brain

The brain has three major divisions: the hindbrain, the midbrain and the forebrain (Figure 19.7).

The **hindbrain**, which runs from the top of the spinal cord into the midbrain, is the most primitive area of the brain and contains the brainstem, where the pons and medulla oblongata are located. These areas of the brain control basic, vital functions, such as the respiratory centres, which control breathing; the cardiovascular centres, which regulate blood pressure; the chemoreceptor trigger zone and emetic zone, which control vomiting; the swallowing centre, which coordinates the complex swallowing reflex; and the reticular activating system (RAS), which controls arousal and awareness of stimuli and contains the sleep centre. The RAS filters the billions of incoming messages, selecting only the most significant for response. When levels of serotonin become high in the RAS, the system shuts down and sleep occurs. The medulla absorbs serotonin from the RAS; when the levels are low enough, consciousness or arousal results.

The cranial nerves (see Figure 19.7), which also emerge from the hindbrain, involve *specific* senses (sight, smell, hearing, balance, taste) and some muscle activity of the head and neck (eg, chewing, eye movement). The cerebellum – a part of the brain that looks like a ball of wool and lies behind the other parts of the hindbrain – coordinates the motor function that regulates posture, balance and voluntary muscle activity.

The **midbrain** contains the thalamus, the hypothalamus and the limbic system (see Figure 19.7). The thalamus sends direct information into the cerebrum to transfer sensations, such as cold, heat, pain, touch and muscle sense. The hypothalamus, which is poorly protected by the blood–brain barrier, acts as a major sensor for activities in the body. Areas of the hypothalamus are responsible for temperature control, water balance, appetite and fluid balance. In addition, the hypothalamus plays a central role in the endocrine system and in the autonomic nervous system.

The **limbic system** is an area of the brain that contains high levels of three neurotransmitters: adrenaline, noradrenaline and serotonin. Stimulation of this area, which appears to be responsible for the expression of emotions, may lead to anger, pleasure, motivation, stress and so on. This part of the brain seems to be largely responsible for the 'human' aspect of brain function. Drug therapy aimed at alleviating emotional disorders such as depression and anxiety often involves attempting to alter the levels of adrenaline, noradrenaline and serotonin.

The **forebrain** is made up of two cerebral hemispheres joined together by an area called the corpus callosum. These two hemispheres contain the sensory neurons, which receive nerve impulses, and the motor neurons, which send them. They also contain areas that coordinate speech and communication and seem to be the area where learning takes place (see Figure 19.7). Different areas of the brain appear to be responsible for receiving and sending information to specific areas of the body. When the brain is viewed at autopsy, it looks homogeneous, but scientists have mapped the general areas that are responsible for sensory response, motor function and other functions (see Figure 19.8). In conjunction with the cerebellum, groups of ganglia or nerve cell bodies called the basal ganglia, located at the bottom of the brain, make up the extrapyramidal motor system. This system coordinates motor activity for unconscious activities such as posture and gait.

Anatomy of the spinal cord

The spinal cord is made up of 31 pairs of spinal nerves. Each spinal nerve has two components or roots. These mixed nerve parts include a sensory fibre (called the dorsal root) and a motor fibre (called the ventral root). The spinal sensory fibres bring information into the CNS from the periphery. The motor fibres cause movement or reaction.

Functions of the central nervous system

The brain is responsible for coordinating reactions to the constantly changing external and internal environment. In all animals, the function of this organ is essentially the same. The human component involving emotions, learning and conscious response takes the human nervous system beyond a simple reflex system and complicates the responses seen to any stimulus.

Sensory functions

Millions of sensory impulses are constantly streaming into the CNS from peripheral receptors. Many of these impulses go directly to specific areas of the brain designated to deal with input from particular areas of the body or from the senses. The responses that occur as a result of these stimuli can be altered by efferent neurons that respond to emotions through the limbic system, to learned responses stored in the cerebral cortex or to autonomic input mediated through the hypothalamus.

The intricacies of the human brain can change the response to a sensation depending on the situation.

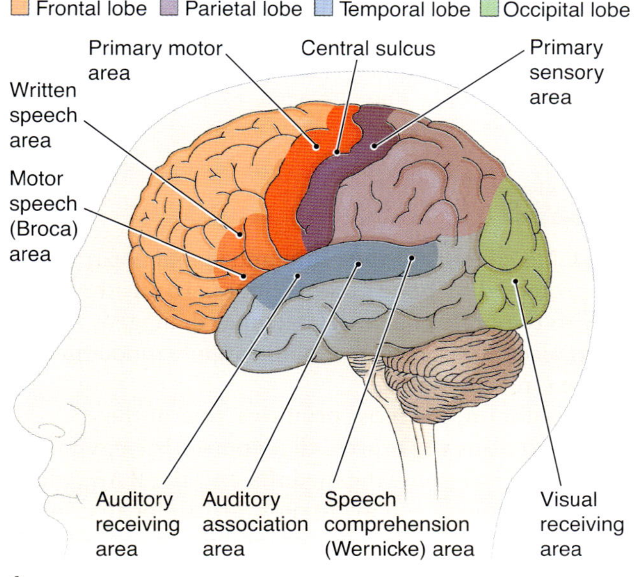

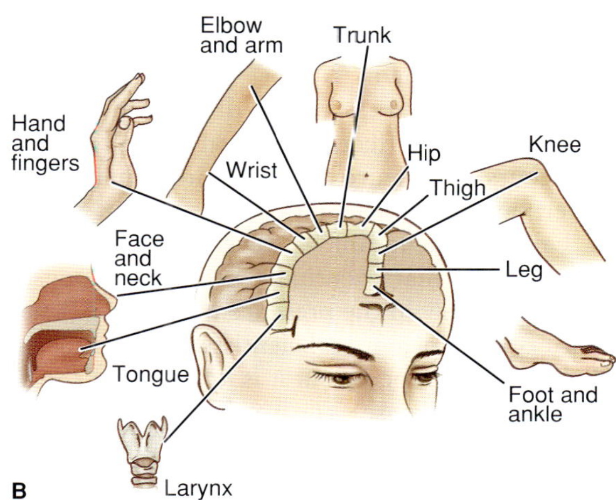

FIGURE 19.8 Functional areas of the brain. **A**. Topographical organisation of functions of control and interpretation in the cerebral cortex. **B**. Areas of the brain that control specific areas of the body. Size indicates relative distribution of control.

People may react differently to the same stimulus. For example, if an individual drops a can on their foot, the physiological response is one of pain and a stimulation of the sympathetic branch of the autonomic nervous system. If the person is alone or in a very comfortable environment (eg, fixing dinner at home), they may scream, swear or jump around. However, if that person is in the company of other people (eg, a cooking teacher working with a class), they may be much more dignified and quiet, even though the physiological effect on the body is the same.

Motor functions

The sensory nerves that enter the brain react with related motor nerves to cause a reaction mediated by muscles or glands. The motor impulses that leave the cortex are further regulated or coordinated by the pyramidal system, which coordinates voluntary movement, and the extrapyramidal system, which coordinates unconscious motor activity that regulates control of position and posture. For example, some drugs may interfere with the extrapyramidal system and cause tremors, shuffling gait and lack of posture and position stability. Motor fibres from the cortex cross to the other side of the spinal cord before emerging to interact with peripheral effectors. In this way, motor stimuli coming from the right side of the brain affect motor activity on the left side of the body. For example, an area of the left cortex may send an impulse down to the spinal cord that reacts with an interneuron, crosses to the other side of the spinal cord and causes a finger on the right hand to twitch.

Intellectual and emotional functions

The way that the cerebral cortex uses sensory information is not clearly understood, but research has demonstrated that the two hemispheres of the brain process information in different ways. The right side of the brain is the more artistic side, concerned with forms and shapes, and the left side is more analytical, concerned with names, numbers and processes. Why the two hemispheres are different and how they develop differently is not known.

When learning takes place, distinct layers of the cerebral cortex are affected, and an actual membrane change occurs in a neuron to store information in the brain permanently. Learning begins as an electrical circuit called an **engram**, a reverberating circuit of action potentials that eventually becomes a long-term, permanent memory in the presence of the proper neurotransmitters and hormones. Scientists do not understand exactly how this happens, but it is known that the nerve requires oxygen, glucose and sleep to process an engram into a permanent memory, and during that processing structural changes occur to the cells involved in the engram. This reverberating circuit is responsible for short-term memory. When people have decreased blood supply to the brain, short-term memory may be lost, and they are not able to remember new things. Because they are unable to remember new things, the brain falls back on long-term, permanent memory for daily functioning. For example, a person may be introduced to a care provider and have no recollection of the person 2 hours later and yet be able to recall the events of several years ago vividly.

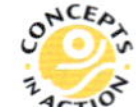

Neurological: Stroke

Several substances appear to affect learning. Antidiuretic hormone (ADH), which is released during reactions to stress, is one such substance. Although too much stress prevents learning, feeling slightly stressed may increase a person's ability to learn. A person who is a little nervous about upcoming surgery, for example, seems to display a better mastery of facts about the surgery and postoperative procedures than a person who is very stressed and scared or one who appears to show no interest or concern. Oxytocin is another substance that seems to increase actual learning. Because childbirth is the only known time that oxytocin levels increase, the significance of this is not understood. Midwives should know that women in labour will very likely remember the smallest details about the whole experience and should use whatever opportunity is made available to carry out teaching.

In addition, the limbic system appears to play an important role in how a person learns and reacts to stimuli. The emotions associated with a memory as well as with the present have an impact on stimulus response. The placebo effect is a documented effect of the mind on drug therapy: if a person perceives that a drug will be effective, it is much more likely to actually be effective. This effect, which uses the actions of the cerebrum and the limbic system, can have a tremendous impact on drug response. Events that are perceived as stressful by some people may be seen as positive by other people.

KEY POINTS

- The CNS consists of the brain and spinal cord, which are protected by bone and meninges. To ensure blood flow to the brain if a vessel becomes damaged, the brain also has a protective blood supply moderated by the circle of Willis.
- The hindbrain, the most primitive area of the brain, contains the centres that control basic, vital functions. The pons, the medulla and the RAS, which regulates arousal and awareness, are all located in the hindbrain. The cerebellum, which helps to coordinate motor activity, is found at the back of the hindbrain.
- The midbrain consists of the hypothalamus, the thalamus and the limbic system. The limbic system

is responsible for the expression of emotion, and the thalamus and hypothalamus coordinate internal and external responses and direct information into the cerebral cortex.
- The cerebral cortex consists of two hemispheres, which regulate the communication between sensory and motor neurons and are the sites of thinking and learning.

CLINICAL SIGNIFICANCE OF DRUGS THAT ACT ON THE NERVOUS SYSTEM

The features of the human nervous system, including the complexities of the human brain, sometimes make it difficult to predict the exact reaction of a particular person to a given drug. When a drug is used to affect the nervous system, the occurrence of many systemic effects is always a possibility because the nervous system affects the entire body. The chapters in this section address the individual classes of drugs used to treat disorders of the nervous system, including their adverse effects. An understanding of the actions of specific drugs makes it easier to anticipate what therapeutic and adverse effects might occur. In addition, nurses and midwives should consider all of the learned, cultural and emotional aspects of a person's situation in an attempt to provide optimal therapeutic benefit and minimal adverse effects.

CHAPTER SUMMARY

- Although nerves do not reproduce, they can regenerate injured parts if the soma and axon hillock remain intact.
- Efferent nerves take information out of the CNS to effector sites; afferent nerves are sensory nerves that take information into the CNS.
- When the transmission of action potentials reaches the axon terminal, it causes the release of chemicals called neurotransmitters, which cross the synaptic cleft to stimulate an effector cell, which can be another nerve, a muscle or a gland.
- A neurotransmitter must be produced by a nerve (each nerve can produce only one kind); it must be released into the synapse when the nerve is stimulated; it must react with a very specific receptor site to cause a reaction; and it must be immediately broken down or removed from the synapse so that the cell can be ready to be stimulated again.
- Much of the drug therapy in the nervous system involves receptor sites and the release or reuptake and breakdown of neurotransmitters.
- The CNS consists of the brain and spinal cord, which are protected by bone and meninges. To ensure blood flow to the brain if a vessel becomes damaged, the brain also has a protective blood supply moderated by the circle of Willis.
- The hindbrain, the most primitive area of the brain, contains the centres that control basic, vital functions. The pons, the medulla and the reticular activating system (RAS), which regulates arousal and awareness, are all located in the hindbrain. The cerebellum, which helps to coordinate motor activity, is found at the back of the hindbrain.
- The midbrain consists of the hypothalamus, the thalamus and the limbic system. The limbic system is responsible for the expression of emotion, and the thalamus and hypothalamus coordinate internal and external responses and direct information into the cerebral cortex.
- The cerebral cortex consists of two hemispheres, which regulate the communication between sensory and motor neurons and are the sites of thinking and learning.
- The mechanisms of learning and processing learned information are not understood. Emotion-related factors influence the human brain, which handles stimuli and responses in complex ways.
- Much remains to be learned about the human brain and how drugs influence it. The actions of many drugs that have known effects on human behaviour are not understood.

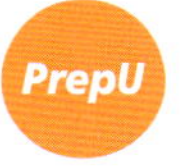

Knowing your strengths and weaknesses helps you to study more effectively. Take a PrepU Practice Quiz to find out how you measure up!

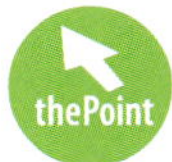

ONLINE RESOURCES

An extensive range of additional resources to enhance teaching and learning and to facilitate understanding of this chapter may be found online at the text's accompanying website, located on thePoint at http://thepoint.lww.com. These include Watch and Learn videos, Concepts in Action animations, journal articles, review questions, case studies, discussion topics and quizzes.

BIBLIOGRAPHY

Barrett, K. E. & Ganong, W. F. (2010). *Ganong's Review of Medical Physiology* (23rd edn). New York: McGraw-Hill.

Goodman, L. S., Brunton, L. L., Chabner, B. & Knollmann, B. C. (2011). *Goodman and Gilman's Pharmacological Basis of Therapeutics* (12th edn). New York: McGraw-Hill.

Guyton, A. & Hall, J. (2011). *Textbook of Medical Physiology* (12th edn). Philadelphia: Saunders Elsevier.

Parpura, V. & Hayden, P. (2008). *Astrocytes in the Physiology of the Nervous System*. New York: Springer.

Porth, C. (2011). *Essentials of Pathophysiology: Concepts of Altered Health States* (3rd edn). Philadelphia: Lippincott Williams & Wilkins.

Porth, C. (2009). *Pathophysiology: Concepts of Altered Health States* (8th edn). Philadelphia: Lippincott Williams & Wilkins.

Strominger, N. L., Demarest, R. J., Laemle, L. B. (2012). *Noback's Human Nervous System* (7th edn). Totowa, NJ: Humana Press.

CHECK YOUR UNDERSTANDING

Answers to the questions in this chapter can be found in Appendix A at the back of this book.

MULTIPLE CHOICE

Select the best answer to the following.

1. The cerebellum:
   a. initiates voluntary muscle movement.
   b. helps regulate the tone of skeletal muscles.
   c. if destroyed, would result in the loss of all voluntary skeletal activity.
   d. contains the centres responsible for the regulation of body temperature.
2. At those regions of the nerve membrane where myelin is present, there is:
   a. low resistance to electrical current.
   b. high resistance to electrical current.
   c. high conductance of electrical current.
   d. energy loss for the cell.
3. The nerve synapse:
   a. is not resistant to electrical current.
   b. cannot become exhausted.
   c. has a synaptic cleft.
   d. transfers information at the speed of electricity.
4. Which of the following could result in the initiation of an action potential?
   a. depolarising the membrane
   b. decreasing the extracellular potassium concentration
   c. increasing the activity of the sodium–potassium active transport system
   d. stimulating the nerve with a threshold electrical stimulus during the absolute refractory period of the membrane
5. Neurotransmitters are:
   a. produced in the muscle to communicate with nerves.
   b. the chemicals used to stimulate or suppress effectors at the nerve synapse.
   c. usually found in the diet.
   d. non-specific in their action on various nerves.
6. The limbic system is an area of the brain that:
   a. is responsible for coordination of movement.
   b. is responsible for the special senses.
   c. is responsible for the expression of emotions.
   d. controls sleep.
7. The most primitive area of the brain, the brainstem, contains areas responsible for:
   a. vomiting, swallowing, respiration, arousal and sleep.
   b. learning.
   c. motivation and memory.
   d. taste, sight, hearing and balance.
8. A clinical indication of poor blood supply to the brain, particularly to the higher levels where learning takes place, would be:
   a. loss of long-term memory.
   b. loss of short-term memory.
   c. loss of coordinated movement.
   d. insomnia.

MULTIPLE RESPONSE

Select all that apply.

1. In explaining the importance of a constant blood supply to the brain, the nurse or midwife would tell the student which of the following?
   a. Energy is needed to maintain nerve membranes and cannot be produced without oxygen.
   b. Carbon dioxide must constantly be removed to maintain the proper pH.
   c. Little glucose is stored in nerve cells, so a constant supply is needed.
   d. The brain needs a constant supply of insulin and thyroid hormone.
   e. The brain swells easily and needs the blood supply to reduce swelling.
   f. Circulating aldosterone levels maintain the fluid balance in the brain.
2. The blood–brain barrier could be described by which of the following?
   a. It is produced by the cells that make up the meninges.
   b. It is regulated by the microglia in the CNS.
   c. It is weaker in certain parts of the brain.
   d. It is uniform in its permeability throughout the CNS.
   e. It is an anatomical structure that can be punctured.
   f. It is more likely to block the entry of proteins into the CNS.

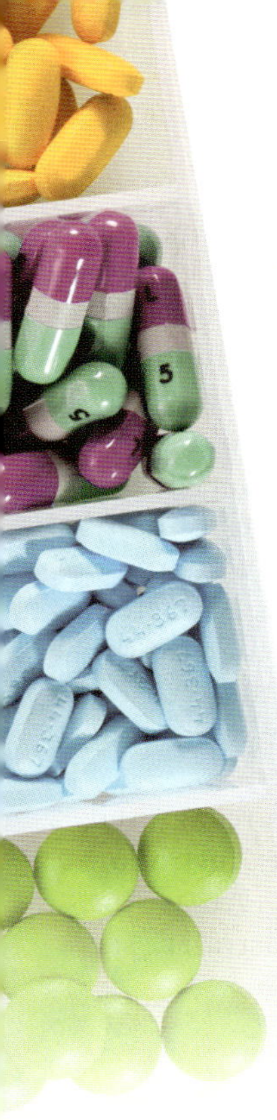

Anxiolytic and hypnotic agents

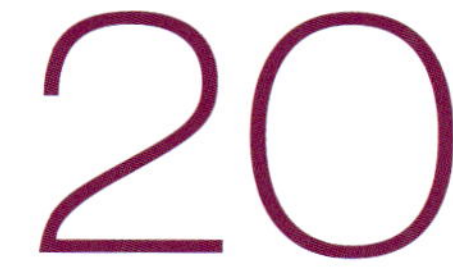

Learning objectives

On completing this chapter you should be able to:

1. Define the states that are affected by anxiolytic or hypnotic agents.
2. Describe therapeutic actions, indications, pharmacokinetics, contraindications, most common adverse reactions and important drug–drug interactions associated with each class of anxiolytic or hypnotic agent.
3. Discuss the use of anxiolytic or hypnotic agents across the lifespan.
4. Compare and contrast the prototype drugs for each class of anxiolytic or hypnotic drug with the other drugs in that class.
5. Outline care considerations and teaching needs for people receiving each class of anxiolytics or hypnotic agent.

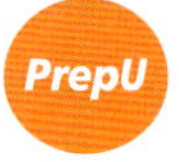

Test your current knowledge of anxiolytic and hypnotic agents with a PrepU Practice Quiz!

Glossary of terms

anxiety: unpleasant feeling of tension, fear or nervousness in response to an environmental stimulus, whether real or imaginary

anxiolytic: drug used to depress the central nervous system (CNS); prevents the signs and symptoms of anxiety

barbiturate: former mainstay drug used for the treatment of anxiety and for sedation and sleep induction; associated with potentially severe adverse effects and many drug–drug interactions, which makes it less desirable than some of the newer agents

benzodiazepine: drug that acts in the limbic system and the reticular activating system (RAS) to make gamma-aminobutyric acid (GABA), an inhibitory neurotransmitter, more effective, causing interference with neuron firing; depresses CNS to block the signs and symptoms of anxiety, and may cause sedation and hypnosis in higher doses

hypnosis: extreme sedation resulting in CNS depression and sleep

hypnotic: drug used to depress the CNS; causes sleep

sedation: loss of awareness of, and reaction to, environmental stimuli

sedative: drug that depresses the CNS; produces a loss of awareness of, and reaction to, the environment

BENZODIAZEPINES USED AS ANXIOLYTICS
alprazolam
bromazepam
clobazam
(P) diazepam
lorazepam
oxazepam
temazepam
triazolam

BARBITURATE USED AS ANXIOLYTIC–HYPNOTIC
(P) phenobarbital (phenobarbitone)

OTHER ANXIOLYTIC AND HYPNOTIC DRUGS
buspirone
chloral hydrate
dexmedetomidine
promethazine
alimemazine (trimeprazine)
zopiclone
zolpidem

The drugs discussed in this chapter are used to alter an individual's responses to environmental stimuli. They have been called **anxiolytics** because they can prevent feelings of tension or fear; **sedatives** because they can calm people and make them unaware of their environment; **hypnotics** because they can cause sleep; and minor tranquillisers because they can produce a state of tranquillity in anxious individuals. In the past, a given drug would simply be used at different doses to yield each of these effects. Further research into how the brain reacts to outside stimuli has resulted in the increased availability of specific agents that produce particular goals and avoid unwanted adverse effects. Use of these drugs also varies across the lifespan (Box 20.1).

STATES AFFECTED BY ANXIOLYTIC AND HYPNOTIC DRUGS

Anxiety

Anxiety is a feeling of tension, nervousness, apprehension or fear that usually involves unpleasant reactions to a stimulus, whether actual or unknown. Anxiety is often accompanied by signs and symptoms of the sympathetic stress reaction (see Chapter 29), which may include sweating, fast heart rate, rapid breathing and elevated blood pressure. Mild anxiety, a not uncommon reaction, may serve as a stimulus or motivator in some situations. A person who feels anxious about being alone in a poorly lit parking lot at night may be motivated to take extra safety precautions. When anxiety becomes overwhelming or severe, it can interfere with the activities of daily living and lead to medical problems related to chronic stimulation of the sympathetic nervous system. A severely anxious person may, for example, be afraid to leave the house or to interact with other people. In these cases, treatment is warranted. Anxiolytic drugs are drugs that are used to lyse or break the feeling of anxiety.

Both severe and chronic anxiety are recognised mental illnesses. Mental health is one of the Australian government's nine National Health Priority Areas; for more information on mental health in Australia, see www.aihw.gov.au/mental-health.

Sedation

The loss of awareness and reaction to environmental stimuli is termed **sedation**. This condition may be desirable in people who are restless, nervous, irritable or

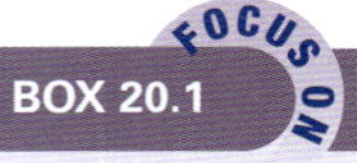

BOX 20.1 Drug therapy across the lifespan

Anxiolytic and hypnotic agents

CHILDREN

Use of anxiolytic and hypnotic drugs with children is challenging. The response of the child to the drug may be unpredictable; inappropriate aggressiveness, crying, irritability and tearfulness are common.

Of the benzodiazepines, only clonazepam and diazepam have established paediatric dosages. Some of the others are used in paediatric settings, and dosage may be calculated using age and weight.

The barbiturates, being older drugs, have established paediatric dosages. These drugs must be used with caution because of the often unexpected responses. Children must be monitored very closely for CNS depression and excitability.

Chloral hydrate is approved for use in children. The potential for adverse effects and the unpleasant taste and odour make the drug less desirable as a sleep agent. The antihistamines diphenhydramine, alimemazine (trimeprazine) and promethazine are more popular for use in helping to calm children and to induce rest and sleep. Care must be taken to assess for possible dried secretions and effects on breathing. Dosage must be calculated carefully.

ADULTS

Adults using these drugs for the treatment of insomnia need to be cautioned that they are for short-term use only. The reason for the insomnia should be sought (eg, medical, hormonal or anxiety problems). Other methods for helping to induce sleep – established routines, quiet activities before bed, a back-rub or warm bath – should be encouraged before drugs are prescribed. Adults receiving anxiolytics also may need referrals for counselling and diagnosis of possible causes. Adults should be advised to avoid driving and making legal decisions when taking these drugs.

Liver function should be evaluated before and periodically during therapy.

PREGNANCY AND BREASTFEEDING

These drugs are contraindicated during pregnancy and breastfeeding because of the potential for adverse effects on the fetus and possible sedation of the baby. The antihistamines, which have not been associated with congenital malformations, may be the safest to use, with caution, if an anxiolytic or hypnotic drug must be used.

OLDER ADULTS

Older people may be more susceptible to the adverse effects of these drugs, from unanticipated CNS effects to increased sedation, dizziness, and even hallucinations. Dosages of all of these drugs should be reduced and the person should be monitored very closely for toxic effects and to provide safety measures if CNS effects do occur.

Baseline liver and renal function tests should be performed, and these values should be monitored periodically for any changes that would indicate a need to decrease dosage further or to stop the drug.

Non-drug measures to reduce anxiety and to help induce sleep are important with older people. The person should be screened for physical problems, neurological deterioration, or depression, which could contribute to the insomnia or anxiety.

overreacting to stimuli. Although sedation is anxiolytic, it may frequently lead to drowsiness. For example, sedative-induced drowsiness is a concern for outpatients who need to be alert and responsive in their normal lives. On the other hand, this tiredness may be desirable for people who are about to undergo surgery or other procedures and who are receiving medical support. The choice of an anxiolytic drug depends on the situation in which it will be used, keeping the related adverse effects in mind.

Hypnosis

Extreme sedation results in further CNS depression and sleep, or **hypnosis**. Hypnotics are used to help people fall asleep by causing sedation. Drugs that are effective hypnotics act on the reticular activating system (RAS) and block the brain's response to incoming stimuli. Hypnosis, therefore, is the extreme state of sedation, in which the person no longer senses or reacts to incoming stimuli.

BENZODIAZEPINES USED AS ANXIOLYTICS

Benzodiazepines, the most frequently used anxiolytic drugs, prevent anxiety without causing much associated sedation. In addition, they are less likely to cause physical dependence than many of the older sedatives/hypnotics that are used to relieve anxiety. Table 20.1 lists the available benzodiazepines, including common indications

TABLE 20.1 *DRUGS IN FOCUS* Benzodiazepines* used as anxiolytics

Drug name	Dosage/route	Usual indications
alprazolam (*Alprax, Kalma*)	1.5–4.5 mg/day PO	Anxiety; panic attack **Onset:** 30 minutes **Duration:** 4–6 hours **Special considerations:** taper after long-term therapy
bromazepam (*Lexotan*)	Adult: 3–12 mg PO tds	Anxiety, agitation **Onset:** 0.5–4 hours **Duration:** 12–24 hours
clobazam (*Frisium*)	Adult: 10–30 mg PO daily in single or divided dose	Acute anxiety, sleep disturbance **Onset:** 1–4 hours **Duration:** 17–49 hours
(P) diazepam (*Valium*)	Adults: 5–40 mg/day; ambulatory patients: 2 mg tid or 5 mg in the evening and 2 mg bd–tid Elderly, debility: 2 mg twice daily or half usual adult dose Paediatric (6 months–3 years): 1–6 mg/day Paediatric (4–14 years): 4–12 mg/day	Anxiety; alcohol withdrawal, muscle relaxant; antiepileptic; antitetanus, preoperative anxiolytic **Onset:** 5–60 minutes **Duration:** 3 hours **Special considerations:** monitor injection sites; drug of choice if route change is anticipated; taper after long-term therapy
lorazepam (*Ativan*)	1–10 mg/day PO in divided doses	Anxiety; anxiolytic **Onset:** 1–30 minutes **Duration:** 12–24 hours **Special considerations:** reduce dosage of narcotics given with this drug
oxazepam (*Serepax*)	Adults: mild to moderate anxiety: 7.5–15 mg 3–4 times daily; severe anxiety, depression associated with anxiety/agitation, alcohol withdrawal: 15–30 mg 3–4 times daily	Anxiety; alcohol withdrawal **Onset:** slow **Duration:** 2–4 hours **Special considerations:** preferred for elderly
temazepam (*Normison*)	10–30 mg PO at bedtime	Hypnotic; treatment of insomnia **Onset:** varies **Duration:** 4–6 hours **Special considerations:** taper after long-term therapy
triazolam (*Hypam*)	0.125–0.5 mg PO at bedtime	Hypnotic; treatment of insomnia **Onset:** varies **Duration:** 2–4 hours **Special considerations:** monitor liver and renal function, full blood count (FBC); taper after long-term therapy

*Onset of action and duration are important in selecting the correct drug for a particular use.

BOX 20.2 FOCUS ON Calculations

A 3-year-old boy weighing 25 kg is prescribed chloral hydrate as a hypnotic at bedtime. The order reads: 50 mg/kg/day PO at bedtime. The drug comes in a syrup form as 1 g/10 mL. How much syrup would you give as the bedtime dose?

First, figure out what the correct dose would be:

$$50 \text{ mg/kg} \times 25 \text{ kg} = 1250 \text{ mg}$$

Set up the equation using the available form and prescribed dose, remembering to convert grams to milligrams

$$\frac{1250}{1000} \times \frac{10}{1} = 12.5 \text{ mL}$$

Because this is a child, it is good practice to ask another nurse to calculate the correct dosage and then compare your work, so you can independently check the accuracy of your calculations.

and specific information about each drug. The benzodiazepines used as anxiolytics include alprazolam (*Alprax, Kalma*), bromazepam (*Lexotan*) (not available in New Zealand), clobazam (*Frisium*), diazepam (*Valium*), lorazepam (*Ativan*), oxazepam (*Serepax*), temazepam (*Normison*, *Temaze*) and triazolam (*Hypam*). Box 20.2 provides an exercise in calculating the dose for a child receiving a sedative/hypnotic.

Therapeutic actions and indications

The benzodiazepines are indicated for the treatment of the following conditions: anxiety disorders, alcohol withdrawal, hyperexcitability and agitation, and pre-operative relief of anxiety and tension to aid in balanced anaesthesia. These drugs act in the limbic system and the RAS to make GABA more effective, causing interference with neuron firing (Figure 20.1). GABA stabilises the postsynaptic cell. This leads to an anxiolytic effect at doses lower than those required to induce sedation and hypnosis. The exact mechanism of action is not clearly understood. Benzodiazepines reduce muscle spasm by a central action that is independent of their sedative effect. As increased muscle tone is a common feature of anxiety states and may contribute to the aches and pains, including headaches that often trouble anxious people, the relaxant effect of benzodiazepines may, therefore, be clinically useful.

Pharmacokinetics

The benzodiazepines are well absorbed from the gastrointestinal (GI) tract, with peak levels achieved in 30 minutes to 2 hours. They bind strongly to plasma protein and their high lipid solubility causes the drug to accumulate gradually in body fat, crossing the placenta and entering breast milk. The benzodiazepines are metabolised extensively in the liver and are eventually excreted as glucoronide conjugates in the urine. Several benzodiazepines are converted into active metabolites, such as *N*-desmthyldiazepam, which can have a half-life of as long as 60 hours and which accounts for the tendency of many benzodiazepines to produce cumulative effects and long hangovers when given at regular intervals. People with liver disease must receive a smaller dose and be monitored closely. Excretion is primarily through the urine.

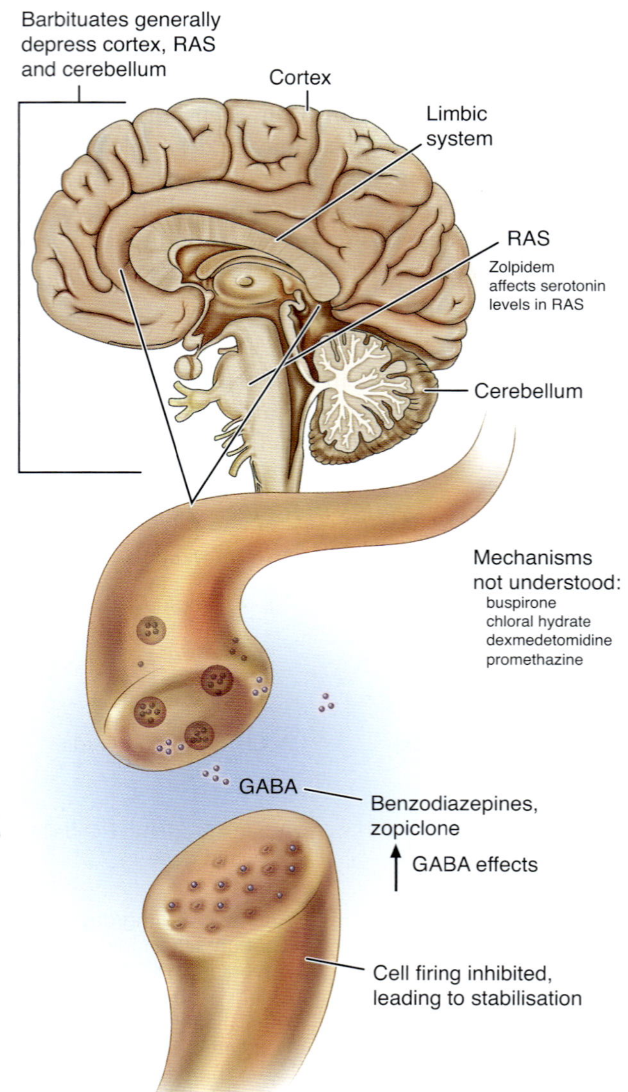

FIGURE 20.1 Sites of action of the benzodiazepines, barbiturates and other anxiolytics.

Contraindications and cautions

Contraindications to benzodiazepines include allergy to any benzodiazepine; psychosis, *which could be exacerbated by sedation*; and acute narrow-angle glaucoma, shock, coma or acute alcoholic intoxication, *all of which could be exacerbated by the depressant effects of these drugs.*

In addition, these sedative/hypnotics are contraindicated in pregnancy *because a predictable syndrome of cleft lip or palate, inguinal hernia, cardiac defects, microcephaly or pyloric stenosis occurs when they are taken in the first trimester.* Neonatal withdrawal syndrome may also result. Breastfeeding is also a contraindication *because of potential adverse effects on the neonate (eg, sedation).*

Use with caution in elderly or debilitated people *because of the possibility of unpredictable reactions* and in cases of renal or hepatic dysfunction, *which may alter the metabolism and excretion of these drugs, resulting in direct toxicity. If possible, hypnotics should be avoided in the elderly, because they are at greater risk of becoming ataxic and confused, leading to falls and injury.* Dose adjustments usually are needed for such people. See the New Zealand Medicines Formulary http://nzformulary.org.

Dependence and tolerance (i.e. a gradual escalation of dose needed to produce the required effect) occurs with chronic use of all benzodiazepines therefore stopping treatment after weeks or months causes increased symptoms of anxiety, together with tremor and dizziness. Addiction (i.e. severe psychological dependence which outlasts the physical withdrawal syndrome) which can occur with many drugs of abuse is not a major problem with benzodiazepines.

Adverse effects

The adverse effects of benzodiazepines are associated with the impact of these drugs on the central and peripheral nervous systems. Nervous system effects include sedation, drowsiness, depression, lethargy, blurred vision, headaches, apathy, light-headedness and confusion. In addition, mild paradoxical excitatory reactions may occur during the first 2 weeks of therapy. Benzodiazepines may occasionally cause marked respiratory depression and facilities for its treatment are therefore essential. The drug flumazenil is used to antagonise the effects of benzodiazepines (refer to Box 20.3).

Several other kinds of adverse effects may occur. GI conditions such as dry mouth, constipation, nausea, vomiting and elevated liver enzyme levels may result. Cardiovascular problems may include hypotension, hypertension, arrhythmias, palpitations and respiratory difficulties. Haematological conditions such as blood dyscrasias and anaemia are possible. Genitourinary (GU) effects include urinary retention and hesitancy, loss of libido and changes in sexual functioning. Because phlebitis, local reactions and thrombosis may occur at local injection sites, such sites should be monitored. Abrupt cessation of these drugs may lead to a withdrawal syndrome characterised by nausea, headache, vertigo, malaise and nightmares.

Prototype summary: diazepam

Indications: management of anxiety disorders, acute alcohol withdrawal, muscle relaxation, treatment of tetanus, antiepileptic adjunct in status epilepticus, preoperative relief of anxiety and tension.

Actions: acts in the limbic system and reticular formation to potentiate the effects of GABA, an inhibitory neurotransmitter; may act in spinal cord and supraspinal sites to produce muscle relaxation.

Pharmacokinetics:

Route	Onset	Peak	Duration
Oral	30–60 min	1–2 hours	3 hours
IM	15–30 min	30–45 min	3 hours
IV	1–5 min	30 min	15–60 min
Rectal	Rapid	1.5 hours	3 hours

$T_{1/2}$: 20–80 hours, metabolised in the liver, excreted in urine.

Adverse effects: mild drowsiness, depression, lethargy, apathy, fatigue, restlessness, bradycardia, tachycardia, constipation, diarrhoea, incontinence, urinary retention, changes in libido, drug dependence with withdrawal syndrome.

Clinically important drug–drug interactions

The risk of CNS depression increases if benzodiazepines are taken with alcohol or other CNS depressants, so such combinations should be avoided. In addition, the effects of benzodiazepines increase if they are taken with cimetidine, oral contraceptives or disulfiram. If any one of these drugs is used with benzodiazepines, people should be monitored and the appropriate dose adjustments made.

Finally, the impact of benzodiazepines may be decreased if they are given with theophyllines or ranitidine. If either of these drugs is used, dose adjustment may be necessary.

Care considerations for people receiving benzodiazepines

Assessment: history and examination

- Assess for contraindications or cautions: known allergies to benzodiazepines *to prevent hypersensitivity reactions*; impaired liver or kidney function, *which could alter the metabolism and excretion of a particular drug*; any condition that might be exacerbated by the depressant effects of the drugs (eg, glaucoma, coma, psychoses, shock, acute alcohol intoxication); and pregnancy and breastfeeding.

- Assess for baseline status before beginning therapy *to check for occurrence of any potential adverse effects*. Assess for the following: temperature and weight; skin colour and lesions; affect, orientation, reflexes and vision; pulse, blood pressure and perfusion; respiratory rate, adventitious sounds and presence of chronic pulmonary disease; and bowel sounds on abdominal examination.
- Perform laboratory tests, including renal and liver function tests and FBC.

Refer to the Critical thinking scenario for a full discussion of care for a person dealing with anxiety.

Implementation with rationale

- Do not administer intra-arterially *because serious arteriospasm and gangrene could occur.* Monitor injection sites carefully for local reactions to institute treatment as soon as possible.
- Do not mix intravenous (IV) drugs in solution with any other drugs *to avoid potential drug–drug interactions.*
- Give parenteral forms only if oral forms are not feasible or available, and switch to oral forms, *which are safer and less likely to cause adverse effects*, as soon as possible.
- Give IV drugs slowly *because these agents have been associated with hypotension, bradycardia and cardiac arrest.*
- Arrange to reduce the dose of narcotic analgesics in people receiving a benzodiazepine *to decrease potentiated effects and sedation.*
- Maintain people who receive parenteral benzodiazepines in bed for a period of at least 3 hours. Do not permit ambulatory people to operate a motor vehicle after an injection *to ensure safety.*
- Monitor hepatic and renal function, as well as FBC, during long-term therapy *to detect dysfunction and to arrange to taper and discontinue the drug if dysfunction occurs.*
- Taper dose gradually after long-term therapy, especially in individuals with epilepsy. *Acute withdrawal could precipitate seizures in these people. It may also cause withdrawal syndrome.*
- Provide comfort measures *to help people tolerate drug effects*, such as having them void before dosing, instituting a bowel program as needed, giving food with the drug if GI upset is severe, providing environmental control (lighting, temperature, stimulation), taking safety precautions (use of side rails, assistance with ambulation) and aiding orientation.
- Provide thorough teaching, including drug name, prescribed dose, measures for avoidance of adverse effects and warning signs that may indicate possible problems. Instruct people about the need for periodic monitoring and evaluation *to enhance knowledge about drug therapy and to promote compliance.*
- Offer support and encouragement *to help the person cope with the diagnosis and the drug regimen.*
- If necessary, use flumazenil (Box 20.3), the benzodiazepine antidote, *for the treatment of overdose.*

Evaluation

- Monitor response to the drug (alleviation of signs and symptoms of anxiety; sleep; sedation).
- Monitor for adverse effects (sedation, hypotension, cardiac arrhythmias, hepatic or renal dysfunction, blood dyscrasias).
- Evaluate the effectiveness of the teaching plan (person can give the drug name, dosage, possible adverse effects to watch for, specific measures to help avoid adverse effects and the importance of continued follow-up).
- Monitor the effectiveness of comfort measures and compliance with the regimen.

BOX 20.3 A benzodiazepine antidote

Flumazenil (*Anexate*), a benzodiazepine antidote, acts by inhibiting the effects of the benzodiazepines at GABA receptors. It is used for three purposes: to treat benzodiazepine overdose, to reverse the sedation caused by benzodiazepines that are used as adjuncts for general anaesthesia, and to reverse sedation produced for diagnostic tests or other medical procedures.

Flumazenil, which is available for IV use only, is injected into the tubing of a running IV. The drug has a rapid onset of action that peaks 5–10 minutes after administration. It is metabolised in the liver. Because this drug has a half-life of about 1 hour, it may be necessary to repeat injections of flumazenil if a long-acting benzodiazepine was used.

People who receive flumazenil should be monitored continually, and life-support equipment should be readily available. If the person has been taking a benzodiazepine for a long period, administration of flumazenil may precipitate a rapid withdrawal syndrome that necessitates supportive measures. Headache, dizziness, vertigo, nausea and vomiting may be associated with use of flumazenil.

CRITICAL THINKING SCENARIO

Benzodiazepines

THE SITUATION

P.P., a 43-year-old mother of three teenage sons, comes to the outpatient department for a routine physical examination. Results are unremarkable except for blood pressure of 145/90, pulse rate of 98 and apparent tension – she is jittery, avoids eye contact and sometimes appears teary-eyed. She says that she is having some problems dealing with 'life in general'. Her sons present many stresses and her husband, who is busy with his career, has little time to deal with issues at home. When he *is* home, he is very demanding. In addition, she thinks she is beginning menopause and is having trouble coping with the idea of menopause as well as with some of the symptoms. Overall, she feels lonely and has no outlet for her anger, tension or stress. A health care provider, who reassures P.P. that this problem is common in women of her age, prescribes the benzodiazepine diazepam (*Valium*) to help P.P. deal with her anxiety.

CRITICAL THINKING

What sort of crisis intervention would be most appropriate for P.P.?
What care interventions are helpful at this point?
What non-drug interventions might be helpful?
What other support systems could be used to help P.P. deal with all that is going on in her life?
Think about the overwhelming problems that P.P. has to deal with on a daily basis and how the anxiolytic effects of diazepam might change her approach to these problems. Could the problems actually get worse?
Develop a care plan for the long-term care of P.P.

DISCUSSION

Anxiolytics are useful for controlling the unpleasant signs and symptoms of anxiety. The diazepam prescribed for P.P. may provide some immediate relief, enabling her to survive the 'crisis' period and plan changes in her life in general. However, the associated drowsiness and sedation may make coping with the problems in her life even more difficult. She should be taught the adverse effects of diazepam, the warning signs of serious adverse effects and the health problems to report.

A follow-up evaluation should be scheduled. Additional meetings with the same health care provider are important for the long-term solution to P.P.'s anxiety. Her need for drug therapy should be re-evaluated once she can discover other support systems and develop other ways of coping. Although anxiolytic therapy may be beneficial initially, it will not solve the problems that are causing anxiety, and in this case, the causes for the anxiety are specific. The anxiolytic should be considered only as a short-term aid.

Unlike P.P., many people in severe crisis do not consciously identify the many causes of stress, or stressors. However, P.P. has identified a list of factors that makes her life stressful. This facilitates the development of coping strategies. She may find the following support systems helpful:

- Referral to a counsellor and involvement of the entire family in identifying problems and ways to deal with them.
- Support groups for women in various stages of life (eg, entering menopause, mothers of children who are entering the teens). Just having the opportunity to discuss problems and explore ways of dealing with them helps many people.

CARE GUIDE FOR P.P.: DIAZEPAM

Assessment: history and examination

Allergies to diazepam, psychoses, acute narrow angle glaucoma, acute alcohol intoxication, impaired liver or kidney function, pregnancy, breastfeeding, concurrent use of alcohol, omeprazole, cimetidine, disulfiram, oral contraceptives, theophylline, ranitidine
CV: blood pressure, pulse, perfusion
CNS: orientation, affect, reflexes, vision
Skin: colour, lesions, texture
Respiratory: respiration, adventitious sounds
GI: abdominal examination, bowel sounds
Laboratory tests: hepatic and renal function tests, FBC

Implementation

Provide comfort and safety measures, small meals, drug with food if GI upset occurs, bowel program as needed; taper dosage after long-term use; reduce dosage if other medications include narcotics; lower dose with renal or hepatic impairment.
Provide support and reassurance to deal with drug effects.
Provide teaching regarding drug, dosage, adverse effects, safety precautions and unusual symptoms to report.

Evaluation

Evaluate drug effects: relief of signs and symptoms of anxiety.
Monitor for adverse effects, particularly sedation, dizziness, insomnia, blood dyscrasia, GI upset, hepatic or renal dysfunction, cardiovascular effects.
Monitor for drug–drug interactions.
Evaluate effectiveness of teaching program.
Evaluate effectiveness of comfort and safety measures.

TEACHING FOR P.P.

- The drug that has been prescribed for you is called diazepam or *Valium*. It belongs to a class of drugs called benzodiazepines, which are used to relieve tension and nervousness. Exactly how the drug works is not completely understood, but it does relax muscle spasms, relieve insomnia and promote calm. Common side effects of this drug include:
  - *Dizziness and drowsiness:* avoid driving or performing hazardous or delicate tasks that require concentration if these effects occur.
  - *Nausea, vomiting and weight loss:* small frequent meals may help to relieve nausea. If weight loss occurs, monitor the loss; if the loss is extensive, consult your health care provider. Do not take this drug with antacids.
  - *Constipation or diarrhoea:* these reactions usually pass with time. If they do not, consult with your health care provider for appropriate therapy.
  - *Vision changes, slurred speech, unsteadiness:* these effects also subside with time. Take extra care in your activities for the first few days. If these reactions do not go away after 3 or 4 days, consult your health care provider.
- Report any of the following conditions to your health care provider: *rash, fever, sore throat, insomnia, depression, clumsiness or nervousness.*
- Tell any doctor, nurse or other health care provider involved in your care that you are taking this drug.
- Keep this drug and all medications safely away from children or pets.
- Avoid the use of over-the-counter medications or herbal therapies while you are taking this drug. If you think that you need one of these products, consult with your health care provider about the best choice because many of these products can interfere with your medication.
- Avoid alcohol while you are taking this drug. Combining alcohol and a benzodiazepine can cause serious problems.
- If you have been taking this drug for a prolonged time, do not stop taking it suddenly. Your body will need time to adjust to the loss of the drug, and the dosage will need to be reduced gradually to prevent serious problems. When discontinuing use of this drug, tell your health care provider if the following occurs: trembling, muscle cramps, sweating, irritability, confusion or seizures.

KEY POINTS

- Anxiety is a feeling of tension, nervousness, apprehension or fear. In the extreme, anxiety may produce physiological manifestations and may interfere with activities of daily life. Anxiolytic drugs, such as the benzodiazepines, depress the CNS to diminish these feelings.
- CNS depressants, such as sedatives, block the awareness of and reaction to environmental stimuli. They induce drowsiness, as do hypnotic drugs, which also depress the CNS and inhibit neuronal arousal.
- Hypnotics react with GABA-inhibitory sites to depress the CNS. They can cause drowsiness, lethargy and other CNS effects.

BARBITURATES USED AS ANXIOLYTIC/HYPNOTICS

The **barbiturates** were once the sedative/hypnotic drugs of choice. Not only is the likelihood of sedation and other adverse effects greater with these drugs than with newer sedative/hypnotic drugs, but the risk of addiction and dependence is also greater. For these reasons, newer anxiolytic drugs have replaced barbiturates in most instances. The only barbiturate used as an anxiolytic/hypnotic in Australia and New Zealand is phenobarbital (phenobarbitone).

Therapeutic actions and indications

The barbiturates are general CNS depressants that inhibit neuronal impulse conduction in the ascending RAS, depress the cerebral cortex, alter cerebellar function and depress motor output (see Figure 20.1). Thus, they can cause sedation, hypnosis, anaesthesia and, in extreme cases, coma. In general, barbiturates are indicated for the relief of the signs and symptoms of anxiety and for sedation, insomnia, pre-anaesthesia and the treatment of seizures (Table 20.2). Parenteral forms, which reach peak levels faster and have a faster onset of action, may be used for the treatment of acute manic reactions and many forms of seizures (see Chapter 23).

Pharmacokinetics

The barbiturates are absorbed well, reaching peak levels in 20–60 minutes. They are metabolised in the liver to varying degrees, depending on the drug, and excreted in the urine. The longer-acting barbiturates tend to be metabolised more slowly and excreted to a greater degree unchanged in the urine. The barbiturates are known to induce liver enzyme systems, increasing the metabolism of the barbiturate broken down by that system, as well as that of any other drug that may be metabolised by that enzyme system. People with hepatic or renal dysfunction require lower doses of the drug to avoid toxic effects and should be monitored closely. Barbiturates are lipid soluble; they readily cross the placenta and enter breast milk.

TABLE 20.2 DRUGS IN FOCUS Barbiturate used as anxiolytic–hypnotic

Drug name	Dosage/route	Usual indications
Ⓟ Phenobarbital (phenobarbitone) sodium (generic)	Adult: 30–120 mg/day PO, slowly IV or IM Paediatric: 1–6 mg/kg/day PO or 1–3 mg/kg/day slowly IV or IM	Sedative–hypnotic; control of seizures Onset: 10–60 minutes Duration: 4–16 hours Special considerations: taper gradually after long-term use; give IV slowly; monitor injection sites

Contraindications and cautions

Contraindications to barbiturates include allergy to any barbiturate and a previous history of addiction to sedative/hypnotic drugs *because the barbiturates are more addictive than most other anxiolytics*. Other contraindications are latent or manifest porphyria, *which may be exacerbated*; marked hepatic impairment or nephritis, *which may alter the metabolism and excretion of these drugs*; and respiratory distress or severe respiratory dysfunction, *which could be exacerbated by the CNS depression caused by these drugs*. Pregnancy is a contraindication *because of potential adverse effects on the fetus*; congenital abnormalities have been reported with barbiturate use.

Use with caution in people with acute or chronic pain *because barbiturates can cause paradoxical excitement, masking other symptoms*; with seizure disorders *because abrupt withdrawal of a barbiturate can precipitate status epilepticus*; and with chronic hepatic, cardiac or respiratory diseases, *which could be exacerbated by the depressive effects of these drugs*. Care should be taken with breastfeeding women *because of the potential for adverse effects on the infant*.

Prototype summary: phenobarbital (phenobarbitone)

Indications: sedation, short-term treatment of insomnia, long-term treatment of tonic–clonic seizures and cortical focal seizures, emergency control of certain acute convulsive episodes, pre-anaesthetic.

Actions: inhibits conduction in the ascending RAS; depresses the cerebral cortex; alters cerebellar function; depresses motor output; can produce excitation, sedation, hypnosis, anaesthesia and deep coma; and has anticonvulsant activity.

Pharmacokinetics:

Route	Peak	Onset	Duration
Oral	15 min	30–60 min	10–16 hours
IM		10–30 min	4–6 hours
IV	up to 15 min	5 min	4–6 hours

$T_{1/2}$: 79 hours; metabolised in the liver, excreted in urine.

Adverse effects: somnolence, agitation, confusion, hyperkinesias, ataxia, vertigo, CNS depression, hallucinations, bradycardia, hypotension, syncope, nausea, vomiting, constipation, diarrhoea, hypoventilation, apnoea, withdrawal syndrome, rash.

Adverse effects

As previously stated, the adverse effects caused by barbiturates are more severe than those associated with other, newer sedatives/hypnotics. For this reason, barbiturates are no longer considered the mainstay for the treatment of anxiety. In addition, the development of physical tolerance and psychological dependence is more likely with the barbiturates than with other anxiolytics.

The most common adverse effects are related to general CNS depression. CNS effects may include drowsiness, somnolence, lethargy, ataxia, vertigo, a feeling of a 'hangover', thinking abnormalities, paradoxical excitement, anxiety and hallucinations. GI signs and symptoms such as nausea, vomiting, constipation, diarrhoea and epigastric pain may occur. Associated cardiovascular effects may include bradycardia, hypotension (particularly with IV administration) and syncope. Serious hypoventilation may occur, and respiratory depression and laryngospasm may also result, particularly with IV administration. Hypersensitivity reactions, including rash, serum sickness and Stevens–Johnson syndrome, which is sometimes fatal, may also occur.

Clinically important drug–drug interactions

Increased CNS depression results if these agents are taken with other CNS depressants, including alcohol, antihistamines and other tranquillisers. If other CNS depressants are used, dose adjustments are necessary.

There is often an altered response to phenytoin if it is combined with barbiturates; evaluate the person frequently if this combination cannot be avoided. If barbiturates are combined with monoamine oxidase (MAO) inhibitors, increased serum levels and effects occur. If the older sedatives/hypnotics are combined with MAO inhibitors, people should be monitored closely and necessary dose adjustments made.

In addition, because of an enzyme-induction effect of barbiturates in the liver, the following drugs may not be as effective as desired: oral anticoagulants, digoxin, tricyclic antidepressants (TCAs), corticosteroids, oral contraceptives, oestrogens, paracetamol, metronidazole, carbamazepine, beta blockers, griseofulvin, theophyllines and doxycycline. If these agents are given in combination with barbiturates, people should be monitored closely; frequent dose adjustments may be necessary to achieve the desired therapeutic effect.

Care considerations for people receiving barbiturates

Assessment: history and examination

- Assess for contraindications or cautions: known allergies to barbiturates *to prevent hypersensitivity reactions* or a history of addiction to sedative/hypnotic drugs *to avert a similar problem with these drugs*; impaired hepatic or renal function *that could alter the metabolism and excretion of the drug*; cardiac dysfunction or respiratory dysfunction; seizure disorders, *which could be exacerbated by these drugs*; acute or chronic pain disorders, *which should be evaluated before using these drugs*; and pregnancy or breastfeeding, *which would indicate a need for caution when using these drugs.*
- Assess for baseline status *before beginning therapy and for the occurrence of any potential adverse effects.* Assess the following: temperature and weight; blood pressure and pulse, including perfusion; skin colour and lesions; affect, orientation and reflexes; respiratory rate and adventitious sounds; and bowel sounds.

Implementation with rationale

- Do not administer these drugs intra-arterially *because serious arteriospasm and gangrene could occur.* Monitor injection sites carefully *for local reactions.*
- Do not mix IV drugs in solution with any other drugs *to avoid potential drug–drug interactions.*
- Give parenteral forms only if oral forms are not feasible or available, and switch to oral forms as soon as possible *to avoid serious reactions or adverse effects.*
- Give IV medications slowly *because rapid administration may cause cardiac problems.*
- Provide standby life-support facilities *in case of severe respiratory depression or hypersensitivity reactions.*
- Taper dose gradually after long-term therapy, especially in people with epilepsy. Acute withdrawal *may precipitate seizures or cause withdrawal syndrome in these individuals.*
- Provide comfort measures *to help people tolerate drug effects*, including small, frequent meals; access to bathroom facilities; bowel program as needed; consuming food with the drug if GI upset is severe; and environmental control, safety precautions, orientation and appropriate skin care as needed.
- Provide thorough teaching, including drug name, prescribed dosage, measures for avoidance of adverse effects, and warning signs that may indicate possible problems. Instruct people about the need for periodic monitoring and evaluation *to enhance knowledge about drug therapy and to promote compliance.*
- Offer support and encouragement *to help the person cope with the diagnosis and the drug regimen.*

Evaluation

- Monitor response to the drug (alleviation of signs and symptoms of anxiety, sleep, sedation, reduction in seizure activity).
- Monitor for adverse effects (sedation, hypotension, cardiac arrhythmias, hepatic or renal dysfunction, skin reactions, dependence).
- Evaluate the effectiveness of the teaching plan (person can give the drug name, dosage, possible adverse effects to watch for, specific measures to help avoid adverse effects and the importance of continued follow-up).
- Monitor the effectiveness of comfort measures and compliance with the regimen.

KEY POINTS

- Barbiturates are an older class of drugs used as anxiolytics, sedatives and hypnotics. Because they are associated with potentially serious adverse effects and interact with many other drugs, they are less desirable than the benzodiazepines or other anxiolytics.

OTHER ANXIOLYTIC AND HYPNOTIC DRUGS

Other drugs are used to treat anxiety or to produce hypnosis that do not fall into either the benzodiazepine or the barbiturate group. See Table 20.3 for a list of other anxiolytic/hypnotic drugs, including usual

TABLE 20.3 DRUGS IN FOCUS Other anxiolytic/hypnotic drugs

Drug name	Usual indications
alimemazine (trimeprazine) (*Vallergan*)	Oral drug for sedation in children **Special considerations:** major component of dosage should be given at bedtime, or if daytime doses are ordered, give directly after meals
buspirone (*Buspar*)	Oral drug for anxiety disorders; off-label use; signs and symptoms of premenstrual syndrome **Special considerations:** may cause dry mouth, headache; use with caution in people with hepatic or renal impairment and in elderly people
chloral hydrate (generic)	Administered PO or PR for nocturnal sedation, preoperative sedation **Special considerations:** withdraw gradually over 2 weeks in people maintained for weeks or months
dexmedetomidine (*Precedex*)	IV drug used for newly intubated and mechanically ventilated people in the intensive care unit **Special considerations:** do not use longer than 24 hours; monitor person continually
promethazine (*Phenergan*)	PO, IM, or IV use to decrease the need for postoperative pain relief and for preoperative sedation **Special considerations:** an antihistamine; monitor injection sites carefully; monitor people for thickened respiratory secretions and breathing difficulties, a problem that can cause concern after anaesthesia
zolpidem (*Stilnox*)	Oral drug for short-term treatment of insomnia **Special considerations:** dispense the least amount possible to depressed and/or suicidal people; withdraw gradually if used for prolonged period; person should take before bed and devote 4–8 hours to sleep; use with caution in people with hepatic or renal impairment; elderly people are especially sensitive to these drugs – administer a lower dose and monitor these people carefully
zopiclone (*Imovane*)	Oral drug for the treatment of insomnia **Special considerations:** tablet must be swallowed whole; instruct the person to take this drug just before bed and allow 8 hours for sleep

indications and special considerations. Such medications include the following:

- Antihistamines (promethazine [*Phenergan*] and alimemazine [trimeprazine] [*Vallergan*]) can be very sedating in some people. They are used as preoperative medications and postoperatively to decrease the need for narcotics.
- Buspirone (*Buspar*) (not available in Australia) is an antianxiety agent, has no sedative, anticonvulsant or muscle relaxant properties, and its mechanism of action is unknown. However, it reduces the signs and symptoms of anxiety without many of the CNS effects and severe adverse effects associated with other anxiolytic drugs. It is rapidly absorbed from the GI tract, metabolised in the liver and excreted in urine.
- Chloral hydrate (generic) is frequently used to produce nocturnal sedation or preoperative sedation. Its mechanism of action is unknown. It is rapidly absorbed from the GI tract and metabolised in the liver and kidney for excretion in the bile and urine.
- Dexmedetomidine (*Precedex*) is given IV at a starting dose of 1 microgram/kg over 10 minutes and then a controlled infusion for up to 24 hours. It is used for the sedation of newly intubated and mechanically ventilated people in an intensive care unit.
- Zopiclone (*Imovane*) is an agent used to treat insomnia. It is thought to react with GABA sites near benzodiazepine receptors. It is rapidly absorbed, metabolised in the liver and excreted in the urine.
- Zolpidem (*Stilnox*) (not available in New Zealand) is used for the short-term treatment of insomnia. It is thought to work by affecting serotonin levels in the sleep centre near the RAS. It is metabolised in the liver and excreted in the urine.

CHAPTER SUMMARY

- Anxiolytics, or minor tranquillisers, are drugs used to treat anxiety by depressing the CNS. When given at higher doses, these drugs may be sedatives or hypnotics.
- Sedatives block the awareness of, and reaction to, environmental stimuli, resulting in associated CNS depression that may cause drowsiness, lethargy and other effects. This action can be beneficial when a person is very excited or afraid.
- Hypnotics further depress the CNS, particularly the RAS, to inhibit neuronal arousal and induce sleep.
- Benzodiazepines are a group of drugs used as anxiolytics. They react with GABA-inhibitory sites to depress the CNS. They can cause drowsiness, lethargy and other CNS effects.

- Barbiturates are an older class of drugs used as anxiolytics, sedatives and hypnotics. Because they are associated with potentially serious adverse effects and interact with many other drugs, they are less desirable than the benzodiazepines or other anxiolytics.
- Buspirone, an anxiolytic drug, does not cause sedation or muscle relaxation. Because of the absence of CNS effects, it is much preferred in certain circumstances (eg, when a person must drive, go to work or maintain alertness).
- Newer hypnotic agents act in the RAS to affect serotonin levels (zolpidem – not available in New Zealand).

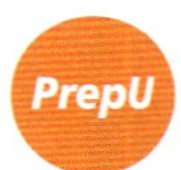

Knowing your strengths and weaknesses helps you to study more effectively. Take a PrepU Practice Quiz to find out how you measure up!

ONLINE RESOURCES

An extensive range of additional resources to enhance teaching and learning and to facilitate understanding of this chapter may be found online at the text's accompanying website, located on thePoint at http://thepoint.lww.com. These include Watch and Learn videos, Concepts in Action animations, journal articles, review questions, case studies, discussion topics and quizzes.

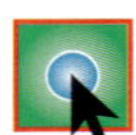

WEB LINKS

Health care providers and students may want to consult the following web resources:

www.beyondblue.org.au
Beyond Blue

BIBLIOGRAPHY

Goodman, L. S., Brunton, L. L., Chabner, B. & Knollmann, B. C. (2011). *Goodman and Gilman's Pharmacological Basis of Therapeutics* (12th edn). New York: McGraw-Hill.

Kyrios, M., Mouding, R. & Nedeljkovic, M. (2011). Anxiety disorders – Assessment and management in general practice. *Australian Family Physician, 40*, 370–374.

Lampe, L. (2013). Drug treatment for anxiety. *Australian Prescriber, 36*, 186–189.

McKenna, L. & Mirkov, S. (2019). *McKenna's Drug Handbook for Nursing and Midwifery* (8th edn). Sydney: Wolters Kluwer Health Australia.

O'Brien, P. G. & Fleming, L. (2012). Recognizing anxiety disorders. *Nurse Practitioner, 37(10)*, 35–42.

Olson, L. G. (2008). Hypnotic hazards: Adverse effects of zolpidem and other z-drugs. *Australian Prescriber, 31*, 146–149.

Parcells, D. A. (2010). Women's mental health nursing: Depression, anxiety and stress during pregnancy. *Journal of Psychiatric & Mental Health Nursing, 17*, 813–820.

Porth, C. M. (2011). *Essentials of Pathophysiology: Concepts of Altered Health States* (3rd edn). Philadelphia: Lippincott Williams & Wilkins.

Porth, C. M. (2009). *Pathophysiology: Concepts of Altered Health States* (8th edn). Philadelphia: Lippincott Williams & Wilkins.

Rang, H. P., Dale, M. M., Ritter, J. M., Flower, R. J. & Henderson, G. (2011). *Rang & Dale's Pharmacology* (7th edn). Edinburgh: Churchill Livingstone.

CHECK YOUR UNDERSTANDING

Answers to the questions in this chapter can be found in Appendix A at the back of this book.

MULTIPLE CHOICE

Select the best answer to the following.

1. Drugs that are used to alter a person's response to the environment are called:
   a. hypnotics.
   b. sedatives.
   c. antiepileptics.
   d. anxiolytics.
2. The benzodiazepines are the most frequently used anxiolytic drugs because:
   a. they are anxiolytic at doses much lower than those needed for sedation or hypnosis.
   b. they can also be stimulating.
   c. they are more likely to cause physical dependence than older anxiolytic drugs.
   d. they do not affect any neurotransmitters.

3. Barbiturates cause liver enzyme induction, which could lead to:
   a. rapid metabolism and loss of effectiveness of other drugs metabolised by those enzymes.
   b. increased bile production.
   c. CNS depression.
   d. the need to periodically lower the barbiturate dose to avoid toxicity.

4. A person who could benefit from an anxiolytic drug for short-term treatment of insomnia would not be prescribed:
   a. zolpidem.
   b. chloral hydrate.
   c. buspirone.
   d. zopiclone.

5. Anxiolytic drugs block the awareness of, and reaction to, the environment. This effect would not be beneficial:
   a. to relieve extreme fear.
   b. to moderate anxiety related to unknown causes.
   c. in treating a person who must drive a vehicle for a living.
   d. in treating a person who is experiencing a stress reaction.

6. Mr Jones is the chief executive officer of a large company and has been experiencing acute anxiety attacks. His physical examination was normal and he was diagnosed with anxiety. Considering his occupation and his need to be alert and present to large groups on a regular basis, the following anxiolytic would be a drug of choice for Mr Jones:
   a. phenobarbital (phenobarbitone).
   b. diazepam.
   c. oxazepam.
   d. buspirone.

7. The benzodiazepines react with:
   a. GABA-receptor sites in the RAS to cause inhibition of neural arousal.
   b. noradrenaline-receptor sites in the sympathetic nervous system.
   c. acetylcholine-receptor sites in the parasympathetic nervous system.
   d. monoamine oxidase to increase noradrenaline breakdown.

8. A child is prescribed phenobarbital preoperatively to relieve anxiety and produce sedation. After giving the injection, you should assess the child for:
   a. acute Stevens–Johnson syndrome.
   b. bone marrow depression.
   c. paradoxical excitement.
   d. withdrawal syndrome.

MULTIPLE RESPONSE

Select all that apply.

1. In assessing a person who is experiencing anxiety, the nurse or midwife would expect to find which of the following?
   a. rapid breathing
   b. rapid heart rate
   c. fear and apprehension
   d. constricted pupils
   e. decreased abdominal sounds
   f. hypotension

2. A woman has a long history of anxiety and has always responded well to diazepam. She has just learned that she is pregnant and feels very anxious. She would like a prescription for diazepam to get her through her early anxiety. What rationale would the nurse or midwife use in explaining why this is not recommended?
   a. This drug is known to cause a predictable syndrome of birth defects, including cleft lip and pyloric stenosis.
   b. Babies born to mothers taking benzodiazepines may progress through a neonatal withdrawal syndrome.
   c. Cardiac defects and small brain development may occur if this drug is taken in the first trimester.
   d. This drug almost always causes loss of the pregnancy.
   e. The hormones the body produces during pregnancy will make you unresponsive to diazepam.
   f. This drug could have adverse effects on your baby; we should explore non-drug measures to help you deal with the anxiety.

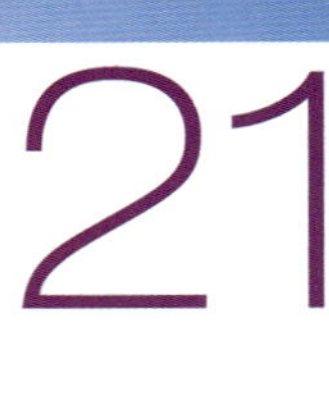

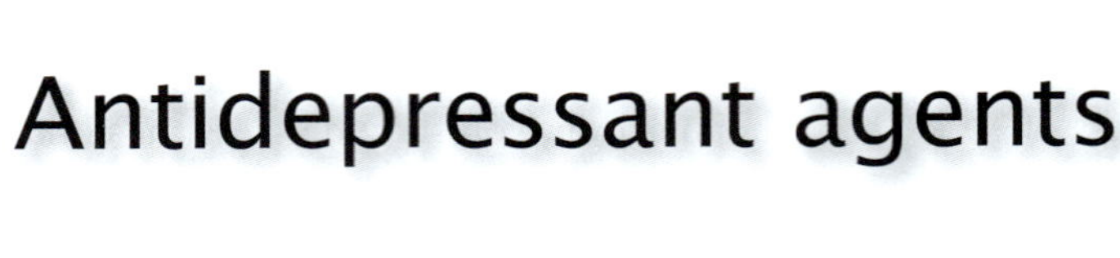

21 Antidepressant agents

Learning objectives

On completing this chapter you should be able to:

1. Describe the biogenic theory of depression.
2. Describe the therapeutic actions, indications, pharmacokinetics, contraindications, most common adverse reactions and important drug–drug interactions associated with each class of antidepressant.
3. Discuss the use of antidepressants across the lifespan.
4. Compare and contrast the prototype drugs for each class of antidepressant with the other drugs in that class and with drugs in the other classes of antidepressants.
5. Outline the care considerations and teaching needs for people receiving each class of antidepressant.

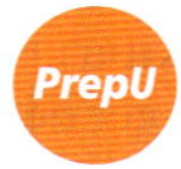

Test your current knowledge of antidepressant agents with a PrepU Practice Quiz!

Glossary of keys terms

affect: feeling that a person experiences when they respond emotionally to the environment

biogenic amine: one of the neurotransmitters noradrenaline, serotonin or dopamine; it is thought that a deficiency of these substances in key areas of the brain results in depression

depression: affective disorder in which a person experiences sadness that is much more severe and longer lasting than is warranted by the event that seems to have precipitated it, with a more intense mood; the condition may not even be traceable to a specific event or stressor

monoamine oxidase (MAO) inhibitor: drug that prevents the enzyme monoamine oxidase from breaking down noradrenaline, leading to increased noradrenaline levels in the synaptic cleft; relieves depression and also causes sympathomimetic effects

selective serotonin reuptake inhibitor (SSRI): drug that specifically blocks the reuptake of serotonin and increases its concentration in the synaptic cleft; relieves depression and is not associated with anticholinergic or sympathomimetic adverse effects

tricyclic antidepressant (TCA): drug that blocks the reuptake of noradrenaline and serotonin; relieves depression and has anticholinergic and sedative effects

tyramine: an amine found in food that causes vasoconstriction and raises blood pressure; ingesting foods high in tyramine while taking an MAO inhibitor poses the risk of a severe hypertensive crisis

TRICYCLIC ANTIDEPRESSANTS
- amitriptyline
- clomipramine
- dosulepin (dothiepin)
- doxepin
- (P) imipramine
- nortriptyline

MONOAMINE OXIDASE INHIBITORS
- (P) phenelzine
- tranylcypromine

SELECTIVE SEROTONIN REUPTAKE INHIBITORS
- citalopram
- duloxetine
- escitalopram
- (P) fluoxetine
- fluvoxamine
- paroxetine
- sertraline

OTHER ANTIDEPRESSANTS
- agomelatine
- bupropion
- desvenlafaxine
- mianserin
- mirtazapine
- moclobemide
- reboxetine
- venlafaxine

When you ask people how they feel, they may say 'pretty good' or 'not so great'. People's responses are usually appropriate to what is happening in their lives, and they describe themselves as being in a good mood or a bad mood. Some days are better than others.

Affect is a term that is used to refer to people's feelings in response to their environment, whether positive and pleasant or negative and unpleasant. All people experience different affective states at various times in their lives. These states of mind, which change in particular situations, usually do not last very long and do not often involve extremes of happiness or depression. If a person's mood goes far beyond the usual normal 'ups and downs', they are said to have an affective disorder. Mental health is a National Priority Area for the Australian Government so is an important area for nurses and midwives to understand and be able to respond to (AIHW, 2018).

DEPRESSION AND ANTIDEPRESSANTS

Depression is a very common affective disorder involving feelings of sadness that are much more severe and longer lasting than the suspected precipitating event, and the mood of affected individuals is much more intense. The depression may not even be traceable to a specific event or stressor (i.e. there are no external causes). People who are depressed may have little energy, sleep disturbances, lack of appetite, limited libido and inability to perform activities of daily living. They may describe overwhelming feelings of sadness, despair, hopelessness and disorganisation.

In many cases, the depression is never diagnosed, and the person is treated for physical manifestations of the underlying disease, such as fatigue, malaise, obesity, anorexia, or alcoholism and drug dependence. Clinical depression is a disorder that can interfere with a person's family life, job and social interactions. Left untreated, it can produce multiple physical problems that can lead to further depression or, in extreme cases, even suicide.

Biogenic amine theory of depression

Research on the development of the drugs known to be effective in relieving depression led to formulation of the current hypothesis regarding the cause of depression. Scientists have theorised that depression results from a deficiency of **biogenic amines** in key areas of the brain; these biogenic amines include noradrenaline, dopamine and serotonin (5-hydroxytryptamine, 5HT). Both noradrenaline and 5HT are released throughout the brain by neurons that react with multiple receptors to regulate arousal, alertness, attention, moods, appetite and sensory processing. Deficiencies of these neurotransmitters may develop for three known reasons. First, monoamine oxidase (MAO) may break them down to be recycled or restored in the neurons. Second, rapid fire of the neurons may lead to their depletion. Third, the number or sensitivity of postsynaptic receptors may increase, thus depleting neurotransmitter levels.

Depression may also occur as a result of other, as yet unknown, causes. This condition may be a syndrome that reflects either activity or lack of activity in a number of sites in the brain, including the arousal centre (reticular activating system [RAS]), the limbic system and basal ganglia.

Drug therapy

The use of agents that alter the concentration of neurotransmitters in the brain is the most effective means of treating depression with drugs. The antidepressant drugs used today counteract the effects of neurotransmitter deficiencies in three ways. First, they may inhibit the effects of MAO, leading to increased noradrenaline or 5HT in the synaptic cleft. Second, they may block reuptake by the releasing nerve, leading to increased neurotransmitter levels in the synaptic cleft. Third, they may regulate receptor sites and the breakdown of neurotransmitters, leading to an accumulation of neurotransmitter in the synaptic cleft.

Antidepressants may be classified into three groups: the tricyclic antidepressants (TCAs), the MAO inhibitors and the selective serotonin reuptake inhibitors (SSRIs). Other drugs that are used as antidepressants similarly increase the synaptic cleft concentrations of these neurotransmitters (see Figure 21.1). For information on how antidepressants affect people from young to old, see Box 21.1.

TRICYCLIC ANTIDEPRESSANTS

The **tricyclic antidepressants** (**TCAs**), including the amines, secondary amines and tetracyclics, all reduce the reuptake of 5HT and noradrenaline into nerves. Because all TCAs are similarly effective, the choice of TCA depends on individual response to the drug and tolerance of adverse effects. A person who does not respond to one TCA may respond to another drug from this class. TCAs that are available include the amines amitriptyline (*Endep*, *Amitrip*), clomipramine (*Anafranil*, *Placil*), dosulepin hydrochloride, dothiepin (*Dothep*), doxepin (*Deptran*, *Sinequan*), imipramine (*Tofranil*) and the secondary amines such as nortriptyline (*Allegron*). Table 21.1 shows the relative frequency of the occurrence of adverse effects by specific type of TCA.

Therapeutic actions and indications

The TCAs inhibit presynaptic reuptake of the neurotransmitters 5HT and noradrenaline, which leads to an

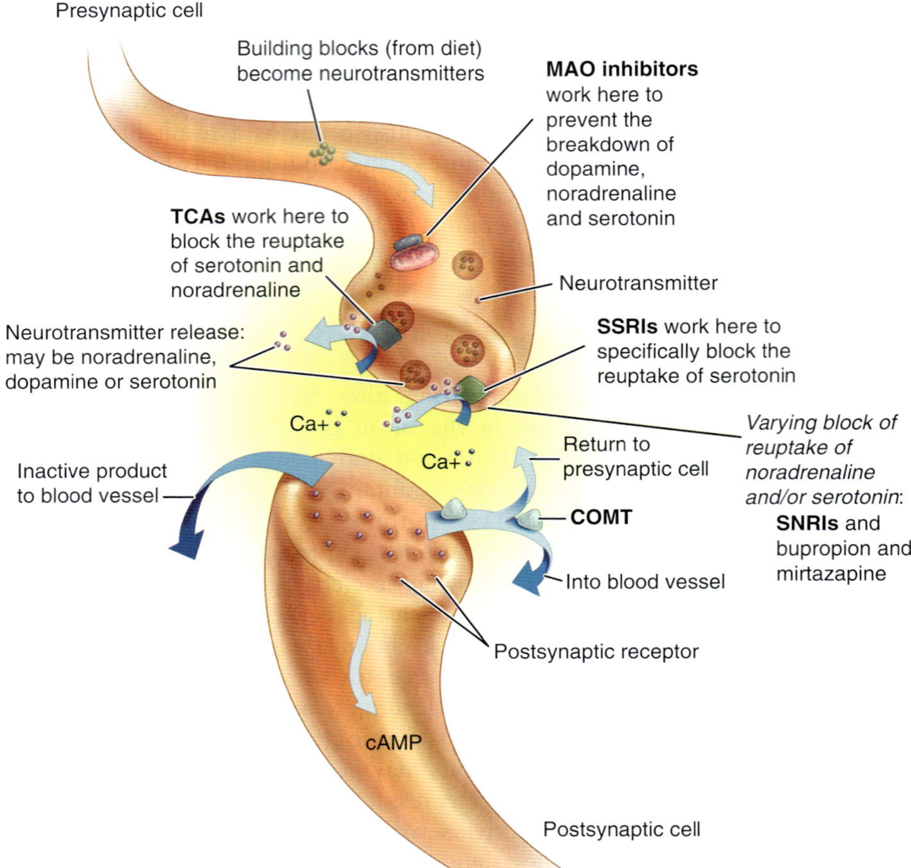

FIGURE 21.1 Sites of action for the antidepressants: monoamine oxidase (MAO) inhibitors, tricyclic antidepressants (TCAs), selective serotonin reuptake inhibitors (SSRIs), serotonin–noradrenaline reuptake inhibitors (SNRIs), and other agents, cyclic adenosine monophosphate (cAMP) and catecholamine-O-methyltransferase (COMT).

BOX 21.1 FOCUS ON Drug therapy across the lifespan

Antidepressant agents

CHILDREN

Use of antidepressant drugs with children poses a challenge. The response of the child to the drug may be unpredictable, and the long-term effects of many of these agents are not clearly understood. Studies have not shown efficacy in using these drugs to treat depression in children and also indicate that there may be an increase in suicidal ideation and suicidal behaviour when antidepressants are used to treat depression in children.

Of the TCAs, clomipramine, imipramine and nortriptyline have established paediatric doses in children older than 6 years. Children should be monitored closely for adverse effects, and dose changes should be made as needed.

MAO inhibitors should be avoided in children if at all possible because of the potential for drug–food interactions and the serious adverse effects.

The SSRIs can cause serious adverse effects in children. Fluvoxamine and sertraline have established paediatric dose guidelines for the treatment of obsessive–compulsive disorders. Fluoxetine is widely used to treat depression in adolescents, and a 2000 survey of off-label uses of drugs showed that it was being used in children as young as 6 months. Dosage regimens must be established according to the child's age and weight, and a child receiving an antidepressant should be monitored very carefully. Underlying medical reasons for the depression should be ruled out before antidepressant therapy is begun. Again, these children should be monitored for any suicidal ideation.

ADULTS

Adults using these drugs should have medical causes for their depression ruled out before therapy is begun. Thyroid disease, hormonal imbalance and cardiovascular disorders can all lead to the signs and symptoms of depression.

The person needs to understand that the effects of drug therapy may not be seen for 4 weeks and that it is important to continue the therapy for at least that long.

PREGNANCY AND BREASTFEEDING

These drugs should be used very cautiously during pregnancy and breastfeeding because of the potential

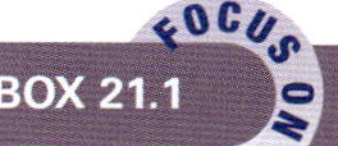

BOX 21.1 Drug therapy across the lifespan *(continued)*

for adverse effects on the fetus and possible neurological effects on the baby. Use should be reserved for situations in which the benefits to the mother far outweigh the potential risks to the neonate.

OLDER ADULTS

Older people may be more susceptible to the adverse effects of these drugs, from unanticipated central nervous system (CNS) effects to increased sedation, dizziness and even hallucinations. Antidepressants have been recognised as a contributory factor to falls due to sedation, insomnia, nocturia, impaired postural reflexes, orthostatic hypotension, cardiac rhythm and conduction disorders, and movement disorders. Doses of all of these drugs need to be reduced and the person monitored very closely for toxic effects. Safety measures should be provided if CNS effects do occur.

People with hepatic or renal impairment should be monitored very closely while taking these drugs. Decreased doses may be needed. Because many older people also have renal or hepatic impairment, they need to be screened carefully.

TABLE 21.1 *DRUGS IN FOCUS* Tricyclic antidepressants

Drug name	Common side effects				Usual dosage
	Sedation	Anticholinergic	Hypotension	Cardiovascular	
Amines					
amitriptyline (*Endep, Amitrip*)	++++	++++	++++	++	75–150 mg/day PO
clomipramine (*Anafranil, Placil*)	+++	+++	+++	+++	25–50 mg PO bd or tds
dosulepin (dothiepin) (*Dothep*)	+++ Central nervous system adverse effects are common, particularly in the elderly, and include anxiety, dizziness, agitation, confusion, sleep disturbances, irritability, and paraesthesia; drowsiness is associated with some of the tricyclic antidepressants ... not sedation www.nzf.org.nz/nzf_2252.html?searchterm=dothiepin	+++	+++	++++ See Medsafe report of prolongation of QT intervals www.medsafe.govt.nz/profs/PUArticles/December2013QTProlongationAndAntidepressants.htm	Adult initially 75 mg (elderly 50–75 mg) daily in divided doses or as a single dose at bedtime, increased gradually as necessary to 150 mg daily (elderly 75 mg may be sufficient); up to 200 mg daily in some circumstances (eg, hospital use) Capsules are 25 mg
doxepin (*Deptran, Sinequan*)	+++	+++	++	++	10–100 mg PO tid
Ⓟ imipramine (*Tofranil*)	++	++	+++	++	Adult: 50–200 mg/day PO Paediatric (5–8 years): 20–30 mg/day Paediatric (> 12 years): 25–75 mg/day Maximum 2.5 mg/kg/day

Continued on following page

TABLE 21.1 DRUGS IN FOCUS Tricyclic antidepressants *(continued)*

Drug name	Common side effects				Usual dosage
	Sedation	Anticholinergic	Hypotension	Cardiovascular	
Secondary amines					
nortriptyline (*Allegron*)	+	+	+	+	Adults: 25 mg tid–qid to a maximum of 100 mg/day Elderly: 25–50 mg/day in divided doses

+ + + +, marked effects; + + +, moderate effects; + +, mild effects; +, negligible effects.

accumulation of these neurotransmitters in the synaptic cleft and increased stimulation of the postsynaptic receptors. The exact mechanism of action in decreasing depression is not known but is thought to be related to the accumulation of noradrenaline and 5HT in certain areas of the brain.

TCAs are indicated for the relief of symptoms of depression. The sedative effects of these drugs may make them more effective in people whose depression is characterised by anxiety and sleep disturbances. They are effective for treating enuresis in children older than 6 years (see Box 21.1). Some of these drugs are being investigated for the treatment of chronic, intractable pain. In addition, the TCAs are anticholinergic. Clomipramine is now also approved for use in the treatment of obsessive–compulsive disorders (OCDs).

Pharmacokinetics

The TCAs are well absorbed from the gastrointestinal (GI) tract, reaching peak levels in 2–4 hours. They are highly bound to plasma proteins and are lipid soluble; this allows them to be distributed widely in the tissues, including the brain. TCAs are metabolised in the liver and excreted in the urine, with relatively long half-lives, ranging from 8 to 46 hours. The TCAs cross the placenta and enter breast milk (see Contraindications and cautions).

Contraindications and cautions

One contraindication to the use of TCAs is the presence of allergy to any of the drugs in this class *because of the risk of hypersensitivity reactions*. Other contraindications include recent myocardial infarction (MI) *because of the potential occurrence of reinfarction or extension of the infarct with the cardiac effects of the drug*; myelography within the previous 24 hours or in the next 48 hours *because of a possible drug–drug interaction with the dyes used in these studies*; and concurrent use of an MAO inhibitor *because of the potential for serious adverse effects or toxic reactions*. In addition, pregnancy and breastfeeding are contraindications *because of the potential for adverse effects in the fetus and neonate*; TCAs should not be used unless the benefit to the mother clearly outweighs the potential risk to the neonate.

Caution should be used with TCAs in people with pre-existing cardiovascular (CV) disorders *because of the cardiac stimulatory effects of the drug* and with *any condition that would be exacerbated by the anticholinergic effects*, such as angle-closure glaucoma, urinary retention, prostate hypertrophy, or GI or genitourinary (GU) surgery. Care should also be taken with people with mental health problems, *who may exhibit a worsening of psychoses or paranoia*, and those with manic–depressive disorder, *who may shift to a manic stage*. There is a black box warning on all of the TCAs bringing attention to a risk of suicidality, especially in children and adolescents; caution should be used, and the amount of drug dispensed at any given time should be limited with people who are potentially suicidal. In addition, caution is necessary in people with a history of seizures *because the seizure threshold may be decreased secondary to stimulation of the receptor sites* and in elderly people. The presence of hepatic or renal disease, *which could interfere with metabolism and excretion of these drugs and lead to toxic levels*, also necessitates caution and the need for a lower dose of the drug.

Adverse effects

The adverse effects of TCAs are associated with the effects of the drugs on the CNS and on the peripheral nervous system. Sedation, sleep disturbances, fatigue, hallucinations, disorientation, visual disturbances, difficulty in concentrating, weakness, ataxia and tremors may occur. Limited quantities of tricyclic antidepressants should be prescribed at any one time because their cardiovascular and epileptogenic effects are dangerous in overdosage. In particular, overdosage with dosulepin (dothiepin) and amitriptyline is associated with a relatively high rate of fatality.

Use of TCAs may lead to GI anticholinergic effects, such as dry mouth, constipation, nausea, vomiting, anorexia, increased salivation, cramps and diarrhoea. Resultant GU effects may include urinary retention and hesitancy, loss of libido and changes in sexual functioning. CV effects such as orthostatic hypotension, hypertension, arrhythmias, MI, angina, palpitations and stroke may also pose problems. Miscellaneous reported effects include alopecia, weight gain or loss, flushing, chills and nasal congestion.

These adverse effects may be intolerable to some people, who then stop taking the particular TCA. Abrupt cessation of all TCAs causes a withdrawal syndrome characterised by nausea, headache, vertigo, malaise and nightmares (see Box 21.2).

Prototype summary: imipramine

Indications: relief of symptoms of depression; enuresis in children older than 6 years; off-label consideration – control of chronic pain.

Actions: inhibits presynaptic reuptake of noradrenaline and serotonin; anticholinergic at CNS and peripheral receptors; sedating.

Pharmacokinetics:

Route	Onset	Peak
Oral	Varies	2–4 hours

$T_{1/2}$: 8–16 hours, metabolised in the liver, excreted in the urine.

Adverse effects: sedation, anticholinergic effects, confusion, anxiety, orthostatic hypotension, dry mouth, constipation, urinary retention, rash, bone marrow depression.

Clinically important drug–drug interactions

If TCAs are given with cimetidine, fluoxetine or ranitidine, an increase in TCA levels results, with an increase in both therapeutic and adverse effects, especially anticholinergic conditions. People should be monitored closely, and appropriate dose reductions should be made.

Other drug combinations may also pose problems. The combination of TCAs and oral anticoagulants leads to higher serum levels of the anticoagulants and increased risk of bleeding. Blood tests should be done frequently, and appropriate dose adjustments in the oral anticoagulant should be made.

If TCAs are combined with sympathomimetics or clonidine, the risk of arrhythmias and hypertension is increased. This combination should be avoided, especially in people with underlying cardiovascular disease.

BOX 21.2 Antidepressant discontinuation syndrome

Antidepressant discontinuation syndrome may occur within 5 days of stopping treatment with antidepressant drugs; symptoms are usually mild and self-limiting (lasting for 1–2 weeks), but in some cases may be severe. Tricyclic antidepressants MAO inhibitors and antidepressants with a shorter half-life, such as paroxetine and venlafaxine, are associated with a higher risk of discontinuation symptoms. The risk of discontinuation symptoms is also increased if the antidepressant is stopped suddenly after regular administration for 8 weeks or more. Symptoms can also occur after a reduction in dose or omission of a dose. The dose should preferably be reduced gradually over about 4 weeks (fluoxetine is an exception to this rule due to its long half-life), or longer if discontinuation symptoms emerge (up to 6 months in people who have been on long-term maintenance treatment). Many people will continue to have symptoms despite a slow withdrawal. Antimuscarinic agents may assist with tricyclic antidepressant withdrawal.

Source: New Zealand Formulary, www.nzf.org.nz/nzf_2225.html#nzf_2230

The combination of TCAs with MAO inhibitors leads to a risk of severe hyperpyretic crisis with severe convulsions, hypertensive episodes and death. This combination should be avoided. Although TCAs and MAO inhibitors have been used together in selected individuals who do not respond to a single agent, the risk of severe adverse effects is very high.

Care considerations for people receiving tricyclic antidepressants

Assessment: history and examination

- Assess for any known allergies to these drugs *to avoid hypersensitivity reactions*; impaired liver or kidney function, *which could alter metabolism and excretion of the drug*; glaucoma, benign prostatic hypertrophy, cardiac dysfunction, GI obstruction, surgery or recent MI, *all of which could be exacerbated by the effects of the drug*; and pregnancy or breastfeeding *to avoid potential adverse effects on the fetus or baby.*
- Assess whether the person has a history of seizure disorders or a history of psychiatric problems or suicidal thoughts, or myelography within the past 24 hours or in the next 48 hours, or is taking an MAO inhibitor, *to avoid potentially serious adverse reactions.*

- Assess temperature and weight; skin colour and lesions; affect, orientation and reflexes; vision; blood pressure, including orthostatic blood pressure; pulse and perfusion; respiratory rate and adventitious sounds; and bowel sounds on abdominal examination. *This determines baseline status before beginning therapy and for any potential adverse effects*. Also obtain an electrocardiogram, as well as renal and liver function tests.

Implementation with rationale

- Limit drug access if the person is suicidal *to decrease the risk of overdose*.
- Maintain the initial dose for 4–8 weeks *to evaluate the therapeutic effect*.
- Administer parenteral forms of the drug only if oral forms are not feasible or available; switch to an oral form, *which is less toxic and associated with fewer adverse effects*, as soon as possible.
- Administer a major portion of the dose at bedtime if drowsiness and anticholinergic effects are severe *to decrease the risk of injury. Elderly people may not be able to tolerate larger doses*.
- Reduce dose if minor adverse effects occur, and discontinue the drug slowly if major or potentially life threatening adverse effects occur *to ensure safety*.
- Provide comfort measures *to help the person tolerate drug effects*. These measures may include voiding before dosing, instituting a bowel program as needed, taking food with the drug if GI upset is severe and environmental control (lighting, temperature, stimuli).
- Provide thorough teaching, including drug name, prescribed dosage, measures for avoidance of adverse effects and warning signs that may indicate possible problems. Instruct the person about the need for periodic monitoring and evaluation *to enhance knowledge about drug therapy and to promote compliance*.
- Offer support and encouragement *to help the person cope with the diagnosis and the drug regimen*.

Evaluation

- Monitor response to the drug (alleviation of signs and symptoms of depression).
- Monitor for adverse effects (sedation, anticholinergic effects, hypotension, cardiac arrhythmias, suicidal thoughts).
- Evaluate the effectiveness of the teaching plan (person can give the drug name, dosage, possible adverse effects to watch for, specific measures to help avoid adverse effects and importance of continued follow-up).
- Monitor the effectiveness of comfort measures and compliance with the regimen.

KEY POINTS

- Affect is a term that refers to the feelings that people experience when they respond emotionally.
- Depression is an affective disorder characterised by inappropriate sadness, despair and hopelessness.
- According to the biogenic amine theory, depression is caused by a brain deficiency of the biogenic amines. Antidepressant drugs are thought to raise the level of the biogenic amines.
- Antidepressant discontinuation syndrome may occur within 5 days of stopping treatment with antidepressant drugs; symptoms are usually mild and self-limiting (lasting for 1–2 weeks), but in some cases may be severe.

MONOAMINE OXIDASE INHIBITORS

Monoamine oxidase (MAO) inhibitors (Table 21.2) irreversibly inhibit MAO, an enzyme found in nerves and other tissues (including the liver), to break down the biogenic amines noradrenaline, dopamine and 5HT, and relieve depression. At one time, MAO inhibitors were used more often, but now they are used rarely because they require a specific dietary regimen to prevent toxicity. There are some people, however, who only seem to respond to these particular drugs, so they remain available. Agents still in use include the reversible MAO type A inhibitor moclobemide (*Amira, Aurorix*), and non-selective MAO inhibitors phenelzine (*Nardil*), and tranylcypromine (*Parnate*). The choice of an MAO inhibitor depends on the prescriber's experience and individual response. A person who does not respond to one MAO inhibitor may respond to another.

Therapeutic actions and indications

Blocking the breakdown of the biogenic amines noradrenaline, dopamine and 5HT allows these amines to accumulate in the synaptic cleft and in neuronal storage vesicles, causing increased stimulation of the postsynaptic receptors. It is thought that this increased stimulation of the receptors causes relief of depression. The MAO inhibitors are generally indicated for treatment of the signs and symptoms of depression in people who cannot tolerate or do not respond to other, safer, antidepressants (see Table 21.2).

Pharmacokinetics

The MAO inhibitors are well absorbed from the GI tract, reaching peak levels in 2–3 hours. They are metabolised in the liver primarily by acetylation and are excreted in the urine. People with liver or renal impairment and those known as 'slow acetylators' may require

TABLE 21.2 DRUGS IN FOCUS Monoamine oxidase (MAO) inhibitors

Drug name	Dosage/route	Usual indications
(P) phenelzine (*Nardil*)	15 mg PO tds; maintenance 15 mg/day PO	Treatment of depression not responsive to other agents
tranylcypromine (*Parnate*)	Adults only: 10 mg morning and afternoon; add further 10 mg at midday if no response after 2 weeks; adjust according to response; maximum 30 mg/day	Treatment of adult reactive depression

lowered doses to avoid exaggerated effects of the drugs. The MAO inhibitors cross the placenta and enter breast milk (see Contraindications and cautions).

Contraindications and cautions

Contraindications to the use of MAO inhibitors include allergy to any of these antidepressants *because of the risk of hypersensitivity reactions*; phaeochromocytoma *because the sudden increases in noradrenaline levels could result in severe hypertension and CV emergencies*; CV disease, including hypertension, coronary artery disease, angina and congestive heart failure, *which could be exacerbated by increased noradrenaline levels*; and known abnormal CNS vessels or defects *because the potential increase in blood pressure and vasoconstriction associated with higher noradrenaline levels could precipitate a stroke*. A history of headaches may also be a contraindication.

Other contraindications include renal or hepatic impairment, *which could alter the metabolism and excretion of these drugs and lead to toxic levels*, and myelography within the past 24 hours or in the next 48 hours *because of the risk of severe reaction to the dye used in myelography. MAO inhibitors may cause idiosyncratic hepatotoxicity if used in people with hepatic impairment*

In addition, caution should be used with people with mental health problems, *who could be overstimulated or shift to a manic phase as a result of the stimulation associated with MAO inhibitors*, and in people with seizure disorders or hyperthyroidism, *both of which could be exacerbated by the stimulation of these drugs*. There is a black box warning on all drugs of this class to bring awareness to a possible risk of suicidality, especially with children and adolescents, in people using these drugs. Care should also be taken with individuals who are soon to undergo elective surgery *because of the potential for unexpected effects with noradrenaline accumulation during the stress reaction*, and with women who are pregnant or breastfeeding *because of potential adverse effects on the fetus and neonate;* these drugs should be used during pregnancy and breastfeeding only if the benefit to the mother clearly outweighs the potential risk to the neonate.

Adverse effects

The MAO inhibitors are associated with more adverse effects, more of which are fatal, than most other antidepressants. The effects relate to the accumulation of *noradrenaline* in the synaptic cleft. Dizziness, excitement, nervousness, mania, hyperreflexia, tremors, confusion, insomnia, agitation and blurred vision may occur.

MAO inhibitors can cause liver toxicity. MAO inhibitors may cause idiosyncratic hepatotoxicity if used in people with hepatic impairment. Other GI effects can include nausea, vomiting, diarrhoea or constipation, anorexia, weight gain, dry mouth and abdominal pain. Urinary retention, dysuria, incontinence and changes in sexual function may also occur. Cardiovascular effects can include orthostatic hypotension, arrhythmias, palpitations, angina and the potentially fatal hypertensive crisis. This last condition is characterised by occipital headache, palpitations, neck stiffness, nausea, vomiting, sweating, dilated pupils, photophobia, tachycardia and chest pain. It may progress to intracranial bleeding and fatal stroke.

MAO inhibitors are associated with discontinuation symptoms on cessation of therapy. Symptoms include agitation, irritability, ataxia, movement disorders, insomnia, drowsiness, vivid dreams, cognitive impairment and slowed speech. Symptoms occasionally experienced when discontinuing MAO inhibitors include hallucinations and paranoid delusions. If possible MAO inhibitors should be withdrawn slowly.

Clinically important drug–drug interactions

Drug interactions of MAO inhibitors with other antidepressants include hypertensive crisis, coma and severe convulsions with TCAs and a potentially life-threatening serotonin syndrome with SSRIs. A period of 6 weeks should elapse after stopping an SSRI before beginning therapy with an MAO inhibitor.

If MAO inhibitors are given with other sympathomimetic drugs (eg, methyldopa, guanethidine), sympathomimetic effects increase. Combinations with insulin or oral hypoglycaemic agents result in additive hypoglycaemic effects. People who receive these combinations must be monitored closely, and appropriate dose adjustments should be made.

Clinically important drug–food interactions

Tyramine and other pressor amines that are found in food, which are normally broken down by MAO enzymes in the GI tract, may be absorbed in high concentrations in the presence of non-selective MAO inhibitors, resulting in increased blood pressure. In addition, tyramine causes the release of stored *noradrenaline* from nerve terminals, which further contributes to high blood pressure and hypertensive crisis. People who take non-selective MAO inhibitors should avoid the tyramine-containing foods listed in Table 21.3.

Prototype summary: phenelzine

Indications: treatment of people with depression who are unresponsive to other antidepressive therapy or in whom other antidepressive therapy is contraindicated.

Actions: irreversibly inhibits MAO, allowing noradrenaline, serotonin and dopamine to accumulate in the synaptic cleft; this accumulation is thought to be responsible for the clinical effects.

Pharmacokinetics:

Route	Onset	Duration
Oral	Slow	48–96 hours

$T_{1/2}$: unknown; metabolised in the liver, excreted in urine.

Adverse effects: dizziness, vertigo, headache, overactivity, hyperreflexia, tremors, mania, weakness, drowsiness, fatigue, sweating, orthostatic hypotension, constipation, diarrhoea, dry mouth, oedema, anorexia, potential for hypertensive crisis.

Care considerations for people receiving monoamine oxidase inhibitors

Assessment: history and examination

- Assess for any known allergies to these drugs *to avoid hypersensitivity reactions*; impaired liver or kidney function *that could alter the metabolism and excretion of the drug*; cardiac dysfunction; GI or GU obstruction, *which could be exacerbated by the drug*; surgery, including elective surgery, *because the effects of changes in noradrenaline levels are unpredictable following surgery*; seizure disorders; psychiatric conditions or suicidality; and occurrence of myelography within the past 24 hours or in the next 48 hours *to avoid the possibility of severe reactions.*
- Determine whether women are pregnant or breastfeeding *because these drugs should not be used during pregnancy or breastfeeding.*
- Assess temperature and weight; skin colour and lesions; affect, orientation, and reflexes; vision; blood pressure, including orthostatic blood pressure; pulse and perfusion; respiratory rate and adventitious sounds; and bowel sounds on abdominal examination *to determine baseline status and for any potential adverse effects before beginning therapy.* Also obtain an electrocardiogram and renal and liver function tests.

Implementation with rationale

- Limit drug access to a potentially suicidal person *to decrease the risk of overdose.*
- Monitor the person for 2–4 weeks *to ascertain the onset of the full therapeutic effect.*
- Monitor blood pressure and orthostatic blood pressure carefully *to arrange for a slower increase*

TABLE 21.3 Tyramine-containing foods

Foods high in tyramine	Foods with moderate amounts of tyramine	Foods with low amounts of tyramine
Aged cheeses: Cheddar cheese, blue cheese, Swiss cheese, Camembert Aged or fermented meats, fish or poultry: chicken pâté, beef liver pâté, caviar Brewer's yeast, Vegemite, Marmite, Bonox Broad beans Red wines: Chianti, Burgundy, sherry, vermouth Soy sauce, tofu, banana peels Smoked or pickled meats, fish or poultry: herring, sausage, corned beef, salami, pepperoni	Meat extracts: consommé, bouillon Pasteurised light and pale beer Avocados	Distilled liquors: vodka, gin, Scotch, rye Cheeses: american, mozzarella, cottage cheese, cream cheese Chocolate Fruits: figs, raisins, grapes, pineapple, oranges Sour cream Yoghurt

in dose as needed for people who show a tendency towards hypotension.

- Monitor liver function before and periodically during therapy and *arrange to discontinue the drug at the first sign of liver toxicity.*
- Discontinue drug and monitor the person carefully at any complaint of severe headache *to decrease the risk of severe hypertension and cerebrovascular effects.*
- Have an adrenergic blocker on standby *as treatment in case of hypertensive crisis.*
- Provide comfort measures *to help the person tolerate drug effects.* These include voiding before dosing, instituting a bowel program as needed, taking food with the drug if GI upset is severe and environmental control (lighting, temperature, decreased stimulation).
- Provide a list of potential drug–food interactions that can cause severe toxicity *to decrease the risk of a serious drug–food interaction.* Provide a diet that is low in tyramine-containing foods.
- Provide thorough teaching, including drug name, prescribed dosage, measures for avoidance of adverse effects and warning signs that may indicate possible problems. Instruct the person about the need for periodic monitoring and evaluation *to enhance knowledge about drug therapy and to promote compliance.*
- Offer support and encouragement *to help the person cope with the disease and the drug regimen.*

Evaluation

- Monitor response to the drug (alleviation of signs and symptoms of depression).
- Monitor for adverse effects (sedation, sympathomimetic effects, hypotension, cardiac arrhythmias, GI disturbances, hypertensive crisis).
- Evaluate the effectiveness of the teaching plan (person can give the drug name, dosage, possible adverse effects to watch for, specific measures to help avoid adverse effects, importance of continued follow-up and importance of avoiding foods high in tyramine).
- Monitor the effectiveness of comfort measures and compliance with the regimen.

KEY POINTS

- The MAO inhibitors prevent the breakdown of noradrenaline and 5HT by monoamine oxidase, leading to an increased level of these biogenic amines in the synaptic cleft. This accumulation of the amines is thought to relieve the signs and symptoms of depression.
- People taking MAO inhibitors need to avoid foods high in tyramine to prevent serious increases in blood pressure and hypertensive crises.

SELECTIVE SEROTONIN REUPTAKE INHIBITORS

Selective serotonin reuptake inhibitors (SSRIs) (Table 21.4), the newest large group of antidepressant drugs, specifically block the reuptake of 5HT, with little to no known effect on noradrenaline. Because SSRIs do not have the many adverse effects associated with TCAs and MAO inhibitors, they are a better choice for many people. SSRIs include fluoxetine (*Prozac*), the first SSRI; citalopram (*Cipramil*); escitalopram (*Lexapro*), fluvoxamine (not available in New Zealand) (*Luvox*); paroxetine (*Aropax*); and sertraline (*Xydep*, *Zoloft*).

Therapeutic actions and indications

The action of SSRIs blocking the reuptake of 5HT increases the levels of 5HT in the synaptic cleft and may contribute to the antidepressant and other effects attributed to these drugs.

SSRIs are indicated for the treatment of depression, OCDs, panic attacks, bulimia, premenstrual dysphoric disorder (PMDD), posttraumatic stress disorders, social phobias and social anxiety disorders. A period of up to 4 weeks is necessary for realisation of the full therapeutic effect. People may respond well to one SSRI and yet show little or no response to another one. The choice of drug depends on the indications and individual response. Box 21.3 provides more information. Ongoing investigations are focusing on the use of these antidepressant drugs in the treatment of other psychiatric disorders (see Table 21.4).

Pharmacokinetics

The SSRIs are well absorbed from the GI tract, metabolised in the liver and excreted in the urine and faeces. The half-life varies widely with the drug being used.

Contraindications and cautions

The SSRIs are contraindicated in the presence of allergy to any of these drugs *because of the risk of hypersensitivity reactions.* Caution should be used in people with impaired renal or hepatic function *that could alter the metabolism and excretion of the drug, leading to toxic effects,* or with diabetes, *which could be exacerbated by the stimulating effects of these drugs.* Caution should also be used with people who are severely depressed or suicidal, especially children and adolescents, *because*

TABLE 21.4 DRUGS IN FOCUS Selective serotonin reuptake inhibitors

Drug name	Dosage/route	Usual indications
citalopram (*Cipramil*)	20 mg/day PO bd, up to 60 mg/day may be needed	Treatment of depression in adults has also been used to treat panic disorder, premenstrual dysphoric disorder (PMDD), obsessive-compulsive disorders (OCDs), social phobias, trichotillomania and posttraumatic stress disorders
duloxetine (*Cymbalta*)	30 mg/day PO, up to 120 mg/day if needed	Treatment of major depressive disorder and management of neuropathic pain associated with diabetic peripheral neuropathy
escitalopram (*Lexapro*)	10 mg/day PO as a single dose; 10–20 mg/day PO maintenance	Treatment of major depressive disorder, maintenance of people with major depressive disorder and generalised anxiety disorder
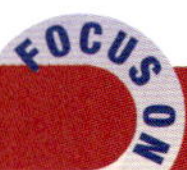 fluoxetine (*Prozac, Lovan*)	20–80 mg/day PO in the am; do not exceed 60 mg/day; reduce dose with hepatic impairment; also available in a 90 mg, once-a-week formulation	Treatment of depression, bulimia, OCDs, panic disorders, PMDD in adults; also under investigation for treatment of other psychiatric disorders, including obesity, alcoholism, chronic pain and various neuropathies
fluvoxamine (*Luvox*)	Adult: 50 mg PO at bedtime to a maximum of 300 mg/day; reduce dose with hepatic impairment Paediatric (8–17 years): 25 mg PO at bedtime; do not exceed 200 mg/day	Treatment of OCDs; also under investigation for treatment of depression, bulimia, panic disorder and social phobia
paroxetine (*Aropax*)	10–20 mg/day PO; do not exceed 60 mg/day; reduce dose in hepatic or renal dysfunction and with the elderly	Treatment of depression, OCDs, PMDD, posttraumatic stress reaction, social anxiety disorders, general anxiety disorders and various panic disorders in adults; also under investigation for treatment of chronic headache, diabetic neuropathy and hot flushes
sertraline (*Xydep, Zoloft*)	Adult: 50–200 mg/day PO; reduce dose with hepatic dysfunction, OCD Paediatric: 25–50 mg/day PO based on age and severity of OCD	Treatment of depression, OCDs, social anxiety disorder, posttraumatic stress disorder, panic disorders and PMDD

FOCUS ON Safe medication administration

***Look-alike, sound-alike medications**: when administering medications, confusion about similar drug names may present a hazard, for example with* Celica *(citalopram) and* Celebrex *(celecoxib). Use caution. Serious adverse effects have been reported, as well as important loss of therapeutic effects, when the wrong drug is given. If any of these drugs is ordered for a person, make sure you know the indication for the drug, as well as the generic name of the prescribed drug.*

of a risk of increased suicidality. The SSRIs have been associated with congenital abnormalities in animal studies and should be used during pregnancy only if the benefits to the mother clearly outweigh the potential risks to the fetus. The SSRIs enter breast milk and can cause adverse effects in the baby, so a different method of feeding should be selected if an SSRI is required by the mother.

In New Zealand, none of the SSRIs have ever been licensed for use in those aged less than 18 years (however, it is recognised that off-label use occurs in this age group). All NZ data sheets (information provided for medicine prescribers) for all SSRIs currently state that 'Safety and effectiveness in children has not been established'. All but fluoxetine and sertraline go further to state that 'use is not recommended in children'.

Adverse effects

The adverse effects associated with SSRIs, which are related to the effects of increased 5HT levels, include CNS effects such as headache, drowsiness, dizziness, insomnia, anxiety, tremor, agitation and seizures. GI effects such as nausea, vomiting, diarrhoea, dry mouth,

Prototype summary: fluoxetine

Indications: treatment of depression, OCDs, bulimia, PMDD, panic disorders; off-label uses include chronic pain, alcoholism, neuropathies, obesity.

Actions: inhibits CNS neuronal reuptake of serotonin, with little effect on noradrenaline and little affinity for cholinergic, histaminic or alpha-adrenergic sites.

Pharmacokinetics:

Route	Onset	Peak
Oral	Slow	6–8 hours

$T_{1/2}$: 2–4 weeks; metabolised in the liver, excreted in urine and faeces.

Adverse effects: headache, nervousness, insomnia, drowsiness, anxiety, tremor, dizziness, sweating, rash, nausea, vomiting, diarrhoea, dry mouth, anorexia, sexual dysfunction, upper respiratory infections, weight loss, fever.

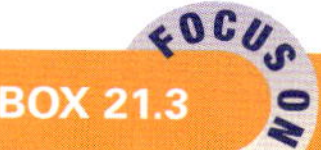

BOX 21.3 Cultural considerations

The popularity of *Prozac*

A rise in the diagnosis of depression began in the 1990s, with that decade's fast-paced lifestyle, high-stress jobs, explosion of information, and rapid change. Many people who have high expectations of both themselves and others are overworked and overstimulated to a point at which they become clinically depressed.

There is now a selection of relatively safe and non-toxic drugs that can be used to treat depression – the selective serotonin reuptake inhibitors (SSRIs). For several years, the SSRIs remained in the top-selling category of prescription drugs. Fluoxetine (*Prozac*), in particular, has been the subject of numerous talk shows, books and movies. In many ways, *Prozac* was the 'in' drug of the 1990s. This societal phenomenon put pressure on health care providers to prescribe a drug even if it was not appropriate to a given person's situation. In some instances, people just wanted the drug that helped their friend. They may not have been willing to listen to their health care provider or to take the time to be properly diagnosed; they just wanted an SSRI. *Prozac* is not the solution to everyone's problem, and it is often difficult to explain this fact to a person. It also may be hard to get the person to understand that this drug is not a quick fix; it takes 4–6 weeks to achieve full therapeutic effectiveness.

It is important to remember the powerful effects of the media on health care-seeking behaviour. As more and more drugs are advertised in magazines and on television, people are becoming aware of options and 'cures' that they might like to try. Education is a tricky yet important part of any health care intervention and an extremely important aspect of health care in our society.

BOX 21.4 Serotonin syndrome

The use of SSRIs has been linked to a condition called serotonin syndrome or serotonin toxicity. Serotonin syndrome is potentially life threatening, as it can result in excessive serotonergic activity at the central and peripheral serotonin receptors. The excessive serotonergic activity is caused by using excessive doses of a single serotonergic drug, or from the use of a combination of serotonergic drugs acting on the same receptors or even from switching between antidepressants without adequate 'wash-out period'. Antidepressant drugs eg, SSRIs and clomipramine, lithium, St John's wort, pethidine, tramadol and linezolid are examples of drugs likely to cause serotonin syndrome.

Source: www.nzf.org.nz/nzf_2287.html

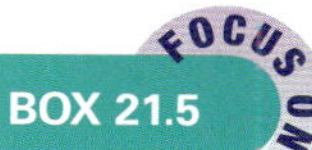

BOX 21.5 The evidence

Childhood suicide and antidepressants

In 2004, the Australian Government Adverse Drug Reactions Advisory Committee (ADRAC) reviewed U.S. Food and Drug Administration (FDA) and UK Committee on Safety of Medicines (CSM) reports around increased risk of suicidal behaviour in children being treated with SSRIs. It was concluded that there was evidence that SSRIs could increase risk of suicidal ideation, attempts and self-harm. ADRAC recommended that use of SSRIs in children or adolescents should only be considered in the full context of the person's overall management. This includes caution and careful monitoring of behaviour and compliance, and should include cognitive behavioural therapy if available. The choice to prescribe SSRIs needs to include consideration of published trial data, product information and manufacturer warnings about use in children and adolescents. Finally, it is advised that SSRIs should not be abruptly stopped in these groups. See www.tga.gov.au/use-ssri-antidepressants-children-and-adolescents-october-2004.

anorexia and constipation. Changes in taste often occur, as do GU effects, including painful menstruation, cystitis, sexual dysfunction, urgency and impotence. Respiratory changes may include cough, dyspnoea, upper respiratory infections and pharyngitis. Other reported effects are sweating, rash, fever and pruritus. Recent studies have linked the incidence of suicidal ideation and suicide attempts to the use of these drugs in children and adolescents (see Box 21.5).

Clinically important drug–drug interactions

Because of the risk of serotonin syndrome if SSRIs are used with MAO inhibitors, this combination should be avoided, and at least 2–4 weeks should be allowed between use of the two types of drugs if a person is switching from one to the other. In addition, the use of SSRIs with TCAs results in increased therapeutic and toxic effects. If these combinations are used, people should be monitored closely, and appropriate dose adjustments should be made. For more information see Box 21.6.

BOX 21.6 FOCUS ON Herbal and alternative therapies

People being treated with SSRIs are at an increased risk of developing a severe reaction, including serotonin syndrome, as well as an increased sensitivity to light if they are also taking St John's wort. Because this herbal therapy is often used to self-treat depression, it is important to forewarn any person who is taking an SSRI not to combine it with taking St John's wort.

Also caution people that there is an increased risk of seizures if evening primrose is used with antidepressants, and people should be cautioned against this combination. Interactions have also been reported when antidepressants are combined with ginkgo, ginseng and valerian. People should be cautioned against using these herbs while taking antidepressants.

Care considerations for people receiving selective serotonin reuptake inhibitors

Assessment: history and examination

- Assess for any known allergies to SSRIs *to avoid hypersensitivity reactions*; severe depression or suicidality, *which could be exacerbated by these drugs*; impaired liver or kidney function, *which could alter metabolism and excretion of the drug*; and diabetes mellitus. Find out whether women are pregnant or breastfeeding *because caution should be used in these situations and drug use limited.*
- Assess temperature and weight; skin colour and lesions; affect, orientation and reflexes; vision; blood pressure and pulse; respiratory rate and adventitious sounds; and bowel sounds on abdominal examination *for baseline status before beginning therapy and for any potential adverse effects*. Also obtain renal and liver function tests.
- *Refer to Critical thinking scenario for a full discussion of care for a person who is dealing with depression.*

Implementation with rationale

- Arrange for lower dose in elderly people and in those with renal or hepatic impairment *because of the potential for severe adverse effects.*
- Monitor the person for up to 4 weeks *to ascertain the onset of full therapeutic effect before adjusting dose.*
- Establish suicide precautions for severely depressed people and limit the quantity of the drug dispensed *to decrease the risk of overdose.*
- Administer the drug once a day in the morning *to achieve optimal therapeutic effects*. If dose is increased or if the person is having severe GI effects, the dose can be divided. Serious name confusion has been reported with some of the SSRIs (see Focus on safe medication administration in the section Contraindications and cautions).
- Suggest that the person use barrier contraceptives *to prevent pregnancy while taking this drug because serious fetal abnormalities can occur.*
- Provide comfort measures *to help the person tolerate drug effects*. These may include voiding before dosing, instituting a bowel program as needed, taking food with the drug if GI upset is severe or environmental control (lighting, temperature, stimuli).
- Provide thorough teaching, including the drug name, prescribed dosage, measures for avoidance of adverse effects and warning signs that may indicate possible problems. Instruct people about the need for periodic monitoring and evaluation *to enhance knowledge about drug therapy and to promote compliance.*
- Offer support and encouragement *to help the person cope with the disease and the drug regimen.*

Evaluation

- Monitor response to the drug (alleviation of signs and symptoms of depression, OCD, bulimia, panic disorder).
- Monitor for adverse effects (sedation, dizziness, GI upset, respiratory dysfunction, GU problems, skin rash, serotonin syndrome).
- Evaluate the effectiveness of the teaching plan (person can give the drug name, dosage, possible adverse effects to watch for, specific measures to help avoid adverse effects, importance of continued follow-up and importance of avoiding pregnancy).
- Monitor the effectiveness of comfort measures and compliance with the regimen.

KEY POINTS

- The SSRIs prevent the reuptake of serotonin into the presynaptic nerve, leading to an accumulation of these biogenic amines in the synaptic cleft. This accumulation causes increased stimulation of the postsynaptic nerve and may be responsible for the antidepressant effects of these drugs.
- The SSRIs are not associated with many of the CNS, CV and anticholinergic effects of other antidepressants.

CRITICAL THINKING SCENARIO

Selective serotonin reuptake inhibitors

THE SITUATION

D.J., a 46-year-old married woman, complains of weight gain, malaise, fatigue, sleeping during the day, loss of interest in daily activities and bouts of crying for no apparent reason. On examination, she weighs 4 kilograms more than the standard weight for her height; all other findings are within normal limits. In conversation with a nurse, D.J. says that in the past 10 months, several events have occurred. She lost both of her parents, her only child graduated from high school and went away to university, her nephew died of renal failure, her only sister learned she had metastatic breast cancer, and she lost her job as a day care provider when the client family moved out of town. In addition, the family cat of 17 years was diagnosed with terminal leukaemia. D.J. is prescribed fluoxetine (*Prozac*) and is given an appointment with a counsellor.

CRITICAL THINKING

What nursing interventions are appropriate at this time? What sort of crisis intervention would be most appropriate? *Balance the benefits of pointing out all of the losses and points of grief that you detect in D.J.'s story with the risks of upsetting her strained coping mechanisms.* What can D.J. expect to experience as a result of the SSRI therapy? How can you help D.J. cope during the lengthy period it takes to reach therapeutic effect? What other future interventions should be planned with D.J.?

DISCUSSION

Many people in severe crisis do not consciously identify the many things that are causing them stress. They have developed coping mechanisms to help them survive and cope with their day-to-day activities. D.J. seems to have reached her limit and exhibits many of the signs and symptoms of depression. However, it is important to make sure that she does not have some underlying medical condition that could be contributing to her complaints. Because of her age, she may also be perimenopausal, which could account for some of her problems.

It is hoped that the fluoxetine, an SSRI, will enable D.J. to regain her ability to cope and her normal affect. The drug should give her brain a chance to reach a new biochemical balance. Before she begins taking the fluoxetine, she should receive a written sheet listing the pertinent drug information, adverse effects to watch for, warning signs to report, and a telephone number to call in case she has questions later or just needs to talk. The written information is especially important because she may not remember drug-related discussions or instructions clearly.

Once the SSRI reaches therapeutic levels, which can take as long as 4 weeks, D.J. may start to feel like her 'old self' and may be strong enough to begin dealing with all her grief. She may recover from her need for the SSRI over time, and use of the medication can then be discontinued.

CARE GUIDE FOR D.J.: FLUOXETINE

Assessment: history and examination

Allergies to fluoxetine or any other antidepressant SSRI; renal or hepatic dysfunction; pregnancy or breastfeeding; diabetes

Concurrent use of TCAs, cyproheptadine, lithium, MAO inhibitors, benzodiazepines, alcohol, other SSRIs

CV: blood pressure, pulse

CNS: orientation, affect, reflexes, vision

Skin: colour, lesions, texture

Respiratory: respiration, adventitious sounds

GI: abdominal examination, bowel sounds

Laboratory tests: hepatic and renal function tests

Implementation

Administer drug in the morning; divide doses if GI upset occurs.

Provide comfort and safety measures such as side rails; provide small meals; facilitate voiding before dosing; give pain medication as needed; suggest barrier contraceptive; limit dosage with people who are potentially suicidal; lower dose with renal or hepatic impairment.

Provide support and reassurance to help D.J. deal with drug effects (4-week delay in full effectiveness).

Provide teaching regarding drug dosage, adverse effect conditions to report and the need to use barrier contraceptives.

Evaluation

Evaluate drug effects: relief of signs and symptoms of depression.

Monitor for adverse effects: sedation, dizziness, insomnia; respiratory dysfunction; GI upset; GU problems; rash.

Monitor for drug–drug interactions.

Evaluate effectiveness of teaching program.

Evaluate effectiveness of comfort and safety measures.

TEACHING FOR D.J.

- The drug that has been prescribed is called a selective serotonin reuptake inhibitor or SSRI. SSRIs change the concentration of serotonin in specific areas of the brain. An increase in serotonin level is believed to relieve depression.
- The drug should be taken once a day in the morning. If your dosage has been increased or if you are having stomach upset, the dose may be divided.

- It may take as long as 4 weeks before you feel the full effects of this drug. Continue to take the drug every day during that time so that the concentration of the drug in your body eventually reaches effective levels.
- Common side effects of SSRIs include the following:
  - *Dizziness, drowsiness, nervousness and insomnia:* if these effects occur, avoid driving or performing hazardous or delicate tasks that require concentration.
  - *Nausea, vomiting and weight loss:* small frequent meals may help. Monitor your weight loss; if it becomes excessive, consult your health care provider.
  - *Sexual dysfunction and flu-like symptoms:* these effects may be temporary. Consult with your health care provider if these conditions become bothersome.
- Report any of the following conditions to your health care provider: rash mania, seizures and severe weight loss.
- Tell your doctors, nurses and other health care providers that you are taking this drug. Keep this drug and all medications out of the reach of children and pets. Do not take this drug during pregnancy because severe fetal abnormalities could occur. The use of barrier contraceptives is recommended while you are taking this drug. If you think that you are pregnant or would like to become pregnant, consult with your health care provider.

SEROTONIN–NORADRENALINE REUPTAKE INHIBITORS (SNRIS)

A major advantage of the SSIRs, SNRIs and other antidepressants is the lack of anticholinergic, cardiovascular and other adverse effects, which were a major limitation of the TCAs.

Desvenlafaxine (*Pristiq*) (not available in New Zealand) blocks the reuptake of noradrenaline and 5HT. It is readily absorbed from the GI tract, reaching peak levels in 7.5 hours. It is metabolised in the liver and excreted through urine within about 72 hours. It passes into breast milk and should not be used by breastfeeding women. It should be used in pregnancy only if the benefit clearly outweighs the risk. It is taken orally, once a day.

Duloxetine (*Cymbalta*) is selectively inhibits 5HT and noradrenaline reuptake and also weakly inhibits dopamine reuptake. It is metabolised in the liver and most of the metabolites are excreted in the urine. Nausea has been reported as the most common adverse event. It is contraindicated in patients with liver disease and those drinking alcohol, as fatal cases of liver failure have been reported. Lower doses are used in patients with end-stage renal disease.

Venlafaxine (*Efexor*) mildly blocks the reuptake of noradrenaline, 5HT and dopamine and has fewer adverse CNS effects than other antidepressants. Its popularity has increased with the introduction of an extended-release form that does away with the multiple daily doses that are required with the regular form. Venlafaxine is readily absorbed from the GI tract, extensively metabolised in the liver and excreted in urine. Adequate studies have not been done in pregnancy and breastfeeding, and it should be used during those times only if the benefit to the mother clearly outweighs the potential risk to the neonate.

OTHER ANTIDEPRESSANTS

Some other effective antidepressants do not fit into any of the three groups that have been discussed in this chapter. These drugs have varying effects on noradrenaline, 5HT and dopamine. Although it is not known how their actions are related to clinical efficacy, these agents may be most effective in treating depression in people who do not respond to other antidepressants. They may even be used before MAO inhibitors or TCAs, which have many more adverse effects. As with the other antidepressants, these drugs have a black box warning to be alert for the possibility of increased suicidality, especially in children and adolescents, whenever the drugs are used. Other antidepressants include the following (see Table 21.5 for usual indications):

- Agomelatine (*Valdoxan*) (not available in New Zealand) is a melatonergic antidepressant used in the treatment of major depressive disorder. The drug is metabolised in the liver and excreted through urine. The drug does cross the placenta and enters breast milk, so it should only be used during pregnancy and breastfeeding if the benefit outweighs the potential risk to the neonate. This drug is associated with CNS effects, as well as GI effects including nausea, dry mouth and abdominal pain.
- Bupropion (*Zyban*) weakly blocks the reuptake of noradrenaline, 5HT and dopamine. At lower doses, this drug is effective in smoking cessation and is indicated as a short-term adjunctive therapy for the treatment of nicotine dependence in people committed to quitting smoking, in conjunction with counselling for smoking cessation. It is well absorbed from the GI tract, metabolised in the liver and excreted in the urine. Zyban tablets should be swallowed whole

TABLE 21.5 DRUGS IN FOCUS SNRIs and other antidepressants

Drug name	Dosage/route	Usual indications
agomelatine (*Valdoxan*)	25 mg PO at night; maximum 50 mg/day	Treatment of major depression in adults, including relapse prevention
bupropion (*Zyban*)	150 mg PO bd in sustained-release form; maximum 300 mg/day	Smoking cessation
desvenlafaxine (*Pristiq*)	50 mg/day PO with or without food; range 50–200 mg/day	Treatment of major depressive disorder in adults
mianserin (*Lumin*)	30 mg/day in three divided doses, maximum 120 mg/day	Treatment of major depression in adults
mirtazapine (*Avanza*)	15 mg/day PO, may be increased to a maximum of 60 mg/day; reduce dose in elderly people and those with renal or hepatic dysfunction	Treatment of depression in adults
moclobemide (*Amira*)	300–600 mg PO daily in two divided doses	Treatment of major depression in adults
reboxetine (*Edronax*)	4 mg PO bd, up to 10 mg/day	Treatment of major depression in adults
duloxetine (*Cymbalta*)	Adults: major depressive disorder, 60 mg PO once daily; generalised anxiety disorder, initially 30 mg PO once daily, up to a maximum of 120 mg PO once daily	Treatment of major depressive disorder and generalised anxiety disorder
venlafaxine (*Efexor XR*)	75 mg/day PO in divided doses, to 375 mg/day; 75 mg/day PO sustained-release formulation to a maximum 225 mg/day; reduce dose with hepatic and renal impairment	Treatment and prevention of depression in generalised anxiety disorder; social anxiety disorder; decreases addictive behaviour

and not crushed or chewed, as this may lead to an increased risk of adverse effects, including seizures. There are no adequate studies done in pregnancy, and the drug should be used during pregnancy only if the benefits to the mother clearly outweigh the potential risks to the fetus. Bupropion does enter breast milk and should not be used by breastfeeding women. The drug is available in a sustained-release formulation which some people find to be more convenient.

- Mianserin (*Lumin*) is a tetracyclic antidepressant, related to other TCAs, used to manage major depression and has effective sedative properties. Mianserin blocks alpha$_2$ adrenoceptors blocking reuptake of noradrenaline, and interacts with serotonin receptors. Mianserin has a half-life of 21–61 hours. It is rapidly absorbed and excreted in the urine and faeces. Little is known about its effects in pregnancy and breastfeeding, and it should be used during those times only if the benefit to the mother clearly outweighs the potential risk to the neonate.
- Mirtazapine (*Avanza*) is rapidly absorbed from the GI tract, extensively metabolised in the liver and excreted in the urine. Mirtazapine has a half-life of 20–40 hours. How its many anticholinergic effects relate to its antidepressive effects is not known. Little is known about its effects in pregnancy and breastfeeding, and it should be used during those times only if the benefit to the mother clearly outweighs the potential risk to the neonate.
- Reboxetine (*Edronax*) is a newer noradrenaline reuptake inhibitor used for managing major depression. It is rapidly absorbed with a half-life of 12 hours. Reboxetine is metabolised in the liver and excreted in the urine. Little is known about its effects in pregnancy and breastfeeding, and it should be used during those times only if the benefit to the mother clearly outweighs the potential risk to the neonate.

CHAPTER SUMMARY

- Depression is a very common affective disorder; it is associated with many physical manifestations and is often misdiagnosed. It could be that depression is caused by a series of events that are not yet understood.
- Antidepressant drugs – TCAs, MAO inhibitors, SSRIs and SNRIs – increase the concentrations of the biogenic amines in the brain.
- Selection of an antidepressant depends on individual drug response and tolerance of associated adverse effects. The adverse effects of TCAs are sedating and anticholinergic; those of MAO inhibitors are CNS related and sympathomimetic. The adverse effects of SSRIs are fewer, but they do cause CNS changes.
- Other antidepressants with unknown mechanisms of action are also effective in treating depression.

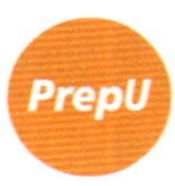

Knowing your strengths and weaknesses helps you to study more effectively. Take a PrepU Practice Quiz to find out how you measure up!

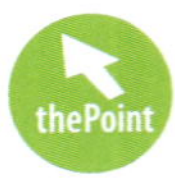

ONLINE RESOURCES

An extensive range of additional resources to enhance teaching and learning and to facilitate understanding of this chapter may be found online at the text's accompanying website, located on thePoint at http://thepoint.lww.com. These include Watch and Learn videos, Concepts in Action animations, journal articles, review questions, case studies, discussion topics and quizzes.

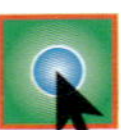

WEB LINKS

Health care providers and students may want to consult the following web resources:

www.aihw.gov.au/mental-health
Australian Institute of Health and Welfare, National Priority Area – Mental Health.

www.beyondblue.org.au
Beyond Blue – The National Depression Initiative.

www.nationaldrugstrategy.gov.au
Australian Government National Drug Strategy.

BIBLIOGRAPHY

Anderson C. & Roy, T. (2013). Patient experiences of taking antidepressants for depression: A secondary qualitative analysis. *Research in Social & Administrative Pharmacy, 9*, 884–902.

Australian Institute of Health and Welfare (AIHW). (2018). *Mental health*. Retrieved August 2019 from https://www.aihw.gov.au/getmedia/1838295a-5588-4747-9515-b826a5ab3d5a/aihw-aus-221-chapter-3-12.pdf.aspx

Buist, A. (2008). Treatment of perinatal depression. *Australian Prescriber, 31*, 36–39.

Casey, G. (2013). Antidepressants: Their role in treating depression. *Kai Tiaki Nursing New Zealand, 19(8)*, 20–24.

Goodman, L. S., Brunton, L. L., Chabner, B. & Knollmann, B. C. (2011). *Goodman and Gilman's Pharmacological Basis of Therapeutics* (12th edn). New York: McGraw-Hill.

Lampe, L. (2005). Antidepressants: Not just for depression. *Australian Prescriber, 28*, 91–93.

McKenna, L. & Mirkov, S. (2019). *McKenna's Drug Handbook for Nursing & Midwifery* (8th edn). Sydney: Wolters Kluwer Health Australia.

Porth, C. M. (2011). *Essentials of Pathophysiology: Concepts of Altered Health States* (3rd edn). Philadelphia: Lippincott Williams & Wilkins.

Porth, C. M. (2009). *Pathophysiology: Concepts of Altered Health States* (8th edn). Philadelphia: Lippincott Williams & Wilkins.

Rahman, S. Z., Basilakis, J., Rahmadi, A., Lujic, S., Musgrave, I., Jorm, L., Hau, P. & Munch, G. (2013). Use of serotonergic antidepressants and St John's wort in older Australians: A population-based cohort study. *Australasian Psychiatry, 21(3)*, 262–266.

Williams, A. V. (2007). Antidepressants in pregnancy and breastfeeding. *Australian Prescriber, 30*, 125–127.

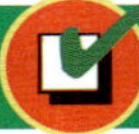

CHECK YOUR UNDERSTANDING

Answers to the questions in this chapter can be found in Appendix A at the back of this book.

MULTIPLE CHOICE

Select the best answer to the following.

1. The biogenic amine theory of depression states that depression is a result of:
   a. an unpleasant childhood.
   b. GABA inhibition.
   c. deficiency of noradrenaline, dopamine or 5HT in key areas of the brain.
   d. blockages within the limbic system, which controls emotions and affect.

2. When teaching a person receiving tricyclic antidepressants (TCAs), it is important to remember that TCAs are associated with many anticholinergic adverse effects. Teaching about these drugs should include anticipation of:
   a. increased libido and increased appetite.
   b. polyuria and polydipsia.
   c. urinary retention, arrhythmias and constipation.
   d. hearing changes, cataracts and nightmares.

3. Adverse effects may limit the usefulness of TCAs with some people. Care interventions that could alleviate some of the unpleasant aspects of these adverse effects include:
   a. always administering the drug when the person has an empty stomach.
   b. reminding the person not to void before taking the drug.
   c. increasing the dose to override the adverse effects.
   d. taking the major portion of the dose at bedtime to avoid experiencing drowsiness and the unpleasant anticholinergic effects.

4. You might question an order for an MAO inhibitor as a first step in the treatment of depression, remembering that these drugs are reserved for use in cases in which there has been no response to other agents because:
   a. MAO inhibitors can cause hair loss.
   b. MAO inhibitors are associated with potentially serious drug–food interactions.
   c. MAO inhibitors are mostly recommended for use in people undergoing surgery.
   d. MAO inhibitors are more expensive than other agents.
5. A woman is being treated for depression and is started on a regimen of *Prozac* (fluoxetine). She calls you 10 days after the drug therapy has started to report that nothing has changed and she wants to try a different drug. You should:
   a. tell her to try sertraline (*Zoloft*) because some people respond to one SSRI and not another.
   b. ask her to try a few days without the drug to see whether there is any difference.
   c. add an MAO inhibitor to her drug regimen to get an increased antidepressant effect.
   d. encourage her to keep taking the drug as prescribed because it usually takes up to 4 weeks to see the full antidepressant effect.
6. The drug of choice for a person with a documented obsessive–compulsive disorder who is also suffering from depression and occasional panic disorder would be:
   a. citalopram.
   b. paroxetine.
   c. fluvoxamine.
   d. fluoxetine.
7. Venlafaxine (*Efexor*) is an antidepressant that might be very effective for use in people who:
   a. have proven to be responsive to other antidepressants.
   b. can tolerate multiple side effects.
   c. are reliable at taking multiple daily dosings.
   d. have not responded to other antidepressants and would benefit from once-a-day dosing.
8. Depression is an affective disorder that is:
   a. always precipitated by a specific event.
   b. most common in people with head injuries.
   c. characterised by overwhelming sadness, despair and hopelessness.
   d. very evident and easy to diagnose in the clinical setting.

MULTIPLE RESPONSE

Select all that apply.

1. Depression is a very common affective disorder that strikes many people. In assessing a person who might be experiencing depression, the nurse or midwife would expect to find which of the following?
   a. lack of energy
   b. hyperactivity
   c. sleep disturbances
   d. libido problems
   e. confusion
   f. decreased reflexes
2. A person reports that he thinks he is taking an antidepressant, but he is not sure. In reviewing his medication history, which of the following drugs would be considered antidepressants?
   a. tetracyclic drugs
   b. cholinergics
   c. SSRIs
   d. MAO inhibitors
   e. angiotensin II–receptor blockers (ARBs)
   f. benzodiazepines

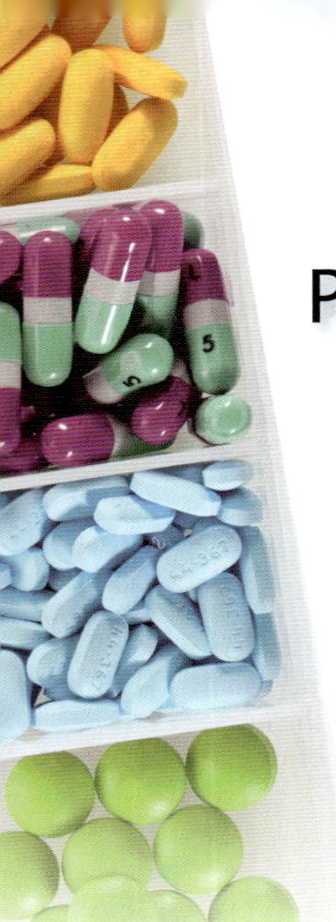

22 Psychotherapeutic agents

Learning objectives

On completing this chapter you should be able to:

1. Define the term psychotherapeutic agent and list conditions that psychotherapeutic agents are used to treat.
2. Describe the therapeutic actions, indications, pharmacokinetics, contraindications, most common adverse reactions and important drug–drug interactions associated with each class of psychotherapeutic agent.
3. Discuss the use of psychotherapeutic agents across the lifespan.
4. Compare and contrast the prototype drugs for each class of psychotherapeutic agent with other drugs in that class and with drugs in the other classes of psychotherapeutic agents.
5. Outline the care considerations and teaching needs for people receiving each class of psychotherapeutic agents.

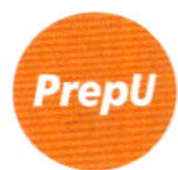

Test your current knowledge of psychotherapeutic agents with a PrepU Practice Quiz!

Glossary of key terms

antipsychotic: drug used to treat disorders involving thought processes; dopamine-receptor blocker that helps affected people to organise their thoughts and respond appropriately to stimuli

attention-deficit disorder: behavioural syndrome characterised by an inability to concentrate for longer than a few minutes and excessive activity

bipolar disorder: behavioural disorder that involves extremes of depression alternating with hyperactivity and excitement

major tranquilliser: former name of antipsychotic drugs; the name is no longer used because it implies that the primary effect of these drugs is sedation, which is no longer thought to be the desired therapeutic action

mania: state of hyperexcitability; one phase of bipolar disorders, which alternate between periods of severe depression and mania

narcolepsy: mental disorder characterised by daytime sleepiness and periods of sudden loss of wakefulness

neuroleptic: a drug with many associated neurological adverse effects that is used to treat disorders that involve thought processes (eg, schizophrenia)

schizophrenia: the most common type of psychosis; characteristics include hallucinations, paranoia, delusions, speech abnormalities and affective problems

ANTIPSYCHOTIC/NEUROLEPTIC DRUGS

Typical antipsychotics

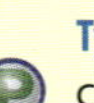 chlorpromazine
droperidol
haloperidol
periciazine
prochlorperazine
zuclopenthixol

Atypical antipsychotics

amisulpride
aripiprazole
brexiprazole
clozapine
lurasidone
olanzapine
paliperidone
quetiapine
risperidone
ziprasidone

ANTIMANIC DRUGS

aripiprazole
asenapine
carbamazepine
lamotrigine
lithium
olanzapine
risperidone
quetiapine
valproic acid
ziprasidone

CENTRAL NERVOUS SYSTEM STIMULANTS

atomoxetine
caffeine
dexamfetamine
guanfacine
lisdexamfetamine
methylphenidate
modafinil

The drugs discussed in this chapter are used to treat psychoses – perceptual and behavioural disorders. These psychotherapeutic agents are targeted at thought processes rather than affective states. Although they do not cure any psychotic disorders, psychotherapeutic agents do help both adults and children to function in a more acceptable manner and carry on activities of daily living (Box 22.1).

MENTAL DISORDERS AND THEIR CLASSIFICATION

Mental disorders were once attributed to environmental influences and life experiences such as poor parenting or trauma. Mental disorders are now thought to be caused by some inherent dysfunction within the brain that leads to abnormal thought processes and responses. Most theories attribute these disorders to some sort of chemical imbalance in specific areas within the brain. Diagnosis of a mental disorder is often based on distinguishing characteristics as described in the *Diagnostic and Statistical Manual of Mental Disorders*, 5th edition (DSM-V). Because no diagnostic laboratory tests are available, assessment and response must be carefully evaluated to determine the basis of a particular problem. Selected disorders are discussed here.

Schizophrenia, the most common type of psychosis, can be very debilitating and prevents affected individuals from functioning in society. Characteristics of schizophrenia include hallucinations, paranoia, delusions, speech abnormalities and affective problems. This disorder, which seems to have a very strong genetic association, may reflect a fundamental biochemical abnormality.

Mania, with its associated bipolar illness (i.e. manic-depressive illness), is characterised by periods of extreme overactivity and excitement. **Bipolar disorder** involves extremes of depression alternating with hyperactivity and excitement. This condition may reflect a biochemical imbalance followed by overcompensation on the part of neurons and their inability to re-establish stability.

Narcolepsy is characterised by daytime sleepiness and sudden periods of loss of wakefulness. This disorder

BOX 22.1 FOCUS ON Drug therapy across the lifespan

Psychotherapeutic agents

CHILDREN

Many of these agents are used in children, often in combination with other central nervous system (CNS) drugs in an attempt to control symptoms and behaviour. Long-term effects of many of these agents are not known and parents should be informed of this fact.

Of the antipsychotics, chlorpromazine, haloperidol, prochlorperazine and risperidone are the only ones with established paediatric regimens. Aripiprazole has doses for children 13–17 years of age. The dose is often higher than that required for adults. The child should be monitored carefully for adverse effects and developmental progress.

Lithium does not have a recommended paediatric dose and the drug should not ordinarily be used in children. If it is used, the dose should be carefully calculated from the child's age and weight, and the child should be monitored very closely for renal, CNS, cardiovascular and endocrine function.

The CNS stimulants are often used in children to manage various attention-deficit disorders. Caution should be used with extended-release preparations because they differ markedly in timing and effectiveness. The child should be assessed carefully and challenged periodically for the necessity of continuing the drug.

ADULTS

Adults using these drugs should be under regular care and should be monitored regularly for adverse effects. The QT_c interval should be evaluated before ziprasidone is prescribed and periodically during use.

People receiving lithium should be encouraged to maintain hydration and salt intake. They need to understand the importance of periodic monitoring of serum lithium levels.

PREGNANCY AND BREASTFEEDING

These drugs should be used very cautiously during pregnancy and breastfeeding because of the potential for adverse effects on the fetus or neonate. A woman maintained on one of these drugs needs to be counselled about the risk to the fetus versus the risk of returning symptoms if the drug is stopped. Use should be reserved for situations in which the benefits to the mother far outweigh the potential risks to the neonate. Women of childbearing age who need to take lithium should be advised to use barrier contraceptives while taking the drug because of the potential for serious congenital abnormalities.

OLDER ADULTS

Older people may be more susceptible to the adverse effects of these drugs and increased risk of falls. All doses need to be reduced and people monitored very closely for toxic effects and to provide safety measures if CNS effects do occur. They should not be used to control behaviour with dementia.

People with renal impairment should be monitored very closely while taking lithium. Decreased doses may be needed. Because many older people may also have renal impairment, they need to be screened carefully. They should maintain hydration and salt intake, which can be a challenge with some older people.

Prolongation of the QT_c interval can cause *torsades de pointes*, a life-threatening, polymorphic ventricular tachycardia. Prolongation of the QT_c interval is associated with the use of risperidone, haloperidol, clozapine, thioridazine, ziprasidone and droperidol. It may be a concern in people who are taking other drugs that prolong the QT_c such as antibiotics, antifungals or antiarrhythmics and in patients with coronary disease and in the elderly. Careful screening and monitoring should be done if these drugs are needed for such people.

may reflect problems with stimulation of the brain by the reticular activating system (RAS) or problems with response to that stimulation.

Attention-deficit disorders involve various conditions characterised by an inability to concentrate on one activity for longer than a few minutes and a state of hyperkinesis. These conditions are usually diagnosed in school-aged children but can occur in adults.

ANTIPSYCHOTIC/NEUROLEPTIC DRUGS

The **antipsychotic** drugs, which are essentially dopamine-receptor blockers, are used to treat disorders that involve thought processes. Because of their associated neurological adverse effects, these medications are also called **neuroleptic** agents. At one time, these drugs were known as **major tranquillisers**. However, that name is no longer used because the primary action of these drugs is not sedation but a change in neuron stimulation and response (Figure 22.1).

Antipsychotics are classified as either typical or atypical: typical antipsychotics include chlorpromazine (*Largactil*), haloperidol (*Serenace*), periciazine (*Neulactil*), prochlorperazine (*Stemetil*) and zuclopenthixol (*Clopixol*). Atypical antipsychotics include amisulpride (*Solian*), aripiprazole (*Abilify*), brexiprazole (*Rexulti*) clozapine (*Clozaril*), lurasidone (Latuda) olanzapine (*Lanzek, Zyprexa*), paliperidone (*Invega*), quetiapine (*Delucon, Seroquel*), risperidone (*Ozidal, Risperdal*) and ziprasidone (*Zeldox*). Atypical antipsychotics are better tolerated than the typical antipsychotics, effectively treating psychoses at doses that do not induce extrapyramidal adverse effects (dystonia, parkinsonism, akathisia and irreversible tardive dyskinesia). Table 22.1 lists both typical and atypical

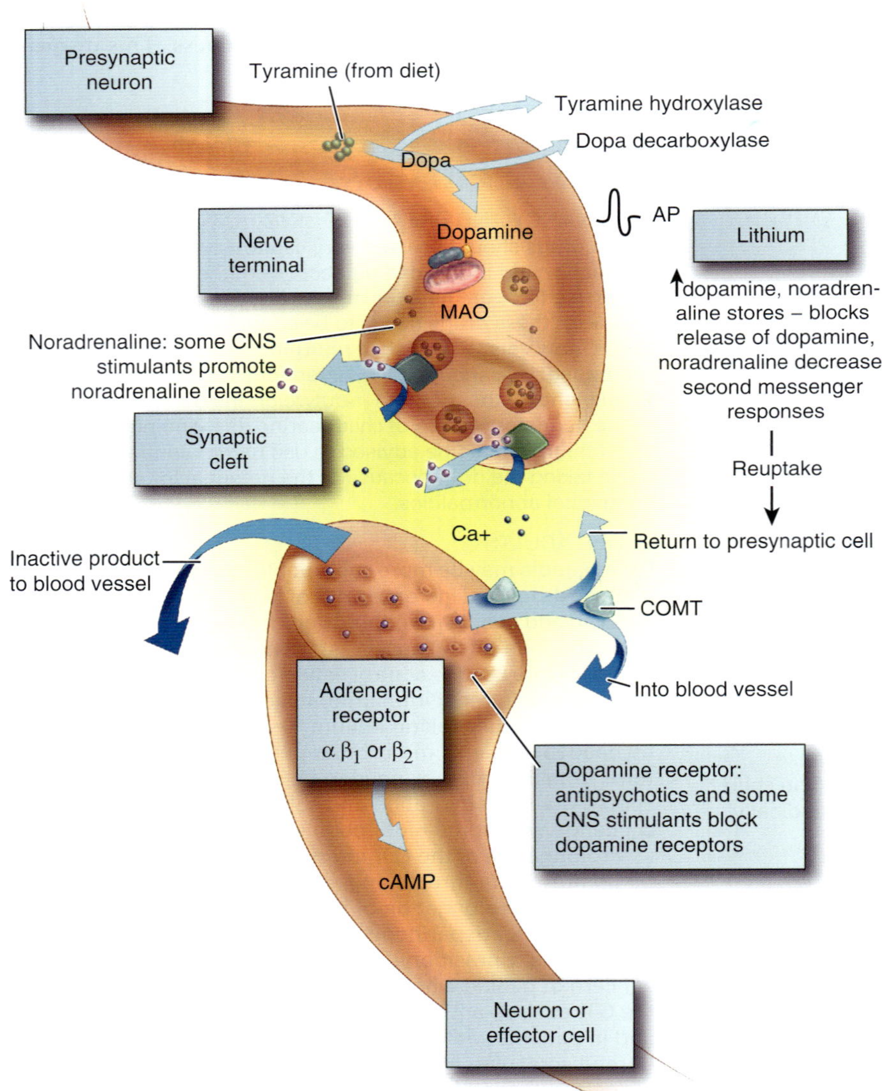

FIGURE 22.1 Sites of action of the drugs used to treat mental disorders: antipsychotics, central nervous system stimulants, lithium.

TABLE 22.1 DRUGS IN FOCUS Antipsychotic/neuroleptic drugs

Drug name	Potency	Common side effects				Usual dosage
		Sedation	Anticholinergic	Hypotension	Extrapyramidal	
Typical antipsychotics						
(P) chlorpromazine (*Largactil*)	Low	++++	+++	+++	++	Adult: 25 mg IM for acute episode, may be repeated; switch to 25–50 mg PO tds Paediatric: < 5 years: 0.5 mg/kg PO; may repeat tid–qid
haloperidol (*Serenace*)	High	+	+/–	+	++++	Adult: 1–15 mg/day PO Elderly: 1–3 mg/day PO Paediatric (3–12 years): for Tourette syndrome and behavioural syndromes, 0.5–3 mg (0.25–1.5 mL) per day (Serenace liquid is recommended); maintenance dose 0.05 mL (0.025 mL/kg) per day
periciazine (*Neulactil*)	Moderate	+++	+++	++++	+	Adult: 15–30 mg daily in 2 divided doses up to 75 mg/day Elderly: initially 15–30 mg/day in divided doses
prochlorperazine (*Stemetil*)	Low	+	++	+	+++	For nausea and vomiting but may also be used for migraine, schizophrenia (particularly in the chronic stage) and acute mania Adult: 5–10 mg PO tds–qid (10–20 mg IM for acute states); or 20–25 mg/day PR Elderly: reduce dose Paediatric: 2.5 mg PO tds
zuclopenthixol (*Clopixol*)	High	+++	+	+++	++++	Adult: 10–50 mg/day in divided doses, increase if necessary by 10–20 mg every 2–3 days to 75 mg; higher doses may be required; usual maintenance for schizophrenia and other psychoses, 20–40 mg/day Acuphase injection: 50–150 mg (1–3 mL) IM repeated if necessary, preferably at intervals of 2–3 days Depot injection: 200–400 mg (1–2 mL) IM every 2–4 weeks Elderly or debilitated: initially quarter to half usual adult dose

Continued on following page

TABLE 22.1 DRUGS IN FOCUS Antipsychotic/neuroleptic drugs *(continued)*

Drug name	Potency	Common side effects: Sedation	Anticholinergic	Hypotension	Extrapyramidal	Usual dosage
Atypical antipsychotics						
amisulpride (*Solian*)	High	++	++	+	+	Adult: 400–800 mg/day in two divided doses, adjusted according to response; maximum 1.2 g/day
aripiprazole (*Abilify*)	Medium	+	+	++	+	Adult: 10–15 mg PO up to 30 mg/day
(P) clozapine (*Clopine, Clozaril*)	Low	++++	++	+++	+/–	Adult: initially 12.5 mg 1–2 times daily on day 1; 25 mg 1–2 times daily on day 2; if well tolerated may increase slowly by 25–50 mg increments up to 300 mg/day within 2–3 weeks up to 900 mg/day; regular white blood cell and absolute neutrophil counts weekly during the first 18 weeks, and at least every 4 weeks thereafter. Monitoring must continue throughout treatment and for 4 weeks after complete discontinuation
olanzapine (*Zyprexa, Zyprexa Zydis*)	High	++++	++	+++	+	Adult: 5–10 mg/day PO, up to 20 mg/day PO for bipolar mania. Rapid-dispersing wafers disperse in mouth
paliperidone (*Invega*)	Medium	+	+	++	++	Adult: 6 mg/day PO; maximum dose 12 mg/day Renal impairment: maximum dose 3 mg/day
quetiapine (*Seroquel, Seroquel XR*)	Medium	++++	++	++	+/–	Adult: initially 25 mg PO bd, up to 300–400 mg/day; 400–800 mg/day PO (extended release [XR]) Elderly, hepatic impairment or hypotensives: reduce dose and titrate very slowly
risperidone (*Risperdal*)	High	+++	+	++	++	Adult: 1 mg PO bd up to 10 mg/day or 25 mg IM once every 2 weeks Paediatric: experience is lacking in children < 15 years with schizophrenia Elderly, renally impaired or hypotensive: 0.5 mg PO bd initially, titrate slowly

TABLE 22.1 DRUGS IN FOCUS Antipsychotic/neuroleptic drugs *(continued)*

Drug name	Potency	Common side effects				Usual dosage
		Sedation	Anticholinergic	Hypotension	Extrapyramidal	
ziprasidone (*Zeldox*)	Medium	+++	++	+	+	Adult: 20–80 mg PO bd; rapid control of as-stated behaviour: 10–20 mg IM, maximum dose 40 mg/day IM; monitor QTc intervals

Each plus sign indicates increased incidence of the given adverse effect.

BOX 22.2 Neuroleptic malignant syndrome

Neuroleptic malignant syndrome is a rare but potentially fatal adverse effect of all antipsychotic drugs. This includes symptoms such as hyperthermia, fluctuating level of consciousness, muscle rigidity, autonomic dysfunction with pallor, tachycardia, labile blood pressure, sweating and urinary incontinence. People who presents with neuroleptic malignant syndrome should seek specialist medical assessment immediately, as admission to a medical intensive care facility may be necessary. Symptoms usually last for 5–7 days after the drug is discontinued.

antipsychotic agents, including the specific type and the occurrence of sedation and other adverse effects.

Therapeutic actions and indications

The typical antipsychotic drugs block dopamine receptors, preventing the stimulation of the post-synaptic neurons by dopamine. They also depress the RAS, limiting the stimuli coming into the brain. They also have anticholinergic, antihistamine and alpha-adrenergic blocking effects, all related to the blocking of the dopamine-receptor sites. Newer atypical antipsychotics block both dopamine and serotonin receptors. This dual action may help to alleviate some of the unpleasant neurological effects and depression associated with the typical antipsychotics (see Table 22.1).

The antipsychotics are indicated for schizophrenia and for manifestations of other psychotic disorders, including hyperactivity, combative behaviour and severe behavioural problems in children (short-term control); some of them are also approved for the treatment of bipolar disorder. Chlorpromazine, one of the older antipsychotics, is also used to decrease preoperative restlessness and apprehension, to treat intermittent porphyria, as an adjunct in the treatment of tetanus and to control nausea, vomiting and intractable hiccups. Haloperidol is frequently used to treat acute psychiatric situations and is available for intravenous (IV) use when prolonged parenteral therapy is required because of swallowing difficulties or the acuity of the behavioural problems. Prochlorperazine is also frequently used to control severe nausea and vomiting associated with surgery and chemotherapy. It has the advantage of being available in oral, rectal and parenteral forms. Aripiprazole, one of the newer atypical antipsychotics, has been found to be effective in treating schizophrenia, major depressive disorder and bipolar disorders and has been used parenterally for the treatment of acute agitation associated with these disorders. Olanzapine and ziprasidone are also used for bipolar disorders and parenterally to treat acute agitation. Quetiapine is also approved for short-term treatment of acute manic episodes associated with bipolar disease. Risperidone is used frequently to treat irritability and aggression associated with autistic disorders in children and adolescents, as well as for acute manic episodes of bipolar disease. Any of these drugs may be effective in a particular person; the selection of a specific drug depends on the desired potency and tolerance of the associated adverse effects. A person who does not respond to one drug may react successfully to another agent. (Responses may also vary because of cultural issues [Box 22.3].) To determine the best therapeutic regimen for a particular person, it may be necessary to try more than one drug.

Pharmacokinetics

The antipsychotics are erratically absorbed from the gastrointestinal (GI) tract, depending on the drug and the preparation of the drug. Intramuscular doses provide four to five times the active dose as oral doses, and caution is required if one is switching between routes. The antipsychotics are widely distributed in the tissues and are often stored there, being released for up to 6 months after the drug is stopped. They are metabolised in the liver and excreted through the bile and urine. Children tend to metabolise these drugs faster than do adults and elderly people, who tend to metabolise them more slowly, making it necessary to carefully monitor these people and adjust doses as needed. Clinical effects may not be seen for several weeks and people should be encouraged to continue taking the drugs even if they see no immediate effectiveness. The antipsychotics cross the

FOCUS ON

BOX 22.3 Cultural considerations

Antipsychotic drugs

The ways in which people in certain cultural groups respond to antipsychotic drugs – either physiologically or emotionally – may vary. Therefore, when a pharmacological regimen is incorporated into overall care, health care providers must consider and respect an individual's cultural beliefs and needs.

- African Americans respond more rapidly to antipsychotic medications and have a greater risk for development of disfiguring adverse effects, such as tardive dyskinesia. Consequently, these people should be started off at the lowest possible dose and monitored closely. African Americans also display a higher red blood cell plasma lithium ratio than Caucasians do and they report more adverse effects from lithium therapy. These people should be monitored closely because they have a higher potential for lithium toxicity at standard therapeutic ranges.
- People in Asian countries, such as India, Turkey, Malaysia, China, Japan and Indonesia, receive lower doses of neuroleptics and lithium to achieve the same therapeutic response as seen in people in Australia and New Zealand. This may be related to these individuals' lower body mass as well as metabolic differences.
- Arab people metabolise antipsychotic medications more slowly than Asian people do and may require lower doses to achieve the same therapeutic effects as in Caucasians.
- Individuals in some cultures use herbs and other folk remedies, and the use of herbs may interfere with the metabolism of Western medications. The nurse or midwife should carefully assess for herbal use and be aware of potential interactions.

BOX 22.4 Antipsychotic drugs and the older person

In prescribing for the elderly, the balance between risks and benefit should be considered before prescribing antipsychotic drugs. In elderly adults with dementia, antipsychotic drugs are associated with a small increased risk of mortality and an increased risk of stroke or transient ischaemic attack. Furthermore, elderly adults are particularly susceptible to postural hypotension and to hyperthermia and hypothermia in hot or cold weather. It is recommended that antipsychotic drugs should not be used in elderly adults to treat mild psychotic symptoms. Initial doses of antipsychotic drugs in the elderly should be reduced (to half the adult dose or less), taking into account factors such as the person's weight, comorbidity and concomitant medication. Treatment should be reviewed regularly.

placenta and enter breast milk (see Contraindications and cautions).

Contraindications and cautions

Antipsychotic drugs are contraindicated in the presence of underlying diseases *that could be exacerbated by the dopamine-blocking effects of these drugs*. They are also contraindicated in the following conditions, *which can be exacerbated by the drugs*: CNS depression, circulatory collapse, Parkinson's disease, coronary disease, severe hypotension, bone marrow suppression and blood dyscrasias. Prolongation of the QT_c interval is a contraindication to the use of ziprasidone, which can further prolong the QT_c interval, *leading to increased risk of serious cardiac arrhythmias*. Antipsychotics are contraindicated for use in elderly people with dementia *because this use is associated with an increased risk of cardiovascular events and death*. In 2005, the U.S. Food and Drug Administration (FDA) issued a public health advisory regarding the use of antipsychotics after postmarketing studies showed that when these drugs were used to control behavioural symptoms of dementia in older adults, the people being treated experienced increased rates of cardiovascular events and death. None of these drugs is approved for this use, but it was common practice in many settings to use them, off-label, to establish behavioural control of people with dementia. Antipsychotics now have a black-box warning on the prescribing information outlining this safety information and contraindication.

Caution should be used in the presence of medical conditions *that could be exacerbated by the anticholinergic effects of the drugs*, such as glaucoma, peptic ulcer and urinary or intestinal obstruction. In addition, care should be taken in people with seizure disorders *because the threshold for seizures could be lowered*; in people with thyrotoxicosis *because of the possibility of severe neurosensitivity*; and in people with active alcoholism *because of potentiation of the CNS depression*.

Other situations that warrant caution include myelography within the last 24 hours or scheduled within the next 48 hours *because severe neuron reaction to the dye used in these tests can occur*, and pregnancy or breastfeeding *because of the potential of adverse effects on the fetus or neonate*. Antipsychotic agents should be used only if the benefit to the mother clearly outweighs the potential risk to the fetus or baby. Because children are more apt to develop dystonia from the drugs, *which could confuse the diagnosis of Reye syndrome*, caution should be used with children younger than 12 years of age who have a CNS infection or chickenpox. *The use of antipsychotics may result in bone marrow suppression, leading to blood dyscrasias*, so care should be taken with people who are immunosuppressed and those who have cancer.

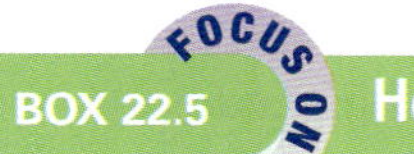

BOX 22.5 Herbal and alternative therapies

Evening primrose

People with schizophrenia should be advised to avoid the use of evening primrose. This herb has been associated with increased symptoms and CNS hyperexcitability.

Adverse effects

The adverse effects associated with the antipsychotic drugs are related to their dopamine-blocking, anticholinergic, antihistamine and alpha-adrenergic activities. The most common CNS effects are sedation, weakness, tremor, drowsiness, extrapyramidal side effects (EPS), pseudoparkinsonism, dystonia, akathisia, tardive dyskinesia and potentially irreversible neuroleptic malignant syndrome. Anticholinergic effects include dry mouth, nasal congestion, flushing, constipation, urinary retention, impotence, glaucoma, blurred vision and photophobia. Cardiovascular (CV) effects, which are probably related to the dopamine-blocking effects, include hypotension, orthostatic hypotension, cardiac arrhythmias, congestive heart failure and pulmonary oedema. Cases of myocarditis, some of which have been fatal, and cardiomyopathy have been reported in patients on clozapine. Ziprasidone is associated with prolongation of the QT_c interval, which could lead to serious or even fatal cardiac arrhythmias. People receiving this drug should have a baseline and periodic electrocardiogram (ECG) during therapy. In late 2003, the FDA issued a requirement that all of the atypical antipsychotics include warnings that there is a risk for the development of diabetes mellitus when these drugs are used. Consequently, when people are maintained on any of the atypical antipsychotics, they should be monitored regularly for the signs and symptoms of diabetes mellitus.

Respiratory effects such as laryngospasm, dyspnoea and bronchospasm may also occur. The phenothiazines (chlorpromazine, prochlorperazine and promethazine) often turn the urine pink to reddish-brown as a result of their excretion. Although this effect may cause great concern to the person, it has no clinical significance. In addition, bone marrow suppression is a possibility with some antipsychotic agents.

Clinically important drug–drug interactions

Because the combination of antipsychotics with beta blockers may lead to an increase in the effect of both drugs, this combination should be avoided if possible. Antipsychotic–alcohol combinations result in an increased risk of CNS depression, and antipsychotic–anticholinergic combinations lead to increased anticholinergic effects, so dose adjustments are necessary. People who take either of these combinations should be monitored closely for adverse effects and supportive measures should be provided. People should not take ziprasidone with any other drug that is associated with prolongation of the QT_c interval.

Prototype summary: chlorpromazine

Indications: management of manifestations of psychotic disorders; relief of preoperative restlessness; adjunctive treatment of tetanus; acute intermittent porphyria; severe behavioural problems in children; control of hiccups, nausea and vomiting.

Actions: blocks postsynaptic dopamine receptors in the brain; depresses those parts of the brain involved in wakefulness and emesis; anticholinergic; antihistaminic; alpha-adrenergic blocking.

Pharmacokinetics:

Route	Onset	Peak	Duration
Oral	30–60 min	2–4 hours	4–6 hours
Intra-muscular	10–15 min	15–20 min	4–6 hours

$T_{1/2}$: 2 hours, then 30 hours; metabolised in the liver, excreted in the urine.

Adverse effects: drowsiness, insomnia, vertigo, extrapyramidal symptoms, orthostatic hypotension, photophobia, blurred vision, dry mouth, nausea, vomiting, anorexia, urinary retention, photosensitivity.

Prototype summary: clozapine

Indications: management of severely ill people with schizophrenia who are unresponsive to standard drugs; reduction of risk of recurrent suicidal behaviour in people with schizophrenia or schizoaffective disorder.

Actions: blocks dopamine and serotonin receptors; depresses the RAS; anticholinergic; antihistaminic; alpha-adrenergic blocking.

Pharmacokinetics:

Route	Onset	Peak	Duration
Oral	Varies	1–6 hours	Weeks

$T_{1/2}$: 4–12 hours; metabolised in the liver, excreted in the urine and faeces.

Adverse effects: drowsiness, sedation, seizures, dizziness, syncope, headache, tachycardia, nausea, vomiting, fever, neuroleptic malignant syndrome.

Care considerations for people receiving antipsychotic/neuroleptic drugs

Assessment: history and examination

- Assess for *contraindications or cautions for the use of the drug* including any known allergies to these drugs, severe CNS depression, circulatory collapse, coronary disease including prolonged QT_c interval, brain damage, severe hypotension, glaucoma, respiratory depression, urinary or intestinal obstruction, thyrotoxicosis, seizure disorder, bone marrow suppression, pregnancy or breastfeeding and myelography within the last 24 hours or scheduled in the next 48 hours. In children younger than 12 years of age, screen for CNS infections.
- Assess temperature; skin colour and lesions; CNS orientation, affect, reflexes and bilateral grip strength; bowel sounds and reported output; pulse, auscultation and blood pressure, including orthostatic blood pressure; respiration rate and adventitious sounds; and urinary output *to determine baseline status before beginning therapy and for any potential adverse effects.* Also obtain liver and renal function tests, thyroid function tests, ECG if appropriate and full blood count (FBC).

Refer to the Critical thinking scenario for a full discussion of care for a person who is prescribed antipsychotic drugs.

Implementation with rationale

- Do not allow the person to crush or chew sustained-release capsules, *which will speed up their absorption and may cause toxicity.*
- If administering parenteral forms, keep person recumbent for 30 minutes *to reduce the risk of orthostatic hypotension.*
- Consider warning the person or their guardians about the risk of development of tardive dyskinesias with continued use *so they are prepared for that neurological change.*
- Monitor FBC *to arrange to discontinue the drug at signs of bone marrow suppression.*
- Monitor blood glucose levels with long-term use *to detect the development of glucose intolerance.*
- Arrange for gradual dose reduction after long-term use. *Abrupt withdrawal has been associated with gastritis, nausea, vomiting, dizziness, arrhythmias and insomnia.*
- Provide positioning of legs and arms *to decrease the discomfort of dyskinesias.*
- Provide sugarless lozenges and ice chips *to increase secretions* and frequent mouth care *to prevent dry mouth from becoming a problem.*
- Encourage person to void before taking a dose *if urinary hesitancy or retention is a problem.*
- Provide safety measures such as side rails and assistance with ambulation if CNS effects or orthostatic hypotension occurs *to prevent injury.*
- Provide for vision examinations *to determine ocular changes and arrange appropriate dose change.*
- Provide thorough teaching, including drug name, prescribed dosage, measures for avoidance of adverse effects, cautions that it may take weeks to see the desired clinical effects, warning signs that may indicate possible problems and the need for monitoring and evaluation *to enhance knowledge about drug therapy and to promote compliance.* (Refer to Critical thinking scenario.) Warn person that urine may have a pink to reddish-brown colour.
- Offer support and encouragement *to help the person to cope with the drug regimen.*

Evaluation

- Monitor response to the drug (decrease in signs and symptoms of psychotic disorder).
- Monitor for adverse effects (sedation, anticholinergic effects, hypotension, extrapyramidal effects, bone marrow suppression).
- Evaluate the effectiveness of the teaching plan (person can give the drug name and dosage, possible adverse effects to watch for, specific measures to prevent adverse effects and warning signs to report).
- Monitor the effectiveness of comfort measures and compliance with the regimen.

KEY POINTS

- Mental disorders are thought-process disorders that may be caused by some inherent dysfunction within the brain. A psychosis is a thought disorder and schizophrenia is the most common psychosis in which delusions and hallucinations are hallmarks.
- Antipsychotic drugs are dopamine-receptor blockers that are effective in helping people to organise thought patterns and to respond appropriately to stimuli.
- Antipsychotics can cause hypotension, anticholinergic effects, sedation and extrapyramidal effects, including parkinsonism, ataxia, tremors and neuroleptic malignant syndrome.

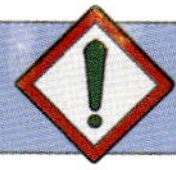

CRITICAL THINKING SCENARIO

Antipsychotic drugs

THE SITUATION

B.A., a 36-year-old, single professional woman, was diagnosed with chronic schizophrenia when she was in high school. Her condition has been well controlled with chlorpromazine *(Largactil)* and she is able to maintain steady employment, live in her own home and carry on a fairly active social life. At her last evaluation, she appeared to be developing bone marrow suppression and her doctor decided to try to taper the drug dosage. As the dosage was being lowered, B.A. became withdrawn and listless, missed several days of work and cancelled most of her social engagements. Afraid of interacting with people, she stayed in bed most of the time. She reported having thoughts of death and paranoid ideation about her neighbours that she was beginning to think might be true.

CRITICAL THINKING

What care interventions are appropriate at this time?
What supportive measures might be useful to help B.A. cope with this crisis and allow her to function normally again?
What happens to brain chemistry after long-term therapy with phenothiazines?
What drug options should be tried?
Are there any other options that might be useful?

DISCUSSION

Schizophrenia is not a disorder that can be resolved simply with proper counselling. B.A., an educated woman with a long history of taking phenothiazines, realises the necessity of drug therapy to correct the chemical imbalance in her brain. She may need a high-potency antipsychotic to return her to the level of functioning she had reached before experiencing this setback. Her knowledge of her individual responses can be used to help select an appropriate drug and dosage. Her experiences may also facilitate her care planning and new drug regimen.

B.A. will need support to cope with problems at work – from her inability to go in to work, to coping with feelings about not meeting her social obligations, to finding the motivation to get up and become active again. She might do well with behaviour modification techniques that give her some control over her activities and allow her to use her knowledge and experience with her own situation to her advantage in forming a new medical regimen. She may need support in explaining her problem to her employer and her social contacts in ways that will help her avoid the prejudice associated with mental illness and will allow her every opportunity to return to her regular routine as soon as she can.

Because it may take several months to find the drug or drugs that will bring B.A. back to a point of stabilisation, it is important to have a consistent, reliable health care team in place to support her through this stabilisation period. She should have a reliable contact person to call when she has questions and when she needs support.

CARE GUIDE FOR B.A.: ANTIPSYCHOTIC/NEUROLEPTIC DRUGS

Assessment: history and examination

Allergies to any of these drugs; CNS depression; CV disease; pregnancy or breastfeeding; myelography; glaucoma; hypotension; thyrotoxicosis; seizures
Concurrent use of anticholinergics, barbiturate anaesthetics, alcohol, pethidine, beta blockers, adrenaline (epinephrine), noradrenaline (norepinephrine)
CV: blood pressure, pulse, orthostatic blood pressure
CNS: orientation, affect, reflexes, vision
Skin: colour, lesions, texture
Respiratory: respiration, adventitious sounds
GI: abdominal examination, bowel sounds
Laboratory tests: thyroid, liver and renal function tests, FBC

Implementation

Give drug in the evening; do not allow person to chew or crush sustained-release capsules
Provide comfort and safety measures: facilitate individuals to void before dosing; raise side rails; provide sugarless lozenges, mouth care; institute safety measures if CNS effects occur; position person to relieve dyskinesia discomfort; taper dosage after long-term therapy.
Provide support and reassurance to help person cope with drug effects.
Teach person about drug, dosage, adverse effects, conditions to report and precautions.

Evaluation

Evaluate drug effects: relief of signs and symptoms of psychotic disorders.
Monitor for adverse effects: sedation, dizziness, insomnia; anticholinergic effects; extrapyramidal effects; bone marrow suppression; skin rash.
Monitor for drug–drug interactions as listed.
Evaluate effectiveness of teaching program.
Evaluate effectiveness of comfort and safety measures.

TEACHING FOR B.A.

- The drugs that are useful for treating schizophrenia are called antipsychotic or neuroleptic drugs. These drugs affect the activities of certain chemicals in your brain and are used to treat certain mental disorders.

- Drugs in this group should be taken exactly as prescribed. Because these drugs affect many body systems, it is important that you have medical checkups regularly.
- Common effects of these drugs include:
  - *Dizziness, drowsiness and fainting:* avoid driving or performing hazardous or delicate tasks that require concentration if these occur. Change position slowly. The dizziness usually passes after 1–2 weeks of drug use.
  - *Pink or reddish urine (with phenothiazines):* these drugs sometimes cause urine to change colour. Do not be alarmed by this change; it does not mean that your urine contains blood.
  - *Sensitivity to light:* bright light might hurt your eyes and sunlight might burn your skin more easily. Wear sunglasses and protective clothing when you must be out in the sun.
  - *Constipation:* consult with your health care provider if this becomes a problem.
- Report any of the following conditions to your health care provider: *sore throat, fever, rash, tremors, weakness and vision changes.*
- Tell any doctor, nurse, midwife or other health care provider that you are taking this drug.
- Keep this drug and all medications out of the reach of children.
- Avoid the use of alcohol or other depressants while you are taking this drug. You also may want to limit your use of caffeine if you feel very tense or cannot sleep.
- Avoid the use of over-the-counter drugs while you are on this drug. Many of them contain ingredients that could interfere with the effectiveness of your drug. If you feel that you need one of these preparations, consult with your health care provider about the most appropriate choice.
- Take this drug exactly as prescribed. If you run out of medicine or find that you cannot take your drug for any reason, consult your health care provider. After this drug has been used for a period of time, additional adverse effects may occur if it is suddenly stopped. This drug dosage will need to be tapered over time.

ANTIMANIC DRUGS

Mania, at the opposite pole from depression, occurs in individuals with bipolar disorder, who experience a period of depression followed by a period of mania. The cause of mania is not understood, but it is thought to be an overstimulation of certain neurons in the brain. The mainstay for treatment of mania has always been lithium (*Lithicarb*, *Quilonum*). Today, many other drugs are used successfully in treating bipolar disorders, including asenapine (*Saphris*), aripiprazole (*Abilify*), carbamazepine (*Tegretol, Teril*), olanzapine (*Zyprexa*, *Zyprexa Zydis*), risperidone (*Ozidal, Risperdal*), quetiapine (*Seroquel*), valproic acid (*Epilim, Valprease, Valpro*) and ziprasidone (*Zeldox*), which are atypical antipsychotics; and lamotrigine (*Lamictal*), an antiepileptic agent discussed in greater detail in Chapter 23. These new approvals were the first advances since the 1970s in the treatment of bipolar disorder (see Table 22.2).

Lithium salts (*Lithicarb*, *Quilonum*) are taken orally for the management of manic episodes and prevention of future episodes. These very toxic drugs can cause severe CNS, renal and pulmonary problems that may lead to death. Despite the potential for serious adverse effects, lithium is used with caution because it is consistently effective in the treatment of mania. The therapeutically effective serum level is 0.6–1.2 mmol/L.

Therapeutic actions and indications

Lithium functions in several ways. It alters sodium transport in nerve and muscle cells; inhibits the release of noradrenaline and dopamine, but not serotonin, from stimulated neurons; increases the intraneuronal stores of noradrenaline and dopamine slightly; and decreases intraneuronal content of second messengers. This last mode of action may allow it to selectively modulate the responsiveness of hyperactive neurons that might contribute to the manic state. Although the biochemical actions of lithium are known, the exact mechanism of action in decreasing the manifestations of mania are not understood.

Pharmacokinetics

Lithium is readily absorbed from the GI tract, reaching peak levels in 30 minutes to 3 hours. It follows the same distribution pattern in the body as water. It slowly crosses the blood–brain barrier. Lithium is excreted from the kidney, although about 80% is reabsorbed. During periods of sodium depletion or dehydration, the kidney reabsorbs more lithium into the serum, often leading to toxic levels. Therefore, people must be encouraged to maintain hydration while taking this drug. Lithium crosses the placenta and enters breast milk, and has been associated with congenital abnormalities (see Contraindications and cautions).

Contraindications and cautions

Lithium is contraindicated in the presence of hypersensitivity to lithium. In addition, it is contraindicated in the following conditions: significant renal or cardiac disease *that could be exacerbated by the toxic effects of the drug*; a history of leukaemia; metabolic disorders, including sodium depletion; dehydration; and diuretic

TABLE 22.2 DRUGS IN FOCUS Antimanic drugs

Drug name	Dosage/route	Usual indications
aripiprazole (*Abilify*)	10–30 mg/day PO	Treatment of acute manic and mixed episodes of bipolar disorders
lamotrigine (*Lamictal*)	25 mg/day PO up to 200 mg/day	Long-term maintenance of people with bipolar disorders; decreases occurrence of acute mood episodes
(P) lithium salts (*Lithicarb, Quilonum SR*)	400–1200 mg/day based on serum lithium levels	Treatment of manic episodes of manic-depressive or bipolar illness; maintenance therapy to prevent or diminish the frequency and intensity of future manic episodes; currently being studied for improvement of neutrophil counts in people with cancer chemotherapy–induced neutropenia and as prophylaxis of cluster headaches and migraine headaches; not recommended for children < 12 years
olanzapine (*Zyprexa, Zyprexa Zydis*)	10 mg/day PO; range 5–20 mg/day	Management of acute manic episodes associated with bipolar disorder, in combination with lithium or valproate, or as monotherapy
quetiapine (*Seroquel*)	50 mg PO bd, titrate to a maximum 800 mg/day	Adjunct or monotherapy for the treatment of manic episodes associated with bipolar disorder
ziprasidone (*Zeldox*)	40 mg PO bd with food; maximum 80 mg bd; or 10–20 mg IM up to a maximum dose of 40 mg/day	Treatment of acute manic and mixed episodes of bipolar disorders

use *because lithium depletes sodium reabsorption and severe hyponatraemia may occur.* (Hyponatraemia leads to lithium retention and toxicity.) Pregnancy and breastfeeding are also contraindications *because of the potential for adverse effects on the fetus or neonate;* breastfeeding should be discontinued while using lithium and women of childbearing age should be advised to use birth control while taking this drug. Caution should be used in any condition *that could alter sodium levels,* such as protracted diarrhoea or excessive sweating; with suicidal or impulsive individuals; and in people who have infection with fever, *which could be exacerbated by the toxic effects of the drug.*

Adverse effects

The adverse effects associated with lithium are directly related to serum levels of the drug.

- *Serum levels of less than 1.5 mmol/L*: CNS problems, including lethargy, slurred speech, muscle weakness and fine tremor; polyuria, which relates to renal toxicity; and beginning of gastric toxicity, with nausea, vomiting and diarrhoea.
- *Serum levels of 1.5–2 mmol/L*: intensification of all of the foregoing reactions, with ECG changes.
- *Serum levels of 2–2.5 mmol/L*: possible progression of CNS effects to ataxia, clonic movements, hyperreflexia and seizures; possible CV effects such as severe ECG changes and hypotension; large output of dilute urine secondary to renal toxicity; fatalities secondary to pulmonary toxicity.
- *Serum levels greater than 2.5 mmol/L*: complex multiorgan toxicity, with a significant risk of death.

Clinically important drug–drug interactions

Some drug–drug combinations should be avoided. A lithium–haloperidol combination may result in an encephalopathic syndrome, consisting of weakness, lethargy, confusion, tremors, extrapyramidal symptoms, leucocytosis and irreversible brain damage (see Box 22.6).

If lithium is given with carbamazepine, increased CNS toxicity may occur and a lithium–iodide salt combination results in an increased risk of hypothyroidism. People who receive either of these combinations should be monitored carefully. In addition, a thiazide diuretic–lithium combination increases the risk of lithium toxicity because of the loss of sodium and increased retention of lithium. If this combination is used, the dose of lithium should be decreased and the person should be monitored closely.

In the following instances, the serum lithium level should be monitored closely and appropriate dose adjustments made. With the combination of lithium and some urine-alkalinising drugs, including antacids, there is a possibility of decreased effectiveness of lithium. If lithium is combined with indometacin or with some non-steroidal anti-inflammatory drugs, higher plasma levels of lithium occur. Most cases of lithium intoxication occur

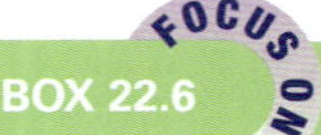

BOX 22.6 Herbal and alternative therapies

Psyllium

People being treated with lithium should be encouraged not to use the herbal therapy psyllium, which is used to treat constipation and to lower cholesterol levels. If this agent is combined with lithium, the absorption of the lithium may be blocked and the person will not receive therapeutic levels. If the person feels a need for a drug to relieve constipation or is concerned about cholesterol levels, they should be encouraged to discuss alternative measures with the health care provider.

as a complication of long-term therapy and are caused by reduced excretion of the drug because of a variety of factors including dehydration, deterioration of renal function, infections, and co-administration of diuretics or NSAIDs (or other drugs that interact).

Prototype summary: lithium

Indications: treatment of manic episodes of bipolar, manic-depressive illness.

Actions: alters sodium transport in nerve and muscle cells; inhibits the release of noradrenaline and dopamine, but not serotonin, from stimulated neurons; increases the intraneuronal stores of noradrenaline and dopamine slightly; and decreases the intraneuronal content of second messengers.

Pharmacokinetics:

Route	Onset	Peak	Duration
Oral	Unknown	0.5–3 hours	8–12 hours
Oral, extended release	Unknown	4–12 hours	12–18 hours

$T_{1/2}$: 24 hours; excreted in the urine.

Adverse effects: CNS problems, including lethargy, slurred speech, muscle weakness and fine tremor; polyuria, gastric toxicity, with nausea, vomiting and diarrhoea progressing; CV collapse, coma; adverse effects are related to serum drug levels.

Care considerations for people receiving lithium

Assessment: history and examination

- Assess for *contraindications or cautions for the use of the drug*, including any known allergies to lithium; renal or CV disease; dehydration; sodium depletion, use of diuretics, protracted sweating or diarrhoea; suicidal or impulsive people with severe depression; pregnancy or breastfeeding; and infection with fever.
- Assess temperature; skin colour and lesions; CNS orientation, affect and reflexes; bowel sounds and reported output; pulse, auscultation and blood pressure, including orthostatic blood pressure; respiration rate and adventitious sounds; and urinary output *for baseline status before beginning therapy and for any potential adverse effects.* Also obtain liver and renal function tests, thyroid function tests, FBC and baseline ECG, and obtain serum lithium levels as appropriate.

Implementation with rationale

- Administer drug cautiously, with daily monitoring of serum lithium levels, to people with significant renal or CV disease, dehydration or debilitation, as well as those taking diuretics, *to monitor for toxic levels and to arrange for appropriate dose adjustment.*
- Administer drug with food or milk *to alleviate GI irritation if GI upset is severe.*
- Arrange to decrease dose after acute manic episodes. *Lithium tolerance is greatest during acute episodes and decreases when the acute episode is over.*
- Ensure that the person maintains adequate intake of salt and fluid *to decrease toxicity.*
- Monitor person's clinical status closely, especially during the initial stages of therapy, *to provide appropriate supportive management as needed.*
- Arrange for small, frequent meals, sugarless lozenges to suck and frequent mouth care, *to increase secretions and decrease discomfort as needed.*
- Provide safety measures such as side rails and assistance with ambulation if CNS effects occur *to prevent injury.*
- Provide thorough teaching, including drug name, prescribed dosage, measures for avoidance of adverse effects, cautions that it may take time to see the desired therapeutic effects, warning signs that may indicate possible problems and the need to avoid pregnancy while taking lithium *to enhance knowledge about drug therapy and to promote compliance.*
- Offer support and encouragement *to help the person to cope with the drug regimen.*

Evaluation

- Monitor response to the drug (decreased manifestations and frequency of manic episodes).

- Monitor for adverse effects (CV toxicity, renal toxicity, GI upset, respiratory complications).
- Evaluate effectiveness of the teaching plan (person can give the drug name and dosage and describe the possible adverse effects to watch for, specific measures to help avoid adverse effects, warning signs to report and the need to avoid pregnancy).
- Monitor effectiveness of comfort measures and compliance with the regimen.

KEY POINTS

- Lithium, a membrane stabiliser, is the standard antimanic drug. Because it is a very toxic salt, serum levels must be carefully monitored to prevent severe toxicity.
- Many other CNS drugs, including many of the atypical antipsychotics, are now approved for use in bipolar disorder. Many people respond to a combination of these drugs to control their bipolar signs and symptoms.

CENTRAL NERVOUS SYSTEM STIMULANTS

CNS stimulants are used clinically to treat both attention deficit disorders and narcolepsy. Paradoxically, these drugs calm hyperkinetic children and help them to focus on one activity for a longer period. They also redirect and excite the arousal stimuli from the RAS (Figure 22.2; see also Figure 22.1). The CNS stimulants

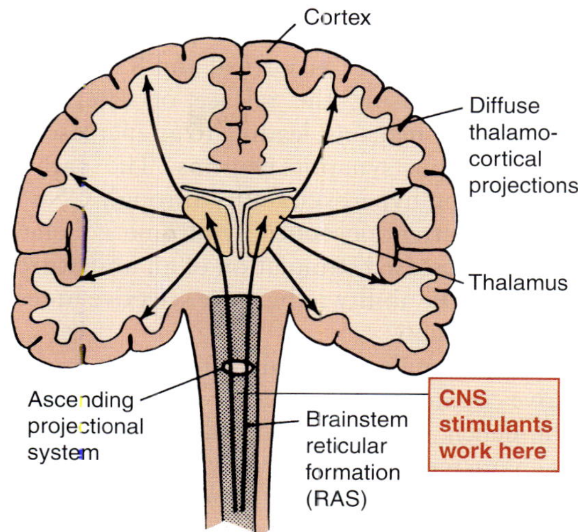

FIGURE 22.2 Site of action of the central nervous system (CNS) stimulants in the reticular activating system (RAS).

that are used to treat attention-deficit disorder and narcolepsy include methylphenidate (*Ritalin*, *Concerta* and others); dexamfetamine (generic); lisdexamfetamine (*Vyvanse*); modafinil (*Modavigil*), which is not associated with many of the systemic stimulatory effects of some of the other CNS stimulants; as well as the newer drugs guanfacine (*Intuniv*), an alpha-adrenergic agonist, and atomoxetine (*Strattera*), a serotonin–noradrenaline reuptake inhibitor with anticholinergic effects but without the CV and stimulatory effects, making it preferable in people who cannot tolerate the systemic stimulatory effects (see Table 22.3). Caffeine (*No Doz*, *Cafnea*) is also used as a CNS stimulant.

TABLE 22.3 DRUGS IN FOCUS Central nervous systems stimulants

Drug name	Dosage/route	Usual indications
atomoxetine (*Strattera*)	Adults and children > 70 kg: 40 mg/day PO, slowly increase to a target daily dose of 80 mg Children ≤ 70 kg: 0.5 mg/kg/day, increase to a target daily dose of 1.2 mg/kg/day Hepatic impairment: decrease dose by 50%	Treatment of attention-deficit/hyperactivity disorders as part of a total treatment program
dexamfetamine (generic)	Narcolepsy: 5–60 mg/day PO in divided doses Attention-deficit disorders: 2.5–5 mg/day PO taken in the morning	Treatment of narcolepsy, attention-deficit disorders, behavioural syndromes
(P) methylphenidate (*Ritalin*, *Concerta* and others)	Adult: 10–60 mg/day PO in divided doses, depending on preparation Paediatric: 5 mg PO bd; increase gradually, do not exceed 60 mg/day	Treatment of attention-deficit disorders and other behavioural syndromes associated with hyperactivity, as well as narcolepsy; currently available in various forms allowing for dosing one, two or three times a day
modafinil (*Modavigil*)	200–400 mg/day PO as a single dose; reduce dose with hepatic impairment and in the elderly	Treatment of narcolepsy in adults, for improving wakefulness in various sleep disorders and for improving wakefulness in people with obstructive sleep apnoea/hypopnoea syndrome

Therapeutic actions and indications

The CNS stimulants act as cortical and RAS stimulants, possibly by increasing the release of catecholamines from presynaptic neurons, leading to an increase in stimulation of the postsynaptic neurons. The paradoxical effect of calming hyperexcitability through CNS stimulation seen in attention-deficit syndrome is believed to be related to increased stimulation of an immature RAS, which leads to the ability to be more selective in response to incoming stimuli.

The CNS stimulants are indicated, as part of a comprehensive treatment program, for the treatment of attention-deficit syndromes, including behavioural syndromes characterised by hyperactivity and distractibility, as well as for narcolepsy and improvement of wakefulness in people with various sleep disorders.

Pharmacokinetics

These drugs are rapidly absorbed from the GI tract, reaching peak levels in 2–4 hours. They are metabolised in the liver and excreted in the urine, with half-lives ranging from 2 to 15 hours, depending on the drug. Safety for use during pregnancy and breastfeeding has not been established; during those periods, these drugs should be used only if the benefit to the mother clearly outweighs the potential risk to the fetus or neonate.

Contraindications and cautions

The CNS stimulants are contraindicated in the presence of known allergy to the drug, *which could lead to hypersensitivity reactions*. Other contraindications include the following conditions: marked anxiety, agitation or tension and severe fatigue or glaucoma, *which could be exacerbated by the CNS stimulation caused by these drugs*; cardiac disease, *which could be aggravated by the stimulatory effects of these drugs, making it important to rule out congenital heart problems*; and pregnancy and breastfeeding *because of the potential for adverse effects on the fetus or neonate.*

Caution should be used in people with a history of seizures, *which could be potentiated by the CNS stimulation*; in people with a history of drug dependence, including alcoholism, *because these drugs may result in physical and psychological dependence*; and in people with hypertension, *which could be exacerbated by the stimulatory effects of these drugs.*

Adverse effects

The adverse effects associated with these drugs are related to the CNS stimulation they cause. CNS effects can include nervousness, insomnia, dizziness, headache, blurred vision and difficulty with accommodation. GI effects such as anorexia, nausea and weight loss may occur. CV effects can include hypertension, arrhythmias and angina. Skin rashes are a common reaction to some of these drugs. Physical and psychological dependence may also develop. Because CNS stimulants have this effect, the drugs are controlled substances. Atomoxetine, which does not show dependence development, is not a controlled substance. The adverse effects associated with this drug are mainly anticholinergic (dry mouth, constipation, nausea, urinary hesitancy).

Clinically important drug–drug interactions

The combination of a CNS stimulant with a monoamine oxidase (MAO) inhibitor leads to an increased risk of adverse effects and increased toxicity and should be avoided if possible.

In addition, the combination of CNS stimulants with tricyclic antidepressants or phenytoin leads to a risk of increased drug levels. People who receive such a combination should be monitored for toxicity.

Ⓟ Prototype summary: methylphenidate

Indications: narcolepsy and attention-deficit disorder.

Actions: mild cortical stimulant with CNS actions similar to those of amphetamines.

Pharmacokinetics:

Route	Onset	Peak	Duration
Oral	Varies	1–3 hours	4–6 hours

$T_{1/2}$: 1–3 hours; metabolised in the liver; excreted in the urine.

Adverse effects: nervousness, insomnia, increased or decreased pulse rate and blood pressure, tachycardia, loss of appetite, nausea, abdominal pain.

Care considerations for people receiving central nervous system stimulants

Assessment: history and examination

- Assess for *contraindications or cautions for the use of the drug*, including any known allergies to the drug; glaucoma, anxiety, tension, fatigue or seizure disorder; cardiac disease and hypertension; pregnancy or breastfeeding; a history of leukaemia; and a history of drug dependency, including alcoholism.
- Assess temperature; skin colour and lesions; CNS orientation, affect and reflexes; ophthalmic examination; bowel sounds and reported output; pulse, auscultation and blood pressure, including orthostatic blood pressure; respiration rate and adventitious sounds; and urinary output

to determine baseline status before beginning therapy and for any potential adverse effects. Also obtain an FBC.

Implementation with rationale

- Ensure proper diagnosis of behavioural syndromes and narcolepsy *because these drugs should not be used until underlying medical causes of the problem are ruled out.*
- Arrange to interrupt the drug periodically in children who are receiving the drug for behavioural syndromes *to determine whether symptoms recur and therapy should be continued.*
- Arrange to dispense the least amount of drug possible *to minimise the risk of overdose and abuse.*
- Administer drug before 6 p.m. *to reduce the incidence of insomnia.*
- Monitor weight, FBC and ECG *to ensure early detection of adverse effects and proper interventions.*
- Consult with the school nurse or counsellor *to ensure comprehensive care of school-aged children receiving CNS stimulants* (Box 22.7).
- Provide safety measures such as side rails and assistance with ambulation if CNS effects occur *to prevent injury.*
- Provide thorough teaching, including drug name, prescribed dosage, the need to secure the drug as a controlled substance, measures for avoidance of adverse effects, warning signs that may indicate possible problems and the need for monitoring and evaluation *to enhance knowledge about drug therapy and to promote compliance.* Offer support and encouragement to help the person to cope with the drug regimen.

Evaluation

- Monitor response to the drug (decrease in manifestations of behavioural syndromes, decrease in daytime sleep and narcolepsy).
- Monitor for adverse effects (CNS stimulation, CV effects, rash, physical or psychological dependence, GI dysfunction).
- Evaluate effectiveness of the teaching plan (person can give the drug name and dosage, name possible adverse effects to watch for and specific measures to help avoid adverse effects and describe the need for follow-up and evaluation).
- Monitor effectiveness of comfort measures and compliance with the regimen.

KEY POINTS

- An attention-deficit disorder is a behavioural syndrome characterised by hyperactivity and a short attention span.
- Narcolepsy is a disorder characterised by daytime sleepiness and sudden loss of wakefulness.
- CNS stimulants, which stimulate cortical levels and the RAS to increase RAS activity, are used to treat attention-deficit disorders and narcolepsy. These drugs improve concentration and the ability to filter and focus incoming stimuli.

BOX 22.7 FOCUS ON **The evidence**

School nursing and Ritalin administration

In the last several years, the number of school children receiving diagnoses of attention-deficit disorder or minimal brain dysfunction and being prescribed methylphenidate (*Ritalin*) has increased dramatically. Because this drug needs to be given two or three times each day, it has become the responsibility of the school nurse to dispense the drug during the day. Some school nurses reportedly spend between 50% and 70% of their time administering these drugs and completing the necessary paperwork. In 2000–2001, several long-acting formulations of methylphenidate became available.

Methylphenidate (*Concerta*) is available in an extended-release tablet in 18, 27, 36 and 54 mg strengths. Methylphenidate (*Ritalin*) is available in long-acting capsules as 10 mg, 20 mg, 30 mg, and 40 mg. This form is suggested for dosing every 12 hours. The advantage of these extended-release forms is expected to be a decrease in the number of students who must see the nurse for medication during the school day and, perhaps, a decrease in the stigma that may be associated with needing this drug.

The school nurse has additional responsibilities besides administering the drug. The school nurse is responsible for assessing children's response to the drug and for coordinating the teacher's and health care providers' input into each individual case, including the incidence of adverse effects and the appropriateness of the drug therapy. The nurse should:

- Ensure that the proper diagnosis is made before supporting the use of the drug.
- Constantly evaluate and work with the primary health care provider to regularly challenge children without the drug to see whether the drug is doing what is expected or whether the child is maturing and no longer needs the drug therapy.

The school nurse needs to be prepared to be an advocate for the best therapeutic intervention for a particular child. Because long-term methylphenidate therapy is associated with many adverse effects, use of the drug should not be taken lightly.

CHAPTER SUMMARY

- Schizophrenia, the most common psychosis, is characterised by delusions, hallucinations and inappropriate responses to stimuli.
- Mania is a state of hyperexcitability, one pole of bipolar disorder.
- An attention-deficit disorder is a behavioural syndrome characterised by hyperactivity and a short attention span.
- Narcolepsy is a disorder characterised by daytime sleepiness and sudden loss of wakefulness.
- Lithium, a membrane stabiliser, is the standard antimanic drug. Because it is a very toxic salt, serum levels must be carefully monitored to prevent severe toxicity. Many other CNS drugs are now approved for use in bipolar disorder.
- CNS stimulants, which stimulate cortical levels and the RAS to increase RAS activity, are used to treat attention-deficit disorders and narcolepsy. These drugs improve concentration and the ability to filter and focus incoming stimuli.

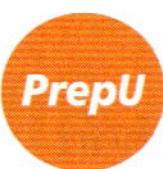

Knowing your strengths and weaknesses helps you to study more effectively. Take a PrepU Practice Quiz to find out how you measure up!

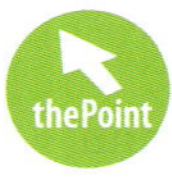

ONLINE RESOURCES

An extensive range of additional resources to enhance teaching and learning and to facilitate understanding of this chapter may be found online at the text's accompanying website, located on thePoint at http://thepoint.lww.com. These include Watch and Learn videos, Concepts in Action animations, journal articles, review questions, case studies, discussion topics and quizzes.

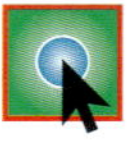

WEB LINKS

Health care providers and students may want to consult the following web resources:

www.aihw.gov.au/reports-data/health-welfare-services/mental-health-services/overview
Australian Institute of Health and Welfare, National Health Priority Area – Mental Health.

https://www1.health.gov.au/internet/main/publishing.nsf/Content/mental-strat
Australian Government National Mental Health Strategy.

BIBLIOGRAPHY

American Psychiatric Association, (2013). *Diagnostic and Statistical Manual of Mental Disorders* (5th edn). www.dsm5.org.

Australian Institute of Health and Welfare (AIHW). (2013). Mental health, www.aihw.gov.au/mental-health.

Blake, T. (2012). Three medication pathways for bipolar disorder. *Nursing, 42(5)*, 28–35.

Caplan, G. (2011). Managing delirium in older patients. *Australian Prescriber, 34*, 16–18.

Fulde, G. (2011). Managing aggressive and violent patients. *Australian Prescriber, 34*, 115–118.

Goodman, L. S., Brunton, L. L., Chabner, B. & Knollmann, B. C. (2011). *Goodman and Gilman's Pharmacological Basis of Therapeutics* (12th edn). New York: McGraw-Hill.

Hazell, P. (2005). Prescribing psychotropic medication to children in general practice. *Australian Prescriber, 28*, 116–118.

Kennedy, D. (2007). Antipsychotic drugs in pregnancy and breastfeeding. *Australian Prescriber, 30*, 162–163.

Lambert, T. (2011). Managing the metabolic adverse effects of antipsychotic drugs in patients with psychosis. *Australian Prescriber, 34*, 97–99.

McKenna, L. & Mirkov, S. (2019). *McKenna's Drug Handbook for Nursing & Midwifery* (8th edn). Sydney: Wolters Kluwer Health Australia.

Nguyen, L. (2008). Lithium I: The basics. *Journal of Emergency Nursing, 34(3)*, 268–269.

Porth, C. M. (2011). *Essentials of Pathophysiology: Concepts of Altered Health States* (3rd edn). Philadelphia: Lippincott Williams & Wilkins.

Porth, C. M. (2009). *Pathophysiology: Concepts of Altered Health States* (8th edn). Philadelphia: Lippincott Williams & Wilkins.

Vance, A. (2008). A current treatment approach for attention deficit hyperactivity disorder. *Australian Prescriber, 31*, 129–132.

CHECK YOUR UNDERSTANDING

Answers to the questions in this chapter can be found in Appendix A at the back of this book.

MULTIPLE CHOICE

Select the best answer to the following.

1. Mental disorders are now thought to be caused by some inherent dysfunction within the brain that leads to abnormal thought processes and responses. They include:
   a. depression.
   b. anxiety.
   c. seizures.
   d. schizophrenia.
2. Antipsychotic drugs are basically:
   a. serotonin reuptake inhibitors.
   b. noradrenaline blockers.
   c. dopamine-receptor blockers.
   d. acetylcholine stimulators.
3. Adverse effects associated with antipsychotic drugs are related to the drugs' effects on receptor sites and can include:
   a. insomnia and hypertension.
   b. dry mouth, hypotension and glaucoma.
   c. diarrhoea and excessive urination.
   d. increased sexual drive and improved concentration.
4. Lithium toxicity can be dangerous. Individual assessment to evaluate for appropriate lithium levels would look for:
   a. serum lithium levels greater than 3 mmol/L.
   b. serum lithium levels greater than 4 mmol/L.
   c. serum lithium levels less than 1.5 mmol/L.
   d. undetectable serum lithium levels.
5. A 6-year-old boy is starting a regimen of Ritalin (methylphenidate) to control an attention-deficit disorder. Family teaching should include which of the following?
   a. This drug can be shared with other family members who might seem to need it.
   b. This drug may cause insomnia, weight loss and GI upset.
   c. Do not alert the school nurse to the fact that this drug is being taken because the child could have problems later on.
   d. This drug should not be stopped for any reason for several years.
6. Antipsychotic drugs are also known as neuroleptic drugs because:
   a. they cause numerous neurological effects.
   b. they frequently cause epilepsy.
   c. they are also minor tranquillisers.
   d. they are the only drugs known to directly affect nerves.
7. Attention-deficit disorders (the inability to concentrate or focus on an activity) and narcolepsy (sudden episodes of sleep) are both most effectively treated with the use of:
   a. neuroinhibitors.
   b. dopamine-receptor blockers.
   c. major tranquillisers.
   d. CNS stimulants.
8. Haloperidol (*Serenace*) is a potent antipsychotic that is associated with:
   a. severe extrapyramidal effects.
   b. severe sedation.
   c. severe hypotension.
   d. severe anticholinergic effects.

MULTIPLE RESPONSE

Select all that apply.

1. Before administering lithium to a person, the nurse or midwife should check for the concomitant use of which of the following drugs, which could cause serious adverse effects?
   a. ibuprofen
   b. haloperidol
   c. thiazide diuretics
   d. antacids
   e. voriconazole
   f. theophylline
2. Dyskinesias are a common side effect of antipsychotic drugs. Care interventions for the person receiving antipsychotic drugs should include which of the following?
   a. Positioning to decrease discomfort of dyskinesias.
   b. Implementing safety measures to prevent injury.
   c. Encouraging the person to chew tablets to prevent choking.
   d. Careful teaching to alert the person and family about this adverse effect.
   e. Applying ice to the joints to prevent damage.
   f. Puréeing all food to decrease the risk of aspiration.

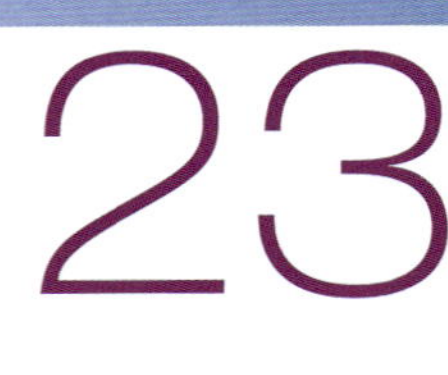

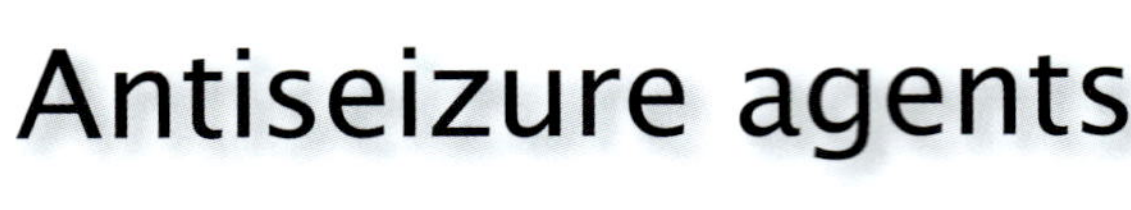

23 Antiseizure agents

Learning objectives

On completing this chapter you should be able to:

1. Define the terms generalised seizure, tonic–clonic seizure, absence seizure, partial seizure and status epilepticus.
2. Describe the therapeutic actions, indications, pharmacokinetics, contraindications, most common adverse reactions and important drug–drug interactions associated with each class of antiseizure agents.
3. Discuss the use of antiepileptic drugs across the lifespan.
4. Compare and contrast the prototype drugs for each class of antiepileptic drug with the other drugs in that class and with drugs from the other classes.
5. Outline the care considerations and teaching needs for people receiving each class of antiepileptic agents.

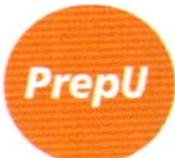
Test your current knowledge of antiseizure agents with a PrepU Practice Quiz!

Glossary of key terms

absence seizure: type of generalised seizure that is characterised by sudden, temporary loss of consciousness, sometimes with staring or blinking for 3–5 seconds; formerly known as a petit mal seizure

antiepileptic: drug used to treat the abnormal and excessive energy bursts in the brain that are characteristic of epilepsy

convulsion: tonic–clonic muscular reaction to excessive electrical energy arising from nerve cells in the brain

epilepsy: collection of various syndromes, all of which are characterised by seizures

generalised seizure: seizure that begins in one area of the brain and rapidly spreads throughout both hemispheres

partial seizures: also called focal seizures; seizures involving one area of the brain that do not spread throughout the entire organ

seizure: sudden discharge of excessive electrical energy from nerve cells in the brain

status epilepticus: state in which seizures rapidly recur; most severe form of generalised seizure

tonic–clonic seizure: type of generalised seizure that is characterised by serious clonic–tonic muscular reactions and loss of consciousness, with exhaustion and little memory of the event on waking; formerly known as a grand mal seizure

DRUGS FOR TREATING GENERALISED SEIZURES

Hydantoins
- (P) phenytoin

Trioxanes
- paraldehyde

Barbiturates and barbiturate-like drugs
- (P) phenobarbital (phenobarbitone)
- primidone

Benzodiazepines
- clobazam
- clonazepam
- (P) diazepam
- midazolam

Succinimides
- (P) ethosuximide

Drugs that modulate the inhibitory neurotransmitter GABA
- acetazolamide
- sodium valproate
- vigabatrin
- zonisamide

DRUGS FOR TREATING PARTIAL SEIZURES
- carbamazepine
- gabapentin
- lacosamide
- lamotrigine
- levetiracetam
- oxcarbazepine
- pregabalin
- tiagabine
- topiramate

Epilepsy, the most prevalent of the neurological disorders, is not a single disease but a collection of different syndromes characterised by the same feature: sudden discharge of excessive electrical energy from nerve cells located within the brain, which leads to a **seizure**. In some cases, this release stimulates motor nerves, resulting in convulsions, with tonic–clonic muscle contractions that have the potential to cause injury, tics or spasms. Other discharges may stimulate autonomic or sensory nerves and cause very different effects, such as a barely perceptible, temporary lapse in consciousness or a sympathetic reaction. Because epilepsy involves a loss of control, it can be very frightening to people when they are first diagnosed (Box 23.1).

The treatment of epilepsy varies widely, depending on the exact problem and its manifestations. The drugs that are used to manage epilepsy are called **antiepileptics**, or antiseizure agents, and are sometimes referred to as anticonvulsants; however, because not all types of epilepsy involve **convulsions**, this term is not generally applicable. The drug of choice for any given situation depends on the type of epilepsy, the person's age (Box 23.2), specific characteristics such as cultural variations (Box 23.3) and tolerance for associated adverse effects. Drugs can be used to treat more than one type of seizure. Table 23.1 lists drugs and the types of seizures that they can be used to treat.

NATURE OF SEIZURES

The form that a particular seizure takes depends on the location of the cells that initiate the electrical discharge and the neural pathways that are stimulated by the initial volley of electrical impulses. For the most part, epilepsy seems to be caused by abnormal neurons that are very sensitive to stimulation or over-respond for some reason. These neurons do not appear to be different from other neurons in any other way. Seizures caused by these abnormal cells are called primary seizures because no underlying cause can be identified. In some cases, however, outside factors – head injury, drug overdose, environmental exposure and so on – may precipitate seizures. Such seizures are often referred to as secondary seizures.

Classification of seizures

Accurate diagnosis of seizure type is very important for determining the correct medication to prevent future seizures while causing the fewest problems and adverse effects. Seizures were formerly categorised as grand mal (tonic–clonic seizures) or petit mal (absence seizures), but the International Classification of Seizures currently refers to seizures in a more systematic approach (based on the description of symptoms and characteristics), grouping them into two main categories: generalised or

BOX 23.1 FOCUS ON **Individual and family teaching**

Teaching and counselling people with epilepsy

Epilepsy, with its stigma, is frightening to people who know little about the disease. This condition has long been associated with some sort of brain dysfunction or possession by the devil or evil spirits. In some eras, exorcism was the first choice of treatment for a person with a seizure disorder. A person who receives a diagnosis of epilepsy must deal with this stigma as well as the significance of the diagnosis. What does having epilepsy mean? Individuals who are newly diagnosed with epilepsy must consider restrictions on their independence as well as the prospect of chronic therapy for control of this problem.

In our society, the ability to be readily mobile – to drive to appointments, work or religious obligations – is very important to many people. In most cases, the driving privileges of affected individuals are revoked, at least temporarily. The conditions for recovering the licence vary with the diagnosis and the laws of each Australian state or territory and in New Zealand.

The person who is newly diagnosed with epilepsy has to cope not only with the stigma of epilepsy, but also with the loss of a driver's licence. The nurse may be in the best position to help the person adjust to both of these problems through education and referrals to community resources. Thorough teaching should include the following:

- Explanations of old stigmas.
- Ways in which people may react to the diagnosis.
- Ways in which people can educate family, friends and employers about the realities of the condition and its treatment.
- Actions to take if a seizure happens so that no injuries occur and no panic develops.
- Information about the availability of public transportation.
- The importance of encouraging people with epilepsy to carry or wear a MedicAlert identification, to alert any emergency carers to their condition and to what drugs they are taking if they are not able to speak for themselves.
- Contact information regarding other community support services.

Many communities have epilepsy support groups that can supply information on valuable resources as well as updated facts about the laws in each area. While people are first adjusting to epilepsy and its implications, it may help to put them in contact with such organisations. The local chapter of Epilepsy Australia may be able to offer support groups, lists of resources and support. Individuals with epilepsy should have several options for getting around without feeling that they are being a burden or an imposition.

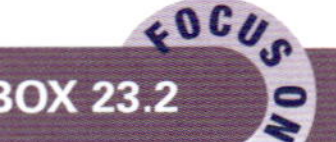

BOX 23.2 Drug therapy across the lifespan

Antiseizure agents

CHILDREN

Antiepileptic drugs can have an impact on a child's learning and social development. Children may also be more sensitive to the sedating effects of some of these drugs. Children should be monitored very closely and often require a switch to a different agent or dosage adjustments based on their response.

Newborns (1–10 days of age) respond best to intramuscular phenobarbital (phenobarbitone) if an antiepileptic is needed.

Older children (2 months to 6 years of age) absorb and metabolise many of these drugs more quickly than adults do and require a larger dosage per kilogram to maintain therapeutic levels. Careful calculation of drug dosage using both weight and age are important in helping the child to receive the best therapeutic effect with the least toxicity. After the age of 10–14 years, many of these drugs can be given in the standard adult dose.

Parents of children receiving these drugs should receive consistent support and education about the seizure disorder and the medications being used to treat it. Many communities have local support groups that can offer lots of educational materials and support programs. It is a very frightening experience to watch your child have a tonic–clonic seizure and parents should be supported with this in mind.

ADULTS

Adults using these drugs should be under regular care and should be monitored routinely for adverse effects. They should be encouraged to carry or wear a Medic-Alert identification to alert emergency personnel that antiepileptic drugs are being taken. Adults also need education and support to deal with the old stigma of seizures as well as the lifestyle changes and drug effects that they may need to cope with.

PREGNANCY AND BREASTFEEDING

Most of these drugs have been associated with fetal abnormalities in animal studies. Some of them are clearly associated with predictable congenital effects in humans. Women of childbearing age should be encouraged to use contraceptives while taking these drugs. If a pregnancy does occur, or if a woman taking one of these drugs desires to become pregnant, the importance of the drug to the mother should be weighed against the potential risk to the fetus. Stopping an antiepileptic can precipitate seizures that could cause anoxia and its related problems for the mother and the baby. Women who are breastfeeding should be encouraged to find another way of feeding the baby to avoid the sedating and central nervous system (CNS) effects that the drugs can have on the infant.

OLDER ADULTS

Older people may be more susceptible to the adverse effects of these drugs. Dosages of all of these drugs may need to be reduced, and the person should be monitored very closely for toxic effects and to provide safety measures if CNS effects do occur.

People with renal or hepatic impairment should be monitored very closely. Baseline renal and liver function tests should be done and dosages adjusted as appropriate. Serum levels of the drug should be monitored closely in such cases to prevent serious adverse effects.

The older person should also be encouraged to wear or carry Medic-Alert identification in case there is an emergency and they are not able to communicate information about the drug or disorder.

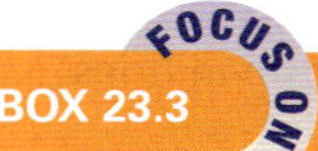

BOX 23.3 Cultural considerations

Altered metabolism of antiseizure agents

Because of differences in liver enzyme functioning among Arabs and Asians, people in these ethnic groups may not metabolise antiseizure agents in the same way as people in other ethnic groups. They may require not only lower doses to achieve the same therapeutic effects, but also frequent dose adjustment.

Nurses and midwives need to be aware that the therapeutic range for people in these ethnic groups may differ from standard norms and that these people may be more apt to show adverse or toxic reactions to antiepileptic drugs at lower doses. As with all medications, the lowest possible dose should be used. Serum drug levels should be closely monitored and titrated carefully and slowly to achieve the maximum benefits with the fewest adverse effects.

TABLE 23.1 Antiepileptic drug therapy grouped by seizure class

Seizures	Generalised seizures (except status epilepticus)	Status epilepticus
Carbamazepine	Carbamazepine	Clonazepam
Clonazepam	Clobazam	Diazepam
Gabapentin	Clonazepam	Lorazepam
Lacosamide	Ethosuximide	Midazolam
Lamotrigine	Lamotrigine	Phenobarbital (phenobarbitone)
Levetiracetam	Levetiracetam	Phenytoin
Oxcarbazepine	Oxcarbazepine	Propofol
Phenytoin	Phenytoin	
Pregabalin	Sodium valproate	
Sodium valproate	Topiramate	
Tiagabine	Vigabatrin	
Topiramate	Zonisamide	
Zonisamide		

Adpted from Aschenbrenner, D. S. & Venable, S. J. (2008). *Drug Therapy in Nursing* (3rd edn). Philadelphia: Lippincott Williams & Wilkins, p. 331.

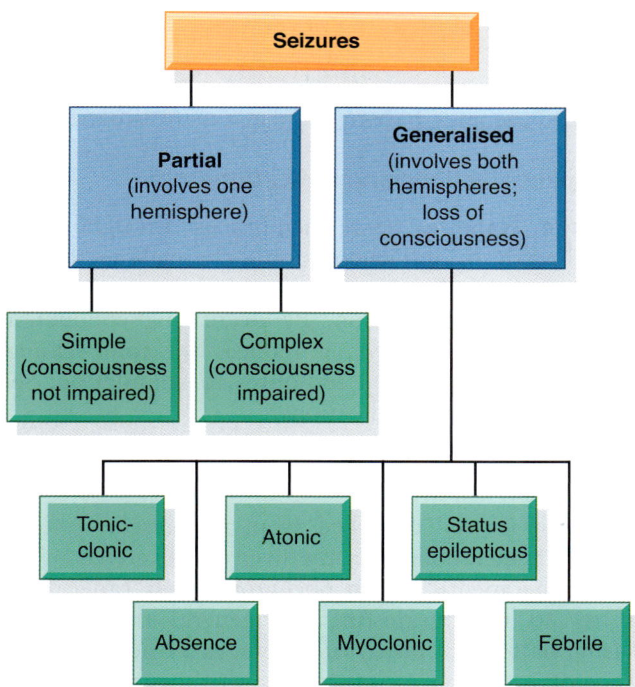

FIGURE 23.1 Classification of seizures. [From Aschenbrenner, D. S. & Venable, S. J. (2008). *Drug Therapy in Nursing* (3rd edn). Philadelphia: Lippincott Williams & Wilkins; p. 332, Figure 21.2.]

partial seizures. Each of these categories can be further subdivided (see Figure 23.1).

Generalised seizures

Generalised seizures begin in one area of the brain and rapidly spread throughout both hemispheres. People who have a generalised seizure usually experience a loss of consciousness resulting from this massive electrical activity throughout the brain.

Generalised seizures are further classified into the following seven types:

1. **Tonic–clonic seizures** involve dramatic tonic–clonic muscle contractions (involuntary muscle contraction followed by relaxation appearing as an aggressive spasm), loss of consciousness and a recovery period characterised by confusion and exhaustion.
2. **Absence seizures** involve abrupt, brief (3- to 5-second) periods of loss of consciousness. Absence seizures occur commonly in children, starting at about 3 years of age, and frequently disappear by puberty. Absence seizures do not usually involve muscle contractions.
3. Myoclonic seizures involve short, sporadic periods of muscle contractions that last for several minutes. They are relatively rare and are often secondary seizures.
4. Febrile seizures are related to very high fevers and usually involve tonic–clonic seizures. Febrile seizures most frequently occur in children; they are usually self-limited and do not reappear.
5. Jacksonian seizures are seizures that begin in one area of the brain and involve one part of the body, and then progressively spread to other parts of the body; they can develop into generalised tonic–clonic seizures.
6. Psychomotor seizures are complex seizures that involve sensory, motor and psychic components. They usually begin with a loss of consciousness and people have no memory of the event. People may exhibit automatic movements, emotional outbursts, and motor or psychological disturbances.
7. **Status epilepticus**, potentially the most dangerous of seizure conditions, is a state in which seizures rapidly recur again and again with no recovery between seizures.

Partial seizures

Partial seizures, or focal seizures, are so called because they involve one area of the brain, usually originating from one site or focus and do not spread throughout the entire organ. The presenting symptoms depend on exactly where in the brain the excessive electrical discharge is occurring. Partial seizures can be further classified as follows:

- Simple partial seizures, which occur in a single area of the brain and may involve a single muscle movement or sensory alteration.
- Complex partial seizures, which involve a series of reactions or emotional changes and complex sensory changes such as hallucinations, mental distortion, changes in personality, loss of consciousness and loss of social inhibitions. Motor changes may include involuntary urination, chewing motions, diarrhoea and so on. The onset of complex partial seizures usually occurs by the late teens.

KEY POINTS

- Epilepsy is characterised by seizures that result from sudden discharge of excessive electrical energy from nerve cells in the brain.
- There are two major categories of seizures: generalised and partial seizures.
- Generalised seizures include the following types: tonic–clonic, absence, myoclonic, febrile, Jacksonian, psychomotor and rapid recurring (status epilepticus).
- Partial seizures may be simple or complex.

DRUGS FOR TREATING GENERALISED SEIZURES

Drugs typically used to treat generalised seizures stabilise the nerve membranes by blocking channels in the cell membrane or altering receptor sites. Because they work generally on the CNS, sedation and other CNS effects often result. Various drugs are used to treat generalised seizures, including a hydantoin, barbiturates, barbiturate-like drugs, benzodiazepines, succinimides and gamma-aminobutyric acid (GABA) inhibitors. These drugs affect the entire brain and reduce the chance of sudden electrical outburst. Associated adverse effects are often related to total brain stabilisation (Figure 23.2).

Absence seizures, another type of generalised seizure, may require drugs that are different from those used to treat or prevent other types of generalised seizures. The succinimides and drugs that modulate the inhibitory neurotransmitter GABA are most frequently used (see Table 23.2).

HYDANTOINS

The currently available hydantoin in Australia and New Zealand is phenytoin (*Dilantin*). Because hydantoins are generally less sedating than many other antiepileptics, phenytoin may be the drug of choice for people who are not willing to tolerate sedation and drowsiness. It does have significant adverse effects; thus, less toxic drugs, such as benzodiazepines, have replaced it in many situations.

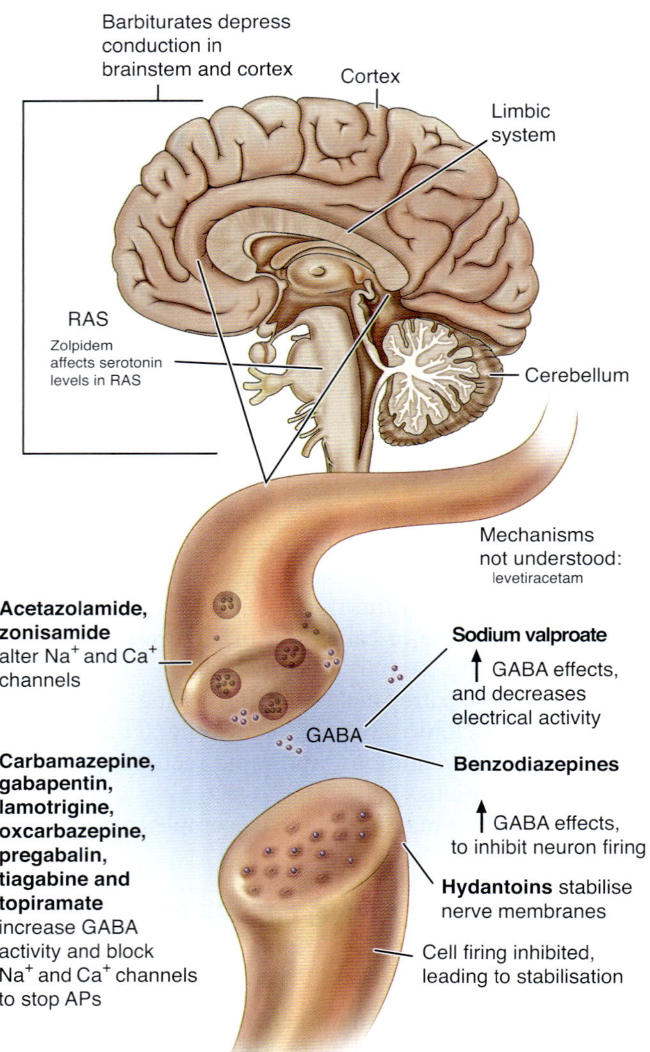

FIGURE 23.2 Sites of action of drugs used to treat various types of epilepsy. AP, action potential; GABA, gamma-aminobutyric acid; RAS, reticular activating system.

Therapeutic actions and indications

Phenytoin stabilises nerve membranes throughout the CNS directly by influencing ionic channels in the cell membrane, thereby decreasing excitability and hyperexcitability to stimulation. By decreasing conduction through nerve pathways, it reduces the tonic–clonic, muscular and emotional responses to stimulation. See Table 23.2 for usual indications.

Pharmacokinetics

Phenytoin is well absorbed from the gastrointestinal (GI) tract, metabolised in the liver and excreted in the urine. Therapeutic serum phenytoin levels range from 10 to 20 micrograms/mL. In general the reported plasma half-life of phenytoin averages 22 hours, with a range of 7–42 hours. Steady-state therapeutic levels are achieved at least 7–10 days (5–7 half-lives) after initiation of therapy with recommended doses of 300 mg/day. Conventionally, with drugs following linear kinetics the half-life is used to determine the dose rate, drug accumulation and the time to reach steady state. Phenytoin, however, demonstrates non-linear kinetics and therefore the half-life is affected by the degree of absorption, saturation of metabolic pathways, dose and the degree of metabolic enzyme induction. This results in considerable inter- and intra-individual variability in phenytoin pharmacokinetics.

As phenytoin is highly protein bound, free phenytoin levels may be altered in people whose protein binding characteristics differ from normal. Protein binding may be lower in neonates and infants with hyperbilirubina; it may also be altered in people with hypoalbuminaemia, uraemia or acute trauma and in pregnancy. Phenytoin is available in oral (also available in paediatric formulation eg, syrup) and parenteral forms.

Contraindications and cautions

Phenytoin is generally contraindicated in the presence of allergy *to avoid hypersensitivity reactions*. These agents are associated with specific birth defects and should not be used in pregnancy or breastfeeding unless the risk of seizures outweighs the potential risk to the fetus. In such cases, the mother should be informed of the potential risks. The risk of taking a woman with a seizure disorder off an antiepileptic drug that has stabilised her condition may be greater than the risk of the drug to the fetus. Discontinuing the drug could result in status epilepticus, which has a high risk of hypoxia for the mother and the fetus. Research has not been able to show the effects

TABLE 23.2 **DRUGS IN FOCUS** **Drugs for treating generalised seizures***

Drug name	Dosage/route	Usual indications
Hydantoin		
Ⓟ phenytoin (*Dilantin*)	Adult, status epilepticus: loading dose of 10–15 mg/kg IV at a rate not exceeding 50 mg/min, followed by maintenance doses of 100 mg orally or IV every 6–8 hours Neonates/paediatric, status epilepticus: loading dose of 10–20 mg/kg IV at a rate not exceeding 1–3 mg/kg/min, maximum 50mg/min Monitor serum levels – therapeutic serum levels are 10–20 micrograms/mL (40–80 micromol/L). After initial dose, determine plasma levels and adjust dosage to 4–8 mg/kg/day PO in 2–3 doses, depending on blood levels. Paediatric dosage forms available include *Dilantin Chewable Infatabs* and *Dilantin Paediatric Suspension*	Treatment of tonic–clonic seizures, prevention of status epilepticus and treatment of seizures after neurosurgery
Barbiturates and barbiturate-like drugs		
Ⓟ phenobarbital (phenobarbitone) (generic)	Adult: 60–240 mg/day PO (up to 350 mg/day); 100–300 mg IM or IV for acute episodes; may be repeated up to 600 mg/day; reduce dose with elderly and with renal or hepatic impairment Paediatric: 1–6 mg/kg/day PO; status epilepticus: 10–20 mg/kg IM (loading dose) then 1–6 mg/kg/day	Long-term treatment of tonic–clonic seizures localised in the cortex; treatment of cortical focal seizures, simple partial seizures, febrile seizures; used as a sedative/hypnotic; emergency control of status epilepticus and acute seizures associated with eclampsia, tetanus and other conditions
primidone (*Mysoline*)	Individualise dose in 2 divided doses. Initially 125 mg in evening, increase by 125 mg/day q 3 days to 500 mg/day then by 250 mg/day (adults) or 125 mg/day (children < 9 years) q 3 days. Usual maintenance, individuals > 9 years: 750–1500 mg/day; 6–9 years: 750–1000 mg/day; 2–5 years: 500–750 mg/day; < 2 years: 250–500 mg/day	Alternative choice in treatment of tonic–clonic, partial, febrile and refractory seizures; may be combined with other agents to treat seizures that cannot be controlled by any other antiseizure agents
Benzodiazepines		
clobazam (*Frisium*)	Paediatric > 4 years: initially 5 mg PO daily in single or divided doses; maintenance dose 0.3–1.0 mg/kg/day. Reduced dosage in people with renal or hepatic impairment	Adjunctive therapy in partial or generalised epilepsy
clonazepam (*Rivotril*)	Adult: initially 1.5 mg/day PO, maintenance (after 2–4 weeks) in 3–4 divided doses, usual dose 4–8 mg/day; up to a maximum 20 mg/day Children up to 10 years or 30 kg: initially 0.01–0.03 mg/kg PO daily (not to exceed 0.05 mg/kg daily) in 2–3 divided doses. Increased by 0.25–0.5 mg every 3 days to maximum maintenance dosage of 0.1–0.2 mg/kg daily. Children 10–16 years: 1.0–1.5 mg/day given in 2–3 divided doses, increased by 0.25–0.5 mg every 3 days until the individual maintenance dose (usually 3–6 mg/day) is reached	Treatment of absence and myoclonic seizures; administered to people who do not respond to succinimides; being studied for use in the treatment of panic attacks, restless leg movements during sleep, hyperkinetic dysarthria, acute manic episodes, multifocal tic disorders, neuralgias and as an adjunct in the treatment of schizophrenia

Continued on following page

TABLE 23.2 DRUGS IN FOCUS Drugs for treating generalised seizures* *(continued)*

Drug name	Dosage/route	Usual indications
Benzodiazepines *(continued)*		
Ⓟ diazepam (*Stesolid Rectal Tubes, Valium*)	Adult: 2–10 mg PO bd to qid or 10–20 mg PR repeated once only, if required, after 5 min, or 2–20 mg IM or IV Elderly or debilitated people: 2–2.5 mg PO daily to bd; or 2–5 mg IM or IV Paediatric: 1–2.5 mg PO tds to qid; or, children 1–6 years: 5 mg PR once; children 7–12 years: 10 mg PR once, PR doses may be repeated, if required, once only after 5 min, or 0.3–0.5 mg/kg PR with a repeat in 4–12 hours if needed, or 0.25 mg/kg IV over 3 min, may repeat in 15–30 min for up to 3 doses Status epilepticus and severe recurrent convulsive seizures: slow IV administration is preferred Infants > 30 days and children < 5 years: 0.2–0.5 mg slowly every 2–5 min up to a maximum of 5 mg Children ≥ 5 years: 1 mg every 2–5 minutes up to a maximum of 10 mg; repeat in 2–4 hours if necessary; EEG monitoring of the seizure may be helpful	Treatment of severe convulsions, clonic–tonic seizures, status epilepticus; treatment of alcohol withdrawal and tetanus; relieves tension, preoperative anxiety; being studied for use in treatment of panic attacks; this drug is no longer used for long-term management of epilepsy
Succinimides		
Ⓟ ethosuximide (*Zarontin*)	Adult and paediatric: 20–30 mg/kg/day in 2 divided doses	Drug of choice for treatment of absence seizures
Drugs that modulate the inhibitory neurotransmitter gamma-aminobutyric acid		
acetazolamide (*Diamox*)	250–1000 mg/day PO in divided doses; 250 mg PO daily if used with other antiepileptics Children: 8–30 mg/kg/day in divided doses; maximum 750 mg/day	Treatment of absence seizures, especially in children with open-angle and secondary glaucoma; to decrease oedema associated with heart failure and drug use; and as a prophylaxis and for mountain sickness
sodium valproate (*Epilim*)	Initially, 600 mg/day. Maximum 2.5 g/day Paediatric: use extreme caution, determine dose by age and weight	Drug of choice for myoclonic seizures; second-choice drug for treatment of absence seizures; also effective in mania, migraine headaches and complex partial seizures
vigabatrin (*Sabril*)	Initially, 1000–4000 mg/day PO	Treatment of epilepsy not well controlled by other antiepileptic drugs
zonisamide (*Zonegran*)	Adults (> 16 years): 100 mg PO daily up to 500 mg/day	Adjunct for treatment of absence seizures

*A trioxane, paraldehyde, is still used rarely to treat generalised seizures.

of even a minor seizure during pregnancy on the fetus, making it important to prevent seizures during pregnancy if at all possible. Women of childbearing age should be urged to use barrier contraceptives while taking these drugs. If a pregnancy does occur, the woman should receive educational materials and counselling.

Caution should be used with elderly or debilitated people, *who may respond adversely to the CNS depression*, and with people who have impaired renal or liver function *which may interfere with drug metabolism and excretion*. People with hepatic impairment are at risk for increased toxicity from phenytoin. Other contraindications include coma, depression or psychoses, *which could be exacerbated by the generalised CNS depression*. Abrupt withdrawal of phenytoin in people with epilepsy may precipitate status epilepticus, hence any need for dosage reduction, discontinuation or substitution of alternative antiepileptic medication should be implemented gradually.

Adverse effects

The most common adverse effects relate to CNS depression and its effects on body function: depression, confusion, drowsiness, lethargy, fatigue, constipation, dry mouth, anorexia, cardiac arrhythmias and changes in blood pressure, urinary retention and loss of libido.

Specifically, phenytoin may cause severe liver toxicity, bone marrow suppression, gingival hyperplasia and potentially serious dermatological reactions (eg, hirsutism, Stevens–Johnson syndrome), all of which are directly related to cellular toxicity.

Clinically important drug–drug interactions

Because the risk of CNS depression is increased with phenytoin taken with alcohol, people should be advised not to drink alcohol while they are taking these agents. Always consult a drug reference before any drug is added to or withdrawn from a therapeutic regimen that involves any of these agents. Box 23.4 describes a hazardous drug–herbal therapy interaction associated with antiepileptic medications.

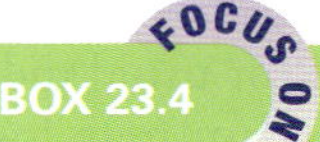

BOX 23.4 Herbal and alternative therapies

People being treated for epilepsy should be advised not to use the herb evening primrose because it increases the risk of having seizures. People being treated with barbiturates or phenytoin should be advised not to use ginkgo, which could cause serious adverse effects.

Prototype summary: phenytoin

Indications: control of tonic–clonic and psychomotor seizures; prevention of seizures during neurosurgery; control of status epilepticus.

Actions: stabilises neuronal membranes and prevents hyperexcitability caused by excessive stimulation; limits the spread of seizure activity from an active focus; has cardiac antiarrhythmic effects similar to those of lidocaine (lignocaine).

Pharmacokinetics:

Route	Onset	Peak	Duration
Oral	Slow	2–12 hours	6–12 hours
IV	1–2 hours	Rapid	12–24 hours

$T_{1/2}$: 6–24 hours; metabolised in the liver, excreted in the urine.

Adverse effects: nystagmus, ataxia, dysarthria, slurred speech, mental confusion, dizziness, fatigue, tremor, headache, dermatitis, Stevens–Johnson syndrome, nausea, gingival hyperplasia, liver damage, haematopoietic complications, sometimes fatal.

BARBITURATES AND BARBITURATE-LIKE DRUGS

Barbiturates and barbiturate-like drugs include phenobarbital (phenobarbitone) (generic) and primidone (*Mysoline* [not available in New Zealand]). These drugs are associated with significant CNS depression.

Therapeutic actions and indications

The barbiturates and barbiturate-type drugs inhibit impulse conduction in the ascending reticular activating system (RAS), depress the cerebral cortex, alter cerebellar function and depress motor nerve output. They stabilise nerve membranes throughout the CNS directly by influencing ionic channels in the cell membrane, thereby decreasing excitability and hyperexcitability to stimulation. By decreasing conduction through nerve pathways, they reduce the tonic–clonic, muscular and emotional responses to stimulation. Phenobarbital depresses conduction in the lower brainstem and the cerebral cortex, as well as depressing motor conduction.

Pharmacokinetics

Phenobarbital, which is available in oral and parenteral forms, is well absorbed from the GI tract, metabolised in the liver and excreted in the urine. This drug has very low lipid solubility, giving it a slow onset and a very long duration of activity. The plasma half-life is 90–100 hours in adults, and 65–70 hours in children, but is greatly prolonged in neonates. The therapeutic serum level range is 15–40 micrograms/mL.

Primidone, available only as an oral agent, is well absorbed from the GI tract, metabolised in the liver to phenobarbital metabolites and excreted in the urine. It tends to have a longer half-life than phenobarbital. The therapeutic serum levels are 5–12 micrograms/mL. Barbiturates readily cross the placenta and, if administered IV, fetal blood concentrations are approximately equal to maternal serum concentrations. Phenobarbital is excreted into breast milk.

Contraindications and cautions

Contraindications and cautions for barbiturates are the same as those discussed for hydantoins. Phenobarbital should not be administered to elderly people who exhibit nocturnal confusion or restlessness from sedative hypnotic drugs or to persons who are known to be, or are likely to become, dependent on sedative hypnotic medications.

Adverse effects

The most common adverse effects associated with barbiturates relate to CNS depression and its effects on body function: depression, confusion, drowsiness, lethargy, fatigue, constipation, dry mouth, anorexia, cardiac arrhythmias and changes in blood pressure, urinary retention and loss of libido. Because barbiturates and barbiturate-like drugs depress nerve function, they can produce sedation, hypnosis, anaesthesia and deep coma. The degree of depression is dose related. At doses below those needed to cause hypnosis, these drugs block seizure activity.

In addition, phenobarbital may be associated with physical dependence and withdrawal syndrome. The drug has also been linked to severe dermatological reactions and the development of drug tolerance related to changes in drug metabolism over time.

Clinically important drug–drug interactions

Because the risk of CNS depression is increased when barbiturates are taken with alcohol, people should be advised not to drink alcohol while they are taking these agents. Always consult a drug reference before any drug is added or withdrawn from a therapeutic regimen that involves any of these agents.

Prototype summary: phenobarbital (phenobarbitone)

Indications: long-term treatment of generalised tonic–clonic and cortical focal seizures; emergency control of certain acute convulsive episodes (status epilepticus, tetanus, eclampsia, meningitis); anticonvulsant treatment of generalised tonic–clonic seizures and focal seizures (parenteral).

Actions: general CNS depressant; inhibits impulse conduction in the ascending RAS; depresses the cerebral cortex; alters cerebellar function; depresses motor output; and can produce excitation, sedation, hypnosis, anaesthesia and deep coma.

Pharmacokinetics:

Route	Onset	Duration
Oral	30–60 min	10–16 hours
IM, SC	10–30 min	4–6 hours
IV	5 min	4–6 hours

$T_{1/2}$: 79 hours; metabolised in the liver, excreted in the urine.

Adverse effects: somnolence, insomnia, vertigo, nightmares, lethargy, nervousness, hallucinations, insomnia, anxiety, dizziness, bradycardia, hypotension, syncope, nausea, vomiting, constipation, diarrhoea, hypoventilation, respiratory depression, tissue necrosis at injection site, withdrawal syndrome.

Benzodiazepines

Some benzodiazepines are used as antiepileptic agents. These include clobazam (*Frisium*), clonazepam (*Rivotril*, *Paxam*), diazepam (*Valium*), and midazolam (*Midazolam Injection*, *Hypnovel*).

Therapeutic actions and indications

The benzodiazepines may potentiate the effects of GABA, an inhibitory neurotransmitter that stabilises nerve cell membranes. These drugs, which appear to act primarily in the limbic system and the RAS, also cause muscle relaxation and relieve anxiety without affecting cortical functioning substantially. The benzodiazepines stabilise nerve membranes throughout the CNS to decrease excitability and hyperexcitability to stimulation. By decreasing conduction through nerve pathways, they reduce the tonic–clonic, muscular and emotional responses to stimulation. In general, these drugs have limited toxicity and are well tolerated by most people. (See Chapter 20 for the use of benzodiazepines as sedatives and anxiolytics.) See Table 23.2 for usual indications for each of these agents. Clonazepam may lose its effectiveness within 3 months (affected individuals may respond to dose adjustment).

Pharmacokinetics

Diazepam is available in oral, rectal and parenteral forms. Diazepam has a biphasic elimination curve, the terminal half-life being 1–2 days. It is extensively protein-bound. Diazepam is metabolised in the liver and the following active metabolites are produced: desmethyldiazepam, methyloxazepam, oxazepam and temazepam. The metabolites are then eliminated by the kidneys in either their free or conjugated form. The half-life of diazepam is prolonged in individuals with kidney or liver disease. Diazepam and its active metabolites show significant accumulation during multiple dosage regimens. Steady state plasma concentrations are attained in 5 days to 2 weeks, as some of its metabolites take several days to weeks to be eliminated.

Clonazepam, on the other hand, is quickly and almost completely absorbed after oral administration. Peak plasma concentrations are reached in most cases within 1–4 hours after an oral dose. The absorption half-life is around 25 minutes. Bioavailability is 90% after oral administration. The mean elimination half-life is 30–40 hours. The elimination half-life and clearance values in neonates are of the same order of magnitude as those reported for adults.

Clonazepam is now available in liquid form, making it a good choice for people who have difficulty swallowing capsules or tablets. These agents are well absorbed from the GI tract, metabolised in the liver and excreted in the urine. They have a long half-life of 18–50 hours.

Contraindications and cautions

Contraindications for benzodiazepines are the same as those discussed for phenytoin.

Adverse effects

The most common adverse effects associated with benzodiazepines relate to CNS depression and its effects on body function: depression, confusion, drowsiness, lethargy, fatigue, constipation, dry mouth, anorexia, cardiac arrhythmias and changes in blood pressure, urinary retention and loss of libido. Benzodiazepines may be associated with physical dependence and withdrawal syndrome. In infants and young children clonazepam may cause increased production of saliva and bronchial secretions. Therefore special attention must be paid to maintaining patency of the airways. The dosage of clonazepam must be carefully adjusted to individual requirements in people: with pre-existing disease of the respiratory system (eg, chronic obstructive pulmonary disease); with pre-existing disease of the liver; undergoing treatment with other centrally acting medications or anti-convulsant (antiepileptic) agents (see Clinically important drug–drug interactions). Like all medicines of this type, clonazepam may, depending on dosage, administration and individual susceptibility, modify the person's reactions (eg, driving ability, behaviour in traffic).

 **Prototype summary: diazepam**

Indications: management of anxiety disorders; acute alcohol withdrawal; muscle relaxant; treatment of tetanus; adjunct in status epilepticus and severe recurrent convulsive seizures; preoperative relief of anxiety and tension; management of epilepsy in people who require intermittent use to control bouts of increased seizure activity.

Actions: acts in the limbic system and reticular formation; potentiates the effects of GABA; has little effect on cortical function.

Pharmacokinetics:

Route	Onset	Peak	Duration
Oral	30–60 min	1–2 hours	3 hours
IM	15–30 min	30–45 min	3 hours
IV	1–5 min	30 min	15–60 min
Rectal	Rapid	1.5 hours	3 hours

$T_{1/2}$: 20–80 hours; metabolised in the liver, excreted in the urine.

Adverse effects: drowsiness, sedation, depression, lethargy, apathy, fatigue, disorientation, bradycardia, tachycardia, paradoxical excitatory reactions, constipation, diarrhoea, incontinence, urinary retention, drug dependence with withdrawal syndrome.

Clinically important drug–drug interactions

Because the risk of CNS depression is increased when benzodiazepines are taken with alcohol, people should be advised not to drink alcohol while they are taking these agents. Always consult a drug reference before any drug is added or withdrawn from a therapeutic regimen that involves any of these agents.

Succinimides

The currently available succinimide is ethosuximide (*Zarontin*). Ethosuximide is most frequently used to treat absence seizures, a form of generalised seizure.

Therapeutic actions and indications

Although the exact mechanism of action is not understood, ethosuximide suppresses the abnormal electrical activity in the brain that is associated with absence seizures. The action may be related to activity in inhibitory neural pathways in the brain (see Figure 23.2). It is indicated for the control of absence seizures (see Table 23.2).

Pharmacokinetics

Ethosuximide is available for oral use. This drug crosses the placenta and enters breast milk (see Contraindications and cautions). Ethosuximide is readily absorbed from the GI tract, reaching peak levels in 1–7 hours. It is metabolised in the liver and excreted in the urine. The half-life of ethosuximide is 30 hours in children and 60 hours in adults. The established therapeutic serum level for ethosuximide is 40–100 micrograms/mL.

Contraindications and cautions

Ethosuximide is contraindicated in the presence of allergy *to avoid hypersensitivity reactions*. Caution should be used with ethosuximide in people with intermittent porphyria, *which could be exacerbated by the adverse effects of the drug*, and those with renal or hepatic disease, *which could interfere with the metabolism and excretion of the drug and lead to toxic levels*. Use during pregnancy should be discussed with the woman because of the potential for adverse effects on the fetus. Another method of feeding the baby should be used if one of these drugs is needed during breastfeeding.

Blood dyscrasias, including some with a fatal outcome, have been reported to be associated with use of ethosuximide; therefore, periodic blood counts should be performed. If signs and/or symptoms of infection (eg, sore throat, fever) develop, blood count determinations should be considered at that point.

Adverse effects

Ethosuximide has relatively few adverse effects compared with many other antiepileptic drugs. Many of the adverse effects associated with the succinimides are related to their depressant effects in the CNS. These may include depression, drowsiness, fatigue, ataxia, insomnia, headache and blurred vision. Decreased GI activity with nausea, vomiting, anorexia, weight loss, GI pain and constipation or diarrhoea may also occur. Bone marrow suppression, including potentially fatal pancytopenia, and dermatological reactions such as pruritus, urticaria, alopecia and Stevens–Johnson syndrome may occur as a result of direct chemical irritation of the skin and bone marrow.

Clinically important drug–drug interactions

Use of ethosuximide with primidone may cause a decrease in serum levels of primidone. People should be monitored and appropriate dose adjustments made if these two agents are used together.

 **Prototype summary: ethosuximide**

Indications: control of absence seizures.

Actions: may act in inhibitory neuronal systems; suppresses the electroencephalographic pattern associated with absence seizures; reduces frequency of attacks.

Pharmacokinetics:

Route	Peak
Oral	3–7 hours

$T_{1/2}$: 30 hours (children), 60 hours (adults); metabolised in the liver, excreted in the urine and bile.

Adverse effects: drowsiness, ataxia, dizziness, irritability, nervousness, headache, blurred vision, pruritus, Stevens–Johnson syndrome, nausea, vomiting, epigastric pain, anorexia, diarrhoea and pancytopenia.

OTHER DRUGS FOR TREATING ABSENCE SEIZURES

Three other drugs that are used in the treatment of absence seizures do not fit into a specific drug class (Table 23.2). These include acetazolamide (*Diamox*, *Glaumox*), sodium valproate (*Epilim*) and zonisamide (*Zonegran*) (not available in New Zealand).

Therapeutic actions and indications

Sodium valproate reduces abnormal electrical activity in the brain and may also increase GABA activity at inhibitory receptors. Acetazolamide – a sulfonamide – alters electrolyte movement, stabilising nerve cell membranes. Another sulfonamide – zonisamide – is a newer agent that inhibits voltage-sensitive sodium and calcium channels, thus stabilising nerve cell membranes and modulating calcium-dependent presynaptic release of excitatory neurotransmitters. See Table 23.2 for usual indications related to these drugs.

Pharmacokinetics

Sodium valproate, available for oral and IV use, is readily absorbed from the GI tract, reaching peak levels in 1–4 hours. It is metabolised in the liver and excreted in the urine, with a half-life of 6–16 hours.

Acetazolamide, which can be given orally or IV, is readily absorbed from the GI tract and is excreted unchanged in the urine with a half-life of 2.5–6 hours.

Zonisamide, an oral drug, is well absorbed from the GI tract, reaching peak levels in 2–6 hours. It is primarily excreted unchanged in the urine, with a half-life of 63 hours.

Contraindications and cautions

These drugs are contraindicated with known allergy to any component of the drug. The sulfonamides are also contraindicated with known allergy to antibacterial sulfonamides and thiazide diuretics *to avoid hypersensitivity reactions*. When it is discontinued, zonisamide should be tapered over 2 weeks because of a risk of precipitating seizures. People who take this drug should be very well hydrated *because of risk of developing renal calculi*.

Caution should be used in people with hepatic or renal impairment, *which could alter metabolism and excretion of the drug*. These drugs should not be used during pregnancy or breastfeeding unless the benefit clearly outweighs the risk to the fetus or neonate *because of the potential for serious adverse effects on the baby*.

Cross-sensitivity between acetazolamide, sulfonamides and other sulphonamide derivatives is possible. Acetazolamide is contraindicated in individuals with marked liver disease or impairment of liver function, including cirrhosis, because of the risk of development of hepatic encephalopathy.

Adverse effects

Sodium valproate is associated with liver toxicity. All of these drugs cause CNS effects related to CNS suppression – weakness, fatigue, drowsiness, dizziness and paraesthesias. Acetazolamide and zonisamide may cause rash and dermatological changes. Zonisamide is associated with bone marrow suppression, renal calculi development and GI upset.

Clinically important drug–drug interactions

Acetazolamide increases the serum levels of tricyclic antidepressants and amphetamines and may increase salicylate toxicity when given with salicylates. Sodium valproate can increase serum levels and potential toxicity of phenobarbital (phenobarbitone), ethosuximide, diazepam, primidone and zidovudine. If any of these drugs are used in combination, the person should be monitored carefully and doses adjusted appropriately.

Breakthrough seizures have been reported when sodium valproate is combined with phenytoin, and extreme care should be taken if this combination must be used.

Zonisamide levels and toxicity are increased if it is combined with carbamazepine, and the person should be monitored and zonisamide dose reduced as needed.

Care considerations for people receiving drugs for treating generalised seizures

The information that follows primarily relates to drug therapy with hydantoins and succinimides, acetazolamide, sodium valproate and zonisamide. See Chapter 20 for care considerations for people receiving barbiturates or benzodiazepines.

Assessment: history and examination

- Assess for contraindications or cautions to the use of hydantoins, including known history of allergy to hydantoins *to avoid hypersensitivity reactions*; cardiac arrhythmias, hypotension, diabetes, coma or psychoses, *which could be exacerbated by the use of the drug*; history of renal or hepatic dysfunction *that might interfere with drug metabolism or excretion*; and current status related to pregnancy and breastfeeding.
- Assess for contraindications or cautions to the use of succinimides, including any known allergies to these drugs; history of intermittent porphyria, *which could be exacerbated by these drugs*; history of renal or hepatic dysfunction *that might interfere with drug metabolism or excretion*; and current status related to pregnancy or breastfeeding.
- Obtain a description of seizures, including onset, aura, duration and recovery, *to determine type of seizure and establish a baseline.*
- Perform a physical assessment *to establish baseline data for determining the effectiveness of therapy and the occurrence of any potential adverse effect.*
- Inspect the skin for colour and lesions *to determine evidence of possible skin effects*; assess pulse and blood pressure and auscultate the heart *to evaluate for possible cardiac effects*; assess level of orientation, affect, reflexes and bilateral grip strength *to evaluate any CNS effects*; monitor bowel sounds and urine output *to determine possible GI or genitourinary (GU) effects*; and evaluate gums and mucous membranes *to establish baseline and monitor changes associated with adverse effects.*
- Obtain a baseline electroencephalogram if appropriate *to evaluate brain function.*
- Assess the person's renal and liver function, including renal and liver function tests, *to determine appropriateness of therapy and determine the need for possible dose adjustment.*

Refer to the Critical thinking scenario for a full discussion of care for a person who is being prescribed antiepileptic drugs.

Implementation with rationale

- Discontinue the drug at any sign of hypersensitivity reaction, liver dysfunction or severe skin rash *to limit reaction and prevent potentially serious reactions.*
- Administer the drug with food *to alleviate GI irritation if GI upset is a problem.*
- Monitor for adverse effects and provide appropriate supportive care as needed *to help the person cope with these effects.*
- Monitor full blood count (FBC) before and periodically during therapy *to detect bone marrow suppression early and provide appropriate interventions.*
- Discontinue the drug if skin rash, bone marrow suppression or unusual depression or personality changes occur *to prevent the development of more serious adverse effects.*
- Discontinue the drug slowly, and never withdraw the drug quickly, *because rapid withdrawal may precipitate absence seizures.*
- Monitor for drug–drug interactions *to arrange to adjust doses appropriately if any drug is added to, or withdrawn from, the drug regimen.*
- Arrange for counselling for women of childbearing age who are taking these drugs. *Because these drugs have the potential to cause serious damage to the fetus,* women should understand the risk of birth defects and use barrier contraceptives to avoid pregnancy.
- Offer support and encouragement *to help the person cope with the drug regimen.*
- Provide thorough teaching, including drug name and prescribed dosage, as well as measures for avoidance of adverse effects and warning signs that may indicate possible problems *to enhance knowledge about drug therapy and to promote compliance*; and the need for periodic blood tests *to evaluate blood counts to reduce the risk of infection and for drug levels to evaluate therapeutic effectiveness and minimise the risk for toxicity.*
- Suggest the wearing or carrying of a MedicAlert bracelet *to alert emergency workers and health care providers about the use of an antiepileptic drug.*

Evaluation

- Monitor response to the drug (decrease in incidence or absence of seizures; serum drug levels within the therapeutic range); evaluate for therapeutic blood levels (40–100 micrograms/mL) for ethosuximide *to ensure the most appropriate dose of the drug.*

- Monitor for adverse effects (CNS changes, GI depression, urinary retention, arrhythmias, blood pressure changes, liver toxicity, bone marrow suppression, severe dermatological reactions).
- Evaluate the effectiveness of the teaching plan (person can give the drug name and dosage and name possible adverse effects to watch for and specific measures to prevent them; person is aware of the risk of birth defects and the need to carry information about the diagnosis and use of this drug).
- Monitor the effectiveness of comfort measures and compliance with the regimen.

KEY POINTS

- Drugs used to treat generalised seizures include the hydantoins, barbiturates and benzodiazepines.
- Drugs used to treat absence seizures – a particular type of generalised seizure – include the hydantoins, succinimides, acetazolamide, sodium valproate and zonisamide.
- All of these drugs stabilise nerve membranes throughout the CNS to decrease excitability and hyperexcitability to stimulation.
- Adverse effects associated with these drugs reflect the CNS depression – lethargy, somnolence, fatigue, dry mouth, constipation and dizziness. Serious liver, bone marrow and dermatological problems can occur with specific drugs.

CRITICAL THINKING SCENARIO

Antiepileptic drugs

THE SITUATION

J.M., an athletic, 18-year-old high-school student, experienced his first seizure during maths class. He seemed attentive and alert, and then he suddenly slumped to the floor with a full tonic–clonic (grand mal) seizure. The other students were frightened and did not know what to do. Fortunately, the teacher was familiar with seizures and quickly reacted to protect J.M. from hurting himself and to explain what was happening.

J.M. was diagnosed with idiopathic generalised epilepsy with tonic–clonic (grand mal) seizures. The combination of phenytoin and phenobarbital (phenobarbitone) that he began taking made him quite drowsy during the day. These drugs were unable to control the seizures, and he had three more seizures in the next month – one at school and two at home. J.M. is now undergoing re-evaluation for possible drug adjustment and counselling.

CRITICAL THINKING

What teaching implications should be considered when meeting with J.M.? *Consider his age and the setting of his first seizure.*

What problems might J.M. encounter in school and in athletics related to the diagnosis and the prescribed medication? *Consider measures that may help him avoid some of the unpleasant side effects related to this particular drug therapy. Driving a car may be a central social focus in the life of an older high-school student.*

What problems can be anticipated and confronted before they occur concerning laws that forbid individuals with newly diagnosed epilepsy from driving?

Develop a teaching protocol for J.M. How will you involve the entire family in the teaching plan?

DISCUSSION

On their first meeting, it is important for the health care professional to establish a trusting relationship with J.M. and his family. J.M., who is at a sensitive stage of development, requires a great deal of support and encouragement to cope with the diagnosis of epilepsy as well as the need for drug therapy. He may need to vent his feelings and concerns and discuss how he can re-enter school without worrying about having a seizure in class. The health care professional should implement a thorough drug teaching program, including a description of warning signs to watch for that should be reported to a health care professional. J.M. should be encouraged to take the following preventive measures:

- Have frequent oral hygiene to protect the gums.
- Avoid operating dangerous machinery or performing tasks that require alertness while drowsy and confused.
- Pace activities as much as possible to help deal with any fatigue and malaise.
- Take the drugs with meals if GI upset is a problem.

This information should be given to both J.M. and his family in written form for future reference, along with the name of a health care professional and a telephone number to call with questions or comments. The importance of continuous medication to suppress the seizures should be stressed. The adverse effects of many of these drugs make it difficult for some people to remain compliant with their drug regimen.

After the discussion with J.M., the health care professional should meet with his family members, who also need support and encouragement to deal with his diagnosis and its implications. They need to know what seizures are, how the prescribed antiepileptic drugs affect the seizures, what they can do when seizures occur, and complete information about the drugs he must take and their anticipated effects. In addition, it is important to work with family members to determine whether any particular thing precipitated the seizures. In other words, was there any warning or aura? This may help with adjustment of drug dosages or avoidance of certain situations or stimuli that precipitate seizures. Family members should be encouraged to report and record any seizure activity that occurs.

Most states and territories do not permit individuals with newly diagnosed epilepsy to drive, and states have varying regulations about the return of the driver's licence after a seizure-free interval. In New Zealand drivers are prohibited from driving for 12 months after a seizure. Driving may then be allowed once the epilepsy is considered to be under control. If driving makes up a major part of J.M.'s social activities, this news may be even more unacceptable than his diagnosis. J.M. and his family should be counselled and helped to devise other ways of getting to places and coping with this restriction. J.M. may be interested in referral to a support group for teens with similar problems, where he can share ideas, support and frustrations.

J.M.'s condition is a chronic one that will require continual drug therapy and evaluation. He will need periodic reteaching and should have the opportunity to ask additional questions and to vent his feelings. J.M. should be encouraged to wear or carry a MedicAlert tag so that emergency medical personnel are aware of his diagnosis and the medications he is taking.

CARE GUIDE FOR J.M.: ANTIEPILEPTIC AGENTS

Assessment: history and examination

Allergies to any of these drugs; hypotension; arrhythmias; bone marrow suppression; coma; psychoses; pregnancy or breastfeeding; hepatic or renal dysfunction

Concurrent use of sodium valproate, cimetidine, disulfiram, isoniazid, sulfonamides, diazoxide, folic acid, rifampicin, sucralfate, theophylline, primidone, paracetamol

CV: blood pressure, pulse, peripheral perfusion

CNS: orientation, reflexes, affect, strength, EEG

Skin: colour, lesions, texture, temperature

GI: abdominal evaluation, bowel sounds

Respiratory: respiration, adventitious sounds

Laboratory tests: FBC, liver and renal function tests

Implementation

Discontinue drug at first sign of liver dysfunction or skin rash.

Provide comfort and safety measures: positioning; give with meals; skin care.

Provide support and reassurance to cope with diagnosis, restrictions and drug effects.

Provide teaching regarding drug name, dosage, side effects, symptoms to report and the need to wear MedicAlert information; other drugs to avoid.

Evaluation

Evaluate drug effects: decrease in incidence and frequency of seizures; serum drug levels within therapeutic range.

Monitor for adverse effects: CNS effects (multiple); bone marrow suppression; rash, skin changes; GI effects – nausea, anorexia; arrhythmias.

Monitor for drug–drug interactions: increased depression with CNS depressants, alcohol; drugs as listed.

Evaluate effectiveness of the teaching program.

Evaluate effectiveness of comfort/safety measures.

Teaching for J.M.

- The drugs that are being evaluated for you are called antiepileptic agents. They are used to stabilise abnormal cells in the brain that have been firing excessively and causing seizures.
- The timing of these doses is very important. To be effective, this drug must be taken regularly.
- Do not stop taking this drug suddenly. If for any reason you are unable to continue taking the drug, notify your health care provider at once. This drug must be slowly withdrawn when its use is discontinued.
- Common effects of these drugs include:
  - *Fatigue, weakness, and drowsiness:* try to space activities evenly throughout the day and allow rest periods to avoid these effects. Take safety precautions and avoid driving or operating dangerous machinery if these conditions occur.
  - *Headaches and difficulty sleeping:* these usually disappear as your body adjusts to the drug. If they persist and become too uncomfortable, consult with your health care provider.
  - *Gastrointestinal upset, loss of appetite, and diarrhoea or constipation:* taking the drug with food or eating small, frequent meals may help alleviate this problem.
- Report any of the following conditions to your health care provider: *skin rash, severe nausea and vomiting, impaired coordination, yellowing of the eyes or skin, fever, sore throat, personality changes, and unusual bleeding or bruising.*
- It is advisable to wear or carry a Medic-Alert warning so that any person who takes care of you in an emergency will know that you are taking this drug.
- Tell any doctor, nurse or other health care provider involved in your care that you are taking this drug.
- Keep this drug and all medications out of the reach of children.
- Do not take any other drug, including over-the-counter medications and alcohol, without consulting with your health care provider. Many of these preparations interact with the drug and could cause adverse effects.
- Report and record any seizure activity that you have while you are taking this drug.
- Take this drug exactly as prescribed. Regular medical follow-up, which may include blood tests, will be necessary to evaluate the effects of this drug on your body.

DRUGS FOR TREATING PARTIAL SEIZURES

Partial seizures may be simple (involving only a single muscle or reaction) or complex (involving a series of reactions or emotional changes). Drugs used in the treatment of partial seizures include carbamazepine (*Tegretol*, *Teril*), gabapentin (*Neurontin*), lacosamide (*Vimpat*), lamotrigine (*Lamictal*), levetiracetam (*Keppra*), oxcarbazepine (*Trileptal*), pregabalin (*Lyrica*), tiagabine (*Gabitril*) and topiramate (*Topamax*) (see Table 23.3). Some of the drugs used to treat generalised seizures have also been found to be useful in treating partial seizures (see Table 23.1).

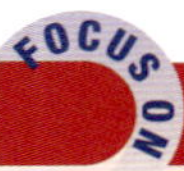

Safe medication administration

Name confusion has been reported between Keppra *(levetiracetam) and* Kaletra *(lopinavir/ritonavir), an HIV antiviral combination drug. Both drugs come in a liquid form, and confusion has been reported in the administration of the two drugs, causing serious adverse effects. Use extreme caution when administering these drugs.*

Therapeutic actions and indications

The drugs used to control partial seizures stabilise nerve membranes in either of two ways – directly, by altering sodium and calcium channels, or indirectly, by increasing the activity of GABA, an inhibitory neurotransmitter, and thereby decreasing excessive activity (see Figure 23.2). Carbamazepine and oxcarbazepine are used as monotherapy, and the remaining drugs are used as adjunctive therapy (see Table 23.3 for usual indications for each agent). Each of the drugs used for treating partial seizures has a slightly different mechanism of action.

Carbamazepine is chemically related to the tricyclic antidepressants. It has the ability to inhibit polysynaptic responses and to block sodium channels to prevent the formation of repetitive action potentials in the abnormal focus.

Gabapentin (*Neurontin*) inhibits polysynaptic responses and blocks stimulus increases in certain situations. However, the mechanism by which gabapentin exerts its anticonvulsant action is unknown. Gabapentin is structurally related to the neurotransmitter GABA but its mechanism of action is different from that of several other medications that interact with GABA synapses including valproate, barbiturates, benzodiazepines, GABA transaminase inhibitors, GABA reuptake inhibitors, GABA agonists and GABA prodrugs.

Lamotrigine and lacosamide may inhibit voltage-sensitive sodium and calcium channels, stabilise nerve cell membranes and modulate calcium-dependent presynaptic release of excitatory neurotransmitters. Levetiracetam is a newer drug, and its mechanism of action is not understood; its antiepileptic action does not seem to be associated with any known mechanisms of inhibitory or excitatory neurotransmission. (See also the Focus on safe medication administration for information about potentially serious name confusion that has occurred with levetiracetam.)

Oxcarbazepine's exact mechanism of action is also unknown. It inhibits voltage-sensitive sodium channels, stabilising hyperexcited nerve cell membranes. It also increases potassium conductance and modulates calcium-dependent presynaptic release of excitatory neurotransmitters. Any or all of these effects may be responsible for the antiseizure effects of the drug.

Pregabalin has a high binding affinity for voltage-gated calcium channels in the cerebrovascular system. It seems to modulate the calcium function in these neurons, leading to a decreased release of neurotransmitters into the synaptic cleft and a decrease in cell activity. Pregabalin does not show affinity for receptor sites or alter responses associated with the action of several common drugs for treating seizures or pain. Pregabalin does not interact with either GABA-A or GABA-B receptors; it is not converted metabolically into GABA or a GABA agonist; it is not an inhibitor of GABA uptake or degradation. Tiagabine (not available in New Zealand) binds to GABA reuptake receptors, causing an increase in GABA levels in the brain. Because GABA is an inhibitory neurotransmitter, the result is a stabilising of nerve membranes and a decrease in excessive activity.

Topiramate blocks sodium channels in neurons with sustained depolarisation and increases GABA activity, inhibiting nerve activity. Topiramate increases the frequency at which GABA activates GABA-A receptors, and enhances the ability of GABA to induce a flux of chloride ions into neurons, suggesting that topiramate potentiates the activity of this inhibitory neurotransmitter. This effect is not blocked by flumazenil, a benzodiazepine antagonist, nor does topiramate increase the duration of the channel opening time, which differentiates topiramate from barbiturates that modulate GABA-A receptors.

Pharmacokinetics

These drugs are all given orally. Levetiracetam is also available for IV use.

Carbamazepine is absorbed from the GI tract and metabolised in the liver by the cytochrome P450 system. It is excreted in the urine with a half-life of 25–65 hours.

Gabapentin is well absorbed from the GI tract and widely distributed in the body. It is excreted unchanged in the urine, with a half-life of 5–7 hours.

Lamotrigine and lacosamide are rapidly absorbed from the GI tract, metabolised in the liver and primarily excreted in the urine. The half-life of lamotrigine is approximately 25 hours.

Levetiracetam is rapidly absorbed from the GI tract, reaching peak levels in 1 hour. It goes through very little metabolism, with most of the drug being excreted unchanged in the urine, with a half-life of 6–8 hours.

TABLE 23.3 DRUGS IN FOCUS Drugs for treating partial seizures

Drug name	Dosage/route	Usual indications
(P) carbamazepine (*Tegretol*)	Adults and children > 15 years: initially 100–200 mg PO once or twice daily increased slowly to 400 mg bd–tid. Maximum 2000 mg/day. Monitor serum levels Paediatric (> 12 years): adult doses, do not exceed 1000 mg/day Paediatric (6–15 years): initially 100 mg PO daily in 2 divided doses, increasing by 100 mg/day in 3–4 divided doses at weekly intervals until optimal control is obtained. Maximum 1000 mg/day. Recommended maintenance doses are, 6–10 years: 400–600 mg/day; 11–15 years: 600–1000 mg/day Paediatric (< 6 years): initially 20–60 mg/day in divided doses increased up to 60 mg/day every 3–7 days. Maximum 600 mg/day. Monitor serum levels	Drug of choice for treatment of partial seizures and tonic–clonic seizures; treatment of trigeminal neuralgia, bipolar disorder
gabapentin (*Neurontin*)	Adult: 900–1800 mg/day PO in divided doses tds Paediatric (3–12 years): day 1: 10 mg/kg; day 2: 20 mg/kg; day 3: 30 mg/kg; usual range: 25–35 mg/kg/day in 3 divided doses. Maximum 40–50 mg/kg/day	Used as adjunct in treating partial seizures; treatment of postherpetic pain in adults and children ages 3–12 years of age; has orphan drug status for the treatment of amyotrophic lateral sclerosis; treatment of pain, migraines, bipolar disorders, tremors of multiple sclerosis and nerve-generated pain states
lacosamide (Vimpat)	Adults: 50–200 mg PO or IV bd up to 600 mg/day Paediatric (> 50 kg), as add-on therapy: 50–200 mg PO or IV bd	Used as adjunct in treating partial seizures with or without secondary generalisation
lamotrigine (*Lamictal*)	Adults and children > 12 years: initially 25 mg once a day for 2 weeks, followed by 50 mg once a day for 2 weeks. Thereafter, dose should be increased by a maximum of 50–100 mg every 1–2 weeks until optimal response is achieved. Usual maintenance does to achieve optimal response is 100–200 mg/day given once a day or as 2 divided doses Paediatric (2–12 years), as add-on therapy with valproate: 0.15 mg/kg/day for 2 weeks, followed by 0.3 mg/kg/day for 2 weeks. Usual maintenance dose is 1–5 mg/kg/day given once a day or as a divided dose, with a maximum of 200 mg/day	Used as adjunct or for monotherapy in treating partial seizures and in treatment of seizures associated with Lennox–Gastaut syndrome in adults and children ≥ 2 years of age; long-term treatment of bipolar disorders
levetiracetam (*Keppra*)	Adult: 250–3000 mg/day PO in divided doses Paediatric (4–16 years): initially 10 mg/kg PO bd to a maximum of 30 mg/kg bd	Newer drug approved for adjunctive treatment of partial seizures in adults and children ≥ 4 years of age; in 2007, it was also approved for the treatment of primary generalised tonic–clonic seizures in adults and treatment of children ≥ 6 years of age with idiopathic generalised epilepsy; being studied for use in absence seizures, myoclonic seizures and drug-resistant seizures of multiple types
oxcarbazepine (*Trileptal*)	Adult: initially 600 mg/day PO in 2 divided doses up to a maximum of 2400 mg/day Paediatric (4–16 years): 8–10 mg/kg/day PO in 2 divided doses, maximum 60 mg/kg/day	Used for monotherapy or adjunctive therapy in treatment of partial seizures in adults and children 4–16 years of age; also being studied as an alternative treatment of bipolar disorders

Continued on following page

TABLE 23.3 **DRUGS IN FOCUS** **Drugs for treating partial seizures *(continued)***

Drug name	Dosage/route	Usual indications
pregabalin (*Lyrica*)	Epilepsy, neuropathic pain: 150–600 mg/day PO in divided doses Postherpetic neuralgia: 75–150 mg PO tds	Used for adjunctive treatment of adults with partial-onset seizures; management of neuropathic pain associated with diabetic peripheral neuropathy and postherpetic neuralgia; fibromyalgia
tiagabine (*Gabitril*)	Adults and paediatrics (> 12 years): initially 7.5–15 mg/day PO in three divided doses, up to 30–50 mg/day PO	Used as adjunct in treating partial seizures in and in children 12–18 years of age
topiramate (*Topamax*)	Adults, epilepsy (monotherapy): 25 mg at night for ≥ 1 week, increased by 25–50 mg/day at weekly intervals to 100 mg/day; maximum 500–1000 mg/day. Paediatric (2–16 years): 0.5–1 mg/kg at night for 1 week, increased by 0.5–1 mg/kg/day at weekly intervals to 3–6 mg/kg/day; maximum 500 mg/day	Used as adjunct in treating partial seizures in adults and children 2–16 years of age; also approved for treatment of tonic–clonic seizures, for prevention of migraine headaches, and as adjunct therapy in Lennox–Gastaut syndrome; being studied for use in cluster headaches, infantile spasms, alcohol dependence, bulimia nervosa and weight loss

Oxcarbazepine is completely absorbed from the GI tract and extensively metabolised in the liver. It is excreted in the urine, with a half-life of 2 and then 9 hours.

Pregabalin is rapidly absorbed orally, reaching peak levels in 1.5 hours. It is not metabolised but is eliminated unchanged in the urine, with a half-life of 6.3 hours.

Tiagabine is rapidly absorbed from the GI tract, reaching peak levels in 45 minutes. It is metabolised in the liver by the cytochrome P450 system. It is excreted in the urine, with a half-life of 4–7 hours.

Topiramate is rapidly absorbed from the GI tract, reaching peak levels in 2 hours. It is widely distributed and is excreted unchanged in the urine.

Contraindications and cautions

Contraindications to the drugs used to control partial seizures include the following conditions: presence of any known allergy to the drug; bone marrow suppression, *which could be exacerbated by the drug effects*; and severe hepatic dysfunction, *which could be exacerbated and could interfere with the metabolism of the drugs*.

Carbamazepine, gabapentin and oxcarbazine have been shown to be dangerous to a fetus and should not be used during pregnancy. Women of childbearing age should be advised to use contraception. These drugs enter breast milk and can cause serious adverse effects in the baby. If any of these drugs is needed during breastfeeding, another method of feeding the baby should be used.

There are no clear studies about the effects of lamotrigine, levetiracetam, pregabalin, tiagabine or topiramate use during pregnancy and breastfeeding. Therefore, these drugs should not be used during pregnancy or breastfeeding unless the benefits to the mother clearly outweigh potential adverse effects in the fetus or neonate. Men considering fathering a child should be advised that, in animal studies, males receiving pregabalin had decreased fertility and associated birth defects in offspring.

Caution should also be used in the following situations: with renal or hepatic dysfunction, *which could alter the metabolism and excretion of the drugs*; and with renal stones, *which could be exacerbated by the effects of some of these agents.*

Adverse effects

The most frequently occurring adverse effects associated with the drugs used for partial seizures relate to the CNS depression that results. The following conditions may occur: drowsiness, fatigue, weakness, confusion, headache and insomnia; GI depression, with nausea, vomiting and anorexia; and upper respiratory infections. These antiepileptics can also be directly toxic to the liver and the bone marrow, causing dysfunction. The exact effects of each drug vary. Antiepileptics have been associated with dizziness and somnolence, which may increase the occurrence of falls in the elderly.

People with renal dysfunction are more likely to experience toxic effects of levetiracetam, and the dose for these individuals needs to be decreased accordingly.

The adverse effects most commonly seen with pregabalin are related to CNS depression – tremor, dizziness, somnolence and visual changes. This drug does have a controlled substance rating as Category V. It can cause feelings of wellbeing and euphoria. Because of this, its use should be limited in people who have a history of abuse of medications or alcohol.

A reduced dose of topiramate is recommended for people with renal impairment. The drug has also been associated with marked CNS depression. Tiagabine has also been associated with serious skin rash.

Clinically important drug–drug interactions

If any of these drugs is taken with other CNS depressants or alcohol, a potential for increased CNS depression exists. Caution people to avoid alcohol while taking drugs for partial seizures or to take extreme precautions if such combinations cannot be avoided.

In addition, numerous drug–drug interactions are associated with carbamazepine. Always consult a drug reference whenever a drug is added or withdrawn from a carbamazepine-containing regimen. Dose adjustments may be necessary.

Oxcarbazepine (*Trileptal*) is an inhibitor of CYP2C19. Therefore, interactions could arise when co-administering high doses of oxcarbazepine with medicinal products that are metabolised by CYP2C19 (eg, phenobarbital [phenobarbitone], phenytoin).

Ⓟ Prototype summary: carbamazepine

Indications: treatment of seizure disorders, including partial seizures with complex patterns; tonic–clonic seizures; mixed seizures; trigeminal neuralgia.

Actions: inhibits polysynaptic responses and blocks post-tetanic potentiations; mechanism of action is not understood; related to the tricyclic antidepressants.

Pharmacokinetics:

Route	Onset	Peak
Oral	Slow	4–5 hours
Extended release oral	Slow	3–12 hours

$T_{1/2}$: 25–65 hours, then 12–17 hours; metabolised in the liver, excreted in the urine and faeces.

Adverse effects: drowsiness, ataxia, dizziness, nausea, vomiting, CV complications, hepatitis, haematological disorders, Stevens–Johnson syndrome.

Care considerations for people receiving drugs to treat partial seizures

Assessment: history and examination

- Assess for contraindications and cautions: any known allergies to these drugs *to avoid hypersensitivity reactions*; history of bone marrow suppression or renal stones, *which could be exacerbated by these drugs*; history of renal or hepatic dysfunction *that might interfere with drug metabolism and excretion*; and current status of pregnancy or breastfeeding, *which are contraindicated or require caution when using these drugs*.
- Perform a physical assessment to establish baseline data for determining the effectiveness of therapy and the occurrence of any *potential adverse effects*.
- Inspect the skin for colour and lesions *to determine evidence of possible skin effects*; assess pulse and blood pressure and auscultate the heart *to evaluate for possible cardiac effects*; assess level of orientation, affect, reflexes and bilateral grip strength *to evaluate any CNS effects*; monitor bowel sounds and urine output *to determine possible GI or GU effects*.
- Obtain a baseline electroencephalogram if appropriate *to evaluate brain function*.
- Assess the person's renal and liver function, including renal and liver function tests, *to determine the appropriateness of therapy and determine the need for possible dose adjustment*.
- Monitor the results of laboratory tests such as urinalysis and FBC with differential *to identify changes in bone marrow function*.

Implementation with rationale

- Administer the drug with food *to alleviate GI irritation if GI upset is a problem*.
- Monitor FBC before and periodically during therapy *to detect and prevent serious bone marrow suppression*.
- Protect the person from exposure to infection *if bone marrow suppression occurs*.
- Discontinue the drug if skin rash, bone marrow suppression, unusual depression or personality changes occur *to prevent further serious adverse effects*.
- Discontinue the drug slowly, and never withdraw the drug quickly, *because rapid withdrawal may precipitate seizures*.
- Arrange for counselling for women of childbearing age who are taking these drugs. *Because these drugs have the potential to cause serious damage to the fetus*, women should understand the risk of birth defects and use barrier contraceptives to avoid pregnancy.
- Evaluate for therapeutic blood levels of carbamazepine (4–12 micrograms/mL) *to ensure that the most effective dose is being used*.
- Provide safety measures to protect the person from injury or falls *if CNS changes occur*.
- Provide teaching, including drug name and prescribed dosage, as well as measures for avoidance of adverse effects, warning signs that may indicate possible problems and the need for periodic laboratory testing and monitoring and evaluation *to enhance knowledge about drug therapy and to promote compliance*.
- Suggest that the person wear or carry a MedicAlert bracelet *to alert emergency workers and health care providers about the use of an antiepileptic drug*.
- Offer support and encouragement *to help the person cope with the drug regimen*.

Evaluation

- Monitor response to the drug (decrease in incidence or absence of seizures).

- Monitor for adverse effects (CNS changes, GI depression, bone marrow suppression, severe dermatological reactions, liver toxicity, renal stones).
- Evaluate the effectiveness of the teaching plan (person can give the drug name and dosage and name possible adverse effects to watch for and specific measures to prevent them; person is aware of the risk of birth defects and the need to carry information about the diagnosis and use of this drug).

KEY POINTS

- Drugs used in the treatment of partial seizures include drugs that stabilise the nerve membrane by altering electrolyte movement or increasing GABA activity.
- Some of the drugs used to treat generalised seizures have also been found to be useful in treating partial seizures.
- Adverse effects associated with the use of drugs used in treating partial seizures include CNS depressive effects and dermatological disorders.

CHAPTER SUMMARY

- Epilepsy is a collection of different syndromes, all of which have the same characteristic: a sudden discharge of excessive electrical energy from nerve cells located within the brain. This event is called a seizure.
- Seizures can be divided into two groups: generalised and partial (focal).
- Generalised seizures can be further classified as: tonic–clonic (grand mal); absence (petit mal); myoclonic; febrile; and status epilepticus (rapidly recurrent).
- Partial (focal) seizures can be further classified as simple or complex.
- Drug treatment depends on the type of seizure that the person has experienced and the toxicity associated with the available agents.
- Drug treatment is directed at stabilising the overexcited nerve membranes and/or increasing the effectiveness of GABA, an inhibitory neurotransmitter.
- Adverse effects associated with antiepileptics (eg, insomnia, fatigue, confusion, GI depression, bradycardia) reflect the CNS depression caused by the drugs.
- People being treated with an antiepileptics should be advised to wear or carry a MedicAlert notification to alert emergency medical professionals to their epilepsy and their use of antiepileptics drugs.
- People being treated with antiepileptics are often on long-term therapy, which requires compliance with their drug regimen and restrictions associated with their disorder and the drug effects.

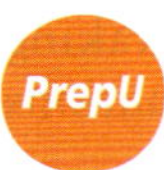

Knowing your strengths and weaknesses helps you to study more effectively. Take a PrepU Practice Quiz to find out how you measure up!

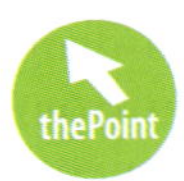

ONLINE RESOURCES

An extensive range of additional resources to enhance teaching and learning and to facilitate understanding of this chapter may be found online at the text's accompanying website, located on thePoint at http://thepoint.lww.com. These include Watch and Learn videos, Concepts in Action animations, journal articles, review questions, case studies, discussion topics and quizzes.

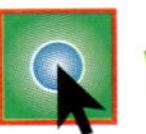

WEB LINKS

Health care providers and students may want to consult the following web resources:

www.epilepsy.org.au
Information about epilepsy research and treatment.

www.epilepsyaustralia.net
Epilepsy Australia.

BIBLIOGRAPHY

Adab, N. (2006). Birth defects and epilepsy medication. *Expert Review of Neurotherapeutics, 6(6)*, 833–845.

Al-aqeel, S. & Al-sabhan, J. (2011). Strategies for improving adherence to antiepileptic drug treatment in patients with epilepsy. *Cochrane Database of Systematic Reviews, 1*, CD008312.

Aschenbrenner, D. S. & Venable, S. J. (2008). *Drug Therapy in Nursing* (3rd edn), Philadelphia: Lippincott Williams & Wilkins.

Bingham, E. (2011). Care of older people with epilepsy. *Nursing Older People, 23(1)*, 24–28.

Farrell, M. & Dempsey, J. (2014). *Smeltzer & Bare's Textbook of Medical-Surgical Nursing* (3rd edn). Sydney: Lippincott Williams & Wilkins.

Goodman, L. S., Brunton, L. L., Chabner, B. & Knollmann, B. C. (2011). *Goodman and Gilman's Pharmacological Basis of Therapeutics* (12th edn). New York: McGraw-Hill.

McKenna, L. & Mirkov, S. (2019). *McKenna's Drug Handbook for Nursing and Midwifery* (8th edn). Sydney: Wolters Kluwer Health Australia.

Ng, Y-T. & Magandu, R. (2013). Status epilepticus in childhood. *Journal of Paediatrics and Child Health, 49(6)*, 432–437.

Porth, C. M. (2011). *Essentials of Pathophysiology: Concepts of Altered Health States* (3rd edn). Philadelphia: Lippincott Williams & Wilkins.

Porth, C. M. (2009). *Pathophysiology: Concepts of Altered Health States* (8th edn). Philadelphia: Lippincott Williams & Wilkins.

Ruth, D. J. & Barnett, J. (2013). Epilepsy in pregnancy. *Journal of Perinatal & Neonatal Nursing, 27(3)*, 217–224.

CHECK YOUR UNDERSTANDING

Answers to the questions in this chapter can be found in Appendix A at the back of this book.

MULTIPLE CHOICE

Select the best answer to the following.

1. When teaching a group of students about epilepsy, which of the following should the nurse or midwife include?
   a. always characterised by grand mal seizures
   b. only a genetic problem
   c. the most prevalent neurological disorder
   d. the name given to one brain disorder
2. Which of the following would the nurse or midwife be least likely to include as a type of generalised seizure?
   a. petit mal seizures
   b. febrile seizures
   c. grand mal seizures
   d. complex seizures
3. Which instruction would the nurse or midwife encourage a person receiving an antiepileptic drug to do?
   a. Give up their driver's licence.
   b. Wear or carry a MedicAlert identification.
   c. Take antihistamines to help dry up secretions.
   d. Keep the diagnosis a secret to avoid prejudice.
4. Drugs that are commonly used to treat grand mal seizures include:
   a. barbiturates, benzodiazepines and hydantoins.
   b. barbiturates, antihistamines and local anaesthetics.
   c. hydantoins and phenobarbital (phenobarbitone).
   d. benzodiazepines and sodium valproate.
5. The drug of choice for the treatment of absence seizures is:
   a. sodium valproate.
   b. phenytoin.
   c. clonazepam.
   d. ethosuximide.
6. Focal or partial seizures:
   a. start at one point and spread quickly throughout the brain.
   b. are best treated with benzodiazepines.
   c. involve only part of the brain.
   d. are easily diagnosed and recognised.
7. One drug that is used alone in the treatment of partial seizures is:
   a. carbamazepine.
   b. topiramate.
   c. lamotrigine.
   d. gabapentin.
8. Treatment of epilepsy is directed at:
   a. blocking the transmission of nerve impulses into the brain.
   b. stabilising overexcited nerve membranes.
   c. blocking peripheral nerve terminals.
   d. thickening the meninges to dampen brain electrical activity.

MULTIPLE RESPONSE

Select all that apply.

1. A person has been stabilised on phenytoin (*Dilantin*) for several years and has not experienced a grand mal seizure in more than 3 years. The person decides to stop the drug because it no longer seems to be needed. In counselling the person, the nurse or midwife should include which of the following points?
   a. He will always need this drug.
   b. This drug needs to be slowly tapered to avoid potentially serious adverse effects.
   c. He is probably correct and the drug is not needed.
   d. The drug should not be stopped until appropriate blood tests are done.
   e. Stopping the drug suddenly could precipitate seizures because the nerves will be more sensitive.
   f. His insurance company won't cover any problems that might occur if he stops the drug without doctor's approval.
2. The most common adverse effects associated with antiepileptic therapy reflect the depression of the CNS. In assessing a person on antiepileptic therapy, the nurse or midwife would monitor the person for which of the following?
   a. hypertension
   b. insomnia
   c. confusion
   d. GI depression
   e. increased salivation
   f. tachycardia

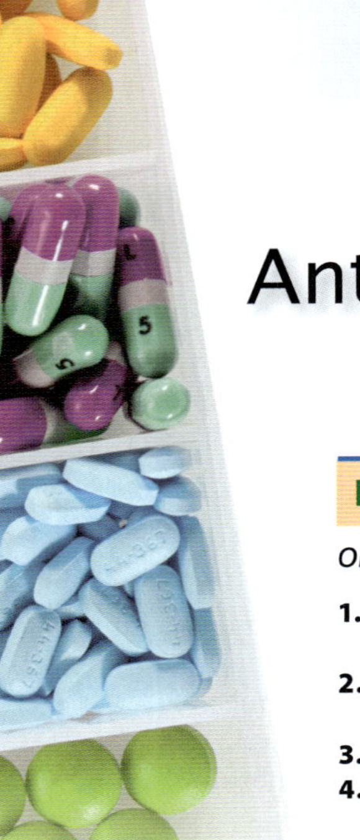

24 Antiparkinsonian agents

Learning objectives

On completing this chapter you should be able to:

1. Describe the current theory of the cause of Parkinson disease and correlate this with the clinical presentation of the disease.
2. Describe the therapeutic actions, indications, pharmacokinetics, contraindications, most common adverse reactions and important drug–drug interactions associated with antiparkinsonian agents.
3. Discuss the use of antiparkinsonian agents across the lifespan.
4. Compare and contrast the prototype drugs for each class of antiparkinsonian agents with the other drugs in that class and with drugs from the other classes that are used to treat the disease.
5. Outline the care considerations and teaching needs for people receiving each class of antiparkinsonian agents.

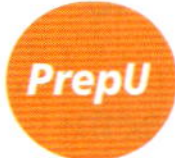

Test your current knowledge of antiparkinsonian agents with a PrepU Practice Quiz!

Glossary of key terms

anticholinergic: drug that opposes the effects of acetylcholine at acetylcholine-receptor sites

bradykinesia: difficulty in performing intentional movements and extreme slowness and sluggishness; characteristic of Parkinson disease

corpus striatum: part of the brain that reacts with the substantia nigra to maintain a balance of suppression and stimulation

dopaminergic: drug that increases the effects of dopamine at receptor sites

Parkinson disease: debilitating disease, characterised by progressive loss of coordination and function, which results from the degeneration of dopamine-producing cells in the substantia nigra

parkinsonism: Parkinson disease–like extrapyramidal symptoms that are adverse effects associated with particular drugs or brain injuries

substantia nigra: a part of the brain rich in dopamine and dopamine receptors; site of degenerating neurons in Parkinson disease

DOPAMINERGIC AGENTS
- amantadine
- apomorphine
- bromocriptine
- carbidopa–levodopa
- (P) levodopa
- levodopa–benserazide
- levodopa–carbidopa–entacapone
- pramipexole
- ropinirole
- rotigotine

ANTICHOLINERGIC AGENTS
- trihexyphenidyl (benzhexol)
- benzatropine
- (P) biperiden

ADJUNCTIVE AGENTS
- entacapone
- rasagiline
- safinamide
- selegiline
- tolcapone

In the 1990s, several prominent figures – including former heavyweight boxing champion Muhammad Ali and actor Michael J. Fox – revealed that they had **Parkinson disease**, a progressive, chronic neurological disorder. In general, Parkinson disease may develop in people of any age, but it usually affects those who are past middle age and entering their 60s or even later years. Therefore, the occurrence of Parkinson disease in these well-known individuals who were relatively young at the time of diagnosis is that much more interesting. The cause of the condition is not known.

At this time, there is no cure for Parkinson disease. Therapy is aimed at management of signs and symptoms to provide optimal functioning for as long as possible.

PARKINSON DISEASE AND PARKINSONISM

Lack of coordination is characteristic of Parkinson disease. Rhythmic tremors develop, insidiously at first. In some muscle groups, these tremors lead to rigidity, and in others weakness. Affected people may have trouble maintaining position or posture, and they may develop the condition known as **bradykinesia**, marked by difficulties in performing intentional movements and extreme slowness or sluggishness.

As Parkinson disease progresses, walking becomes a problem; a shuffling gait is a hallmark of the condition. In addition, people may drool, and their speech may be slow and slurred. As the cranial nerves are affected, they may develop a mask-like expression. Parkinson disease does not affect the higher levels of the cerebral cortex, so a very alert and intelligent person may be trapped in a progressively degenerating body.

Parkinsonism is a term used to describe the Parkinson disease–like extrapyramidal symptoms that are adverse effects associated with particular drugs or brain injuries. People typically exhibit tremors and bradykinesia.

Pathophysiology

Although the cause of Parkinson disease is not known, it is known that the signs and symptoms of the disease relate to damaged neurons in the basal ganglia of the brain. Theories about the cause of the degeneration of these neurons range from viral infection, blows to the head, brain infection, atherosclerosis and exposure to certain drugs and environmental factors.

Even though the actual cause is not known, the mechanism that causes the signs and symptoms of Parkinson disease is understood. In a part of the brain called the **substantia nigra**, a dopamine-rich area, nerve cell bodies begin to degenerate. This process results in a reduction of the number of impulses sent to the **corpus striatum** in the basal ganglia. This area of the brain, in conjunction with the substantia nigra, helps to maintain muscle tone not related to any particular movement. The corpus striatum is connected to the substantia nigra by a series of neurons that use gamma-aminobutyric acid (GABA), an inhibitory neurotransmitter. The substantia nigra sends nerve impulses back into the corpus stratum using the inhibitory neurotransmitter dopamine. The two areas then mutually inhibit activity in a balanced manner.

Higher neurons originating in the cerebral cortex secrete acetylcholine (an excitatory neurotransmitter) in the area of the corpus striatum to coordinate intentional movements of the body. When dopamine decreases in the area, a chemical imbalance occurs that allows the cholinergic or excitatory cells to dominate. This affects the functioning of the basal ganglia and the cortical and cerebellar components of the extrapyramidal motor system. The extrapyramidal system is one that provides coordination for unconscious muscle movements, including those that control position, posture and movement. The result of this imbalance in the motor system is apparent as the manifestations of Parkinson disease (Figure 24.1).

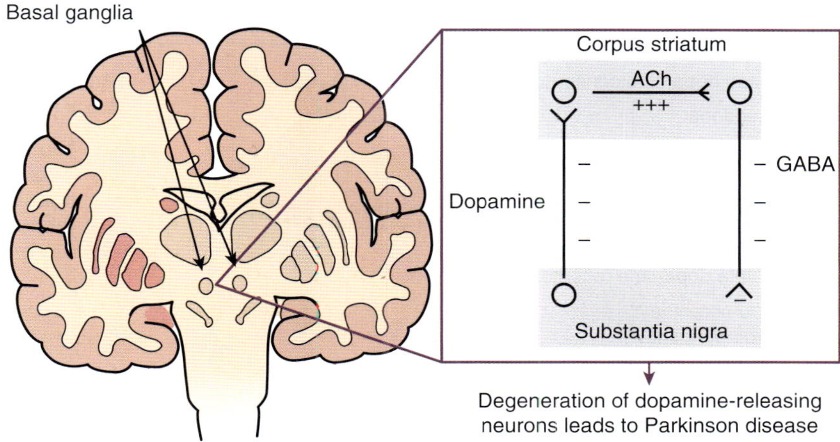

FIGURE 24.1 Schematic representation of the degeneration of neurons that leads to Parkinson disease. Cells in the corpus striatum send impulses to the substantia nigra using gamma-aminobutyric acid (GABA) to inhibit activity. In turn, the substantia nigra sends impulses to the corpus striatum, using dopamine, to inhibit activity. Cortical areas use acetylcholine (ACh) to stimulate intentional movements.

Treatment

At this time, there is no treatment that arrests the neuron degeneration of Parkinson disease and the eventual decline in the person's function. Surgical procedures involving the basal ganglia have been tried with varying success at prolonging the degeneration caused by this disease. Drug therapy remains the primary treatment.

Therapy is aimed at restoring the balance between the declining levels of dopamine, which has an inhibitory effect on the neurons in the basal ganglia, and the now-dominant cholinergic neurons, which are excitatory. This may help to reduce the signs and symptoms of parkinsonism and restore normal function for a time (Figure 24.2).

Total management of care in individuals with Parkinson disease presents a challenge. People should be encouraged to be as active as possible, to perform exercises to prevent the development of skeletal deformities and to attend to their care as long as they can. Both the person and their family need instruction about following drug protocols and monitoring adverse effects, as well as encouragement and support for coping with the progressive nature of the disease (Box 24.1). Because of the degenerative effects of this disease, individuals may experience episodes of depression or emotional upset. Psychological support, as well as physical support, is a crucial aspect of care.

KEY POINTS

- Parkinson disease is a progressive nervous system disease characterised by tremors, changes in posture and gait and a mask-like facial expression.
- The loss of dopamine-secreting cells results in a loss of the inhibitory dopamine effect and is thought to be responsible for Parkinson disease.

DOPAMINERGIC AGENTS

Dopaminergics – drugs that increase the effects of dopamine at receptor sites – have been proven to be even more effective than anticholinergics in the treatment of parkinsonism (see Table 24.1). Dopaminergic agents include amantadine (*Symmetrel*), apomorphine (*Apomine*), bromocriptine (*Parlodel*), carbidopa–levodopa (*Sinemet*), levodopa–benserazide (*Madopar*), levodopa–carbidopa–entacapone (*Stalevo*), pramipexole (*Sifrol*), ropinirole (*Appese*, *Repreve*) and rotigotine (*Neupro*).

Therapeutic actions and indications

Dopamine does not cross the blood–brain barrier. Therefore, other drugs that act like dopamine or increase dopamine concentrations indirectly must be used to increase dopamine levels in the substantia nigra or to directly stimulate the dopamine receptors in that area. This action helps to restore the balance between the inhibitory and stimulating neurons. Dopaminergic agents are effective as long as enough intact neurons remain in the substantia nigra to respond to increased levels of dopamine. After the neural degeneration has progressed beyond a certain point, these agents are no longer effective.

The dopaminergics are indicated for the relief of the signs and symptoms of idiopathic Parkinson disease

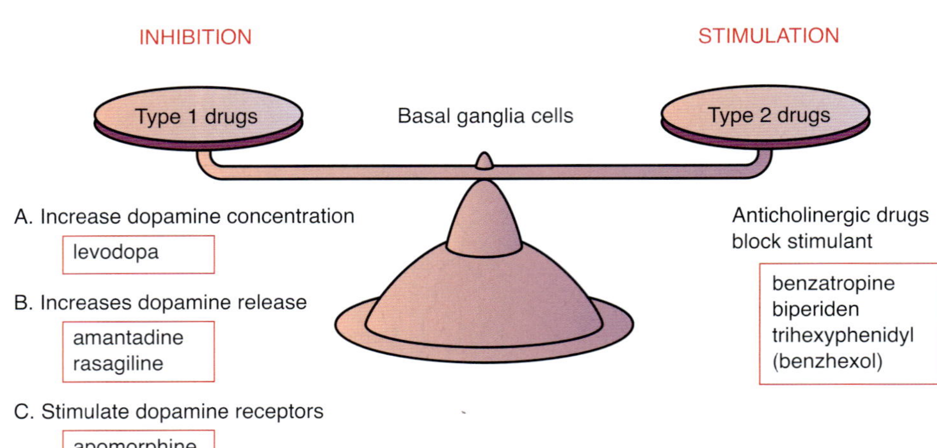

FIGURE 24.2 Drug therapy in treating Parkinson disease is aimed at achieving a balance between the stimulating cholinergic effects and the inhibitory effects of dopamine in the basal ganglia. Type 1 drugs affect dopamine and are inhibitory. Type 2 drugs block cholinergic effects, preventing stimulation.

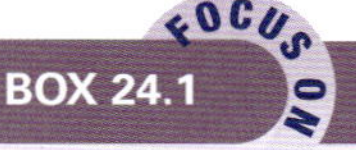

BOX 24.1 **Drug therapy across the lifespan**

Antiparkinsonian agents

CHILDREN

The safety and effectiveness of most of these drugs has not been established in children. The incidence of Parkinson disease in children is very small. Children do, however, experience parkinsonian symptoms as a result of drug effects.

ADULTS

The eventual dependence and lack of control that accompany Parkinson disease are devastating to all people and their families but may be particularly overwhelming to individuals in their prime of life who value high degrees of autonomy, self-determination and independence. Although these characteristics are not associated with any particular ethnic group, they are valued more highly among certain cultures than others. It is important for the health care professional to assess all families with sensitivity to determine what convictions they hold and plan care accordingly.

Adults diagnosed with Parkinson disease require extensive teaching, support and help coping with the disease as well as with the effects of the drugs.

With the increasing interest in herbal and alternative therapies, it is important to stress the need to inform the health care provider about any other treatment being used. Vitamin B6 can pose a serious problem for people who are taking some of these drugs.

PREGNANCY AND BREASTFEEDING

Women of childbearing age should be advised to use contraception when they are on these drugs. If a pregnancy does occur, or is desired, they need counselling about the potential for adverse effects. Women who are breastfeeding should be encouraged to find another method of feeding the baby because of the potential for adverse drug effects on the baby.

OLDER ADULTS

Although Parkinson disease may affect individuals of any age, gender or nationality, the frequency of the disease increases with age. This debilitating condition, which affects more men than women, may be one of many chronic problems associated with ageing.

The drugs that are used to manage Parkinson disease are associated with more adverse effects in older people with long-term problems. Both anticholinergic and dopaminergic drugs aggravate glaucoma, benign prostatic hypertrophy, constipation, cardiac problems and chronic obstructive pulmonary diseases. Special precautions and frequent follow-up visits are necessary for older people with Parkinson disease, and their drug dosages may need to be adjusted frequently to avoid serious problems. In many cases, other agents are given to counteract the effects of these drugs, and people then have complicated drug regimens with many associated adverse effects and problems. Consequently, it is essential for these people to have extensive written drug-teaching protocols.

(see Table 24.1 for usual indications for each of these agents). Levodopa is the mainstay of treatment for Parkinson disease. This precursor of dopamine crosses the blood–brain barrier and is converted into dopamine. In this way, it acts like a replacement therapy. Although levodopa is almost always given in combination form with carbidopa as a fixed-dose combination drug (*Sinemet*), other drugs besides carbidopa may be used (see Adjunctive agents). When used with carbidopa, the enzyme dopa decarboxylase is inhibited in the periphery, diminishing the metabolism of levodopa in the gastrointestinal (GI) tract and in peripheral tissues, thereby leading to higher levels crossing the blood–brain barrier. Because the carbidopa decreases the amount of levodopa needed to reach a therapeutic level in the brain, the dose of levodopa can be decreased, which reduces the incidence of adverse side effects.

Amantadine is an antiviral drug that also seems to increase the release of dopamine, being effective as long as there is a possibility of more dopamine release.

Apomorphine is a newer adjunctive therapy for Parkinson disease that directly binds with postsynaptic dopamine receptors. Similar to apomorphine, bromocriptine and pramipexole act as direct dopamine agonists on dopamine-receptor sites in the substantia nigra. Because bromocriptine does not depend on cells in the area to biotransform it or to increase the release of already produced dopamine, it may be effective longer than levodopa or amantadine.

Ropinirole and rotigotine directly stimulate dopamine receptors. They are also used to treat restless legs syndrome.

Pharmacokinetics

The dopaminergics are usually given orally and are generally well absorbed from the GI tract and widely distributed in the body. Apomorphine, however, must be given subcutaneously. The dopaminergics are metabolised in the liver and peripheral cells and excreted in the urine. They cross the placenta and enter breast milk.

Contraindications and cautions

The dopaminergics are contraindicated in the presence of any known allergy to the drug or drug components *to prevent hypersensitivity reactions*, and in angle-closure glaucoma, *which could be exacerbated by these drugs*. Dopaminergics enter breast milk and should not be used during breastfeeding because of the potential for adverse effects in the baby. In addition, levodopa is contraindicated in people with history or presence of suspicious skin lesions *because this drug has been associated with the development of melanoma*.

TABLE 24.1 DRUGS IN FOCUS **Dopaminergic agents**

Drug name	Dosage/route	Usual indications
amantadine (*Symmetrel*)	100 mg PO bd; doses > 200 mg/day may provide some additional relief but may also be associated with increasing toxicity. Maximum 400 mg/day	Antiviral; treatment of idiopathic and drug-induced parkinsonism in adults
apomorphine (*Apomine*)	After determining threshold dose, administer continuous SC infusion of apomorphine by portable syringe driver. Dose should be titrated to the patient's response. Infusion rates can be started at 1 mg/hour then increased as necessary. Maximum daily dose should in general not exceed 200 mg/day. Infusions should be run for waking hours only	Intermittent treatment of hypomobility 'off' episodes of advanced Parkinson disease
bromocriptine (*Parlodel*)	1.25 mg PO bd; titrate up to 5–40 mg/day in divided doses	Treatment of idiopathic Parkinson disease; may be beneficial in later stages when response to levodopa decreases
carbidopa–levodopa (*Sinemet*)	1 tablet Sinemet 25/100 (25 mg carbidopa with 100 mg levodopa) PO tds up to a maximum of 8 tablets a day. When more levodopa is required, Sinemet 25/250 should be substituted for Sinemet 25/100. If necessary, the dosage of Sinemet 25/250 may be increased by 1 tablet every day or every other day to a maximum of 8 tablets a day.	Treatment of idiopathic Parkinson disease
levodopa–benserazide (*Madopar*)	125 mg PO tds increased to 500–1000 mg/day in 3–4 divided doses	Treatment of idiopathic Parkinson disease
levodopa–carbidopa–entacapone (Stalevo)	Individualised up to maximum levodopa 1500 mg/day	Treatment of idiopathic Parkinson disease with fluctuating motor status
pramipexole (*Sifrol*)	0.125 mg PO tds, titrate up to 1.5 mg PO tds	Treatment of idiopathic Parkinson disease
ropinirole (*Appese, Repreve*)	0.25 mg PO; titrate up to maximum dose of 4 mg/day	Treatment of idiopathic Parkinson disease in early stages and in later stages when combined with levodopa; treatment of restless legs syndrome
rotigotine (*Neupro*)	Patch applied once daily	Treatment of idiopathic Parkinson disease

Administer dopaminergic agents cautiously with people who have *any condition that could be exacerbated by dopamine-receptor stimulation*, such as cardiovascular disease, including myocardial infarction, arrhythmias and hypertension; bronchial asthma; history of peptic ulcers; urinary tract obstruction; and psychiatric disorders. Care is also necessary during pregnancy *because these drugs cross the placenta and could adversely affect the fetus*, and in people with renal and hepatic disease, *which could interfere with the metabolism and excretion of the drug.* Closely monitor cardiac status in people receiving apomorphine because of the associated risk for hypotension and prolonged QT interval.

Adverse effects

The adverse effects associated with the dopaminergics usually result from stimulation of dopamine receptors. Central nervous system (CNS) effects may include anxiety, nervousness, headache, malaise, fatigue, confusion, mental changes, blurred vision, muscle twitching and ataxia. Peripheral effects may include anorexia, nausea, vomiting, dysphagia, and constipation or diarrhoea; cardiac arrhythmias, hypotension and palpitations; bizarre breathing patterns; urinary retention; and flushing, increased sweating and hot flushes. Bone marrow depression and hepatic dysfunction have also been reported.

Clinically important drug–drug interactions

If dopaminergics are combined with monoamine oxidase (MAO) inhibitors, therapeutic effects increase and a risk of hypertensive crisis exists. The MAO inhibitor should be stopped 14 days before beginning therapy with a dopaminergic.

The combination of levodopa with vitamin B6 or with phenytoin may lead to decreased efficacy of the levodopa (see Critical thinking scenario). Reduced effectiveness of both drugs may also result if dopaminergics are combined with dopamine antagonists. In addition, people who take dopaminergics should be cautioned to avoid over-the-counter vitamins; if such medications are used, the person should be monitored closely because a decrease in dopaminergic effectiveness can result.

Prototype summary: levodopa

Indications: treatment of parkinsonism and Parkinson disease.

Actions: precursor of dopamine, which is deficient in parkinsonism; crosses the blood–brain barrier, where it is converted to dopamine and acts as a replacement neurotransmitter; effective for 2–5 years in relieving the symptoms of Parkinson disease.

Pharmacokinetics:

Route	Onset	Peak	Duration
Oral	Varies	0.5–2 hours	5 hours

$T_{1/2}$: 1–3 hours; metabolised in the liver, excreted in the urine.

Adverse effects: adventitious movements, ataxia, increased hand tremor, dizziness, numbness, weakness, agitation, anxiety, anorexia, nausea, dry mouth, dysphagia, urinary retention, flushing, cardiac irregularities.

Care considerations for people receiving dopaminergic agents

Assessment: history and examination

- Assess for contraindications or cautions: any known allergies to these drugs to *avoid hypersensitivity reactions*; GI depression or obstruction, urinary hesitancy or obstruction, benign prostatic hypertrophy or glaucoma, *which may be exacerbated by these drugs*; cardiac arrhythmias, hypertension or respiratory disease, *which may be exacerbated by dopamine-receptor stimulation*; current status of pregnancy or breastfeeding, *which are cautions or contraindications to use of the drug*; and renal or hepatic dysfunction, *which could interfere with the drug's excretion or metabolism*.
- Perform a physical assessment *to determine baseline status before beginning therapy, to determine the effectiveness of drug therapy and to monitor for any potential adverse effects*.
- Inspect the skin for evidence of skin lesions or history of melanoma if the person is to receive levodopa, *which could cause or exacerbate melanoma*.
- Assess for a history of prolonged QT interval and obtain an electrocardiogram if apomorphine is to be administered *to avoid further prolonged QT interval and serious arrhythmias*.
- Assess level of orientation and neurological status, including affect, reflexes, bilateral grip strength, gait, tremors and spasticity, *to evaluate any CNS effects*.
- Auscultate lungs and assess respiratory status *to evaluate for changes that could be exacerbated by the drug's effect*.
- Monitor pulse, blood pressure and cardiac output *to evaluate for possible adverse effects*.
- Auscultate bowel sounds to evaluate GI motility *to assess for adverse effects*.
- Assess urine output and palpate bladder *to determine adequate bladder and renal function*.
- Monitor the results of laboratory tests, such as liver and renal function studies, *to determine need for possible dose adjustment*, and full blood count (FBC) with differential *to evaluate for possible bone marrow suppression*.

Implementation with rationale

- Arrange to decrease the dose of the drug if therapy has been interrupted for any reason *to prevent systemic dopaminergic effects*.
- Evaluate disease progress and signs and symptoms periodically and record *for reference of disease progress and drug response*.
- Give the drug with meals *to alleviate GI irritation if GI upset is a problem*.
- Monitor bowel function and institute a bowel program *if constipation is severe*.
- Ensure that the person voids before taking the drug *if urinary retention is a problem*.
- Monitor urinary output, palpate bladder and check for residual urine *if urinary retention becomes a problem*.
- Establish safety precautions if CNS or vision changes occur *to prevent injury*.
- Monitor hepatic, renal and haematological tests periodically during therapy *to detect early signs of dysfunction and consider re-evaluation of drug therapy*.
- Provide support services and comfort measures as needed *to improve compliance*.
- Provide thorough teaching about topics such as the drug name and prescribed dose, measures to help avoid adverse effects, warning signs that may indicate problems, and the need for periodic monitoring and evaluation *to enhance knowledge about drug therapy and to promote compliance*.

- Offer support and encouragement *to help the person cope with the disease and drug regimen.*

Evaluation

- Monitor response to the drug (improvement in signs and symptoms of Parkinson disease).
- Monitor for adverse effects (CNS changes, urinary retention, GI depression, tachycardia, increased sweating, flushing).
- Evaluate the effectiveness of the teaching plan (person can give the drug name and dosage, name possible adverse effects to watch for and specific measures to prevent them and discuss the importance of continued follow-up).
- Monitor the effectiveness of support measures and compliance with the regimen.

KEY POINTS

- Dopaminergic drugs are used to increase the effects of dopamine at receptor sites, restoring the balance of neurotransmitters in the basal ganglia.
- The adverse effects associated with these drugs are related to the systemic effects of dopamine, increased heart rate, increased blood pressure, decreased GI activity and urinary retention.
- Levodopa is the standard dopaminergic used to treat parkinsonism and Parkinson disease. Several other dopaminergics are now used as adjuncts to levodopa to increase the dopamine effects as long as possible.

ANTICHOLINERGIC AGENTS

Anticholinergics (Table 24.2) are drugs that oppose the effects of acetylcholine at receptor sites in the substantia nigra and the corpus striatum, thus helping to restore

CRITICAL THINKING SCENARIO

Effects of vitamin B6 intake on levodopa levels

THE SITUATION

S.S., a 58-year-old man with well-controlled Parkinson disease, presents with severe nausea, anorexia, fainting spells and heart palpitation. He has been maintained on levodopa for the Parkinson disease and he claims to have followed his drug regimen religiously.

According to S.S. the only change in his lifestyle has been the addition of several health foods and vitamins. His daughter, who recently returned from her first year at university, has begun a new health regimen, including natural foods and plenty of supplemental vitamins. She was so enthusiastic about her new approach that everyone in the family agreed to give this diet a try.

CRITICAL THINKING

Based on S.S.'s signs and symptoms, what has probably occurred?

In Parkinson disease, is it possible to differentiate a deterioration of illness from a toxic reaction to a drug?

What care implications should be considered when teaching S.S. and his family about the effects of vitamin B6 on levodopa levels?

In what ways can the daughter cope with her role in this crisis?

Develop a new care plan for S.S. that involves all family members and that includes drug teaching.

DISCUSSION

The presenting symptoms reflect an increase in Parkinson's symptoms, as well as an increase in peripheral dopamine reactions (eg, palpitations, fainting, anorexia, nausea). It is necessary to determine whether the problem involves a further degeneration in the neurons in the substantia nigra or the particular medication that S.S. has been taking. In many people, responsiveness to levodopa is lost as neural degeneration continues.

The explanation of the new lifestyle – full of grains, natural foods and vitamins – alerts the nurse to the possibility of excessive vitamin B6 intake. In reviewing the vitamin bottles and some of the food packages supplied by S.S., it seems that too much vitamin B6, which speeds the conversion of levodopa to dopamine before it can cross the blood–brain barrier, might be the reason the person's symptoms recurred.

The status of S.S.'s Parkinson disease should be evaluated, and then he can be restarted on levodopa. The smallest dose possible should be used initially, with gradual increases to achieve the maximum benefit with the fewest side effects. It would be wise to consider combining the drug with carbidopa to prevent some of S.S.'s recent problems.

In addition, S.S. should receive thorough drug teaching in written form for future reference. The need to avoid vitamin B6 should be emphasised. The entire family should be involved in an explanation of what happened and how this situation can be avoided in the future. Because the daughter may feel guilty about her role, she should have the opportunity to discuss her feelings and explore the positive impact of healthy food on nutrition and quality of life. This situation can serve as a good teaching example for staff, as well as present them with an opportunity to review drug therapy in Parkinson disease and the risks and benefits of more extreme diets.

CARE GUIDE FOR S.S.: LEVODOPA

Assessment: history and examination

Allergies to levodopa; chronic obstructive pulmonary disease (COPD); dysrhythmias, hypotension, hepatic or renal dysfunction; psychoses; peptic ulcer; glaucoma

Concurrent use of MAO inhibitors, phenytoin, pyridoxine, papaverine or tricyclic antidepressants (TCAs)

Focus physical examination on:

CV: blood pressure, pulse rate, peripheral perfusion, electrocardiogram results

CNS: orientation, affect, reflexes, grip strength

Renal: output, bladder palpation

GI: abdominal examination, bowel sounds

Respiratory: respiration, adventitious sounds

Laboratory tests: renal and liver function tests, FBC

Implementation

Ensure safe and appropriate administration of drug.

Provide comfort and safety: slow positioning changes; assess orientation, provide pain medication as needed; give drug with food; administer with carbidopa; have person void before each dose.

Provide support and reassurance to deal with disease and drug effects.

Instruct the person regarding drug dose, effects and adverse symptoms to report.

Evaluation

Evaluate drug effects: relief of signs and symptoms of Parkinson disease.

Monitor for adverse effects: CNS effects; renal changes, urinary retention; GI effects (constipation); increased sweating or flushing.

Monitor for drug–drug interactions: hypertensive crisis with MAO inhibitors, decreased effects with vitamin B6 or phenytoin.

Evaluate the effectiveness of the teaching program.

Evaluate the effectiveness of comfort and safety measures.

TEACHING FOR S.S.

- The drug that has been prescribed is called levodopa. It increases the levels of dopamine in the central areas of the brain and helps to reduce the signs and symptoms of Parkinson disease.
- Often, this drug is combined with another drug, which allows the correct levels of levodopa to reach the brain.
- People who take this drug must have their individual dose needs adjusted over time.
- Common effects of this drug include:
  - *Fatigue, weakness and drowsiness*: try to space activities evenly through the day; allow rest periods to avoid these side effects. Take safety precautions and avoid driving or operating dangerous machinery if these conditions occur.
  - *Dizziness, fainting*: change position slowly to avoid dizzy spells.
  - *Increased sweating, darkened urine*: this is a normal reaction. Avoid very hot environments.
  - *Headaches, difficulty sleeping*: these usually pass as the body adjusts to the drug. If they become too uncomfortable and persist, consult with your health care provider.
- Report any of the following to your health care provider: *uncontrolled movements of any body part, chest pain or palpitations, depression or mood changes, difficulty in voiding, or severe or persistent nausea and vomiting.*
- Be aware that vitamin B6 interferes with the effects of levodopa. If you feel that you need a vitamin product, consult with your health care provider about using an agent that does not contain vitamin B6.
- Avoid eating large quantities of health foods that contain vitamin B6, such as grains and brans. If you are taking a carbidopa–levodopa combination, these precautions are not as important.
- Tell any doctor, nurse or other health care provider involved in your care that you are taking this drug.
- Keep this drug and all medications out of the reach of children.
- Do not overexert yourself when you begin to feel better. Pace yourself.
- Take this drug exactly as directed, and schedule regular medical checkups to evaluate its effects.

chemical balance in the area. Anticholinergics used to treat Parkinson disease include benzatropine (*Benztrop*), biperiden (*Akineton*) (not available in New Zealand) and trihexyphenidyl (benzhexol) (*Artane*) (not available in New Zealand).

Therapeutic actions and indications

The anticholinergics used to treat parkinsonism are synthetic drugs that have been developed to have a greater affinity for cholinergic receptor sites in the CNS than for those in the peripheral nervous system. However, they still block, to some extent, the cholinergic receptors that are responsible for stimulation of the parasympathetic nervous system's postganglionic effectors. This blockage is associated with the adverse effects (see Chapter 33), including slowed motility and secretions, with dry mouth and constipation, urinary retention, blurred vision and dilated pupils.

TABLE 24.2 DRUGS IN FOCUS Anticholinergic agents

Drug name	Dosage/route	Usual indications
trihexyphenidyl (benzhexol) (*Artane*)	1–10 mg PO daily in 3 divided doses before meals	Adjunctive treatment of parkinsonism and drug-induced extrapyramidal reactions
benzatropine (*Benztrop*)	0.5–6 mg/day PO may be needed; 1–2 mg IM or IV; reduce dose in older people	Adjunctive treatment of parkinsonism, and drug-induced parkinsonism resulting from drug effects
(P) biperiden (*Akineton*)	Initially 1 mg bd, then increase to 1–4 mg PO tds or qid	Adjunctive treatment of parkinsonism, and drug-induced parkinsonism resulting from drug effects

Anticholinergic drugs are indicated for the treatment of parkinsonism, whether idiopathic, atherosclerotic or postencephalitic, and for the relief of symptoms of extrapyramidal disorders associated with the use of some drugs, including phenothiazines. Although these drugs are not as effective as levodopa in the treatment of advancing cases of the disease, they may be useful as adjunctive therapy and for people who no longer respond to levodopa. See Table 24.2 for usual indications.

Pharmacokinetics

The anticholinergic drugs are variably absorbed from the GI tract, reaching peak levels in 1–4 hours. They are metabolised in the liver and excreted by cellular pathways. All of them cross the placenta and enter breast milk (see Contraindications and cautions). Benzatropine and biperiden are available in oral and intramuscular/intravenous forms. Trihexyphenidyl (benzhexol) is only available in an oral form.

Contraindications and cautions

Anticholinergics are contraindicated in the presence of allergy to any of these agents *to avoid hypersensitivity reactions.* In addition, they are contraindicated in narrow-angle glaucoma, GI obstruction, genitourinary (GU) obstruction and prostatic hypertrophy, *all of which could be exacerbated by the peripheral anticholinergic effects of these drugs*, and in myasthenia gravis, *which could be exacerbated by the blocking of acetylcholine-receptor sites at neuromuscular synapses.* The safety and efficacy for use in children have not been established.

Administer these agents cautiously in the following conditions: tachycardia and other dysrhythmias and hypertension or hypotension *because the blocking of the parasympathetic system may cause a dominance of sympathetic stimulatory activity*, and hepatic dysfunction, *which could interfere with the metabolism of the drugs and lead to toxic levels.* They should be used during pregnancy and breastfeeding only if the benefit to the mother clearly outweighs the potential risk to the fetus or neonate. In addition, use caution in individuals who work in hot environments *because reflex sweating may be blocked, placing the individuals at risk for heat prostration.*

Adverse effects

The use of anticholinergics for Parkinson disease and parkinsonism is associated with CNS effects that relate to the blocking of central acetylcholine receptors, such as disorientation, confusion and memory loss. Agitation, nervousness, delirium, dizziness, light-headedness and weakness may also occur.

Anticipated peripheral anticholinergic effects include dry mouth, nausea, vomiting, paralytic ileus and constipation related to decreased GI secretions and motility. In addition, other adverse effects may occur, including tachycardia, palpitations and hypotension related to the blocking of the suppressive cardiac effects of

(P) Prototype summary: biperiden

Indications: adjunctive therapy for Parkinson disease; relief of symptoms of extrapyramidal disorders (parkinsonism).

Actions: acts as an anticholinergic, principally in the CNS, returning balance to the basal ganglia and reducing the severity of rigidity, akinesia and tremors; peripheral anticholinergic effects help to reduce drooling and other secondary effects of parkinsonism.

Pharmacokinetics:

Route	Onset	Peak	Duration
Oral	1 hours	1–1.5 hours	6–12 hours
IM	15 min	Unknown	Unknown

$T_{1/2}$: 18.4–24.3 hours; metabolised in the liver.

Adverse effects: disorientation, confusion, memory loss, nervousness, light-headedness, dizziness, depression, blurred vision, mydriasis, dry mouth, constipation, urinary retention, urinary hesitation, flushing, decreased sweating.

the parasympathetic nervous system; urinary retention and hesitancy related to a blocking of bladder muscle activity and sphincter relaxation; blurred vision and photophobia related to pupil dilation and blocking of lens accommodation; and flushing and reduced sweating related to a blocking of the cholinergic sites that stimulate sweating and blood vessel dilation in the skin.

Clinically important drug–drug interactions

When these anticholinergic drugs are used with other drugs that have anticholinergic properties, including the tricyclic antidepressants and the phenothiazines, there is a risk of potentially fatal paralytic ileus and an increased risk of toxic psychoses. If such combinations must be given, monitor people closely and implement supportive measures. Dose adjustments are often necessary. In addition, when antipsychotic drugs are combined with anticholinergics, a risk for decreased antipsychotic therapeutic effectiveness may occur, possibly as a result of a central antagonism of the two agents.

Care considerations for people receiving anticholinergic agents

Assessment: history and examination

- Assess for contraindications or cautions: any known allergies to these drugs *to avoid hypersensitivity reactions*; GI depression or obstruction, urinary hesitancy or obstruction, benign prostatic hypertrophy or glaucoma, *which may be exacerbated by the peripheral anticholinergic effect of the drug*; cardiac arrhythmias, hypertension or hypotension, *which may be increased due to the dominance of sympathetic stimulatory activity due to blockage of parasympathetic activity*; myasthenia gravis, *which may be exacerbated by blockage of acetylcholine receptors*; current status related to pregnancy or breastfeeding *due to risk of fetal or infant adverse effects*; hepatic dysfunction, *which could interfere with drug metabolism and increase risk for toxicity*; and exposure to a hot environment, *which may block the individual's reflex sweating.*
- Perform a physical assessment *to determine baseline data for determining the effectiveness of the drug and the occurrence of adverse effects associated with drug therapy.*
- Assess level of orientation and neurological status, including affect, reflexes, bilateral grip strength, gait, tremors and spasticity, *to evaluate any CNS effects.*
- Monitor pulse, blood pressure and cardiac output *to evaluate for possible adverse effects related to blocking of suppressive action on the heart.*
- Auscultate bowel sounds *to evaluate GI motility and detect possible indications of paralytic ileus.*
- Assess urine output and palpate bladder *to determine adequate renal and bladder function.*
- Monitor the results of laboratory tests such as renal and liver function tests *to determine the need for possible dose adjustment and identify potential toxic effects.*

Implementation with rationale

- Arrange to decrease dose or discontinue the drug *if dry mouth becomes so severe that swallowing becomes difficult.* Provide sugarless lozenges to suck and frequent mouth care to help with this problem.
- Give drug with caution and arrange for a decrease in dose in hot weather or with exposure to hot environments *because people are at increased risk for heat prostration because of decreased ability to sweat.*
- Give drug with meals if GI upset is a problem, before meals if dry mouth is a problem and after meals if drooling occurs and the drug causes nausea *to facilitate compliance with drug therapy.*
- Monitor bowel function and institute a bowel program *if constipation is severe.*
- Ensure that the person voids before taking the drug; monitor urinary output and palpate for bladder distension and residual urine *if urinary retention is a problem.*
- Establish safety precautions if CNS or vision changes occur *to prevent injury.*
- Provide thorough teaching about topics such as the drug name and prescribed dose, measures to help avoid adverse effects, warning signs that may indicate problems and the need for periodic monitoring and evaluation *to enhance knowledge about drug therapy and to promote compliance.*
- Offer support and encouragement *to help the person cope with the progressive nature of the disease and long-term drug regimen.*

Evaluation

- Monitor response to the drug (improvement in signs and symptoms of Parkinson disease or parkinsonism).
- Monitor for adverse effects (CNS changes, urinary retention, GI slowing, tachycardia, decreased sweating, flushing).
- Evaluate the effectiveness of the teaching plan (person can give the drug name and dosage, name possible adverse effects to watch for and

specific measures to prevent them and discuss the importance of continued follow-up).

- Monitor the effectiveness of support measures and compliance with the regimen.

KEY POINTS

- Anticholinergic agents are used to suppress the stimulatory effects of acetylcholine in the substantia nigra, bringing balance into the control of movement.
- The adverse effects associated with the anticholinergic drugs are related to blocking of the acetylcholine in the parasympathetic nervous system – dry mouth, constipation, urinary retention, increased heart rate, decreased sweating.

ADJUNCTIVE AGENTS

Adjunctive agents used to improve response to traditional therapy include entacapone (*Comtan*), rasagiline (*Azilect*) (not available in New Zealand), tolcapone (*Tasmar*) (not available in Australia) and selegiline (*Eldepryl, Selgene*). See Table 24.3 for additional information.

Entacapone is used with carbidopa–levodopa to increase the plasma concentration and duration of action of levodopa. It does this by inhibiting catechol-O-methyl transferase (COMT), a naturally occurring enzyme that eliminates catecholamines, including dopamine. It is given with the carbidopa–levodopa at a dose of 200 mg PO, with a maximum of eight doses a day. It is readily absorbed from the GI tract, metabolised in the liver and excreted in urine and faeces. Women of childbearing age should be encouraged to use barrier contraceptives while taking this drug, which crosses the placenta and could have adverse effects on the fetus.

Rasagiline is an irreversible MAO type B selective inhibitor and its mechanism of action in Parkinson disease is not understood. It is believed that MAO inhibition leads to elevated dopamine levels and promotes increased extracellular dopamine levels in the striatum. It is rapidly absorbed with peak levels achieved in approximately half an hour. It undergoes hepatic metabolism after GI absorption and is excreted in the urine and faeces. Being a MAO inhibitor, there is a risk of development of hypertensive crisis. When combined with antidepressant treatment, there is an increased risk of serotonin syndrome. As prolactin secretion is blocked, rasagiline may inhibit breastfeeding.

Tolcapone works in a similar way with carbidopa–levodopa to further increase plasma levels of levodopa. Tolcapone also blocks the enzyme COMT, which is responsible for the breakdown of dopamine. Because this drug has been associated with fulminant and potentially fatal liver damage, it is contraindicated in the presence of liver disease. Tolcapone is reserved for use in later stages of Parkinson disease, when carbidopa–levodopa is losing its effectiveness. It undergoes hepatic metabolism after GI absorption and is excreted in the urine and faeces. It is given in doses of 100 or 200 mg PO three times a day, up to a maximum of 600 mg/day. Women of childbearing age should be encouraged to use barrier contraceptives while taking this drug, which crosses the placenta and could have adverse effects on the fetus.

Selegiline is used with carbidopa–levodopa after people have shown signs of deteriorating response to this treatment. Its mechanism of action is not understood. It does irreversibly inhibit MAO, which has an important role in the breakdown of catecholamines, including dopamine. The maximum daily dose of the drug is 10 mg, and the dose of levodopa needs to be reduced when this drug is started. It is well absorbed from the GI tract, extensively metabolised in the liver and excreted in urine. It is not known whether this drug crosses the placenta, but it should be used in pregnancy only if the benefits to the mother clearly outweigh any potential risks to the fetus.

TABLE 24.3 DRUGS IN FOCUS Adjunctive antiparkinsonian drugs

Drug name	Dosage/route	Usual indications
entacapone (*Comtan*)	200 mg PO taken with levodopa–carbidopa, maximum of 10 doses (2000 mg) a day	Adjunctive treatment of idiopathic Parkinson disease with levodopa–carbidopa for people who are experiencing 'wearing off' of drug effects
rasagiline (*Azilect*)	1 mg PO once daily with or without levodopa	Adjunctive treatment or treatment of idiopathic Parkinson disease
selegiline (*Selgene, Eldepryl*)	5 mg PO bd (at breakfast and lunch); attempt to decrease levodopa–carbidopa dose after 2–3 days	Adjunctive treatment of idiopathic Parkinson disease with levodopa–carbidopa in people whose response to that therapy has decreased
tolcapone (*Tasmar*)	100 mg PO tds; maximum daily dose 600 mg	Adjunctive treatment of idiopathic Parkinson disease with levodopa–carbidopa

Because of the risk of MAO inhibitor–induced hypertensive effects, people should be urged to immediately report severe headache and any other unusual symptoms which they have not experienced before.

Care considerations for people receiving adjunctive agents

Care considerations for people receiving the drugs listed in this section are similar to those for people receiving the dopaminergic drugs. Details related to each individual drug can be found in the specific drug monograph in your drug guide.

KEY POINTS

- Adjunctive drugs are used to increase the responsiveness of the cells to dopamine. They act to decrease the breakdown of dopamine, leaving it on the receptor for longer periods of time.
- Adjunctive drugs are only used in combination with carbidopa–levodopa and are usually reserved for use when the person stops responding adequately to traditional therapy.

CHAPTER SUMMARY

- Parkinson disease is a progressive, chronic neurological disorder for which there is no cure.
- Loss of dopamine-secreting neurons in the substantia nigra is characteristic of Parkinson disease. Destruction of dopamine-secreting cells leads to an imbalance between excitatory cholinergic cells and inhibitory dopaminergic cells.
- Signs and symptoms of Parkinson disease include tremor, changes in posture and gait, slow and deliberate movements (bradykinesia) and eventually drooling and changes in speech.
- Drug therapy for Parkinson disease is aimed at restoring the dopamine–acetylcholine balance. The signs and symptoms of the disease can be managed until the degeneration of neurons is so extensive that a therapeutic response no longer occurs.
- Anticholinergic drugs are used to block the excitatory cholinergic receptors and dopaminergic drugs are used to increase dopamine levels or to directly stimulate dopamine receptors.
- Many adverse effects are associated with the drugs used for treating Parkinson disease, including CNS changes, anticholinergic effects when using the anticholinergics (atropine-like or parasympathetic blocking effects) and dopamine stimulation (sympathetic-type effects) in the peripheral nervous system when using the dopaminergics.

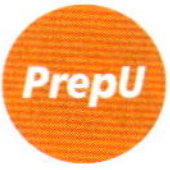

Knowing your strengths and weaknesses helps you to study more effectively. Take a PrepU Practice Quiz to find out how you measure up!

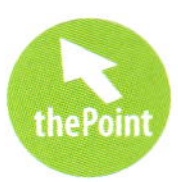

ONLINE RESOURCES

An extensive range of additional resources to enhance teaching and learning and to facilitate understanding of this chapter may be found online at the text's accompanying website, located on thePoint at http://thepoint.lww.com. These include Watch and Learn videos, Concepts in Action animations, journal articles, review questions, case studies, discussion topics and quizzes.

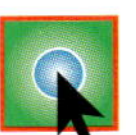

WEB LINKS

Health care providers and students may want to consult the following web resources:

www.parkinsons.org.au
Parkinson's Australia. Information on parkinsonism, ataxia and related disorders, including support groups, research and treatment.

www.parkinsons.org.nz
Parkinson's New Zealand. Information on parkinsonism, ataxia and related disorders, including support groups, research and treatment.

BIBLIOGRAPHY

Cranwell-Bruce, L. A. (2010). Drugs for Parkinson's disease. *MEDSURG Nursing, 19(6)*, 347–355.

Daley, D. J., Myint, P. K., Gray, R. J. & Deane, K. H. (2012). Systematic review on factors associated with medication non-adherence in Parkinson's disease. *Parkinsonism & Related Disorders, 18(10)*, 1053–1061.

Farrell, M. & Dempsey, J. (2014). *Smeltzer & Bare's Textbook of Medical-Surgical Nursing* (3rd edn). Sydney: Lippincott Williams & Wilkins.

Goodman, L. S., Brunton, L. L., Chabner, B. & Knollmann, B. C. (2011). *Goodman and Gilman's Pharmacological Basis of Therapeutics* (12th edn). New York: McGraw-Hill.

Hallett, P. F. & Standaert, D. G. (2004). Rationale for and use of NMDA receptor antagonists in Parkinson's disease. *Pharmacology and Therapeutics*, 102, 155–174.

McKenna, L. & Mirkov, S. (2019). *McKenna's Drug Handbook for Nursing and Midwifery* (8th edn). Sydney: Wolters Kluwer Health Australia.

Porth, C. M. (2011). *Essentials of Pathophysiology: Concepts of Altered Health States* (3rd edn). Philadelphia: Lippincott Williams & Wilkins.

Porth, C. M. (2009). *Pathophysiology: Concepts of Altered Health States* (8th edn). Philadelphia: Lippincott Williams & Wilkins.

Selbach, A. & Silburn, P. (2012). Management of Parkinson's disease. *Australian Prescriber, 35*, 183–188.

Turnbull, G. I. & Millar, J. (2006). A proactive physical management model of Parkinson's disease. *Topics in Geriatric Rehabilitation, 22*, 162–171.

Wright, J. & Walker, J. (2013). Medication adherence in Parkinson's. *British Journal of Nursing, 22(12)*, 686–699.

CHECK YOUR UNDERSTANDING

Answers to the questions in this chapter can be found in Appendix A at the back of this book.

MULTIPLE CHOICE

Select the best answer to the following.

1. Parkinson disease is a progressive, chronic neurological disorder that is usually:
   a. associated with severe head injury.
   b. associated with chronic diseases.
   c. associated with old age.
   d. known to affect people of all ages with no known cause.
2. Parkinson disease reflects an imbalance between inhibitory and stimulating activity of nerves in the:
   a. reticular activating system.
   b. cerebellum.
   c. basal ganglia.
   d. limbic system.
3. The main underlying problem with Parkinson disease seems to be a decrease in the neurotransmitter:
   a. acetylcholine.
   b. noradrenaline.
   c. dopamine.
   d. serotonin.
4. Anticholinergic drugs are effective in early Parkinson disease. They act:
   a. to block stimulating effects of acetylcholine in the brain to bring activity back into balance.
   b. to block the signs and symptoms of the disease, making it more acceptable.
   c. to inhibit dopamine effects in the brain and increase neuron activity
   d. to increase the effectiveness of the inhibitory neurotransmitter GABA.
5. A person receiving an anticholinergic drug for Parkinson disease is planning a winter trip to Tahiti. The temperature in Tahiti is 20°C warmer than at home. What precautions should the person be urged to take?
   a. Take the drug with plenty of water to stay hydrated.
   b. Reduce dose and take precautions to reduce the risk for heat stroke.
   c. Wear sunglasses and use sunscreen because of photophobia that will develop.
   d. Avoid drinking the water to prevent gastric distress.
6. Replacing dopamine in the brain would seem to be the best treatment for Parkinson disease. This is difficult because dopamine:
   a. is broken down in gastric acid.
   b. is not available in drug form.
   c. cannot cross the blood–brain barrier.
   d. is used peripherally before reaching the brain.
7. A person taking levodopa and over-the-counter megavitamins might experience:
   a. cure from Parkinson disease.
   b. return of Parkinson's symptoms.
   c. improved health and wellbeing.
   d. a resistance to viral infections.
8. A person who has been diagnosed with Parkinson disease for many years and whose symptoms were controlled using *Sinemet* has started to exhibit increasing signs of the disease. Possible treatment might include:
   a. increased exercise program.
   b. addition of benzatropine to the drug regimen.
   c. combination therapy with an anticholinergic drug.
   d. changes in diet to eliminate vitamin B6.

MULTIPLE RESPONSE

Select all that apply.

1. A person asks the nurse to explain parkinsonism to him. Which of the following possible causes of parkinsonism might be included in the explanation?
   a. adverse effect of drug therapy
   b. brain injury
   c. viral infection
   d. dementia
   e. bacterial infection
   f. birth defect
2. No therapy is available that will stop the loss of neurons and the eventual decline of function in people with Parkinson disease. As a result, care should involve which of the following interventions?
   a. regular exercises to slow loss of function
   b. supportive education as drugs fail and new therapy is needed
   c. community and family support networking
   d. discontinuation of drug therapy to test for a cure
   e. special vitamin therapy to slow the loss of the neurons
   f. explanations of the adjunctive drug therapy that may be used

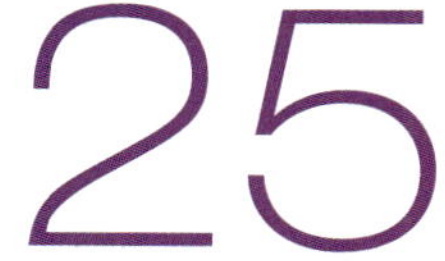

Muscle relaxants

Learning objectives

On completing this chapter you should be able to:

1. Describe a spinal reflex and discuss the pathophysiology of muscle spasm and muscle spasticity.
2. Describe the therapeutic actions, indications, pharmacokinetics, contraindications, most common adverse reactions and important drug–drug interactions associated with the centrally acting and the direct-acting skeletal muscle relaxants.
3. Discuss the use of muscle relaxants across the lifespan.
4. Compare and contrast the prototype drugs baclofen and dantrolene with other muscle relaxants in their classes.
5. Outline the care considerations, including important teaching points for people receiving muscle relaxants.

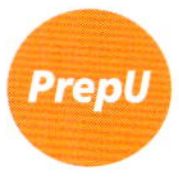
Test your current knowledge of muscle relaxants with a PrepU Practice Quiz!

Glossary of key terms

basal ganglia: lower area of the brain, associated with coordination of unconscious muscle movements that involve movement and position

cerebellum: lower portion of the brain, associated with coordination of muscle movements, including voluntary motion, as well as extrapyramidal control of unconscious muscle movements

extrapyramidal tract: cells from the cortex and subcortical areas, including the basal ganglia and the cerebellum, which coordinate unconsciously controlled muscle activity; allows the body to make automatic adjustments in posture or position and balance

hypertonia: state of excessive muscle response and activity

interneuron: neuron in the central nervous system (CNS) that communicates with other neurons, not with muscles or glands

pyramidal tract: fibres within the CNS that control precise, intentional movement

spasticity: sustained muscle contractions

spindle gamma loop system: simple reflex arcs that involve sensory receptors in the periphery that respond to stretch and spinal motor nerves and cause muscle fibre contraction: responsible for maintaining muscle tone and keeping an upright position against the pull of gravity

CENTRALLY ACTING SKELETAL MUSCLE RELAXANTS

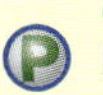 baclofen
diazepam
orphenadrine

DIRECT-ACTING SKELETAL MUSCLE RELAXANTS

botulinum toxin type A
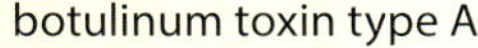
Ⓟ dantrolene

Many injuries and accidents result in local damage to muscles or the skeletal anchors of muscles. These injuries may lead to muscle spasm and pain, which may be of long duration and may interfere with normal functioning. Damage to central nervous system (CNS) neurons may cause a permanent state of muscle **spasticity** – sustained muscle contractions – as a result of loss of nerves that help to maintain balance in controlling muscle activity.

Neuron damage, whether temporary or permanent, may be treated with skeletal muscle relaxants. Most skeletal muscle relaxants work in the brain and spinal cord, where they interfere with the cycle of muscle spasm and pain. However, the botulinum toxins and dantrolene enter muscle fibres directly. See Box 25.1 for discussion of the use of these muscle relaxants in various age groups.

NERVES AND MOVEMENT

Posture, balance and movement are the result of a constantly fluctuating sequence of muscle contraction and relaxation. The nerves that regulate these actions are the spinal motor neurons. These neurons are influenced by higher-level brain activity in the lower areas of the brain, the **cerebellum** (associated with conscious muscle movements) and **basal ganglia** (associated with unconscious muscle movements). This brain activity provides coordination of contractions, and the cerebral cortex allows conscious thought to regulate movement.

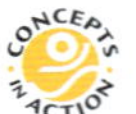

Nutritional: Muscle contraction

Spinal reflexes

The spinal reflexes are the simplest nerve pathways that monitor movement and posture (see Figure 25.1). Spinal reflexes can be simple, involving an incoming sensory neuron and an outgoing motor neuron, or more complex, involving **interneurons** that communicate with the related centres in the brain. Simple reflex arcs involve sensory receptors in the periphery and spinal motor nerves. Such reflex arcs make up what is known as the **spindle gamma loop system**; they respond to stretch receptors or spindles on muscle fibres to cause a muscle fibre contraction that relieves the stretch. In this system, nerves from stretch receptors form a synapse with gamma nerves in the spinal cord, which send an impulse to the stretched muscle fibres to stimulate their contraction. These reflexes are responsible for maintaining muscle tone and keeping an upright position against the pull of gravity and are important in helping venous return when the contracting muscle fibres massage veins

BOX 25.1 FOCUS ON **Drug therapy across the lifespan**

Skeletal muscle relaxants

CHILDREN

The safety and effectiveness of most of these drugs have not been established in children. Agents have been used, with adjustments to the adult dosage based on the child's age and weight.

Baclofen is often used to relieve the muscle spasticity associated with cerebral palsy. A carer needs intensive education in the use of the intrathecal infusion pump and how to monitor the child for therapeutic as well as adverse effects.

Dantrolene is used to treat upper motor neuron spasticity in children. The dosage is based on body weight and increases over time. The child should be screened regularly for CNS and gastrointestinal (GI) toxicity, including hepatic toxicity.

ADULTS

Adults being treated for acute musculoskeletal pain should be cautioned to avoid driving and to take safety precautions against injury because of the related CNS effects, including dizziness and drowsiness.

Adults complaining of muscle spasm pain that may be related to anxiety often respond very effectively to diazepam, which is a muscle relaxant and anxiolytic.

PREGNANCY AND BREASTFEEDING

Women of childbearing age should be advised to use contraception when they are taking these drugs. If a pregnancy does occur, or is desired, they need counselling about the potential for adverse effects. Women who are breastfeeding should be encouraged to find another method of feeding the baby because of the potential for adverse drug effects on the baby.

Premenopausal women are also at increased risk for the hepatotoxicity associated with dantrolene and should be monitored very closely for any change in hepatic function and given written information about the prodrome syndrome that often occurs with hepatic toxicity.

OLDER ADULTS

Older people are more likely to experience the adverse effects associated with these drugs – CNS, gastrointestinal and cardiovascular. Because older people often also have renal or hepatic impairment, they are also more likely to have toxic levels of the drug related to changes in metabolism and excretion.

If dantrolene is required for an older person, lower doses and more frequent monitoring are needed to assess for potential cardiac, respiratory and liver toxicity.

Older women who are receiving hormone replacement therapy are at the same risk for development of hepatotoxicity as premenopausal women and should be monitored accordingly.

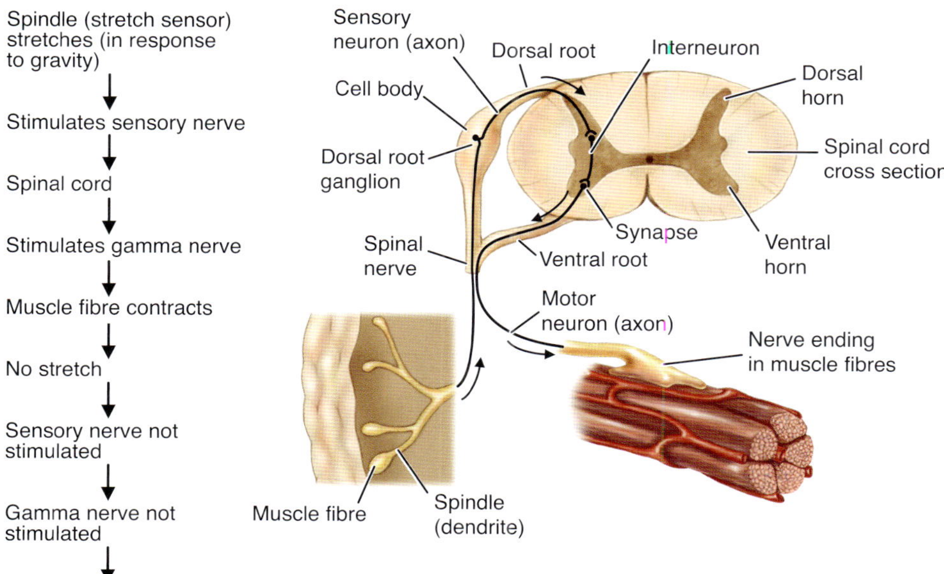

FIGURE 25.1 Reflex arc showing the pathway of impulses. The spindle gamma loop reflex arc: the relaxing and contracting of muscle fibres causes muscle tone and ability to stand upright and promotes venous return.

to help move the blood towards the heart. Other spinal reflexes may involve synapses with interneurons within the spinal cord, which adjust movement and response based on information from higher brain centres to coordinate movement and position.

Brain control

Many areas within the brain influence the spinal motor nerves. Areas of the brainstem, the basal ganglia and the cerebellum modulate spinal motor nerve activity and help to coordinate activity among various muscle groups, thereby allowing coordinated movement and control of body muscle motions. Nerve areas within the cerebral cortex allow conscious, or intentional, movement. Nerves within the cortex send signals down the spinal cord, where they cross to the opposite side of the spinal cord before sending out nerve impulses to cause muscle contraction. In this way, each side of the cortex controls muscle movement on the opposite side of the body.

Different fibres control different types of movements. Those fibres that control precise, intentional movement make up the **pyramidal tract** within the CNS. The **extrapyramidal tract** is composed of cells from the cerebral cortex, as well as those from several subcortical areas, including the basal ganglia and the cerebellum. This tract modulates or coordinates unconsciously controlled muscle activity, and allows the body to make automatic adjustments in posture or position and balance. The extrapyramidal tract controls lower-level, or crude, movements.

NEUROMUSCULAR ABNORMALITIES

All of the areas mentioned work together to allow for a free flow of impulses into and out of the CNS to coordinate posture, balance and movement. When injuries, diseases and toxins affect the normal flow of information into and out of the CNS motor pathways, many clinical signs and symptoms may develop, ranging from simple muscle spasms to spasticity – or sustained muscle spasm – and paralysis.

Muscle spasm

Muscle spasms often result from injury to the musculoskeletal system – for example, overstretching a muscle, wrenching a joint or tearing a tendon or ligament. These injuries can cause violent and painful involuntary muscle contractions. It is thought that these spasms are caused by the flood of sensory impulses coming to the spinal cord from the injured area. These impulses can be passed through interneurons to spinal motor nerves, which stimulate an intense muscle contraction. The contraction cuts off blood flow to the muscle fibres in the injured area, causing lactic acid to accumulate, resulting in pain. The new flood of sensory impulses caused by the pain may lead to further muscle contraction, and a vicious cycle may develop (see Figure 25.2).

Muscle spasticity

Muscle spasticity is the result of damage to neurons within the CNS rather than injury to peripheral

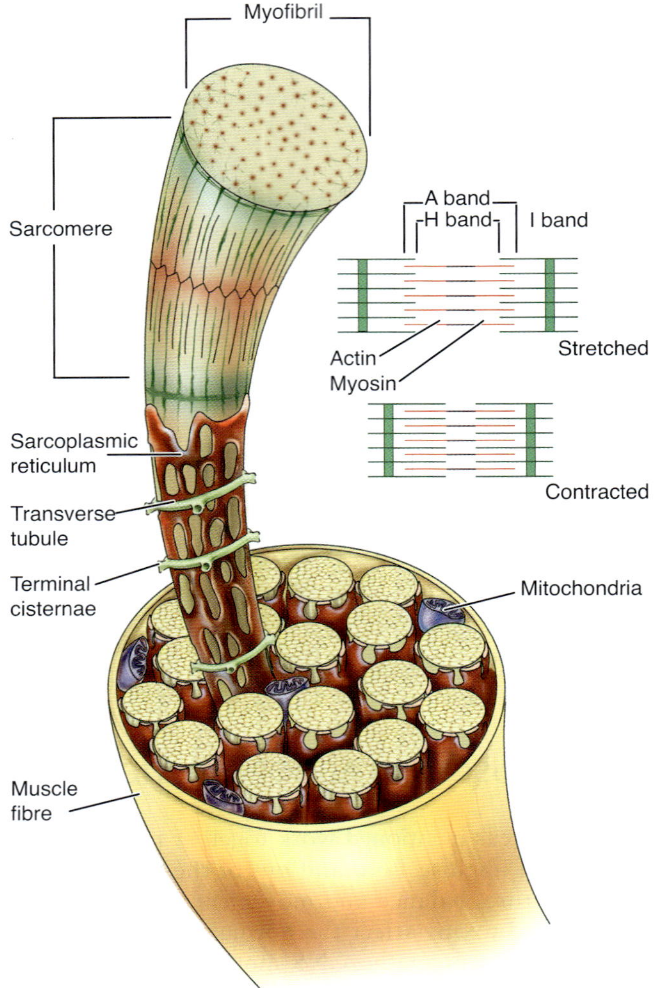

FIGURE 25.2 When stimulation stops, calcium ions are actively transported back into the sarcoplasmic reticulum, resulting in decreased calcium ions in the sarcoplasm. The removal of calcium ions restores the inhibitory action of troponin–tropomyosin; cross-bridge action is impossible in this state.

structures. Because the spasticity is caused by nerve damage in the CNS, it is a permanent condition. Spasticity may result from an increase in excitatory influences or a decrease in inhibitory influences within the CNS. The interruption in the balance among all of these higher influences within the CNS may lead to excessive stimulation of muscles, or **hypertonia**, in opposing muscle groups at the same time, a condition that may cause contractures and permanent structural changes. This control imbalance also results in a loss of coordinated muscle activity.

For example, the signs and symptoms of cerebral palsy and paraplegia are related to the disruption in the nervous control of the muscles. The exact presentation of any chronic neurological disorder depends on the specific nerve centres and tracts that are damaged and how the control imbalance is manifested.

KEY POINTS

- Movement and muscle control are regulated by spinal reflexes and the upper CNS, including the basal ganglia, cerebellum and cerebral cortex.
- Spinal reflexes can be simple, involving an incoming sensory neuron and an outgoing motor neuron, or more complex, involving interneurons that communicate with the related centres in the brain.
- The pyramidal tract in the cerebellum coordinates intentional muscle movement, and the extrapyramidal tract in the cerebellum and basal ganglia coordinates involuntary muscle activity.
- Muscle or skeletal damage may send a multitude of stimuli to the spinal cord and result in muscle spasms or extended contraction.
- Damaged motor neurons can cause muscle spasticity and impaired movement and coordination.

CENTRALLY ACTING SKELETAL MUSCLE RELAXANTS

Centrally acting skeletal muscle relaxants (Table 25.1) include baclofen (*Lioresal*) and orphenadrine (*Norflex*). Diazepam (*Valium*), a drug widely used as an anxiety agent (see Chapter 20), has also been shown to be an effective centrally acting skeletal muscle relaxant. It may be advantageous in situations in which anxiety may be precipitating the muscle spasm.

Other measures in addition to these drugs should be used to alleviate muscle spasm and pain. Such modalities as rest of the affected muscle, heat applications to increase blood flow to the area to remove the pain-causing chemicals, physical therapy to return the muscle to normal tone and activity, and anti-inflammatory agents (including non-steroidal anti-inflammatory drugs [NSAIDs]) if the underlying problem is related to injury or inflammation may help. This may be aided by use of a combined product such as orphenadrine and paracetamol (*Norgesic*).

Therapeutic actions and indications

The centrally acting skeletal muscle relaxants work in the CNS to interfere with the reflexes that are causing the muscle spasm. Because these drugs lyse or destroy spasm, they are often referred to as spasmolytics. Although the exact mechanism of action of these skeletal muscle relaxants is not known, it is thought to involve action in the upper or spinal interneurons. The primary indication for the use of centrally acting skeletal muscle agents is the relief of discomfort associated with acute, painful musculoskeletal conditions as an adjunct to rest, physical therapy and other measures.

TABLE 25.1 DRUGS IN FOCUS Centrally acting skeletal muscle relaxants

Drug name	Dosage/route	Usual indications
(P) baclofen (*Lioresal*)	Adults: initially 5 mg PO tid increasing every 3 days to 30–75 mg/day. Via intrathecal infusion pump, dosage individualised according to response Paediatric: dosing complex – see manufacturer's instructions	Treatment of muscle spasticity associated with neuromuscular diseases such as multiple sclerosis, muscle rigidity and spinal cord injuries
diazepam (*Valium*)	2–10 mg deep IM or slow IV injection q 3–4 hours, 10–60 mg PO daily	Treatment of muscle spasm or spasticity, including cerebral palsy
orphenadrine (*Norflex*)	100 mg PO bd (maximum 300 mg/day)	Relief of discomfort of acute musculoskeletal conditions in adults

Because these drugs work in the upper levels of the CNS, possible depression must be anticipated with their use. See Table 25.1 for usual indications for each of these agents.

Pharmacokinetics

Baclofen is available in oral and intrathecal forms and can be administered via a delivery pump for the treatment of central spasticity. Baclofen is not metabolised but, like the other skeletal muscle relaxants, it is excreted in the urine.

Contraindications and cautions

Centrally acting skeletal muscle relaxants are contraindicated in the presence of any known allergy to any of these drugs and with skeletal muscle spasms resulting from rheumatic disorders. In addition, baclofen should not be used to treat any spasticity that contributes to locomotion, upright position or increased function. *Blocking this spasticity results in loss of these functions.* All centrally acting skeletal muscle relaxants should be used cautiously in the following circumstances: with a history of epilepsy *because the CNS depression and imbalance caused by these drugs may exacerbate the seizure disorder*; with cardiac dysfunction *because muscle function may be depressed*; with any condition marked by muscle weakness, *which the drugs could make much worse*; and with hepatic or renal dysfunction, *which could interfere with the metabolism and excretion of the drugs, leading to toxic levels.* No good studies exist regarding the effects of these agents during pregnancy and breastfeeding; therefore, use should be limited to those situations in which the benefit to the mother clearly outweighs any potential risk to the fetus or neonate.

Adverse effects

The most frequently seen adverse effects associated with these drugs relate to the associated CNS depression: drowsiness, fatigue, weakness, confusion, headache and insomnia. Gastrointestinal disturbances, which may be linked to CNS depression of the parasympathetic reflexes, include nausea, dry mouth, anorexia and constipation. In addition, hypotension and arrhythmias may occur, again as a result of depression of normal reflex arcs. Urinary frequency, enuresis and feelings of urinary urgency reportedly may occur.

Clinically important drug–drug interactions

If any of the centrally acting skeletal muscle relaxants are taken with other CNS depressants or alcohol, CNS depression may increase. People should be cautioned to avoid alcohol while taking these muscle relaxants; if this combination cannot be avoided, they should take extreme precautions.

(P) Prototype summary: baclofen

Indications: alleviation of signs and symptoms of spasticity; may be of use in spinal cord injuries or spinal cord diseases.

Actions: gamma-aminobutyric acid (GABA) analogue; exact mechanism of action is not understood; inhibits monosynaptic and polysynaptic spinal reflexes; CNS depressant.

Pharmacokinetics:

Route	Onset	Peak	Duration
Oral	1 hours	2 hours	4–8 hours
Intrathecal	30–60 min	4 hours	4–8 hours

$T_{1/2}$: 3–4 hours; not metabolised; excreted in the urine.

Adverse effects: transient drowsiness, dizziness, weakness, fatigue, constipation, headache, insomnia, hypotension, nausea, urinary frequency.

Care considerations for people receiving centrally acting skeletal muscle relaxants

Assessment: history and examination

- Assess for contraindications or cautions for the use of the drug, including any known allergies, *to prevent hypersensitivity reactions*; cardiac depression, epilepsy, muscle weakness or rheumatic disorder, *which could be exacerbated by the effects of these drugs*; pregnancy or breastfeeding, *which would be contraindications to use of the drugs*; and renal or hepatic dysfunction, *which alter metabolism and excretion of the drugs.*
- Assess temperature; skin colour and lesions; CNS orientation, affect, reflexes, bilateral grip strength and spasticity evaluation; bowel sounds and reported output; and liver and renal function tests *to determine baseline status before beginning therapy and for any potential adverse effects.*

Implementation with rationale

- Provide additional measures to relieve discomfort – heat, rest for the muscle, NSAIDs, positioning – *to augment the effects of the drug at relieving the musculoskeletal discomfort.*
- Discontinue drug at any sign of hypersensitivity reaction or liver dysfunction *to prevent severe toxicity.*
- If using baclofen, taper the drug slowly over 1–2 weeks *to prevent the development of psychoses and hallucinations.* Use baclofen cautiously in people whose spasticity contributes to mobility, posture or balance *to prevent loss of this function.*
- If person is receiving baclofen through a delivery pump, the person should understand the pump, the reason for frequent monitoring and how to adjust the dose and program the unit *to enhance knowledge and promote compliance.*
- Monitor respiratory status *to evaluate adverse effects and arrange for appropriate dose adjustment or discontinuation of the drug.*
- Provide thorough teaching, including drug name, prescribed dosage, measures for avoidance of adverse effects, warning signs that may indicate possible problems and the need for monitoring and evaluation *to enhance knowledge about drug therapy and to promote compliance.*
- Offer support and encouragement *to help the person cope with the drug regimen.*

Evaluation

- Monitor response to the drug (improvement in muscle spasm and relief of pain; improvement in muscle spasticity).
- Monitor for adverse effects (CNS changes, GI depression, urinary urgency).
- Evaluate the effectiveness of the teaching plan (person can give the drug name and dosage, name possible adverse effects to watch for and specific measures to prevent them and describe, if necessary, proper intrathecal administration).
- Monitor the effectiveness of comfort measures and compliance with the regimen.

KEY POINTS

- The centrally acting skeletal muscle relaxants interfere with the reflexes that are causing the muscle spasm.
- The centrally acting skeletal muscle relaxants cause central CNS depression, and the adverse effects associated with them are related to the CNS depression (insomnia, dizziness, confusion, anticholinergic effects).
- The centrally acting muscle relaxants are used for the relief of discomfort associated with acute, painful musculoskeletal conditions as an adjunct to rest, physical therapy and other measures.

DIRECT-ACTING SKELETAL MUSCLE RELAXANTS

The direct-acting skeletal muscle relaxants enter the muscle to prevent muscle contraction directly. Direct-acting skeletal muscle relaxants (Table 25.2) include dantrolene (*Dantrium*) and botulinum toxin type A (*Botox, Dysport*).

Therapeutic actions and indications

Dantrolene directly affects peripheral muscle contraction and has become important in the management of spasticity associated with neuromuscular diseases. Dantrolene acts within skeletal muscle fibres, interfering with the release of calcium from the muscle tubules (see Figure 25.2). This action prevents the fibres from contracting. Dantrolene does not interfere with neuromuscular transmissions, and it does not affect the surface membrane of skeletal muscle. Botulinum toxin A binds directly to the receptor sites of motor nerve terminals and inhibits the release of acetylcholine, leading to local muscle paralysis. This drug is injected locally and used to paralyse or prevent the contractions of specific muscle groups.

Long-term use of dantrolene commonly results in a decrease of the amount and intensity of required care. Continued long-term use is justified as long as the drug reduces painful and disabling spasticity. This agent is

TABLE 25.2 DRUGS IN FOCUS Direct-acting skeletal muscle relaxants

Drug name	Dosage/route	Usual indications
botulinum toxin type A (*Botox, Dysport*)	Botulinum doses are complex. It is licenced for many conditions. Brands are not interchangeable. See manufacturer's instructions	Improvement of appearance in glabellar (frown) lines associated with corrugator or procerus muscle activity in adults; treatment of cervical dystonia; approved in 2004 for treatment of strabismus and blepharospasm associated with dystonia in people ≥ 12 years of age; treatment of severe primary axillary hyperhidrosis (sweating) when injected into the axillary area
(P) dantrolene (*Dantrium*)	Adult: initially 25 mg PO; increase based on spinal cord injuries; prevention and management of response to a maximum 400 mg/day for spasticity Paediatric: initially 0.5 mg/kg PO bd, increasing to tid–qid to a maximum of 2 mg/kg tid. Maximum 50 mg qid	Management of upper motor neuron–associated muscle spasticity such as spinal cord injury, myasthenia gravis, cerebral palsy, multiple sclerosis, muscular dystrophy, polio, tetanus, quadriplegia and amyotrophic lateral sclerosis (ALS); prevention or treatment of malignant hyperthermia – a state of intense muscle contraction prophylaxis in susceptible people who must undergo anaesthesia and after acute episodes to prevent recurrence

not used for the treatment of muscle spasms associated with musculoskeletal injury or rheumatic disorders. Table 25.2 presents additional information about these agents, including usual indications.

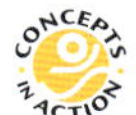

Nutritional: Calcium in muscles

Pharmacokinetics

Dantrolene is used in oral or parenteral forms. Dantrolene is slowly absorbed from the GI tract and metabolised in the liver with a half-life of 4–8 hours. Excretion is through the urine. Dantrolene crosses the placenta and was found to be embryotoxic in animal studies. Use should be reserved for those situations in which the benefit to the mother clearly outweighs the risk to the fetus. Dantrolene enters breast milk and is contraindicated for use during breastfeeding. Safety for use in children younger than 5 years of age has not been established; because the long-term effects are not known, careful consideration should be given to use of the drug in children.

The botulinum toxins are not generally absorbed systemically, and there is no pharmacokinetic information available.

Contraindications and cautions

Dantrolene is contraindicated in the presence of any known allergy to the drug. It is also contraindicated in the following conditions: spasticity that contributes to locomotion, upright position or increased function, *which would be lost if that spasticity were blocked*; active hepatic disease, *which might interfere with metabolism of the drug and because of known liver toxicity*; and breastfeeding *because the drug may cross into breast milk and cause adverse effects in the infant.* The botulinum toxins are contraindicated in the presence of allergy to any component of the drug or with active infection at the site of the injection *because injecting the drug could aggravate the infection.*

Caution should be used with dantrolene in the following circumstances: in women and in all people older than 35 years *because of increased risk of potentially fatal hepatocellular disease* (Box 25.2); in people with a history of liver disease or previous dysfunction, *which could make the liver more susceptible to cellular toxicity;* in people with respiratory depression, *which could be exacerbated by muscular weakness;* in people with cardiac disease *because cardiac muscle depression may be a risk;* and during pregnancy *because of the potential for adverse effects on the fetus.* Caution should be used with the botulinum toxins with any peripheral neuropathic disease; with neuromuscular disorders, *which could be exacerbated by the effects of the drug*; with pregnancy and breastfeeding; and with any known cardiovascular disease.

Adverse effects

The most frequently seen adverse effects associated with dantrolene relate to drug-caused CNS depression: drowsiness, fatigue, weakness, confusion, headache and insomnia, and visual disturbances. GI disturbances may be linked to direct irritation or to alterations in smooth muscle function caused by the drug-induced calcium

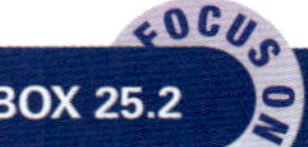

BOX 25.2 Gender considerations

Understanding the risks of liver damage with dantrolene

Dantrolene (Dantrium) is associated with potentially fatal hepatocellular injury. When liver damage begins to occur, people often experience a prodrome, or warning syndrome, which includes anorexia, nausea and fatigue. The incidence of such hepatic injury is greater in women and in individuals older than 35 years of age.

In women, a combination of dantrolene and oestrogen seems to affect the liver, thus posing a greater risk. Women of all ages may be at increased risk, because those entering menopause may be taking hormone replacement therapy. People older than 35 years of age are at increasing risk of liver injury because of the changing integrity of the liver cells that comes with age and exposure to toxins over time.

If a particular woman needs dantrolene for relief of spasticity, she should not be taking any oestrogens (eg, oral contraceptives, hormone replacement therapy) and she should be monitored closely for any sign of liver dysfunction. For safer relief of spasticity in these women, baclofen may be helpful.

effects. Such adverse GI effects may include GI irritation, diarrhoea, constipation and abdominal cramps. Dantrolene may also cause direct hepatocellular damage and hepatitis that can be fatal. Urinary frequency, enuresis and feelings of urinary urgency reportedly occur, and crystalline urine with pain or burning on urination may result. In addition, several unusual adverse effects may occur, including acne, abnormal hair growth, rashes, photosensitivity, abnormal sweating, chills and myalgia.

The botulinum toxins have been associated with anaphylactic reactions; with headache, dizziness, muscle pain and paralysis; and with redness and oedema at the injection site. Adverse effects associated with use of botulinum toxin type A for cosmetic purposes include headache, respiratory infections, flu-like syndrome and droopy eyelids in severe cases. Pain, redness and muscle weakness have also been reported. The reactions tend to be temporary, but there have been reports of reactions that lasted several months.

Clinically important drug–drug interactions

If dantrolene is combined with oestrogens, the incidence of hepatocellular toxicity is apparently increased. If possible, this combination should be avoided. If the botulinum toxins are used with other drugs that interfere with neuromuscular transmission – neuromuscular junction (NMJ) blockers, lincosamides, magnesium sulphate, anticholinesterases, suxamethonium chloride or colistimethate sodium – or with aminoglycosides, there is a risk of additive effects. If any of these must be given in combination, extreme caution should be used.

Prototype summary: dantrolene

Indications: control of clinical spasticity resulting from upper motor neuron disorders; preoperatively to prevent or attenuate the development of malignant hyperthermia in susceptible people; IV for management of fulminant malignant hyperthermia.

Actions: interferes with the release of calcium from the sarcoplasmic reticulum within skeletal muscles, preventing muscle contraction; does not interfere with neuromuscular transmission.

Pharmacokinetics:

Route	Onset	Peak	Duration
Oral	Slow	4–6 hours	8–10 hours
IV	Rapid	5 hours	6–8 hours

$T_{1/2}$: 9 hours (oral), 4–8 hours (IV); excreted in the urine.

Adverse effects: drowsiness, dizziness, weakness, fatigue, diarrhoea, hepatitis, myalgia, tachycardia, transient blood pressure changes, rash, urinary frequency.

Care considerations for people receiving a direct-acting skeletal muscle relaxant

Assessment: history and examination

- Assess for contraindications or cautions for the use of the drug including any known allergies *to prevent hypersensitivity reactions*; cardiac depression; epilepsy; muscle weakness; respiratory depression, *which could be exacerbated by the effects of these drugs*; pregnancy and breastfeeding, *which require cautious use*; renal or hepatic dysfunction, *which could alter the metabolism and excretion of the drug*; and local infections (if using botulinum toxins) *to prevent exacerbation of the infections.*
- Assess temperature; skin colour and lesions; CNS orientation, affect, reflexes, bilateral grip strength and spasticity; respiration and adventitious sounds; pulse, electrocardiogram (ECG) and cardiac output; bowel sounds and reported output; and liver and renal function tests *to determine baseline status before beginning therapy and for any potential adverse effects.*
- *Refer to the Critical thinking scenario for a full discussion of care for a person who is receiving a direct-acting skeletal muscle relaxant.*

Implementation with rationale

- Discontinue the drug at any sign of liver dysfunction. *Early diagnosis of liver damage may prevent permanent dysfunction. Arrange for the drug to be discontinued if signs of liver damage appear.* A prodrome, with nausea, anorexia and fatigue, is present in 60% of people with evidence of hepatic injury.
- Do not administer botulinum toxins into any area with an active infection *because of the risk of exacerbation of the infection.*
- Monitor intravenous access sites for potential extravasation *because the drug is alkaline and very irritating to tissues.*
- Institute other supportive measures (eg, ventilation, anticonvulsants as needed, cooling blankets) for the treatment of malignant hyperthermia *to support the person through the reaction.*
- Periodically discontinue the drug for 2–4 days *to monitor therapeutic effectiveness.* A clinical impression of exacerbation of spasticity indicates a positive therapeutic effect and justifies continued use of the drug.
- Establish a therapeutic goal before beginning oral therapy (eg, to gain or enhance the ability to engage in a therapeutic exercise program; to use braces; to accomplish transfer manoeuvres) *to promote compliance and a sense of success with therapy.*
- Discontinue the drug if diarrhoea becomes severe *to prevent dehydration and electrolyte imbalance.* The drug may be restarted at a lower dose.
- Provide thorough teaching, including drug name, prescribed dosage, measures for avoidance of adverse effects, warning signs that may indicate possible problems and the need for monitoring and evaluation *to enhance knowledge about drug therapy and to promote compliance.*
- Offer support and encouragement to help the person cope with the drug regimen.

Evaluation

- Monitor response to the drug (improvement in spasticity, improvement in movement and activities; improvement in dystonia, facial lines, sweating with botulinum toxins).
- Monitor for adverse effects (CNS changes, diarrhoea, liver toxicity, urinary urgency).
- Evaluate the effectiveness of the teaching plan (person can give the drug name and dosage, possible adverse effects to watch for and specific measures to prevent adverse effects, and therapeutic goals).
- Monitor the effectiveness of comfort measures and compliance with the regimen.

KEY POINTS

- Centrally acting skeletal muscle relaxants are used to relieve the effects of muscle spasm. Dantrolene, a direct-acting skeletal muscle relaxant, is used to control spasticity and prevent malignant hyperthermia.
- Botulinum toxin type A is used to improve the appearance of moderate to severe glabellar lines and to treat cervical dystonia, severe primary axillary hyperhidrosis, and strabismus and blepharospasm associated with dystonia.

CRITICAL THINKING SCENARIO

Skeletal muscle relaxants for cerebral palsy

THE SITUATION

L.G. is 26 years old. He was diagnosed with cerebral palsy shortly after his birth. He lives in the community in a group home with six other affected people. Two adult carers provide supervision. In the past few months, L.G.'s spasticity has progressed severely, making it impossible for him to carry on his daily activities without extensive assistance.

Following a clinical evaluation, his health care team suggests trying a course of dantrolene therapy. After learning about the risks of dantrolene-related hepatic dysfunction, L.G. decides that the benefits of dantrolene therapy are more important to him than the risks of hepatotoxicity. The health care team proceeds with a complete physical examination, including liver enzyme analysis. Therapy begins and a clinic staff member schedules L.G. for a visit by a community nurse in 4 days.

CRITICAL THINKING

What basic principles must be included in the care plan for L.G. for the visiting nurses? *Think about the importance of including the adult carers in any teaching or evaluation programs. Consider specific problems that could develop that L.G. would be unable to handle on his own.*

What therapeutic goals might the nurse set with L.G. and his carer? How might these be evaluated?

What additional drug-related information should be posted in the group home and reviewed with L.G. and his carers?

DISCUSSION

In the first visit to the home, the nurse needs to establish a relationship with L.G. and his carers. They should all realise that drug therapy, and other measures, are needed to help L.G. attain his full potential and make use of his existing assets. Step-by-step therapeutic goals should be established and written down for future reference. Small reachable goals, such as partially dressing himself, walking to the table for meals, and managing parts of his daily hygiene routine are best at the beginning. Written goals provide a good basis for future evaluation when drug therapy is stopped briefly to determine its therapeutic effectiveness. It also helps L.G. to see progress and improvement.

In addition, the nurse should perform a complete examination to obtain baseline data. The person should be asked about any noticeable changes or problems since starting the drug. If improvement appears to have occurred, the dosage may be slowly increased until the optimal level of functioning has been achieved. The nurse is in a position to evaluate this and report it to the primary carer.

While in the home, the nurse can also evaluate resources and environmental limitations and suggest improvements (eg, use of leg braces). L.G. and his carers should receive a drug teaching card that includes a telephone number to call with questions or concerns; warning signs of liver disease; and a list of findings to report. The nurse should discuss anticipated appointments for liver function tests to ensure that L.G. can keep the appointments. The health care team should work closely with L.G. to maximise his involvement in his care and to minimise unnecessary problems and confusion. Because the treatment involves a long-term commitment, a good working relationship among all members of the health care team is important to ensure continuity of care and optimal results.

CARE GUIDE FOR L.G.: MUSCLE RELAXANTS

Assessment: history and examination

Concentrate the health history on allergies to any skeletal muscle relaxants, respiratory depression, muscle weakness, hepatic or renal dysfunction, and concurrent use of verapamil or alcohol.

Focus the physical examination on the following:

CV: blood pressure pulse rate, peripheral perfusion, ECG

CNS: orientation, affect, reflexes, grip strength

Skin: colour, lesions, texture, temperature

GI: abdominal examination, bowel sounds

Respiratory: respiration, adventitious sounds

Laboratory tests: renal and hepatic function

Implementation

Discontinue drug at first sign of liver dysfunction.

Provide comfort and safety measures: positioning, orientation, safety measures, pain medication as needed.

Provide support and reassurance to help L.G. deal with spasticity and drug effects.

Teach L.G. about drug, dosage, drug effects and symptoms of reportable serious adverse effects.

Evaluation

Evaluate drug effects: relief of spasticity, improved daily function.

Monitor for adverse effects: multiple CNS effects, respiratory depression, rash, skin changes, GI problems (diarrhoea, hepatotoxicity), urinary urgency or weakness.

Monitor for drug–drug interactions: myocardial suppression with verapamil or alcohol.

Evaluate effectiveness of teaching program.

TEACHING FOR L.G.

- The drug prescribed for you is a direct-acting skeletal muscle relaxant called dantrolene (*Dantrium*). This drug makes spastic muscles relax. Because this drug may cause liver damage, it is important that you have regular medical check-ups.
- Common side effects of skeletal muscle relaxants, such as dantrolene, include:
  - *Fatigue, weakness and drowsiness:* try to pace activities evenly throughout the day and allow rest periods to avoid discouraging side effects. If they become too severe, consult your health care provider.
  - *Dizziness and fainting:* change position slowly to avoid dizzy spells. If these effects should occur, avoid activities that require coordination and concentration.
  - *Diarrhoea:* be sure to be near bathroom facilities if this occurs. This effect usually subsides after a few weeks.
- Report any of the following to your health care provider: *fever, chills, rash, itching, changes in the colour of your urine or stool, or a yellowish tint to the eyes or skin.*
- Keep this drug and all medications out of the reach of children.
- Do not overexert yourself when you begin to feel better. Pace yourself.
- Take this drug exactly as directed and schedule regular medical checkups to evaluate the effects of this drug on your body.

CHAPTER SUMMARY

- Upper-level controls of muscle activity include the pyramidal tract in the cerebellum, which regulates coordination of intentional muscle movement, and the extrapyramidal tract in the cerebellum and basal ganglia, which coordinates crude movements related to unconscious muscle activity.
- Damage to a muscle or anchoring skeletal structure may result in the arrival of a flood of impulses to the spinal cord. Such overstimulation may lead to a muscle spasm or a state of increased contraction.
- Damage to motor neurons can cause muscle spasticity, with a lack of coordination between muscle groups and loss of coordinated activity, including the ability to perform intentional tasks and maintain posture, position and locomotion.
- Centrally acting skeletal muscle relaxants are used to relieve the effects of muscle spasm. Dantrolene, a direct-acting skeletal muscle relaxant, is used to control spasticity and prevent malignant hyperthermia.
- Botulinum toxin type A is used to improve the appearance of moderate to severe glabellar lines and to treat cervical dystonia, severe primary axillary hyperhidrosis, and strabismus and blepharospasm associated with dystonia.

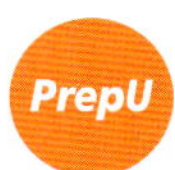

Knowing your strengths and weaknesses helps you to study more effectively. Take a PrepU Practice Quiz to find out how you measure up!

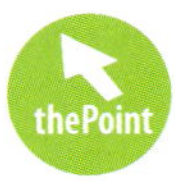

ONLINE RESOURCES

An extensive range of additional resources to enhance teaching and learning and to facilitate understanding of this chapter may be found online at the text's accompanying website, located on thePoint at http://thepoint.lww.com. These include Watch and Learn videos, Concepts in Action animations, journal articles, review questions, case studies, discussion topics and quizzes.

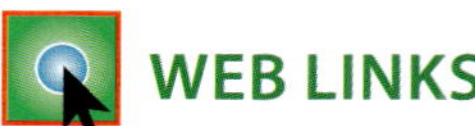

WEB LINKS

Health care providers and students may want to consult the following web resources:

www.cerebralpalsy.org.au
The Cerebral Palsy Alliance. Information on research and support services for people with cerebral palsy.

www.cpaustralia.com.au
Cerebral Palsy Australia. Information on research and support services for people with cerebral palsy.

BIBLIOGRAPHY

Aslan, A., Cemek, M., Buyukokuroglu, M. E., Altunbas, K., Bas, O., Yurumez, Y. & Cosar, M. (2009). Dantrolene can reduce secondary damage after spinal cord injury. *European Spine Journal, 18*, 1442–1451.

Bhimani, R. (2008). Intrathecal baclofen therapy in adults and guideline for clinical nursing care. *Rehabilitation Nursing, 33(3)*, 110–116.

Darlington, A. B. (2010). The Botox© phenomenon. *Plastic Surgical Nursing, 30(1)*, 22–26.

Drummer, O. H. (2008). The role of drugs in road safety. *Australian Prescriber, 31*, 33–35.

Farrell, M. & Dempsey, J. (2014). *Smeltzer & Bare's Textbook of Medical-Surgical Nursing* (3rd edn). Sydney: Lippincott Williams & Wilkins.

Goodman, L. S., Brunton, L. L., Chabner, B. & Knollmann, B. C. (2011). *Goodman and Gilman's Pharmacological Basis of Therapeutics* (12th edn). New York: McGraw-Hill.

McKenna, L. & Mirkov, S. (2019). *McKenna's Drug Handbook for Nursing and Midwifery* (8th edn). Sydney: Wolters Kluwer Health Australia.

Mitchell-Brown, F. (2012). Malignant hyperthermia: Turn down the heat. *Nursing, 42(5)*, 38–45.

Porth, C. M. (2011). *Essentials of Pathophysiology: Concepts of Altered Health States* (3rd edn). Philadelphia: Lippincott Williams & Wilkins.

Porth, C. M. (2009). *Pathophysiology: Concepts of Altered Health States* (8th edn). Philadelphia: Lippincott Williams & Wilkins.

Scheinberg, A. (2009). Clinical use of botulinum toxin. *Australian Prescriber, 32*, 39–42.

CHECK YOUR UNDERSTANDING

Answers to the questions in this chapter can be found in Appendix A at the back of this book.

MULTIPLE CHOICE

Select the best answer to the following.

1. A muscle spasm often results from:
   a. damage to the basal ganglia.
   b. central nervous system damage.
   c. injury to the musculoskeletal system.
   d. chemical imbalance within the CNS.
2. Muscle spasticity is the result of:
   a. direct damage to a muscle cell.
   b. overstretching of a muscle.
   c. tearing of a ligament.
   d. damage to neurons within the CNS.
3. Signs and symptoms of tetanus, which includes severe muscle spasm, are best treated with:
   a. baclofen.
   b. diazepam.
   c. orphenadrine.
   d. botulinum toxin A.
4. The drug of choice for a person experiencing severe muscle spasms and pain precipitated by anxiety is:
   a. orphenadrine.
   b. baclofen.
   c. diazepam.
   d. botulinum toxin A.
5. Dantrolene (*Dantrium*) differs from the other skeletal muscle relaxants because:
   a. it acts in the highest levels of the CNS.
   b. it is used to treat muscle spasms as well as muscle spasticity.
   c. it cannot be used to treat neuromuscular disorders.
   d. it acts directly within the skeletal muscle fibre and not within the CNS.
6. The use of neuromuscular junction blockers may sometimes cause a condition known as malignant hyperthermia. The drug of choice for prevention or treatment of this condition is:
   a. baclofen.
   b. diazepam.
   c. dantrolene.
   d. orphenadrine.
7. Dantrolene is associated with potentially fatal cellular damage. If a person's condition is being managed with dantrolene, the person should:
   a. have repeated FBCs during therapy.
   b. have renal function tests done monthly.
   c. be monitored for signs of liver damage and have liver function tests done regularly.
   d. have a thorough eye examination before and periodically during therapy.

MULTIPLE RESPONSE

Select all that apply.

1. Spasmolytics, or centrally acting muscle relaxants, block the reflexes in the central nervous system that lead to spasm. While a person is taking one of these drugs, which of the following interventions should be implemented?
   a. rest for the affected muscle
   b. heat to the affected area
   c. ice packs to the affected area
   d. use of anti-inflammatory agents
   e. body temperature check every 2 hours to watch for malignant hyperthermia
   f. positioning to decrease pain and spasm
2. Muscle relaxants would be used in which of the following circumstances?
   a. to treat spasticity related to spinal cord injury
   b. to treat spasticity that contributes to locomotion, upright position or increase in function
   c. to treat spasticity that is related to toxins, such as tetanus
   d. to treat spasticity that is a result of neuromuscular degeneration
   e. to reduce the severity of head position associated with cervical dystonia
   f. to reduce the appearance of frown lines (glabellar lines)

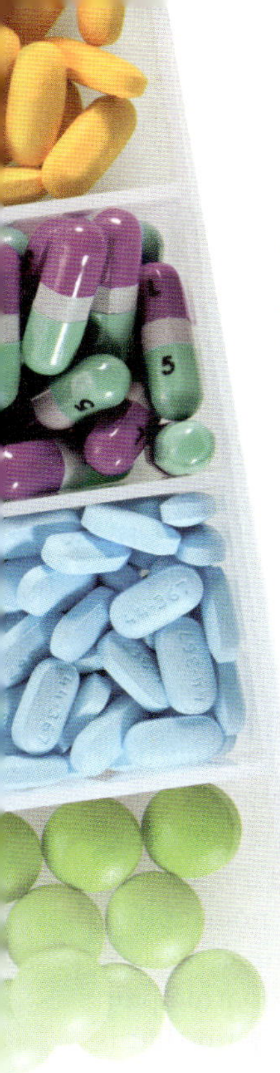

Opioids, opioid antagonists and antimigraine agents

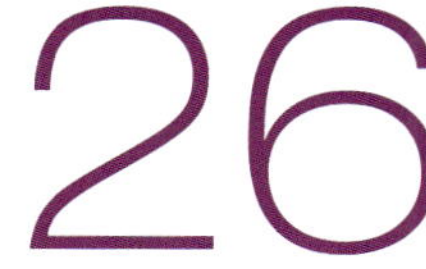

Learning objectives

On completing this chapter you should be able to:

1. Outline the gate theory of pain and explain therapeutic ways to block pain using the gate theory.
2. Describe the therapeutic actions, indications, pharmacokinetics, contraindications, most common adverse reactions and important drug–drug interactions associated with opioids and antimigraine agents.
3. Discuss the use of the different classes of opioids, opioid antagonists and antimigraine agents across the lifespan.
4. Compare and contrast the prototype drugs morphine, naloxone, ergotamine and sumatriptan with other drugs in their respective classes.
5. Outline the care considerations, including important teaching points, for people receiving an opioid, an opioid antagonist or an antimigraine drug.

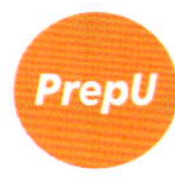

Test your current knowledge of opioids, opioid antagonists and antimigraine agents with a PrepU Practice Quiz!

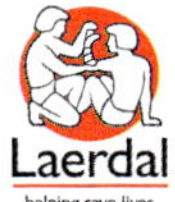

Simulation-based learning

On completion of the chapter, consider the scenario of Doris Bowman (Part 2) who arrives in the recovery room after undergoing major abdominal surgery and is complaining of pain. Consider Doris' pain management in this case. How might the concepts learnt in this chapter apply more broadly to postoperative pain management?

Then, work through the second scenario of Marilyn Hughes (Part 2) who has had a recent fall. Consider how the concepts learnt in this chapter relating to pain management apply to her case.

Glossary of key terms

A fibres: large-diameter nerve fibres that carry peripheral impulses associated with touch and temperature to the spinal cord

A-delta fibres: small-diameter nerve fibres that carry peripheral impulses associated with pain to the spinal cord

C fibres: unmyelinated, slow-conducting fibres that carry peripheral impulses associated with pain to the spinal cord

ergot derivative: drug that causes a vascular constriction in the brain and the periphery; relieves or prevents migraine headaches but is associated with many adverse effects

gate control theory: theory that states that the transmission of a nerve impulse can be modulated at various points along its path by descending fibres from the brain that close the 'gate' and block transmission of pain information and by A fibres that are able to block transmission in the dorsal horn by closing the gate for transmission for the A-delta and C fibres

migraine headache: headache characterised by severe, unilateral, pulsating head pain associated with systemic effects, including GI upset and sensitisation to light and sound; related to a hyperperfusion of the brain from arterial dilation

opioid agonists: drugs that react at opioid-receptor sites to stimulate the effects of the receptors

opioid agonists–antagonists: drugs that react at some opioid-receptor sites to stimulate their activity and at other opioid-receptor sites to block activity

opioid antagonists: drugs that block the opioid-receptor sites; used to counteract the effects of opioids or to treat an overdose of opioids

opioid receptors: receptor sites on nerves that react with endorphins and encephalins, which are receptive to opioid drugs

opioids: drugs, originally derived from opium, that react with specific opioid receptors throughout the body

pain: a sensory and emotional experience associated with actual or potential tissue damage

spinothalamic tract: nerve pathway from the spine to the thalamus along which pain impulses are carried to the brain

triptan: selective serotonin-receptor blocker that causes a vascular constriction of cranial vessels; used to treat acute migraine attacks

OPIOIDS
Opioid agonists
alfentanil
codeine
fentanyl
hydromorphone
methadone
(P) morphine
oxycodone
pethidine
remifentanil
tapentadol
tramadol

Opioid agonists–antagonists
buprenorphine

Opioid antagonists
(P) naloxone
naltrexone

ANTIMIGRAINE AGENTS
Ergot derivatives
(P) ergotamine

Triptans
eletriptan
naratriptan
rizatriptan
(P) sumatriptan
zolmitriptan

Pain, by definition, is a sensory and emotional experience associated with actual or potential tissue damage. The perception of pain is part of the clinical presentation in many disorders and is one of the hardest sensations for people to cope with during the course of a disease or dysfunction. The drugs involved in the management of severe pain, whether acute or chronic, are discussed in this chapter. These agents all work in the central nervous system (CNS) – the brain and the spinal cord – to alter the way that pain impulses arriving from peripheral nerves are processed. These agents can change the perception and tolerance of pain. Two major types of drugs are considered here: the opioids – the opium derivatives that are used to treat many types of pain; and the antimigraine drugs, which are reserved for the treatment of migraine headache, a type of severe headache. Opioid antagonists, which are used to block the effects of the opioids in cases of overdose, are also discussed.

PAIN

Pain is described as an unpleasant sensation and emotional experience. In many ways it is a subjective experience. The physiological processes that cause pain are perceived and reacted to in different ways because of learned experiences, cultural differences and environmental stimuli. Pain occurs whenever tissues are damaged. The injury to cells releases many chemicals, including kinins and prostaglandins, which stimulate specific sensory nerves. Pain can be acute or chronic. Acute pain occurs in response to recent tissue damage or injury. This type of pain makes a person aware of an injury and should lead to measures to care for the injury and teaches the person to avoid similar situations that could cause this pain. Chronic pain is constant or intermittent pain that keeps occurring long past the time the injured area would be expected to heal. Chronic pain can cause a stress reaction, interrupt much-needed sleep and interfere with all of the activities of daily living. Pain can also be classified by location. 'Where does it hurt?' is a common question in assessing pain. Sometimes the location of the pain is a direct indicator of where the tissue damage has occurred. In some cases so-called referred pain occurs. A person experiencing pain from damage to the heart muscle may actually feel the pain in the neck or jaw. The sensation of pain is experienced in a different area of the body. Referred pain often follows predictable pathways, which helps health care providers figure out where the injury has occurred. Pain can be further classified by originating source as nociceptive, neuropathic or psychogenic. Nociceptive pain is caused by a direct stimulus to a pain receptor. Neuropathic pain is caused by nerve injury. Psychogenic pain is pain that is associated with emotional, psychological or behavioural stimuli.

Pain impulse transmission and perception

Two small-diameter sensory nerves, called the **A-delta and C fibres**, respectively, respond to stimulation by generating nerve impulses that produce pain sensations. The A-delta fibres are small, myelinated fibres that respond quickly to acute pain. The C fibres are unmyelinated and are slow conducting. Pain impulses from the skin, subcutaneous tissues, muscles and deep visceral structures are conducted to the dorsal, or posterior, horn of the spinal cord on these fibres. In the spinal cord, these nerves form synapses with spinal cord nerves that then send impulses to the brain (Figure 26.1).

In addition, large-diameter sensory nerves enter the dorsal horn of the spinal cord. These so-called **A fibres** do not transmit pain impulses; instead, they transmit sensations associated with touch and temperature. The A fibres, which are larger and conduct impulses more rapidly than do the smaller fibres, can actually block the ability of the smaller fibres to transmit their signals to the secondary neurons in the spinal cord. The dorsal horn, therefore, can be both excitatory and inhibitory with regard to pain impulses that are transmitted from the periphery.

The impulses reaching the dorsal horn are transmitted upwards towards the brain by a number of specific ascending nerve pathways. These pathways run from the spinal cord into the thalamus, where they form synapses with various nerve cells that transmit the information to the cerebral cortex, along the **spinothalamic tracts.** According to the **gate control theory**, the transmission of these impulses can be modulated or adjusted all along these tracts. All along the spinal cord, the interneurons can act as 'gates' by blocking the ascending transmission of pain impulses. It is thought that the gates can be closed by stimulation of the larger A fibres and by descending impulses coming down the spinal cord from higher levels in such areas as the cerebral cortex, the limbic system and the reticular activating system.

The inhibitory influence of the higher brain centres on the transmission of pain impulses helps to explain much of the mystery associated with pain. Several factors, including learned experiences, cultural expectations, individual tolerance and the placebo effect, can activate the descending inhibitory nerves from the upper CNS. These other factors need to be considered and incorporated into pain management strategies, which usually involve the use of drugs. For example, the placebo effect, stress reduction, acupuncture and back rubs (which stimulate the A fibres) can all play important roles in the effective management of pain.

Pain receptors

Opioid receptors are receptor sites that respond to naturally occurring peptides, the endorphins and the encephalins. These receptor sites are found in the CNS, on nerves in the periphery and on cells in the gastrointestinal (GI) tract. In the brainstem, opioid receptors help to control blood pressure, pupil diameter, GI secretions and the chemoreceptor trigger zone (CTZ) that regulates nausea and vomiting, cough and respiration. In the spinal cord and thalamus, these receptors help to integrate and relate incoming information about pain. The endorphins and encephalins normally modulate the pain information coming into the brain. Endorphins are released during stress to block the sensation of pain. Professional athletes may be injured during an important game and have no sensation of pain or injury because their stress reaction is highly activated, and the endorphins are blocking pain transmission into the brain. In the hypothalamus, stimulation of the opioid receptors may interrelate the endocrine and neural responses to pain. In the limbic system, the receptors incorporate emotional aspects of pain and response to pain. At peripheral nerve sites, they may block the release of neurotransmitters that are related to pain and inflammation.

Pain perception

Many factors play a role in a person's perception of pain. Past experience has a big impact on how pain is

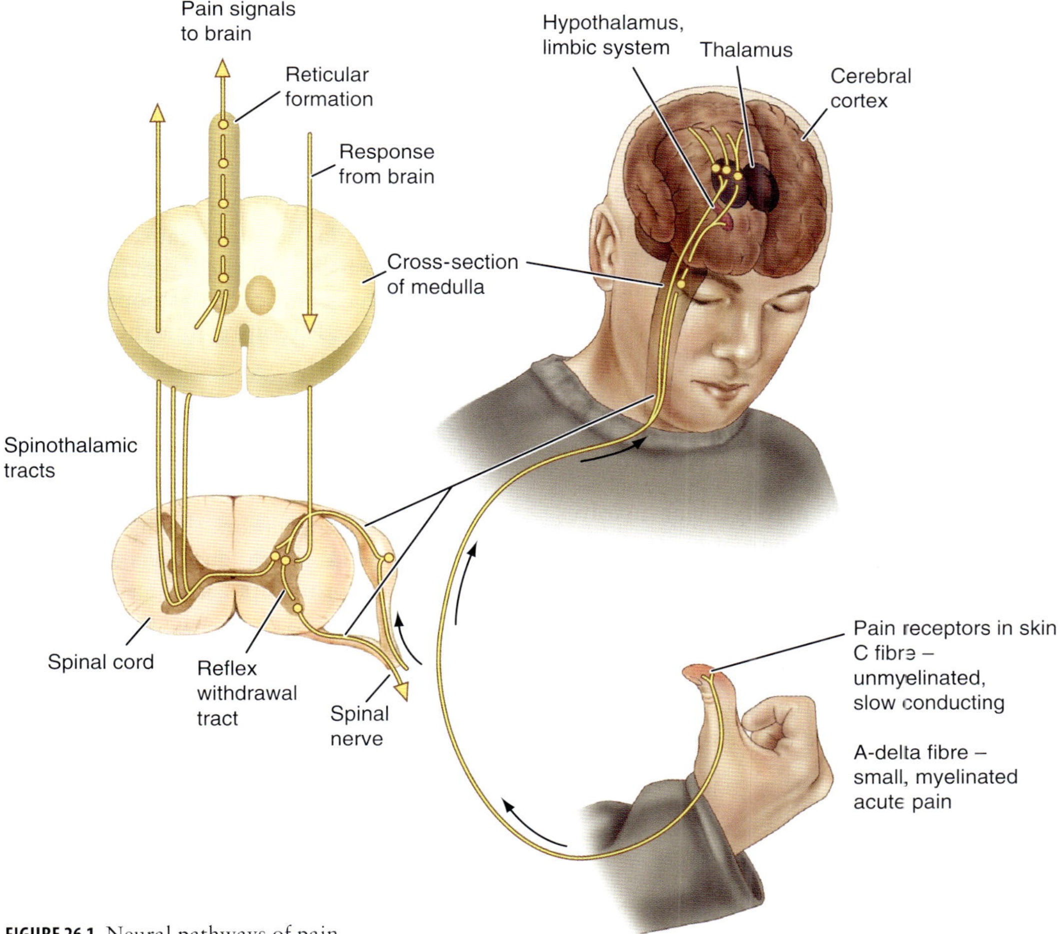

FIGURE 26.1 Neural pathways of pain.

perceived. Having experienced pain in the past, a person may fear the intensity it could reach and the overall impact of that pain. Learned response to pain also plays a large role. Children learn the accepted response to painful stimuli when growing up. Some children are taught to ignore pain and deal with it without showing emotion. Some children learn that reacting to pain can lead to much-wanted attention. The environmental setting in which the pain occurs also has an influence on perception and response to pain. A parent may not be willing to admit pain when the children are present, feeling that the role of the parent is to be strong. If you cut your finger when you are alone, you may perceive pain and react loudly. If you cut your finger when you are surrounded by young children, you may show no reaction and just go on with your activity. These varied influences on pain perception and response often make it very difficult to effectively evaluate and manage pain.

Pain management

Accurately assessing pain can lead to effective pain management. Because so many factors play a role in pain perception and it is very subjective, assessment has to depend on the person's report of pain. Health care providers often use a scale system to evaluate an individual's pain. Individuals may be asked to rank their pain on a scale from 0 to 10, with 0 being no pain and 10 being the worst possible pain. Some pain scales use drawings of faces and ask the person to pick the face that most reflects the pain they feel. Numerous methods, both non-pharmacological and pharmacological, may be used to manage pain. Non-pharmacological treatments can include warmth, massage, positioning, acupuncture or meditation. Pharmacological methods often include the use of non-steroidal anti-inflammatory drugs (NSAIDs) or paracetamol (Chapter 16) for tissue-related pain or atypical antipsychotics or other CNS depressants for the treatment of neurogenic pain. These methods can be used individually or in combination. The goal is to achieve maximum pain relief.

One major method of pain management involves the use of **opioids**. The opioids, or narcotics, were first derived from the opium plant. Although most opioids are now synthetically prepared, their chemical structure resembles that of the original plant alkaloids. All drugs in this class are similar, in that they occupy specific opioid receptors in the CNS. Their actions in the body are related to the stimulation of the various opioid receptors that they occupy.

KEY POINTS

- When tissue is injured, various chemicals are released and pain results.
- A-delta and C fibres carry pain impulses to the spinal cord.
- According to the gate control theory of pain, impulses travel from the spine to the cortex via tracts that can be modulated along the way at specific gates. These gates can be closed to block the transmission of pain impulses by descending nerves from the upper CNS, which relate to emotion, culture, placebo effect and stress, and by large diameter sensory A fibres, which are associated with touch.
- Endogenous endorphins and encephalins react with opioid receptors to regulate the transmission of pain.
- Opioids are derived from the opium plant; they bind to opioid receptors to relieve pain and promote feelings of wellbeing or euphoria.

OPIOIDS

The opioid drugs used vary with the type of opioid receptors with which they react. This accounts for a change in pain relief, as well as a variation in the side effects that can be anticipated. Four types of opioid receptors have been identified: mu (μ), kappa (κ), beta (β) and sigma (σ). The mu-receptors are primarily pain-blocking receptors. Besides analgesia, mu-receptors also account for respiratory depression, a feeling of euphoria, decreased GI activity, pupil constriction and the development of physical dependence. The kappa-receptors are associated with some analgesia and with pupillary constriction, sedation and dysphoria. The beta-receptors react with encephalins in the periphery to modulate pain transmission. The sigma-receptors cause pupillary dilation and may be responsible for the hallucinations, dysphoria and psychoses that can occur with opioid use. The administration of opioids requires specific considerations related to age (Box 26.1).

OPIOID AGONISTS

The **opioid agonists** (Table 26.1) are drugs that react with the opioid receptors throughout the body to cause analgesia, sedation or euphoria (Figure 26.2). Anticipated effects other than analgesia are mediated by the types of opioid receptors affected by each drug. Because of the potential for the development of physical dependence while taking these drugs, the opioid agonists are classified as controlled substances. The degree of control is determined by the relative ability of each drug to cause physical dependence. Opioid agonists include alfentanil (*Rapifen*), codeine (generic), fentanyl (*Abstral*, *Actiq*, *Durogesic*, *Sublimaze*), hydromorphone (*Dilaudid*, *Jurnista*), methadone (*Biodone*, *Physeptone*), morphine (*Anamorph*, *Sevredol*, *MS Contin* and others), oxycodone (*Endone*, *OxyContin*, *Oxynorm*, *Proladone*), pethidine (generic), remifentanil (*Ultiva*), tapentadol (*Palexia SR*) (not available in New Zealand) and tramadol (*Durotram XR*, *Lodam*, *Tramal* and others).

Therapeutic actions and indications

The opioid agonists act at specific opioid-receptor sites in the CNS to produce analgesia, sedation and a sense of wellbeing. These preparations are also used as antitussives and as adjuncts to general anaesthesia to produce rapid analgesia, sedation and respiratory depression. Indications for opioid agonists include relief of severe acute or chronic pain, preoperative medication, analgesia during anaesthesia and specific individual indications, depending on their receptor affinity. (See Table 26.1 for usual indications for each opioid agonist.) Accurate calculation of a dose is crucial to prevent overdosing.

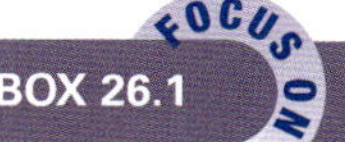

BOX 26.1 Drug therapy across the lifespan

Opioids

CHILDREN

The safety and effectiveness of many of these drugs have not been established in children. If an opioid is used, the dose should be calculated very carefully, and the child should be monitored closely for the adverse effects associated with opioid use.

Opioids that have an established paediatric dose include codeine, fentanyl (but not transdermal fentanyl), hydrocodone, pethidine and morphine. Oxycodone is not recommended for children.

Methadone is not recommended as an analgesic in children. If a child older than 16 years of age requires an opioid agonist–antagonist, buprenorphine–naloxone is the preparation of choice. Naloxone is the drug of choice for reversal of opioid effects and opioid overdose in children.

ADULTS

Adults being treated for acute pain should be reassured that the risk of addiction to an opioid during treatment is remote. They should be encouraged to ask for pain medication before the pain is acute, to get better coverage for their pain. Many institutions allow people to self-regulate intravenous drips to control their pain postoperatively.

PREGNANCY AND BREASTFEEDING

The opioids are contraindicated or should only be used with caution during pregnancy because of the potential for adverse effects on the fetus. These drugs enter breast milk and can cause opioid effects in the baby, so caution should be used during breastfeeding. Morphine and pethidine are often used for analgesia for labour. The mother should be monitored closely for adverse reactions, and, if the drug is used over a prolonged labour, the newborn infant should be monitored for opioid effects such as respiratory depression. Naloxone should be readily available for the baby if the mother has received an opioid in the hours immediately before the birth.

OLDER ADULTS

Elderly people should be specifically asked whether they require pain medication. Because many older people can recall a time when nurses were able to spend more time with people, they may tend to believe that the nurse will meet their needs.

Older people are more likely to experience the adverse effects associated with these drugs, including CNS, GI and cardiovascular (CV) effects.

Because older people often have renal or hepatic impairment, they are also more likely to have toxic levels of the drug related to changes in metabolism and excretion. The older person should have safety measures in effect – side rails, call light, assistance to ambulate – when receiving one of these drugs in the hospital setting.

TABLE 26.1 *DRUGS IN FOCUS* Opioids

Drug name	Dosage/route	Usual indications
Opioid agonists		
alfentanil (*Rapifen*)	Spontaneous ventilation: 7 micrograms/kg by slow IV injection Controlled ventilation: 20–50 micrograms/kg by slow IV injection	Analgesic supplement and anaesthetic induction agent in inpatient surgery
codeine (generic)	Adults (for pain): 30–60 mg (usual 30 mg) every 4–6 hours, maximum 300 mg/day Adults (antitussive): 15–30 mg q 6–8 hours Child (antitussive): 0.25–0.5 mg/kg/dose q 6–8 hours, maximum 240 mg/day, maximum duration 3 days Codeine tablets 30 mg are contraindicated in children < 12 years	Relief of mild to moderate pain; relief of coughing induced by mechanical or chemical irritation of the respiratory tract

Continued on following page

TABLE 26.1 DRUGS IN FOCUS Opioids *(continued)*

Drug name	Dosage/route	Usual indications
Opioid agonists *(continued)*		
fentanyl (*Abstral, Actiq, Duragesic, Sublimaze*)	Injection: adults, 50–100 micrograms (elderly 25–50 micrograms) IM 30–60 min preoperatively, then 25–50 micrograms IM or IV maintenance Children > 2 years, 2–3 micrograms/kg/dose IV (general anaesthesia), 0.5–1 microgram/kg IV, maximum 50 micrograms/dose (procedural sedation, analgesia) Sublingual tablets: adults, initially 100 micrograms to a maximum of 800 micrograms/dose Orally dissolving tablets: adults, initially 100 micrograms, to a maximum of 800 micrograms/dose Lozenges: adults, initially 200 micrograms, increasing to a maximum of 1200 micrograms/dose Patches: adults, 12 micrograms every 72 hours or by calculation from previous day's opiate dose, increasing or decreasing as necessary. Not for children < 12 years. Use caution in individuals < 18 years	Injection only: for analgesia before, during and after surgery Transdermal patch is for management of persistent chronic pain in opioid-tolerant patients Sublingual tablets, orally dissolving tablets and lozenges should only be administered to opioid-tolerant patients for persistent cancer pain Patients can be considered opioid tolerant if they take at least 60 mg oral morphine daily, at least 25 micrograms of transdermal fentanyl per hour, at least 30 mg of oxycodone daily, at least 8 mg of oral hydromorphone daily or an equianalgesic dose of another opioid for a week or longer
hydromorphone (*Dilaudid, Jurnista*)	Immediate-release tablets (*Dilaudid*), adults: starting dose 2–4 mg every 4 hours, then titrate according to response Prolonged release (*Jurnista*), adults: starting dose 4–8 mg every 24 hours. Do not give more than once in 24 hours. Titrate at every fourth dose. Parenteral, adults: 1–2 mg every 4–6 hours (IM, SC) or 0.5–1 mg by slow IV over 2–3 minutes	Relief of moderate to severe pain in adults
methadone (*Biodone, Physeptone*)	Pain management, adults: 5–10 mg SC, IM, PO q 6–8 hours Opioid addiction: initially 10–20 mg/day, increasing by a maximum 5–10 mg/day or 30 mg/week; maintenance: 30–50 mg/day (maximum 80 mg/day)	Relief of severe pain; detoxification and temporary maintenance treatment of opioid addiction in adults
(P) morphine sulfate (*Anamorph, Kapanol, m-Eslon, MS Contin, Sevredol*)	Adult: 5–20 mg IM or SC or 15–30 mg PO q 4–6 hours Paediatric, > 2 years: 0.1–0.2 mg/kg/dose (maximum 15 mg) 4-hourly IM or SC, or 0.2–0.5 mg/kg/dose (maximum 5 mg) PO 4–6-hourly, or 0.3–0.6 mg/kg/dose (sustained release) PO 12-hourly	Relief of moderate to severe chronic and acute pain; preoperatively and postoperatively and during labour
oxycodone (*OxyContin, Oxynorm, Endone, Proladone*)	Immediate release: initially 5 mg PO q 6 hours, titrate according to response Controlled release: initially 10 mg PO q 12 hours, increasing as necessary Suppository: 30 mg PR q 6–8 hours as needed	Relief of moderate to severe pain in adults
pethidine (generic)	Adult: 25–100 mg IM, SC or 25–50 mg slow IV q 3–4 hours Paediatric: 0.5–2 mg/kg IM or SC q 3–4 hours (maximum 100 mg)	Relief of moderate to severe pain, preoperative analgesia and support of anaesthesia, and obstetrical analgesia
remifentanil (*Ultiva*)	Adult and children > 2 years: dose determined by general anaesthetic being used	Analgesic for use during general anaesthesia **Special considerations:** must be under the direct supervision of anaesthesia practitioner

TABLE 26.1 **DRUGS IN FOCUS** **Opioids *(continued)***

Drug name	Dosage/route	Usual indications
Opioid agonists *(continued)*		
tapentadol (*Palexia IR, Palexia SR*)	Adult: initially 50–100 mg every 4–6 hours increasing as needed to a maximum of 600 mg/day	Relief of moderate to severe chronic pain
tramadol (*Durotram XR, Tramal, Tramal SR*)	Adult, immediate release: 50–100 mg 2–3 times daily increasing to a maximum of 400 mg/day; sustained release: 100–200 mg twice daily increasing to a maximum of 400 mg/day	Relief of moderate to moderately severe pain **Special considerations:** limit use in people with a history of addictions
Opioid agonists–antagonists		
buprenorphine (*Norspan, Temgesic*)	200–400 micrograms SL q 6–8 hours, 300–600 micrograms IM or IV q 6–8 hours or 1 transdermal patch every 7 days	Treatment of mild to moderate pain
Opioid antagonists		
(P) naloxone (*Narcan*)	Adult, opioid overdose: initially 0.4–2 mg SC IM but preferably IV; may repeat every 2–3 min to a maximum of 10 mg Paediatric: 0.01 mg/kg IV, IM or SC Neonatal: 0.01 mg/kg IV, IM or SC q 2–3 minutes	Diagnosis of opioid overdose, reversal of opioid effects
naltrexone (*ReVia*)	Adult: 50 mg/day PO for up to 12 weeks	Adjunct treatment of alcohol or opioid dependence in adults

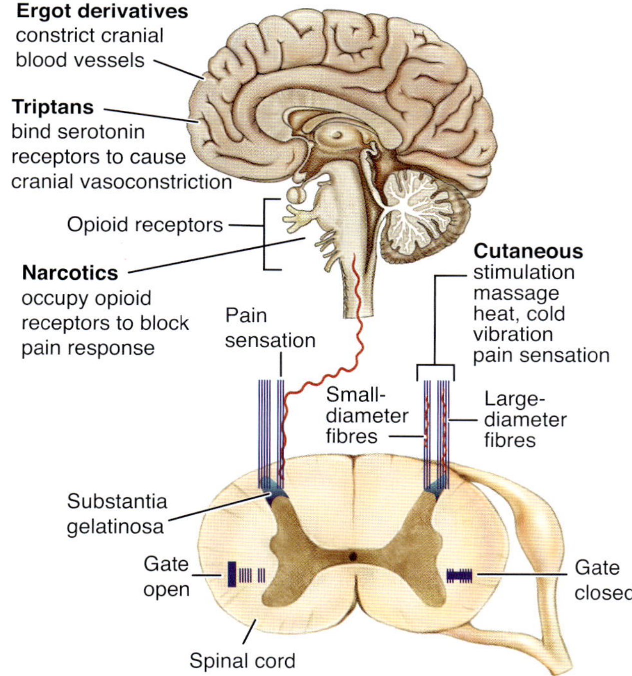

FIGURE 26.2 Sites of action. Opioid agonists occupy opioid receptors to block pain response. Ergot derivatives constrict cranial blood vessels and triptans bind serotonin receptors to cause cranial vasoconstriction.

In deciding which opioid to use in any particular situation, it is important to consider all of the aspects of the person's condition and to select the drug that will be most effective in each situation with the fewest adverse effects. Each person is different, and their response to a drug is also different (Box 26.2). For example, if an analgesic that is long acting but not too sedating is desired for an outpatient, hydromorphone might fit those objectives. Fentanyl, which is available for injection, is also available as a lozenge for treating breakthrough pain, as a transdermal patch and in an ionic delivery system, which activates the release of the drug as needed for treating breakthrough pain in people with cancer. See the Critical thinking scenario for information about using morphine to relieve pain.

Pharmacokinetics

Intravenous (IV) administration is the most reliable way to achieve therapeutic levels of opioids. Intramuscular (IM) and subcutaneous (SC) administration offer varying rates of absorption, and absorption is slower in females than in males because of the normal fat content of female muscles and tissue. These drugs undergo hepatic metabolism and are generally excreted in the urine and bile. Half-life periods vary widely, depending on the drug being used. These agents cross the placenta and are known to enter breast milk.

Contraindications and cautions

The opioid agonists are contraindicated in the following conditions: presence of any known allergy to any opioid agonist *to avoid hypersensitivity reactions*; diarrhoea caused by toxic poisons *because depression of GI activity could lead to increased absorption and toxicity*; and after biliary surgery or surgical anastomoses

BOX 26.2 Differences in responses to opioid therapy

Because of physical and cultural differences among various ethnic groups, people from certain groups respond differently to particular medications. Nurses should keep in mind that people in some ethnic groups are genetically predisposed to metabolise medications differently. For example, people of Arabian descent may not achieve the same pain relief from opioids as people in other ethnic groups; their inborn differences in metabolism may require larger doses to achieve therapeutic effects.

Some African American people seem to have a decreased sensitivity to the pain-relieving qualities of some opioids, although the reason for this is unknown. Moreover, increasing the dosage of these medications may not increase the level of pain relief and actually may be toxic. In such cases, another class of medication might be used to 'boost' the pain-relieving qualities of the opioid.

Among some immigrant and first-generation Asian Americans, it may not be socially acceptable to show strong emotion, such as that associated with pain. The sensitive nurse will frequently ask such people if they are comfortable or require additional medication.

Although many of these studies were done on American people, ethnic minority groups (eg, people of Asian descent, people from the Middle East) are increasing in New Zealand and Australia. Therefore, health care providers will need to carefully monitor opioid responses of people from ethnic minority groups.

because of the adverse effects associated with slowed GI activity due to opioids.

Opioids are classified as pregnancy category C, therefore their use is not recommended during pregnancy. If used during pregnancy or labour they may cause withdrawal symptoms and/or respiratory depression in the newborn infant. Many sources recommend waiting 4–6 hours after receiving an opioid before breastfeeding the baby if an opioid is needed for pain control.

Caution should be used in people with respiratory dysfunction, *which could be exacerbated by the respiratory depression caused by these drugs*; recent GI or genitourinary (GU) surgery, acute abdomen or ulcerative colitis, *which could become worse with the depressive effects of the opioids*; head injuries, alcoholism, delirium tremens or cerebral vascular disease, *which could be exacerbated by the CNS effects of the drugs*; liver or renal dysfunction, *which could alter the metabolism and excretion of the drugs*; and during pregnancy, labour or breastfeeding *because of potential adverse effects on the fetus or neonate, including respiratory depression.*

Adverse effects

The most frequently seen adverse effects associated with opioid agonists relate to their effects on various opioid receptors. Respiratory depression with apnoea, cardiac arrest and shock may result from opioid-induced respiratory centre depression. Orthostatic hypotension is commonly seen with some opioids. Gastrointestinal

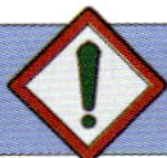

CRITICAL THINKING SCENARIO

Using morphine to relieve pain

THE SITUATION

L.M., a 25-year-old businessman, was in a car crash and suffered a fractured pelvis, a fractured left tibia, a fractured right humerus, and multiple contusions and abrasions. For the first 2 days after surgery to reduce the fractures, L.M. was heavily sedated. As healing progressed, he was taught to use a patient-controlled analgesia (PCA) system using morphine. PCA provides a baseline, constant infusion of morphine and gives the person control of the system to add bolus doses of morphine if they feel that pain is not being controlled. The system prevents overdose by locking out extra doses until a specific period of time has elapsed. L.M. became agitated when he was not able to give himself a bolus because the appropriate time between boluses had not elapsed. The nurse working with L.M. noted an increase in blood pressure, pulse and respiration. L.M. had no fever. He did seem very anxious and rated his pain at 10. The nurse tried several non-pharmacological measures to alleviate the pain and spent time talking with L.M. and reassuring him. By day 5, L.M. was switched to an oral morphine and plans were made to wean him from the opioids.

CRITICAL THINKING

What basic principles must be included in the care plan for L.M.? *Think about the difficult position the floor nurse is in when L.M. begins demanding pain relief before the prescribed time limit.*

What implications will L.M.'s agitation have on the way that the staff respond to him and on other people in the area?

What other measures could be used to help relieve pain and make the opioid more effective?

What plans could the health care team make with L.M. to give him more control over his situation and increase the chances that the pain relief will be effective?

DISCUSSION

In assessing L.M.'s response to drug therapy, you suspect that the morphine was not providing the desired therapeutic effect. Numerous research studies have shown that, in general, the dose of opioids prescribed for acute pain relief provides inadequate analgesic coverage. It could be that the dose of morphine ordered for L.M. was just not sufficient to relieve his pain. This person has many causes of acute pain and will heal more quickly if the pain is managed better. He has requested more drugs because the dose is too small or the intervals between doses are too long to effectively relieve his pain. Other measures may be successful in helping the morphine relieve the pain. Back rubs, environmental controls to decrease excessive stimuli (eg, noise, lighting, temperature, interruptions) and stress reduction may all be useful. Discussing the possibility of increasing the drug dose with the doctor would be appropriate.

L.M. may be very anxious about his injuries, and the opportunity to vent his feelings and concerns may alleviate some of the tension associated with pain. He may fear that if he does not cover the pain before it gets too bad, it will be very hard to get any pain relief. The staff can work on this concern and figure out a way to reassure him.

The health care team should try to discuss the concerns with L.M., including the concern about physical dependency. L.M. is a businessman and may respond positively to having some input into his care; he may even offer suggestions as to how he could cope better and adjust to his situation. Cortical impulses can close gates as effectively as descending inhibitory pathways, and stimulation of the cortical pathways through education and active involvement should be considered an important aspect of pain relief. Because L.M.'s injuries are extensive, a long-term approach should be taken to his care. The sooner that L.M. can be involved, the better the situation will be for everyone involved.

CARE GUIDE FOR L.M.: OPIOIDS

Assessment: history and examination

Assess history of allergies to any opioid drug, respiratory depression, GI or biliary surgery, hepatic or renal dysfunction, alcoholism or convulsive disorders.

Focus the physical examination on the following:

CV: blood pressure, pulse rate, peripheral perfusion, ECG

CNS: orientation, affect, reflexes, grip strength

Skin: colour, lesions, texture, temperature

GI: abdominal examination, bowel sounds

Respiratory: respiration, adventitious sounds

Laboratory tests: renal and liver function tests

Implementation

Provide an opioid antagonist and facilities for assisted ventilation during IV administration.

Provide comfort and safety measures: orientation, accurate timing of doses, monitoring for extravasation and additional measures for pain relief to increase effects.

Provide support and reassurance to deal with drug effects and addiction potential.

Provide teaching about the drug, dosage, drug effects and symptoms of serious reactions to report.

Evaluation

Evaluate drug effects: relief of pain, sedation.

Monitor for adverse effects: CNS effects (multiple), respiratory depression, rash, skin changes, GI depression, constipation.

Monitor drug–drug interactions: increased respiratory depression, sedation, coma with barbiturate anaesthetics, monoamine oxidase inhibitors, phenothiazines.

Evaluate the effectiveness of the teaching program.

Evaluate the effectiveness of comfort and safety measures.

TEACHING FOR L.M.

- An opioid is used to relieve pain. Do not hesitate to take this drug if you feel uncomfortable. Remember that it is important to use the drug before the pain becomes severe and thus more difficult to treat.
- Common effects of these drugs include:
  - *Constipation*: your health care provider will suggest appropriate measures to alleviate this common problem.
  - *Dizziness, drowsiness and visual changes*: if any of these occur, avoid driving, operating complex machinery or performing delicate tasks. If these effects occur in the hospital, the side rails on the bed may be raised for your protection.
  - *Nausea and loss of appetite*: taking the drug with food may help. Lying quietly until these sensations pass may also help to alleviate this problem.
- Report any of the following to your health care provider: *severe nausea or vomiting, skin rash, or shortness of breath or difficulty breathing.*
- Avoid the use of alcohol, antihistamines and other over-the-counter drugs while taking this drug. Many of these drugs could interact with this opioid.
- Tell any doctor, nurse, dentist or other health care provider involved in your care that you are taking this drug.
- Keep this drug and all medications out of the reach of children.
- Do not take any leftover medication for other disorders and do not let anyone else take your medication.
- Take this drug exactly as prescribed. Regular medical follow-up is necessary to evaluate the effects of this drug on your body.

BOX 26.3 Laxative for dealing with opioid-induced constipation

One of the most uncomfortable side effects of opioid use is constipation. Frequently, when ordering an opioid for pain, a prescriber will also order a laxative to avert serious constipation discomfort. When a person is on long-term opioids for controlling pain in cases of cancer or in hospice settings where palliative care uses opioids to make people comfortable, constipation can be a real problem. In 2008, methylnaltrexone bromide (*Relistor*) was approved for the treatment of opioid-induced constipation in people who are receiving palliative care and who no longer respond to traditional laxatives. *Relistor* is a peripherally acting, mu-specific opioid antagonist. It blocks the mu-receptors responsible for constipation related to opioid use. *Relistor* is given by SC injection once each day. It is rapidly absorbed from the tissues, reaching peak levels in 30 minutes. It is excreted primarily unchanged in the urine, with a half-life of 8 hours. The adverse effects associated with the drug are related to the increase in GI activity that occurs – diarrhoea, abdominal pain, flatulence and nausea.

Prototype summary: morphine

Indications: relief of moderate to severe acute or chronic pain; preoperative medication; component of combination therapy for severe chronic pain; intraspinal to reduce intractable pain.

Actions: acts as an agonist at specific opioid receptors in the CNS to produce analgesia, euphoria and sedation.

Pharmacokinetics:

Route	Onset	Peak	Duration
Oral	Varies	60 min	5–7 hours
SC	Rapid	50–90 min	5–7 hours
IM	Rapid	30–60 min	5–6 hours
IV	Immediate	20 min	5–6 hours

$T_{1/2}$: 1.5–2 hours; metabolised in the liver, excreted in the urine and bile.

Adverse effects: light-headedness, dizziness, sedation, nausea, vomiting, dry mouth, constipation, ureteral spasm, respiratory depression, apnoea, circulatory depression, respiratory arrest, shock, cardiac arrest.

effects such as nausea, vomiting, constipation and biliary spasm may occur as a result of CTZ stimulation and negative effects on GI motility. Box 26.3 discusses a drug approved to treat opioid-induced constipation. Neurological effects such as light-headedness, dizziness, psychoses, anxiety, fear, hallucinations, pupil constriction and impaired mental processes may occur as a result of the stimulation of CNS opioid receptors in the cerebrum, limbic system and hypothalamus. GU effects, including ureteral spasm, urinary retention, hesitancy and loss of libido, may be related to direct receptor stimulation or to CNS activation of sympathetic pathways. In addition, sweating and dependence (both physical and psychological) are possible, more so with some agents than with others.

Clinically important drug–drug interactions

When opioid agonists are given with barbiturate general anaesthetics or with some phenothiazines and MAO inhibitors, the likelihood of respiratory depression, hypotension and sedation or coma is increased. If these drug combinations cannot be avoided, individuals should be monitored closely and appropriate supportive measures taken.

Opioid agonists–antagonists

The **opioid agonists–antagonists** (Table 26.1) stimulate certain opioid receptors but block other such receptors. These drugs, which have less abuse potential than the pure opioid agonists, exert a similar analgesic effect as morphine. Like morphine, they may cause sedation, respiratory depression and constipation. They have also been associated with more psychotic-like reactions, and they may even induce a withdrawal syndrome in people who have been taking opioids for a long period.

The only available opioid agonist–antagonist currently is buprenorphine (*Norspan*).

Therapeutic actions and indications

The opioid agonists–antagonists act at specific opioid-receptor sites in the CNS to produce analgesia, sedation, euphoria and hallucinations. In addition, they block opioid receptors that may be stimulated by other opioids. These drugs have three functions: (1) relief of moderate to severe pain; (2) adjuncts to general anaesthesia; and (3) relief of pain during labour and delivery. See Table 26.1 for usual indications for each opioid agonist–antagonist agent.

Pharmacokinetics

Opioid agonists–antagonists are readily absorbed after IM administration and reach peak levels rapidly when given IV. They are metabolised in the liver and excreted in urine or faeces. They are known to cross the placenta and enter breast milk.

Buprenorphine is available for use in IM and IV forms.

Contraindications and cautions

Opioid agonists–antagonists are contraindicated in the presence of any known allergy to any opioid agonist-antagonist *to avoid hypersensitivity reactions*.

Caution should be used in cases of physical dependence on an opioid *because a withdrawal syndrome may be precipitated*; the opioid antagonistic properties can block the analgesic effect and intensify the pain. Opioid agonists–antagonists may be desirable for relieving chronic pain in people who are susceptible to opioid dependence, but extreme care must be used if they are switched directly from an opioid agonist to one of these drugs.

Caution should also be exercised in the following conditions: chronic obstructive pulmonary disease or other respiratory dysfunction, *which could be exacerbated by respiratory depression*; acute myocardial infarction (MI), documented coronary artery disease (CAD) or hypertension, *which could be exacerbated by the cardiac stimulatory effects of these drugs*; and renal or hepatic dysfunction, *which could interfere with the metabolism and excretion of the drug*.

There are no adequate studies regarding their effects during pregnancy. They should be used during pregnancy only if the benefit to the mother clearly outweighs the risk to the fetus *because of potential adverse effects on the neonate, including respiratory depression*. They can be used to relieve pain during labour and delivery, which provides a short-term exposure to the fetus. They are known to enter breast milk and should be used with caution during breastfeeding *because of the potential for adverse effects on the baby*.

Adverse effects

The most frequently seen adverse effects associated with opioid agonists–antagonists relate to their effects on various opioid receptors. Respiratory depression with apnoea and suppression of the cough reflex is associated with the respiratory centre depression. Nausea, vomiting, constipation and biliary spasm may occur as a result of CTZ stimulation and the negative effects on GI motility. Light-headedness, dizziness, psychoses, anxiety, fear, hallucinations and impaired mental processes may occur as a result of the activation of CNS opioid receptors in the cerebrum, limbic system and hypothalamus. GU effects, including ureteral spasm, urinary retention, hesitancy and loss of libido, may be related to direct receptor stimulation or to CNS activation of sympathetic pathways. Although sweating and dependence, both physical and psychological, are possible, their occurrence is considered less likely than with opioid agonists.

Clinically important drug–drug interactions

When opioid agonists–antagonists, like opioid agonists, are given with barbiturate general anaesthetics, the likelihood of respiratory depression, hypotension, and sedation or coma increases. If this combination cannot be avoided, individuals should be monitored closely and appropriate supportive measures taken.

Use of opioid agonists–antagonists in people who have previously received any opioid puts these individuals at risk for increased adverse effects, including respiratory depression. When such a sequence of drugs is used, individuals will require support and monitoring.

Care considerations for people receiving opioid agonists and opioid agonists–antagonists

Assessment: history and examination

- Assess for contraindications or cautions: any known allergies to these drugs *to avoid hypersensitivity reactions*; respiratory dysfunction, *which may be exacerbated by the respiratory depression caused by these drugs*; MI or CAD, *which could be exacerbated by the effects of these drugs*; renal or hepatic dysfunction, *which might interfere with drug metabolism or excretion*; current status of pregnancy and breastfeeding, *which require cautious use of the drugs*; diarrhoea caused by toxic poisons *because depression of GI activity could lead to increased absorption and toxicity*; and after biliary surgery or surgical anastomoses *because of the adverse effects associated with slowed GI activity due to opioids*.
- Perform a pain assessment with the person *to establish baseline status and evaluate the effectiveness of drug therapy*.
- Perform a physical assessment *to establish baseline status before beginning therapy, determine drug effectiveness and evaluate for any potential adverse effects*.
- Assess orientation, affect, reflexes and pupil size *to evaluate any CNS effects*; monitor respiratory rate and auscultate lungs for adventitious sounds *to evaluate respiratory effects*.
- Monitor pulse, blood pressure and cardiac output *to evaluate for cardiac effects*.
- Palpate abdomen for distension and auscultate bowel sounds *to monitor for GI effects*; assess urine output and palpate for bladder distension *to evaluate for GU effects*.
- Monitor the results of laboratory tests such as liver and renal function tests *to determine the need for possible dose adjustment and identify toxic drug effects*.

Implementation with rationale

- Perform baseline and periodic pain assessments *to monitor drug effectiveness and provide appropriate changes in pain management protocol as needed.*

- Have an opioid antagonist and equipment for assisted ventilation readily available when administering the drug IV *to provide support in case of severe reaction.*
- Monitor injection sites for irritation and extravasation *to provide appropriate supportive care if needed.*
- Monitor timing of analgesic doses. *Prompt administration may provide a more acceptable level of analgesia and lead to quicker resolution of the pain.*
- Use extreme caution when injecting these drugs into any body area that has poor perfusion or shock *because absorption may be delayed, and after repeated doses an excessive amount is absorbed all at once.*
- Use additional measures to relieve pain (eg, back rubs, stress reduction, hot packs, ice packs) *to increase the effectiveness of the opioid being given and reduce pain.*
- Monitor respiratory status before beginning therapy and periodically during therapy *to monitor for potential respiratory depression.*
- Institute comfort and safety measures, such as side rails and assistance with ambulation, *to ensure safety*; bowel program as needed *to treat constipation*; environmental controls *to decrease stimulation*; and small, frequent meals *to relieve GI distress if GI upset is severe.*
- Reassure individuals that the risk of addiction is minimal. *Most people who receive these drugs for medical reasons do not develop dependency syndromes.*
- Offer support and encouragement *to help the person cope with the drug regimen.*
- Provide thorough teaching, including drug name, prescribed dose and schedule of administration; measures for avoidance of adverse effects; warning signs that may indicate possible problems; safety measures such as avoiding driving, getting assistance with ambulation, avoiding making important decisions or signing important papers; and the need for monitoring and evaluation *to enhance the person's knowledge about drug therapy and to promote compliance.*

Evaluation

- Monitor the person's response to the drug (relief of pain, sedation).
- Monitor for adverse effects (CNS changes, GI depression, respiratory depression, arrhythmias, hypertension).
- Evaluate the effectiveness of the teaching plan (person can give the drug name and dosage and describe possible adverse effects to watch for, specific measures to prevent them and warning signs to report).
- Monitor the effectiveness of comfort measures and compliance with the regimen.

OPIOID ANTAGONISTS

The **opioid antagonists** (Table 26.1) are drugs that bind strongly to opioid receptors but do not activate them. They block the effects of the opioid receptors and are often used to block the effects of too many opioids in the system. The opioid antagonists in use include naloxone (*Narcan*) and naltrexone (*Naltraccord [New Zealand only], ReVia*).

Therapeutic actions and indications

The opioid antagonists block opioid receptors and reverse the effects of opioids, including respiratory depression, sedation, psychomimetic effects and hypotension.

These agents are indicated for reversal of the adverse effects of opioid use, including respiratory depression and sedation, and for treatment of opioid overdose. (See Table 26.1 for usual indications for each opioid antagonist agent.) The opioid antagonists do not have an appreciable effect in most people, but individuals who are addicted to opioids experience the signs and symptoms of withdrawal when receiving these drugs rapidly.

Pharmacokinetics

Opioid antagonists may be administered parenterally (SC, IM or IV) or orally. These drugs are well absorbed after injection and are widely distributed in the body. They undergo hepatic metabolism and are excreted primarily in the urine.

Contraindications and cautions

Opioid antagonists are contraindicated in the presence of any known allergy to any opioid antagonist *to avoid hypersensitivity reactions.* Caution should be used in the following circumstances: during pregnancy and breastfeeding *because of potential adverse effects on the fetus and neonate*; with opioid addiction *because of the precipitation of a withdrawal syndrome*; and with CV disease, *which could be exacerbated by the reversal of the depressive effects of opioids.*

Adverse effects

The most frequently seen adverse effects associated with these drugs relate to the blocking effects of the opioid receptors. The most common effect is an acute opioid abstinence syndrome that is characterised by nausea, vomiting, sweating, tachycardia, hypertension, tremulousness and feelings of anxiety. A naloxone challenge should be administered before giving naltrexone to help to avoid acute reactions.

CNS excitement and reversal of analgesia are especially common after surgery. CV effects related to the reversal of the opioid depression can include tachycardia, blood pressure changes, dysrhythmias and pulmonary oedema.

Drug–drug interactions

To reverse the effects of buprenorphine larger doses of opioid antagonists may be needed.

 **Prototype summary: naloxone**

Indications: complete or partial reversal of opioid depression; diagnosis of suspected opioid overdose.

Actions: pure opioid antagonist; reverses the effects of the opioids, including respiratory depression, sedation and hypotension.

Pharmacokinetics:

Route	Peak	Onset	Duration
IV	Unknown	2 min	4–6 hours
IM, SC	Unknown	3–5 min	4–6 hours

$T_{1/2}$: 30–81 minutes; metabolised in the liver, excreted in the urine.

Adverse effects: acute opioid abstinence syndrome (nausea, vomiting, sweating, tachycardia, fall in blood pressure), hypotension, hypertension, pulmonary oedema.

Care considerations for people receiving opioid antagonists

Assessment: history and examination

- Assess for contraindications or cautions: any known allergies to these drugs *to avoid hypersensitivity reactions*; history of opioid addition, *which may lead to opioid abstinence syndrome*; history of MI or CAD, *which may be exacerbated by the reversal of opioid depression*; and current status of pregnancy and breastfeeding, *which require cautious use of these drugs.*
- Perform a physical assessment to establish *baseline status before beginning therapy and for any potential adverse effects.*
- Assess the person's neurological status, including level of orientation, affect, reflexes and pupil size, *to evaluate CNS effects*; monitor respiratory rate and auscultate lungs for adventitious sounds *to evaluate respiratory status.*
- Monitor vital signs, including pulse and blood pressure, *to identify changes and risks to the CV system.*
- Obtain an ECG as appropriate *to evaluate for cardiac effects.*

Implementation with rationale

- Maintain open airway and provide artificial ventilation and cardiac massage as needed *to support the person.* Administer vasopressors as needed *to manage opioid overdose.*
- Administer naloxone challenge before giving naltrexone *because of the serious risk of acute withdrawal.*
- Provide continuous monitoring, *adjusting the dose as needed, during treatment of acute overdose.*
- Provide comfort and safety measures *to help the person cope with the withdrawal syndrome.*
- Ensure that people receiving naltrexone have been opioid free for 7–10 days *to prevent severe withdrawal syndrome.* Check urine opioid levels if there is any question.
- If the person is receiving naltrexone as part of a comprehensive opioid or alcohol withdrawal program, advise the individual to wear or carry a MedicAlert warning *so that health care personnel know how to treat the person in an emergency.*
- Institute comfort and safety measures, such as side rails and assistance with ambulation, *to ensure safety;* institute a bowel program as needed *for treatment of constipation*; use environmental controls *to decrease stimulation*; and provide small, frequent meals *to relieve GI irritation if GI upset is severe.*
- Offer support and encouragement *to help the person cope with the effects of the drug regimen.*
- Provide thorough teaching, including drug name and prescribed dosage; measures to avoid adverse effects; warning signs to report immediately that may indicate possible problems; safety measures such as avoiding driving, avoiding making important decisions and having a responsible person available for assistance; and the importance of continued monitoring and evaluation *to enhance knowledge about drug therapy and to promote compliance.*

Evaluation

- Monitor response to the drug (reversal of opioid effects, treatment of alcohol dependence).
- Monitor for adverse effects (CV changes, arrhythmias, hypertension).

- Evaluate the effectiveness of the teaching plan (person can give the drug name and dosage and describe possible adverse effects to watch for, specific measures to prevent them and warning signs to report).
- Monitor the effectiveness of comfort measures and compliance with the regimen.

KEY POINTS

- Opioid agonists react with opioid-receptor sites to stimulate their activity.
- Opioid agonists–antagonists react with some opioid-receptor sites to stimulate activity and block other opioid-receptor sites.
- Opioid antagonists are used to treat opioid overdose or to reverse unacceptable adverse effects.

MIGRAINE HEADACHES

The term **migraine headache** is used to describe several different syndromes, all of which include severe, throbbing headaches on one side of the head. This pain can be so severe that it can cause widespread disturbances, affecting GI and CNS function, including mood and personality changes.

Migraine headaches should be distinguished from cluster headaches and tension headaches (Box 26.4). Cluster headaches usually begin during sleep and involve sharp, steady eye pain that lasts 15–90 minutes, with sweating, flushing, tearing and nasal congestion. Tension headaches, which usually occur at times of stress, feel like a dull band of pain around the entire head and last from 30 minutes to 1 week. They are accompanied by anorexia, fatigue and a mild intolerance to light or sound.

Migraines are generally classified as common or classic. Common migraines, which occur without an aura, cause severe, unilateral, pulsating pain that is frequently accompanied by nausea, vomiting and sensitivity to light and sound. Such migraine headaches are often aggravated by physical activity. Classic migraines are usually preceded by an aura – a sensation involving sensory or motor disturbances – that usually occurs about half an hour before the pain begins. The pain and adverse effects are the same as those of the common migraine.

It is believed that the underlying cause of migraine headaches is cranial arterial dilation. Headaches accompanied by an aura are associated with hypoperfusion of the brain during the aura stage, followed by reflex cranial arterial dilation and hyperperfusion. The underlying cause and continued state of cranial arterial dilation are not clearly understood, but they may be related to the release of bradykinins or serotonin, or as a response to other hormones and chemicals.

BOX 26.4 FOCUS ON **Gender considerations**

Headache distribution

Headaches are distributed in the general population in a definite gender-related pattern. For example:

- Migraine headaches are three times more likely to occur in women than men.
- Cluster headaches are more likely to occur in men than in women.
- Tension headaches are more likely to occur in women than in men.

There is some speculation that the female predisposition to migraine headaches may be related to the vascular sensitivity to hormones. Some women can directly associate migraine occurrence with periods of fluctuations in their menstrual cycle. The introduction of the triptan class of antimigraine drugs has been beneficial for many of these women.

ANTIMIGRAINE AGENTS

For many years, the one standard treatment for migraine headaches was acute analgesia, often involving an opioid, together with control of lighting and sound and the use of ergot derivatives. In the late 1990s, a new class of drugs, the triptans, was found to be extremely effective in treating migraine headaches without the adverse effects associated with ergot derivative use. However, because these newer agents are also associated with many systemic adverse effects, their usefulness is limited in some people (see Box 26.5). Table 26.2 includes additional information about each class of antimigraine agents.

ERGOT DERIVATIVES

The **ergot derivatives** cause constriction of cranial blood vessels and decrease the pulsation of cranial arteries. As a result, they reduce the hyperperfusion of the basilar artery vascular bed.

Available ergot derivatives include ergotamine (*Cafergot*) (no longer available in Australia).

Therapeutic actions and indications

The ergot derivatives block alpha-adrenergic and serotonin-receptor sites in the brain to cause a constriction of cranial vessels, a decrease in cranial artery pulsation and a decrease in the hyperperfusion of the basilar artery bed (see Figure 26.2). These drugs are indicated for the prevention or abortion of migraine or vascular headaches. Ergotamine, the prototype drug in this class,

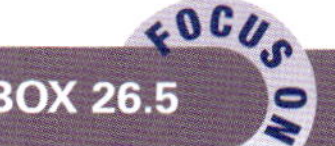

BOX 26.5 FOCUS ON **Drug therapy across the lifespan**

Antimigraine agents

CHILDREN

None of the drugs used to treat migraines is recommended for use in children. The ergot derivatives can have many adverse effects in children, and there is not enough clinical experience with triptans to recommend them for use in children under 12 years for naratriptan and sumatriptan and under 17 years for the others.

ADULTS

Adults requesting treatment for migraine headaches should be carefully evaluated before one of the antimigraine drugs is used to ensure that the headache being treated is of the type that can benefit from these drugs.

PREGNANCY AND BREASTFEEDING

The ergots and the triptans are contraindicated during pregnancy because of the potential for adverse effects in the mother and fetus. Women of childbearing age should be advised to use contraception while they are taking these drugs. Women who are breastfeeding should be encouraged to find another method of feeding the baby because of the potential for adverse drug effects on the baby.

OLDER ADULTS

Older adults are more likely to have chronic diseases such as CV disease or renal or hepatic impairment that would be exacerbated by the antimigraine drugs. They should be used with extreme caution in older adults. The older adult should be encouraged to take the least amount of the drug possible and should be monitored closely for any sign of chest pain, MI or acute vascular changes. Safety measures are extremely important with the older adult. If the person is in an institutional setting, side rails, assistance with moving and careful monitoring should be used.

was the mainstay of migraine headache treatment before the development of triptans. (See Table 26.2 for usual indications for each drug.)

Pharmacokinetics

The ergot derivatives are rapidly absorbed from many routes, with an onset of action ranging from 15 to 30 minutes. They are metabolised in the liver and primarily excreted in the bile.

Ergotamine is administered orally or rectally for rapid absorption.

Contraindications and cautions

Ergot derivatives are contraindicated in the following circumstances: presence of allergy to ergot preparations *to avoid hypersensitivity reactions*; CAD, hypertension or peripheral vascular disease, *which could be exacerbated by the CV effects of these drugs*; impaired liver function, *which could alter the metabolism and excretion of these drugs*; and pregnancy or breastfeeding *because of the potential for adverse effects on the fetus and neonate*. Ergotism (vomiting, diarrhoea, seizures) has been reported in affected infants.

TABLE 26.2 *DRUGS IN FOCUS* Antimigraine agents

Drug name	Dosage/route	Usual indications
Ergot derivatives		
(P) ergotamine (*Cafergot*)	2 tablets PO up to 6 tablets/day	Prevention and abortion of migraine attacks in adults
Triptans		
eletriptan (*Relpax*)	Initially, 40 mg PO; repeat after 2 hours if needed Maximum 160 mg/day	Treatment of acute migraines in adults
naratriptan (*Naramig*)	2.5 mg PO; may repeat in 4 hours if needed; maximum 5 mg in 2 hours	Treatment of acute migraines in adults
rizatriptan (*Maxalt*)	10 mg SL; may repeat in 2 hours; do not exceed 30 mg in 24 hours	Treatment of acute migraines in adults; orally disintegrating tablet may be useful if there is difficulty swallowing
(P) sumatriptan (*Clustran, Imigran, Sumagran, SumaPen*)	50–100 mg PO at first sign of headache, may repeat in 2 hours (maximum 300 mg in 24 hours); by nasal spray in one nostril: may repeat in 2 hours (do not exceed 40 mg/day)	Treatment of acute migraines, cluster headaches in adults
zolmitriptan (*Zomig*)	2.5 mg PO; may repeat in 2 hours; do not exceed 10 mg/day	Treatment of acute migraines in adults

Caution should be used in two instances: with pruritus, *which could become worse with drug-induced vascular constriction*, and with malnutrition *because ergot derivatives stimulate the CTZ and can cause severe GI reactions, possibly worsening malnutrition*.

Prototype summary: ergotamine

Indications: prevention or abortion of vascular headaches.

Actions: constricts cranial blood vessels, decreases pulsation of cranial arteries and decreases hyperperfusion of the basilar artery vascular bed; mechanism of action is not understood.

Pharmacokinetics:

Route	Onset	Peak
Oral	Rapid	0.5–3 hours

$T_{1/2}$: 2.7 hours, then 21 hours; metabolised in the liver, excreted in the faeces.

Adverse effects: numbness, tingling in the fingers and toes, muscle pain in the extremities, pulselessness or weakness in the legs, praecordial distress, tachycardia, bradycardia, ergotism (nausea, vomiting, diarrhoea, severe thirst, hypoperfusion, chest pain, confusion).

Adverse effects

The adverse effects of ergot derivatives can be related to the drug-induced vascular constriction. CNS effects include numbness, tingling of extremities and muscle pain; CV effects such as pulselessness, weakness, chest pain, arrhythmias, localised oedema and itching and MI may also occur. In addition, the direct stimulation of the CTZ can cause GI upset, nausea, vomiting and diarrhoea. Ergotism, a syndrome associated with the use of these drugs, causes nausea, vomiting, severe thirst, hypoperfusion, chest pain, blood pressure changes, confusion, drug dependency (with prolonged use) and a drug-withdrawal syndrome.

Clinically important drug–drug interactions

If these drugs are combined with beta blockers, the risk of peripheral ischaemia and gangrene is increased. Such combinations should be avoided.

TRIPTANS

The **triptans** class of drugs cause cranial vascular constriction and relief of migraine headache pain in many people. These drugs are not associated with the vascular and GI effects of the ergot derivatives. The triptan of choice for a particular individual depends on personal experience and other pre-existing medical conditions. A person may have a poor response to one triptan and respond well to another.

Available triptans include eletriptan (*Relpax*) (not available in New Zealand), naratriptan (*Naramig*), rizatriptan (*Maxalt*), sumatriptan (*Clustran*, *Imigran*, *Sumagran*, *SumaPen*) and zolmitriptan (*Zoltrip*, *Zomig*).

Therapeutic actions and indications

The triptans bind to selective serotonin-receptor sites to cause vasoconstriction of cranial vessels, relieving the signs and symptoms of migraine headache (see Figure 26.2). They are indicated for the treatment of acute migraine and are not used for prevention of migraines. (See Table 26.2 for usual indications for each of the triptans.)

Sumatriptan, the first drug of this class, is used for the treatment of acute migraine attacks and for the treatment of cluster headaches in adults. It can be given orally, SC or by nasal spray.

Naratriptan, rizatriptan and zolmitriptan are used orally only for the treatment of acute migraines. Rizatriptan and zolmitriptan are also available as fast-dissolving tablets.

Pharmacokinetics

The triptans are rapidly absorbed from many sites; they are metabolised in the liver (sumatriptan by MAO) and are primarily excreted in the urine. They cross the placenta and have been shown to be toxic to the fetus in animal studies. They also enter breast milk. The safety and efficacy of use in children have not been established.

Contraindications and cautions

Triptans are contraindicated with any of the following conditions: allergy to any triptan *to avoid hypersensitivity reactions*; pregnancy *because of the possibility of severe adverse effects on the fetus*; and active CAD, *which could be exacerbated by the vessel-constricting effects of these drugs*. These drugs should be used with caution in elderly people *because of the possibility of underlying vascular disease*; in individuals with risk factors for CAD; in breastfeeding women *because of the possibility of adverse effects on the infant*; and in people with renal or hepatic dysfunction, *which could alter the metabolism and excretion of the drug*. Rizatriptan seems to have more angina-related effects, and it is not recommended for people with a history of CAD, *which could be exacerbated by its cardiac effects*.

Adverse effects

The adverse effects associated with the triptans are related to the vasoconstrictive effects of the drugs. CNS effects may include numbness, tingling, burning sensation, feelings of coldness or strangeness, dizziness, weakness, myalgia and vertigo. GI effects such as dysphagia and abdominal discomfort may occur. CV effects can be severe and include blood pressure alterations and tightness or pressure in the chest.

Clinically important drug–drug interactions

Combining triptans with ergot-containing drugs results in a risk of prolonged vasoactive reactions. There is a risk of severe adverse effects if these drugs are used within 2 weeks after discontinuation of an MAO inhibitor *because of the increased vasoconstrictive effects that occur.* If triptans are to be given, it is imperative that the person has not received an MAO inhibitor in more than 2 weeks.

 **Prototype summary: sumatriptan**

Indications: treatment of acute migraine; treatment of cluster headaches (SC route).

Actions: binds to serotonin receptors to cause vasoconstrictive effects on cranial blood vessels.

Pharmacokinetics:

Route	Onset	Peak	Duration
Nasal spray	Varies	5–20 min	Unknown
Oral	1–1.5 hours	2–4 hours	Up to 24 hours
SC	Rapid	1–5 hours	Up to 24 hours

$T_{1/2}$: 115 minutes; metabolised in the liver, excreted in the urine.

Adverse effects: dizziness, vertigo, weakness, myalgia, blood pressure alterations, tightness or pressure in the chest, injection-site discomfort, tingling, burning sensations, numbness.

Care considerations for people receiving antimigraine agents

Assessment: history and examination

- Assess for contraindications or cautions: any known allergies to any components of the drugs *to avoid hypersensitivity reactions*; history of MI, CAD or hypertension, *which may be exacerbated by the drug*; hepatic or renal dysfunction, *which could alter the metabolism and excretion of the drug*; pruritus or malnutrition, *which could be exacerbated by ergot derivatives*; and current status of pregnancy and breastfeeding, *which would be cautions to the use of these drugs.*
- Perform a physical assessment *to establish baseline status before beginning therapy, determine drug effectiveness and evaluate for any potential adverse effects.*
- Assess neurological status, including level of orientation, affect and reflexes, *to evaluate CNS effects of the drugs.*
- Monitor for complaints of extremity numbness and tingling *to identify effects on vascular constriction.*
- Inspect the skin for localised oedema, itching or breakdown with ergot derivatives *to evaluate potential dermatological effects.*
- Assess vital signs, including pulse rate and blood pressure; obtain an ECG as appropriate *to evaluate cardiac status for changes.*
- Monitor the results of laboratory tests, including liver and renal function tests, *to determine the need for dose adjustment and identify possible toxic effects.*

Implementation with rationale

- Administer the drug to relieve acute migraines; *these drugs are not used for prevention.*
- Administer at the first sign of a headache and do not wait until it is severe, *to improve therapeutic effectiveness.*
- Arrange for safety precautions if CNS or visual changes occur *to prevent injury.*
- Provide comfort and safety measures, such as environmental controls and stress reduction, *for the relief of headache.* Provide additional pain relief as needed.
- Monitor the blood pressure of any person with a history of CAD, and discontinue the drug if any sign of angina or prolonged hypertension occurs, *to prevent severe vascular effects.*
- Offer support and encouragement *to help the individual cope with the disorder and associated drug regimen.*
- Provide thorough teaching, including drug name, prescribed dose and schedule for administration; measures to avoid adverse effects; warning signs that may indicate possible problems; signs of ergotism if taking ergot derivatives; safety measures such as avoiding driving and avoiding overdose; and importance of follow-up monitoring and evaluation *to enhance the person's knowledge about drug therapy and to promote compliance.*

Evaluation

- Monitor the person's response to the drug (relief of acute migraine headaches).
- Monitor for adverse effects (CV changes, arrhythmias, hypertension, CNS changes).
- Evaluate the effectiveness of the teaching plan (person can give the drug name and dosage and

describe possible adverse effects to watch for, specific measures to prevent them and warning signs to report).

- Monitor the effectiveness of comfort measures and compliance with the regimen.

KEY POINTS

- Migraine headaches are severe, throbbing headaches on one side of the head that may be associated with an aura or warning syndrome. These headaches are thought to be caused by cranial arterial dilation and hyperperfusion of the brain vessels.
- Treatment of migraines may involve either ergot derivatives or triptans. Ergot derivatives cause vasoconstriction and are associated with sometimes severe systemic vasoconstrictive effects, whereas triptans, a newer class of selective serotonin-receptor blockers, cause CNS vasoconstriction but are not associated with as many adverse systemic effects.

CHAPTER SUMMARY

- Pain occurs any time that tissue is injured and various chemicals are released. The pain impulses are carried to the spinal cord by small-diameter A-delta and C fibres, which form synapses with interneurons in the dorsal horn of the spinal cord.
- Opioid receptors found throughout various tissues in the body react with endogenous endorphins and encephalins to modulate the transmission of pain impulses.
- Opioids, derived from the opium plant, react with opioid receptors to relieve pain. In addition, they lead to constipation, respiratory depression, sedation and suppression of the cough reflex; they also stimulate feelings of wellbeing or euphoria.
- Because opioids of all kinds are associated with the development of physical dependency, they are controlled substances.
- The effectiveness and adverse effects associated with specific opioids are associated with their particular affinity for various types of opioid receptors.
- Opioid agonists react with opioid-receptor sites to stimulate their activity.
- Opioid agonists–antagonists react with some opioid-receptor sites to stimulate activity and block other opioid-receptor sites. These drugs are not as addictive as pure opioid agonists.
- Opioid antagonists, which work to reverse the effects of opioids, are used to treat opioid overdose or to reverse unacceptable adverse effects.
- Migraine headaches are severe, throbbing headaches on one side of the head that may be associated with an aura or warning syndrome. These headaches are thought to be caused by arterial dilation and hyperperfusion of the brain vessels.
- Treatment of migraines may involve either ergot derivatives or triptans. Ergot derivatives cause vasoconstriction and are associated with sometimes severe systemic vasoconstrictive effects, whereas triptans, a newer class of selective serotonin-receptor blockers, cause CNS vasoconstriction but are not associated with as many adverse systemic effects.

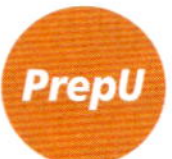

Knowing your strengths and weaknesses helps you to study more effectively. Take a PrepU Practice Quiz to find out how you measure up!

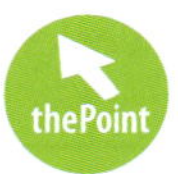

ONLINE RESOURCES

An extensive range of additional resources to enhance teaching and learning and to facilitate understanding of this chapter may be found online at the text's accompanying website, located on thePoint at http://thepoint.lww.com. These include Watch and Learn videos, Concepts in Action animations, journal articles, review questions, case studies, discussion topics and quizzes.

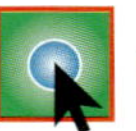

WEB LINKS

Health care providers and students may want to consult the following web resources:

http://headacheaustralia.org.au
Headache Australia. Information on headache, including migraine and headache management.

www.neurological.org.nz/disorders/migraine
Neurological Foundation of New Zealand. Information on migraine, management and support.

www.who.int/cancer/palliative/painladder/en
World Health Organization cancer pain ladder.

BIBLIOGRAPHY

Beggs, S. (2008). Paediatric analgesia. *Australian Prescriber, 31*, 63–65.

Farrell, M. & Dempsey, J. (2014). *Smeltzer & Bare's Textbook of Medical-Surgical Nursing* (3rd edn). Sydney: Lippincott Williams & Wilkins.

Goodman, L. S., Brunton, L. L., Chabner, B. & Knollmann, B. C. (2011). *Goodman and Gilman's Pharmacological Basis of Therapeutics* (12th edn). New York: McGraw-Hill.

Junquist, C. R., Karan, S. & Perlis, M. L. (2011). Risk factors for opioid-induced excessive respiratory depression. *Pain Management Nursing, 12(3)*, 180–187.

Lange, S. E. (2011). Primary headache disorders in the emergency department. *Advanced Emergency Nursing Journal, 33(3)*, 237–251.

Matzo, M. & Dawson, K. A. (2013). Opioid-induced neurotoxicity. *American Journal of Nursing, 113(10)*, 51–56.

McDonough, M. (2013). Opioid treatment of opioid addiction. *Australian Prescriber, 36*, 83–87.

McKenna, L. & Mirkov, S. (2019). *McKenna's Drug Handbook for Nursing and Midwifery* (8th edn). Sydney: Wolters Kluwer Health Australia.

Pierce, M. (2013). Oral triptans and nausea: Treatment considerations in migraine. *Headache, 53*(suppl1), 17–20.

Porth, C. M. (2011). *Essentials of Pathophysiology: Concepts of Altered Health States* (3rd edn). Philadelphia: Lippincott Williams & Wilkins.

Porth, C. M. (2009). *Pathophysiology: Concepts of Altered Health States* (8th edn). Philadelphia: Lippincott Williams & Wilkins.

Roberts, L. J. (2008). Managing acute pain in patients with an opioid abuse or dependence disorder. *Australian Prescriber, 31*, 133–135.

Stark, R. J. & Stark, C. D. (2008). Migraine prophylaxis. *Medical Journal of Australia, 189(5)*, 283–288.

Steefel, L. & Novak, D. (2012). When tension headaches become chronic. *The Nurse Practitioner, 37(11)*, 24–30.

CHECK YOUR UNDERSTANDING

Answers to the questions in this chapter can be found in Appendix A at the back of this book.

MULTIPLE CHOICE

Select the best answer to the following.

1. According to the gate control theory, pain:
   a. is caused by gates in the CNS.
   b. can be blocked or intensified by gates in the CNS.
   c. is caused by gates in peripheral nerve sensors.
   d. cannot be affected by learned experiences.
2. Opioid receptors are found throughout the body:
   a. only in people who have become addicted to opiates.
   b. in increasing numbers with chronic pain conditions.
   c. to incorporate pain perception and blocking.
   d. to initiate the release of endorphins.
3. Most opioids are controlled substances because they:
   a. are very expensive.
   b. can cause respiratory depression.
   c. can be addictive.
   d. can be used only in a hospital setting.
4. Injecting an opioid into an area of the body that is chilled can be dangerous because:
   a. an abscess will form.
   b. the injection will be very painful.
   c. an excessive amount may be absorbed all at once.
   d. opioids are inactivated by cold temperatures.
5. Proper administration of an ordered opioid:
   a. can lead to addiction.
   b. should be done promptly to prevent increased pain and the need for larger doses.
   c. would include holding the drug as long as possible until the person really needs it.
   d. should rely on the person's request for medication.
6. Migraine headaches:
   a. occur during sleep and involve sweating and eye pain.
   b. occur with stress and feel like a dull band around the entire head.
   c. often occur when drinking coffee.
   d. are throbbing headaches on one side of the head.
7. The triptans are a class of drugs that bind to selective serotonin-receptor sites and cause:
   a. cranial vascular dilation.
   b. cranial vascular constriction.
   c. clinical depression.
   d. nausea and vomiting.
8. The only triptan that has been approved for use in treating cluster headaches as well as migraines is:
   a. naratriptan.
   b. rizatriptan.
   c. sumatriptan.
   d. zolmitriptan.

MULTIPLE RESPONSE

Select all that apply.

1. Opioids are drugs that react with opioid receptors throughout the body. Which of the following would the health care provider expect to find when assessing a person who was taking an opioid?
   a. hypnosis
   b. sedation
   c. analgesia
   d. euphoria
   e. orthostatic hypotension
   f. increased salivation
2. The health care provider would expect to administer an opioid as the analgesic of choice for which people?
   a. a person with severe postoperative pain
   b. a person with severe chronic obstructive pulmonary disease and difficulty breathing
   c. a person with severe, chronic pain
   d. a person with ulcerative colitis
   e. a person with recent biliary surgery
   f. a person with cancer and severe bone pain

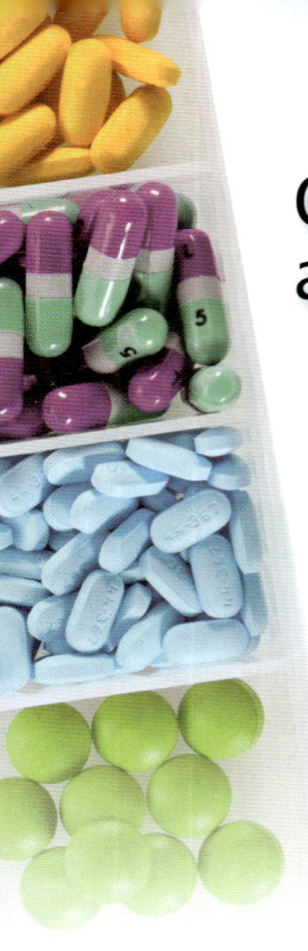

General and local anaesthetic agents

27

Learning objectives

On completing this chapter you should be able to:

1. Describe the concept of balanced anaesthesia.
2. Describe the actions and uses of local anaesthesia.
3. Describe the therapeutic actions, indications, pharmacokinetics, contraindications, most common adverse reactions and important drug–drug interactions associated with general and local anaesthetics.
4. Outline the preoperative and postoperative needs of a person receiving general or local anaesthesia.
5. Compare and contrast the prototype drugs thiopental, midazolam, nitrous oxide and lidocaine (lignocaine) with other drugs in their respective classes.
6. Outline the care considerations, including important teaching points, for people receiving general and local anaesthetics.

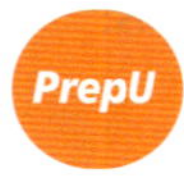

Test your current knowledge of general and local anaesthetic agents with a PrepU Practice Quiz!

Glossary of key terms

amnesia: loss of memory of an event or procedure
anaesthetic: drug used to cause complete or partial loss of sensation
analgesia: loss of pain sensation
balanced anaesthesia: use of several different types of drugs to achieve the quickest, most effective anaesthesia with the fewest adverse effects
general anaesthesia: use of drugs to induce a loss of consciousness, amnesia, analgesia and loss of reflexes to allow performance of painful surgical procedures
induction: time from the beginning of anaesthesia until achievement of surgical anaesthesia
local anaesthesia: use of powerful nerve blockers that prevents depolarisation of nerve membranes, blocking the transmission of pain stimuli and, in some cases, motor activity
plasma esterase: enzyme found in plasma that immediately breaks down ester-type local anaesthetics
premedication: medication administered before surgery to facilitate sedation and general anaesthesia
unconsciousness: loss of awareness of one's surroundings
volatile liquid: liquid that is unstable at room temperature and releases vapours; used as an inhaled general anaesthetic, usually in the form of a halogenated hydrocarbon

GENERAL ANAESTHETIC AGENTS

Barbiturate anaesthetics
- thiopental (P)

Non-barbiturate general anaesthetics
- droperidol
- ketamine
- midazolam (P)
- propofol

Anaesthetic gas
- nitrous oxide (P)

Volatile liquids
- desflurane
- isoflurane (P)
- methoxyflurane
- sevoflurane

LOCAL ANAESTHETIC AGENTS

Esters
- tetracaine (amethocaine)
- benzocaine

Amides
- bupivacaine
- cinchocaine
- levobupivacaine
- lidocaine (lignocaine) (P)
- mepivacaine
- prilocaine
- ropivacaine

Anaesthetics are drugs that are used to cause complete or partial loss of sensation. The anaesthetics can be subdivided into general and local anaesthetics, depending on their site of action. General anaesthetics are central nervous system (CNS) depressants used to produce loss of pain sensation and consciousness. Local anaesthetics are drugs used to cause loss of pain sensation and feeling in a designated area of the body without the systemic effects associated with severe CNS depression. This chapter discusses various general and local anaesthetics. Box 27.1 highlights information about using anaesthetics with various age groups.

GENERAL ANAESTHESIA

General anaesthesia involves the administration of a combination of several different general anaesthetic agents to achieve the following goals: **analgesia**, or loss of pain perception; **unconsciousness**, or loss of awareness of one's surroundings; and **amnesia**, or inability to recall what took place. Ideally, the drugs are combined to achieve the best effects with the fewest adverse effects. In addition, general anaesthesia also blocks the body reflexes. Blockage of autonomic reflexes prevents involuntary reflex response to body injury that might compromise a person's cardiac, respiratory, gastrointestinal (GI) and immune status. Blockage of muscle reflexes prevents jerking movements that might interfere with the success of the surgical procedure.

Risk factors associated with general anaesthesia

Widespread CNS depression, which is not without risks, occurs with general anaesthesia. In addition, all other body systems are affected. Because of the wide systemic effects, people must be evaluated for factors that may increase their risk. These factors include the following:

- *CNS factors*: underlying neurological disease (eg, epilepsy, stroke, myasthenia gravis) that presents a

BOX 27.1 FOCUS ON Drug therapy across the lifespan

Anaesthetic agents

CHILDREN

Children are at greater risk for complications after anaesthesia – laryngospasm, bronchospasm, aspiration and even death. They require very careful monitoring and support, and the anaesthetist needs to be very skilled at calculating dosage and balance during the procedure. Propofol is widely used for diagnostic tests and short procedures in children older than 3 years of age because of its rapid onset and metabolism and generally smooth recovery. Sevoflurane has a minimal impact on intracranial pressure and allows a very rapid induction and recovery with minimal sympathetic reaction. It is still quite expensive, however, which may limit its use. The dosage of anaesthetics may need to be higher in children, and that factor will be considered by the anaesthetist.

Care after general anaesthesia should include support and reassurance; assessment of the child for any skin breakdown related to immobility, and safety precautions until full recovery has occurred.

Local anaesthetics are used in children in much the same way that they are used in adults.

Bupivacaine does not have established doses for children younger than 12 years of age. Benzocaine should not be used in children younger than 1 year of age.

When topically applying a local anaesthetic, it is important to remember that there is greater risk of systemic absorption and toxicity with infants.

Tight nappies can act like occlusive dressings and increase systemic absorption. Children need to be cautioned not to bite themselves when receiving dental anaesthesia.

ADULTS

Adults require a considerable amount of teaching and support when receiving anaesthetics, including what will happen, what they will feel, how it will feel when they recover and the approximate time to recovery.

Adults should be monitored closely until fully recovered from general anaesthetics and should be cautioned to prevent injury when receiving local anaesthetics. It is important to remember to reassure and talk to adults who may be aware of their surroundings yet unable to speak.

PREGNANCY AND BREASTFEEDING

Most of the general anaesthetics are not recommended for use during pregnancy because of the potential risk to the fetus. Short-onset and local anaesthetics are frequently used at delivery. Use of a regional or other local anaesthetic is usually preferred if surgery is needed during pregnancy. During breastfeeding, it is recommended that the mother wait 4–6 hours to feed the baby after the anaesthetic is used.

OLDER ADULTS

Older people are more likely to experience the adverse effects associated with these drugs, including CNS, cardiovascular and dermatological effects. Thinner skin and the possibility of decreased perfusion to the skin makes them especially susceptible to skin breakdown during immobility. Because older people often also have renal or hepatic impairment, they are also more likely to have toxic levels of the drug related to changes in metabolism and excretion. The older person should have safety measures in effect, such as siderails, a call bell and assistance to ambulate; special efforts to provide skin care to prevent skin breakdown are especially important with older skin. The older person may require longer monitoring and regular orienting and reassuring. After general anaesthesia, it is very important to promote vigorous deep breathing and coughing to decrease the risk of pneumonia.

risk of abnormal reaction to the CNS-depressing and muscle-relaxing effects of these drugs.
- *Cardiovascular factors*: underlying vascular disease, coronary artery disease or hypotension, which put people at risk for severe reactions to anaesthesia, such as hypotension and shock, arrhythmias and ischaemia.
- *Respiratory factors*: obstructive pulmonary disease (eg, asthma, chronic obstructive pulmonary disease, bronchitis), which can complicate the delivery of gas anaesthetics, as well as the intubation and mechanical ventilation that must be used in most cases of general anaesthesia.
- *Renal and hepatic function*: conditions that interfere with the metabolism and excretion of anaesthetics (eg, acute renal failure, hepatitis) and could result in prolonged anaesthesia and the need for continued support during recovery. Toxic reactions to the accumulation of abnormally high levels of anaesthetic agents may even occur.

Balanced anaesthesia

With the wide variety of drugs available, the therapeutic effects required need to be balanced with the potential for adverse effects. This is accomplished by **balanced anaesthesia** – the combining of several drugs, each with a specific effect, to achieve analgesia, muscle relaxation, unconsciousness and amnesia rather than using one drug. Balanced anaesthesia commonly involves the following agents:

- *Preoperative medications*, which may include the use of anticholinergics that decrease secretions to facilitate intubation and prevent bradycardia associated with neural depression.
- *Sedative–hypnotics* to relax the person, facilitate amnesia and decrease sympathetic stimulation.
- *Antiemetics* to decrease the nausea and vomiting associated with the slowing of GI activity.
- *Antihistamines* to decrease the chance of allergic reaction and help to dry up secretions.
- *Opioids* to aid analgesia and sedation.

Many of these drugs are given before the general anaesthetic is administered as **premedication** to facilitate the process. Some are continued during surgery to aid the general anaesthetic, allowing therapeutic effects at lower doses. For example, people may receive a neuromuscular-junction (NMJ) blocker (Chapter 28) to stop muscle activity and a rapid-acting intravenous general anaesthetic to induce anaesthesia, and then a gas general anaesthetic to balance the anaesthetic effect during the procedure and allow for easier recovery. Careful selection of appropriate general anaesthetic agents, along with monitoring and support of the person, helps to alleviate many problems relating to general anaesthesia.

Administration of general anaesthesia

General anaesthesia is delivered by a specialist doctor (anaesthetist) trained in the delivery of these potent drugs along with intubation, mechanical ventilation and full life support. During the delivery of anaesthesia, the person can go through predictable stages (Figure 27.1), referred to as the depth of anaesthesia:

Stage 1, the analgesia stage, refers to the loss of pain sensation, with the person still conscious and able to communicate.

Stage 2, the excitement stage, is a period of excitement and often combative behaviour, with many signs of sympathetic stimulation (eg, tachycardia, increased respirations and blood pressure changes).

Stage 3, surgical anaesthesia, involves relaxation of skeletal muscles, return of regular respirations, and progressive loss of eye reflexes and pupil dilation. Surgery can be safely performed in stage 3.

Stage 4, medullary paralysis, is very deep CNS depression with loss of respiratory and vasomotor centre stimuli, in which death can occur rapidly. If a person reaches this level, the anaesthesia has become too intense and the situation is critical.

General anaesthesia administration is also divided into three phases: induction, maintenance and recovery.

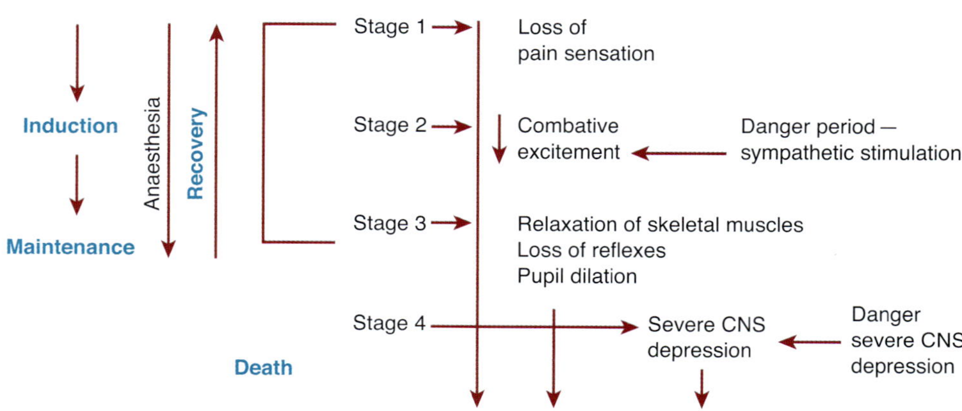

FIGURE 27.1 Stages of general anaesthesia.

Induction

Induction is the period from the beginning of anaesthesia until stage 3, or surgical anaesthesia, is reached. The danger period for many people during induction is stage 2 because of the systemic stimulation that occurs. Often a rapid-acting anaesthetic is used to move quickly through this phase and into stage 3. NMJ blockers may be used during induction to facilitate intubation, which is necessary to support the person with mechanical ventilation during anaesthesia (see Chapter 28).

Maintenance

Maintenance is the period from stage 3 until the surgical procedure is complete. A slower, more predictable anaesthetic, such as a gas anaesthetic, may be used to maintain the anaesthesia once the person is in stage 3.

Recovery

Recovery is the period from discontinuation of the anaesthetic until the person has regained consciousness, movement and the ability to communicate. During recovery, the person requires continuous monitoring for any adverse effects of the drugs used and to ensure support of the person's vital functions as necessary.

KEY POINTS

- General anaesthesia produces analgesia, amnesia and unconsciousness.
- General anaesthesia places the person at risk for problems because of its extensive CNS depression and widespread effects on other body systems.
- Balanced anaesthesia involves the administration of several drugs rather than a single drug to achieve analgesia, muscle relaxation, unconsciousness and amnesia.
- Induction of anaesthesia is the period ranging from administration of the anaesthetic to the point of surgical anaesthesia.

GENERAL ANAESTHETIC AGENTS

Several different types of drugs are used as general anaesthetics. These include barbiturate and non-barbiturate anaesthetics, gas anaesthetics and volatile liquids. See Table 27.1 for a list of general anaesthetic agents along with the anticipated adverse effects of these drugs.

BARBITURATE ANAESTHETICS

The barbiturate anaesthetics (Table 27.1) are intravenous drugs used to induce rapid anaesthesia, which is then maintained with an inhaled drug. The available drug in this group is thiopental (*Pentothal*).

Therapeutic actions and indications

Thiopental is a barbiturate that is used for induction of anaesthesia, particularly in intravenous anaesthetics. Because it has no analgesic properties, the person may need additional analgesics after surgery.

Pharmacokinetics

Thiopental has a very rapid onset of action, usually within 10–30 seconds, and an ultra-short recovery period of 5–8 minutes. Induction is generally smooth and rapid, but dose-related cardiovascular and respiratory depression can occur. Waking from a moderate dose of thiopental is rapid because the drug redistributes into other tissues, particularly fat. However, metabolism is slow and sedative effects can persist for 24 hours. Repeated doses have a cumulative effect and recovery is much slower.

Contraindications and cautions

The drug should not be used until the anaesthetist and staff are ready and equipped for intubation and respiratory support *because of the rapid onset and because the drug can cause respiratory depression and apnoea*. The drug should not be used during pregnancy or breastfeeding unless the benefit clearly outweighs the potential risk to the fetus or neonate *because of the CNS depressive effects of this drug. This drug is lipophilic and can be rapidly absorbed through the placental barrier.*

Adverse effects

The adverse effects associated with this drug are related to the suppression of the CNS, with decreased pulse, hypotension, suppressed respirations and decreased GI activity. Nausea and vomiting after recovery are common.

 **Prototype summary: thiopental**

Indications: induction of anaesthesia, maintenance of anaesthesia; induction of a hypnotic state.

Actions: depresses the CNS to produce hypnosis and anaesthesia without analgesia.

Pharmacokinetics:

Route	Onset	Duration
IV	1 min	20–30 min

$T_{1/2}$: 3–8 hours; metabolised in the liver, excreted in the urine.

Adverse effects: emergence delirium, headache, restlessness, anxiety, cardiovascular depression, respiratory depression, apnoea, salivation, hiccups, skin rashes.

TABLE 27.1 DRUGS IN FOCUS General anaesthetic agents

Drug name	Onset	Recovery	Analgesia	Systems alert[a] CV	Resp	CNS	GI	Renal	Hepatic
Barbiturate anaesthetics									
thiopental (*Pentothal*)	10–30 seconds	3–8 minutes	none	—	—	—	—	—	—
Non-barbiturate general anaesthetics									
droperidol (*Droleptan*)	3–10 minutes	2–4 hours	—	++	—	+	—	+	+
ketamine (*Ketalar*)	30 seconds	45 minutes	+	++	—	+++	—	—	—
midazolam (*Hypnovel*)	15 minutes	30 minutes	+	—	+++	—	++	—	—
propofol (*Diprivan, Fresofol, Provive*)	30–60 seconds	25–10 minutes	+	++	+	++	—	—	—
Anaesthetic gas									
nitrous oxide (blue cylinder)	1–2 minutes	rapid	++++	+++	+	+	—	—	—
Volatile liquids									
desflurane (*Suprane*)	1–2 minutes	15–20 minutes	+	—	++++	—	—	—	—
isoflurane (*Aerrane, Forthane*)	1–2 minutes	15–20 minutes	+	++	+	—	+	—	—
methoxyflurane (*Penthrox*)	10–30 seconds	rapid	++++	+	+	+	+	++	++
sevoflurane (*Sevorane*)	30 seconds	10 minutes	+	—	++	—	—	—	—

[a]Systems alert indicates physiological systems with anticipated adverse effects to these drugs. When drugs are selected, the individual's condition and potential for serious problems with these adverse effects should be considered.
—, no effect; +, mild effect; ++, moderate effect; +++, strong effect; ++++, powerful effect

Clinically important drug–drug interactions

Caution must be used when barbituates are used with any other CNS suppressants. They can cause decreased effectiveness of theophylline, oral anticoagulants, beta blockers, corticosteroids, hormonal contraceptives, metronidazol and carbamazepine. Combinations of barbiturate anaesthetics and opioids may produce apnoea more commonly than occurs with other analgesics.

NON-BARBITURATE ANAESTHETICS

The other parenteral drugs used for intravenous administration in anaesthesia are non-barbiturates, with a wide variety of effects. Such anaesthetics include droperidol (*Droleptan*), ketamine (*Ketalar*), midazolam (*Hypnovel*) and propofol (*Diprivan*). (See Table 27.1.)

Therapeutic action and indications

Midazolam is the prototype non-barbiturate anaesthetic. It is a very potent amnesiac. These drugs are thought to act in the reticular activating system (RAS) and limbic system to potentiate the effects of gamma-aminobutyric acid (GABA). Midazolam's amnesiac effects occur at doses below those needed to cause sedation. It is widely used to produce amnesia or sedation for many diagnostic, therapeutic and endoscopic procedures. Midazolam can also be used to induce anaesthesia and to provide continuous sedation for people who are intubated and those being mechanically ventilated. Droperidol produces marked sedation and produces a state of mental detachment. It also has antiemetic effects, reducing the incidence of nausea and vomiting in surgical and diagnostic procedures. Ketamine has been associated with a bizarre state of unconsciousness in which the person appears to be awake but is unconscious and cannot feel pain. This drug, which causes sympathetic stimulation with increase in blood pressure and heart rate, may be helpful in situations when cardiac depression is dangerous. Propofol is often used for short procedures because it has a very rapid clearance and produces much less of a hangover effect and allows for quick recovery. It is also used to maintain people on mechanical ventilation.

Pharmacokinetics

Midazolam has a rapid onset but does not reach peak effectiveness for 30–60 minutes. Droperidol has an onset of action within 3 minutes and an ultra-short recovery period. Ketamine has an onset of action within 30 seconds and a very slow recovery period (45 minutes). Propofol is a very short-acting anaesthetic with a rapid onset of action of 30–60 seconds; duration of anaesthesia after a single dose is 3–10 minutes.

Contraindications and cautions

Midazolam is more likely to cause nausea and vomiting than are some of the other anaesthetics, and so it should be used with caution in any person who could be compromised by vomiting. It has been associated with respiratory depression and respiratory arrest, and so life support equipment should be readily available whenever it is used. Droperidol should be used with caution in individuals with renal or hepatic failure and should be used with extreme care in people with prolonged QT intervals or who are at risk for prolonged QT intervals.

Adverse effects

People receiving any general anaesthetic are at risk for skin breakdown because they will not be able to move. Care must be taken to prevent decubitus ulcer formation. People receiving midazolam should be monitored for respiratory depression and CNS suppression. During the recovery period, droperidol may cause hypotension, chills, hallucinations and drowsiness. It may also cause QT prolongation, which puts the person at risk for serious cardiac arrhythmias. Ketamine crosses the blood–brain barrier and can cause hallucinations, dreams and psychotic episodes. Propofol often causes local burning on injection. It can cause bradycardia, hypotension and, in extreme cases, pulmonary oedema.

Clinically important drug–drug interactions

If ketamine and isoflurane are used in combination, severe cardiac depression with hypotension and bradycardia may occur. If these agents must be used together, the person should be monitored closely. Droperidol should not be used with other drugs that prolong the QT interval. If this combination is necessary, the person should be monitored continuously. Ketamine may also potentiate the muscular-blocking action of NMJ blockers, and the person may require prolonged periods of respiratory support. Midazolam is associated with increased toxicity and length of recovery when used in combination with inhaled anaesthetics, other CNS depressants, opioids, propofol or thiopental. If any of these agents are used in combination, careful balancing of drug doses is necessary.

 **Prototype summary: midazolam**

Indications: sedation, anxiolysis and amnesia before diagnostic, therapeutic or endoscopic procedures; induction of anaesthesia; continuous sedation of intubated people.

Actions: acts mainly at the limbic system and RAS; potentiates the effects of GABA; has little effect on cortical function; exact mechanism of action is not understood.

Pharmacokinetics:

Route	Onset	Peak	Duration
Oral	30–60 min	12 hours	2–6 hours
IM	15 min	30 min	2–6 hours
IV	3–5 min	< 30 min	2–6 hours

$T_{1/2}$: 1.8–6.8 hours; metabolised in the liver, excreted in the urine.

Adverse effects: transient drowsiness, sedation, drowsiness, lethargy, apathy, fatigue, disorientation, restlessness, constipation, diarrhoea, incontinence, urinary retention, bradycardia, tachycardia, phlebitis at IV injection site.

ANAESTHETIC GASES

Like all inhaled drugs, anaesthetic gases enter the bronchi and alveoli, rapidly pass into the capillary system (because gases flow from areas of higher concentration to areas of lower concentration) and are transported to the heart to be pumped throughout the body. These gases have a very high affinity for fatty tissue, and they are lipophilic, including the lipid membrane of the nerves in the CNS. The gases pass quickly into the brain and cause severe CNS depression. Once the person is in stage 3 of anaesthesia, the anaesthetist regulates the amount of gas that is delivered to ensure that it is sufficient to keep the person unconscious but not enough to cause severe CNS depression. This is done by decreasing the concentration of the gas that is flowing into the bronchi, creating a concentration gradient that results in the movement of gas in the opposite direction – out of the tissues and back to expired air.

Nitrous oxide is an anaesthetic gas (provided in a blue cylinder). (See Table 27.1.)

Therapeutic actions and indications

Nitrous oxide is a very potent analgesic. However, it is the weakest of the gas anaesthetics and the least toxic. It moves so quickly in and out of the body that it can actually accumulate and cause pressure in closed body compartments such as the sinuses. Because nitrous oxide is such a potent analgesic, it is used frequently for dental surgery and during labour. It does not cause muscle relaxation. Nitrous oxide is usually combined with other agents for anaesthetic use.

Pharmacokinetics

All of these agents have a rapid onset of action, usually within 1–2 minutes, and a rapid recovery period. Timing of recovery depends on the other drugs being used.

Contraindications and cautions

Nitrous oxide can block the reuptake of oxygen after surgery and cause hypoxia. Because of this reaction, it is always given in combination with oxygen. Susceptible individuals should be monitored for signs of hypoxia, chest pain and stroke.

Adverse effects

As with other general anaesthetics, people need to be monitored for skin integrity when they are not able to move for periods of time. Nitrous oxide can cause acute sinus and middle ear pain, bowel obstruction and pneumothorax because it so rapidly moves into and accumulates in closed spaces. Because nitrous oxide inactivates vitamin B12, people should also be monitored for low vitamin B12 levels, including neurological, immune and haematological complications.

Clinically important drug–drug interactions

Caution should be used if these drugs are combined with any other drug that causes CNS depression. If halothane and ketamine are used in combination, severe cardiac depression with hypotension and bradycardia may occur. If these agents must be used together, the person should be monitored closely.

VOLATILE LIQUIDS

Inhaled anaesthetics also can be **volatile liquids** – liquids that are unstable at room temperature and release gases.

 **Prototype summary: nitrous oxide**

Indications: induction and maintenance of anaesthesia.

Actions: depresses the CNS to produce anaesthesia and analgesia.

Pharmacokinetics:

Route	Onset	Duration
IV	1–2 min	20 min

$T_{1/2}$: minutes; the rise time of alveolar concentrations is faster than for any other anaesthetic agent, and elimination is faster than for any other anaesthetic; it is not metabolised but is excreted in the lungs.

Adverse effects: cardiovascular depression, respiratory depression, apnoea, earache, sinus pain, vomiting, malignant hyperthermia.

These gases are then inhaled by the person. Therefore, volatile liquids act like gas anaesthetics.

Most of the volatile liquids in use are halogenated hydrocarbons such as desflurane (*Suprane*), isoflurane (*Aerrane, Forthane*), methoxyflurane (*Penthrox*) and sevoflurane (*Sevorane*). (See Table 27.1.)

Therapeutic actions and indications

Desflurane is widely used in outpatient surgery because of its rapid onset and quick recovery time.

Isoflurane is widely used to maintain anaesthesia after inductions. It can cause muscle relaxation.

Sevoflurane is used in outpatient surgery as an induction agent and is rapidly cleared for quick recovery.

Pharmacokinetics

Desflurane and isoflurane have a rapid onset – also within 1–2 minutes – and rapid recovery – usually within 15–20 minutes. Sevoflurane, the newest of the volatile liquids, has a very rapid onset of action – within 30 seconds – and a very rapid clearance – lasting only about 10 minutes. These drugs are all cleared through the lungs.

Contraindications and cautions

Desflurane use should be avoided in people with respiratory problems and in those with increased sensitivity *because of its irritation to the airways and tendency to cause respiratory depression*. In addition, it is not recommended for induction in children *because of its irritation of the airways*. Isoflurane and sevoflurane should be used with caution in individuals with respiratory depression *to avoid severe respiratory depression*. All of these drugs have the potential to trigger malignant hyperthermia and should be used with caution in any individual at high risk for developing it *to avoid development of malignant hyperthermia*. Dantrolene, the preferred treatment for malignant hyperthermia, should be readily available whenever any of these drugs is used. These drugs should be avoided in pregnancy and breastfeeding unless the benefit clearly outweighs the risk to the fetus or baby *because of the CNS depressive effects of the drugs*.

Adverse effects

Desflurane is associated with a collection of respiratory reactions, including cough, increased secretions and laryngospasm. Isoflurane is associated with hypotension, hypercapnoea, muscle soreness and a bad taste in the mouth, but it does not cause cardiac arrhythmias or respiratory irritation, as do some other volatile liquids.

Clinically important drug–drug interactions

Caution should be used when any of these drugs is combined with other CNS suppressants.

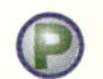 **Prototype summary: isoflurane**

Indications: induction and maintenance of general anaesthesia.

Actions: depresses the CNS, causing anaesthesia; relaxes muscles; sensitises the myocardium to the effects of adrenaline (epinephrine) and noradrenaline (norepinephrine).

Pharmacokinetics:

Route	Onset	Peak	Duration
Inhaled	Rapid	Rapid	End of inhalation

$T_{1/2}$: unknown; minimally metabolised in the liver, excreted in the urine.

Adverse effects: disorientation, restlessness, bradycardia, tachycardia, hypoxia, acidosis, malignant hyperthermia, hyperkalaemia, respiratory depression, apnoea, dyspnoea, arrhythmias, hepatic injury, ileus, shivering.

BOX 27.2 Adverse reactions

Volatile liquid anaesthetics can trigger malignant hyperthermia and are contraindicated in those susceptible to malignant hyperthermia. They can increase cerebrospinal pressure and should be used with caution in those with raised intracranial pressure. They can also cause hepatotoxicity in those sensitised to halogenated anaesthetics. In children with neuromuscular disease, inhalational anaesthetics are very rarely associated with hyperkalaemia, resulting in cardiac arrhythmias and death. Cardiorespiratory depression, hypotension and arrhythmias are common adverse effects of volatile liquid anaesthetics.

Care considerations for people receiving general anaesthetic agents

Assessment: history and examination

- Assess for contraindications or cautions: any known allergies to general anaesthetics *to avoid hypersensitivity reactions*; impaired liver or kidney function, *which might interfere with drug metabolism and excretion*; myasthenia gravis or cardiac or respiratory disease, *which may be exacerbated by the depressive effects of the drug*; personal or family history of malignant hyperthermia, *which may be triggered by the use of general anaesthetics*.
- Perform a physical assessment, including weighing the person, *to determine the appropriate dosing of the drug and to establish a baseline status before beginning therapy and evaluate for any potential adverse effects*.
- Assess the person's neurological status, including level of consciousness, affect, reflexes and pupil size and reaction, and evaluate muscle tone and response, *to monitor CNS depression and provide appropriate support as needed*.
- Monitor vital signs, including temperature, pulse and blood pressure, for changes, and auscultate lung and heart sounds *to monitor for adverse effects of the drugs*.
- Obtain an electrocardiogram (ECG) *to evaluate for underlying cardiac problems that may be exacerbated by the drug*.
- Assess skin colour and lesions *to monitor for potential skin breakdown resulting from paralysis and immobility while under anaesthesia*.
- Auscultate abdomen for bowel sounds *to evaluate GI motility*.
- Monitor the results of laboratory tests, including renal and liver function tests, *to determine the possible need for a reduction in dose and evaluate for possible toxicity*.

Implementation with rationale

- Keep in mind that the drug must be administered by trained personnel (usually an anaesthetist) *because of the potential risks associated with its use*.
- Have emergency equipment to maintain airway and provide mechanical ventilation readily available *when person is not able to maintain respiration because of CNS depression*.
- Monitor temperature *for prompt detection and treatment of malignant hyperthermia*. Maintain dantrolene on standby.

- Monitor pulse, respiration, blood pressure, ECG and cardiac output continually during administration *to assess systemic response to CNS depression and provide appropriate support as needed.*
- Monitor temperature and reflexes *because dose adjustment may be needed to alleviate potential problems and to maximise overall benefit with the least toxicity.*
- Institute safety precautions, such as side rails, and monitor person until the recovery phase is complete and the person is conscious and able to move and communicate *to ensure safety.*
- Provide comfort measures *to help the person tolerate drug effects.* Provide pain relief as appropriate, along with reassurance and support *to deal with the effects of anaesthesia and loss of control,* skin care and turning *to prevent skin breakdown* and supportive care *for conditions such as hypotension and bronchospasm.*
- Offer support and encouragement *to help the person cope with the procedure and the drugs being used.*
- Provide the following preoperative teaching, *realising that most individuals who receive the drug will be unconscious or will be receiving teaching about a particular procedure:*
  - information about the anaesthetic (eg, what to expect, rate of onset, time to recovery)
  - medications that may be used preoperatively
  - effects of the medication on the person preoperatively
  - measures to maintain the person's safety preoperatively and during recovery
  - how the person will feel during the recovery phase
  - signs and symptoms to report during recovery and afterward.

Evaluation

- Monitor response to the drug (analgesia, loss of consciousness).
- Monitor for adverse effects (respiratory depression, hypotension, bronchospasm, slowed GI activity, skin breakdown, malignant hyperthermia).
- Evaluate the effectiveness of the teaching plan (person can relate anticipated effects of the drug and the recovery process).
- Monitor the effectiveness of comfort and safety measures.

KEY POINTS

- General anaesthetics must be administered by doctors or anaesthetists trained in their administration and prepared to provide constant monitoring and life support measures to assist the person when the CNS is depressed.
- General anaesthetics include barbiturates and non-barbiturate drugs, which are administered parenterally, and anaesthetic gases and volatile liquids, which are administered through inhalation.
- People receiving general anaesthetics must be constantly monitored because the CNS depression can cause respiratory arrest, cardiovascular reactions including hypotension and alterations in GI activity that can lead to nausea and vomiting.

LOCAL ANAESTHESIA

Local anaesthesia refers to a loss of sensation in limited areas of the body. It can be achieved by several different methods: topical administration, infiltration, field block, nerve block and intravenous regional anaesthesia.

Topical administration

Topical local anaesthesia involves the application of a cream, lotion, ointment or drop of a local anaesthetic to traumatised skin to relieve pain. It can also involve applying these forms to the mucous membranes in the eye, nose, throat, mouth, urethra, anus or rectum to relieve pain or to anaesthetise the area to facilitate a medical procedure. Although systemic absorption is rare with topical application, it can occur if there is damage or breakdown of the tissues in the area.

Infiltration

Infiltration local anaesthesia involves injecting the anaesthetic directly into the tissues to be treated (eg, sutured, drilled, cut). This injection brings the anaesthetic into contact with the nerve endings in the area and prevents them from transmitting nerve impulses to the brain.

Field block

Field block local anaesthesia involves injecting the anaesthetic all around the area that will be affected by the procedure or surgery. This is more intense than infiltration anaesthesia because the anaesthetic agent comes in contact with all of the nerve endings surrounding the area. This type of block is often used for tooth extractions.

Nerve block

Nerve block local anaesthesia involves injecting the anaesthetic at some point along the nerve or nerves that run to and from the region in which the loss of pain sensation or muscle paralysis is desired. These blocks are not performed in the surgical field, but at some distance from the field. They involve a greater area with potential for more adverse effects. Several types of nerve blocks are possible:

- Peripheral nerve block: blockage of the sensory and motor aspects of a particular nerve for relief of pain or for diagnostic purposes.
- Central nerve block: injection of anaesthetic into the roots of the nerves in the spinal cord.
- Epidural anaesthesia: injection of the drug into the epidural space where the nerves emerge from the spinal cord.
- Caudal block: injection of anaesthetic into the sacral canal, below the epidural area.
- Spinal anaesthesia: injection of anaesthetic into the spinal subarachnoid space.

Intravenous regional local anaesthesia

Intravenous regional local anaesthesia involves carefully draining all of the blood from the person's arm or leg, securing a tourniquet to prevent the anaesthetic from entering the general circulation, and then injecting the anaesthetic into the vein of the arm or leg. This technique is used for very specific surgical procedures.

LOCAL ANAESTHETIC AGENTS

Local anaesthetic agents (Table 27.2) are used primarily to prevent the person from feeling pain for varying periods of time after the agents have been administered in the peripheral nervous system. In increasing concentrations, local anaesthetics can also cause loss of the following sensations (in this sequence): temperature, touch, proprioception (position sense) and skeletal muscle tone. If these other aspects of nerve function are progressively lost, recovery occurs in the reverse order of the loss.

The local anaesthetics are very powerful nerve blockers, and it is very important that their effects be limited to a particular area of the body. They should not be absorbed systemically. Systemic absorption could produce toxic effects on the nervous system and the heart (eg, severe CNS depression, cardiac arrhythmias).

TABLE 27.2 *DRUGS IN FOCUS* Local anaesthetic agents

Drug name	Onset	Duration	Administration	Special considerations
Esters				
tetracaine (amethocaine) (*Minims Amethocaine Eye Drops*)	10–20 seconds	10–20 minutes	Eye	Eye should be protected from rubbing or contamination
benzocaine (*Cepacaine*)	1 minute	30–60 minutes	Skin, mucous membranes	Avoid tight bandages with skin preparation
Amides				
bupivacaine (*Marcain*)	5–20 minutes	2–7 hours	Local, epidural, dental, caudal, subarachnoid, sympathetic, retrobulbar	Do not use Bier Block – deaths have occurred
cinchocaine (*Proctosedyl, Rectinol, Scheriproct*)	< 15 minutes	3–4 hours	Skin, mucous membranes	Monitor for local reactions
levobupivacaine (*Chirocaine*)	8–20 minutes	7–10 hours	Local nerve block, epidural	Use cautiously in individuals with cardiovascular conditions
(P) lidocaine (lignocaine) (*EMLA, Xylocaine, Ziagel*)	5–15 minutes	30–90 minutes	Caudal, epidural, spinal cervical, dental, skin, mucous membrane, topical patch	Short acting, preferred for short procedures; danger if absorbed systemically
mepivacaine (*Scandonest*)	5–10 minutes	0.5 hours	Dental procedures	Advise person to take care with hot drinks
prilocaine (*Citanest*)	1–15 minutes	0.5–3 hours	Nerve block, dental	Advise people not to bite themselves
ropivacaine (*Naropin*)	1–5 minutes	2–6 hours	Nerve block, epidural, caudal	Avoid rapid infusion; offers good pain management postop and OB

Local anaesthetics are classified as esters or amides. The agent of choice depends on the method of administration, the length of time for which the area is to be anaesthetised and consideration of potential adverse effects. Esters include benzocaine (*Cepacaine*) and tetracaine (amethocaine) (generic). Amides include bupivacaine (*Marcain*), cinchocaine (*Proctosedyl, Rectinol, Scheriproct*), levobupivacaine (*Chirocaine*), lidocaine (lignocaine) (*Xylocaine*), mepivacaine (*Scandonest*), prilocaine (*Citanest*) and ropivacaine (*Naropin*).

Therapeutic actions and indications

Local anaesthetics work by causing a temporary interruption in the production and conduction of nerve impulses. They affect the permeability of nerve membranes to sodium ions, which normally infuse into the cell in response to stimulation. By preventing the sodium ions from entering the nerve, they stop the nerve from depolarising. A particular section of the nerve cannot be stimulated, and nerve impulses directed towards that section are lost when they reach that area.

The way in which a local anaesthetic is administered helps to increase its effectiveness by delivering it directly to the area that is causing or will cause the pain, thereby decreasing systemic absorption and related toxic effects (Figure 27.2). Local anaesthetics are indicated for infiltration anaesthesia, peripheral nerve block, spinal anaesthesia and the relief of local pain.

Pharmacokinetics

The ester local anaesthetics are broken down immediately in the plasma by enzymes known as **plasma esterases**. The amide local anaesthetics are metabolised more slowly in the liver, and serum levels of these drugs (i.e. active metabolites) can increase and lead to toxicity.

Contraindications and cautions

The local anaesthetics are contraindicated with any of the following conditions: history of allergy to any one of these agents or to parabens *to avoid hypersensitivity reactions*; heart block, *which could be greatly exacerbated with systemic absorption*; shock, *which could alter the local delivery and absorption of these drugs*; and decreased plasma esterases, *which could result in toxic levels of the ester-type local anaesthetics*.

They should be used during pregnancy and breastfeeding only if the benefit outweighs any potential risk to the fetus or neonate that could occur if the drug is inadvertently absorbed systemically *because of the suppressive effects on nerves*.

Adverse effects

The adverse effects of these drugs may be related to their local blocking of sensation (eg, skin breakdown, self-injury, biting oneself). Loss of skin integrity is always a problem if the person is unable to move, and care must

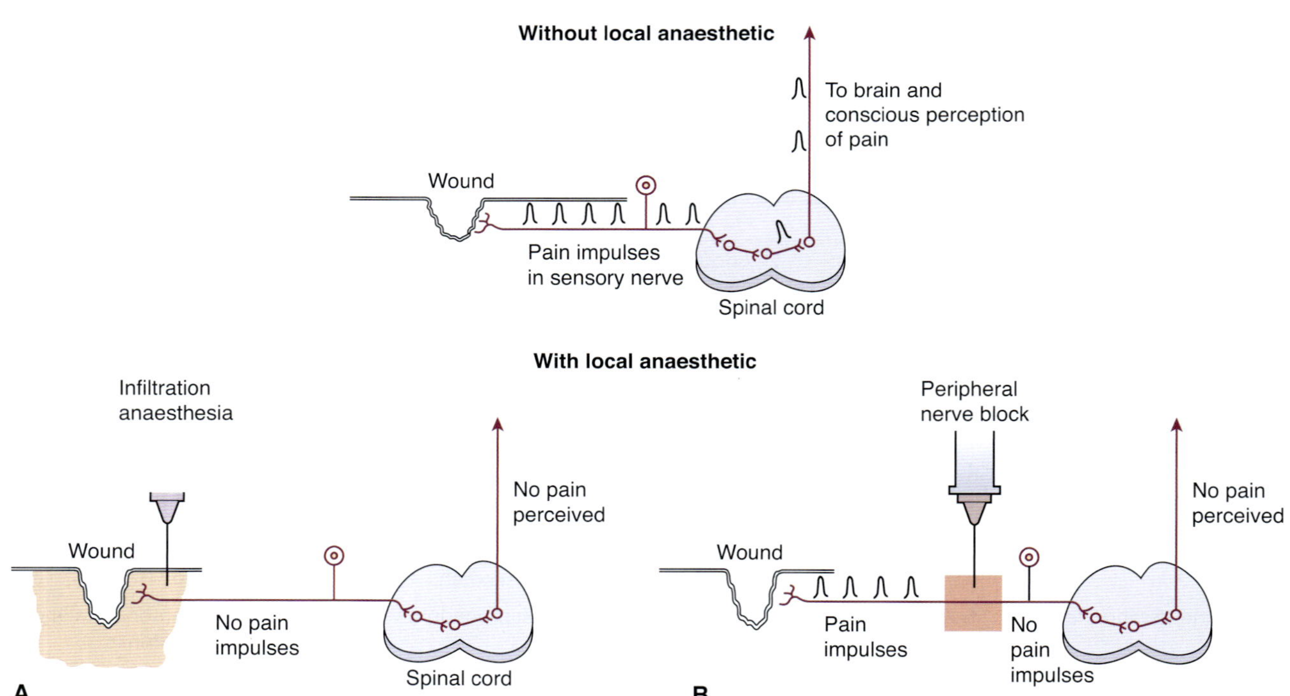

FIGURE 27.2 Mechanism of action of local anaesthetics. **Top.** An injury produces pain impulses (action potentials) that are conducted and transmitted in an area of the brain in which pain is perceived. **A.** Conduction of the pain impulse has been blocked by infiltration anaesthetics at the site of the injury. **B.** A nerve block at some distance from the injury. Local anaesthetics block the movement of sodium into the nerve and prevent nerve depolarisation, stopping the transmission of the pain impulse.

be taken to prevent skin breakdown. Other problematic effects are associated with the route of administration and the amount of drug that is absorbed systemically. These effects are related to the blockade of nerve depolarisation throughout the system. Effects that may occur include CNS effects such as headache (especially with epidural and spinal anaesthesia), restlessness, anxiety, dizziness, tremors, blurred vision and backache; GI effects such as nausea and vomiting; cardiovascular effects such as peripheral vasodilation, myocardial depression, arrhythmias and blood pressure changes, all of which may lead to fatal cardiac arrest; and respiratory arrest.

Clinically important drug–drug interactions

When local anaesthetics and succinylcholine are given together, increased and prolonged neuromuscular blockade occurs. There is also less risk of systemic absorption and increased local effects if these drugs are combined with adrenaline (epinephrine).

 **Prototype summary: lidocaine (lignocaine)**

Indications: infiltration anaesthesia, peripheral and sympathetic nerve blocks, central nerve blocks, spinal and caudal anaesthesia, topical anaesthetic for skin or mucous membrane disorders.

Actions: blocks the generation and conduction of action potentials in sensory nerves by reducing sodium permeability, reducing the height and rate of rise of the action potential, increasing the excitation threshold and slowing the conduction velocity.

Pharmacokinetics:

Route	Onset	Peak	Duration
IM	5–10 min	5–15 min	2 hours
Topical	Not generally absorbed systemically		

$T_{1/2}$: 10 minutes, then 1.5–3 hours; metabolised in the liver, excreted in the urine.

Adverse effects: headache, backache, hypotension, urinary retention, urinary incontinence, pruritus, seizures; when locally applied: burning, stinging, swelling, tenderness.

Care considerations for people receiving local anaesthetic agents

Assessment: history and examination

- Assess for contraindications and cautions: any known allergies to these drugs or to parabens *to avoid hypersensitivity reactions*; impaired liver function, *which could alter metabolism and clearance of the drug*; low plasma esterases, *which could lead to toxicity of esters*; heart block, *which could be exacerbated by the drug effects*; shock *to prevent altered local delivery and absorption*; and current status of pregnancy or breastfeeding, *which are cautions to the use of the drug.*
- Perform a physical assessment *to establish a baseline status before beginning therapy and for any potential adverse effects.*
- Inspect site for local anaesthetic application *to ensure integrity of the skin and to prevent inadvertent systemic absorption of the drug.*
- Assess the person's neurological status, including level of orientation, reflexes, pupil size and reaction, muscle tone and response and sensation, *to evaluate the effectiveness of the drug and monitor for potential toxic neurological effects.*
- Monitor vital signs, including temperature, pulse and blood pressure, and assess respiratory rate and auscultate lungs for adventitious sounds *to identify changes and possible systemic absorption.*
- Monitor laboratory test results, such as liver function tests and plasma esterases (if appropriate), *to determine possible need for dose adjustment.*
- Refer to the Critical thinking scenario for a full discussion of care for a person who is receiving local anaesthesia.

Implementation with rationale

- Have emergency equipment readily available *to maintain airway and provide mechanical ventilation if needed.*
- Ensure that drugs for managing hypotension, cardiac arrest and CNS alterations are readily available *in case of severe reaction and toxicity.*
- Ensure that the person receiving spinal anaesthesia or epidural anaesthesia are well hydrated and remain lying down for up to 12 hours after the anaesthesia *to minimise headache.*
- Establish safety precautions *to prevent injury during the time that the person has a loss of sensation and/or mobility.*
- Provide meticulous skin care to the site of administration *to reduce the risk of breakdown.*
- Provide comfort measures *to help the person tolerate drug effects.* Provide pain relief, as well as skin care and turning *to prevent skin breakdown,* and supportive care for hypotension *to prevent shock or serious hypoxia.*
- Offer support and encouragement *to help the person cope with the procedure and drugs being used.*

- Provide thorough teaching, including anaesthetic to be given, method for administration, activities involved with administering and monitoring the drug, and safety precautions.

Evaluation

- Monitor the person's response to the drug (loss of feeling in designated area).
- Monitor for adverse effects (respiratory depression, blood pressure changes, arrhythmias, GI upset, skin breakdown, injury, CNS alterations).
- Evaluate the effectiveness of the teaching plan (the person can relate the anticipated effects of the drug and the recovery process).

KEY POINTS

- Local anaesthetics block the depolarisation of nerve membranes, preventing the transmission of pain sensations and motor stimuli.
- Local anaesthetics are administered to deliver the drug directly to the desired area and to prevent systemic absorption, which could lead to serious interruption of nerve impulses and response.
- Ester-type local anaesthetics are immediately destroyed by plasma esterases. Amide local anaesthetics are destroyed in the liver and have a greater risk of accumulation and systemic toxicity.

CRITICAL THINKING SCENARIO

Local anaesthesia

THE SITUATION

A.M., a 32-year-old male athlete with a history of asthma (which could indicate pulmonary dysfunction), was admitted to the hospital for an inguinal hernia repair. At the person's request, the surgeon elected to use a local anaesthetic employing spinal anaesthesia. Because the extent of the repair was unknown (A.M. had undergone two previous repairs), bupivacaine, a long-acting anaesthetic, was selected. He remained alert (blood pressure 120/64 mmHg, pulse 62 beats/minute, respiration rate 10/minute) and stable throughout the procedure. Two hours after the conclusion of the procedure, A.M. appeared agitated (blood pressure 154/68 mmHg, pulse 88 beats/minute, respiration rate 12/minute). Although he did not complain of discomfort, he did state that he still had no feeling and had only limited movement of his legs.

CRITICAL THINKING

What safety precautions need to be taken?

What interventions should be done at this point?

How could the man be reassured? *Think about the anxiety level of the man – an athlete who elected to have local anaesthesia may have a problem with control and feel somewhat invincible. Consider the anxiety that loss of mobility and sensation in the legs may cause in a person who makes his living as an athlete.*

In addition, consider the expected duration of action of bupivacaine and the rate of return of function.

DISCUSSION

Bupivacaine is a long-acting anaesthetic with effects that may persist for several hours. The timing of the drug's effects should be explained to A.M., and he should be monitored for a period of time to determine whether his agitated state and slightly elevated vital signs are a result of anxiety or an unanticipated reaction to the surgery or the drug. Life-support equipment should be on standby in case his condition is a toxic drug reaction or some unanticipated problem occurring after surgery.

The health care professional is in the best position to perform the following interventions: explaining the effects of the drug and the anticipated recovery schedule; keeping the man as flat as possible to decrease the headache usually associated with spinal anaesthesia; encouraging the man to turn from side to side periodically to allow skin care to be performed and to alleviate the risk of pressure sore development; and staying with the man as much as possible to reassure him, to answer his questions, and to encourage him to talk about his feelings and reaction.

If the agitated state is caused by a stress reaction, the man should return to normal; comfort measures, teaching and reassurance should be provided. An elevated systolic pressure with a normal diastolic pressure often is an indication of a sympathetic stress response. An athlete is more likely than most people to suffer great anxiety and fear if his legs become numb and he is unable to move them. Teaching and comfort measures may be all that is needed to relieve the anxiety and ensure a good recovery.

CARE GUIDE FOR A.M.: LOCAL ANAESTHESIA

Assessment: history and examination

Assess for allergies to local anaesthetics or to parabens, cardiac disorders, vascular problems, hepatic dysfunction; also assess for concurrent use of suxamethonium.

Focus physical examination on the following:
CV: blood pressure, pulse, peripheral perfusion, ECG
CNS: orientation, affect, reflexes, vision
Skin: colour, lesions, texture, sweating
Respiratory: respiration, adventitious sounds
Laboratory tests: liver function tests, plasma esterases

Implementation

Provide comfort and safety measures: positioning, skin care, side rails, pain medication as needed, maintain airway, antidotes on standby.

Provide support and reassurance to deal with loss of sensation and mobility.

Provide teaching about procedure being performed and what to expect.

Provide life support as needed.

Evaluation

Evaluate drug effects: loss of sensation, loss of movement.

Monitor for adverse effects: cardiovascular effects (blood pressure changes, arrhythmias), respiratory depression, GI upset, CNS alterations, skin breakdown, anxiety and fear.

Monitor for drug–drug interactions as indicated for each drug.

Evaluate the effectiveness of the teaching program and comfort and safety measures.

Constantly monitor vital signs and muscular function and sensation as it returns.

TEACHING FOR A.M.

Teaching about local anaesthetics is usually incorporated into the overall teaching plan about the procedure that the man will undergo. Things to highlight with the man would include the following:

- Discussion of the overall procedure:
  - What it will feel like (any numbness, tingling, inability to move, pressure, pain, choking?)
  - Any anticipated discomfort
  - How long it will last
  - Concerns during the procedure: report any discomfort and ask any questions as they arise
- Discussion of the recovery:
  - How long it will take
  - Feelings to expect: tingling, numbness, pressure, itching
  - Pain that will be felt as the anaesthesia wears off
  - Measures to reduce pain in the area
  - Signs and symptoms to report (eg, pain along a nerve route, palpitations, feeling faint, disorientation)

CHAPTER SUMMARY

- General anaesthetics result in analgesia, amnesia and unconsciousness; they also block muscle reflexes that could interfere with a surgical procedure or put the person at risk for harm.
- The use of general anaesthetics involves a widespread CNS depression that could be harmful, especially in people with underlying CNS, cardiovascular or respiratory diseases.
- Anaesthesia proceeds through four predictable stages from loss of sensation to total CNS depression and death.
- Induction of anaesthesia is the period of time from the beginning of anaesthesia administration until the person reaches surgical anaesthesia.
- Balanced anaesthesia involves giving a variety of drugs, including anticholinergics, rapid intravenous anaesthetics, inhaled anaesthetics, NMJ blockers and opioids.
- People receiving general anaesthetics should be monitored for any adverse effects; they need reassurance and safety measures until the recovery of sensation, mobility and the ability to communicate.
- Local anaesthetics block the depolarisation of nerve membranes, preventing the transmission of pain sensations and motor stimuli.
- Local anaesthetics are administered to deliver the drug directly to the desired area and to prevent systemic absorption, which could lead to serious interruption of nerve impulses and response.
- Ester-type local anaesthetics are immediately destroyed by plasma esterases. Amide local anaesthetics are destroyed in the liver and have a greater risk of accumulation and systemic toxicity.
- Care of people receiving general or local anaesthetics should include safety precautions to prevent injury and skin breakdown; support and reassurance to deal with the loss of sensation and mobility; and teaching regarding what to expect, to decrease stress and anxiety.

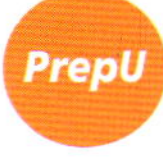

Knowing your strengths and weaknesses helps you to study more effectively. Take a PrepU Practice Quiz to find out how you measure up!

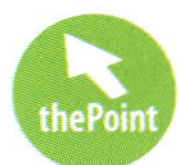

ONLINE RESOURCES

An extensive range of additional resources to enhance teaching and learning and to facilitate understanding of this chapter may be found online at the text's accompanying website, located on thePoint at http://thepoint.lww.com. These include Watch and Learn videos, Concepts in Action animations, journal articles, review questions, case studies, discussion topics and quizzes.

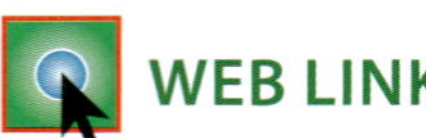

WEB LINKS

Health care providers and students may want to consult the following web resources:

http://allaboutanaesthesia.com.au
Information for people about types of anaesthesia.

www.anzca.edu.au
The Australian and New Zealand College of Anaesthetists.

www.painmanagement.org.au
The Australian Pain Management Association. Information on pain management, research and education.

www.spanza.org.au
The Society for Paediatric Anaesthesia in New Zealand and Australia.

BIBLIOGRAPHY

Armstrong, B., Reid, C., Heath, P., Simpson, H., Kitching, J., Nicholas, J., Chan, L., Taylor, J. & Rush, H. (2009). Rapid sequence induction anaesthesia: A guide for nurses in the emergency department. *International Emergency Nursing*, *17(3)*, 161–168.

Brandis, C. (2011). Alkalinisation of local anaesthetic solutions. *Australian Prescriber*, *34*, 173–175.

Braun, A. R., Leslie, K., Merry, A. F. & Story, D. (2010). What are we telling our patients? A survey of risk disclosure for anaesthesia in Australia and New Zealand, *Anaesthesia & Intensive Care*, *38(5)*, 935–938.

Braun, A. R., Skene, L. & Merry, A. F. (2010). Informed consent for anaesthesia in Australia and New Zealand. *Anaesthesia & Intensive Care*, *38(5)*, 809–822.

Farrell, M. & Dempsey, J. (2014). *Smeltzer & Bare's Textbook of Medical-Surgical Nursing* (3rd edn). Sydney: Lippincott Williams & Wilkins.

Gibbs, N. M. (2013). National anaesthesia mortality reporting in Australia from 1985–2008. *Anaesthesia & Intensive Care*, *41(3)*, 294–310.

Goodman, L. S., Brunton, L. L., Chabner, B. & Knollmann, B. C. (2011). *Goodman and Gilman's Pharmacological Basis of Therapeutics* (12th edn). New York: McGraw-Hill.

McKenna, L. & Mirkov, S. (2019). *McKenna's Drug Handbook for Nursing and Midwifery* (8th edn). Sydney: Wolters Kluwer Health Australia.

Mitchell-Brown, F. (2012). Malignant hyperthermia: Turn down the heat. *Nursing*, *42(5)*, 38–45.

Murtagh, J. E. (2006). Managing painful paediatric procedures. *Australian Prescriber*, *29*, 94–96.

Porth, C. M. (2011). *Essentials of Pathophysiology: Concepts of Altered Health States* (3rd edn). Philadelphia: Lippincott Williams & Wilkins.

Porth, C. M. (2009). *Pathophysiology: Concepts of Altered Health States* (8th edn). Philadelphia: Lippincott Williams & Wilkins.

Sawhney, M. (2012). Epidural analgesia: What nurses need to know. *Nursing*, *42(8)*, 36–42.

Schnabel, A., Poepping, D. M., Kranke, P., Zahn, P. K. & Pogatzki-Zahn, E. M. (2011). Efficacy and adverse effects of ketamine as an additive for paediatric caudal anaesthesia: A quantitative systematic review of randomized controlled trials. *British Journal of Anaesthesia*, *107(4)*, 601–611.

Wild, M. R., Gornall, C. B., Griffiths, D. E. & Curran, J. (2011). Maintenance of anaesthesia with sevoflurane or isoflurane effects on adverse airway events in smokers. *Anaesthesia*, *59(9)*, 891–893.

CHECK YOUR UNDERSTANDING

Answers to the questions in this chapter can be found in Appendix A at the back of this book.

MULTIPLE CHOICE

Select the best answer to the following.

1. The most dangerous period for many people undergoing general anaesthesia is during which stage?
   a. stage 1, when communication becomes difficult
   b. stage 2, when systemic stimulation occurs
   c. stage 3, when skeletal muscles relax
   d. there is no real danger during general anaesthesia

2. Recovery after a general anaesthetic refers to the period of time:
   a. from the beginning of the anaesthesia until the person is ready for surgery.
   b. during the surgery when anaesthesia is maintained at a certain level.
   c. from discontinuation of the anaesthetic until the person has regained consciousness, movement and the ability to communicate.
   d. when the person is in the most danger of CNS depression.

3. While a person is receiving a general anaesthetic, they must be continually monitored because:
   a. the person has no pain sensation.
   b. generalised CNS depression affects all body functions.
   c. the person cannot move.
   d. the person cannot communicate.

4. The teacher determines that teaching about general anaesthetics was successful when the students identify which person as being most qualified to administer general anaesthetics?
   a. clinical supervisor
   b. graduate nurse
   c. trained doctor
   d. surgeon

5. Local anaesthetics are used to block feeling in specific body areas. If given in increasing concentrations, local anaesthetics can cause loss, in order, of the following:
   a. temperature sensation, touch sensation, proprioception and skeletal muscle tone.
   b. touch sensation, skeletal muscle tone, temperature sensation and proprioception.
   c. proprioception, skeletal muscle tone, touch sensation and temperature sensation.
   d. skeletal muscle tone, touch sensation, temperature sensation and proprioception.

MULTIPLE RESPONSE

Select all that apply.

1. Comfort measures that are important for a person receiving a local anaesthetic would include which of the following?
   a. skin care and turning
   b. reassurance over loss of control and sensation
   c. use of antihypertensive agents
   d. use of analgesics as needed
   e. ice applied to the area involved
   f. safety precautions to prevent injury

2. A nurse would anticipate the use of general anaesthetics for which of the following reasons?
   a. to produce analgesia
   b. to produce amnesia
   c. to activate the reticular activating system
   d. to block muscle reflexes
   e. to cause unconsciousness
   f. to prevent nausea

3. Balanced anaesthesia combines different classes of drugs to achieve the best effects with the fewest adverse effects. Balanced anaesthesia usually involves the use of which of the following?
   a. anticholinergics
   b. opioids
   c. sedative/hypnotics
   d. beta-adrenergic blockers
   e. dantrolene
   f. neuromuscular-blocking agents

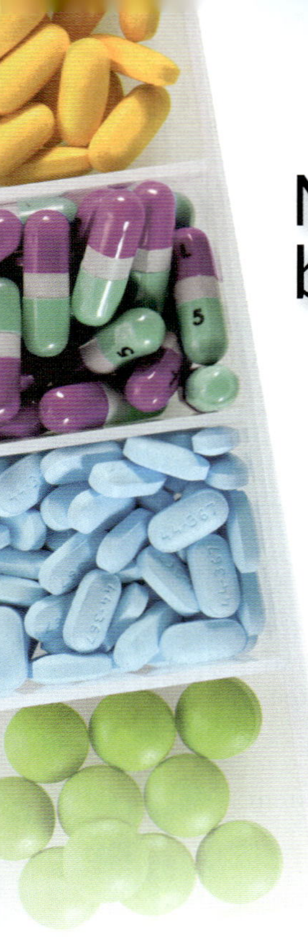

Neuromuscular junction–blocking agents

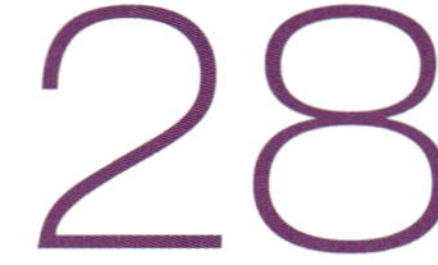

Learning objectives

On completing this chapter you should be able to:

1. Draw and label a neuromuscular junction.
2. Describe the therapeutic actions, indications, pharmacokinetics, contraindications, most common adverse reactions and important drug–drug interactions associated with the depolarising and non-depolarising neuromuscular-junction blockers.
3. Discuss the use of neuromuscular-junction blockers across the lifespan.
4. Compare and contrast the prototype drugs pancuronium and suxamethonium chloride with other neuromuscular-junction blockers.
5. Outline the care considerations, including important teaching points, for people receiving a neuromuscular-junction blocker.

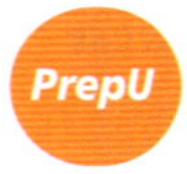
Test your current knowledge of neuromuscular junction blocking agents with a PrepU Practice Quiz!

Glossary of key terms

acetylcholine-receptor site: area on the muscle cell membrane where acetylcholine (ACh) reacts with a specific receptor site to cause stimulation of the muscle in response to nerve activity

depolarising neuromuscular-junction (NMJ) blocker: drug that stimulates a muscle cell, causing it to contract, with no allowance for repolarisation and re-stimulation of the muscle; characterised by contraction and then paralysis

malignant hyperthermia: reaction to some NMJ drugs in susceptible individuals; characterised by extreme muscle rigidity, severe hyperpyrexia, acidosis and, in some cases, death

neuromuscular junction (NMJ): the synapse between a nerve and a muscle cell

non-depolarising neuromuscular-junction (NMJ) blocker: drug that prevents stimulation or depolarisation of the muscle cell; prevents depolarisation and stimulation by blocking the effects of acetylcholine

paralysis: lack of muscle function

sarcomere: functional unit of a muscle cell, composed of actin and myosin molecules arranged in layers to give the unit a striped or striated appearance

sliding filament theory: theory explaining muscle contraction as a reaction of actin and myosin molecules when they are freed to react by the inactivation of troponin after calcium is allowed to enter the cell during depolarisation

NEUROMUSCULAR JUNCTION–BLOCKING AGENTS

Non-depolarising NMJs
atracurium
cisatracurium
mivacurium
(P) pancuronium
rocuronium
vecuronium

Depolarising NMJ
(P) suxamethonium chloride

Nerves communicate with muscles at a synapse called the neuromuscular junction (NMJ). At this point, a nerve stimulates a muscle to contract. If the nerve is not able to communicate with the muscle cell, the muscle will not be able to contract, and paralysis will result. Certain clinical situations require that a person not be able to move muscles, including surgery, diagnostic procedures and mechanical ventilation. Anaesthetics (discussed in Chapter 27) can prevent muscle movement by suppressing function through the central nervous system (CNS), with many systemic complications from this depression. The NMJ-blocking drugs are used to prevent the nerve stimulation at the muscle cell and cause paralysis of the muscle directly without total CNS depression and its many systemic effects.

THE NEUROMUSCULAR JUNCTION

The **neuromuscular junction** is the point at which a motor neuron communicates with a skeletal muscle fibre. The end result is muscular contraction. NMJ-blocking agents affect the normal functioning of muscles by interfering with the normal processes that occur at the junction of the nerve and muscle cell.

The functional unit of a muscle, called a **sarcomere**, is made up of light and dark filaments formed by actin and myosin molecules. These molecules are arranged in orderly stacks that give the sarcomere a striated or striped appearance. Normal muscle function involves the arrival of a nerve impulse at the motor nerve terminal, followed by the release of the neurotransmitter acetylcholine (ACh) into the synaptic cleft. At the **acetylcholine-receptor site** on the effector side of the synapse, ACh interacts with the nicotinic cholinergic receptors, causing depolarisation of the muscle membrane. ACh is then broken down by acetylcholinesterase (an enzyme), freeing the receptor for further stimulation. With stimulation, this depolarisation allows the release of calcium ions, stored in tubules, into the cell. The calcium binds to troponin, a chemical found throughout the sarcomere. This binding of troponin releases the actin and myosin binding sites, allowing them to react with each other. The actin and myosin molecules react with each other again and again, sliding along the filament and making it shorter. This is a contraction of the muscle fibre according to the **sliding filament theory** (Figure 28.1). As the calcium is removed from the cell during repolarisation of the muscle membrane, the troponin is freed and once again prevents the actin and myosin from reacting with each other. The muscle filament then relaxes or slides back to the resting position.

A dynamic balance of excitatory and inhibitory impulses to the muscle results in muscle tone. However, if ACh cannot react with the cholinergic muscle receptor or if the muscle cells cannot repolarise to allow new stimulation and muscle contraction, muscle **paralysis**, or loss of muscle function, occurs.

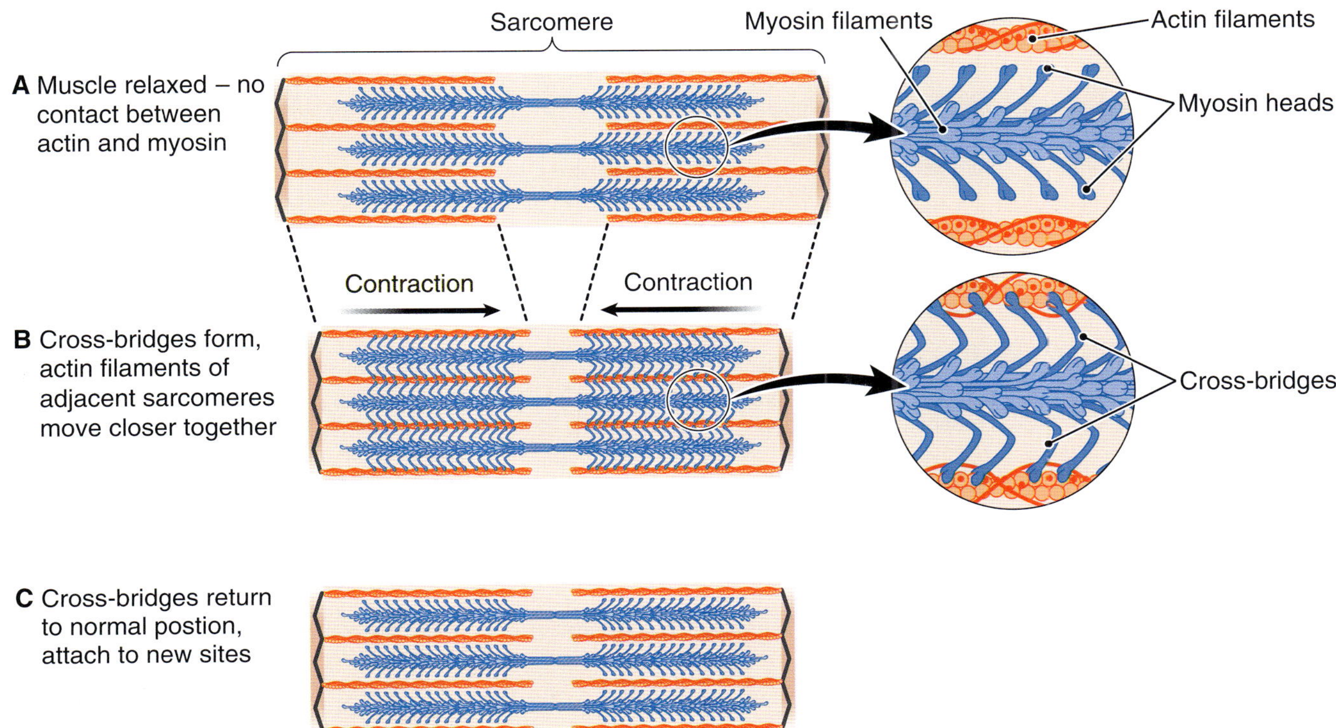

FIGURE 28.1 Sliding filament mechanism of skeletal muscle contraction. **A.** Muscle is relaxed, and there is no contact between the actin and myosin filaments. **B.** Cross-bridges form, and the actin filaments of adjacent sarcomeres are moved closer together as the muscle fibre contracts. **C.** The cross-bridges return to their original position and attach to new sites to prepare for another pull on the actin filaments and further contraction.

KEY POINTS

- The nerves and muscles communicate at the neuromuscular junction (NMJ).
- Acetylcholine (ACh) acts as the neurotransmitter at the NMJ.
- NMJ blockers interfere with muscle function.

NEUROMUSCULAR JUNCTION–BLOCKING AGENTS

Drugs that affect the NMJ can be divided into two types. One type, the **non-depolarising NMJs**, includes those agents that act as antagonists to ACh at the NMJ and prevent depolarisation of muscle cells. The other type, the **depolarising NMJs** (of which there is one drug), act as an ACh agonist at the junction, causing stimulation of the muscle cell and staying on the receptor site, preventing it from repolarising, which results in muscle paralysis with the muscle in a constant, contracted state. Both of these types of drugs are used to cause paralysis for the performance of surgical procedures, endoscopic diagnostic procedures or facilitation of mechanical ventilation. Table 28.1 lists these drugs, their preferred uses and potential problems. Box 28.1 highlights information about using NMJ blockers with various age groups (see also the Critical thinking scenario for care related to an elderly person receiving an NMJ).

NON-DEPOLARISING NEUROMUSCULAR-JUNCTION BLOCKERS

The first non-depolarising NMJ blocker to be discovered was curare, a poison used on the tips of arrows or spears by hunters to paralyse their game. Animals died when their respiratory muscles became paralysed. Because the poison was destroyed by the cooking process or by gastric acid if the meat were eaten raw, it was safe for

TABLE 28.1 DRUGS IN FOCUS Neuromuscular-junction blockers

Drug name	Preferred uses	Special considerations
Non-depolarising neuromuscular-junction blockers		
atracurium (*Tracrium*)	Mechanical ventilation; long duration of action; surgical procedures	Has no effect on pain perception or consciousness; do not use before induction of anaesthesia; bradycardia is more common with this drug; reduce dose in renal failure
cisatracurium (*Nimbex*)	Intermediate action; used for surgical procedures and to facilitate intubation	No known effect on pain perception or consciousness; contains benzyl alcohol, avoid use in neonates
mivacurium (*Mivacron*)	Short duration; mechanical ventilation and tracheal intubation	No effect on pain perception or consciousness
(P) pancuronium (generic)	Surgical procedures; mechanical ventilation	Vagalytic effect, associated with increased heart rate; long-term use for mechanical ventilation, monitor for prolonged adverse effects
rocuronium (*Esmeron*)	Rapid onset; preferred for rapid intubation; short outpatient surgical procedures	No known effect on pain perception or consciousness; may be associated with pulmonary hypertension; use caution with hepatic impairment
vecuronium (*Vecure*)	Short surgical procedures; intubation; mechanical ventilation	May contain benzyl alcohol; avoid use in neonates, can cause fatalities in premature infants; monitor with long-term use during ventilation; if response does not occur with first twitch test, discontinue – may be associated with permanent muscle damage
Depolarising neuromuscular-junction blocker		
suxamethonium chloride (generic)	Surgical procedures; intubation; mechanical ventilation	May cause myalgia secondary to muscle contraction; associated with increased intraocular pressure; increased intragastric pressure, which may cause vomiting; more likely to cause malignant hyperthermia

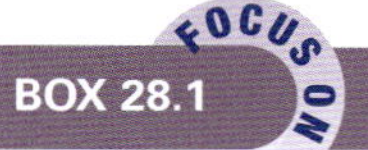

BOX 28.1 Drug therapy across the lifespan

NMJ-blocking agents

CHILDREN

Children require very careful monitoring and support after the use of NMJ blockers. These agents are used by anaesthetists who are skilled in their use and with full support services available.

The non-depolarising NMJs are preferable because of the lack of muscle contraction, with its resultant discomfort on recovery. Suxamethonium chloride is usually preferred when a very short-acting, rapid-onset blocker is needed (eg, for intubation).

ADULTS

Adults need to be monitored closely for full return of muscle function. If suxamethonium chloride is used, they need to be told that they will experience muscle pain and discomfort when the procedure is over.

PREGNANCY AND BREASTFEEDING

The NMJs are used during pregnancy and breastfeeding only if the benefit to the mother outweighs the potential risk to the fetus or neonate.

OLDER ADULTS

Because older people often also have renal or hepatic impairment, they are more likely to have toxic levels of the drug related to changes in metabolism and excretion. The older person should receive special efforts to provide skin care to prevent skin breakdown, which is more likely with older skin. The older person may require longer monitoring and regular orienting and reassuring.

humans. Curare was first purified for clinical use as the NMJ blocker tubocurarine, which has since been replaced with more refined drugs that can control onset and duration of effect. Non-depolarising NMJ blockers include atracurium (*Tracrium*), cisatracurium (*Nimbex*), mivacurium (*Mivacron*), pancuronium (generic), rocuronium (*Esmeron*) and vecuronium (*Vecure*).

Therapeutic actions and indications

Non-depolarising NMJ blockers are used when clinical situations require or desire muscle paralysis (see Table 28.1 for preferred uses). Therapeutically, non-depolarising NMJ blockers:

- Serve as an adjunct to general anaesthetics during surgery when reflex muscle movement could interfere with the surgical procedure or the delivery of gas anaesthesia.
- Facilitate mechanical intubation by preventing resistance to passing of the endotracheal tube and in situations in which people 'fight' or resist the respirator.
- Facilitate various endoscopic diagnostic procedures when reflex muscle reaction could interfere with the procedure.
- Facilitate electroconvulsive therapy when intense skeletal muscle contractions as a result of electric shock could cause the person broken bones or other injury.

Pharmacokinetics

All non-depolarising NMJ blockers are similar in structure to ACh and compete with ACh for the muscle ACh-receptor site (Figure 28.2). As a result, they occupy the muscular cholinergic receptor site and do not allow stimulation to occur. These agents do not cause the activation of muscle cells, and consequently muscle contraction does not occur. Because they are not broken down by acetylcholinesterase, their effect is longer lasting than that of ACh. The non-depolarising NMJ blockers are hydrophilic instead of lipophilic, so they do not readily cross the blood–brain barrier and have little effect on the ACh receptors in the brain.

Non-depolarising NMJs are metabolised in the serum, although metabolism is dependent on the liver to produce the needed plasma cholinesterases. Most of the metabolites are excreted in the urine.

Each non-depolarising NMJ blocker differs in terms of time of onset and duration (Figure 28.3). The drug of choice in any given situation is determined by the procedure being performed, including the estimated time involved.

Contraindications and cautions

Non-depolarising NMJ blockers are contraindicated in the following conditions: known allergy to any of these drugs *to prevent hypersensitivity reactions*; myasthenia gravis *because blocking of the ACh cholinergic receptors aggravates the neuromuscular disease* (which results from destruction of the ACh-receptor sites) *and increases the muscular effects* (see Chapter 32); renal or hepatic disease, *which could interfere with the metabolism or excretion of these drugs, leading to toxic effects*; and pregnancy.

Caution should be used in people with any family or personal history of **malignant hyperthermia**, a serious adverse effect associated with these drugs that is characterised by extreme muscle rigidity, severe hyperpyrexia (fever), acidosis and death in some cases, *because malignant hyperthermia can occur with the use of these drugs*. Caution should also be used in the following circumstances: pulmonary or cardiovascular dysfunction, *which could be exacerbated by the paralysis of the respiratory muscles and resulting changes in perfusion and respiratory function*; altered fluid and electrolyte imbalance, *which could affect membrane stability and subsequent muscular function*; some respiratory conditions *that could be made worse by the histamine release associated with some of these agents*; and breastfeeding *because of the potential for adverse effects on the baby.*

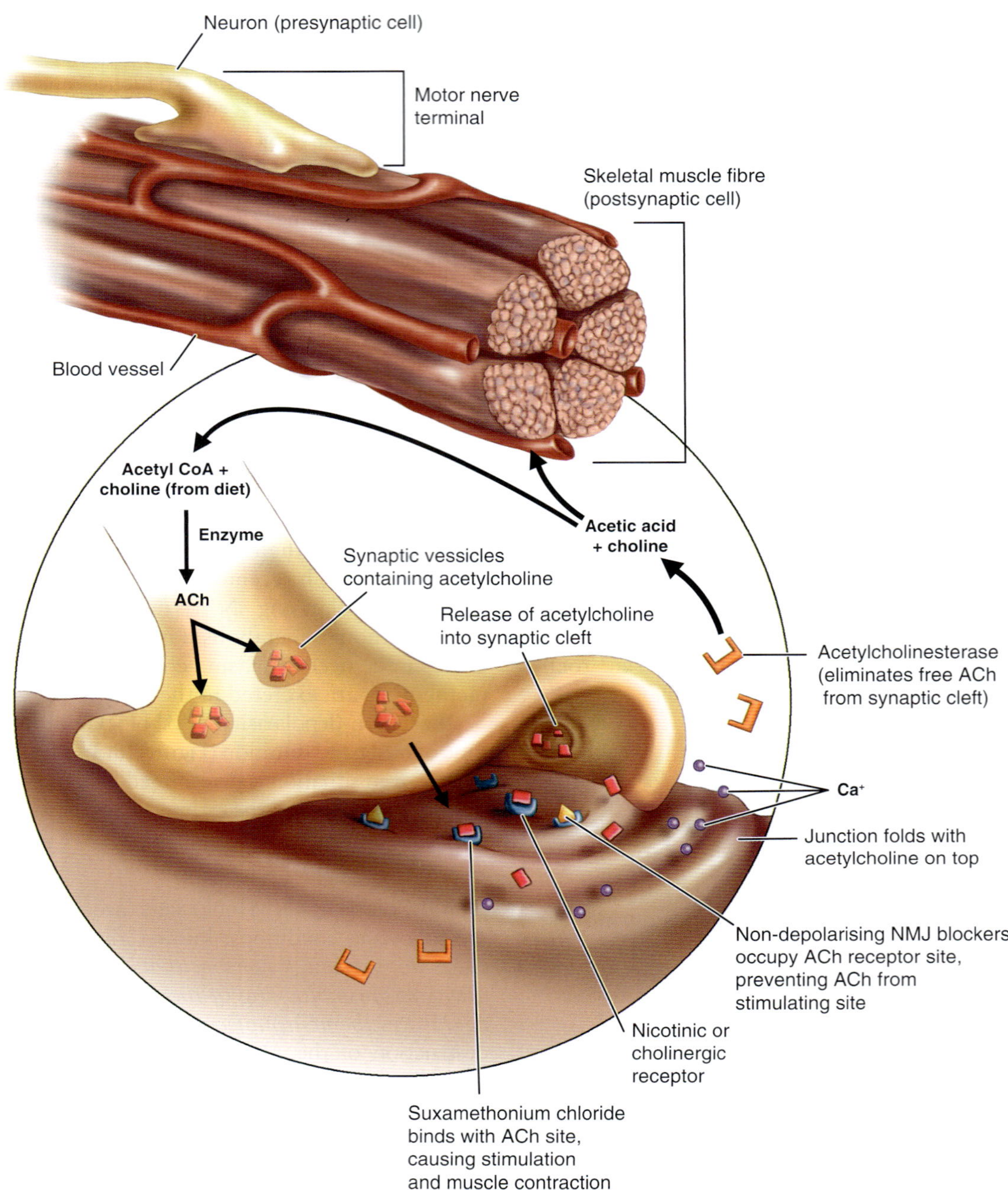

FIGURE 28.2 Sites of action of the NMJ blockers.

Adverse effects

The adverse effects related to the use of non-depolarising NMJ blockers are associated with the paralysis of muscles. Profound and prolonged muscle paralysis is always possible, and people must be supported until they are able to resume voluntary and involuntary muscle movement. When the respiratory muscles are paralysed, depressed respiration, bronchospasm and apnoea are anticipated adverse effects. These agents are never used without an anaesthetist present who can provide assisted ventilatory measures and deliver oxygen under positive pressure. Intubation is an anticipated procedure with these drugs.

The histamine release associated with many of the depolarising NMJ blockers can cause respiratory obstruction with wheezing and bronchospasm. Hypotension and cardiac arrhythmias may occur in individuals who do not adapt to the drugs effectively, use the drugs for prolonged periods, have certain underlying conditions or take certain drugs that are known to affect cardiovascular receptors. Prolonged drug use may also result in gastrointestinal (GI) dysfunction related to paralysis of the muscles in the GI tract; constipation, vomiting, regurgitation and aspiration may occur. Pressure ulcers may develop because the person loses reflex muscle movement that protects the body. Hyperkalaemia may occur as a result of muscle membrane alterations.

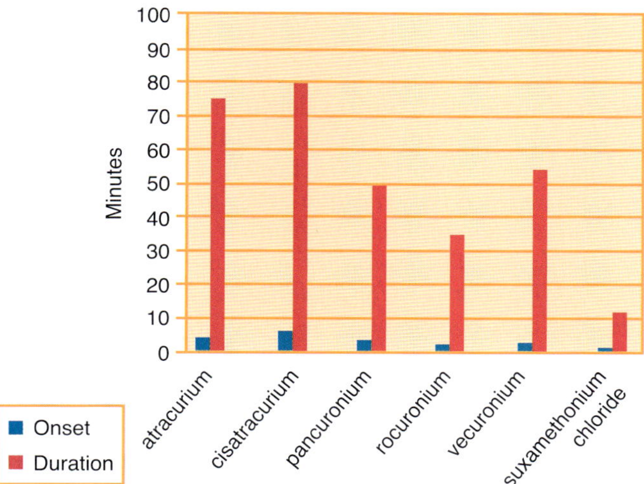

FIGURE 28.3 Onset and duration of non-depolarising NMJ blockers.

Clinically important drug–drug interactions

Many drugs are known to react with the non-depolarising NMJ blockers. Some drug combinations result in an increased neuromuscular effect. Halogenated hydrocarbon anaesthetics such as halothane cause a membrane-stabilising effect, which greatly enhances the paralysis induced by the non-depolarising NMJ blockers. If these drugs are used together for a procedure, dose adjustments are necessary, and individuals should be monitored closely until they recover fully. A combination of non-depolarising NMJ blockers and aminoglycoside antibiotics (eg, gentamicin) also leads to increased neuromuscular blockage. Individuals who receive this drug combination require a lower dose of the non-depolarising NMJ blocker and prolonged support and monitoring after the procedure.

Calcium-channel blockers may also greatly increase the paralysis caused by non-depolarising NMJ blockers because of their effects on the calcium channels in the muscle. If this combination cannot be avoided, the dose of the non-depolarising NMJ agent should be lowered and the person should be monitored closely until complete recovery occurs.

If non-depolarising NMJ blockers are combined with cholinesterase inhibitors, the effectiveness of the non-depolarising NMJ blockers is decreased because of a build-up of ACh in the synaptic cleft. Combination with xanthines (eg, theophylline, aminophylline) could result in reversal of the neuromuscular blockage. Individuals receiving this combination of drugs should be monitored very closely during the procedure for the potential of early arousal and return of muscle function.

Do not mix the drug with any alkaline solutions such as barbiturates because a precipitate may form, making it inappropriate for use.

Medication safety

Neuromuscular junction–blocking agents (NMJ blockers) are high-risk medications and must be segregated, sequestered, and differentiated from other medications, wherever they are stored in the organisation.

- Eliminate the storage of NMJ blockers in areas of the hospital where they are not routinely needed. NMJ blockers must not kept as ward or imprest stock and/or in automated dispensing cabinets (except in operating room/anaesthesia stock).
- Segregate NMJ blockers from all other medications by placing them in separate lidded containers in the refrigerator labelled with auxiliary labels that state: 'WARNING: PARALYSING AGENT – CAUSES RESPIRATORY ARREST – PATIENT MUST BE VENTILATED'

Prototype summary: pancuronium

Indications: as an adjunct to general anaesthesia; to induce skeletal muscle relaxation; to reduce the intensity of muscle contractions in electroconvulsive therapy; to facilitate the care of people undergoing mechanical ventilation.

Actions: occupies the muscular cholinergic receptor site, preventing ACh from reacting with the receptor; does not cause activation of muscle cells; causes a flaccid paralysis.

Pharmacokinetics:

Route	Onset	Duration
IV	4–6 min	120–180 min

$T_{1/2}$: 89–161 minutes; metabolised in the tissues, excreted unchanged in the urine.

Adverse effects: respiratory depression, apnoea, bronchospasm, cardiac arrhythmias.

DEPOLARISING NEUROMUSCULAR-JUNCTION BLOCKER

There is only one agent classified as a depolarising NMJ blocker: suxamethonium chloride, also known as succinylcholine (generic).

Therapeutic actions and indications

Suxamethonium chloride, a depolarising NMJ blocker, attaches to the ACh-receptor site on the muscle cell, causing a prolonged depolarisation of the muscle. This depolarisation causes stimulation of the muscle and muscle contraction (seen as twitching) and then flaccid paralysis. Both effects cause muscles to stop responding to stimuli, and paralysis occurs.

Suxamethonium chloride has a rapid onset and a short duration of action because it is broken down by cholinesterase in the plasma. Unlike endogenous ACh, however, suxamethonium chloride is not broken down instantly. The result is a prolonged contraction of the muscle, which

BOX 28.2 FOCUS ON Cultural considerations

Suxamethonium chloride and paralysis

Suxamethonium chloride is broken down in the body by cholinesterase, an enzyme found in the plasma. Several conditions may cause the body to produce less of this enzyme, including cirrhosis, metabolic disorders, carcinoma, burns, dehydration, malnutrition, hyperpyrexia, thyrotoxicosis, collagen diseases and exposure to neurotoxic insecticides. If plasma cholinesterase levels are low, the serum levels of suxamethonium chloride remain elevated and the paralysis can last much longer than anticipated. These people need support and ventilation for long periods after surgery.

There is also a genetic predisposition to low plasma cholinesterase levels. People should be asked whether they or any family member has a history of either low plasma cholinesterase levels or prolonged recovery from anaesthetics. Alaskan Eskimos belong to such a genetic group, and they are especially likely to suffer prolonged paralysis and inability to breathe for several hours after suxamethonium chloride has been used for surgery. If there is no other drug of choice for these people, special care must be taken to monitor their response and ensure their breathing for an extended postoperative period.

cannot be re-stimulated. Eventually a gradual repolarisation occurs as continually stimulated channels in the cell membrane close. Certain ethnic groups may have a genetic predisposition for a prolongation of paralysis (Box 28.2).

Pharmacokinetics

Like the non-depolarising NMJ blockers, suxamethonium chloride, is metabolised in the serum, although metabolism is dependent on the liver to produce the needed plasma cholinesterases. Individuals with hepatic impairment may experience prolonged effects of this drug. Onset of action is usually within 1 minute, and duration of effect is 10–12 minutes. Most of the metabolites are excreted in the urine. Individuals with renal impairment may be at risk for increased toxicity from the drugs. Suxamethonium chloride crosses the placenta. Effects on breastfeeding are not known.

Contraindications and cautions

The contraindications and cautions for suxamethonium chloride are the same as for non-depolarising NMJ blockers. Suxamethonium chloride is often used during caesarean sections, but accurate timing is necessary to prevent serious effects on the fetus. In addition, suxamethonium chloride should be used with caution in individuals with fractures *because the muscle contractions it causes might lead to additional trauma*; in individuals with narrow-angle glaucoma or penetrating eye injuries *because intraocular pressure increases*; and in individuals with paraplegia or spinal cord injuries, *which could cause loss of potassium from the overstimulated cells and hyperkalaemia.*

Extreme caution is necessary in the presence of genetic or disease-related conditions causing low plasma cholinesterase levels, such as cirrhosis, metabolic disorders, carcinoma, burns, dehydration, malnutrition, hyperpyrexia, thyroid toxicosis, collagen diseases and exposure to neurotoxic insecticides. *Low plasma cholinesterase levels may result in a very prolonged paralysis because suxamethonium chloride is not broken down in the plasma and continues to stimulate the receptor site, leading to a need for prolonged support after use of the drug is discontinued.*

Adverse effects

The adverse effects of suxamethonium chloride are the same as those for non-depolarising NMJ blockers. In addition, suxamethonium chloride is associated with muscle pain related to the initial muscle contraction reaction. A non-depolarising NMJ blocker may be given first to prevent some of these contractions and the associated discomfort. Aspirin also alleviates much of this pain after the procedure. Malignant hyperthermia, which may occur in susceptible individuals, is a very serious condition characterised by massive muscle contraction, sharply elevated body temperature, severe acidosis and, if uncontrolled, death. This reaction is most likely with suxamethonium chloride, and treatment involves dantrolene (see Chapter 25) to inhibit the muscle effects of the NMJ blocker.

Clinically important drug–drug interactions

Potential drug–drug interactions for suxamethonium chloride are the same as for the non-depolarising NMJ blockers.

Prototype summary: suxamethonium chloride

Indications: as an adjunct to general anaesthesia; to facilitate endotracheal intubation; to induce skeletal muscle relaxation during surgery or mechanical ventilation.

Actions: combines with ACh receptors at the motor endplate to produce depolarisation; this inhibits neuromuscular transmission, causing a flaccid paralysis.

Pharmacokinetics:

Route	Onset	Duration
IV	30–60 secs	4–6 min

$T_{1/2}$: 2–3 minutes; metabolised in the tissues, excreted unchanged in the urine.

Adverse effects: muscle pain, related to the contraction of the muscles as a first reaction; respiratory depression, apnoea.

Care considerations for people receiving NMJ blocking agents

Assessment: history and examination

- Assess for contraindications or cautions: any known allergies to these drugs *to avoid hypersensitivity reactions*; impaired liver or kidney function, *which might interfere with metabolism or excretion of the drug*; myasthenia gravis, *which may be exacerbated by the use of this drug*; impaired cardiac or respiratory function, *which may be worsened due to the drug's effect on respiratory muscles and change in perfusion*; personal or family history of malignant hyperthermia, *which may increase the person's risk for this condition*; fractures, *which might lead to additional trauma with administration of suxamethonium chloride*; narrow-angle glaucoma *because an increase in intraocular pressure can occur with suxamethonium chloride*; paraplegia, *which might lead to potassium imbalance with administration of suxamethonium chloride*; and current status of pregnancy or breastfeeding.
- Perform a physical assessment *to establish baseline status before beginning therapy and evaluation for any potential adverse effects.*
- Assess the person's neurological status, including level of orientation, affect, reflexes, pupil size and reactivity, and muscle tone and response, *to monitor drug effects and recovery.*
- Monitor respiratory rate and auscultate lung sounds for evidence of adventitious sounds *to evaluate effects on respiratory muscles and monitor for adverse reactions.*
- Monitor vital signs, including temperature, pulse rate and blood pressure, *to identify changes.*
- Auscultate the abdomen for evidence of bowel sounds *to monitor effects on GI muscles and recovery.*
- Inspect the skin for colour and evidence of pressure areas or breakdown, *which could result when movement ceases.*
- Monitor the results of laboratory tests, including liver function tests, *to determine the need for possible dose adjustment and serum electrolyte levels to determine potential cautions to the use of the drugs.*
- Refer to the Critical thinking scenario for a full discussion of care for an elderly person who is receiving suxamethonium chloride.

Implementation with rationale

- Be aware that administration of the drug should be performed by trained personnel (usually an anaesthetist) *because of the potential for serious adverse effects and the need for immediate ventilatory support.*
- Ensure that emergency supplies and equipment are readily available *to maintain airway and provide mechanical ventilation.*
- Do not mix the drug with any alkaline solutions such as barbiturates *because a precipitate may form, making it inappropriate for use.*
- Test the person's response and recovery periodically if the drug is being given over a long period to maintain mechanical ventilation. *Discontinue the drug if response does not occur or is greatly delayed.*
- Monitor the person's temperature *for prompt detection and treatment of malignant hyperthermia*; have dantrolene readily available *for treatment of malignant hyperthermia if it should occur.*
- Arrange for a small dose of a non-depolarising NMJ blocker before the use of suxamethonium chloride *to reduce the adverse effects associated with muscle contraction.*
- Ensure that a cholinesterase inhibitor is readily available *to overcome excessive neuromuscular blockade caused by non-depolarising NMJ blockers.*
- Have a peripheral nerve stimulator on standby *to assess the degree of neuromuscular blockade, if appropriate.*
- Provide comfort measures *to help the person tolerate drug effects*, such as pain relief as appropriate; reassurance, support and orientation *for conscious individuals unable to move or communicate*; skin care and turning *to prevent skin breakdown*; and supportive care *for emergencies such as hypotension and bronchospasm.*
- Monitor the person's response closely (blood pressure, temperature, pulse, respiration, reflexes) to determine effectiveness; expect dose adjustment *to ensure the greatest therapeutic effect with minimal risk of toxicity.*
- Provide thorough preoperative teaching about this drug *because most people who receive the drug will be receiving teaching about a particular procedure and will be unconscious when the drug is given.* Teaching includes drug to be given, method for administration, effects of the drug (i.e. what to expect) and safety precautions.
- Offer support and encouragement *to help the person to cope with drug effects.*

Evaluation

- Monitor person's response to the drug (adequate muscle paralysis).

- Monitor for adverse effects (respiratory depression, hypotension, bronchospasm, GI slowdown, skin breakdown, fear related to helplessness and inability to communicate).
- Evaluate effectiveness of the teaching plan (the person can relate anticipated effects of the drug and the recovery process).
- Monitor the effectiveness of comfort measures and compliance with the regimen.

KEY POINTS

- Non-depolarising NMJ blockers prevent ACh from exciting the muscle, and paralysis ensues because the muscle cannot respond.
- Depolarising NMJ blockers cause muscle paralysis by acting like ACh. They excite (depolarise) the muscle and prevent repolarisation and further stimulation. There is only one drug available in this class.

CRITICAL THINKING SCENARIO

Using suxamethonium chloride in an elderly person

THE SITUATION

S.N., an 82-year-old Caucasian woman in very good health, has been admitted to the hospital for an exploratory laparotomy to evaluate a probable abdominal mass. On admission, health care practitioners learned that she had a history of mild hypertension that was well regulated by diuretic therapy. She received a baseline physical examination and preoperative instruction. On the morning of the surgery, it was noted that the anaesthesiologist planned to give her a general anaesthetic and suxamethonium chloride to ensure muscle paralysis.

CRITICAL THINKING

What areas must be considered for S.N.? *Consider the woman's age and associated chronic problems that often occur with ageing. Also consider the support that she has available and potential physical and emotional support that she might need before and after this procedure. Use of a NMJ blocker in the elderly presents some care challenges that may not be seen with younger people.*

What particular care activities should be considered with S.N.? *Because S.N. has been maintained on long-term diuretic therapy, she is at special risk for electrolyte imbalance.*

What, if any, complications could arise if S.N. has electrolyte disturbances before surgery?

DISCUSSION

Before surgery, the preoperative teaching protocol should be reviewed with the woman. S.N. should be advised that she may experience back and neck pain secondary to the muscle contractions caused by suxamethonium chloride and throat pain after the procedure. Reassure her that this is normal and that medication will be made available to alleviate the discomfort. Review deep breathing and coughing; she may need encouragement to clear secretions from her lungs and ensure full inflation. This is usually easier to do if it is a familiar activity. S.N.'s serum electrolytes should be evaluated before surgery because potassium imbalance can cause unexpected effects with suxamethonium chloride. Renal and liver function tests also should be performed to ensure that the dose of the NMJ blocker is not excessive.

During the procedure, S.N.'s cardiac and respiratory status should be monitored carefully for any potential problems; such effects are more common in people with underlying physical problems. Because of S.N.'s age and potential circulatory problems, she should receive meticulous skin care and turning as soon as the procedure allows this kind of movement. She should be turned frequently during the recovery period, and her skin should be checked for any breakdown. Clinical staff must remain close by until she has regained muscle control and the ability to communicate. She should be evaluated for the need for pain medication and position adjustments.

S.N. will require additional teaching about her diagnosis and potential treatment. This should wait until she has regained her full ability to communicate and is able to respond and participate in any discussion that may be held. At that time, she may require emotional support and encouragement. It may be necessary to contact available family or social service agencies regarding her physical and medical needs.

CARE GUIDE FOR S.N.: SUXAMETHONIUM CHLORIDE

Assessment: history and examination

Assess allergies to the drug, and assess for history of respiratory or cardiac disorders, myasthenia gravis, hepatic or renal dysfunction, fractures, and glaucoma.

Concurrent use of aminoglycosides or calcium-channel blockers.

Focus the physical examination on the following:

CV: blood pressure, pulse rate, peripheral perfusion and ECG

CNS: orientation, affect, reflexes and vision

Skin: colour, lesions, texture and sweating

GU: urinary output and bladder tone

GI: abdominal examination

Respiratory: respirations and adventitious sounds

Implementation

Provide comfort and safety measures: positioning, skin care, temperature control, pain medication as needed, maintain airway, ventilate person, have antidotes on standby.

Provide support and reassurance to deal with paralysis and inability to communicate.

Provide teaching about procedure being performed and what to expect.

Assist with life support as needed.

Evaluation

Evaluate drug effects: muscle paralysis.

Monitor for adverse effects: cardiovascular effects (tachycardia, hypotension, respiratory distress, increased respiratory secretions), GI effects (constipation, nausea), skin breakdown, anxiety, fear.

Monitor for drug–drug interactions as indicated.

Evaluate the effectiveness of the teaching program and comfort and safety measures.

Constantly monitor vital signs and watch for return of normal muscular function.

TEACHING FOR S.N.

- Before the surgery is performed, you will be given a drug to paralyse your muscles called a neuromuscular blocking agent. It is important that your muscles do not move at this time because it could interfere with the procedure.
- Common effects of these drugs include complete paralysis:
  - You will not be able to move or to speak while you are receiving this drug.
  - You will not be able to breathe on your own, and you will receive assistance in breathing.
- This drug may not affect your level of consciousness, and it can be very frightening to be unable to communicate with anyone around you. Someone will be with you, will try to anticipate your needs, and will explain what is going on at all times.
- This drug may have no effect on your pain perception. Every effort will be made to make sure that you do not experience pain.
- You will be receiving suxamethonium chloride; with this drug, you may experience back and throat pain related to muscle contractions that occur. You will be able to take aspirin to relieve this discomfort.
- Recovery of your muscle function may take 2–3 hours and someone will be nearby at all times until you have recovered from the paralysis.

CHAPTER SUMMARY

- Motor nerves communicate with muscles at a point called the neuromuscular junction (NMJ), using acetylcholine (ACh) as the neurotransmitter.
- NMJ blockers interfere with muscle function. The two groups of NMJ blockers are non-depolarising and depolarising agents.
- The non-depolarising NMJs include agents that act as antagonists to ACh at the NMJ and prevent depolarisation of muscle cells. The depolarising NMJs act as an ACh agonist at the junction, causing stimulation of the muscle cell and then preventing it from repolarising.
- NMJ blockers are primarily used as adjuncts to general anaesthesia, to facilitate endotracheal intubation, to facilitate mechanical ventilation and to prevent injury during electroconvulsive therapy.
- Adverse effects of NMJ blockers, such as prolonged paralysis, inability to breathe, weakness, muscle pain and soreness, and effects of immobility are related to muscle function blocking.
- Care of people receiving NMJ blockers must include: support and reassurance because communication is decreased with paralysis; vigilant maintenance of airways and respiration; prevention of skin breakdown; and monitoring for return of function.

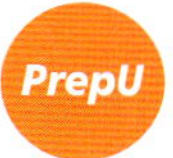

Knowing your strengths and weaknesses helps you to study more effectively. Take a PrepU Practice Quiz to find out how you measure up!

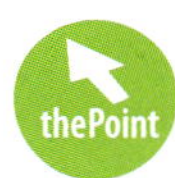

ONLINE RESOURCES

An extensive range of additional resources to enhance teaching and learning and to facilitate understanding of this chapter may be found online at the text's accompanying website, located on thePoint at http://thepoint.lww.com. These include Watch and Learn videos, Concepts in Action animations, journal articles, review questions, case studies, discussion topics and quizzes.

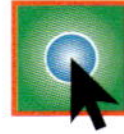

WEB LINKS

Health care providers and students may want to consult the following web resources:

http://allaboutanaesthesia.com.au
Information about anaesthesia and anaesthetics.

www.anzca.edu.au
The Australian and New Zealand College of Anaesthetists.

www.spanza.org.au
The Society for Paediatric Anaesthesia in New Zealand and Australia.

www.ismp.org/sites/default/files/attachments/2019-01/TMSBP-for-Hospitalsv2.pdf
2018-2019 Targeted Medication Safety Best Practices for Hospitals

BIBLIOGRAPHY

Farrell, M. & Dempsey, J. (2014). *Smeltzer & Bare's Textbook of Medical-Surgical Nursing* (3rd edn). Sydney: Lippincott Williams & Wilkins.

Goodman, L. S., Brunton, L. L., Chabner, B. & Knollmann, B. C. (2011). *Goodman and Gilman's Pharmacological Basis of Therapeutics* (12th edn). New York: McGraw-Hill.

Hutton, D. (2011). Emergency preparedness in the OR. Malignant hyperthermia – Part 1. *Plastic Surgical Nursing, 31(1)*, 23–28.

Jaramillo, K. S., Scruth, E. & Cheng, E. (2009). Prolonged paralysis and apnea after receiving a neuromuscular blocking agent: What nurses should know. *American Journal of Critical Care, 18(6)*, 588–591.

McKenna, L. & Mirkov, S. (2019). *McKenna's Drug Handbook for Nursing and Midwifery* (8th edn). Sydney: Wolters Kluwer Health Australia.

Mitchell-Brown, F. (2012). Malignant hyperthermia: Turn down the heat. *Nursing, 42(5)*, 38–45.

Porth, C. M. (2011). *Essentials of Pathophysiology: Concepts of Altered Health States* (3rd edn). Philadelphia: Lippincott Williams & Wilkins.

Porth, C. M. (2009). *Pathophysiology: Concepts of Altered Health States* (8th edn). Philadelphia: Lippincott Williams & Wilkins.

Wadlund, D. L. (2006). Prevention, recognition and management of nursing complications in the intraoperative and postoperative surgical patient. *Nursing Clinics of North America, 41*, 219–229.

CHECK YOUR UNDERSTANDING

Answers to the questions in this chapter can be found in Appendix A at the back of this book.

MULTIPLE CHOICE

Select the best answer to the following.

1. Non-depolarising NMJ blockers:
   a. antagonise acetylcholine to prevent depolarisation of muscle cells.
   b. act as agonists of acetylcholine, leading to depolarisation of muscle cells.
   c. prevent the repolarisation of muscle cells.
   d. are associated with painful muscle contractions on administration.
2. Curare is used as a poison on arrow tips in some cultures. Curare:
   a. is a depolarising NMJ blocker.
   b. causes muscle paralysis in the brain.
   c. is not affected by cooking.
   d. has no clinical use today.
3. Suxamethonium chloride has a more rapid onset of action and a shorter duration of activity than the non-depolarising NMJ blockers because it:
   a. does not bind well to receptor sites.
   b. rapidly crosses the blood–brain barrier and is lost.
   c. is broken down by acetylcholinesterase that is found in the plasma.
   d. is very unstable.
4. When planning the care of a person who is to receive a NMJ blocker, the nurse or midwife would expect which of the following about the person?
   a. Transfer to an intensive care unit would be essential.
   b. Intubation would be necessary to maintain respirations.
   c. He would have no memory of any events.
   d. No adverse effects would occur after the drug is stopped.
5. Malignant hyperthermia can occur with any NMJ blocker, but it most often occurs with suxamethonium chloride. The nurse or midwife would expect to see which drug ordered?
   a. phenobarbitone
   b. pancuronium
   c. dantrolene
   d. diazepam
6. A person's recovery from an NMJ blocker:
   a. is predictable, based on the drug given.
   b. can be affected by genetic enzyme deficiency.
   c. can always be ensured because of the drug half-life.
   d. can be shortened by administration of oxygen.
7. When preparing NMJ blockers for administration, it is important that they:
   a. are not mixed in with any alkaline solutions.
   b. are not exposed to light.
   c. are not mixed with any other drug.
   d. are not mixed with heparin.

MULTIPLE RESPONSE

Select all that apply.

1. The nurse or midwife would expect administration of a NMJ blocker as the drug of choice to accomplish which of the following?
   a. facilitate endotracheal intubation
   b. facilitate mechanical ventilation
   c. prevent injury during electroconvulsive therapy
   d. relieve pain during labour and birth
   e. treat myasthenia gravis
   f. treat a person with a history of malignant hyperthermia

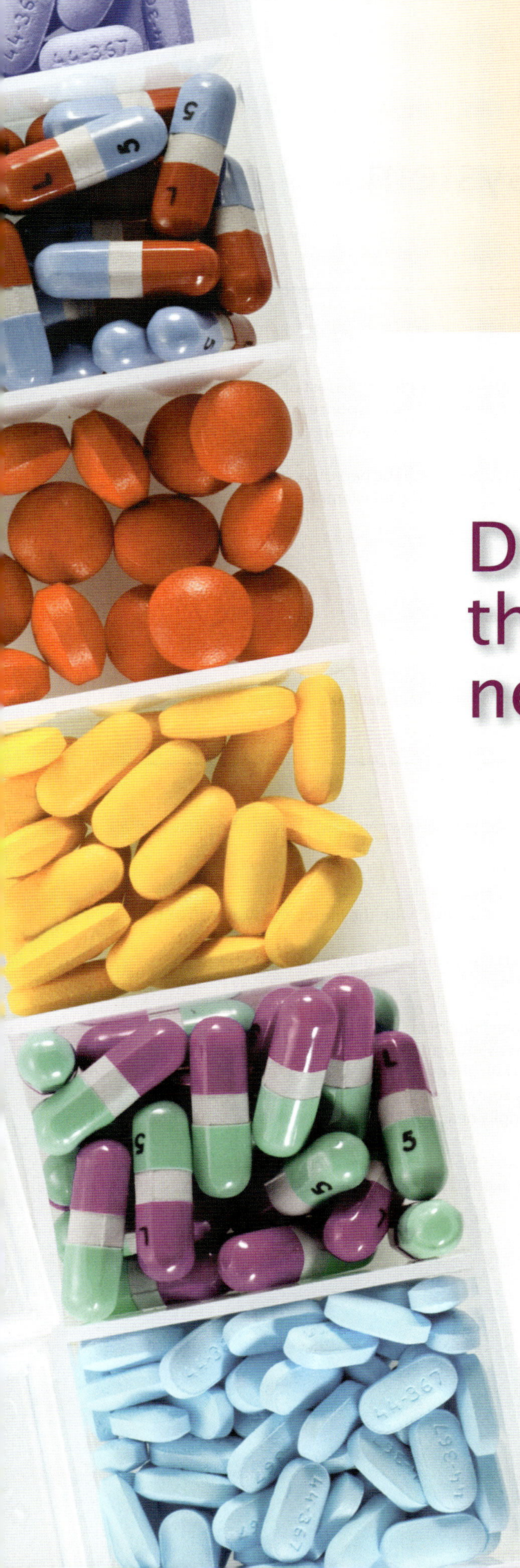

PART 5

Drugs acting on the autonomic nervous system

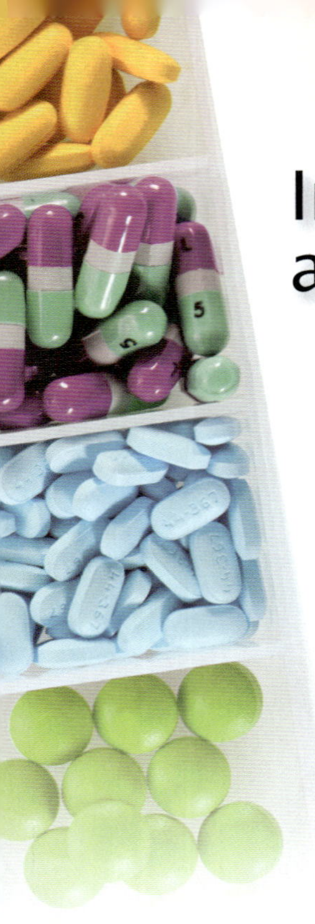

Introduction to the autonomic nervous system

29

Learning objectives

On completing this chapter you should be able to:

1. Describe how the autonomic nervous system differs anatomically from the rest of the nervous system.
2. Outline a sympathetic response and the clinical manifestation of this response.
3. Describe the alpha and beta receptors found within the sympathetic nervous system by sites and actions that follow the stimulation of each kind of receptor.
4. Outline the events that occur with stimulation of the parasympathetic nervous system.
5. Define the terms muscarinic receptor and nicotinic receptor, giving an example of each.

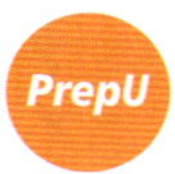

Test your current knowledge of the autonomic nervous system with a PrepU Practice Quiz!

Glossary of key terms

acetylcholinesterase: enzyme responsible for the immediate breakdown of acetylcholine when released from the nerve ending; prevents overstimulation of cholinergic receptor sites

adrenergic receptors: receptor sites on effectors that respond to noradrenaline

alpha receptors (α-receptors): adrenergic receptors that are found in smooth muscles

autonomic nervous system: portion of the central and peripheral nervous systems that, with the endocrine system, functions to maintain internal homeostasis

beta receptors (β-receptors): adrenergic receptors that are found in the heart, lungs and vascular smooth muscle

cholinergic receptors: receptor sites on effectors that respond to acetylcholine

ganglia (pl.; sing. ganglion): groups of closely packed nerve cell bodies

monoamine oxidase (MAO): enzyme that breaks down noradrenaline to make it inactive

muscarinic receptors: cholinergic receptors that also respond to stimulation by muscarine

nicotinic receptors: cholinergic receptors that also respond to stimulation by nicotine

parasympathetic nervous system: 'rest-and-digest' response mediator that contains central nervous system (CNS) cells from the cranium or sacral area of the spinal cord, long preganglionic axons, ganglia near or within the effector tissue and short postganglionic axons that react with cholinergic receptors

sympathetic nervous system: 'fight-or-flight' response mediator; composed of CNS cells from the thoracic or lumbar areas, short preganglionic axons, ganglia near the spinal cord and long postganglionic axons that react with adrenergic receptors

The **autonomic nervous system** (ANS) is sometimes called the involuntary or visceral nervous system because it mostly functions with the person having little conscious awareness of its activity. Working closely with the endocrine system, the ANS helps to regulate and integrate the body's internal functions within a relatively narrow range of normal, on a minute-to-minute basis. The ANS integrates parts of the central nervous system (CNS) and peripheral nervous system to automatically react to changes in the internal and external environments (see Figure 29.1).

STRUCTURE AND FUNCTION OF THE AUTONOMIC NERVOUS SYSTEM

The main nerve centres for the ANS are located in the hypothalamus, the medulla and the spinal cord. Nerve impulses that arise in peripheral structures are carried to these centres by afferent nerve fibres. These integrating centres in the CNS respond by sending out efferent impulses along the autonomic nerve pathways. These impulses adjust the functioning of various internal organs in ways that keep the body's internal environment constant, or homeostatic.

Nerve impulse transmission

Throughout the ANS, nerve impulses are carried from the CNS to the outlying organs by way of a two-neuron system. In most peripheral nervous system activities, the CNS nerve body sends an impulse directly to an effector organ or muscle. The ANS does not send impulses directly to the periphery. Instead, axons from CNS neurons end in **ganglia**, or groups of nerve bodies that are packed together, located outside of the CNS. These ganglia receive information from the preganglionic neuron that started in the CNS and relay that information along postganglionic neurons. The postganglionic neurons transmit impulses to the neuroeffector cells – muscles, glands and organs.

Functions

The ANS works to regulate blood pressure, heart rate, respiration, body temperature, water balance, urinary excretion and digestive functions, among other things. This system exerts minute-to-minute control of body responses, which is balanced by the two divisions of the ANS.

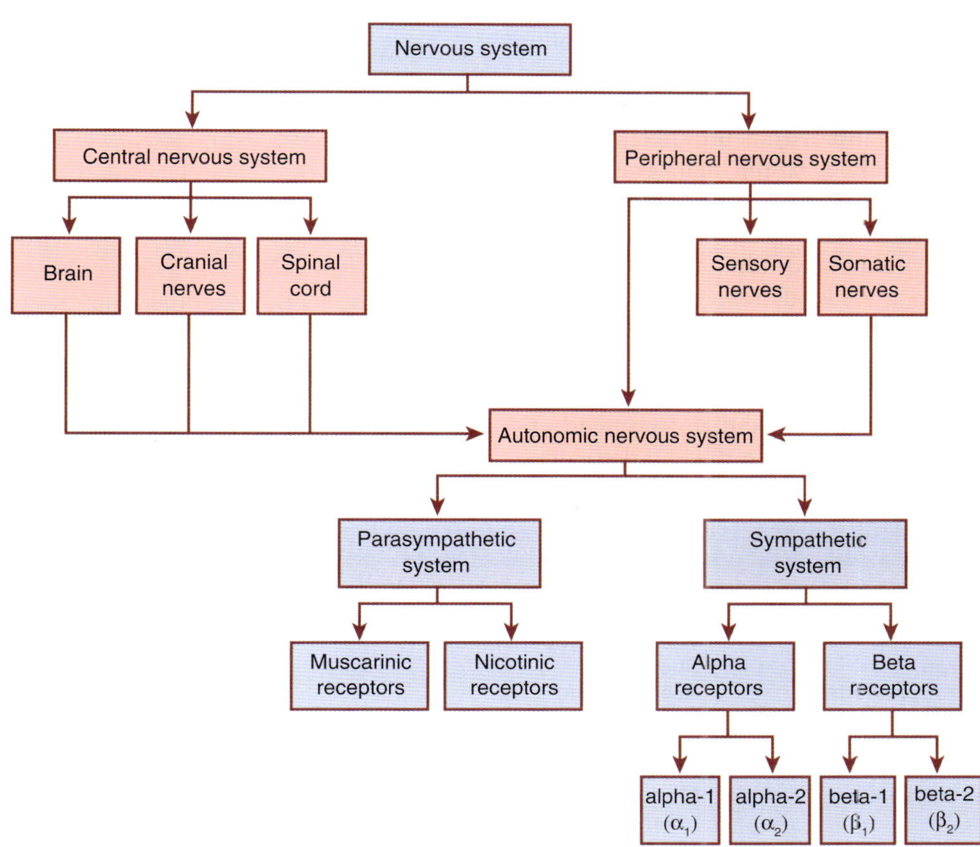

FIGURE 29.1 Organisation of the nervous system.

Divisions

The ANS is divided into two parts: the **sympathetic nervous system** and the **parasympathetic nervous system**. These two parts differ in three basic ways: (1) the location of the originating cells in the CNS, (2) the location of the nerve ganglia and (3) the preganglionic and postganglionic neurons (see Table 29.1 and Figure 29.2).

THE SYMPATHETIC NERVOUS SYSTEM

The sympathetic nervous system (SNS) is sometimes referred to as the 'fight-or-flight' system, or the system responsible for preparing the body to respond to stress. Stress can be either internal, such as cell injury or cell death, or external, such as a perceived or learned reaction to various external situations or stimuli. For the most part, the SNS acts much like an accelerator, speeding things up for action.

Structure and function

The SNS is also called the thoracolumbar system because the CNS cells that originate impulses for this system are located in the thoracic and lumbar sections of the spinal cord. These cells send out short preganglionic fibres that synapse or communicate with nerve ganglia located in chains running alongside the spinal cord. Acetylcholine is the neurotransmitter released by these preganglionic nerves. The nerve ganglia, in turn, send out long postganglionic fibres that synapse with neuroeffectors, using noradrenaline or adrenaline as the neurotransmitter. One of the sympathetic ganglia, on either side of the spinal cord, does not develop postganglionic axons, but produces noradrenaline and adrenaline, which are secreted directly into the bloodstream. These ganglia have evolved into the adrenal medullae (the medulla originates from neural crest cells that migrate from these sympathetic ganglia). When the SNS is stimulated, the chromaffin cells of the adrenal medullae secrete adrenaline and noradrenaline directly into the bloodstream.

When stimulated, the SNS prepares the body to flee or to turn and fight (see Figure 29.3). Cardiovascular activity increases, as do blood pressure, heart rate and blood flow to the skeletal muscles. Respiratory efficiency also increases; bronchi dilate to allow more air to enter with each breath and the respiratory rate increases. Pupils dilate to permit more light to enter the eye, to improve vision in darkened areas (which helps a person to see in order to fight or flee). Sweating increases to dissipate heat generated by the increased metabolic activity.

Piloerection (hair standing on end) also occurs. In lower animals, this important protection mechanism makes the fur stand on end so that an attacking larger animal is often left with a mouthful of fur while the intended victim scurries away. The actual benefit to humans is not known, except that this activity helps to generate heat when the core body temperature is too low.

Stimulation of the SNS causes blood to be diverted away from the gastrointestinal (GI) tract because there is no real need to digest food during a fight-or-flight situation. Subsequently, bowel sounds decrease and digestion slows dramatically; sphincters are constricted and bowel evacuation does not occur. Blood is also diverted away from other internal organs, including the kidneys, resulting in activation of the renin–angiotensin system (Chapter 42) and a further increase in blood pressure and blood volume as water is retained by the kidneys. Sphincters in the urinary bladder are also constricted, precluding urination.

Several other metabolic activities occur that prepare the body to fight or flee. For example, glucose is formed by glycogenolysis, to increase blood glucose levels and provide energy. The hypothalamus causes the secretion of adrenocorticotropic hormone (ACTH), leading to a release of the adrenal hormones, including cortisol, which suppresses the immune and inflammatory reactions to preserve energy that otherwise might be used by these activities. The corticosteroid hormones also block protein production, another energy-saving activity, and increase the release of glucose to provide energy. Aldosterone, also released with adrenal stimulation, retains sodium and water and causes the excretion of potassium in the urine. The hypothalamus also causes the release of thyroid-stimulating hormone (TSH), which stimulates

TABLE 29.1 Comparison of the sympathetic and parasympathetic nervous systems

Characteristic	Sympathetic	Parasympathetic
CNS nerve origin	Thoracic, lumbar spinal cord	Cranium, sacral spinal cord
Preganglionic neuron	Short axon	Long axon
Preganglionic neurotransmitter	Acetylcholine	Acetylcholine
Ganglia location	Next to spinal cord	Within or near effector organs
Postganglionic neuron	Long axon	Short axon
Postganglionic neurotransmitter	Noradrenaline, adrenaline	Acetylcholine
Neurotransmitter terminator	Monoamine oxidase (MAO), catechol-*O*-methyltransferase (COMT)	Acetylcholinesterase
General response	Fight or flight	Rest and digest

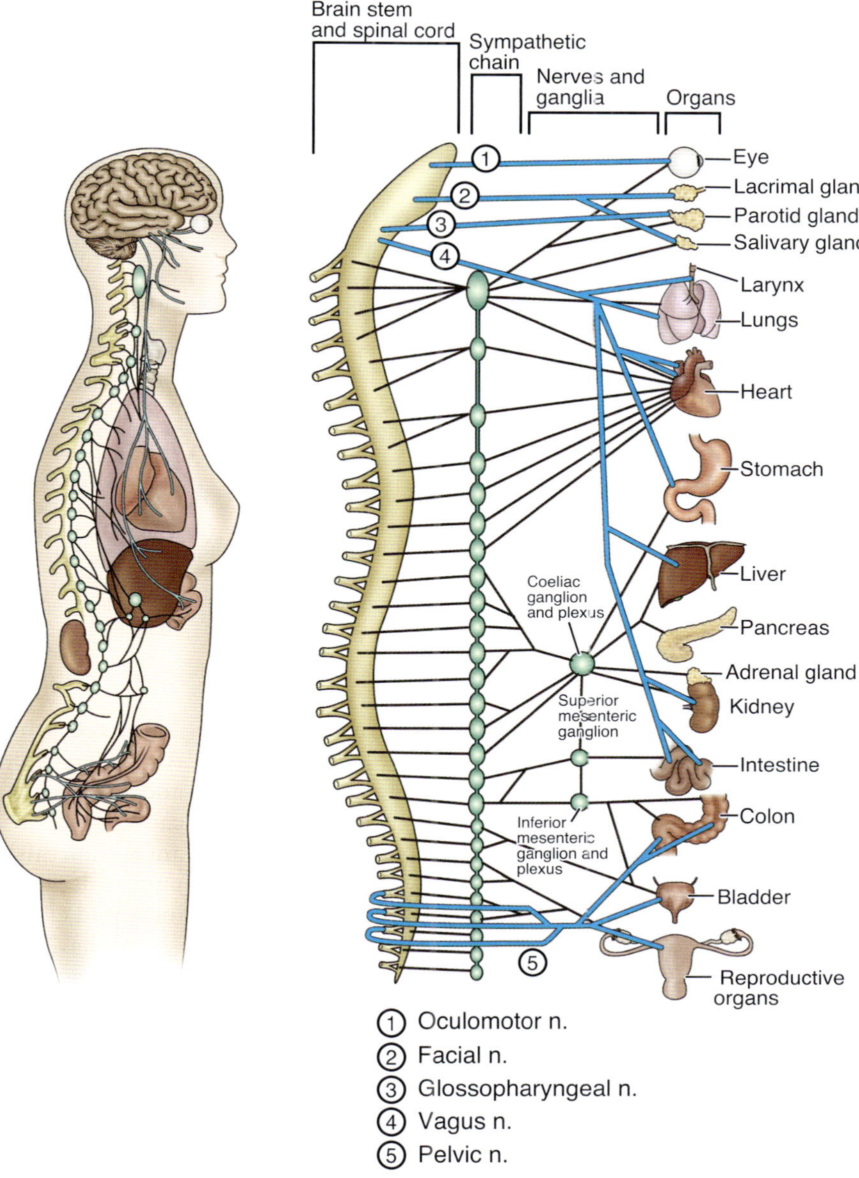

FIGURE 29.2 The autonomic nervous system. The sympathetic, or thoracolumbar, division sends relatively short preganglionic fibres to the chains of paravertebral ganglia and to certain outlying ganglia. The second cell, or postganglionic cell, sends relatively long postganglionic fibres to the organs it innervates. The parasympathetic, or craniosacral, division sends long preganglionic fibres that synapse with a second nerve cell in ganglia located close to or within the organs that are then innervated by short postganglionic fibres.

the production and release of thyroid hormone, which increases metabolism and the efficient use of energy. Together, all of these activities prepare the body to flee or to fight more effectively. When overstimulated, however, they can lead to system overload and a variety of disorders.

Adrenergic response

Sympathetic postganglionic nerves that synthesise, store and release noradrenaline are referred to as adrenergic nerves. Adrenergic nerves are also found within the CNS. The chromaffin cells of the adrenal medulla are also adrenergic because they synthesise, store and release noradrenaline, as well as adrenaline.

Noradrenaline synthesis and storage

Noradrenaline belongs to a group of structurally related chemicals called catecholamines that also includes dopamine, serotonin and adrenaline. Noradrenaline is made by the nerve cells using tyrosine, which is obtained in the diet. Dihydroxyphenylalanine (dopa) is produced by nerves, using tyrosine from the diet and other chemicals. With the help of the enzyme dopa decarboxylase, the dopa is converted to dopamine, which in turn is converted to noradrenaline in adrenergic cells. The noradrenaline is then stored in granules or storage vesicles within the cell. These vesicles move down the nerve axon to the terminals of the axon, where they line up along the cell membrane. To be an adrenergic nerve, the nerve must contain all of the enzymes and

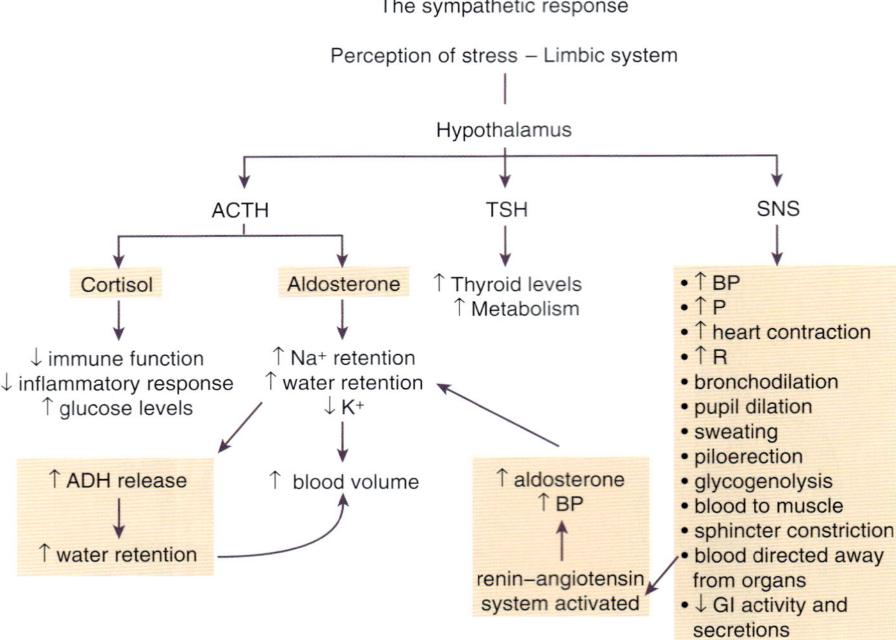

FIGURE 29.3 The 'fight-or-flight' response: the sympathetic stress reaction. ACTH, adrenocorticotropic hormone; ADH, antidiuretic hormone; BP, blood pressure; GI, gastrointestinal; P, pulse; R, respiratory rate; SNS, sympathetic nervous system; TSH, thyroid-stimulating hormone.

building blocks necessary to produce noradrenaline (see Figure 29.4).

Noradrenaline release

When the nerve is stimulated, the action potential travels down the nerve axon and arrives at the axon terminal (see Chapter 19). The action potential then depolarises the axon membrane. This action allows calcium into the nerve, causing the membrane to contract and the storage vesicles to fuse with the cell membrane, releasing their load of noradrenaline into the synaptic gap or cleft. The noradrenaline travels across the very short gap to very specific adrenergic receptor sites on the effector cell on the other side of the synaptic gap.

Adrenergic receptors

Adrenergic receptors can be stimulated by the neurotransmitter released from the axon in the immediate vicinity and they can be further stimulated by circulating noradrenaline and adrenaline secreted directly into the bloodstream by the adrenal medulla. The receptor sites that react with neurotransmitters at adrenergic sites have been classified as **alpha receptors** and **beta receptors**. These receptors are further classified as alpha-1 (α_1)-, alpha-2 (α_2)-, beta-1 (β_1)- and beta-2 (β_2)-receptors (see Table 29.2). It is thought that receptors may respond to different concentrations of noradrenaline or different ratios of noradrenaline and adrenaline. Different drugs that are known to affect the SNS may affect parts of the sympathetic response, but not all of it, because they are designed to stimulate specific adrenergic receptors.

Alpha receptors

Alpha-1 receptors are found in blood vessels, in the iris and in the urinary bladder. In blood vessels, they can cause vasoconstriction and increase peripheral resistance, thus raising blood pressure. In the iris, they cause pupil dilation. In the urinary bladder, they cause the increased closure of the internal sphincter.

Alpha-2 receptors are located on nerve membranes and act as modulators of noradrenaline release. When noradrenaline is released from a nerve ending, it crosses the synaptic cleft to react with its specific receptor site. Some of it also flows back to react with the alpha receptor on the nerve membrane. This causes a reflex decrease in noradrenaline release. In this way, the Alpha-2 receptor helps to prevent overstimulation of effector sites. These receptors are also found on the beta cells in the pancreas, where they help to moderate the insulin release stimulated by SNS activation.

Beta receptors

Beta-1 receptors are found in cardiac tissue, where they can stimulate increased myocardial activity and increased heart rate. They are also responsible for increased lipolysis or breakdown of fat for energy in peripheral tissues. Beta-2 receptors are found in the smooth muscle in blood vessels, in the bronchi, in the periphery and in uterine muscle. In blood vessels, beta$_2$ stimulation leads to vasodilation. Beta-2 receptors also cause dilation in the bronchi. In the periphery, they can cause increased muscle and liver breakdown of glycogen and increased release of glucagon from the alpha cells of the pancreas. Stimulation of Beta-2 receptors in the uterus results in relaxed uterine smooth muscle.

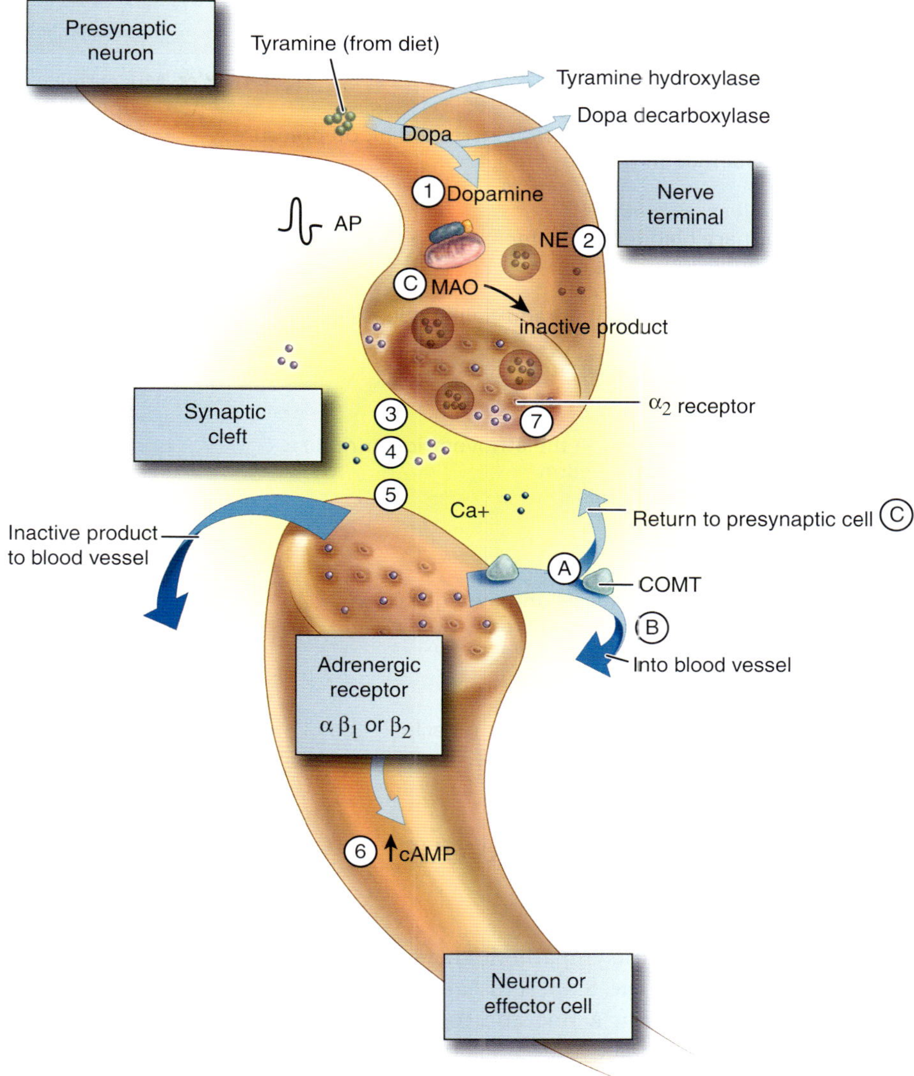

FIGURE 29.4 Sequence of events at an adrenergic synapse. 1. Dopamine, a precursor of noradrenaline (NA), is synthesised from tyrosine in several steps. 2. Dopamine is taken into the storage vesicle and converted to NA. 3. Release of neurotransmitter by an action potential (AP) in the presynaptic nerve. 4. Diffusion of neurotransmitter across synaptic cleft. 5. Combination of neurotransmitter with receptor. The events resulting from NA's occupying of receptor sites depend on the nature of the postsynaptic cell. 6. Interaction of NA with many beta receptors leads to increased synthesis of cyclic adenosine monophosphate (cAMP). 7. Feedback control at alpha-2 receptor leads to decreased NA release from presynaptic neuron. Deactivation of NA occurs by breakdown of NA by the enzyme COMT (**A**) or, most importantly, by reuptake into the presynaptic neuron (**C**), where it may be reused or inactivated by another enzyme, monoamine oxidase (MAO). Some of the neurotransmitter may also diffuse away from the synaptic cleft (**B**).

Termination of response

Once noradrenaline has been released into the synaptic cleft, stimulation of the receptor site is terminated and disposal of any extra noradrenaline, as well as the neurotransmitter that has reacted with the receptor site, must occur. Most of the free noradrenaline molecules are taken up by the nerve terminal that released them in a process called reuptake. This neurotransmitter is then repackaged into vesicles to be released later with nerve stimulation. This is an effective recycling effort by the nerve. Enzymes are also in the area, as well as in the liver, to metabolise or biotransform any remaining noradrenaline or any noradrenaline that is absorbed into circulation. These enzymes are **monoamine oxidase** (MAO) and catechol-O-methyl transferase (COMT).

KEY POINTS

- The autonomic nervous system (ANS), which is divided into two parts – the sympathetic nervous system (SNS) and the parasympathetic nervous system – works with the endocrine system to regulate internal functioning and maintain homeostasis.
- The SNS is responsible for the fight-or-flight response.
- The SNS is composed of CNS cells arising in the thoracic or lumbar area of the spinal cord and long postganglionic axons that react with effector cells. The neurotransmitter used by the preganglionic cells is acetylcholine (ACh); the neurotransmitter used by the postganglionic cells is noradrenaline.
- SNS adrenergic receptors are classified as Alpha-1, Alpha-2, Beta-1 or Beta-2 receptors.

TABLE 29.2 Physiological effects of specific receptor sites in the autonomic nervous system

Sympathetic system	Parasympathetic system
Alpha-1 receptors Vasoconstriction Increased peripheral resistance with increased blood pressure Contracted piloerection muscles Pupil dilation Thickened salivary secretions Closure of urinary bladder sphincter Male sexual emission Alpha-2 receptors Negative feedback control of noradrenaline release from presynaptic neuron Moderation of insulin release from the pancreas Beta-1 receptors Increased heart rate Increased conduction through the atrioventricular node Increased myocardial contraction Lipolysis in peripheral tissues Beta-2 receptors Vasodilation Bronchial dilation Increased breakdown of muscle and liver glycogen Release of glucagon from the pancreas Relaxation of uterine smooth muscle Decreased muscle tone and activity Decreased GI secretions Relaxation of urinary bladder detrusor muscle	Muscarinic receptors Pupil constriction Accommodation of the lens Decreased heart rate Increased GI motility Increased GI secretions Increased urinary bladder contraction Male erection Sweating Nicotinic receptors Muscle contractions Release of noradrenaline from the adrenal medulla Autonomic ganglia stimulation

THE PARASYMPATHETIC NERVOUS SYSTEM

In many areas, the parasympathetic nervous system works in opposition to the SNS. This allows the autonomic system to maintain a fine control over internal homeostasis. For example, the SNS increases heart rate, whereas the parasympathetic system decreases it. Thus, the ANS can influence heart rate by increasing or decreasing sympathetic activity or by increasing or decreasing parasympathetic activity. This is very much like controlling the speed of a car by moving between the accelerator and the brake or combining the two. Whereas the SNS is associated with the stress reaction and expenditure of energy, the parasympathetic system is associated with activities that help the body to store or conserve energy, a 'rest-and-digest' response (see Table 29.3).

Structure and function

The parasympathetic system is sometimes called the craniosacral system because the CNS neurons that originate parasympathetic impulses are found in the cranium (one of the most important being the vagus or tenth cranial nerve) and in the sacral area of the spinal cord (see Figure 29.2). It has long preganglionic axons that meet in ganglia located close to or within the organ to be affected. The postganglionic axon is very short, going directly to the effector cell. The neurotransmitter used by both the preganglionic and the postganglionic neurons is ACh.

Parasympathetic system stimulation results in the following actions:

- Increased motility and secretions in the GI tract to promote digestion and absorption of nutrients.
- Decreased heart rate and contractility to conserve energy and provide rest for the heart.
- Constriction of the bronchi, with increased secretions.
- Relaxation of the GI and urinary bladder sphincters, allowing evacuation of waste products.
- Pupillary constriction, which decreases the light entering the eye and decreases stimulation of the retina.

These activities are aimed at increasing digestion, absorption of nutrients and building of essential proteins, as well as a general conservation of energy.

Cholinergic response

Neurons that use ACh as their neurotransmitter are called cholinergic neurons. There are four basic kinds of cholinergic nerves:

1. All preganglionic nerves in the ANS, both sympathetic and parasympathetic

TABLE 29.3 Comparing the effects of autonomic stimulation

Effector site	Sympathetic reaction	Parasympathetic reaction
Eye structures		
Iris radial muscle	Contraction (pupil dilates)	—
Iris sphincter muscle	—	Contraction (pupil constricts)
Ciliary muscle	—	Contraction (lens accommodates for near vision)
Lacrimal glands	—	↑ Secretions
Heart	↑ Rate, contractility ↑ Atrioventricular conduction	↓ Rate ↓ Atrioventricular conduction
Blood vessels		
Skin, mucous membranes	Constriction	—
Skeletal muscle	Dilation	—
Bronchial muscle	Relaxation (dilation)	Constriction
Gastrointestinal system		
Muscle motility and tone	↓ Activity	↑ Activity
Sphincters	Contraction	Relaxation
Secretions	↓ Secretions	↑ Activity
Salivary glands	Thick secretions	Copious, watery secretions
Gallbladder	Relaxation	Contraction
Liver	Glyconeogenesis	—
Urinary bladder		
Detrusor muscle	Relaxation	Contraction
Trigone muscle and sphincter	Contraction	Relaxation
Sex organs		
Male	Emission	Erection (vascular dilation)
Female	Uterine relaxation	—
Skin structures		
Sweat glands	↑ Sweating	—
Piloerector muscles	Contracted (goosebumps)	—

—, no reaction or response.

2. Postganglionic nerves of the parasympathetic system and a few SNS nerves, such as those that re-enter the spinal cord and cause general body reactions such as sweating
3. Motor nerves on skeletal muscles
4. Cholinergic nerves within the CNS

Acetylcholine synthesis and storage

ACh is an ester of acetic acid and an organic alcohol called choline. Cholinergic nerves use choline, obtained in the diet, to produce ACh. The last step in the production of the neurotransmitter involves choline acetyltransferase, an enzyme that is also produced within cholinergic nerves. Just like noradrenaline, the ACh is produced in the nerve and travels to the end of the axons, where it is packaged into vesicles. To be a cholinergic nerve, the nerve must contain all of the enzymes and building blocks necessary to produce ACh.

Acetylcholine release

The vesicles full of ACh move to the nerve membrane; when an action potential reaches the nerve terminal, calcium entering the cell causes the membrane to contract and secrete the neurotransmitter into the synaptic cleft. The ACh travels across the synaptic cleft and reacts with very specific **cholinergic receptor** sites on the effector cell (see Figure 29.5).

Cholinergic receptors

Cholinergic receptors or ACh receptors are found on organs and muscles. They have been classified as **muscarinic receptors** and **nicotinic receptors**. This classification is based on very early research of the ANS that used muscarine (a plant alkaloid from mushrooms) and nicotine (a plant alkaloid found in tobacco plants) to study the actions of the parasympathetic system.

Muscarinic receptors

As the name implies, muscarinic receptors are receptors that can be stimulated by muscarine. They are found in visceral effector organs, such as the GI tract, bladder and heart, in sweat glands and in some vascular smooth muscle. Stimulation of muscarinic receptors causes pupil constriction, increased GI motility and secretions (including saliva), increased urinary bladder contraction and a slowing of the heart rate.

Nicotinic receptors

Nicotinic receptors are located in the CNS, the adrenal medulla, the autonomic ganglia and the neuromuscular junction. Stimulation of nicotinic receptors causes muscle contractions, autonomic responses such as signs and symptoms of a stress reaction and release of noradrenaline and adrenaline from the adrenal medulla.

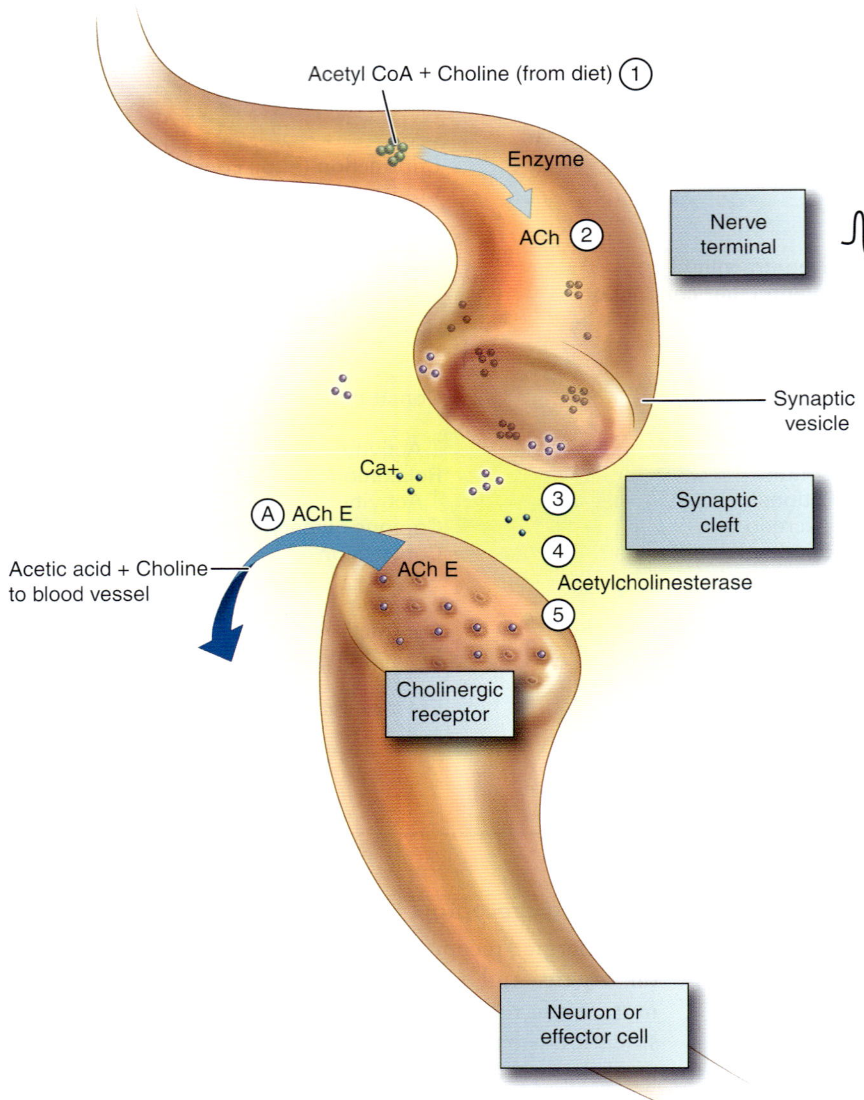

FIGURE 29.5 Sequence of events at a cholinergic synapse. 1. Synthesis of acetylcholine (ACh) from choline (a substance in the diet) and a cofactor (the enzyme is choline acetyltransferase, CoA). 2. Uptake of neurotransmitter into storage (synaptic) vesicle. 3. Release of neurotransmitter by an action potential (AP) in the presynaptic nerve. 4. Diffusion of neurotransmitter across the synaptic cleft. 5. Combination of neurotransmitter with receptor. The events resulting from ACh's occupation of receptor sites depend on the nature of the postsynaptic cell. ACh excites some cells and inhibits others. An enzyme, acetylcholinesterase (AChE), found in the tissues and on the postsynaptic cell, inactivates ACh (**A**). Some of the products diffuse into the circulation, but most of the choline formed is taken up and reused by the cholinergic neuron.

Termination of response

Once the effector cell has been stimulated by ACh, stimulation of the receptor site must be terminated and destruction of any ACh must occur. The destruction of ACh is carried out by the enzyme **acetylcholinesterase**. This enzyme reacts with the ACh to form a chemically inactive compound. The breakdown of the released ACh is accomplished in 1/1000 second and the receptor is vacated, allowing the effector membrane to repolarise and be ready for the next stimulation.

KEY POINTS

- The parasympathetic system, when stimulated, acts as a rest-and-digest response. It increases the digestion, absorption and metabolism of nutrients and slows metabolism and function to save energy.
- The parasympathetic system comprises CNS cells that arise in the cranium and sacral region of the spinal cord, long preganglionic axons that secrete ACh, ganglia located very close to or within the effector tissue and short postganglionic axons that also secrete ACh.
- ACh is made by choline from the diet and packaged into storage vesicles to be released by the cholinergic nerve into the synaptic cleft. ACh is broken down to an inactive form almost immediately by acetylcholinesterase.
- Parasympathetic system receptors are classified as muscarinic or nicotinic, depending on what response they have to these plant alkaloids.

CHAPTER SUMMARY

- The autonomic nervous system (ANS) works with the endocrine system to regulate internal functioning and maintain homeostasis. The two parts of the ANS, the sympathetic nervous system (SNS) and the parasympathetic nervous system, work in opposition to maintain minute-to-minute regulation of the internal environment and to allow rapid response to stress situations.
- The SNS, when stimulated, is responsible for the fight-or-flight response. It prepares the body for immediate reaction to stressors by increasing metabolism, diverting blood to big muscles and increasing cardiac and respiratory function.
- The parasympathetic system, when stimulated, acts as a rest-and-digest response. It increases the digestion, absorption and metabolism of nutrients and slows metabolism and function to save energy.
- The SNS is composed of CNS cells arising in the thoracic or lumbar area of the spinal cord, short preganglionic axons, ganglia located near the spinal cord and long postganglionic axons that react with effector cells. The neurotransmitter used by the preganglionic cells is acetylcholine (ACh); the neurotransmitter used by the postganglionic cells is noradrenaline.
- One SNS ganglion on either side of the spinal cord does not develop postganglionic axons, but instead secretes noradrenaline directly into the bloodstream to travel throughout the body to react with adrenergic receptor sites. These ganglia evolve into the adrenal medulla.
- SNS adrenergic receptors are classified as being Alpha-1, Alpha-2, Beta-1 or Beta-2 receptors based on the effectors that they stimulate.
- ACh is made by choline from the diet and packaged into storage vesicles to be released by the cholinergic nerve into the synaptic cleft. ACh is broken down to an inactive form almost immediately by acetylcholinesterase.
- The parasympathetic system comprises CNS cells that arise in the cranium and sacral region of the spinal cord, long preganglionic axons that secrete ACh, ganglia located very close to or within the effector tissue and short postganglionic axons that also secrete ACh.
- Noradrenaline is made by adrenergic nerves using tyrosine from the diet. It is packaged in storage vesicles that align on the axon membrane and is secreted into the synaptic cleft when the nerve is stimulated. It reacts with specific receptor sites and is then broken down by MAO or COMT to relax the receptor site and recycle the building blocks of noradrenaline.
- Parasympathetic system receptors are classified as muscarinic or nicotinic, depending on what response they have to these plant alkaloids.

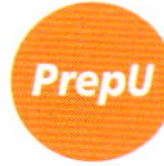

Knowing your strengths and weaknesses helps you to study more effectively. Take a PrepU Practice Quiz to find out how you measure up!

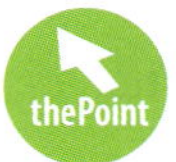

ONLINE RESOURCES

An extensive range of additional resources to enhance teaching and learning and to facilitate understanding of this chapter may be found online at the text's accompanying website, located on thePoint at http://thepoint.lww.com. These include Watch and Learn videos, Concepts in Action animations, journal articles, review questions, case studies, discussion topics and quizzes.

BIBLIOGRAPHY

Barrett, K. E. & Ganong, W. F. (2010). *Ganong's Review of Medical Physiology* (23rd edn). New York: McGraw-Hill.

Davis, G. (2007). The central, peripheral and autonomic nervous system: An overview. *Nurse Prescribing, 5(1)*, 16–21.

Goodman, L. S., Brunton, L. L., Chabner, B. & Knollmann, B. C. (2011). *Goodman and Gilman's Pharmacological Basis of Therapeutics* (12th edn). New York: McGraw-Hill.

Guyton, A. & Hall, J. (2011). *Textbook of Medical Physiology* (12th edn). Philadelphia: Saunders Elsevier.

McCorry, L. K. (2007). Physiology of the Autonomic Nervous System. *American Journal of Pharmaceutical Education, 71(4)*, 78. www.ncbi.nlm.nih.gov/pmc/articles/PMC1959222/.

Porth, C. M. (2011). *Essentials of Pathophysiology: Concepts of Altered Health States* (3rd edn). Philadelphia: Lippincott Williams & Wilkins.

Porth, C. M. (2009). *Pathophysiology: Concepts of Altered Health States* (8th edn). Philadelphia: Lippincott Williams & Wilkins.

Robertson, D., Biaggioni, I., Burnstock, G., Low, P. A. & Paton, F. R. (2012). *Primer on the Autonomic Nervous System* (3rd edn). London: Elsevier.

CHECK YOUR UNDERSTANDING

Answers to the questions in this chapter can be found in Appendix A at the back of this book.

MULTIPLE CHOICE

Select the best answer to the following.

1. When describing the functions of the autonomic nervous system, which of the following would the instructor include?
   a. maintenance of balance and posture
   b. maintenance of the special senses
   c. regulation of integrated internal body functions
   d. coordination of peripheral and central nerve pathways
2. The autonomic nervous system differs from other systems in the CNS in that it:
   a. uses only peripheral pathways.
   b. affects organs and muscles via a two-neuron system.
   c. uses a unique one-neuron system.
   d. bypasses the CNS in all of its actions.
3. If you suspect that a person is very stressed and is experiencing a sympathetic stress reaction, you would expect to find:
   a. increased bowel sounds and urinary output.
   b. constricted pupils and warm, flushed skin.
   c. slow heart rate and decreased systolic blood pressure.
   d. dilated pupils and elevated systolic blood pressure.
4. The nurse determines that the Beta-2 receptors in the sympathetic nervous system have been stimulated by which finding?
   a. increased heart rate
   b. increased myocardial contraction
   c. bronchial dilation
   d. uterine contraction
5. After a postganglionic receptor site has been stimulated, the neurotransmitter must be broken down immediately. The sympathetic system breaks down postganglionic neurotransmitters by using:
   a. liver enzymes and acetylcholinesterase.
   b. acetylcholinesterase and MAO.
   c. COMT and liver enzymes.
   d. MAO and COMT.
6. The parasympathetic nervous system, in most situations, opposes the actions of the sympathetic nervous system, allowing the autonomic nervous system to:
   a. generally have no effect.
   b. maintain a fine control over internal homeostasis.
   c. promote digestion.
   d. respond to stress most effectively.
7. Cholinergic neurons, those using acetylcholine as their neurotransmitter, would be least likely found in:
   a. motor nerves on skeletal muscles.
   b. preganglionic nerves in the sympathetic and parasympathetic systems.
   c. postganglionic nerves in the parasympathetic system.
   d. the adrenal medulla.
8. Stimulation of the parasympathetic nervous system would cause:
   a. slower heart rate and increased GI secretions.
   b. faster heart rate and urinary retention.
   c. vasoconstriction and bronchial dilation.
   d. pupil dilation and muscle paralysis.

MULTIPLE RESPONSE

Select all that apply.

1. The sympathetic nervous system:
   a. is called the thoracolumbar system.
   b. is called the fight-or-flight system.
   c. is called the craniosacral system.
   d. uses acetylcholine as its sole neurotransmitter.
   e. uses adrenaline as its sole neurotransmitter.
   f. is active during a stress reaction.
2. The sympathetic system uses catecholamines at the postganglionic receptors. Which of the following are considered to be catecholamines?
   a. dopamine
   b. noradrenaline
   c. acetylcholine
   d. adrenaline
   e. monoamine oxidase
   f. serotonin

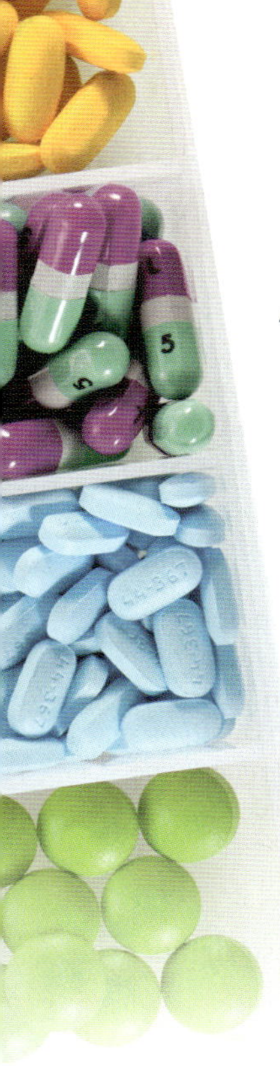

Adrenergic agonists

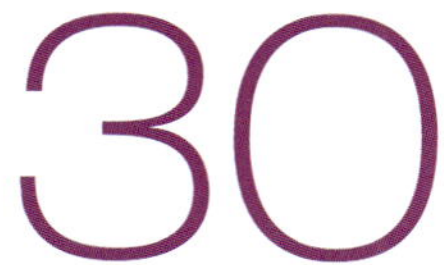

Learning objectives

On completing this chapter you should be able to:

1. Describe two ways that sympathomimetic drugs act to produce effects at adrenergic receptors.
2. Describe the therapeutic actions, indications, pharmacokinetics, contraindications, most common adverse reactions and important drug–drug interactions associated with adrenergic agonists.
3. Discuss the use of adrenergic agents across the lifespan.
4. Compare and contrast the prototype drugs dopamine, phenylephrine and isoprenaline with other adrenergic agonists.
5. Outline the care considerations, including important teaching points, for people receiving an adrenergic agent.

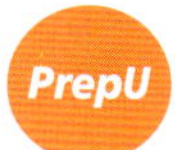

Test your current knowledge of adrenergic agonists with a PrepU Practice Quiz!

Glossary of key terms

adrenergic agonist: a drug that stimulates the adrenergic receptors of the sympathetic nervous system, either directly (by reacting with receptor sites) or indirectly (by increasing noradrenaline [norepinephrine] levels)

alpha agonist: specifically stimulating to the alpha receptors within the sympathetic nervous system, causing body responses seen when the alpha receptors are stimulated

beta agonist: specifically stimulating to the beta receptors within the sympathetic nervous system, causing body responses seen when the beta receptors are stimulated

glycogenolysis: breakdown of stored glucose (glycogen) to increase the blood glucose levels

sympathomimetic: drug that mimics the sympathetic nervous system (SNS) with the signs and symptoms seen when the SNS is stimulated

ALPHA- AND BETA-ADRENERGIC AGONISTS

adrenaline (epinephrine)
dobutamine
(P) dopamine
ephedrine
metaraminol
noradrenaline (norepinephrine)
pseudoephedrine

ALPHA-SPECIFIC ADRENERGIC AGONISTS

clonidine (alpha-2 specific)
(P) phenylephrine

BETA-SPECIFIC ADRENERGIC AGONISTS (Also see beta-adrenergic agonists in Chapter 55)

(P) isoprenaline
salbutamol
salmeterol
terbutaline

An **adrenergic agonist** is also called a **sympathomimetic** drug because it mimics the effects of the sympathetic nervous system (SNS). The therapeutic and adverse effects associated with these drugs are related to their stimulation of adrenergic receptor sites. That stimulation can be either direct, by occupation of the adrenergic receptor, or indirect, by modulation of the release of neurotransmitters from the axon. Some drugs act in both ways. Adrenergic agonists also can affect both the alpha and beta receptors, or they can act at specific receptor sites.

The use of adrenergic agonists varies from ophthalmic preparations for dilating pupils to systemic preparations used to support individuals experiencing shock. They are used in people of all ages (Box 30.1).

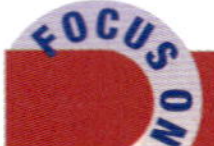

Safe medication administration

Administering ophthalmic medications

Some of the adrenergic agonists are applied in the eye; it is important to review the administration technique. First, wash hands thoroughly. Do not touch the dropper to the eye or to any other surfaces. Have the person tilt their head back or lie down and stare upwards. Gently grasp the lower eyelid and pull the eyelid away from the eyeball. Instill the prescribed number of drops into the lower conjunctival sac and then release the lid slowly (Figure 30.1). Have the person close the eye and look downwards. Apply gentle pressure to the inside corner of the eye for 3–5 minutes. Do not rub the eyeball and do not rinse the dropper. If more than one type of eye drop is being used, wait 5 minutes before administering the next one.

ALPHA- AND BETA-ADRENERGIC AGONISTS

Drugs that are generally sympathomimetic (Figure 30.2) are called **alpha-adrenergic agonists** (alpha agonists) (stimulate alpha receptors) and **beta-adrenergic agonists** (beta agonists) (stimulate beta receptors). These agonists stimulate all of the adrenergic receptors, that is, they affect both alpha and beta receptors (Table 30.1). Agents that affect both alpha- and beta-receptor sites include adrenaline (epinephrine) (*Anapen, EpiPen*), dobutamine (*Dobutrex*), dopamine (generic), ephedrine (generic), metaraminol (generic) and noradrenaline (norepinephrine) (*Levophed*). Several of these drugs are naturally occurring catecholamines.

Subdivision of alpha and beta receptors

There is a further subdivision of adrenergic receptors into alpha-1, alpha-2, beta-1, beta-2 and beta-3 receptors. The alpha-1 receptors are found in the peripheral blood vessels, the eye and the heart. Stimulation of alpha-1 receptors causes vasoconstriction of peripheral blood vessels and contraction of the dilator muscle of the pupil resulting in

BOX 30.1 FOCUS ON **Drug therapy across the lifespan**

Adrenergic agonists

CHILDREN

Children are at greater risk for complications associated with the use of adrenergic agonists, including tachycardia, hypertension, tachypnoea and gastrointestinal (GI) complications. The dosage for these agents needs to be calculated from the child's body weight and age. It is good practice to have a second person check the dosage calculation before administering the drug to avoid potential toxic effects. Children should be carefully monitored and supported during the use of these drugs.

Phenylephrine is often found in over-the-counter (OTC) allergy and cold preparations, and parents need to be instructed to be very careful with the use of these drugs – they should check the labels for ingredients, monitor the recommended dose and avoid combining drugs that contain similar ingredients.

ADULTS

Adults being treated with adrenergic agonists for shock or shock-like states require constant monitoring and dosage adjustments based on their response. People who may be at increased risk for cardiac complications should be monitored very closely and started on a lower dose. Adults using these agents for glaucoma or for seasonal rhinitis need to be cautioned about the use of OTC drugs and alternative therapies that might increase the drug effects and cause serious adverse effects.

PREGNANCY AND BREASTFEEDING

Many of these drugs are used in emergency situations and may be used during pregnancy and breastfeeding. In general, there are no adequate studies about their effects during pregnancy and breastfeeding, and in those situations, they should be used only if the benefit to the mother is greater than the risk to the fetus or neonate.

OLDER ADULTS

Older people are more likely to experience the adverse effects associated with these drugs – central nervous system (CNS), cardiovascular (CV), GI and respiratory. Because older people often have renal or hepatic impairment, they are also more likely to have toxic levels of the drug related to changes in metabolism and excretion. Older people should be started on lower doses of the drugs and should be monitored very closely for potentially serious arrhythmias or blood pressure changes.

They also should be cautioned about the use of OTC drugs and complementary therapies that could increase drug effects and cause serious adverse reactions.

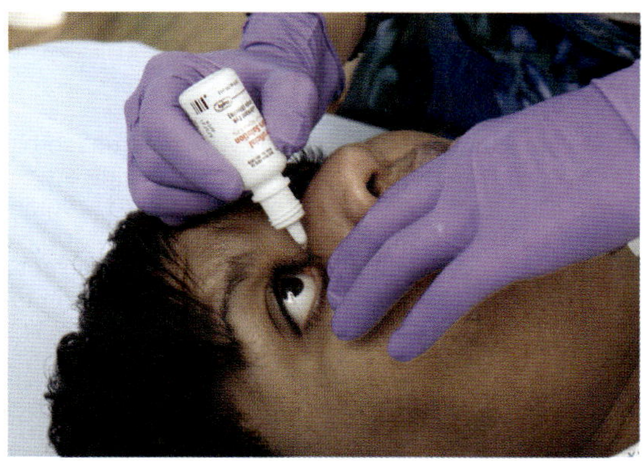

FIGURE 30.1 After gently exposing the lower conjunctival sac, an eyedrop is administered. [From Lynn, P. (2006). *Taylor's clinical nursing skills: A nursing process approach* (2nd edn). Philadelphia: Lippincott Williams & Wilkins, p. 244, Figure 4.]

dilation of the pupil. In the heart, stimulation of alpha-1 receptors increases the contractility of the heart. Beta-1 receptors are also found in the heart and their stimulation causes increased heart rate as well as increased contractility of the heart muscle. Beta-2 receptors on the other hand are found in the lung, the uterus and the liver. A very important function of beta-2 receptors is to cause opening of the airways by dilation of bronchial muscle. Stimulation of beta-2 receptors also results in glycogenolysis and relaxation of the uterus.

Therapeutic actions and indications

The effects of the sympathomimetic drugs are mediated by the adrenergic receptors in target organs: heart rate increases with increased myocardial contractility; bronchioles dilate and respirations increase in rate and depth; blood vessels constrict, causing an increase in blood pressure; intraocular pressure decreases; **glycogenolysis** (breakdown of glucose stores so that the glucose can be

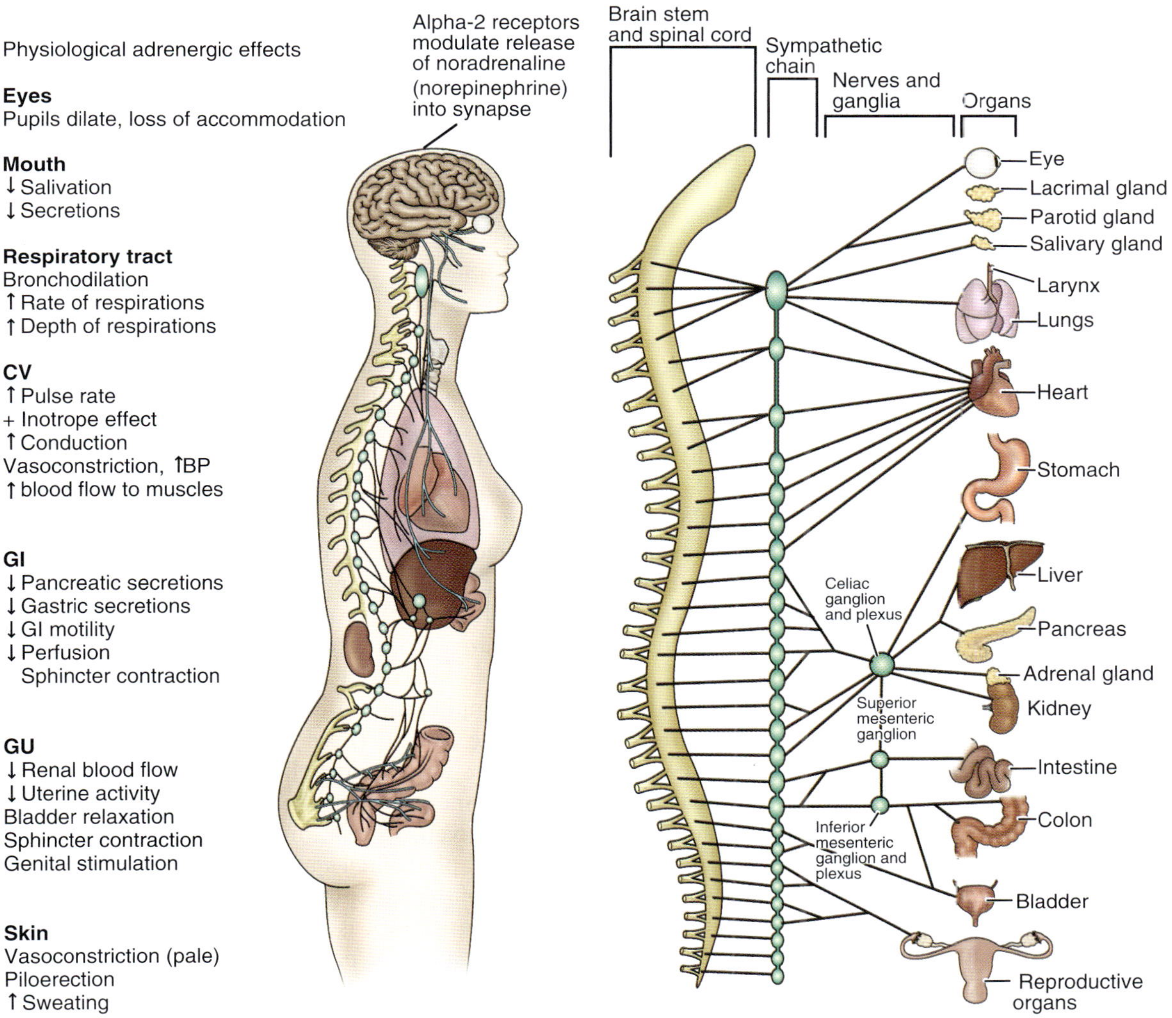

Physiological adrenergic effects

Eyes
Pupils dilate, loss of accommodation

Mouth
↓ Salivation
↓ Secretions

Respiratory tract
Bronchodilation
↑ Rate of respirations
↑ Depth of respirations

CV
↑ Pulse rate
+ Inotrope effect
↑ Conduction
Vasoconstriction, ↑BP
↑ blood flow to muscles

GI
↓ Pancreatic secretions
↓ Gastric secretions
↓ GI motility
↓ Perfusion
Sphincter contraction

GU
↓ Renal blood flow
↓ Uterine activity
Bladder relaxation
Sphincter contraction
Genital stimulation

Skin
Vasoconstriction (pale)
Piloerection
↑ Sweating

Alpha-2 receptors modulate release of noradrenaline (norepinephrine) into synapse

Brain stem and spinal cord
Sympathetic chain
Nerves and ganglia
Organs
Eye
Lacrimal gland
Parotid gland
Salivary gland
Larynx
Lungs
Heart
Stomach
Liver
Pancreas
Adrenal gland
Kidney
Celiac ganglion and plexus
Superior mesenteric ganglion
Intestine
Colon
Inferior mesenteric ganglion and plexus
Bladder
Reproductive organs

FIGURE 30.2 Sympathetic nervous system and physiological effects of adrenergic stimulation. Adrenergic agonists cause stimulation of adrenergic receptors, producing physiological effects associated with sympathetic stimulation. Receptor site–specific adrenergic agonists have more pronounced effect on particular responses.

TABLE 30.1 DRUGS IN FOCUS Alpha- and beta-adrenergic agonists

Drug name	Dosage/route	Usual indications
adrenaline (*EpiPen*)	Adult: 0.5–1 mg IV for acute treatment; 0.3–0.5 mg SC or IM for respiratory distress; EpiPen: IMI into anterolateral thigh Adults ≥ 30 kg: 300 micrograms using autoinjector; may repeat every 5–15 min if symptoms recur or do not subside Children 15–30 kg: 150 micrograms using autoinjector; may repeat after 15 min if symptoms recur or do not subside Paediatric: 5–10 micrograms/kg IV; base dose on age, weight and response; do not repeat more than q 6 hours; topical nasal drops for children > 6 years as needed	Treatment of shock when increased blood pressure and heart contractility are essential; to prolong effects of regional anaesthetic; primary treatment for bronchospasm; as an ophthalmic agent; to produce a local vasoconstriction that prolongs the effects of local anaesthetics
dobutamine (*Dobutrex*)	2.5–10 micrograms/kg/min IV with dose adjusted based on response	Treatment of heart failure
(P) dopamine (generic)	Initially 2–5 micrograms/kg/min IV with incremental increases up to 20–50 micrograms/kg per minute based on response	Treatment of shock
ephedrine (generic)	Adult: 25–50 mg IM, SC or 10–25 mg IV q 5–10 minutes Paediatric: 25–100 mg/m^2 IM or SC in 4–6 divided doses; 3 mg/kg/day in 4–6 divided doses PO, SC or IV for bronchodilation	Treatment of hypotensive episodes
metaraminol (generic)	15–100 mg in 500 mL normal saline or 5% glucose, adjust rate according to blood pressure Paediatric: 0.01 mg/kg IV as a single dose	Prevention and management of acute hypotension
noradrenaline (norepinephrine) (*Levophed*)	8–12 micrograms base/min IV; base rate and dose on response	Treatment of shock; used during cardiac arrest to get sympathetic activity

used as energy) occurs; pupils dilate; and sweating can increase (see Figure 30.2). These drugs are generally indicated for the treatment of hypotensive states or shock, bronchospasm and some types of asthma. Table 30.1 discusses usual indications for each of these agents.

Dopamine, a naturally occurring catecholamine, is the sympathomimetic of choice for the treatment of shock. It stimulates the heart and increases blood pressure but also causes a renal and splanchnic arteriole dilation that increases blood flow to the kidneys. This prevents the diminished renal blood supply and possible renal shutdown that can occur with adrenaline or noradrenaline, which are also naturally occurring catecholamines that interact with both alpha- and beta-adrenergic receptors and are used for the treatment of shock and to stimulate the body after cardiac arrest (see Table 30.1 for additional indications for adrenaline and noradrenaline).

Dobutamine, ephedrine and metaraminol are synthetic catecholamines. Dobutamine, although it acts at both beta-receptor sites, has a preference for beta-1-receptor sites. It is used in the treatment of heart failure because it can increase myocardial contractility without much change in rate and does not increase the oxygen demand of the cardiac muscle, an advantage over all of the other sympathomimetic drugs.

Ephedrine stimulates the release of noradrenaline from nerve endings and acts directly on adrenergic receptor sites. Although ephedrine was once used for situations ranging from the treatment of shock to chronic management of asthma and allergic rhinitis, its use in many areas is declining because of the availability of less toxic drugs with more predictable onset and action.

Many OTC cold products contain ephedrine or pseudoephedrine. These products can be used to produce methamphetamine, an often-abused street drug. By law, the sale of these products is now restricted. The products are found behind the counter at pharmacies, not on open shelves; the amount that can be purchased at any given time is limited and in Australia and New Zealand pharmacies maintain a record of multiple purchases of pseudoephedrine by any one individual.

Metaraminol is very similar to noradrenaline. It is given as a single parenteral injection to manage hypotension by increasing myocardial contractility and causing peripheral vasoconstriction. Its use is limited to situations in which dopamine or noradrenaline cannot be used.

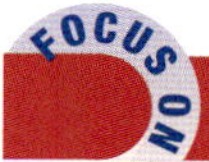

Safe medication administration

Ephedra, a herb that acts like ephedrine, has been in headlines in recent years because people who were using the herb to promote weight loss died suddenly. The U.S. Food and Drug Administration (FDA) has banned ephedra as a drug and in Australia the TGA imposes a restriction on ephedra that stipulates the ephedrine concentration from all ingredients must not exceed 0.001%. Importation to Australia also requires an import permit licence. People should be taught about the potential danger of this product. Any person who is at risk for serious reactions to the stimulatory effects of a sympathomimetic – people with narrow-angle glaucoma, dehydration, cerebral or peripheral vascular disease, cardiac disease or arrhythmias, hypertension, renal dysfunction, thyroid disease, diabetes, prostatic disorders, pregnancy or breastfeeding – should receive direct instruction about the dangers of this product.

Pharmacokinetics

These drugs are generally absorbed rapidly after injection or passage through mucous membranes. They are metabolised in the liver and excreted in the urine. When used in emergency situations, they are given intravenously (IV) to achieve rapid onset of action.

Contraindications and cautions

The alpha and beta agonists are contraindicated in people with known hypersensitivity to any component of the drug *to prevent hypersensitivity reactions*; phaeochromocytoma *because the systemic overload of catecholamines could be fatal*; with tachyarrhythmias or ventricular fibrillation *because the increased heart rate and oxygen consumption usually caused by these drugs could exacerbate these conditions*; with hypovolaemia, *for which fluid replacement would be the treatment for the associated hypotension*; and with halogenated hydrocarbon general anaesthetics (and several industrial solvents), *which sensitise the myocardium to catecholamines and could cause serious cardiac effects.* Caution should be used with any kind of peripheral vascular disease (eg, atherosclerosis, Raynaud disease, diabetic endarteritis), *which could be exacerbated by systemic vasoconstriction.* Because the sympathomimetic drugs stimulate the SNS, they should be used during pregnancy and breastfeeding only if the benefits to the mother clearly outweigh any potential risks to the fetus or neonate.

Adverse effects

The adverse effects associated with the use of alpha- and beta-adrenergic agonists may be associated with the drugs' effects on the sympathetic nervous system: arrhythmias, hypertension, palpitations, angina and dyspnoea related to the effects on the heart and CV system; nausea, vomiting and constipation related to the depressant effects on the GI tract; and headache, sweating, feelings of tension or anxiety and piloerection related to the sympathetic stimulation. Because all of these drugs cause vasoconstriction, care must be taken to avoid extravasation of any infused drug. The vasoconstriction in the area of extravasation can lead to cell death in that area.

Clinically important drug–drug interactions

Increased effects of tricyclic antidepressants and monoamine oxidase (MAO) inhibitors can occur because of the increased noradrenaline levels or increased receptor stimulation that occurs with both drugs. There is an increased risk of hypertension if alpha- and beta-adrenergic agonists are given with any other drugs that cause hypertension, including herbal therapies and OTC preparations (Box 30.2). Any adrenergic agonist will lose effectiveness if combined with any adrenergic antagonist. Monitor the person's drug regimen for appropriate use of the drugs.

 **Prototype summary: dopamine**

Indications: correction of haemodynamic imbalances present in shock.

Actions: acts directly and by the release of noradrenaline (norepinephrine) from sympathetic nerve terminals; mediates dilation of vessels in the renal and splanchnic beds to maintain renal perfusion while stimulating the sympathetic response.

Pharmacokinetics:

Route	Onset	Peak	Duration
IV	1–2 min	10 min	Length of infusion

$T_{1/2}$: 2 minutes; metabolised in the liver, excreted in the urine.

Adverse effects: tachycardia, ectopic beats, anginal pain, hypotension, dyspnoea, nausea, vomiting, headache.

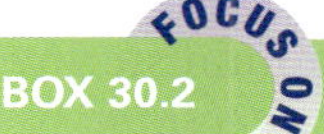

BOX 30.2 Herbal and alternative therapies

People being treated with any adrenergic agonists and who are also taking ma huang, guarana or caffeine are at increased risk for overstimulation, including increased blood pressure, stroke and death. Counsel people to avoid these combinations.

Care considerations for people receiving alpha- and beta-adrenergic agonists

Assessment: history and examination

- Assess for contraindications or cautions: any known allergies to these drugs *to avoid hypersensitivity reactions*; phaeochromocytoma, *which could lead to fatal reactions due to systemic overload of catecholamines*; tachyarrhythmias or ventricular fibrillation, *which could be exacerbated by these drugs*; hypovolaemia, *which would require fluid replacement as treatment for the associated hypotension*; general anaesthesia with halogenated hydrocarbon anaesthetics, *which could lead to serious cardiac effects (similar sensitisation can occur as a result of industrial solvent exposure)*; the presence of vascular disease, *which could be exacerbated with the use of these drugs*; and current status of pregnancy and breastfeeding.
- Perform a physical assessment to establish baseline status *before beginning therapy and during therapy to evaluate for any potential adverse effects and to determine the effectiveness of therapy.*
- Assess vital signs, especially pulse and blood pressure, *to monitor for possible excess stimulation of the cardiac system*; obtain an electrocardiogram (ECG) *to evaluate for possible arrhythmias.*
- Note respiratory rate and auscultate lungs for adventitious sounds *to evaluate effects on bronchi and respiration.*
- Monitor urine output *to evaluate perfusion of the kidneys and therapeutic effects.*
- Monitor the results of laboratory tests, such as renal and liver function tests, *to determine the need for possible dose adjustment* and serum electrolyte levels to *evaluate fluid loss and appropriateness of therapy.*

Refer to Critical thinking scenario for a full discussion of care for a person who is experiencing adrenergic agonist toxicity.

Implementation with rationale

- Use extreme caution in calculating and preparing doses of these drugs *because even small errors could have serious effects.* Always dilute a parenteral drug before use if it is not prediluted *to prevent tissue irritation on injection.*
- Use aseptic no-touch technique when administering ophthalmic or nasal agents *to prevent infection.*
- Monitor people receiving the drug ophthalmically or nasally for all of the systemic effects associated with parenteral administration *to prevent potentially serious adverse effects if the drug is absorbed systemically.*
- Monitor response closely (blood pressure, ECG, urine output, cardiac output) and adjust dose accordingly *to ensure the most benefit with the least amount of toxicity.*
- If extravasation occurs, administer 1 mg diluted terbutaline (1 mg/10 mL) SC once daily into the area of extravasation, followed by topical nitroglycerin 2%, *to preserve tissue*, and monitor for hypotension.
- Provide comfort measures to help the person cope with sympathomimetic effects of the drug; monitor light exposure *to prevent sensitivity to light caused by pupil dilation*, encourage voiding before giving the drug *to alleviate urinary retention caused by sphincter contraction*, monitor bowel function and provide assistance as needed *to deal with GI suppression,* and offer support and relaxation measures *to deal with feelings of tension and anxiety.*
- Provide the following teaching to people using these drugs orally or ophthalmically. Most of these drugs are given in emergency situations and teaching will be based on the person's condition and awareness. Teaching includes:
  - drug name, prescribed dosage and schedule for administration
  - rationale for the drug
  - proper technique for administration
  - measures to prevent or avoid adverse effects
  - need to check with the prescriber before taking any OTC medication
  - warning signs that might indicate a problem
  - importance of avoiding intake of caffeine-containing products
  - need for follow-up monitoring and evaluation

Evaluation

- Monitor the response to the drug (improvement in blood pressure, ocular pressure, bronchial airflow).
- Monitor for adverse effects (CV changes, decreased urine output, headache, GI upset).
- Monitor the effectiveness of comfort measures and compliance with the regimen.
- Evaluate the effectiveness of the teaching plan (person can name the drug, dosage, adverse effects to watch for and specific measures to avoid them).

KEY POINTS

- Adrenergic agonists (sympathomimetics) stimulate the adrenergic receptors in the SNS.
- Alpha- and beta-adrenergic agonists stimulate all of the adrenergic receptors in the SNS. They induce a fight-or-flight response and are frequently used to treat shock.

CRITICAL THINKING SCENARIO

Adrenergic agonist toxicity

THE SITUATION

M.C. is a 26-year-old man who has recently moved from Western Australia to Tasmania. He has been experiencing sinusitis, runny nose and cold-like symptoms for 2 weeks. He appears at an outpatient hospital with complaints of headache, 'jitters', inability to sleep, loss of appetite and a feeling of impending doom. He states that he feels 'on edge' and has not been productive in his job as a watch repairman and jeweller. According to his history, M.C. has been treated with several different drugs for nocturnal enuresis, a persisting childhood problem. Only pseudoephedrine, which he has been taking for 2 years, has been successful (an off-label use of the drug). He has no other significant health problems. He denies any side effects from the use of pseudoephedrine but does admit to self-medicating his nagging cold with OTC preparations – a nasal spray used four times a day and a combination decongestant–pain reliever. A physical examination reveals a pulse of 104 beats/minute, blood pressure 154/86 mmHg, and respiration 16/minute. M.C. appears flushed and slightly diaphoretic.

CRITICAL THINKING

What are the important care implications for M.C.? *Think about the problems that confront a person in a new area seeking health care for the first time.*

What could be causing the problems that M.C. presents with? *The diagnosis of ephedrine overdose was eventually made based on the person's history of OTC drug use and the presenting signs and symptoms.*

Keeping in mind that this diagnosis means that M.C. has an overstimulated sympathetic stress reaction, what other physical problems can be anticipated? *Overwhelming feelings of anxiety and stress are influencing M.C.'s response to work and health care.*

Given this fact, how may the health professional best deal with explaining the problem and how it could have happened – without making the person feel uninformed or that the practice of his former health care provider is being questioned?

What treatment should be planned and what teaching points should be covered for M.C.?

DISCUSSION

The first step in caring for M.C. is establishing a trusting relationship to help alleviate some of the anxiety he is feeling. Being in a new state and seeking health care in a new setting can be very stressful for people under normal circumstances. In M.C.'s case, the sympathomimetic effects of the drugs that he has been taking make him feel even more anxious and jittery.

A careful history will help to determine whether there are any underlying medical problems that could be exacerbated by these drug effects. A review of M.C.'s nocturnal enuresis and the treatments that have been tried will enhance understanding of his former health care and suggest possible implications for further study. This questioning will also reassure M.C. that he is an important member of the health team and that the information he has to offer is valued.

A careful review of the OTC drugs that M.C. has been using will be informative for the person, as well as for the health care providers, who have not actually checked OTC drugs for those specific ingredients, because combining them to ease signs and symptoms often results in toxic levels and symptoms of overdose. Many of these preparations contain sympathomimetics, such as phenylephrine, which will have additive effects to the pseudoephedrine. M.C. will need a full teaching program about the effects of his pseudoephedrine and which OTC drugs to avoid. The treatment for his current problems involves withdrawal of the OTC drugs; when these drug levels fall, the signs and symptoms will disappear. M.C. may also wish to avoid nicotine and caffeine because these stimulants could increase his 'jitters'.

To build trust and ensure that the underlying cause of the problem was drug toxicity, M.C. should receive written instructions that highlight warning signs to report, including chest pain, palpitations and difficulty voiding. He also should be given the health care provider's telephone number with instructions to call the next day and report on his health status. Finally, specimens of nasal discharge should be cultured and antibiotic treatment prescribed, if appropriate.

CARE GUIDE FOR M.C.: ADRENERGIC AGONIST TOXICITY

Assessment: history and examination

Assess the person's history of drug allergies, CV dysfunction, pheochromocytoma, narrow-angle glaucoma, prostatic hypertrophy, thyroid disease or diabetes, as well as concurrent use of MAO inhibitors, tricyclic antidepressants, reserpine, ephedrine or urinary alkalinisers.

Focus the physical examination on the following:

CV: blood pressure, pulse rate, peripheral perfusion and ECG

CNS: orientation, affect, reflexes, peripheral sensation and vision

Skin: colour and temperature
GI: abdominal examination
GU: urine output, bladder percussion and prostate palpation
Respiratory: respiratory rate and adventitious sounds

Implementation

Ensure safe and appropriate administration of the drug.
Provide comfort and safety measures: temperature and lighting control (person may have pupil dilation secondary to sympathetic effects), mouth care and skin care.
Monitor blood pressure, pulse rate and respiratory status throughout drug therapy.
Provide support and reassurance to deal with drug therapy and effects.
Provide teaching about drug name, dosage, side effects, precautions and warning signs to report.

Evaluation

Evaluate drug effects: relief of enuresis.
Monitor for adverse effects: CV effects, dizziness, confusion, headache, rash, difficulty voiding, sweating, flushing and pupillary dilation.
Monitor for drug–drug interactions as indicated.
Evaluate the effectiveness of the teaching program as well as comfort and safety measures.

TEACHING FOR M.C.

- The drug that you have been taking is pseudoephedrine. It is called an adrenergic agonist (or a sympathomimetic drug). Pseudoephedrine acts by mimicking the effects of the sympathetic nervous system, which is the part of your nervous system that is responsible for your response to fear or danger (this is called the 'fight-or-flight' response). Because this drug triggers many effects in the body, you may experience some undesired adverse effects. It is crucial to discuss the effect of the drug with your health care provider and to try to make the effect as tolerable as possible.
- If you have diagnosed prostate problems, it might help to void before taking each dose of the drug.
- Some of the following adverse effects may occur:
  - *Restlessness or shaking*: if these occur, avoid driving, operating machinery or performing delicate tasks.
  - *Flushing or sweating*: avoid warm temperatures and heavy clothing; frequent washing with cool water may help.
  - *Heart palpitations*: if you feel that your heart is beating too fast or skipping beats, sit down for a while and rest. If the feeling becomes too uncomfortable, notify your health care provider.
  - *Sensitivity to light*: avoid glaring lights or wear sunglasses if you are in bright light. Be careful when moving between extremes of light because your vision may not adjust quickly.
- Report any of the following to your health care provider: *difficulty voiding, chest pain, difficulty breathing, dizziness, headache or changes in vision.*
- Do not stop taking this drug suddenly; make sure that you have enough of your prescription. This drug dose should be reduced gradually over 2–4 days when you are instructed to discontinue it by your health care provider.
- Avoid OTC medications, including cold and allergy remedies and diet pills. If you feel that you need one of these, check with your health care provider first.
- Tell any health care provider who takes care of you that you are taking this drug.
- Keep this drug and all medications out of the reach of children. Do not share this drug with other people.

ALPHA-SPECIFIC ADRENERGIC AGONISTS

Alpha-specific adrenergic agonists (Table 30.2), or alpha agonists, are drugs that bind primarily to alpha receptors rather than to beta receptors. Drugs belonging to this class include clonidine (*Catapres*) and phenylephrine (*Abalon*, *Neo-Synephrine*).

Therapeutic actions and indications

Therapeutic effects of the alpha-specific adrenergic agonists result from the stimulation of alpha receptors within the SNS (see Figure 30.2). The uses are varied, depending on the specific drug and the route of administration (Table 30.2).

Phenylephrine, a potent vasoconstrictor and alpha-1-agonist with little or no effect on the heart or bronchi, is used in many combination cold and allergy products. Parenterally it is used to treat shock or shock-like states, to overcome paroxysmal supraventricular tachycardia, to prolong local anaesthesia and to maintain blood pressure during spinal anaesthesia. Topically it is used to treat allergic rhinitis and to relieve the symptoms of otitis media. Ophthalmically it is used to dilate the pupils for eye examination, before surgery or to relieve elevated eye pressure associated with glaucoma. Phenylephrine is found in many cold and allergy products because it is so effective in constricting topical vessels and decreasing the swelling, signs and symptoms of rhinitis.

Clonidine specifically stimulates CNS alpha-2 receptors. This leads to decreased sympathetic outflow from the CNS because the alpha-2 receptors moderate the release of noradrenaline from the nerve axon.

TABLE 30.2 **DRUGS IN FOCUS** **Alpha-specific adrenergic agonists**

Drug name	Dosage/route	Usual indications
clonidine (*Catapres*)	75 micrograms PO bd or tds to maximum 900 micrograms/day; 150–300 micrograms IM or IV in 10 mL normal saline over 5 minutes	Treatment of essential hypertension; chronic pain; to ease opiate withdrawal; used only for adults
(P) phenylephrine (*Abalon, Neo-Synephrine*)	1–10 mg SC or IM or 0.1–0.5 mg IV as a starting dose; 0.5 mg IV by rapid injection to convert tachycardias; eye drops, 1–2 drops in affected eye(s)	Cold and allergies; shock and shock-like states; supraventricular tachycardias; mydriatic, to dilate the pupil in diagnostic or therapeutic procedures; allergic rhinitis; otitis media

Clonidine is available in oral and transdermal forms for use to control hypertension and as an injection for epidural infusion to control pain in people with cancer. Because of its centrally acting effects, clonidine is associated with many more CNS effects (bad dreams, sedation, drowsiness, fatigue, headache) than other sympathomimetics. It can also cause extreme hypotension, heart failure and bradycardia due to its decreased effects of the sympathetic outflow from the CNS.

Pharmacokinetics

These drugs are generally well absorbed and reach peak levels in a short period – 20–45 minutes. They are widely distributed in the body, metabolised in the liver and primarily excreted in the urine. The transdermal form of clonidine is slow release and has a 7-day duration of effects, so it only needs to be replaced once a week. Phenylephrine can be given intramuscularly (IM), subcutaneously (SC), IV, orally and as a nasal or an ophthalmic solution.

Contraindications and cautions

The alpha-specific adrenergic agonists are contraindicated in the presence of allergy to the specific drug *to avoid hypersensitivity reactions*; severe hypertension or tachycardia *because of possible additive effects*; and narrow-angle glaucoma, *which could be exacerbated by arterial constriction*. There are no adequate studies about use during pregnancy and breastfeeding, so use should be reserved for situations in which the benefit to the mother outweighs any potential risk to the fetus or neonate.

They should be used with caution in the presence of CV disease or vasomotor spasm *because these conditions could be aggravated by the vascular effects of the drug*; thyrotoxicosis or diabetes *because of the thyroid-stimulating and glucose-elevating effects of sympathetic stimulation*; or renal or hepatic impairment, *which could interfere with metabolism and excretion of the drug*.

Adverse effects

People receiving these drugs often experience adverse effects that are extensions of the therapeutic effects or other sympathetic stimulatory reactions. CNS effects include feelings of anxiety, restlessness, depression, fatigue, strange dreams and personality changes. Blurred vision and sensitivity to light may occur because of the pupil dilation that occurs when the sympathetic system is stimulated. Cardiovascular effects can include arrhythmias, ECG changes, blood pressure changes and peripheral vascular problems. Nausea, vomiting and anorexia can occur, related to the depressant effects of the SNS on the GI tract. Genitourinary effects can include decreased urinary output, difficulty urinating, dysuria and changes in sexual function related to the sympathetic stimulation of these systems. These drugs should not be stopped suddenly; adrenergic receptors will be very sensitive to catecholamines and sudden withdrawal can lead to tachycardia, hypertension, arrhythmias, flushing and even death. Avoid these effects by tapering the drug over 2–4 days when it is being discontinued. As with other sympathomimetics, if phenylephrine is given IV, care should be taken to avoid extravasation. The vasoconstricting effects of the drug can lead to necrosis and cell death in the area of extravasation.

Clinically important drug–drug interactions

Phenylephrine combined with MAOIs can cause severe hypertension, headache and hyperpyrexia; this combination should be avoided. Increased sympathomimetic effects occur when phenylephrine is combined with tricyclic antidepressants (TCAs); if this combination must be used, the person should be monitored very closely.

Clonidine has a decreased antihypertensive effect if taken with TCAs and a paradoxical hypertension occurs if it is combined with propranolol. If these combinations are used, the person's response should be monitored closely and dose adjustment made as needed.

Any adrenergic agonist will lose effectiveness if combined with any adrenergic antagonist. Monitor the person's drug regimen for appropriate use of the drugs.

Prototype summary: phenylephrine

Indications: treatment of vascular failure in shock or drug-induced hypotension; to overcome paroxysmal supraventricular tachycardia; to prolong spinal anaesthesia; as a vasoconstrictor in regional anaesthesia; to maintain blood pressure during anaesthesia; topically for symptomatic relief of nasal congestion and as adjunctive therapy in middle-ear infections; ophthalmically to dilate pupils and as a decongestant to provide temporary relief of eye irritation.

Actions: powerful postsynaptic alpha-adrenergic receptor stimulant causing vasoconstriction and raising systolic and diastolic blood pressure with little effect on the beta receptors in the heart.

Pharmacokinetics:

Route	Onset	Duration
IV	Immediate	15–20 min
IM, SC	10–15 min	30–120 min
Topically	Very little systemic absorption occurs	

$T_{1/2}$: 47–100 hours; metabolised in the tissues and liver; excreted in urine and bile.

Adverse effects: fear, anxiety, restlessness, headache, nausea, decreased urine formation, pallor.

Care considerations for people receiving alpha-specific adrenergic agonists

Assessment: history and examination

- Assess for contraindications or cautions: any known allergies to the drug *to avoid hypersensitivity reactions*; presence of any CV diseases, *which could be exacerbated by the vascular effects of these drugs;* thyrotoxicosis or diabetes, *which would lead to an increase in thyroid stimulation or glucose elevation*; chronic renal failure, *which could be exacerbated by drug use*; renal or hepatic impairment, *which could interfere with drug excretion or metabolism*; and current status of pregnancy and breastfeeding.
- Perform a physical assessment to establish *baseline status before beginning therapy to determine effectiveness and during therapy to evaluate for any potential adverse effects.*
- Assess level of orientation, affect, reflexes and vision *to monitor for CNS changes related to drug therapy.*
- Monitor blood pressure and pulse, assess peripheral perfusion and obtain ECG, if indicated, *to determine drug effectiveness and evaluate for adverse CV effects.*
- Assess urinary output *to evaluate renal function and monitor for adverse effects of the drug.*
- Evaluate person for nausea and constipation *to assess adverse effects of the drug and establish appropriate interventions.*
- Monitor laboratory test results, such as renal and liver function tests, *to determine drug effects on renal and hepatic systems.*

Implementation with rationale

- Do not discontinue the drug abruptly *because sudden withdrawal can result in rebound hypertension, arrhythmias, flushing and even hypertensive encephalopathy and death*; taper drug over 2–4 days.
- Do not discontinue the drug before surgery; document on the person's chart and monitor blood pressure carefully during surgery. *Sympathetic stimulation may alter the normal response to anaesthesia, as well as recovery from anaesthesia.*
- Monitor blood pressure, orthostatic blood pressure, pulse, rhythm and cardiac output regularly, even with ophthalmic preparations, *to adjust dose or discontinue the drug if CV effects are severe.*
- When giving phenylephrine IV, ensure that an alpha-blocking agent is readily available to counteract the effects *in case severe reaction occurs*; infiltrate any area of extravasation with 1 mg diluted terbutaline (1 mg/10 mL) SC once daily into the area of extravasation, followed by topical nitroglycerin 2%, *to preserve tissue*; monitor for hypotension.
- Arrange for supportive care and comfort measures, including rest and environmental control, *to decrease CNS irritation*; analgesics for headache *to relieve discomfort*; safety measures, such as use of side rails and assistance with ambulation if CNS effects occur, *to protect the person from injury*; and protective measures *if CNS effects are severe.*
- Provide thorough teaching about drug name, dose and schedule for administration; technique for administration if appropriate; measures to prevent potential adverse effects such as voiding before taking the drug and use of bowel training activities if constipation is a problem; safety measures such as avoiding driving and operating dangerous machinery if CNS effects occur, and getting up and down slowly if orthostatic hypotension is an issue;

warning signs of problems; and importance of monitoring and follow-up.

Evaluation

- Monitor response to the drug (improvement in condition being treated).
- Monitor for adverse effects (GI upset, CNS and CV changes).
- Monitor the effectiveness of comfort measures and compliance with the regimen.
- Evaluate the effectiveness of the teaching plan (person can name drug, dosage, adverse effects to watch for and specific measures to avoid them).

KEY POINTS

- alpha-specific adrenergic agonists, such as phenylephrine and clonidine, stimulate only the alpha receptors within the SNS. Clonidine stimulates alpha-2 receptors and is used to treat hypertension because its action blocks the release of noradrenaline (norepinephrine) from nerve axons.
- Care must be taken to prevent extravasation when using IV; the vasoconstrictive properties of the drug can cause necrosis and cell death in the area of extravasation.
- These drugs should be tapered over 2–4 days when discontinued because the adrenergic receptors will be very sensitive and rebound hypertension, tachycardia, arrhythmias and even death can occur.

BETA-SPECIFIC ADRENERGIC AGONISTS

Most of the drugs that belong to the class of beta-specific adrenergic agonists (Table 30.3), or beta agonists, are beta-2-specific agonists and are used to manage and treat bronchial spasm, asthma and other obstructive pulmonary conditions. These drugs, including salbutamol (*Butamol*, *Ventolin*), salmeterol (*Serevent*) and terbutaline, are discussed in Chapter 55, which deals with drugs used to treat obstructive pulmonary diseases. This section specifically addresses isoprenaline (*Isuprel*), which is used as a sympathomimetic for its overall stimulatory properties.

Therapeutic actions and indications

Therapeutic effects of isoprenaline are related to its stimulation of all beta-adrenergic receptors. Desired effects of the drug include increased heart rate, conductivity and contractility; bronchodilation; increased blood flow to skeletal muscles and splanchnic beds; and relaxation of the uterus. Its use has decreased over the years as more specific drugs with less toxicity have been developed to treat the cardiac problems isoprenaline was developed to treat. Some research has shown that isoprenaline exerts a 'coronary steal' effect,

TABLE 30.3 *DRUGS IN FOCUS* Beta-specific adrenergic agonists

Drug name	Dosage/route	Usual indications
(P) isoprenaline (*Isuprel*)	Adult: IV injection, 0.02–0.06 mg; IV infusion, 5 micrograms/minute; 0.2 mg IM or SC Paediatric: 0.1–1.0 micrograms/kg/minute IV has been used	Treatment of shock, cardiac arrest, and certain ventricular arrhythmias; treatment of heart block in transplanted hearts; prevention of bronchospasm during anaesthesia
salbutamol (*Butamol*, *Ventolin*)	Adult: 2–4 mg tds–qid PO, or 1–2 inhalations every 4–6 hours Paediatric, ventolin elixir, 2–6 years: 2.5–5 mL (1–2 mg salbutamol) PO tid–qid 6–12 years: 5 mL (2 mg salbutamol) PO tid–qid > 12 years: 5–10 mL (2–4 mg salbutamol) PO tid–qid Nebules: 2.5–5 mg by inhalation via nebuliser qid	Treatment and prevention of bronchospasm; treatment of acute bronchospasm and exercise-induced bronchospasm when used by inhalation
salmeterol (*Serevent*)	Adults: 1 inhalation twice daily; maximum of 2 inhalations bid Children ≥ 4 years: 1 inhalation bid	Treatment and prevention of bronchial asthma and reversible bronchospasm, including exercise-induced bronchospasm (people ≥ 4 years)
terbutaline (*Bricanyl*)	Adults and children > 12 years: 1–2 inhalations (maximum of 6 inhalations) as required; maximum of 24 inhalations in 24 hours Children 3–12 years: 1–2 inhalations (maximum of 4 inhalations) as required. Maximum of 16 inhalations in 24 hours	Treatment and prevention of bronchial asthma and reversible bronchospasm

diverting blood away from injured or hypoxic areas of the heart muscle, an effect that can increase the size and extent of an evolving myocardial infarction, further decreasing its usefulness in the clinical setting. There are some emergency situations however, that respond well to isoprenaline. See Table 30.3 for usual indications.

Pharmacokinetics

Isoprenaline is rapidly distributed after injection; it is metabolised in the liver and excreted in the urine. The half-life is relatively short – less than 1 hour.

Contraindications and cautions

Isoprenaline is contraindicated in the presence of allergy to the drug or any components of the drug *to avert hypersensitivity reactions*; with pulmonary hypertension, *which could be exacerbated by the effects of the drug*; during anaesthesia with halogenated hydrocarbons, *which sensitise the myocardium to catecholamines and could cause a severe reaction*; with eclampsia, uterine haemorrhage and intrauterine death, *which could be complicated by uterine relaxation or increased blood pressure*; and during pregnancy and breastfeeding *because of potential effects on the fetus or neonate*. Caution should be used with diabetes, thyroid disease, vasomotor problems, degenerative heart disease or history of stroke, *all of which could be exacerbated by the sympathomimetic effects of the drug* and with severe renal impairment, *which could alter the excretion of the drug*.

Prototype summary: isoprenaline

Indications: management of bronchospasm during anaesthesia; vasopressor during shock; adjunct in the management of cardiac standstill and arrest, as well as serious ventricular arrhythmias that require increased inotropic action.

Actions: acts on beta-adrenergic receptors to produce increased heart rate, positive inotropic effect, bronchodilation and vasodilation.

Pharmacokinetics:

Route	Onset	Duration
IV	Immediate	1–2 min

$T_{1/2}$: unknown; metabolised in the tissues.

Adverse effects: restlessness, apprehension, anxiety, fear, cardiac arrhythmias, tachycardia, nausea, vomiting, heartburn, respiratory difficulties, coughing, pulmonary oedema, sweating, pallor.

Adverse effects

People receiving isoprenaline often experience adverse effects related to the stimulation of sympathetic adrenergic receptors. CNS effects include restlessness, anxiety, fear, tremor, fatigue and headache. Cardiovascular effects can include tachycardia, angina, myocardial infarction and palpitations. Pulmonary effects can be severe, ranging from difficulty breathing, coughing and bronchospasm to severe pulmonary oedema. GI upset, nausea, vomiting and anorexia can occur as a result of the slowing of the GI tract with SNS stimulation. Other anticipated effects can include sweating, pupil dilation, rash and muscle cramps.

Clinically important drug–drug interactions

Increased sympathomimetic effects can be expected if this drug is taken with other sympathomimetic drugs. Decreased therapeutic effects can occur if this drug is combined with beta-adrenergic blockers.

Care considerations for people receiving beta-specific adrenergic agonists

Assessment: history and examination

- Assess for contraindications or cautions: any known allergies to any drug or any components of the drug *to avoid possible hypersensitivity reactions*; pulmonary hypertension, which *could be exacerbated by the effects of the drug*; anaesthesia with halogenated hydrocarbons, *which sensitise the myocardium to catecholamines and could cause severe reaction*; eclampsia, uterine haemorrhage and intrauterine death, *which could be complicated by uterine relaxation or increased blood pressure*; diabetes, thyroid disease, vasomotor problems, degenerative heart disease or history of stroke, *all of which could be exacerbated by the sympathomimetic effects of the drugs*; severe renal impairment, *which could interfere with the excretion of the drug*; and current status of pregnancy and breastfeeding.
- Perform a physical assessment to establish a baseline before beginning therapy and during therapy *to determine the drug's effectiveness and identify any potential adverse effects.*
- Assess CV status, including pulse rate and blood pressure, *to evaluate for any CV effects associated with SNS stimulation*; obtain an ECG *to evaluate for changes indicating excessive SNS stimulation.*
- Assess respiratory status and listen for adventitious sounds *to monitor drug effects and assess for any adverse effects.*

- Monitor urine output *to evaluate renal function and kidney perfusion.*
- Monitor laboratory test results, including thyroid function tests, blood glucose levels and renal function, *to monitor drug effects and potential adverse effects.*

Implementation with rationale

- Monitor pulse and blood pressure carefully during administration *to arrange to discontinue the drug at any sign of toxicity.*
- Ensure that a β-adrenergic blocker is readily available when giving parenteral isoprenaline *in case severe reaction occurs.*
- Use minimal doses of isoprenaline needed to achieve desired effects *to prevent adverse effects and maintain safety.*
- Arrange for supportive care and comfort measures, including rest and environmental control, *to relieve CNS effects*; provide analgesics for headache and safety measures if CNS effects occur *to provide comfort and prevent injury*; and avoid overhydration *to prevent pulmonary oedema.*
- Provide thorough teaching, including drug name, dosage and frequency of administration; rationale for administration; monitoring required; anticipated adverse effects, measures to reduce these and warning signs of problems to report immediately.

Evaluation

- Monitor response to the drug (improvement in condition being treated, stabilisation of blood pressure, prevention of preterm labour, cardiac stimulation).
- Monitor for adverse effects (GI upset, CNS changes, respiratory problems).
- Evaluate the effectiveness of the teaching plan (person can name drug, dosage, adverse effects to watch for and specific measures to reduce them).
- Monitor the effectiveness of comfort measures and compliance with the regimen.

KEY POINTS

- Most of the beta-2-specific adrenergic agonists are used to manage and treat asthma, bronchospasm and other obstructive pulmonary diseases.
- Isoprenaline, a non-specific beta-specific adrenergic agent, is used for its sympathomimetic effects to treat shock, cardiac standstill and certain arrhythmias when used systemically; it is especially effective in the treatment of heart block in transplanted hearts.
- Because of its many adverse effects, isoprenaline is reserved for use in emergency situations that do not respond to other, safer therapies.

CHAPTER SUMMARY

- Adrenergic agonists, also called sympathomimetics, are drugs that mimic the effects of the sympathetic nervous system (SNS) and are used to stimulate the adrenergic receptors within the SNS. The adverse effects associated with these drugs are usually also a result of sympathetic stimulation.
- Adrenergic agonists include alpha- and beta-adrenergic agonists, which stimulate both types of adrenergic receptors in the SNS, and alpha-specific and beta-specific adrenergic agonists, which stimulate only alpha or only beta receptors, respectively.
- alpha-specific adrenergic agonists, such as phenylephrine and clonidine, stimulate only the alpha receptors within the SNS. Clonidine specifically stimulates alpha-2 receptors and is used to treat hypertension because its action blocks the release of noradrenaline (norepinephrine) from nerve axons.
- Many of the beta-2-specific adrenergic agonists are used to manage and treat asthma, bronchospasm and other obstructive pulmonary diseases.
- Isoprenaline, a non-specific beta-specific adrenergic, is used to treat shock, cardiac standstill and certain arrhythmias when used systemically; it is especially effective in the treatment of heart block in transplanted hearts.

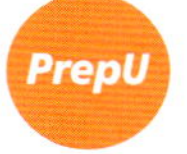

Knowing your strengths and weaknesses helps you to study more effectively. Take a PrepU Practice Quiz to find out how you measure up!

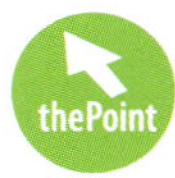

ONLINE RESOURCES

An extensive range of additional resources to enhance teaching and learning and to facilitate understanding of this chapter may be found online at the text's accompanying website, located on thePoint at http://thepoint.lww.com. These include Watch and Learn videos, Concepts in Action animations, journal articles, review questions, case studies, discussion topics and quizzes.

BIBLIOGRAPHY

Farrell, M. & Dempsey, J. (2014). *Smeltzer & Bare's Textbook of Medical-Surgical Nursing* (3rd edn). Sydney: Lippincott Williams & Wilkins.

Goodman, L. S., Brunton, L. L., Chabner, B. & Knollmann, B. C. (2011). *Goodman and Gilman's Pharmacological Basis of Therapeutics* (12th edn). New York: McGraw-Hill.

Lim, A., Hussainy, S. & Abramson, M. J. (2013). Asthma drugs in pregnancy and lactation. *Australian Prescriber, 36,* 150–153.

McKenna, L. & Mirkov, S. (2019). *McKenna's Drug Handbook for Nursing and Midwifery* (8th edn). Sydney: Wolters Kluwer Health Australia.

National Center for Complementary and Alternative Medicine. (2013). Herbs at a Glance: Ephedra. Available at: http://nccam.nih.gov/health/ephedra?nav=gsa.

Porth, C. M. (2011). *Essentials of Pathophysiology: Concepts of Altered Health States* (3rd edn). Philadelphia: Lippincott Williams & Wilkins.

Porth, C. M. (2009). *Pathophysiology: Concepts of Altered Health States* (8th edn). Philadelphia: Lippincott Williams & Wilkins.

Vale, S., Smith, J. & Loh, R. (2012). Safe use of adrenaline autoinjectors. *Australian Prescriber, 35*, 56–58.

Wilmot, L. A. (2010). Shock: Early recognition and management. *Journal of Emergency Nursing, 36(2)*, 134–139.

CHECK YOUR UNDERSTANDING

Answers to the questions in this chapter can be found in Appendix A at the back of this book.

MULTIPLE CHOICE

Select the best answer to the following.

1. The instructor determines that teaching about adrenergic drugs has been successful when the class identifies the drugs as also being called:
   a. sympatholytic agents.
   b. cholinergic agents.
   c. sympathomimetic agents.
   d. anticholinergic agents.
2. The adrenergic agent of choice for treating the signs and symptoms of allergic rhinitis is:
   a. noradrenaline (norepinephrine).
   b. phenylephrine.
   c. dobutamine.
   d. dopamine.
3. An adrenergic agent being used to treat shock infiltrates into the tissue with intravenous administration. Which action would be most appropriate?
   a. Watch the area for any signs of necrosis and report it to the doctor.
   b. Notify the doctor and decrease the rate of infusion.
   c. Administer diluted terbutaline followed by topical nitroglycerin 2%.
   d. Apply ice and elevate the arm.
4. Phenylephrine, an alpha-specific agonist, is found in many cold and allergy preparations. The nurse or midwife instructs the person to be alert for which adverse effects?
   a. urinary retention and pupil constriction
   b. hypotension and slow heart rate
   c. personality changes and increased appetite
   d. cardiac arrhythmias and difficulty urinating
5. Adverse effects associated with adrenergic agonists are related to the generalised stimulation of the sympathetic nervous system and could include:
   a. slowed heart rate.
   b. constriction of the pupils.
   c. hypertension.
   d. increased GI secretions.
6. A person has elected to take an OTC cold preparation that contains phenylephrine. The nurse or midwife would advise the person not to take that drug if the person has:
   a. thyroid or cardiovascular disease.
   b. a cough and runny nose.
   c. chronic obstructive pulmonary disease.
   d. hypotension.

MULTIPLE RESPONSE

Select all that apply.

1. Isoprenaline is a non-specific beta-agonist. The nurse or midwife might expect to administer this drug for which of the following conditions?
   a. preterm labour
   b. bronchospasm
   c. cardiac standstill
   d. shock
   e. heart block in transplanted hearts
   f. heart failure
2. A nurse or midwife would question the order for an adrenergic agonist for a person who is also receiving which of the following:
   a. anticholinergic drugs
   b. halogenated hydrocarbon anaesthetic
   c. beta blockers
   d. benzodiazepines
   e. MAO inhibitors
   f. tricyclic antidepressants

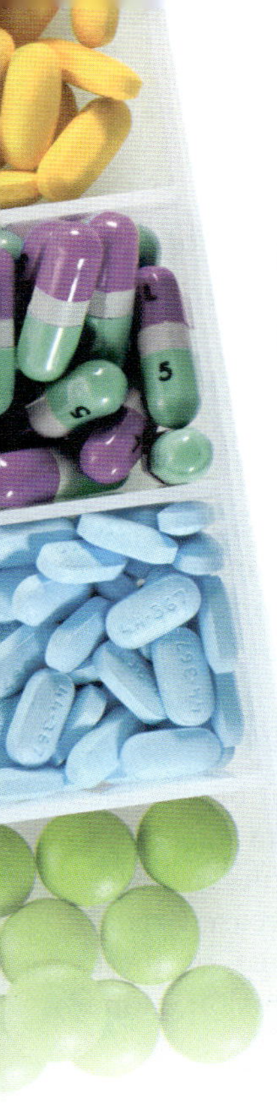

Adrenergic-blocking antagonists

31

Learning objectives

On completing this chapter you should be able to:

1. Describe the effects of adrenergic-blocking agents on adrenergic receptors, correlating these effects with their clinical effects.
2. Describe the therapeutic actions, indications, pharmacokinetics, contraindications and cautions, most common adverse reactions and important drug–drug interactions associated with adrenergic-blocking agents.
3. Discuss the use of adrenergic-blocking agents across the lifespan.
4. Compare and contrast the prototype drugs labetalol, doxazosin, propranolol and atenolol with other adrenergic-blocking agents.
5. Outline the care considerations, including important teaching points, for people receiving an adrenergic-blocking agent.

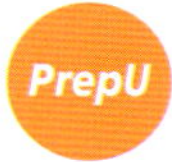

Test your current knowledge of adrenergic-blocking antagonists with a PrepU Practice Quiz!

Glossary of key terms

adrenergic receptor–site specificity: a drug's affinity for only adrenergic-receptor sites; certain drugs may have specific affinity for only alpha- or only beta-adrenergic receptor sites

alpha-1-selective adrenergic-blocking agents: drugs that block the postsynaptic alpha-1-receptor sites, causing a decrease in vascular tone and a vasodilation that leads to a fall in blood pressure; these drugs do not block the presynaptic alpha-2-receptor sites, and therefore the reflex tachycardia that accompanies a fall in blood pressure does not occur

beta adrenergic–blocking agents: drugs that, at therapeutic levels, selectively block the beta receptors of the sympathetic nervous system

beta-1-selective adrenergic-blocking agents: drugs that, at therapeutic levels, specifically block the beta-1 receptors in the sympathetic nervous system while not blocking the beta-2 receptors and resultant effects on the respiratory system

bronchodilation: relaxation of the muscles in the bronchi, resulting in a widening of the bronchi; an effect of sympathetic stimulation

phaeochromocytoma: a tumour of the chromaffin cells of the adrenal medulla that periodically releases large amounts of noradrenaline and adrenaline into the system, with resultant severe hypertension and tachycardia

sympatholytic: a drug that lyses, or blocks, the effects of the sympathetic nervous system

NON-SELECTIVE ADRENERGIC-BLOCKING AGENTS
carvedilol
(P) labetalol

ALPHA-1-SELECTIVE ADRENERGIC-BLOCKING AGENTS
alfuzosin
(P) doxazosin
prazosin
silodosin
tamsulosin
terazosin

NON-SELECTIVE BETA-ADRENERGIC-BLOCKING AGENTS
nebivolol
oxprenolol
pindolol
(P) propranolol
sotalol
timolol

BETA-1-SELECTIVE ADRENERGIC-BLOCKING AGENTS

atenolol
betaxolol
bisoprolol
esmolol
metoprolol

Adrenergic-blocking agents are also called **sympatholytic** drugs because they lyse, or block, the effects of the sympathetic nervous system (SNS). The therapeutic and adverse effects associated with these drugs are related to their **adrenergic receptor–site specificity**, that is, the ability to react with specific adrenergic receptor sites without activating them, thus preventing the typical manifestations of SNS activation. By occupying the adrenergic receptor site, they prevent noradrenaline released from the nerve terminal or from the adrenal medulla from activating the receptor, thus blocking the SNS effects.

The adrenergic blockers have varying degrees of specificity for the adrenergic receptor sites. For example, some can interact with both alpha and beta receptors. Some are specific to alpha receptors, with some being even more specific to just alpha-1 receptors. Other adrenergic blockers interact with both beta-1 and beta-2 receptors, whereas others interact with just either beta-1 or beta-2 receptors. This specificity allows the clinician to select a drug that will have the desired therapeutic effects without the undesired effects that occur when the entire SNS is blocked. In general, however, the specificity of adrenergic-blocking agents depends on the concentration of the drug in the body. Most specificity is lost with higher serum drug levels (see Figure 31.1).

The effects of the adrenergic-blocking agents vary with the age of the person (see Box 31.1). Various alternative and herbal remedies can also affect these drugs (see Box 31.2).

NON-SELECTIVE ADRENERGIC-BLOCKING AGENTS

Drugs that block both alpha- and beta-adrenergic receptors are primarily used to treat cardiac-related conditions. These drugs include carvedilol (*Dilatrend*) and labetalol (*Presolol*, *Trandate*) (see Table 31.1).

Therapeutic actions and indications

Adrenergic-blocking agents competitively block the effects of noradrenaline at alpha and beta receptors throughout the SNS. Subsequently, this results in lower blood pressure, slower pulse rate and increased renal perfusion with decreased renin levels. Most of these drugs are indicated to treat essential hypertension, alone or in combination with diuretics.

Labetalol is a newer drug that is used orally to treat hypertension. It can also be used with diuretics and has been used to treat hypertension associated with **phaeochromocytoma** (tumour of the chromaffin cells of the adrenal medulla, which periodically releases large amounts of noradrenaline and adrenaline into the system) and clonidine withdrawal. Carvedilol is only

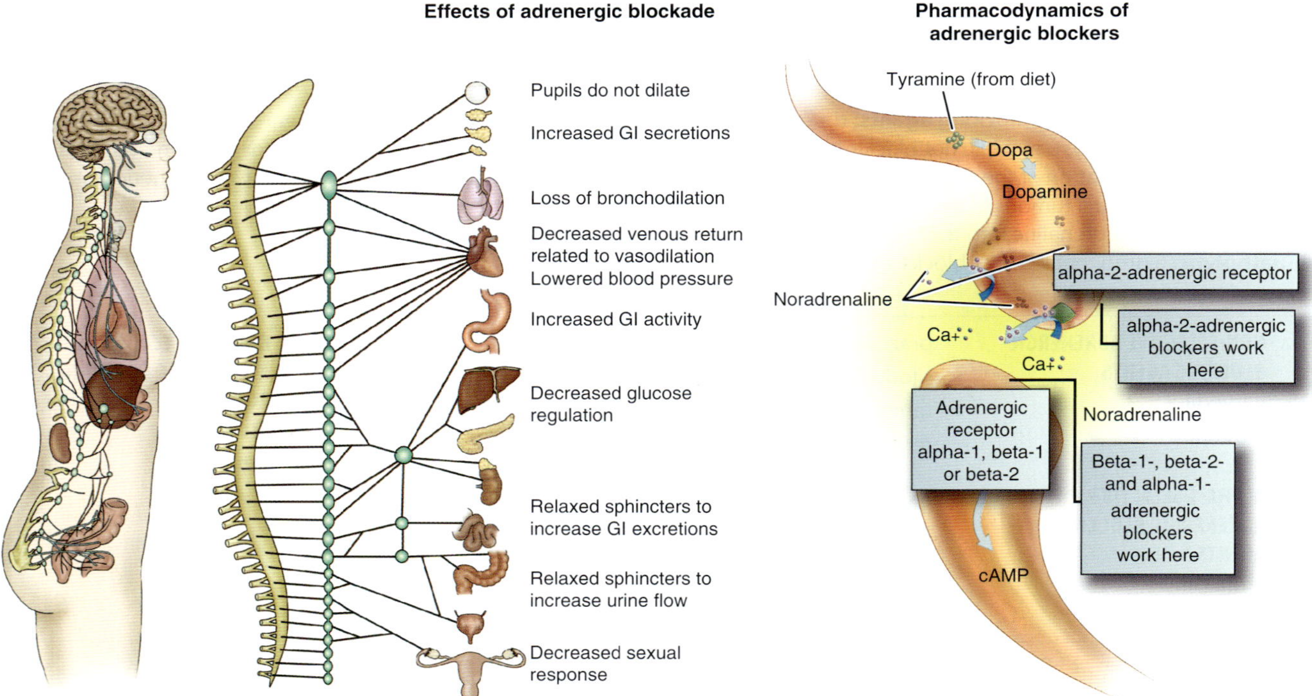

FIGURE 31.1 Site of action of adrenergic receptors and resultant physiological responses. These responses are blocked by adrenergic blockers.

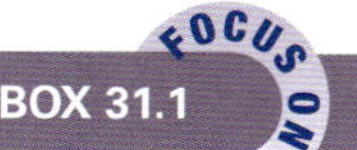

BOX 31.1 Drug therapy across the lifespan

Adrenergic-blocking agents

CHILDREN

Children are at greater risk for complications associated with the use of adrenergic-blocking agents, including bradycardia, difficulty breathing and changes in glucose metabolism. The safety and efficacy for use of these drugs has not been established for children younger than 18 years of age. If one of these drugs is used, the dose for these agents needs to be calculated from the child's body weight and age. It is good practice to have a second person check the dose calculation before administering the drug to avoid potential toxic effects. Only one adrenergic-blocking agent – prazosin, used to treat hypertension – has an established paediatric dose, so it might be the drug to consider when one is needed. Children should be carefully monitored and supported when this drug is given.

ADULTS

Adults being treated with adrenergic-blocking agents should be cautioned about the many adverse effects associated with the drugs. People with diabetes need to be re-educated about ways to monitor themselves for hyperglycaemia and hypoglycaemia because the sympathetic reaction (sweating, feeling tense, increased heart rate, rapid breathing) usually alerts people that there is a problem with their glucose levels. People with severe thyroid disease are also at high risk for serious adverse effects when taking these drugs, and if one of them is needed, the person should be monitored very closely. Propranolol and metoprolol are associated with more central nervous system (CNS) adverse effects than other adrenergic blockers, and people who have CNS complications already or who develop CNS problems while taking an adrenergic blocker might do better with a different agent.

PREGNANCY AND BREASTFEEDING

In general, there are no adequate studies about the effects of adrenergic blockers during pregnancy and breastfeeding, and they should be used only in those situations in which the benefit to the mother is greater than the risk to the fetus or neonate. Adrenergic blockers can affect labour, and babies born to mothers taking these drugs may exhibit adverse cardiovascular (CV), respiratory and CNS effects. Many of these drugs were teratogenic in animal studies. Because of a similar risk of adverse reactions on the baby, breastfeeding mothers should find another way to feed the baby if an adrenergic-blocking drug is needed.

OLDER ADULTS

Older people are more likely to experience the adverse effects associated with these drugs – CNS, CV, GI and respiratory effects. Because older people often also have renal or hepatic impairment, they are more likely to have toxic levels of the drug related to changes in metabolism and excretion. The older person should be started on lower doses of the drugs and should be monitored very closely for potentially serious arrhythmias or blood pressure changes. Bisoprolol is often a drug of choice for older people who require an adrenergic blocker for hypertension because it is not associated with as many problems in the elderly and regular dosing profiles can be used.

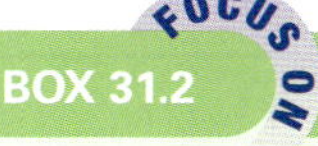

BOX 31.2 Herbal and alternative therapies

People who use alternative therapies as part of their daily regimen should be cautioned about potential increased adrenergic-blocking effects if the following alternative therapies are combined with adrenergic-blocking agents:

- Ginseng, sage – increased antihypertensive effects (risk of hypotension and increased CNS effects)
- Xuan shen, nightshade – slow heart rate (risk of severe bradycardia and reflex arrhythmias)
- Celery, coriander, Di huang, fenugreek, goldenseal, Java plum, xuan seng – lower blood glucose (increased risk of severe hypoglycaemia)
- Saw palmetto – increased urinary tract complications

People who are prescribed an adrenergic-blocking drug should be cautioned about the use of herbs, teas and alternative medicines. If a person feels that one of these agents is needed, the health care provider should be consulted and appropriate precautions should be taken to ensure that the person is able to achieve the most therapeutic effects with the least adverse effects while taking the drug.

available orally and is used to treat hypertension, as well as heart failure and left ventricular dysfunction after myocardial infarction (MI). Table 31.1 shows usual indications for each of these agents.

Pharmacokinetics

These drugs are well absorbed when given orally and are distributed throughout the body when given IV or orally. They are metabolised in the liver and excreted in faeces and urine. The half-life varies with the particular drug and preparation.

Contraindications and cautions

The non-selective adrenergic-blocking agents are contraindicated in individuals with known hypersensitivity to any component of the drug *to avoid potentially serious hypersensitivity reactions*; with bradycardia or heart blocks, *which could be worsened by the slowed heart rate and conduction*; with asthma, *which could be exacerbated by the loss of noradrenaline's effect of* ***bronchodilation***; with shock or heart failure

TABLE 31.1 **DRUGS IN FOCUS** Non-selective adrenergic-blocking agents

Drug name	Dosage/route	Usual indications
carvedilol (*Dilatrend, Vedilol*)	Adult, hypertension: 12.5 mg/day for 2 days then 25 mg/day. Maximum 50 mg/day Adult, heart failure: initially 3.125 mg bd increasing at 2-weekly intervals to 6.25 mg, 12.5 mg and 25 mg bd	Treatment of hypertension and heart failure in adults, alone or as part of combination therapy
(P) labetalol (*Presolol, Trandate*)	100 mg PO bd initially, maintenance 200–400 mg PO bd; maximum 2400 mg/day	Treatment of hypertension, hypertension associated with phaeochromocytoma, and clonidine withdrawal

(HF), *which could become worse with the loss of the sympathetic reaction*; and women who are breastfeeding *because of the potential adverse effects on the neonate*.

These drugs should be used with caution in individuals with diabetes *because the disorder could be aggravated by the blocked sympathetic response and because the usual signs and symptoms of hypoglycaemia and hyperglycaemia are masked with the SNS blockade*. Caution also should be used in people with bronchospasm, *which could progress to respiratory distress due to the loss of noradrenaline's bronchodilating actions*; and in pregnancy *because there are no well-defined studies to evaluate the potential risk to the fetus*. The drugs should only be used if the benefit to the mother clearly outweighs the potential risk to the fetus.

Adverse effects

The adverse effects associated with the use of non-selective adrenergic-blocking agents are usually associated with the drug's effects on the SNS. These effects can include dizziness, paraesthesias, insomnia, depression, fatigue and vertigo, *which are related to the blocking of noradrenaline's effect in the CNS*. Nausea, vomiting, diarrhoea, anorexia and flatulence are *associated with the loss of the balancing sympathetic effect on the gastrointestinal (GI) tract and increased parasympathetic dominance*. Cardiac arrhythmias, hypotension, HF, pulmonary oedema and cerebrovascular accident or stroke, are *related to the lack of stimulatory effects and loss of vascular tone in the CV system*. Bronchospasm, cough, rhinitis and bronchial obstruction are *related to loss of bronchodilation of the respiratory tract and vasodilation of mucous membrane vessels*. Other effects reported include decreased exercise tolerance, hypoglycaemia and rash *related to the sympathetic blocking effects*. Abruptly stopping these drugs after long-term therapy can result in MI, stroke and arrhythmias *related to an increased hypersensitivity to catecholamines that develops when the receptor sites have been blocked*. Carvedilol has been associated with hepatic failure *related to its effects on the liver*.

Clinically important drug–drug interactions

There is increased risk of excessive hypotension if any of these drugs is combined with general anaesthetics in volatile liquid form such as enflurane, halothane or isoflurane. The effectiveness of diabetic agents is increased, leading to hypoglycaemia when such agents are used with these drugs; individuals should be monitored closely and dose adjustments made as needed. In addition, carvedilol has been associated with potentially dangerous conduction system disturbances when combined with verapamil or diltiazem; if this combination is used, the person requires continuous monitoring.

(P) Prototype summary: labetalol

Indications: hypertension, alone or in combination with other drugs; off-label uses – control of blood pressure in phaeochromocytoma, clonidine-withdrawal hypertension.

Actions: competitively blocks alpha- and beta-receptor sites in the SNS, leading to lower blood pressure without reflex tachycardia and decreased renin levels.

Pharmacokinetics:

Route	Onset	Peak	Duration
Oral	Varies	1–2 hours	8–12 hours
IV	Immediate	5 min	5.5 hours

$T_{1/2}$: 6–8 hours, with hepatic metabolism and excretion in the urine.

Adverse effects: dizziness, vertigo, fatigue, gastric pain, flatulence, impotence, bronchospasm, dyspnoea, cough, decreased exercise tolerance.

Care considerations for people receiving non-selective adrenergic-blocking agents

Assessment: history and examination

- Assess for contraindications or cautions: any known allergies to these *to avoid hypersensitivity reactions*; presence of bradycardia or heart blocks, *which could be worsened by the slowing of heart rate and conduction*; asthma or bronchospasm, *which could be exacerbated by the loss of the bronchodilation effect of noradrenaline*; shock or HF, *which could worsen with the loss of the sympathetic reaction*; diabetes, *which could be aggravated by the blocking of the sympathetic response and the masking of the usual signs and symptoms of hypoglycaemia and hyperglycaemia*; and pregnancy or breastfeeding status *because of the potential adverse effects on the fetus or neonate.*
- Perform a physical assessment *to establish baseline data for determining the effectiveness of the drug and the occurrence of any adverse effects associated with drug therapy*; assess the level of orientation and for any complaints of dizziness, paraesthesias or vertigo.
- Monitor vital signs and assess cardiovascular status, including pulse, blood pressure and cardiac output, *to evaluate for possible cardiac effects*; obtain an electrocardiogram (ECG) as ordered *to assess for possible irregularities in rate or rhythm*; assess respiratory rate and auscultate lungs *to determine the presence of any adventitious sounds*; observe for ease of breathing, and report any signs and symptoms of bronchospasm or respiratory distress; and monitor GI activity *to determine the need for interventions to deal with increased activity.*
- Monitor the results of laboratory tests such as renal and liver function studies and electrolyte levels *to determine the need for possible dose adjustment*; monitor blood glucose levels *to evaluate for hyper- or hypoglycaemia.*

Implementation with rationale

- Do not discontinue abruptly after chronic therapy *because hypersensitivity to catecholamines may develop and the person could have a severe reaction*; taper drug slowly over 2 weeks, monitoring the person.
- Consult with the doctor about withdrawing the drug before surgery *because withdrawal is controversial; effects on the sympathetic system after surgery can cause problems.*
- Encourage the person to adopt lifestyle changes, including diet, exercise, smoking cessation and stress reduction, *to aid in lowering blood pressure.*
- Assess heart rate *for changes that might suggest arrhythmias.* Obtain blood pressure in various positions *to assess for orthostatic hypotension.*
- Institute safety precautions especially if the person complains of dizziness, fatigue or vertigo or if orthostatic hypotension occurs *to prevent injury to the person.*
- Monitor GI function and need for increased access to bathroom facilities and need for increased fluid intake *related to diarrhoea.*
- Monitor for any sign of liver failure *to arrange to discontinue the drug if this occurs* (this effect is more likely to happen with carvedilol).
- Offer support and encouragement *to help the person deal with the drug regimen.*
- Provide thorough teaching, including drug name, dosage and schedule for administration; measures to prevent adverse effects and warning signs of problems; the need to avoid herbal or alternative therapies unless allowed by the prescriber; and safety measures, such as changing position slowly and avoiding driving or operating hazardous machinery; and the need for monitoring and evaluation *to enhance knowledge about drug therapy and to promote compliance.*

Evaluation

- Monitor response to the drug (improvement in blood pressure and HF).
- Monitor for adverse effects (CV changes, headache, GI upset, bronchospasm, liver failure).
- Evaluate the effectiveness of the teaching plan (person can name drug, dosage, adverse effects to watch for, specific measures to avoid adverse effects).
- Monitor the effectiveness of comfort measures and compliance with the regimen.

KEY POINTS

- Adrenergic-blocking agents block the effects of the SNS.
- The non-selective adrenergic-blocking agents block all receptors, that is, both alpha and beta receptors.
- Selective adrenergic-blocking agents have specific affinity for alpha or beta receptors or for specific alpha-1-, alpha-2-, beta-1- or beta-2-receptor sites.
- Blocking all of the receptor sites within the SNS results in a lowering of blood pressure.

ALPHA-1-SELECTIVE ADRENERGIC-BLOCKING AGENTS

Alpha-1-selective adrenergic-blocking agents are drugs that have a specific affinity for alpha-1 receptors. These drugs include alfuzosin (*Xatral SR*) (not available in New Zealand), doxazosin (generic; not available in Australia), prazosin (*Minipress*), silodosin (*Urorec*) tamsulosin (*Flomaxtra*) and terazosin (generic) (see Table 31.2).

Therapeutic actions and indications

The therapeutic effects of the alpha-1-selective adrenergic-blocking agents come from their ability to block the postsynaptic alpha-1-receptor sites. This causes a decrease in vascular tone and vasodilation, which leads to a fall in blood pressure. Because these drugs do not block the presynaptic alpha-2-receptor sites, the reflex tachycardia that accompanies a fall in blood pressure does not occur. They also block smooth muscle receptors in the prostate, prostatic capsule, prostatic urethra and urinary bladder neck, which leads to a relaxation of the bladder and prostate, and improved flow of urine in males. These drugs are available in oral form and can be used to treat benign prostatic hypertrophy (BPH) (see Chapter 52 for further discussion on BPH) and hypertension. The drugs may be used alone or as part of a combination therapy. Table 31.2 shows usual indications for each of these agents.

Pharmacokinetics

The alpha-1-selective adrenergic-blocking agents are well absorbed after oral administration and undergo extensive hepatic metabolism. They are excreted in the urine.

Contraindications and cautions

The alpha-1-selective adrenergic-blocking agents are contraindicated in the presence of allergy to any of these drugs *to avoid hypersensitivity reactions* and also with breastfeeding *because the drugs cross into breast milk and could have adverse effects on the neonate.* They should be used cautiously in the presence of HF or renal failure *because their blood pressure–lowering effects could exacerbate these conditions* and with hepatic impairment, *which could alter the metabolism of these drugs.* Caution also should be used during pregnancy *because of the potential for adverse effects on the fetus.*

Adverse effects

The adverse effects associated with the use of these drugs *are usually related to their effects of SNS blockage.* CNS effects include headache, dizziness, weakness, fatigue, drowsiness and depression. Nausea, vomiting, abdominal pain and diarrhoea may occur *as a result of direct effects on the GI tract and sympathetic blocking.* Anticipated cardiovascular effects include arrhythmias, hypotension, oedema, HF and angina. The vasodilation caused by these drugs can also cause flushing, rhinitis, reddened eyes, nasal congestion and priapism.

Clinically important drug–drug interactions

Increased hypotensive effects may occur if these drugs are combined with any other vasodilating or antihypertensive drugs, such as nitrates, calcium-channel blockers and angiotensin-converting enzyme (ACE) inhibitors.

TABLE 31.2 *DRUGS IN FOCUS* Alpha-1-selective adrenergic-blocking agents

Drug name	Dosage/route	Usual indications
alfuzosin (*Xatral SR*)	10 mg/day PO	Treatment of benign prostatic hyperplasia (BPH)
(P) doxazosin (generic)	1 mg/day PO up to 16 mg/day PO for hypertension; 1–8 mg/day PO for BPH	Treatment of hypertension and BPH
prazosin (*Minipress*)	Adult: 1 mg PO bd to tds with maintenance at 3–20 mg/day PO in divided doses	Treatment of hypertension alone or in combination with other drugs
silodosin (*Urorec*)	Adult: 8 mg PO once daily (if renal impairment, start with 4 mg PO daily, increasing to 8 mg PO daily depending on response)	Management of lower urinary tract symptoms associated with BPH
tamsulosin (*Flomaxtra*)	400 micrograms/day PO 30 minutes after the same meal each day	Treatment of BPH
terazosin (generic)	1–5 mg/day PO, preferably at bedtime for hypertension; 10 mg/day PO for BPH	Treatment of hypertension and BPH

Prototype summary: doxazosin

Indications: treatment of mild to moderate hypertension as monotherapy or in combination with other antihypertensives; treatment of BPH.

Actions: reduces total peripheral resistance through alpha blockade; does not affect heart rate or cardiac output; increases high-density lipoproteins while lowering total cholesterol levels.

Pharmacokinetics:

Route	Onset	Peak	Duration
Oral	Varies	2–3 hours	Not known

$T_{1/2}$: 22 hours, with hepatic metabolism and excretion in the bile, faeces and urine.

Adverse effects: headache, fatigue, dizziness, postural dizziness, vertigo, tachycardia, oedema, nausea, dyspepsia, diarrhoea, sexual dysfunction.

Care considerations for people receiving alpha-1-selective adrenergic-blocking agents

Assessment: history and examination

- Assess for contraindications or cautions: any known allergies to either drug *to avoid hypersensitivity reactions*; HF or renal failure, *which could be exacerbated by drug use*; hepatic dysfunction, *which could alter the drug's metabolism*; and current status of pregnancy or breastfeeding *because of unknown or adverse effects to the fetus or neonate.*
- Perform a physical assessment *to establish baseline data for determining the effectiveness of drug therapy and the occurrence of any adverse effects.*
- Monitor the level of orientation, affect and reflexes *to monitor for CNS changes related to drug therapy.*
- Monitor vital signs and assess cardiovascular status, including pulse, blood pressure, peripheral perfusion and cardiac output, *to evaluate for possible cardiac effects*; obtain an ECG as ordered *to assess for possible irregularities in rate or rhythm.*
- Assess renal function, including urinary output, *to evaluate effects on the renal system and assess BPH and its effects on urinary output.*
- Monitor renal and liver function tests *to evaluate potential need for dose adjustment.*

Implementation with rationale

- Monitor blood pressure, pulse, rhythm and cardiac output regularly *to evaluate for changes that may indicate a need to adjust dose or discontinue the drug if cardiovascular effects are severe.*
- Establish safety precautions if CNS effects or orthostatic hypotension occurs *to prevent injury.*
- Arrange for small, frequent meals if GI upset is severe *to relieve discomfort and maintain nutrition.*
- Arrange for supportive care and comfort measures (rest, environmental control, other measures) *to decrease CNS effects*; provide headache medication *to alleviate discomfort*; arrange safety measures if CNS effects occur *to prevent injury.*
- Offer support and encouragement *to help the person deal with the drug regimen.*
- Provide thorough teaching, including drug name, dosage and administration; measures to prevent adverse effects and warning signs to report to the prescriber; safety measures such as changing positions slowly and avoiding driving or operating hazardous machinery; and dietary measures in conjunction with drug therapy to promote blood pressure control or alleviate GI upset *to enhance knowledge about drug therapy and to promote compliance.*
- Offer support and encouragement *to help the person deal with the drug regimen.*

Evaluation

- Monitor response to the drug (lowering of blood pressure).
- Monitor for adverse effects (GI upset, CNS or CV changes).
- Evaluate effectiveness of the teaching plan (person can name drug, dosage, adverse effects to watch for and specific measures to avoid them).
- Monitor the effectiveness of comfort measures and compliance with the regimen.

KEY POINTS

- Alpha-1-selective adrenergic-blocking agents decrease blood pressure by blocking the postsynaptic alpha-1-receptor sites, decreasing vascular tone and promoting vasodilation.
- Alpha-1-selective adrenergic-blocking agents are used to treat hypertension and are often used to treat BPH because of their relaxing effects on the bladder and prostate.

NON-SELECTIVE BETA-ADRENERGIC–BLOCKING AGENTS

The **beta adrenergic–blocking agents** (Table 31.3) are used to treat CV problems (hypertension, angina, migraine headaches) and to prevent reinfarction after MI. These drugs are widely used and include nebivolol (*Nebilet*), oxprenolol (*Corbeton*) (not available in

TABLE 31.3 **DRUGS IN FOCUS** **Non-selective beta-adrenergic-blocking agents**

Drug name	Dosage/route	Usual indications
nebivolol (*Nebilet*)	Initially 5 mg/day PO, increase at 2-week intervals based on person's response; maximum dose 10 mg/day	Treatment of hypertension, alone or as part of combination therapy in adults
oxprenolol (*Corbeton*)	20–40 mg PO bd or tds; up to 320 mg daily depending on individual response	Treatment of angina pectoris, cardiac arrhythmias, hypertension
pindolol (*Visken*)	10–30 mg daily. Doses > 15 mg should be divided into 2–3 daily doses	Treatment of hypertension in adults
(P) propranolol (*Inderal*)	Dose varies widely based on indication; check drug guide for specific information	Treatment of hypertension, angina, idiopathic hypertrophic subaortic stenosis (IHSS)–induced palpitations, angina and syncope, certain cardiac arrhythmias induced by catecholamines or digoxin, phaeochromocytoma; prevention of reinfarction after MI; prophylaxis for migraine headache (which may be caused by vasodilation and is relieved by vasoconstriction, although the exact action is not clearly understood); prevention of stage fright (which is a sympathetic stress reaction to a particular situation); and treatment of essential tremors
sotalol (*Cardol, Sotacor*)	160 mg/day PO in 2 divided doses. Usual range 160–320 mg/day PO	Treatment of potentially life-threatening ventricular arrhythmias; maintenance of normal sinus rhythm in people with atrial fibrillation/flutter
timolol (*Nyogel, Tenopt*)	Eye drops: 1 drop of 0.25% solution bd, increased if necessary to 1 drop of 0.5% solution in the affected eye(s) bd	Treatment of hypertension; prevention of reinfarction after MI; prophylaxis for migraine; in ophthalmic form, reduction of intraocular pressure in open-angle glaucoma

New Zealand), pindolol (*Visken*), propranolol (*Inderal*), sotalol (*Cardol, Sotacor*) and timolol (*Nyogel, Tenopt*). The prototype drug, propranolol, was the first non-selective beta blocker available.

Therapeutic actions and indications

The therapeutic effects of these drugs are related to their competitive blocking of the beta-adrenergic receptors in the SNS. The blockade of the beta receptors in the heart and in the juxtaglomerular apparatus of the nephron accounts for most of the therapeutic benefit. Decreased heart rate, contractility and excitability, as well as a membrane-stabilising effect, lead to a decrease in arrhythmias, a decreased cardiac workload and decreased oxygen consumption. The juxtaglomerular cells are not stimulated to release renin, which further decreases the blood pressure. These effects are useful in treating hypertension and chronic angina and can help to prevent reinfarction after an MI by decreasing cardiac workload and oxygen consumption. Sotalol is used exclusively for treating life-threatening ventricular arrhythmias and to maintain sinus rhythm in individuals with atrial flutter or atrial fibrillation (see Chapter 45).

Propranolol is very effective in blocking all of the beta receptors in the SNS and was one of the first drugs of the class (see Table 31.3 for usual indications). Since the introduction of propranolol, newer and more selective drugs have become available that are not associated with some of the adverse effects seen with total blockade of the SNS beta receptors. Nebivolol is not associated with the variety of adverse effects seen with propranolol use. Oxprenolol blocks autonomic beta-adrenergic receptors, leading to lowering of heart rate, and reduces myocardial demand. Timolol has several recommended uses, which are listed in Table 31.3; timolol is available in an ophthalmic form of the drug for reduction of intraocular pressure in people with open-angle glaucoma. When this drug is used topically, eye muscle relaxation occurs. However, topical use of timolol has been associated with bradycardia, bronchospasm and dyspnoea.

Pharmacokinetics

These drugs are absorbed from the GI tract after oral administration and undergo hepatic metabolism. Food has been found to increase the bioavailability of propranolol, although this effect was not found with other beta adrenergic–blocking agents. Absorption of sotalol is decreased by the presence of food. Propranolol also crosses the blood–brain barrier, but nadolol and sotalol do not, making them a better choice if CNS effects occur with propranolol. These drugs are all excreted in the urine.

Contraindications and cautions

Non-selective beta adrenergic–blocking agents are contraindicated in the presence of allergy to any of these drugs or any components of the drug being used *to avoid hypersensitivity reactions*; with bradycardia or heart blocks, shock or HF, *which could be exacerbated by the cardiac-suppressing effects of these drugs*; with bronchospasm, chronic obstructive pulmonary disease (COPD) or acute asthma, *which could worsen due to the blocking of the sympathetic bronchodilation*; with pregnancy *because teratogenic effects have occurred in animal studies with all of these drugs except sotalol and because neonatal apnoea, bradycardia and hypoglycaemia could occur*; and with breastfeeding *because of the potential effects on the neonate, which could include slowed heart rate, hypotension and hypoglycaemia.* The safety and efficacy for use of these drugs in children have not been established.

These drugs should be used cautiously in individuals with diabetes and hypoglycaemia *because of the blocking of the normal signs and symptoms of hypoglycaemia and hyperglycaemia*; with thyrotoxicosis *because of the adrenergic-blocking effects on the thyroid gland*; or with renal or hepatic dysfunction, *which could interfere with the excretion and metabolism of these drugs.*

Adverse effects

People receiving these drugs often experience adverse effects *related to blockage of beta receptors in the SNS.* CNS effects include headache, fatigue, dizziness, depression, paraesthesias, sleep disturbances, memory loss and disorientation. Cardiovascular effects can include bradycardia, heart block, HF, hypotension and peripheral vascular insufficiency. Pulmonary effects can range from difficulty breathing, coughing and bronchospasm to severe pulmonary oedema and bronchial obstruction. GI upset, nausea, vomiting, diarrhoea, gastric pain and even colitis can occur as a result of unchecked parasympathetic activity and the blocking of the sympathetic receptors. Genitourinary effects can include decreased libido, impotence, dysuria and Peyronie disease. Other effects that can occur include decreased exercise tolerance (individuals often report that their 'get up and go' is gone), hypoglycaemia or hyperglycaemia and liver changes. If these drugs are stopped abruptly after long-term use, there is a risk of angina, MI, hypertension and stroke because the receptor sites become hypersensitive to catecholamines after being blocked by the drugs.

Clinically important drug–drug interactions

A paradoxical hypertension occurs when beta blockers are given with clonidine, and an increased rebound hypertension with clonidine withdrawal may also occur. It is best to avoid this combination.

A decreased antihypertensive effect occurs when beta blockers are given with non-steroidal anti-inflammatory drugs (NSAIDs); if this combination is used, the person should be monitored closely and dose adjustment should be made to achieve the desired control of blood pressure.

An initial hypertensive episode followed by bradycardia may occur if these drugs are given with adrenaline. Peripheral ischaemia may occur if the beta blockers are taken in combination with ergot alkaloids.

When these drugs are given with insulin or other oral hypoglycaemic agents, there is a potential for change in blood glucose levels. The person will also not display the usual signs and symptoms of hypoglycaemia or hyperglycaemia, which are caused by activation of the SNS. Because these effects are blocked, the person will need new indications to alert them to potential problems. If this combination is used, the person should monitor blood glucose levels frequently throughout the day and should be alert to new manifestations indicating glucose imbalance.

Prototype summary: propranolol

Indications: treatment of hypertension, angina pectoris, idiopathic hypertrophic subaortic stenosis (IHSS), supraventricular tachycardia, tremor; prevention of reinfarction after MI; adjunctive therapy in phaeochromocytoma; prophylaxis of migraine headache; management of situational anxiety.

Actions: competitively blocks beta-adrenergic receptors in the heart and juxtaglomerular apparatus; reduces vascular tone in the CNS.

Pharmacokinetics:

Route	Onset	Peak	Duration
Oral	20–30 min	60–90 min	6–12 hours
IV	Immediate	1 min	4–6 hours

$T\text{-}1_{/2}$: 3–5 hours with hepatic metabolism and excretion in the urine.

Adverse effects: allergic reaction, bradycardia, HF, cardiac arrhythmias, cerebrovascular accident, pulmonary oedema, gastric pain, flatulence, impotence, decreased exercise tolerance, bronchospasm.

Care considerations for people receiving non-selective beta-adrenergic-blocking agents

Assessment: history and examination

- Assess for contraindications or cautions: known allergy to any drug or to any components of the drug *to avoid hypersensitivity reactions*; bradycardia or heart blocks, shock or HF, *which could be exacerbated by the cardiac-suppressing effects of these drugs*; bronchospasm, COPD or acute asthma, *which could worsen with blocking of the sympathetic bronchodilation*; diabetes or hypoglycaemia, *which could lead to altered blood glucose levels*; thyrotoxicosis *because of adrenergic-blocking effects on the thyroid gland*; renal or hepatic dysfunction, *which could interfere with the excretion or metabolism of these drugs*; and status of pregnancy and breastfeeding *because of the potential effects on the fetus or neonate.*
- Perform a physical assessment to establish baseline data *for determining the effectiveness of the drug and the occurrence of any adverse effects.*
- Assess level of orientation and sensory function *to evaluate for possible CNS effects.*
- Monitor cardiopulmonary status, including pulse, blood pressure and respiratory rate; auscultate lungs for adventitious breath sounds; obtain an ECG as ordered *to evaluate for changes in heart rate or rhythm*; check colour, sensation, and capillary refill of extremities *to evaluate for possible peripheral vascular insufficiency.*
- Assess abdomen, including auscultating bowel sounds, *to monitor for GI effects.*
- Monitor the results of laboratory tests, such as electrolyte levels, to *monitor for risk of arrhythmias*, adrenal and hepatic function studies, *to determine the need for possible dose adjustment.*
- *Refer to the Critical thinking scenario for a full discussion of care for a person who is receiving beta adrenergic–blocking agents.*

Implementation with rationale

- Do not stop these drugs abruptly after chronic therapy, but taper gradually over 2 weeks *because long-term use of these drugs can sensitise the myocardium to catecholamines, and severe reactions could occur.*
- Continuously monitor any individual receiving an IV form of these drugs *to avert serious complications caused by rapid sympathetic blockade.*
- Monitor blood pressure, pulse, rhythm and cardiac output regularly *to evaluate drug effectiveness and to monitor for changes that may indicate a need to adjust dose or discontinue the drug if cardiovascular effects are severe.*
- Arrange for supportive care and comfort measures (rest, environmental control, other measures) *to relieve CNS effects*; institute safety measures if CNS effects occur *to prevent injury;* provide small, frequent meals and mouth care *to help relieve the discomfort of GI effects*; establish a daily activity program, spacing activities *to help the person deal with activity intolerance.*
- Offer support and encouragement *to help the person deal with the drug regimen.*
- Provide thorough teaching, including drug name, dose and schedule of administration; use of drug with food or meals, if appropriate; possible adverse effects and measures to prevent them; warning signs to report; safety measures, such as changing position slowly, avoiding driving or using hazardous machinery, and pacing activities; and the need for follow-up evaluation and possible changes in dose to achieve therapeutic effectiveness, *to enhance knowledge about drug therapy and to promote compliance.*

Evaluation

- Monitor response to the drug (lowering of blood pressure, decrease in anginal episodes, improvement in condition being treated).
- Monitor for adverse effects (GI upset, CNS changes, respiratory problems, CV effects, loss of libido and impotence).
- Evaluate the effectiveness of the teaching plan (person can name drug, dosage, adverse effects to watch for and specific measures to avoid them).
- Monitor the effectiveness of comfort measures and compliance with the regimen.

KEY POINTS

- Beta blockers are drugs used to block the beta receptors within the SNS. These drugs are used for a wide range of conditions, including hypertension, stage fright, migraines, angina and essential tremors.
- Non-selective blockade of all beta receptors results in a loss of the reflex bronchodilation that occurs with sympathetic stimulation. This limits the use of these drugs in individuals who smoke or have allergic or seasonal rhinitis, asthma or COPD.

CRITICAL THINKING SCENARIO

Non-selective beta blockers (propranolol)

THE SITUATION

M.R., a 59-year-old man, has been seen several times complaining of tremor in his hands that eventually made it very difficult for him to work as a computer programmer. A diagnosis of essential tremor was made, and he was prescribed propranolol (*Inderal*) 40 mg twice daily. M.R. had good effects with the drug and had no further problems until the following June, when acute respiratory distress developed while he was picnicking in a state park with his family. On the way to the emergency room, he suffered an apparent respiratory arrest. He was admitted to the hospital and placed in the respiratory intensive care unit. It was found that M.R. had a history of hay fever and allergic rhinitis during the pollen season but had never experienced such a severe reaction.

CRITICAL THINKING

Why did M.R. have such a severe reaction? What appropriate measures should be taken to ensure that M.R. recovers fully and does not re-experience this event?

What sort of support will M.R. and his family need after going through such a frightening experience? Think about the children who may have witnessed the respiratory arrest and how they should be reassured, depending on their ages. *Think about the support M.R.'s wife may need and the fear that may now be associated with M.R.'s condition. M.R. has been taking propranolol for several months and needs to decide whether he should continue the drug with modifications to his lifestyle or the addition of other drugs to deal with his respiratory issues.*

What kind of teaching program will need to be developed to help M.R. deal with this drug, and its potential adverse effects?

DISCUSSION

Propranolol, a non-selective beta blocker, was prescribed to decrease the tremor he was experiencing. The exact action of this drug to decrease the tremor is thought to be related to its membrane-stabilising properties. The desired therapeutic effect is the reduction of the tremor, but all of the beta-blocking effects will occur and need to be monitored. He did well on the drug until pollen season arrived. That is because propranolol, a non-selective beta blocker, prevented the compensatory bronchodilation that occurs when the SNS is stimulated. When the pollen reacted with M.R.'s airways, causing them to swell and become narrower, his swollen bronchial tubes were unable to allow air to flow through them. The result was bronchial constriction and respiratory distress that, in M.R.'s case, progressed to a respiratory arrest. Before he began taking propranolol, M.R. probably had been effectively compensating for the swelling of the bronchi through bronchodilation and had never experienced such a reaction. There are few other drugs for treating essential tremor. M.R. and his health care providers will need to decide whether the benefit that the drug has brought to him is worth the potential for adverse effects. They might be able to suggest additional drugs to deal with the seasonal allergic reactions to make the use of the propranolol safer for M.R.

M.R. may want to discuss this frightening incident with his health care provider. He also may want to include his family in this discussion. It should be stressed that he did so well up to this point because he had not been exposed to pollen and therefore had not had the problem that brought him into the hospital this time. M.R. probably never reported the occurrence of hay fever to his health care provider when the drug was prescribed because it had never been a problem and probably did not seem significant to him. M.R. and his family should receive support and be encouraged to talk about what happened and how they reacted to it. It is normal to feel frightened and unsure when a loved one is in distress. They should be involved in the discussion of what medical regimen would be most appropriate for M.R. at this point.

CARE GUIDE FOR M.R.: PROPRANOLOL

Assessment: history and examination

Review the person's history for allergy to propranolol, HF, shock, bradycardia, heart block, hypotension, COPD, thyroid disease, diabetes, respiratory impairment, and concurrent use of barbiturates, NSAIDs, piroxicam, sulindac, lidocaine (lignocaine), cimetidine, phenothiazines, clonidine, theophylline and rifampicin.

Focus the physical examination on the following:

CV: blood pressure, pulse, peripheral perfusion, ECG

CNS: orientation, affect, reflexes, vision

Skin: colour, lesions, texture

GU: urinary output, sexual function

GI: abdominal, liver evaluation

Respiratory: respirations, adventitious sounds

Implementation

Ensure safe and appropriate administration of the drug.

Provide comfort and safety measures: assistance/side rails; temperature control; rest periods; mouth care; small, frequent meals.

Monitor blood pressure, pulse, and respiratory status throughout drug therapy.

Taper the drug gradually if it is to be discontinued to decrease the risk of severe hypertension, MI or stroke related to abrupt withdrawal.

Provide support and reassurance to deal with drug effects and discomfort, sexual dysfunction and fatigue.

Provide teaching regarding drug name, dosage, side effects, precautions and warning signs to report.

Evaluation

Evaluate drug effects: blood pressure within normal limits, decrease in essential tremors, stabilised cardiac rhythm.

Monitor for adverse effects: CV effects: HF, block; dizziness, confusion; sexual dysfunction; GI effects; hypoglycaemia; respiratory problems.

Monitor for drug–drug interactions as indicated.

Evaluate the effectiveness of the teaching program.

Evaluate the effectiveness of comfort and safety measures.

TEACHING FOR M.R.

- The drug that has been prescribed for you, propranolol, is a non-selective beta adrenergic–blocking agent. This agent works to prevent certain stimulating activities that normally occur in the body in response to such factors as stress, injury or excitement. It stabilises certain nerve membranes, which helps to decrease your tremor.

  You should learn to take your pulse and monitor it daily, writing the pulse rate on the calendar. Your current pulse rate is 82 beats/minute.
- Never discontinue this medication suddenly. If you find that your prescription is running low, notify your health care provider at once. This drug needs to be tapered over time to prevent severe reactions when its use is discontinued. Some of the following adverse effects may occur:
  - *Fatigue, weakness*: try to stagger your activities throughout the day to allow rest periods.
  - *Dizziness, drowsiness*: if these should occur, take care to avoid driving, operating dangerous machinery or doing delicate tasks. Change position slowly to avoid dizzy spells.
  - *Change in sexual function*: be assured that this is a drug effect and discuss it with your health care provider.
  - *Nausea, diarrhoea*: these gastrointestinal discomforts often diminish with time. If they become too uncomfortable or do not improve, talk to your health care provider.
  - *Dreams, confusion*: these are drug effects. If they become too uncomfortable, discuss them with your health care provider.
- Report any of the following to your health care provider: very slow pulse, need to sleep on more pillows at night, difficulty breathing, swelling in the ankles or fingers, sudden weight gain, mental confusion or personality change, fever or rash.
- Avoid over-the-counter medications, including cold and allergy remedies and diet pills. Many of these preparations contain drugs that could interfere with this medication. If you feel that you need one of these, check with your health care provider first.
- Tell any doctor, nurse, or other health care provider that you are taking these drugs, keep all medications out of the reach of children and do not share these drugs with other people.

BETA-1-SELECTIVE ADRENERGIC-BLOCKING AGENTS

Beta-1-selective adrenergic-blocking agents (Table 31.4) have an advantage over the non-selective beta blockers in some cases. Because they do not usually block beta-2-receptor sites, they do not block the sympathetic bronchodilation that is so important for people with lung diseases or allergic rhinitis. Consequently, these drugs are preferred for individuals who smoke or who have asthma, any other obstructive pulmonary disease or seasonal or allergic rhinitis. These selective beta blockers are also used for treating hypertension, angina and some cardiac arrhythmias. Beta-1-selective adrenergic-blocking agents include atenolol (*Tenormin*), betaxolol (*Betoptic*), bisoprolol (*Bicor, Bispro*), esmolol (*Brevibloc*) and metoprolol (*Betaloc, Lopresor*).

Therapeutic actions and indications

The therapeutic effects of these drugs are related to their ability to selectively block beta-1 receptors in the SNS at therapeutic doses. As a result, these drugs do not block the beta-2 receptors and therefore do not prevent sympathetic bronchodilation. However, the selectivity is lost with doses higher than the recommended range.

The blockade of the beta-1 receptors in the heart and in the juxtaglomerular apparatus accounts for most of the therapeutic benefits. Decreased heart rate, contractility and excitability, as well as a membrane-stabilising effect, lead to a decrease in arrhythmias, decreased cardiac workload and decreased oxygen consumption. The juxtaglomerular cells are not stimulated to release renin, which further decreases blood pressure. These drugs are useful in treating cardiac arrhythmias, hypertension and chronic angina and can help to prevent

TABLE 31.4 DRUGS IN FOCUS Beta-1-selective adrenergic-blocking agents

Drug name	Dosage/route	Usual indications
(P) atenolol (*Tenormin*)	Initially 50 mg/day PO, may be increased to 100 mg/day	Treatment of MI, chronic angina, hypertension in adults (atenolol is more widely used than the other drugs of this class for hypertension)
betaxolol (*Betoptic*)	1 drop in affected eye(s) for glaucoma	Available as ophthalmic agent for treatment of ocular hypertension, open-angle glaucoma
bisoprolol (*Bicor, Bispro*)	Initially 1.25 mg/day PO for 1 week, increased weekly to maximum 10 mg/day PO	Treatment of hypertension in adults, alone or as part of combination therapy
esmolol (*Brevibloc*)	50–200 micrograms/kg per minute IV, with dose based on person's response	Treatment of supraventricular tachycardias (eg, atrial flutter, atrial fibrillation) in adults, and non-compensatory tachycardia when the heart rate must be slowed (IV use only)
metoprolol tartrate (*Lopresor*)	Immediate release tablets: angina, hypertension: 50–100 mg PO once daily or bd. Maximum 400 mg/day in 2–3 divided doses Ampoules: disturbances of cardiac rhythm: 5 mg injected slowly IV (1–2 mg/min) repeated at 5-minute intervals. Maximum 15 mg	Treatment of hypertension; prevention of reinfarction after MI; early acute MI treatment
metoprolol succinate (*Betaloc CR*)	Modified release for chronic heart failure: start at 11.875–23.75 mg/day for 2 weeks, then 47.5 mg/day for 2 weeks, then 95 mg/day for 2 weeks then 190 mg/day as required	Treatment of symptomatic mild to severe chronic heart failure (extended-release preparation only), hypertension; angina pectoris, maintenance treatment after MI, cardiac arrhythmias

reinfarction after an MI by decreasing cardiac workload and oxygen consumption.

Beta-1-selective adrenergic-blocking agents in ophthalmic form are used to decrease intraocular pressure and to treat open-angle glaucoma. The beta-1-selective blocker of choice depends on the condition or combination of conditions being treated and personal experience with the drugs. See Table 31.4 for usual indications for each drug.

Pharmacokinetics

The beta-1-selective adrenergic blockers are absorbed from the GI tract after oral administration, reach peak levels directly with IV infusion and are not usually absorbed when given in ophthalmic form. The bioavailability of metoprolol is increased if it is taken in the presence of food. These drugs are metabolised in the liver and excreted in the urine. Metoprolol readily crosses the blood–brain barrier and may cause more CNS effects than atenolol, which does not cross the barrier.

Contraindications and cautions

The beta-1-selective adrenergic blockers are contraindicated in the presence of allergy to the drug or any components of the drug *to avoid hypersensitivity reactions*; with sinus bradycardia, heart block, cardiogenic shock, HF or hypotension, *all of which could be exacerbated by the cardiac-depressing and blood pressure–lowering effects of these drugs*; and with breastfeeding *because of the potential adverse effects on the neonate*. They should be used with caution in individuals with diabetes, thyroid disease or COPD *because of the potential for adverse effects on these diseases with sympathetic blockade*; and in pregnancy *because of the potential for adverse effects on the fetus*. The safety and efficacy of the use of these drugs in children have not been established.

Adverse effects

People receiving these drugs often experience adverse effects *related to the blocking of beta-1 receptors in the SNS*. CNS effects include headache, fatigue, dizziness, depression, paraesthesias, sleep disturbances, memory loss and disorientation. CV effects can include bradycardia, heart block, HF, hypotension and peripheral vascular insufficiency. Pulmonary effects ranging from rhinitis to bronchospasm and dyspnoea can occur; these effects are not as likely to occur with these drugs as with the non-selective beta blockers. GI upset, nausea, vomiting, diarrhoea, gastric pain and even colitis can occur as a result of unchecked parasympathetic activity and the blocking of the sympathetic receptors. Genitourinary effects can include decreased libido, impotence, dysuria and Peyronie disease. Other effects that can occur include decreased exercise tolerance (people often report that their 'get up and go' is gone), hypoglycaemia or hyperglycaemia, and liver changes that are reflected in increased concentrations of liver enzymes. If these drugs are stopped abruptly after long-term use, there is a risk of severe hypertension, angina, MI and stroke *because the receptor sites become hypersensitive to catecholamines after being blocked by the drug.*

Clinically important drug–drug interactions

A decreased hypertensive effect occurs if these drugs are given with clonidine, NSAIDs, rifampicin or barbiturates. If such a combination is used, the person should be monitored closely and dose adjustment made.

There is an initial hypertensive episode followed by bradycardia if these drugs are given with adrenaline.

Increased serum levels and increased toxicity of IV lidocaine (lignocaine) will occur if it is given with these drugs.

An increased risk for orthostatic hypotension occurs if these drugs are taken with prazosin. If this combination is used, the person must be monitored closely and safety precautions taken.

The selective beta-1 blockers have increased effects if they are taken with verapamil, cimetidine or propylthiouracil. The person should be monitored closely and appropriate dose adjustment made.

(P) Prototype summary: atenolol

Indications: treatment of angina pectoris, hypertension, MI; off-label uses are prevention of migraine headaches, alcohol withdrawal syndrome and supraventricular tachycardias.

Actions: blocks beta-1-adrenergic receptors, decreasing the excitability of the heart, cardiac output and oxygen consumption; decreases renin release, which lowers blood pressure.

Pharmacokinetics:

Route	Onset	Peak	Duration
Oral	Varies	2–4 hours	24 hours
IV	Immediate	5 min	24 hours

$T_{1/2}$: 6–7 hours, with excretion in the bile, faeces and urine.

Adverse effects: allergic reaction, dizziness, bradycardia, HF, arrhythmias, gastric pain, flatulence, impotence, bronchospasm, decreased exercise tolerance.

Care considerations for people receiving beta-1-selective adrenergic-blocking agents

Assessment: history and examination

- Assess for contraindications or cautions: known allergies to any drug or any components of the drug *to avoid hypersensitivity reactions*; bradycardia or heart blocks, shock or HF, *which could be exacerbated by the cardiac-suppressing effects of these drugs*; diabetes, thyroid disease or COPD *to reduce risk of adverse effects on these conditions due to sympathetic blockade*; and current status of pregnancy or breastfeeding *because of the potential effects on the fetus or neonate.*
- Perform a physical assessment to establish baseline status before beginning therapy *to determine the effectiveness of therapy and evaluate for any potential adverse effects.*
- Assess neurological status, including level of orientation and sensation, *to evaluate for CNS effects.*
- Monitor cardiac status, including pulse, blood pressure, and heart rate, *to identify changes*, and obtain an ECG as ordered *to evaluate for changes in heart rate or rhythm.*
- Assess pulmonary status, including respirations, and auscultate lungs for adventitious sounds *to monitor respiratory status.*
- Examine the abdomen and auscultate bowel sounds *to evaluate GI effects.*
- Monitor urine output *to monitor the effectiveness of cardiac output and any changes in renal perfusion.*
- Monitor the results of laboratory tests, including electrolyte levels, *to monitor for risk of arrhythmias*, and renal and hepatic function studies, *to determine the need for possible dose adjustment.*

Implementation with rationale

- Do not stop these drugs abruptly after chronic therapy, but taper gradually over 2 weeks *to prevent the possibility of severe reactions.* Long-term use of these drugs can sensitise the myocardium to catecholamines *and severe reactions could occur.*
- Consult with the doctor about discontinuing these drugs before surgery *because withdrawal of the drug before surgery when the person has been maintained on the drug is controversial.*
- Give oral forms of metoprolol with food *to facilitate absorption.*

- Continuously monitor any individual receiving an IV form of these drugs *to detect severe reactions to sympathetic blockade and to ensure rapid response if these reactions occur.*
- Arrange for supportive care and comfort measures, including rest, environmental control and other measures, *to relieve CNS effects*; safety measures if CNS effects occur, *to protect the person from injury*; small, frequent meals and mouth care *to relieve the discomfort of GI effects*; and an activity program and daily energy management ideas *to help to deal with activity intolerance.*
- Offer support and encouragement *to help the person deal with the drug regimen.*
- Provide thorough teaching, including drug name, dosage and schedule for administration; use of drug with food or meals if appropriate; technique for ophthalmic administration if indicated; potential adverse effects, measures to avoid drug-related problems, and warning signs of problems; safety measures such as changing position slowly and avoiding driving or operating hazardous machinery; and energy conservation measures as appropriate.

Evaluation

- Monitor response to the drug (lowered blood pressure, fewer anginal episodes, lowered intraocular pressure).
- Monitor for adverse effects (GI upset, CNS changes, cardiovascular effects, loss of libido and impotence, potential respiratory effects).
- Evaluate the effectiveness of the teaching plan (person can name drug, dosage, adverse effects to watch for and specific measures to avoid them).
- Monitor the effectiveness of comfort measures and compliance with the regimen.

KEY POINTS

- Beta-1-selective adrenergic-blocking agents do not block the beta-2 receptors that are responsible for bronchodilation and therefore are preferred in individuals with respiratory problems.
- Beta-1-selective adrenergic-blocking agents are used to treat hypertension and angina in extended-release forms and to treat HF.
- All of the adrenergic-blocking drugs must be tapered when they are discontinued after long-term use. The blocking of the receptor sites makes them hypersensitive to catecholamines, and extreme hypertension, angina, MI or stroke could occur.

CHAPTER SUMMARY

- Adrenergic-blocking agents, or sympatholytic drugs, lyse, or block, the effects of the sympathetic nervous system (SNS).
- Both the therapeutic and the adverse effects associated with these drugs are related to their blocking of the normal responses of the SNS.
- The alpha- and beta-adrenergic-blocking agents block all of the receptor sites within the SNS, which results in lower blood pressure, slower pulse and increased renal perfusion with decreased renin levels. These drugs are indicated for the treatment of essential hypertension. They are associated with many adverse effects, including lack of bronchodilation, cardiac suppression and diabetic reactions.
- Selective adrenergic-blocking agents have been developed that, at therapeutic levels, have specific affinity for alpha or beta receptors or for specific alpha-1-, beta-1-, or beta-2-receptor sites. This specificity is lost at levels higher than the therapeutic range.
- Alpha-adrenergic drugs specifically block the alpha receptors of the SNS. At therapeutic levels, they do not block beta receptors.
- Non-specific alpha-adrenergic-blocking agents are used to treat phaeochromocytoma, a tumour of the adrenal medulla.
- Alpha-1-selective adrenergic-blocking agents block the postsynaptic alpha-1-receptor sites, causing a decrease in vascular tone and a vasodilation that leads to a fall in blood pressure without the reflex tachycardia that occurs when the presynaptic alpha-2-receptor sites are also blocked.
- Beta blockers are drugs used to block the beta receptors within the SNS. These drugs are used for a wide range of conditions, including hypertension, stage fright, migraines, angina and essential tremors.
- Blockade of all beta receptors results in a loss of the reflex bronchodilation that occurs with sympathetic stimulation. This limits the use of these drugs in individuals who smoke or have allergic or seasonal rhinitis, asthma or COPD.
- Beta-1-selective adrenergic-blocking agents do not block the beta-2 receptors that are responsible for bronchodilation and therefore are preferred in people with respiratory problems.

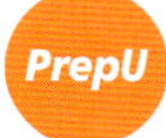

Knowing your strengths and weaknesses helps you to study more effectively. Take a PrepU Practice Quiz to find out how you measure up!

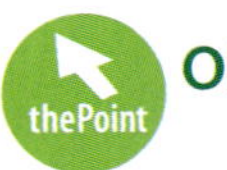

ONLINE RESOURCES

An extensive range of additional resources to enhance teaching and learning and to facilitate understanding of this chapter may be found online at the text's accompanying website, located on thePoint at http://thepoint.lww.com. These include Watch and Learn videos, Concepts in Action animations, journal articles, review questions, case studies, discussion topics and quizzes.

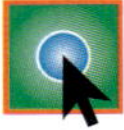

WEB LINKS

Health care providers and students may want to consult the following web resources:

www.heartfoundation.org.au
The Heart Foundation Australia. Information, support groups, diet, exercise and research information on hypertension and other cardiovascular diseases.

www.heartfoundation.org.nz
The National Heart Foundation New Zealand. Information, support groups, diet, exercise and research information on hypertension and other cardiovascular diseases.

BIBLIOGRAPHY

Barrett, K. E. & Ganong, W. F. (2010). *Ganong's Review of Medical Physiology* (23rd edn). New York: McGraw-Hill.

Elsik, M. & Krum, H. (2007). Should beta blockers remain first-line drugs for hypertension? *Australian Prescriber, 30*, 5–7.

Farrell, M. & Dempsey, J. (2014). *Smeltzer & Bare's Textbook of Medical-Surgical Nursing* (3rd edn). Sydney: Lippincott Williams & Wilkins.

Fonseca, V. A. (2010). Effects of beta-blockers on glucose and lipid metabolism. *Current Medical Research & Opinion, 26(3)*, 615–629.

Goodman, L. S., Brunton, L. L., Chabner, B. & Knollmann, B. C. (2011). *Goodman and Gilman's Pharmacological Basis of Therapeutics* (12th edn). New York: McGraw-Hill.

Guyton, A. & Hall, J. (2011). *Textbook of Medical Physiology* (12th edn). Philadelphia: Saunders Elsevier.

McKenna, L. & Mirkov, S. (2019). *McKenna's Drug Handbook for Nursing and Midwifery* (8th edn). Sydney: Wolters Kluwer Health Australia.

Nelson, M. (2010). Drug treatment of elevated blood pressure. *Australian Prescriber, 33*, 108–112.

Porth, C. M. (2011). *Essentials of Pathophysiology: Concepts of Altered Health States* (3rd edn). Philadelphia: Lippincott Williams & Wilkins.

Porth, C. M. (2009). *Pathophysiology: Concepts of Altered Health States* (8th edn). Philadelphia: Lippincott Williams & Wilkins.

Wiysonge, C. S. & Opie, L. H. (2013). β-blockers as initial therapy for hypertension. *JAMA, 310(7)*, 1851–1852.

Wiysonge, C. S., Bradley, H. A, Volmink, J., Mayosi, B. M., Mbewu, A. & Opie, L. H. (2012). Beta-blockers for hypertension. *Cochrane Database of Systematic Reviews*, CD002003.

CHECK YOUR UNDERSTANDING

Answers to the questions in this chapter can be found in Appendix A at the back of this book.

MULTIPLE CHOICE

Select the best answer to the following.

1. Adrenergic-blocking drugs, because of their clinical effects, are also known as:
   a. anticholinergics.
   b. sympathomimetics.
   c. parasympatholytics.
   d. sympatholytics.
2. The nurse or midwife would anticipate administering drugs that generally block all adrenergic receptor sites to treat:
   a. allergic rhinitis.
   b. COPD.
   c. cardiac-related conditions.
   d. premature labour.
3. A person with which of the following would most likely be prescribed an alpha-1-selective adrenergic-blocking agent?
   a. COPD and hypotension
   b. hypertension and BPH
   c. erectile dysfunction and hypotension
   d. shock states and bronchospasm
4. The beta blocker of choice for a person who is hypertensive and has angina is:
   a. nebivolol.
   b. pindolol.
   c. timolol.
   d. sotolol.
5. A nurse or midwife would question an order for beta-1-selective adrenergic blocker for a person with:
   a. cardiac arrhythmias.
   b. hypertension.
   c. cardiogenic shock.
   d. open-angle glaucoma.
6. A smoker who is being treated for hypertension with a beta blocker is most likely receiving:
   a. a non-specific beta blocker.
   b. an alpha-1-specific beta blocker.
   c. beta and alpha blockers.
   d. a beta-1-specific blocker.
7. You would caution a person who is taking an adrenergic blocker:
   a. to avoid exposure to infection.
   b. to stop the drug if they experience flu-like symptoms.
   c. never to stop the drug abruptly.
   d. to avoid exposure to the sun.

MULTIPLE RESPONSE

Select all that apply.

1. A nurse or midwife would question an order for a beta-adrenergic blocker if the person was also receiving what other drugs?
   a. clonidine
   b. ergot alkaloids
   c. aspirin
   d. NSAIDs
   e. triptans
   f. adrenaline (epinephrine)
2. The beta-adrenergic blocker propranolol is approved for a wide variety of uses. Which of the following are approved indications?
   a. migraine headaches
   b. stage fright
   c. bronchospasm
   d. reinfarction after an MI
   e. erectile dysfunction
   f. hypertension

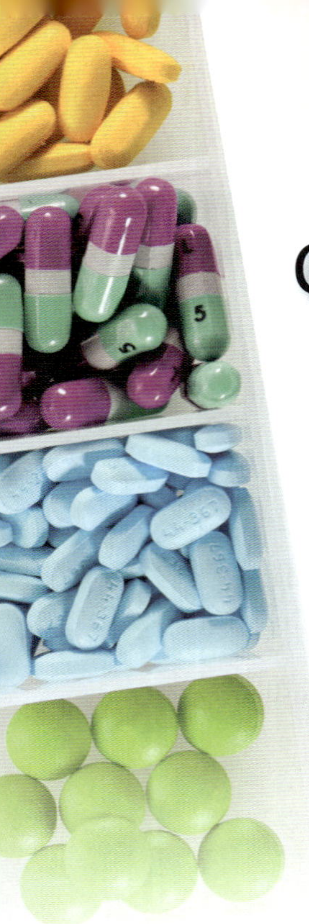

32 Cholinergic agonists

Learning objectives

On completing this chapter you should be able to:

1. Describe the effects of cholinergic receptors, correlating these effects with the clinical effects of cholinergic agonists.
2. Describe the therapeutic actions, indications, pharmacokinetics, contraindications and cautions, most common adverse reactions and important drug–drug interactions associated with the direct- and indirect-acting cholinergic agonists.
3. Discuss the use of cholinergic agonists across the lifespan.
4. Compare and contrast the prototype drugs bethanechol, donepezil and pyridostigmine with other cholinergic agonists.
5. Outline the care considerations, including important teaching points, for people receiving a cholinergic agonist.

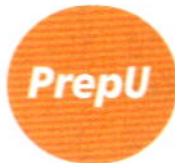

PrepU Test your current knowledge of cholinergic agonists with a PrepU Practice Quiz!

Glossary of key terms

acetylcholinesterase: enzyme responsible for the immediate breakdown of acetylcholine when released from the nerve ending; prevents overstimulation of cholinergic receptor sites

Alzheimer disease: degenerative disease of the cortex with loss of acetylcholine-producing cells and cholinergic receptors; characterised by progressive dementia

cholinergic agonists: responding to acetylcholine; refers to receptor sites stimulated by acetylcholine, as well as neurons that release acetylcholine

miosis: constriction of the pupil; relieves intraocular pressure in some types of glaucoma

myasthenia gravis: autoimmune disease characterised by antibodies to cholinergic receptor sites, leading to destruction of the receptor sites and decreased response at the neuromuscular junction; it is progressive and debilitating, leading to paralysis

nerve gas: irreversible acetylcholinesterase inhibitor used in warfare to cause paralysis and death by prolonged muscle contraction and parasympathetic crisis

parasympathomimetic: mimicking the effects of the parasympathetic nervous system, leading to bradycardia, hypotension, pupil constriction, increased GI secretions and activity, increased bladder tone, relaxation of sphincters and bronchoconstriction

DIRECT-ACTING CHOLINERGIC AGONISTS

- (P) bethanechol
- carbachol
- pilocarpine

INDIRECT-ACTING CHOLINERGIC AGONISTS

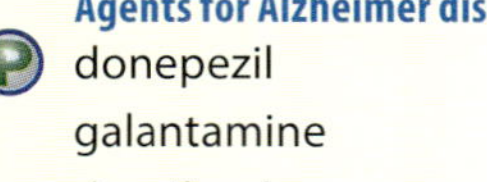

Agents for myasthenia gravis

- edrophonium
- neostigmine
- (P) pyridostigmine

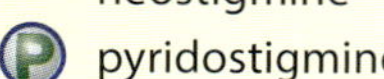

Agents for Alzheimer disease

- (P) donepezil
- galantamine
- rivastigmine

Cholinergic agonists act at the same site as the neurotransmitter acetylcholine (ACh) and increase the activity of the ACh receptor sites throughout the body. Because these sites are found extensively throughout the parasympathetic nervous system, their stimulation produces a response similar to what is seen when the parasympathetic system is activated. As a result, these drugs are often called **parasympathomimetic** because their action mimics the action of the parasympathetic nervous system. Because the action of these drugs cannot be limited to a specific site, their effects can be widespread throughout the body, and they are usually associated with many undesirable systemic effects.

Cholinergic agonists work either directly or indirectly. Direct-acting cholinergic agonists occupy receptor sites for ACh on the membranes of the effector cells of the postganglionic cholinergic nerves, causing increased stimulation of the cholinergic receptor. In contrast, indirect-acting cholinergic agonists cause increased stimulation of the ACh receptor sites by reacting with the enzyme **acetylcholinesterase** and preventing it from breaking down the ACh that was released from the nerve. These drugs produce their effects indirectly by producing an increase in the level of ACh in the synaptic cleft, leading to increased stimulation of the cholinergic receptor site (Figure 32.1). See Box 32.1 for use of these drugs across the lifespan.

DIRECT-ACTING CHOLINERGIC AGONISTS

The direct-acting cholinergic agonists are similar to ACh and react directly with receptor sites to cause the same reaction as if ACh had stimulated the receptor sites. These drugs usually stimulate muscarinic receptors within the parasympathetic system. They are used as systemic agents to increase bladder tone, urinary excretion and gastrointestinal (GI) secretions, and as ophthalmic agents to induce miosis to relieve the increased intraocular pressure of glaucoma (see Table 32.1). Systemic absorption usually does not occur when these drugs are used ophthalmically.

Direct-acting cholinergic agonists include bethanechol (*Urocarb*), carbachol (*Miostat*) and pilocarpine (*Isopto Carpine*). These agents are used infrequently today because of their widespread parasympathetic activity. More-specific and less-toxic drugs are now available and preferred.

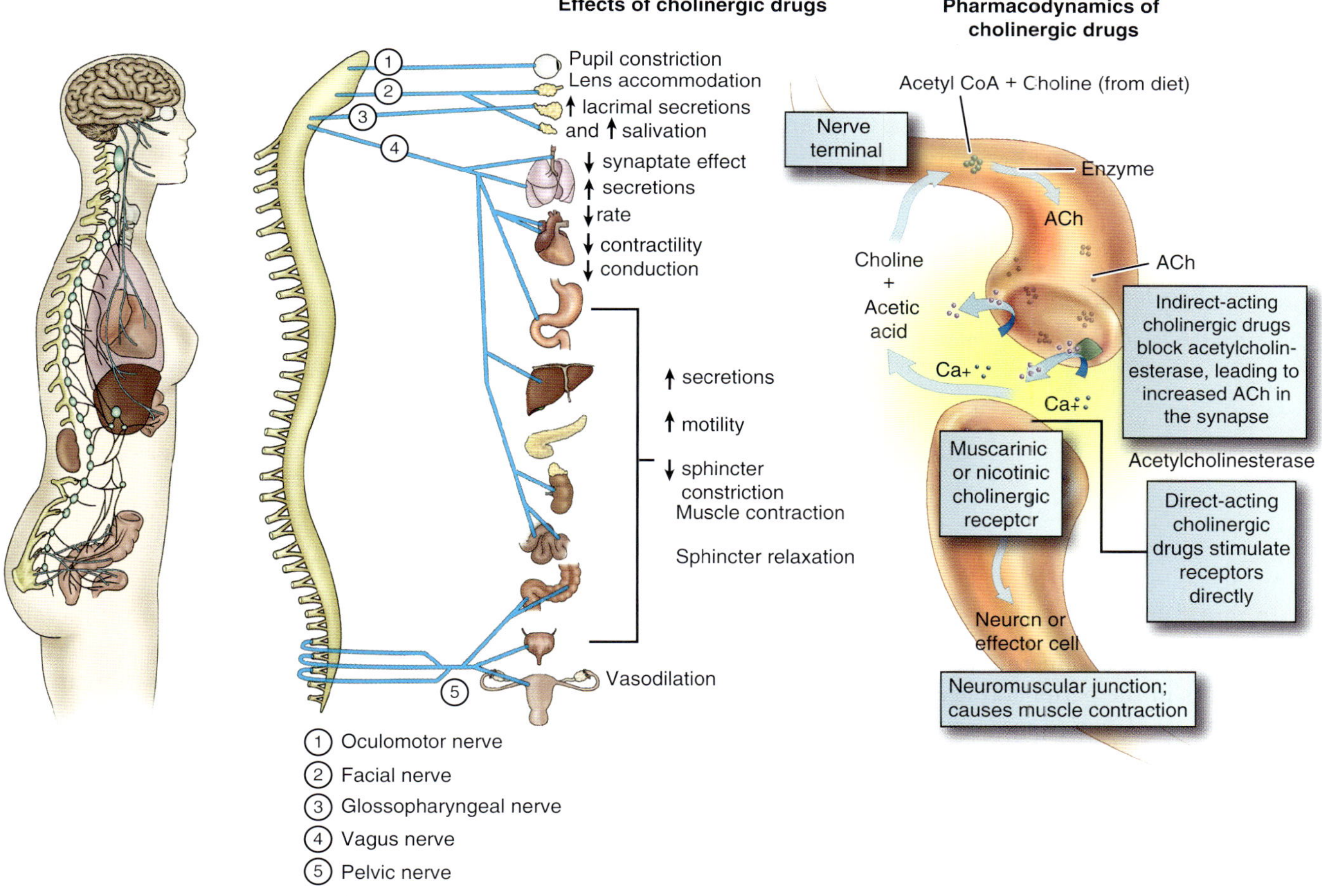

FIGURE 32.1 Pharmacodynamics of cholinergic drugs and associated physiological responses.

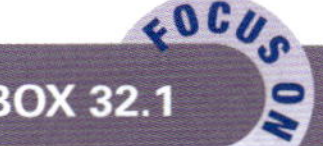

BOX 32.1 Drug therapy across the lifespan

Cholinergic agonists

CHILDREN

Children may be more susceptible to the adverse effects associated with the cholinergic agonists, including GI upset, diarrhoea, increased salivation that could lead to choking, and loss of bowel and bladder control, a problem that could cause stress in the child. Children should be monitored closely if these agents are used and should receive appropriate supportive care.

Bethanechol is approved for the treatment of neurogenic bladder in children older than 8 years of age. Neostigmine and pyridostigmine are used in the control of myasthenia gravis and for reversal of neuromuscular junction blocker effects in children. Care should be taken in determining the appropriate dose based on weight. Edrophonium is used for diagnosis of myasthenia gravis only.

ADULTS

Adults should be cautioned about the many adverse effects that can be anticipated when using a cholinergic agonist. Flushing, increased sweating, increased salivation and GI upset, and urinary urgency often occur. The person also needs to be aware that dizziness, drowsiness and blurred vision may occur, and that driving and operating dangerous machinery should be avoided.

PREGNANCY AND BREASTFEEDING

In general, there are no adequate studies about the effects of these drugs during pregnancy and breastfeeding. Therefore, the cholinergic agonist should be used only in those situations in which the benefit to the mother is greater than the risk to the fetus or neonate. Breastfeeding women who require one of these drugs should find another way to feed the baby.

OLDER ADULTS

Older people are more likely to experience the adverse effects associated with these drugs – central nervous system (CNS), cardiovascular (CV), GI, respiratory and urinary effects. Because older people often have renal or hepatic impairment, they are also more likely to have toxic levels of the drug related to changes in metabolism and excretion.

The older person should be started on lower doses of the drugs and should be monitored very closely for potentially serious arrhythmias or hypotension. Safety precautions should be established if the drug causes dizziness or drowsiness. Special efforts may also be needed to help the person maintain fluid intake and nutrition if the GI effects become uncomfortable. Taking the drug with food and eating several small meals throughout the day may alleviate some of these problems.

TABLE 32.1 DRUGS IN FOCUS Direct-acting cholinergic agonists

Drug name	Dosage/route	Usual indications
(P) bethanechol (*Urocarb*)	10–30 mg PO or SL tds or qid	Treatment of non-obstructive postoperative and postpartum urinary retention, neurogenic bladder atony in adults and children > 8 years; diagnosis and treatment of reflux oesophagitis in adults, and used orally in infants and children for treatment of oesophageal reflux
carbachol (*Miostat*)	Intraocular injection: gently instil ≤ 0.5 mL into anterior chamber before or after suturing; miosis usually maximal within 2–5 minutes	Induction of miosis to relieve increased intraocular pressure of glaucoma; allows surgeons to perform certain surgical procedures
pilocarpine (*Isopto Carpine*)	Instil 1–2 drops in affected eye(s) tid–qid	Induction of miosis to relieve increased intraocular pressure of glaucoma; allows surgeons to perform certain surgical procedures

Therapeutic actions and indications

The direct-acting cholinergic agonists act at cholinergic receptors in the peripheral nervous system to mimic the effects of ACh and parasympathetic stimulation. These parasympathetic effects include slowed heart rate and decreased myocardial contractility, vasodilation, bronchoconstriction and increased bronchial mucus secretion, increased GI activity and secretions, increased bladder tone, relaxation of GI and bladder sphincters, and pupil constriction (see Figure 32.1).

The agent bethanechol, which has an affinity for the cholinergic receptors in the urinary bladder, is available for use orally and subcutaneously to treat non-obstructive postoperative and postpartum urinary retention and to treat neurogenic bladder atony. It directly increases detrusor muscle tone and relaxes the sphincters to improve bladder emptying. Because this drug is not destroyed by acetylcholinesterase, the effects on the receptor site are longer lasting than with stimulation by ACh. See Table 32.1 for additional indications.

The drugs carbachol and pilocarpine are available as ophthalmic agents. They are used to induce **miosis**, or pupil constriction; to relieve the increased intraocular pressure of glaucoma; and to allow surgeons to perform certain surgical procedures.

Pilocarpine, which binds to muscarinic receptors throughout the system, is used to increase secretions in the mouth and GI tract and relieve the symptoms of dry mouth that are in seen in Sjögren syndrome. It is approved for use in adults and is given three times a day, often with meals.

Pharmacokinetics

The direct-acting cholinergic agonists are generally well absorbed after oral administration and have relatively short half-lives, ranging from 1 to 6 hours. The metabolism and excretion of these drugs is not known but is believed to occur at the synaptic level using normal processes similar to the way that ACh is handled. Drugs used topically are not generally absorbed systemically.

Contraindications and cautions

These drugs are used sparingly *because of the potential undesirable systemic effects of parasympathetic stimulation*. They are contraindicated with hypersensitivity to any component of the drug *to avoid hypersensitivity reaction* and in the presence of any condition that would be exacerbated by parasympathetic effects, such as bradycardia, hypotension, vasomotor instability and coronary artery disease, *which could be made worse by the cardiac- and CV-suppressing effects of the parasympathetic system*. Peptic ulcer, intestinal obstruction or recent GI surgery *could be negatively affected by the GI-stimulating effects of the parasympathetic nervous system*. Asthma *could be exacerbated by the increased parasympathetic effect, overriding the protective sympathetic bronchodilation*. Bladder obstruction or impaired healing of sites from recent bladder surgery *could be aggravated by the stimulatory effects on the bladder*. Epilepsy and parkinsonism *could be affected by the stimulation of ACh receptors in the brain*. Caution should be used during pregnancy and breastfeeding *because of the potential adverse effects on the fetus or neonate*.

Adverse effects

Individuals should be cautioned about the potential adverse effects of these drugs. Even if the drug is being given as a topical ophthalmic agent, there is always a possibility that it can be absorbed systemically. The adverse effects associated with these drugs are related to parasympathetic nervous system stimulation. Cardiovascular effects can include bradycardia, heart block, hypotension and even cardiac arrest related to the cardiac-suppressing effects of the parasympathetic nervous system. GI effects can include nausea, vomiting, cramps, diarrhoea, increased salivation and involuntary defecation related to the increase in GI secretions and activity. Dehydration is possible due to the increase in GI motility and resultant diarrhoea. Urinary tract effects can include a sense of urgency related to the stimulation of the bladder muscles and sphincter relaxation. Other effects may include flushing and increased sweating secondary to stimulation of the cholinergic receptors in the sympathetic nervous system.

Clinically important drug–drug interactions

There is an increased risk of cholinergic effects if these drugs are combined or given with acetylcholinesterase inhibitors, such as neostigmine or tacrine. The person should be monitored and appropriate dose adjustments made.

Prototype summary: bethanechol

Indications: acute postoperative or postpartum non-obstructive urinary retention; neurogenic atony of the bladder with retention.

Actions: acts directly on cholinergic receptors to mimic the effects of ACh; increases tone of detrusor muscles and causes emptying of the bladder.

Pharmacokinetics:

Route	Onset	Peak	Duration
Oral	30–90 min	60–90 min	1–6 hours

$T_{1/2}$: metabolism and excretion unknown; thought to be synaptic.

Adverse effects: abdominal discomfort, salivation, nausea, vomiting, sweating, flushing.

Care considerations for people receiving direct-acting cholinergic agonists

Assessment: history and examination

- Assess for contraindications or cautions: known allergies to these drugs *to avoid hypersensitivity reactions*; bradycardia, vasomotor instability, peptic ulcer, obstructive urinary or GI diseases; recent GI or genitourinary (GU) surgery; asthma; parkinsonism or epilepsy, *which could be exacerbated or complicated by parasympathetic stimulation*; and current status of pregnancy and breastfeeding *because of the potential for adverse effects to the fetus or neonate*.
- Perform a physical assessment *to establish a baseline status before beginning therapy*,

to determine the effectiveness of therapy and evaluate for any potential adverse effects.
- Assess vital signs, including pulse and blood pressure, and cardiopulmonary status, including heart and lung sounds, *to evaluate for changes related to CV effects of parasympathetic activity*; obtain an electrocardiogram (ECG) as indicated *to evaluate heart rate and rhythm.*
- Assess abdomen, *auscultating for bowel sounds*; palpate bladder *for distension.*
- Monitor intake and output, noting any complaints of urinary urgency, *to monitor for drug effects on the urinary system.*

Implementation with rationale

- Ensure proper administration of ophthalmic preparations *to increase the effectiveness of drug therapy and minimise the risk of systemic absorption.*
- Administer oral drug on an empty stomach *to decrease nausea and vomiting.*
- Monitor response closely, including blood pressure, ECG, urine output and cardiac output, *and arrange to adjust dose accordingly to ensure the most benefit with the least amount of toxicity.* Maintain a cholinergic blocking drug on standby such as atropine *to use as an antidote for excessive doses of cholinergic drugs* (see Focus on safe medication administration in discussion of Agents for myasthenia gravis in this chapter) *to reverse overdose or counteract severe reactions* (see Chapter 33 for further discussion of atropine).
- Provide safety precautions if the person reports poor visual acuity in dim light *to prevent injury.*
- Monitor urinary output *to evaluate effects on the bladder*; ensure ready access to bathroom facilities *as needed with GI stimulation.*
- Provide thorough teaching, including drug name, dosage and schedule of administration; administration of oral forms before meals or without food; proper administration for ophthalmic preparations as indicated; measures to prevent or minimise adverse effects; need for readily available access to toileting facilities; warning signs of problems; and importance of follow-up and evaluation.

Evaluation

- Monitor response to the drug (improvement in bladder function, increased salivation, miosis).
- Monitor for adverse effects (CV changes, GI stimulation, urinary urgency, respiratory distress).
- Evaluate the effectiveness of the teaching plan (person can name drug, dosage, adverse effects to watch for and specific measures to avoid them, and proper administration of ophthalmic drugs).
- Monitor the effectiveness of comfort and safety measures and compliance with the regimen.

KEY POINTS

- Cholinergic agonists stimulate the parasympathetic nerves, some nerves in the brain and the neuromuscular junction at the same site that ACh does.
- Cholinergic agonists are used topically in the eye to produce miosis (pupillary constriction) and treat glaucoma.
- Systemically, these agents are used to increase bladder tone (eg, postoperative or postpartum) and to increase secretions to relieve dry mouth associated with Sjögren's syndrome.

INDIRECT-ACTING CHOLINERGIC AGONISTS

The indirect-acting cholinergic agonists do not react directly with ACh receptor sites; instead, they react chemically with acetylcholinesterase (the enzyme responsible for the breakdown of ACh) in the synaptic cleft to prevent it from breaking down ACh. As a result, the ACh that is released from the presynaptic nerve remains in the area and accumulates, stimulating the ACh receptors for a longer period of time than normally expected. These drugs work at all ACh receptors, in the parasympathetic nervous system, in the central nervous system (CNS) and at the neuromuscular junction. Most of these drugs bind reversibly to acetylcholinesterase, so their effects pass with time when the acetylcholinesterase is released and allowed to break down ACh. However, there are certain indirect-acting cholinergic agonists that irreversibly bind to acetylcholinesterase. These drugs are not used therapeutically; they have been developed as nerve gas to be used as weapons (Box 32.2). Because these drugs might be encountered in a war situation, it is important to have an antidote readily available to military personnel and any civilian who might be affected. Pralidoxime (currently unavailable in Australia and New Zealand) is an antidote developed for the irreversible indirect-acting cholinergic agonists and is also used to reverse poisoning associated with organophosphate pesticides (Box 32.3).

The reversible indirect-acting cholinergic agonists fall into two main categories: (1) agents used to treat myasthenia gravis; and (2) agents used to treat Alzheimer disease.

■ BOX 32.2 Nerve gas: an irreversible indirect-acting cholinergic agonist

Worldwide events and conflicts over recent decades have made the potential use of nerve gas a major news story. Developed as a weapon, nerve gas is an irreversible acetylcholinesterase inhibitor. The drug is inhaled and quickly spreads throughout the body, where it permanently binds with acetylcholinesterase. This causes an accumulation of ACh at nerve endings and a massive cholinergic response. The heart rate slows and becomes ineffective, pupils and bronchi constrict, the GI tract increases activity and secretions, and muscles contract and remain that way. The muscle contraction soon immobilises the diaphragm, causing breathing to stop. The bodies of people who are killed by nerve gas have a characteristic rigor of muscle contraction.

If an attack using nerve gas is expected, individuals who may be exposed are given intramuscular injections of atropine (to temporarily block cholinergic activity and to activate ACh sites in the central nervous system) and pralidoxime (currently unavailable in Australia and New Zealand) (to free up the acetylcholinesterase to start breaking down ACh). An autoinjection is provided to military personnel who may be at risk. The injector is used to give atropine and then pralidoxime. The injections are repeated in 15 minutes.

If symptoms of nerve gas exposure exist after an additional 15 minutes, the injections are repeated. If symptoms still persist after a third set of injections, medical help should be sought.

■ BOX 32.3 Pralidoxime: antidote for irreversible indirect-acting cholinergic agonists

Pralidoxime (currently unavailable in Australia and New Zealand), an antidote for irreversible acetylcholinesterase-inhibiting drugs, or nerve gas, is given IM or IV to reactivate the acetylcholinesterase that has been blocked by these drugs. Freeing up the acetylcholinesterase allows it to break down accumulated ACh that has overstimulated ACh receptor sites, causing paralysis.

Pralidoxime does not readily cross the blood–brain barrier, and it is most useful for treating peripheral drug effects. It reacts within minutes after injection and should be available for any person receiving indirect-acting cholinergic agonists to treat myasthenia gravis. The person and a significant other should understand when to use the drug and how to administer it.

Pralidoxime is also used with atropine (which does cross the blood–brain barrier and will block the effects of accumulated ACh at CNS sites) to treat organophosphate pesticide poisonings and nerve gas exposure (see Box 32.2), both of which cause inactivation of acetylcholinesterase.

Adverse effects associated with the use of pralidoxime include dizziness, blurred vision, diplopia, headache, drowsiness, hyperventilation and nausea. These effects are also seen with exposure to nerve gas and organophosphate pesticides, so it can be difficult to differentiate drug effects from the effects of the poisoning.

AGENTS FOR MYASTHENIA GRAVIS

Myasthenia gravis is a chronic muscular disease caused by a defect in neuromuscular transmission. It is thought to be an autoimmune disease in which individuals make antibodies to their ACh receptors. These antibodies cause gradual destruction of the ACh receptors, resulting in fewer and fewer receptor sites available for stimulation. ACh is the neurotransmitter that is used at the nerve–muscle synapse. If the ACh receptors are blocked and cannot be stimulated, muscle activity is decreased. The disease is marked by progressive weakness and lack of muscle control, with periodic acute episodes. Some people have a very mild clinical presentation, such as drooping eyelids, and go into remission with no further signs and symptoms for several years. Other individuals have a more severe course of the disease, with progressive skeletal muscle weakness that may confine them to a wheelchair. The disease can further progress to paralysis of the diaphragm, which interferes with breathing and would prove fatal without intervention. Often, during the course of the disease, the person will experience a very intense phase of the disease, called a myasthenic crisis. Management of this crisis can be very challenging.

AGENTS FOR ALZHEIMER DISEASE

Alzheimer disease is a progressive disorder involving neural degeneration in the cortex that leads to a marked loss of memory and of the ability to carry on activities of daily living. Because of this, Alzheimer disease can have very negative effects on the individual and their family (Box 32.4). Dementia, of which Alzheimer disease is one of the common causes, is an area identified by the Australian government as a National Health Priority Area (AIHW, 2013).

The cause of the disease is not yet known, but it is known that there is a progressive loss of ACh-producing neurons and their target neurons in the cortex of the brain. These neurons seem to be related to memory and associations between memories that allow connections between thoughts and stimuli (eg, seeing a face and being able to know that it is a face and to name the person the face belongs to). There are four reversible indirect-acting cholinergic agonists available to slow the progression of this disease. These include donepezil (*Aricept*), galantamine (*Galantyl*, *Reminyl*) and rivastigmine (*Exelon*) (see Table 32.2). In late 2003, an N-methyl-D-aspartate receptor antagonist, memantine (*Ebixa*), was also approved for use in the treatment of Alzheimer disease. This drug works in

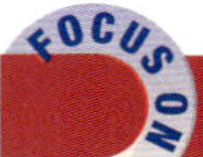

Safe medication administration

Myasthenic crisis versus cholinergic crisis

Myasthenia gravis is an autoimmune disease that runs an unpredictable course throughout the person's life. Often, the disease goes through an intense phase called a myasthenic crisis, marked by extreme muscle weakness and respiratory difficulty.

Because of the variability of the disease and the tendency to have crises and periods of remission, management of the drug dose for a person with myasthenia gravis is a challenge. If a person goes into remission, a smaller dose is needed. If a person has a crisis, an increased dose is needed. To further complicate the clinical picture, the presentation of a cholinergic overdose or cholinergic crisis is similar to the presentation of a myasthenic crisis. The individual with a cholinergic crisis presents with progressive muscle weakness and respiratory difficulty as the accumulation of ACh at the cholinergic receptor site leads to reduced impulse transmission and muscle weakness. This is a crisis when the respiratory muscles are involved.

For a myasthenic crisis, the correct treatment is increased cholinergic drug. However, treatment of a cholinergic crisis requires withdrawal of the drug. The person's respiratory difficulty usually necessitates acute medical attention. At this point, the drug edrophonium can be used as a diagnostic agent to distinguish the two conditions. If the person improves immediately after the edrophonium injection, the problem is a myasthenic crisis, which is improved by administration of the cholinergic drug. If the person gets worse, the problem is probably a cholinergic crisis, and withdrawal of the person's cholinergic drug along with intense medical support is indicated. Atropine helps to alleviate some of the parasympathetic reactions to the cholinergic drug. However, because atropine is not effective at the neuromuscular junction, only time will reverse the drug toxicity.

The person and significant others will need support, teaching and encouragement to deal with the tricky regulation of the cholinergic medication throughout the course of the disease. Health professionals in the acute care setting need to be mindful of the difficulty in distinguishing drug toxicity from the need for more drug – and be prepared to respond appropriately.

The drugs used to help people with this progressive disease are several indirect-acting cholinergic agonists that do not cross the blood–brain barrier and do not effect ACh transmission in the brain (see Table 32.2). These drugs include neostigmine (generic) and pyridostigmine (Mestinon).

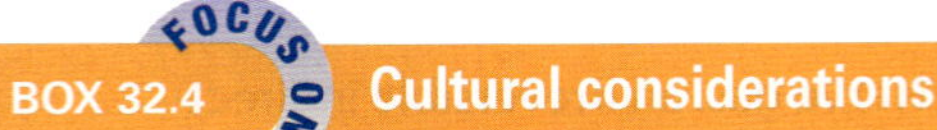

BOX 32.4 Cultural considerations

Alzheimer disease

Alzheimer disease is a chronic, progressive disease on the brain's cortex. Eventually it results in memory loss so severe that the person may not remember how to perform basic activities of daily living and may not recognise close family members. Although Alzheimer disease primarily strikes the elderly, it has a tremendous impact on family members of all ages. For example, adult children of people with Alzheimer disease, many of whom are busy raising children of their own, may find themselves in the role of carers – in essence, becoming parents of their parent. This new role can put tremendous stress on individuals who are trying to struggle with work, family and issues related to their parent's care.

When caring for a person with Alzheimer disease and their family, the health professional must remember that the person's cultural background can affect how the family copes. For example, those who tend to have solid extended families or who are part of communities that offer strong social support and interdependence may be better equipped to deal with caring for the person as the disease progresses. In contrast, families that are more goal and achievement oriented and who value autonomy and independence may find themselves overwhelmed by the person's needs and may require more support and referrals to community resources.

The health professional is in the best position to evaluate the family situation. By approaching each situation as unique and striving to incorporate cultural and social norms into the considerations for care, the health professional can help to ease the family's burden while also maintaining the dignity of the person and the family through this difficult experience.

a unique way to slow the effects of this disease and is the only drug of its class that is available (Box 32.5).

Therapeutic actions and indications

The indirect-acting cholinergic agonists work by reversibly blocking acetylcholinesterase at the synaptic cleft. This blocking allows the accumulation of ACh released from the nerve endings and leads to increased and prolonged stimulation of ACh receptor sites at all of the postsynaptic cholinergic sites. Indirect-acting cholinergic agonists work to relieve the signs and symptoms of myasthenia gravis and increase muscle strength by allowing ACh to accumulate in the synaptic cleft at neuromuscular junctions. Indirect-acting cholinergic agonists that more readily cross the blood–brain barrier and seem to affect mostly the cells in the cortex to increase ACh concentration in the area of the brain where ACh-producing cells are dying, affecting memory and the ability to access and link different memories, are used in the treatment of Alzheimer disease. In addition to usual indications, pyridostigmine has also been approved for military personnel to increase survival after exposure to particular **nerve gases** – irreversible acetylcholinesterase inhibitors used in warfare to cause paralysis and death by prolonged muscle contraction and parasympathetic crisis – and to reverse the effects of non-depolarising neuromuscular-junction blockers used to cause paralysis in surgery. See Table 32.2 for usual indications for each drug.

Pharmacokinetics

Anticholinesterase inhibitors are well absorbed after oral administration and distributed throughout the

TABLE 32.2 DRUGS IN FOCUS Indirect-acting cholinergic agonists

Drug name	Dosage/route	Usual indications
Agents for myasthenia gravis		
edrophonium (generic)	Adult (diagnosis only): 2 mg IV over 15–30 seconds, then 8 mg IV if response was seen or 10 mg IM, repeat with 2 mg IM in 12 hours to rule out false-negative results Paediatric (diagnosis only): 0.5–2 mg IV based on weight, or 2–5 mg IM	Diagnosis of myasthenia gravis
neostigmine (generic)	*Myasthenia gravis control* Adults: 1–2.5 mg/dose IM or SC. Total daily dose 5–20 mg Paediatric IM or SC: 0.2–0.5 mg/dose Neonates: 0.05–0.25 mg IM q 2–4 hours, half an hour before feeding *Antidote for non-depolarising neuromuscular junction blockers (with atropine)* Adults: 0.5–2.5 mg/dose IV with atropine sulfate 0.6–1.2 mg over 1 minute Paediatric: 0.05 mg/kg/dose IV (maximum dose 2.5 mg) with atropine sulfate 0.02 mg/kg/dose	Diagnosis and management of myasthenia gravis; reversal of toxicity from non-depolarising neuromuscular junction–blocking drugs, which are used to paralyse muscles during surgery (see Chapter 28)
(P) pyridostigmine (*Mestinon*)	Adult: 30–120 mg PO bd–qid; usual dose range 5–20 tablets a day Children < 6 years: initial dose 30 mg Children 6–12 years: initial dose 60 mg increased gradually, in increments of 15–30 mg daily, until maximal improvement is obtained. Usual dose range 30–360 mg	Management of myasthenia gravis; antidote to neuromuscular-junction blockers; increases survival after exposure to nerve gas
Agents for Alzheimer disease		
(P) donepezil (*Aricept*)	5–10 mg PO daily at bedtime	Management of Alzheimer dementia, including severe dementia
galantamine (*Galantyl, Reminyl*)	4–12 mg PO bd; reduce dose to 16 mg/day maximum with renal or hepatic impairment; available as an oral solution 4 mg/mL; range 16–32 mg/day; extended-release tablets, range 16–24 mg/day taken as a single dose	Management of mild to moderate Alzheimer dementia delays progression of disease
rivastigmine (*Exelon*)	1.5–6 mg PO bd, based on response and tolerance; transdermal system, one 4.6 mg/24 hours patch placed once a day, maximum 9.5 mg/24 hours	Management of mild to moderate Alzheimer dementia; treatment of dementia related to Parkinson disease

BOX 32.5 Memantine for treating Alzheimer disease

In 2003, the Therapeutic Goods Administration approved a new drug for treating Alzheimer disease. The drug, memantine hydrochloride (*Ebixa, Memanxa*), has been used in Europe for several years and has been reported to slow the memory loss of people with moderate to severe dementia associated with Alzheimer disease. Memantine has a low to moderate affinity for *N*-methyl-D-aspartate (NMDA) receptors with no effects on dopamine, gamma-aminobutyric acid, histamine, glycine or adrenergic-receptor sites. It is thought that persistent activation of the CNS NMDA receptors contributes to the symptoms of Alzheimer disease. By blocking these sites, it is thought that the symptoms are reduced or delayed.

The drug is available in a tablet form and is started at 5 mg/day PO, increasing by 5 mg/day at weekly intervals. The target dose is 20 mg/day given as 10 mg twice daily. Dose reduction should be considered in individuals with renal impairment. Headache, dizziness, fatigue, confusion and constipation are common adverse effects. The drug should not be taken with anything that alkalinises the urine. Affected people and family members need to understand that this drug is not a cure but may offer some extended time with mild symptoms.

body. The sites of metabolism and excretion for all of these drugs are not known. It is thought that they are metabolised at the nerve synapse or in the tissues.

Neostigmine is a synthetic drug that has a strong influence at the neuromuscular junction. Neostigmine has a duration of action of 2–4 hours and therefore must be given every few hours, based on individual response, to maintain a therapeutic level.

Pyridostigmine has a longer duration of action than neostigmine (3–6 hours) and is preferred in some cases for the management of myasthenia gravis because it does not need to be taken as frequently.

Edrophonium is administered intravenously and has a very short duration of action (10–20 minutes). It is an orphan drug currently not approved by TGA and remains an unapproved medicine in New Zealand.

The drugs used to treat Alzheimer disease are well absorbed and distributed through the body. They are metabolised in the liver by the cytochrome P450 system, so caution must be used for individuals with hepatic impairment and for cases in which many interacting drugs are used. The drugs used to treat Alzheimer disease are excreted in the urine.

Galantamine is available as prolonged-release capsules. It has a half-life of 7 hours and is taken twice a day. An extended-release form, recently available, can be taken just once a day. Rivastigmine is available in capsule and solution forms to help with people who have swallowing difficulties, as well as a transdermal patch that is applied once a day. The duration of effects for rivastigmine is 12 hours. Donepezil, with a 70-hour half-life, is available in oral form, as capsules, and as an oral solution. It can be given once-a-day, which is advantageous with a disease that affects memory and the person's ability to remember to take pills throughout the day.

Contraindications and cautions

Anticholinesterase inhibitors are contraindicated in the presence of allergy to any of these drugs *to avoid hypersensitivity reactions*; with bradycardia or intestinal or urinary tract obstruction, *which could be exacerbated by the stimulation of cholinergic receptors*; in pregnancy *because the uterus could be stimulated and labour induced*; and during breastfeeding *because of the potential effects on the baby.*

Caution should be used with *any condition that could be exacerbated by cholinergic stimulation*. Although the effects of these drugs are generally more localised to the cortex and the neuromuscular junction, the possibility of parasympathetic effects must be considered carefully in individuals with asthma, coronary disease, peptic ulcer, arrhythmias, epilepsy or parkinsonism, *which could be exacerbated by the effects of parasympathetic stimulation*. Drugs used to treat Alzheimer disease are metabolised in the liver and excreted in the urine, so caution should be used in the presence of hepatic or renal dysfunction, *which could interfere with the metabolism and excretion of the drugs.*

Adverse effects

The adverse effects associated with agents for treating myasthenia gravis or Alzheimer disease are related to the stimulation of the parasympathetic nervous system. GI effects can include nausea, vomiting, cramps, diarrhoea, increased salivation and involuntary defecation related to the increase in GI secretions and activity due to parasympathetic nervous system stimulation. Cardiovascular effects can include bradycardia, heart block, hypotension and even cardiac arrest, related to the cardiac-suppressing effects of the parasympathetic nervous system. Urinary tract effects can include a sense of urgency related to stimulation of the bladder muscles and sphincter relaxation. Miosis and blurred vision, headaches, dizziness and drowsiness can occur related to CNS cholinergic effects. Other effects may include flushing and increased sweating secondary to stimulation of the cholinergic receptors in the sympathetic nervous system.

Clinically important drug–drug interactions

There may be an increased risk of GI bleeding if these drugs are used with NSAIDs because of the combination of increased GI secretions and the GI mucosal erosion associated with the use of NSAIDs. If this combination is used, the person should be monitored closely for any sign of GI bleeding. The effect of anticholinesterase drugs is decreased if they are taken in combination with any cholinergic drugs because these work in opposition to each other.

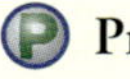

Prototype summary: pyridostigmine

Indications: treatment of myasthenia gravis, antidote for non-depolarising neuromuscular-junction blockers, increased survival after exposure to nerve gas.

Actions: reversible cholinesterase inhibitor that increases the levels of ACh, facilitating transmission at the neuromuscular junction.

Pharmacokinetics:

Route	Onset	Duration
Oral	35–45 min	3–6 hours
IM	15 min	3–6 hours

$T_{1/2}$: 1.9–3.7 hours; metabolism is in the liver and tissue, and excretion is in the urine.

Adverse effects: bradycardia, cardiac arrest, tearing, miosis, salivation, dysphagia, nausea, vomiting, increased bronchial secretions, urinary frequency, and incontinence.

Prototype summary: donepezil

Indications: treatment of mild to moderate Alzheimer disease.

Actions: reversible cholinesterase inhibitor that causes elevated ACh levels in the cortex, which slows the neuronal degradation of Alzheimer disease.

Pharmacokinetics:

Route	Onset	Peak
Oral	Varies	2–4 hours

$T_{1/2}$: 70 hours; metabolism is in the liver, and excretion is in the urine.

Adverse effects: insomnia, fatigue, rash, nausea, vomiting, diarrhoea, dyspepsia, abdominal pain, muscle cramps.

Care considerations for people receiving indirect-acting cholinergic agonists

Assessment: history and examination

- Assess for contraindications or cautions: known allergies to any of these drugs *to avoid hypersensitivity reactions*; arrhythmias, coronary artery disease, hypotension, urogenital or GI obstruction or peptic ulcer, *which could be exacerbated by cholinergic stimulation*; recent GI or GU surgery, *which could limit use of the drugs because of the stimulatory effects of the parasympathetic system, which could aggravate healing*; regular use of NSAIDs, cholinergic drugs or theophylline, *which could cause a drug–drug interaction*; and current status of pregnancy and breastfeeding *because of potential effects to the fetus or neonate.*
- Perform a physical assessment *to establish baseline status before beginning therapy and to determine any potential adverse effects*: assess orientation, affect, reflexes, ability to carry on activities of daily living (Alzheimer drugs) and vision *to monitor for CNS changes related to drug therapy*; blood pressure, pulse, ECG, peripheral perfusion and cardiac output *to monitor the parasympathetic effects on the vascular system*; and urinary output and renal and liver function tests *to monitor drug effects on the renal system and liver, which could change the metabolism and excretion of the drugs.*

Refer to the Critical thinking scenario for a full discussion of care for a person who is receiving indirect-acting cholinergic agonists.

Implementation with rationale

- If the drug is given IV, administer it slowly *to avoid severe cholinergic effects.*
- Maintain atropine sulphate on standby *as an antidote in case of overdose or severe cholinergic reaction.*
- Discontinue the drug if excessive salivation, diarrhoea, emesis or frequent urination becomes a problem *to decrease the risk of severe adverse reactions.*
- Administer the oral drug with meals *to decrease GI upset if it is a problem.*
- Mark the person's chart and notify the surgeon if the person is to undergo surgery *because prolonged muscle relaxation may occur if suxamethonium-type anaesthetics are used.* The person will require prolonged support and monitoring.
- Monitor the person being treated for Alzheimer disease for any progress *because the drug is not a cure and only slows progression*; refer families to supportive services.
- The person who is being treated for myasthenia gravis and significant others should receive instruction in drug administration, warning signs of drug overdose, and signs and symptoms to report immediately *to enhance knowledge about drug therapy and to promote compliance.*
- Arrange for supportive care and comfort measures, including rest, environmental control and other measures, *to decrease CNS irritation*; headache medication *to relieve pain*; safety measures if CNS effects occur *to prevent injury*; protective measures if CNS effects are severe *to prevent injury*; and small, frequent meals if GI upset is severe *to decrease discomfort and maintain nutrition.*
- Provide thorough teaching, including dosage, adverse effects to anticipate and measures to avoid them and warning signs of problems, as well as proper administration for each route used, *to enhance knowledge about drug therapy and to promote compliance.*
- Offer support and encouragement *to help the person deal with the drug regimen.*

Evaluation

- Monitor response to the drug (improvement in condition being treated).
- Monitor for adverse effects (GI upset, CNS changes, CV changes, GU changes).
- Evaluate the effectiveness of the teaching plan (person can name drug, dosage, adverse effects to watch for and specific measures to avoid them and proper administration).
- Monitor the effectiveness of comfort measures and compliance with the regimen.

KEY POINTS

- Myasthenia gravis is an autoimmune disease characterised by antibodies to the ACh receptors. This results in a loss of ACh receptors and eventual loss of response at the neuromuscular junction.
- Acetylcholinesterase inhibitors are used to treat myasthenia gravis because they allow the accumulation of ACh in the synaptic cleft, prolonging stimulation of any ACh sites that remain.
- Alzheimer disease is a progressive dementia characterised by a loss of ACh-producing neurons and ACh receptor sites in the neurocortex.
- Acetylcholinesterase inhibitors that cross the blood–brain barrier are used to manage Alzheimer disease by increasing ACh levels in the brain and slowing the progression of the disease.

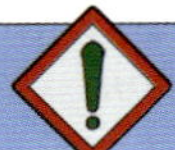

CRITICAL THINKING SCENARIO

Indirect-acting cholinergic agonists

THE SITUATION

A.J., a 75-year-old man with an unremarkable medical history, is seen in the clinic for evaluation of memory loss and confusion. Three years ago, his wife began to notice memory gaps and confusion when A.J. was driving around town. He would get lost only a few blocks from home. The problem has become steadily worse. He was diagnosed with Alzheimer disease after neurological tests and medical evaluation ruled out other causes for his problem. He did not want to take any drugs, but when he heard the diagnosis, he became quite frightened and agreed to try medication. His wife states that she is somewhat concerned about giving him medication because he has sometimes had trouble swallowing and chokes on his food. She excitedly tells A.J. that once he starts the medication, his memory will return and things will be normal again. A.J. is placed on rivastigmine.

CRITICAL THINKING

What could be responsible for A.J.'s symptoms?

What modifications can be made to the prescription to ensure A.J.'s safety if he is having trouble swallowing?

What important information about the disease and the effectiveness of drug therapy needs to be discussed with A.J. and his wife? *Will things return to normal?*

What potential adverse effects can be anticipated with rivastigmine, and how might these effects complicate the situation for A.J. and his wife?

DISCUSSION

Alzheimer disease is a chronic, progressive disease that involves the loss of neurons in the cortex of the brain that are responsible for making connections between different memories. A.J. has had the problem for at least 3 years, and his loss of memory and confusion have become worse over that period of time. Unfortunately, there is nothing available at this time that can stop the loss of neurons or restore the function that has already been lost.

One of the problems that occur with Alzheimer disease is difficulty swallowing. Swallowing is a complex CNS reflex that requires coordination of impulses, and with this disease, the ability to swallow in a coordinated manner is often lost. This can lead to aspiration and pneumonia, which are often the underlying causes of death with Alzheimer disease. Since A.J. already has some difficulty swallowing, it would be important to look into the forms in which rivastigmine is provided. In this case, the drug is available in capsule form and as an oral solution. The oral solution might be suggested because it could be much easier to swallow. As the disease progresses, this drug is also available as a transdermal system, which would eliminate the need to swallow the drug. The status of A.J.'s swallowing should be evaluated before starting therapy and periodically as time goes on to determine how safe the dosage form of the drug is for his particular situation.

A.J. and his wife should receive information on Alzheimer disease and its progression. The drugs available at this time do not reverse the memory loss and they do not cure the disease. A.J.'s wife may be encouraged to monitor A.J.'s behaviour, ability to perform activities of daily living and other significant markers of importance to them. The drug should slow the progression of the disease and it might be helpful to monitor progress to see if the drug is being effective. She might also want to become involved in an Alzheimer support group or organisation, which could provide valuable support, educational materials and access to community resources. This is an overwhelming diagnosis and it might be necessary to approach these individuals over several visits to give them both time to adjust. It is important to always include a family member and provide information in writing for later reference when doing teaching with a person with Alzheimer disease.

Many of the adverse effects associated with the indirect-acting cholinergic agonists are a result of the parasympathetic stimulation caused by these drugs and may complicate A.J.'s care as his disease progresses. GI effects can include increased salivation, which may further add to his difficulty swallowing; nausea and vomiting, which could make it difficult to maintain nutrition; and cramps, diarrhoea and involuntary defecation related to the increase in GI secretions and activity, which could make toileting difficult and add to Mrs. J.'s home care burden. Cardiovascular effects can include bradycardia, heart block and hypotension, which could lead to dizziness and weakness and further complicate safety issues. Urinary tract effects can include a sense of urgency related to stimulation of the bladder muscles and sphincter relaxation, which could lead to incontinence as the person becomes less responsive to normal reflexes. Miosis and blurred vision, headaches, dizziness and drowsiness can occur, further complicating safety issues. The benefits of slowing the progression of the disease often need to be weighed against all of the potential adverse effects that can complicate care and safety.

CARE GUIDE FOR A.J.: INDIRECT-ACTING CHOLINERGIC AGONISTS

Assessment: history and examination

Assess for contraindications or cautions: known allergies to any of the components of this drug, arrhythmias, coronary artery disease, hypotension, urogenital or GI obstruction, peptic ulcer, recent GI or GU surgery, and regular use of NSAIDs, cholinergic drugs or theophylline.

Focus the physical examination on the following:

CNS: orientation, affect, reflexes, memory response, ability to carry out simple commands, vision

CV: blood pressure, pulse, peripheral perfusion, ECG

GI: abdominal exam

GU: urinary output, bladder tone

Respiratory: respirations, adventitious sounds

Skin: colour, temperature, texture

Implementation

Ensure safe and appropriate administration of the drug; monitor the ability to swallow and the appropriateness of dosage form.

Provide comfort and safety measures (eg, physical assistance, raising side rails on the bed); temperature control; pain relief; small, frequent meals.

Monitor cardiac status and urine output throughout drug therapy.

Provide support and reassurance to deal with side effects, discomfort and GI effects.

Provide the individual and the family with teaching regarding drug name, dosage, side effects, precautions and warning signs of serious adverse effects to report.

Evaluation

Evaluate drug effects: slowing of progression of dementia.

Monitor for adverse effects: CV effects – bradycardia, heart block, hypotension; urinary problems; GI effects; respiratory problems.

Monitor for drug–drug interactions.

Evaluate the effectiveness of teaching program and comfort and safety measures.

INDIVIDUAL/FAMILY TEACHING FOR A.J.

- The drug that was ordered for you is called rivastigmine. It is called a cholinergic agonist or a parasympathetic drug because it mimics the effects of the parasympathetic nervous system. Cholinergic drugs get this name because they act at certain nerve–nerve and nerve–muscle junctions in the body that are called cholinergic sites. They use a chemical called acetylcholine (ACh) to carry out their functions. The nerves in your brain that are affected by Alzheimer disease use ACh to help you to remember things and make connections between memories.
- Some of the following adverse effects may occur.
  - *Nausea, vomiting, diarrhoea*: it is wise to be near bathroom facilities after taking your drug. If these symptoms become too severe, consult with your health care provider.
  - *Flushing, sweating*: staying in a cool environment and wearing lightweight clothing may help.
  - *Increased salivation*: this may increase your difficulty in swallowing.
  - *Urgency to void*: maintaining access to a bathroom may relieve some of this discomfort.
  - *Headache*: aspirin or another headache medication (if not contraindicated in your particular case) will help to alleviate this pain.
  - *Changes in vision, dizziness*: these might lead to falls or more confusion.
- Report any of the following to your health care provider: *very slow pulse, light-headedness, fainting, excessive salivation, abdominal cramping or pain, weakness or confusion, blurring of vision, further signs of dementia.*
- Tell any doctor, nurse or other health care provider involved in your care that you are taking this drug.

CHAPTER SUMMARY

- Cholinergic drugs are chemicals that act at the same site as the neurotransmitter acetylcholine (ACh), stimulating the parasympathetic nerves, some nerves in the brain and the neuromuscular junction.
- Direct-acting cholinergic drugs react with the ACh receptor sites to cause cholinergic stimulation.
- Use of direct-acting cholinergic drugs is limited by the systemic effects of the drug. They are used to induce miosis and to treat glaucoma; one agent is available to treat neurogenic bladder and bladder

atony postoperatively or postpartum, and another agent is available to increase GI secretions and relieve the dry mouth of Sjögren syndrome.

- All indirect-acting cholinergic drugs are acetylcholinesterase inhibitors. They block acetylcholinesterase to prevent it from breaking down ACh in the synaptic cleft.
- Cholinergic stimulation by acetylcholinesterase inhibitors is due to an accumulation of the ACh released from the nerve ending.
- Myasthenia gravis is an autoimmune disease characterised by antibodies to the ACh receptors. This results in a loss of ACh receptors and eventual loss of response at the neuromuscular junction.
- Acetylcholinesterase inhibitors are used to treat myasthenia gravis because they allow the accumulation of ACh in the synaptic cleft, prolonging stimulation of any ACh sites that remain.
- Alzheimer disease is a progressive dementia characterised by a loss of ACh-producing neurons and ACh receptor sites in the neurocortex.
- Acetylcholinesterase inhibitors that cross the blood–brain barrier are used to manage Alzheimer disease by increasing ACh levels in the brain and slowing the progression of the disease.
- Side effects associated with the use of these drugs are related to stimulation of the parasympathetic nervous system (bradycardia, hypotension, increased GI secretions and activity, increased bladder tone, relaxation of GI and GU sphincters, bronchoconstriction, pupil constriction) and may limit the usefulness of some of these drugs.

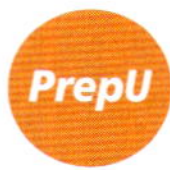

Knowing your strengths and weaknesses helps you to study more effectively. Take a PrepU Practice Quiz to find out how you measure up!

ONLINE RESOURCES

An extensive range of additional resources to enhance teaching and learning and to facilitate understanding of this chapter may be found online at the text's accompanying website, located on thePoint at http://thepoint.lww.com. These include Watch and Learn videos, Concepts in Action animations, journal articles, review questions, case studies, discussion topics and quizzes.

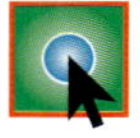

WEB LINKS

Health care providers and patients may want to consult the following web sources:

www.aihw.gov.au/dementia
The Australian Institute of Health and Welfare National Health Priority Area – Dementia.

www.alzheimers.org.au
Information on resources, medical treatments, outreach programs and local support groups involved with Alzheimer disease.

www.myasthenia.org.au
The Australian Myasthenic Association in NSW. Information and resources on myasthenia gravis and treatments.

www.myastheniawa.info
The Myasthenia Gravis Friends and Support Group, Western Australia. Information and resources on myasthenia gravis and treatments.

BIBLIOGRAPHY

Australian Institute of Health and Welfare (AIHW). (2013). Dementia, www.aihw.gov.au/dementia.

Crouch, A. M. (2009). Treating dementia. *Australian Prescriber, 32*, 9–12.

Downey, D. (2008). Pharmacology update. Pharmacologic management of Alzheimer disease. *Journal of Neuroscience Nursing, 40(1)*, 55–59.

Farrell, M. & Dempsey, J. (2014). *Smeltzer & Bare's Textbook of Medical-Surgical Nursing* (3rd edn). Sydney: Lippincott Williams & Wilkins.

Goodman, L. S., Brunton, L. L., Chabner, B. & Knollmann, B. C. (2011). *Goodman and Gilman's Pharmacological Basis of Therapeutics* (12th edn). New York: McGraw-Hill.

Grossberg, G. T., Pejovic, V. & Miller, M. L. (2007). Current strategies for the treatment and prevention of Alzheimer disease. *Primary Psychiatry, 14(8)*, 39–50, 51–54.

Koch, J. A., Steele, M. R. & Koch, L. M. (2013). Myasthenia gravis. *Journal of Gerontological Nursing, 39(12)*, 11–15.

McKenna, L. & Mirkov, S. (2019). *McKenna's Drug Handbook for Nursing and Midwifery* (8th edn). Sydney: Wolters Kluwer Health Australia.

Mestecky, A-M. (2013). Myasthenia gravis. *British Journal of Neuroscience Nursing, 9(3)*, 110–112.

Mitchell, G. (2013). Applying pharmacology to practice: The case of dementia. *Nurse Prescribing, 11(4)*, 185–190.

Porth, C. M. (2011). *Essentials of Pathophysiology: Concepts of Altered Health States* (3rd edn). Philadelphia: Lippincott Williams & Wilkins.

Porth, C. M. (2009). *Pathophysiology: Concepts of Altered Health States* (8th edn). Philadelphia: Lippincott Williams & Wilkins.

Reddel, S. W. (2007). Treatment of myasthenia gravis. *Australian Prescriber, 30*, 156–160.

Varner, M. (2013). Myasthenia gravis and pregnancy. *Clinical Obstetrics & Gynecology, 56(2)*, 372–381.

CHECK YOUR UNDERSTANDING

Answers to the questions in this chapter can be found in Appendix A at the back of this book.

MULTIPLE CHOICE

Select the best answer to the following.

1. Indirect-acting cholinergic agents:
   a. react with ACh receptor sites on the membranes of effector cells.
   b. react chemically with acetylcholinesterase to increase ACh concentrations.
   c. are used to increase bladder tone and urinary excretion.
   d. should be given with food to slow absorption.
2. A person is to receive pilocarpine. The nurse understands that this drug would be most likely used to treat which of the following?
   a. myasthenia gravis
   b. neurogenic bladder
   c. glaucoma
   d. Alzheimer disease
3. Myasthenia gravis is treated with indirect-acting cholinergic agents that:
   a. lead to accumulation of ACh in the synaptic cleft.
   b. block the GI effects of the disease, allowing for absorption.
   c. directly stimulate the remaining ACh receptors.
   d. can be given only by injection because of problems associated with swallowing.
4. A person with myasthenia gravis is no longer able to swallow. Which of the following would the health professional expect the doctor to order?
   a. donepezil
   b. memantine
   c. pyridostigmine
   d. gentamicin
5. Alzheimer disease is marked by a progressive loss of memory and is associated with:
   a. degeneration of dopamine-producing cells in the basal ganglia.
   b. loss of ACh-producing neurons and their target neurons in the CNS.
   c. loss of ACh receptor sites in the parasympathetic nervous system.
   d. increased levels of acetylcholinesterase in the CNS.
6. The nurse would expect to administer donepezil to a person with Alzheimer disease who:
   a. cannot remember family members' names.
   b. is mildly inhibited and can still follow medical dosing regimens.
   c. is able to carry on normal activities of daily living.
   d. has memory problems and would benefit from once-a-day dosing.
7. Adverse effects associated with the use of cholinergic drugs include:
   a. constipation and insomnia.
   b. diarrhoea and urinary urgency.
   c. tachycardia and hypertension.
   d. dry mouth and tachycardia.
8. Nerve gas is an irreversible acetylcholinesterase inhibitor that can cause muscle paralysis and death. An antidote to such an agent is:
   a. atropine.
   b. propranolol.
   c. pralidoxime.
   d. neostigmine.

MULTIPLE RESPONSE

Select all that apply.

1. A nurse is explaining myasthenia gravis to a family. Which of the following points would be included in the explanation?
   a. It is thought to be an autoimmune disease.
   b. It is associated with destruction of ACh receptor sites.
   c. It is best treated with potent antibiotics.
   d. It is a chronic and progressive muscular disease.
   e. It is caused by demyelination of the nerve fibre.
   f. Once diagnosed, it has a 5-year survival rate.
2. A nurse would question an order for a cholinergic drug if the person was also taking which of the following?
   a. theophylline
   b. NSAIDs
   c. cefalosporin
   d. atropine
   e. propranolol
   f. memantine

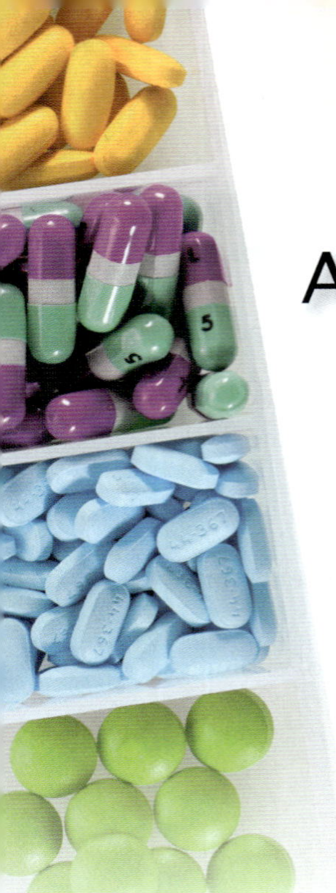

33

Anticholinergic agents

Learning objectives

On completing this chapter you should be able to:

1. Define anticholinergic agents.
2. Describe the therapeutic actions, indications, pharmacokinetics, contraindications and cautions, most common adverse reactions and important drug–drug interactions of anticholinergic agents.
3. Discuss the use of anticholinergic agents across the lifespan.
4. Compare and contrast the prototype drug atropine with other anticholinergic agents.
5. Outline the care considerations, including important teaching points, for people receiving anticholinergic agents.

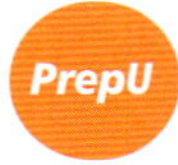

Test your current knowledge of anticholinergic agents with a PrepU Practice Quiz!

Glossary of key terms

anticholinergic: drug that opposes the effects of acetylcholine at acetylcholine receptor sites
belladonna: a plant that contains atropine as an alkaloid; used to dilate the pupils as a fashion statement in the past; used in herbal medicine much as atropine is used today
cycloplegia: inability of the lens in the eye to accommodate to near vision, causing blurring and inability to see near objects
mydriasis: relaxation of the muscles around the pupil, leading to pupil dilation
parasympatholytic: lysing or preventing parasympathetic effects

ANTICHOLINERGIC AGENTS/ PARASYMPATHOLYTICS

- Ⓟ atropine
- benztropine
- biperidem
- cyclopentolate
- glycopyrronium bromide (glycopyrrolate)
- hyoscine
- hyoscyamine
- oxybutynin
- ipratropium
- propantheline
- solifenacin
- tiotropium
- tolterodine
- trihexyphenidyl (benzhexol)

Drugs that are used to block the effects of acetylcholine are called **anticholinergic** drugs. Because this action lyses, or blocks, the effects of the parasympathetic nervous system, they are also called **parasympatholytic** agents. This class of drugs was once very widely used to decrease gastrointestinal (GI) activity and secretions in the treatment of ulcers and to decrease other parasympathetic activities to allow the sympathetic system to become more dominant. Today, more specific and less systemically toxic drugs are available for many of the conditions that would benefit from these effects. Therefore this class of drugs is less commonly used. Atropine is the only widely used anticholinergic drug. Box 33.1 discusses the use of anticholinergics across the lifespan.

ANTICHOLINERGICS/ PARASYMPATHOLYTICS

Anticholinergic agents include atropine (generic), benzatropine (*Benztrop*, *Cogentin*), biperiden (*Akineton*) cyclopentolate (*Cyclogyl*), glycopyrronium bromide (glycopyrrolate) (*Robinul*), hyoscine (also known as

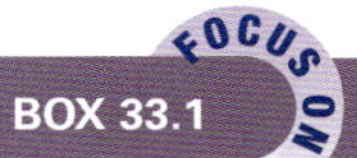

BOX 33.1 **Drug therapy across the lifespan**

Anticholinergic agents/parasympatholytics

CHILDREN

The anticholinergic agents are often used in children. Children are often more sensitive to the adverse effects of the drugs, including constipation, urinary retention, heat intolerance and confusion. If a child is given one of these drugs, the child should be closely watched and monitored for adverse effects, and appropriate supportive measures should be instituted.

ADULTS

Adults need to be made aware of the potential for adverse effects associated with the use of these drugs. They should be encouraged to void before taking the medication if urinary retention or hesitancy is a problem. They should be encouraged to drink plenty of fluids and to avoid hot temperatures because heat intolerance can occur and it will be important to maintain hydration should this happen. Safety precautions may be needed if blurred vision and dizziness occur. The person should be urged not to drive or perform tasks that require concentration and coordination.

PREGNANCY AND BREASTFEEDING

These drugs should not be used during pregnancy because they cross the placenta and could cause adverse effects on the fetus. If the benefit to the mother clearly outweighs the potential risk to the fetus, they should be used with caution. Breastfeeding women should find another method of feeding the baby if an anticholinergic drug is needed because of the potential for serious adverse effects on the baby.

OLDER ADULTS

Older adults are more likely to experience the adverse effects associated with these drugs; dose should be reduced, and the person should be monitored very closely. Because older people are more susceptible to heat intolerance owing to decreased body fluid and decreased sweating, extreme caution should be used when an anticholinergic drug is given. The person should be urged to drink plenty of fluids and to avoid extremes of temperature or exertion in warm temperatures. The older adult is more likely to experience confusion, hallucinations and psychotic syndromes when taking an anticholinergic drug. Safety precautions may be needed if central nervous system (CNS) effects are severe. Older adults may also have renal impairment, making them more likely to have problems excreting these drugs. Further reduction in dose may be needed in the older person who also has renal dysfunction.

scopolamine; *Buscopan*), hyoscyamine (*Donnatab*) (not available in New Zealand), ipratropium (*Atrovent*), oxybutynin (*Ditropan*, *Oxytrol*), propantheline (*Pro-Banthine*), solifenacin (*Vesicare*), tiotropium (*Spiriva*), tolterodine (*Detrusitol*), trihexyphenidyl (benzhexol) (*Artane*) and tiotropium (*Spiriva, Respimat*) (see Table 33.1).

Therapeutic actions and indications

The anticholinergic drugs competitively block the acetylcholine receptors at the muscarinic cholinergic receptor sites that are responsible for mediating the effects of the parasympathetic postganglionic impulses (Figure 33.1). Some are more specific to particular receptors in the respiratory, genitourinary (GU) or GI tracts, making them preferred for treating specific conditions, and others more generally depress the parasympathetic system. When the parasympathetic system is blocked, the effects of the sympathetic system are more prominently seen. These drugs can be used to decrease secretions before anaesthesia; to treat parkinsonism (by blocking the stimulating effects of acetylcholine); to restore cardiac rate and blood pressure after vagal stimulation during surgery; to relieve bradycardia caused by a hyperactive carotid sinus reflex; to relieve pylorospasm and hyperactive bowel; to relax biliary and ureteral colic; to relax bladder detrusor muscles and tighten sphincters; to help to control crying or laughing episodes in people with brain injuries; to relax uterine hypertonicity; to help in the management of peptic ulcer; to control rhinorrhoea associated with hay fever; as an antidote for cholinergic drugs and for poisoning by certain mushrooms; and as an ophthalmic agent to cause mydriasis or cycloplegia in acute inflammatory conditions (Table 33.1). Anticholinergic drugs also are thought to block the effects of acetylcholine in the CNS, which may account for their effectiveness in treating motion sickness.

Atropine, the prototype drug, has been used for many years and is derived from the plant **belladonna.** (Belladonna was once used by fashionable ladies of the European courts to dilate their pupils in an effort to make them more innocent looking and alluring.) Atropine is used to depress salivation and bronchial secretions and to dilate the bronchi, but it can thicken respiratory secretions (causing obstruction of airways). Atropine is also used to inhibit vagal responses in the heart, to relax the GI and GU tracts, to inhibit GI secretions, to cause **mydriasis** or relaxation of the pupil of the eye (also called a mydriatic effect) and to cause **cycloplegia**, or inhibition of the ability of the lens in the eye to accommodate to near vision (also called a cycloplegic effect).

Atropine works by blocking only the muscarinic effectors in the parasympathetic nervous system and the few cholinergic receptors in the sympathetic nervous system (SNS), such as those that control sweating. It acts by competing with acetylcholine for the muscarinic acetylcholine receptor sites. It does not block the nicotinic receptors and therefore has little or no effect at the neuromuscular junction.

TABLE 33.1 DRUGS IN FOCUS Anticholinergic agents/parasympatholytics

Drug name	Dosage/route	Usual indications
(P) atropine (generic)	0.3–0.6 mg IM, SC or IV 1 hour before anaesthesia in conjunction with a narcotic; use caution with older people Paediatric: 0.1–0.4 mg IV, IM or SC based on weight	Decrease secretions, bradycardia, pylorospasm, ureteral colic, relaxing of bladder, emotional lability with head injuries, antidote for cholinergic drugs, pupil dilation
cyclopentolate (*Cyclogyl*)	1 drop into eye; may repeat in 5 minutes	Mydriasis and cyclopegia for diagnostic procedures, preoperative or postoperative
glycopyrronium bromide (glycopyrrolate) (*Robinul, Seebri*)	Adults: 200–400 micrograms (or 4–5 micrograms/kg); maximum 400 micrograms Children 1 month–12 years: 4–8 micrograms/kg; maximum 200 micrograms *Seebri* capsules for inhalation: inhale the content of 1 capsule (50 micrograms) via Breezhaler inhaler	Decrease secretions before anaesthetic or intubation; used orally as an adjunct for treatment of ulcers (although not drug of choice); protects the person from the peripheral effects of cholinergic drugs; reverses neuromuscular blockade Capsules for inhalation: COPD
hyoscine hydrobromide (generic)	Adult: 300–600 micrograms IV, SC or IM 30–60 min before induction of anaesthesia; may be repeated tid–qid; maximum 1 mg Elderly: reduced dosage may be required Paediatric: 6 micrograms/kg, or 200 micrograms/m^2 IM, SC or IV	Preoperative medication to produce sedation and amnesia, inhibit salivation and excessive secretions of the respiratory tract
hyoscine butylbromide (*Buscopan, Gastro-Sooothe*)	20 mg PO qid	Relief of GI tract, renal and biliary spasm, motion sickness
hyoscine hydrobromide with atropine and hyoscyamine (*Donnatab*)	1–2 tabs PO tds or qid	Adjunctive therapy to treat peptic ulcer, overactive GI disorders; neurogenic bladder or cystitis; parkinsonism; biliary or renal colic; to decrease secretions preoperatively; treatment of partial heart block associated with vagal activity; treatment of rhinitis or anticholinesterase poisoning
ipratropium (*Atrovent*)	Adults: 2 puffs tid–qid, up to 4 puffs/dose if needed; 250–500 micrograms qid via nebuliser	Maintenance treatment of bronchospasm associated with chronic obstructive pulmonary disease (COPD); nasal spray for symptomatic relief of perennial and seasonal rhinitis
oxybutynin (*Ditropan, generic, Oxytrol*)	Adult: 5 mg PO bd–tds; maximum 20 mg/day Elderly: 2.5 mg PO bd, increased as necessary Children > 5 years: 5 mg PO bd; maximum 15 mg/day	Therapy of urgency and incontinence that characterise neurogenic bladder disorders and idiopathic detrusor instability
propantheline (*Pro-Banthine*)	15 mg PO tds 30 minutes before meals and 30 mg at night	To decrease GI secretions and stop GI spasms in conditions that would benefit from these actions
tiotropium (*Spiriva, Spririva Respimat*)	Handihaler (capsule with powder for inhalation): 18 micrograms/day; not recommended for children Respimat device, adults and children < 6 years: 5 micrograms (two puffs) once daily	Maintenance treatment of bronchospasm associated with COPD, for long-term use Spiriva Respimat is indicated as add-on maintenance bronchodilator treatment in patients ≥ 6 years with moderate to severe asthma

Ipratropium and tiotropium act more specifically to decrease respiratory secretions and cause bronchodilation. They are used as bronchodilators and to decrease symptoms of upper respiratory irritation. These agents are discussed in Chapter 55. Hyoscyamine acts more specifically on the receptors in the GI tract and is used as an adjunct in the treatment of peptic ulcers, irritable bowel syndrome and GI disorders. These agents are discussed in Chapter 58.

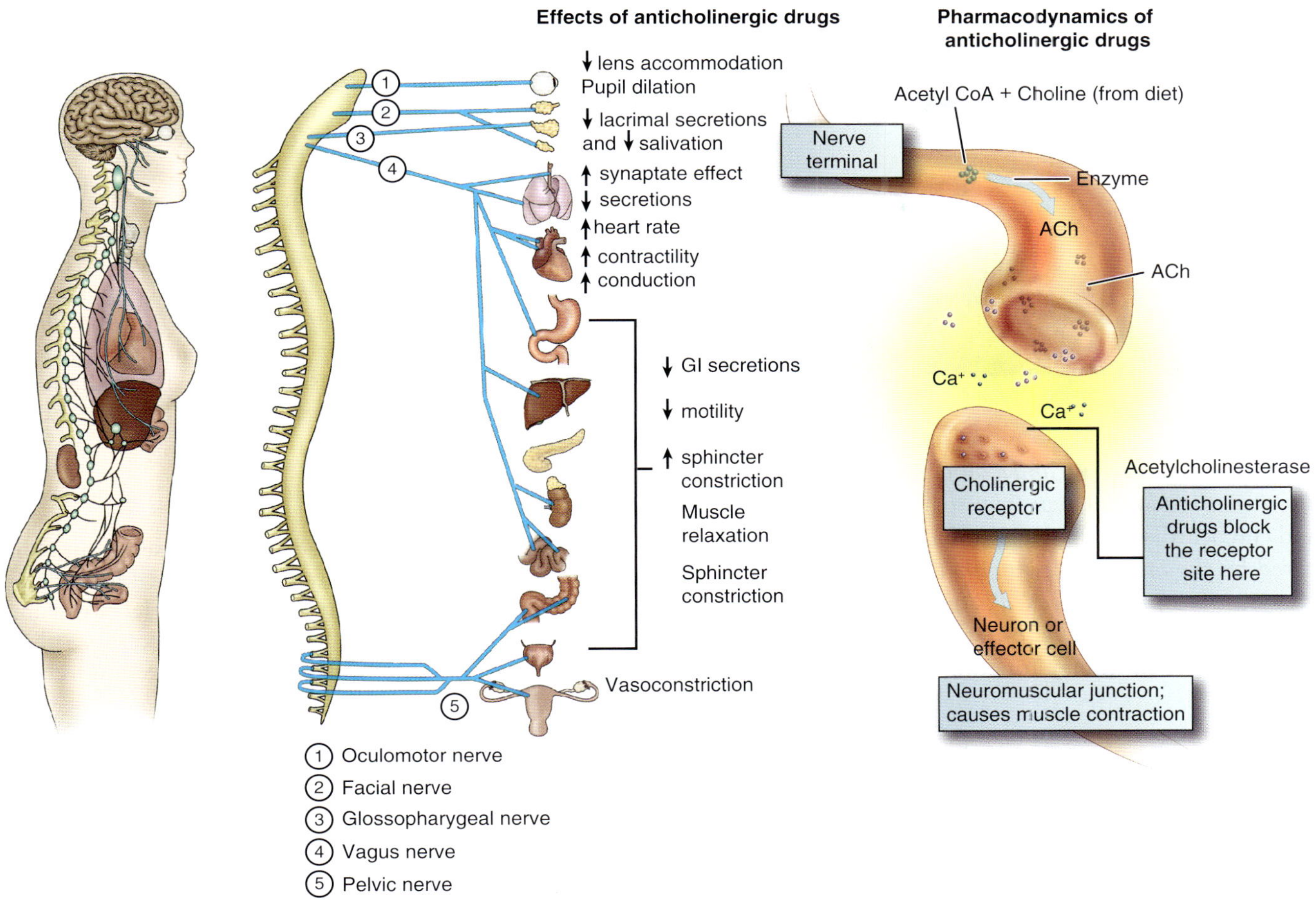

FIGURE 33.1 Pharmacodynamics of anticholinergic drugs and associated physiological responses.

Pharmacokinetics

The anticholinergics are well absorbed after oral and parenteral administration. Atropine is administered through oral (PO), intramuscular (IM), intravenous (IV), subcutaneous (SC) and ophthalmic routes. Propantheline is an oral drug. Glycopyrronium bromide (glycopyrrolate) is available through oral, IM, IV and SC routes. These drugs are widely distributed throughout the body and cross the blood–brain barrier. Their half-lives vary with route and drug. They are excreted in the urine.

Contraindications and cautions

Anticholinergics are contraindicated in the presence of known allergy to any of these drugs *to avoid hypersensitivity reactions*. They are also contraindicated with any condition that could be exacerbated by blockade of the parasympathetic nervous system. These conditions include glaucoma *because of the possibility of increased intraocular pressure with pupil dilation*; stenosing peptic ulcer, intestinal atony and paralytic ileus, *all of which could be exacerbated with a further slowing of GI activity*; prostatic hypertrophy and bladder obstruction, *which could be further compounded by a blocking of*

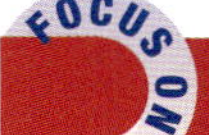

Safe medication administration

Applying dermal patch delivery systems

If a drug has been ordered to be given via a transdermal patch, review the proper technique for applying a transdermal patch. The patch should be applied to a clean, dry, intact and hairless area of the body. Do not shave an area of application – that could abrade the skin and lead to increased absorption. Hair may be clipped if necessary. Peel off the backing without touching the adhesive side of the patch (Figure 33.2). Place the patch at a new site each time to avoid skin irritation or degradation. Be sure to remove the old patch and clean the area when putting on a new transdermal patch. It is important to remember that many transdermal systems contain an aluminised barrier that could cause an electrical charge with arcing, smoke and severe transdermal burns if a defibrillator is discharged over it or if the person has magnetic resonance imaging (MRI). Remove any transdermal patches in the area if a defibrillator is to be used or before the person has an MRI.

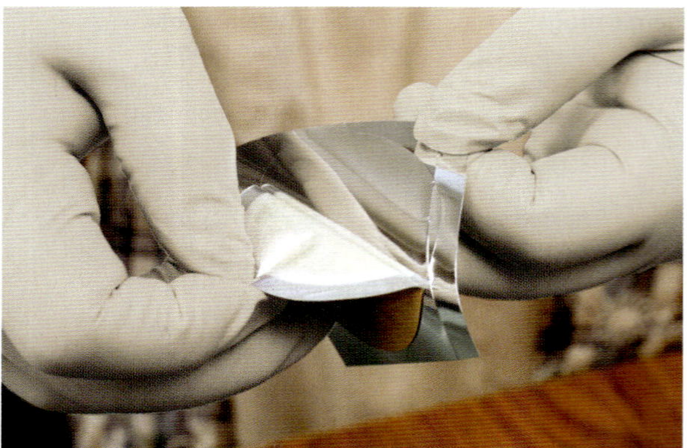

FIGURE 33.2 Carefully remove the backing from the patch without touching the adhesive.

bladder muscle activity and a blocking of sphincter relaxation in the bladder; cardiac arrhythmias, tachycardia and myocardial ischaemia, *which could be exacerbated by the increased sympathetic influence, including tachycardia and increased contractility that occurs when the parasympathetic nervous system is blocked*; impaired liver or kidney function, *which could alter the metabolism and excretion of the drug*; and myasthenia gravis, *which could worsen with further blocking of the cholinergic receptors*. (Low doses of atropine are sometimes used in myasthenia gravis to block unwanted GI and cardiovascular effects of the cholinergic drugs used to treat that condition.)

Caution should be used in women who are breastfeeding *because of possible suppression of breastfeeding*; pregnancy *because of the potential for adverse effects to the fetus*; hypertension *because of the possibility of additive hypertensive effects from the sympathetic system's dominance with parasympathetic nervous system blocking*; and spasticity and brain damage, *which could be exacerbated by cholinergic blockade within the CNS*.

Adverse effects

The adverse effects associated with the use of anticholinergic drugs are caused by the systemic blockade of cholinergic receptors. What are adverse effects in some cases may be the desired therapeutic effects in others (Table 33.2). The intensity of adverse effects is related

TABLE 33.2 Effects of parasympathetic blockade and associated therapeutic uses

Physiological effect	Therapeutic uses
Gastrointestinal Smooth muscle: blocks spasm, blocks peristalsis Secretory glands: decreases acid and digestive enzyme production	Decreases motility and secretory activity in peptic ulcer, gastritis, cardiospasm, pylorospasm, enteritis, diarrhoea, hypertonic constipation
Urinary tract Decreases tone and motility in the ureters and fundus of the bladder; increases tone in the bladder sphincter	Increases bladder capacity in children with enuresis, spastic paraplegics; decreases urinary urgency and frequency in cystitis; antispasmodic in renal colic and to counteract bladder spasm caused by morphine
Biliary tract Relaxes smooth muscle, antispasmodic	Relief of biliary colic; counteracts spasms caused by narcotics
Bronchial muscle Weakly relaxes smooth muscle	Aerosol form may be used in asthma; may counteract bronchoconstriction caused by drugs
Cardiovascular system Increases heart rate (may decrease heart rate at very low doses); causes local vasodilation and flushing	Counteracts bradycardia caused by vagal stimulation, carotid sinus syndrome, surgical procedures; used to overcome heart blocks following MI; used to counteract hypotension caused by cholinergic drugs
Ocular effects Pupil dilation, cycloplegia	Allows ophthalmological examination of the retina, optic disc; relaxes ocular muscles and decreases irritation in iridocyclitis, choroiditis
Secretions Reduces sweating, salivation, respiratory tract secretions	Preoperatively before inhalation anaesthesia; reduces nasal secretions in rhinitis, hay fever; may be used to reduce excessive sweating in hyperhidrosis
Central nervous system Decreases extrapyramidal motor activity Atropine may cause excessive stimulation, psychosis, delirium, disorientation	Decreases tremor in parkinsonism; helps to prevent motion sickness

to drug dose: the more of the drug in the system, the greater are the systemic effects. These adverse effects could include CNS effects, such as blurred vision, pupil dilation and resultant photophobia, cycloplegia and increased intraocular pressure, all of which are related to the blocking of the parasympathetic effects in the eye.

Weakness, dizziness, insomnia, mental confusion and excitement are effects related to cholinergic receptor blockade within the CNS. Dry mouth results from the blocking of GI secretions. Altered taste perception, nausea, heartburn, constipation, bloated feelings and paralytic ileus are related to a slowing of GI activity. Tachycardia and palpitations are possible effects related to blocking of the parasympathetic effects on the heart. Urinary hesitancy and retention are related to the blocking of bladder muscle activity and sphincter relaxation. Decreased sweating and an increased predisposition to heat prostration are related to the inability to cool the body by sweating, a result of blocking of the sympathetic cholinergic receptors responsible for sweating. Suppression of breastfeeding is related to anticholinergic effects in the breasts and in the CNS. The severity of the adverse effects is related to the dose of the drug.

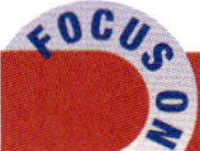

Safe medication administration

Atropine toxicity

Although atropine is used in a large variety of clinical settings (see Table 33.1 for usual indications), this drug can also be a poison, causing severe toxicity. Because it is found in many natural products, including the belladonna plant, and may be present in herbal or alternative therapy products, atropine toxicity can occur inadvertently. Atropine toxicity should be considered whenever a person receiving an anticholinergic drug presents with a sudden onset of bizarre mental and neurological symptoms. Toxicity is dose related and usually progresses as follows:

0.5 mg atropine: slight cardiac slowing, dryness of mouth, inhibition of sweating

1.0 mg atropine: definite mouth and throat dryness, thirst, rapid heart rate, pupil dilation

2.0 mg atropine: rapid heart rate, palpitations; marked mouth dryness; dilated pupils; some blurring of vision

5.0 mg atropine: all of the foregoing and marked speech disturbances; difficulty swallowing; restlessness, fatigue and headache; dry and hot skin; difficulty voiding; reduced intestinal peristalsis

10.0 mg atropine: all of the foregoing symptoms, more marked; pulse rapid and weak; iris nearly gone; vision blurred; skin flushed, hot, dry and scarlet; ataxia; restlessness and excitement; hallucinations; delirium and coma

Treatment is as follows. If the poison was taken orally, immediate gastric lavage should be done to limit absorption. Physostigmine can be used as an antidote, however it is controversial. It can result in serious adverse effects and is only recommended in life-threatening situations. A slow IV injection of 0.5–4 mg (depending on the size of the individual) usually reverses the delirium and coma of atropine toxicity. Physostigmine is metabolised rapidly, so the injection may need to be repeated every 1–2 hours until the atropine has been cleared from the system. Diazepam is the drug of choice if an anticonvulsant is needed. Cool baths and alcohol sponging may relieve the fever and hot skin. In extreme cases, respiratory support may be needed. It is important to remember that the half-life of atropine is 2.5 hours; at extremely high doses, several hours may be needed to clear the atropine from the body.

Clinically important drug–drug interactions

The incidence of anticholinergic effects increases if these drugs are combined with any other drugs with anticholinergic activity, including antihistamines,

Prototype summary: atropine

Indications: to decrease secretions before surgery, treatment of parkinsonism, restoration of cardiac rate and arterial pressure following vagal stimulation, relief of bradycardia and syncope due to hyperactive carotid sinus reflex, relief of pylorospasm, relaxation of the spasm of biliary and ureteral colic and bronchospasm, control of crying and laughing episodes associated with brain lesions, relaxation of uterine hypertonicity, management of peptic ulcer, control of rhinorrhoea associated with hay fever, antidote for cholinergic overdose and poisoning from various mushrooms.

Actions: competitively blocks acetylcholine muscarinic receptor sites, blocking the effects of the parasympathetic nervous system.

Pharmacokinetics:

Route	Onset	Peak	Duration
IM	10–15 min	30 min	4 hours
IV	Immediate	2–4 min	4 hours
SC	Varies	1–2 hours	4 hours
Topical	5–10 min	30–40 min	7–14 days

$T_{1/2}$: 2.5 hours, with metabolism in the liver and excretion in the urine.

Adverse effects: blurred vision, mydriasis, cycloplegia, photophobia, palpitations, bradycardia, dry mouth, altered taste perception, urinary hesitancy and retention, decreased sweating and predisposition to heat prostration (see Focus on safe medication administration for more information about atropine toxicity).

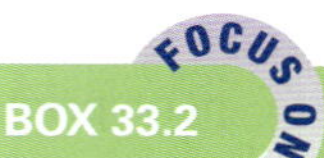

BOX 33.2 Herbal and alternative therapies

The risk of anticholinergic effects can be exacerbated if anticholinergic agents are combined with burdock, rosemary or turmeric used as herbal therapy. Advise people who use herbal therapies to avoid these combinations.

antiparkinsonism drugs, monoamine oxidase (MAO) inhibitors and tricyclic antidepressants (TCAs). If such combinations must be used, the person should be monitored closely and dose adjustments made. People should be advised to avoid over-the-counter products that contain these drugs. The effectiveness of phenothiazines decreases if they are combined with anticholinergic drugs and the risk of paralytic ileus increases. This combination should be avoided. Anticholinergics also may interact with certain herbal therapies (see Box 33.2).

KEY POINTS

- At cholinergic receptor sites, anticholinergic drugs block the effects of acetylcholine. Because they block the effects of the parasympathetic nervous system, they are also known as parasympatholytic drugs.
- When the parasympathetic system is blocked, the pupils dilate, the heart rate rises, and GI activity and urinary bladder tone and function decrease.

Care considerations for people receiving anticholinergic agents

Assessment: history and examination

- Assess for contraindications or cautions: any known allergies to these drugs *to avoid hypersensitivity reactions*; glaucoma; stenosing peptic ulcer, intestinal atony, paralytic ileus, GI obstruction, severe ulcerative colitis and toxic megacolon; prostatic hypertrophy and bladder obstruction; cardiac arrhythmias, tachycardia and myocardial ischaemia, *all of which could be exacerbated by parasympathetic blockade*; impaired liver or kidney function, *which could alter the metabolism and excretion of the drug*; myasthenia gravis, *which could worsen with further blocking of the cholinergic receptors*; pregnancy *because of the potential for adverse effects on the fetus*; breastfeeding *because of possible suppression of breastfeeding*; hypertension *because of the possible additive hypertensive effects*; and muscle spasticity and brain damage, *which could be exacerbated by cholinergic blockade.*

See the Critical thinking scenario to learn more about care for the person who has heart disease and is taking anticholinergic drugs.

- Perform a physical assessment, including a review of all body systems, *to establish baseline status before beginning therapy, determine drug effectiveness and evaluate for any potential adverse effects.*
- Assess neurological status, including level of orientation, affect, reflexes and papillary response, *to evaluate any CNS effects.*
- Monitor vital signs and cardiopulmonary status, including pulse, blood pressure, heart rate and heart sounds; auscultate lung sounds. Obtain an electrocardiogram if ordered *to identify changes in heart rate or rhythm.*
- Assess abdomen; auscultate bowel sounds. Evaluate bowel and bladder patterns; monitor urinary output; palpate bladder for possible distension *to evaluate for GI and GU adverse effects.*
- Monitor the results of laboratory tests, including renal function studies, *to determine need for possible dose adjustment and to identify potential toxicity.*

Implementation with rationale

- Ensure proper administration of the drug *to ensure effective use and decrease the risk of adverse effects (see Focus on safe medication administration).*
- Provide comfort measures *to help the person tolerate drug effects*: sugarless lozenges to suck and frequent mouth care *to alleviate problems associated with dry mouth*; lighting control *to alleviate photophobia*; small and frequent meals *to alleviate GI discomfort*; bowel program, including a high-fibre diet, *to alleviate constipation*; safety precautions, such as side rails if appropriate, assistance with ambulation and advice to avoid driving or operating hazardous machinery *to prevent injury if CNS effects are severe*; analgesics *to relieve pain if headaches occur*; voiding before taking medication *if urinary retention is a problem* (commonly occurs with benign prostatic hyperplasia); and encouraging fluid intake and monitoring heat exposure *because the ability to sweat will be reduced.*
- Monitor response closely, including blood pressure, electrocardiogram, urine output and cardiac output, *for changes that may indicate a need to adjust dose to ensure benefit with the least amount of toxicity.*
- Offer support and encouragement *to help the person deal with the drug regimen.*

- Provide thorough teaching about drug name, dosage and schedule for administration; proper technique for topical application, if appropriate (see Focus on safe medication administration); measures to minimise or prevent adverse effects; safety measures such as avoiding driving, avoiding operating hazardous machinery, staying hydrated and monitoring exposure to heat; dietary recommendations if appropriate; warning signs of problems and the need to report these; and importance of follow-up monitoring and evaluation.

Evaluation

- Monitor response to the drug (improvement in disorder being treated).
- Monitor for adverse effects (cardiovascular changes, GI problems, CNS effects, urinary hesitancy and retention, pupil dilation and photophobia, decrease in sweating and heat intolerance).
- Evaluate the effectiveness of the teaching plan (person can name drug, dosage, adverse effects to watch for and specific measures to avoid them, proper administration of ophthalmic drugs).
- Monitor the effectiveness of comfort measures and compliance with the regimen.

KEY POINTS

- Atropine is the most commonly used anticholinergic drug. It is indicated for a wide variety of conditions and is available in oral, parenteral and topical forms.
- People receiving anticholinergic drugs must be monitored for dry mouth, difficulty swallowing, constipation, urinary retention, tachycardia, pupil dilation and photophobia, cycloplegia and blurring of vision, and heat intolerance caused by a decrease in sweating.

CRITICAL THINKING SCENARIO

Anticholinergic drugs and heart disease

THE SITUATION

E.K., a 64-year-old woman with a long history of heart disease, has experienced repeated bouts of cystitis. The course of her most current infection was marked by severe pain, frequency, urgency and even nocturnal enuresis. She was treated with an antibiotic deemed appropriate after a urine culture and sensitivity test, and she was given oxybutynin to relax her bladder spasms and alleviate some of the unpleasant side effects that she was experiencing. Within the next few days, she plans to travel to a warm climate for the winter and wants any information that she should have before she goes.

CRITICAL THINKING

E.K. presents many care problems. What are the implications of giving an anticholinergic drug to a person with a long history of heart disease?

Repeated bouts of cystitis are not normal; what potential problems should be addressed in this area?

E.K. is about to leave for her winter home in Queensland; what teaching plans will be essential for her if she is taking oxybutynin when she leaves?

What are the medical problems that can arise with people who live in different areas at different times of the year?

Considering her age, what written information should E.K. take with her as she travels?

DISCUSSION

E.K. is doing well with her cardiac problems at the moment, but she could develop problems as a result of the anticholinergic drug that has been prescribed. The anticipated adverse effect of tachycardia could tip the balance in a compensated heart, leading to heart failure or oxygen delivery problems. She will need to be carefully evaluated for the status of her heart disease and potential problems.

E.K. should be further evaluated for the cause of her repeated bouts with cystitis. Does she have a structural problem, a dietary problem, or a simple hygiene problem? She should receive instruction on ways to avoid bladder infections, such as wiping only from front to back, voiding after sexual intercourse, avoiding baths, avoiding citrus juices and other alkaline ash foods that decrease the acidity of the urine and promote bacterial growth, and pushing fluids as much as possible.

E.K. also should be evaluated to establish a baseline for vision, reflexes, the possibility of glaucoma, GI problems, and so on. She should receive thorough teaching about her atropine, especially adverse effects to anticipate, safety measures to take if vision changes occur, and a bowel program that she can follow to avoid constipation.

Because E.K. is leaving a cold climate and travelling to a warm climate, she will need to be warned that oxybutynin decreases sweating. This means that she may be susceptible to heat stroke in the warmer climate. She should be encouraged to take precautions to avoid these problems.

It will be difficult to monitor E.K. while she is away. It should be anticipated that people such as E.K. might have two sets of health care providers who may not communicate with each other. It is important to give E.K. written information about her current diagnosis, including test results; details about her drugs, including dosages; information about the adverse effects she may experience plus ways to deal with them; and ways to avoid cystitis in the future. It may be useful to include a telephone number that E.K. can use or give to her northern health care provider to use if further testing or follow-up is indicated.

CARE GUIDE FOR E.K.: HEART DISEASE

Assessment: history and examination

Assess for a history of allergy to anticholinergic drugs, COPD, narrow-angle glaucoma, myasthenia gravis, bowel or urinary obstruction, tachycardia and recent GI or urinary surgery.

Focus the physical examination on the following:

CV: blood pressure, pulse rate, peripheral perfusion, ECG

CNS: orientation, affect, reflexes, vision

Skin: colour, lesions, texture, sweating

GU: urinary output, bladder tone

GI: abdominal exam

Respiratory: respiratory rate, adventitious sounds

Implementation

Ensure safe and appropriate administration of drug.

Provide comfort and safety measures, including assistance/side rails; temperature control; dark glasses; small, frequent meals; artificial saliva, fluids; sugarless lozenges, mouth care; bowel program.

Provide support and reassurance to deal with drug effects, discomfort and GI effects.

Provide teaching regarding drug name, dosage, adverse effects, precautions and warnings to report.

Monitor blood pressure and pulse rate, and adjust dose as needed.

Evaluation

Evaluate drug effects: pupil dilation, decrease in signs and symptoms being treated.

Monitor for adverse effects: CV effects – tachycardia, heart failure; CNS – confusion, dreams; urinary retention; GI effects – constipation; visual blurring, photophobia.

Monitor for drug–drug interactions as indicated for each drug.

Evaluate effectiveness of teaching program and comfort and safety measures.

TEACHING FOR E.K.

- Anticholinergics are drugs that block or stop the actions of a group of nerves that are part of the parasympathetic nervous system. These drugs may decrease the activity of your GI tract, dilate your pupils, or speed up your heart.
- Some of the following adverse effects may occur:
  - *Dry mouth, difficulty swallowing*: frequent mouth care will help to remove dried secretions and keep the mouth fresh. Sucking on sugarless lollies will help to keep the mouth moist. Taking lots of fluids with meals (unless you are on fluid restriction) will help swallowing.
  - *Blurred vision, sensitivity to light*: if your vision is blurred, avoid driving, operating hazardous machinery, or doing close work that requires attention to detail until your vision returns to normal. Dark glasses will help to protect your eyes from the light.
  - *Retention of urine*: take the drug just after you have emptied your bladder. Moderate your fluid intake while the drug's effects are the highest; if possible, take the drug before bedtime, when this effect will not be a problem.
  - *Constipation*: include fluid and fibre in your diet, and follow any bowel regimen that you may have. Monitor your bowel movements so that appropriate laxatives can be taken if necessary.
  - *Flushing, intolerance to heat, decreased sweating*: this drug blocks sweating, which is your body's way of cooling off. This places you at increased risk for heat stroke. Avoid extremes of temperature, dress coolly on very warm days, and avoid exercise as much as possible.
  - (Report any of the following to your health care provider): *eye pain, skin rash, fever, rapid heartbeat, chest pain, difficulty breathing, agitation or mood changes* (a dose adjustment may help to alleviate this problem).
- Avoid the use of over-the-counter medications, especially for sleep and nasal congestion; avoid antihistamines, diet pills and cold capsules. These products may contain drugs that cause similar anticholinergic effects, which could cause a severe reaction. Consult with your health care provider if you feel that you need medication for symptomatic relief.
- Tell any doctor, nurse or other health care provider involved in your care that you are taking these drugs.
- Keep these drugs, and all medications, out of the reach of children. Do not share these drugs with other people.

CHAPTER SUMMARY

- Anticholinergic drugs, also called parasympatholytic drugs, block the effects of acetylcholine at cholinergic receptor sites, thus blocking the effects of the parasympathetic nervous system.
- Parasympathetic nervous system blockade causes an increase in heart rate, decrease in GI activity, decrease in urinary bladder tone and function, and pupil dilation and cycloplegia.
- These drugs also block cholinergic receptors in the CNS and sympathetic postganglionic cholinergic receptors, including those that cause sweating.
- Many systemic adverse effects associated with the use of anticholinergic drugs are due to the systemic cholinergic blocking effects that also produce the desired therapeutic effect.
- Individuals receiving anticholinergic drugs must be monitored for dry mouth, difficulty swallowing, constipation, urinary retention, tachycardia, pupil dilation and photophobia, cycloplegia and blurring of vision, and heat intolerance caused by a decrease in sweating.

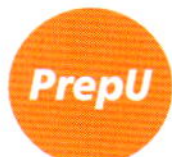

Knowing your strengths and weaknesses helps you to study more effectively. Take a PrepU Practice Quiz to find out how you measure up!

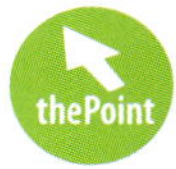

ONLINE RESOURCES

An extensive range of additional resources to enhance teaching and learning and to facilitate understanding of this chapter may be found online at the text's accompanying website, located on thePoint at http://thepoint.lww.com. These include Watch and Learn videos, Concepts in Action animations, journal articles, review questions, case studies, discussion topics and quizzes.

BIBLIOGRAPHY

Farrell, M. & Dempsey, J. (2014). *Smeltzer & Bare's Textbook of Medical-Surgical Nursing* (3rd edn). Sydney: Lippincott Williams & Wilkins.

Goodman, L. S., Brunton, L. L., Chabner, B. & Knollmann, B. C. (2011). *Goodman and Gilman's Pharmacological Basis of Therapeutics* (12th edn). New York: McGraw-Hill.

Graudins, L. V. (2009). Preventing motion sickness in children. *Australian Prescriber, 32*, 61–63.

Kuteesa, W. (2006). Anticholinergic drugs for overactive bladder. *Australian Prescriber, 29*, 22–24.

McKenna, L. & Mirkov, S. (2019). *McKenna's Drug Handbook for Nursing and Midwifery* (8th edn). Sydney: Wolters Kluwer Health Australia.

Porth, C. M. (2011). *Essentials of Pathophysiology: Concepts of Altered Health States* (3rd edn). Philadelphia: Lippincott Williams & Wilkins.

Porth, C. M. (2009). *Pathophysiology: Concepts of Altered Health States* (8th edn). Philadelphia: Lippincott Williams & Wilkins.

Seale, J. P. (2003). Anitcholinergic bronchodilators. *Australian Prescriber, 26*, 33–35.

CHECK YOUR UNDERSTANDING

Answers to the questions in this chapter can be found in Appendix A at the back of this book.

MULTIPLE CHOICE

Select the best answer to the following.

1. Anticholinergic drugs are used:
   a. to allow the sympathetic system to dominate.
   b. to block the parasympathetic system, which is commonly hyperactive.
   c. as the drugs of choice for treating ulcers.
   d. to stimulate GI activity.

2. Atropine and hyoscine work by blocking:
   a. nicotinic receptors only.
   b. muscarinic and nicotinic receptors.
   c. muscarinic receptors only.
   d. adrenergic receptors to allow cholinergic receptors to dominate.

3. Which of the following suggestions would the nurse or midwife make to help a person who is receiving an anticholinergic agent reduce the risks associated with decreased sweating?
   a. covering the head and using sunscreen
   b. ensuring hydration and temperature control
   c. changing position slowly and protecting from the sun
   d. monitoring for difficulty swallowing and breathing

4. Which of the following would the nurse or midwife be least likely to include when developing a teaching plan for a person who is receiving an anticholinergic agent?
   a. encouraging the person to void before dosing
   b. setting up a bowel program to deal with constipation
   c. encouraging the person to use sugarless lozenges to combat dry mouth
   d. performing exercises to increase the heart rate

MULTIPLE RESPONSE

Select all that apply.

1. A nurse or midwife would expect atropine to be used for which of the following?
   a. to depress salivation
   b. to dry up bronchial secretions
   c. to increase the heart rate
   d. to promote uterine contractions
   e. to treat myasthenia gravis
   f. to treat Alzheimer disease

2. Remembering that anticholinergics block the effects of the parasympathetic nervous system, the nurse or midwife would question an order for an anticholinergic drug for people with which of the following conditions?
   a. ulcerative colitis
   b. asthma
   c. bradycardia
   d. inner ear imbalance
   e. glaucoma
   f. prostatic hyperplasia

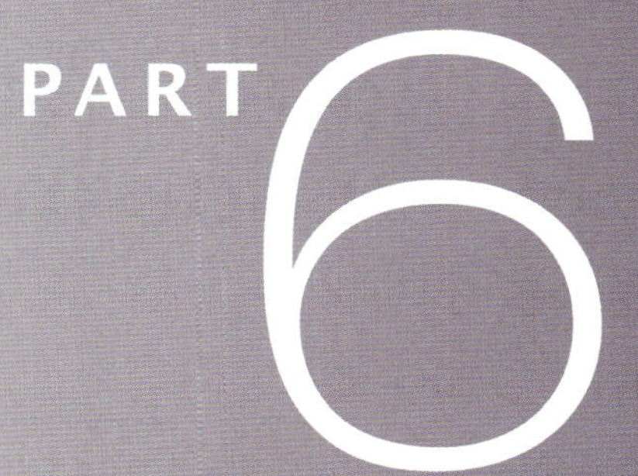

Drugs acting on the endocrine system

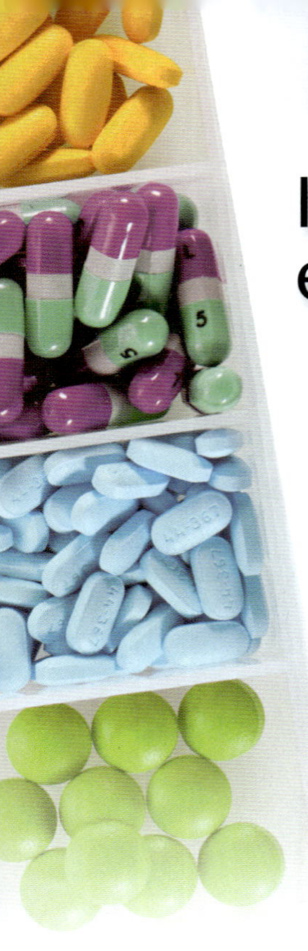

Introduction to the endocrine system

34

Learning objectives

On completing this chapter you should be able to:

1. Label a diagram showing the glands of the traditional endocrine system and list the hormones produced by each.
2. Describe two theories of hormone action.
3. Discuss the role of the hypothalamus as the master gland of the endocrine system, including influences on the actions of the hypothalamus.
4. Outline a negative feedback system within the endocrine system and explain the ways that this system controls hormone levels in the body.
5. Describe the hypothalamic–pituitary axis (HPA) and what would happen if a hormone level was altered within the HPA.

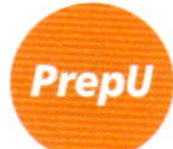

Test your current knowledge of the endocrine system with a PrepU Practice Quiz!

Glossary of key terms

anterior pituitary: lobe of the pituitary gland that produces stimulating hormones, as well as growth hormone, prolactin and melanocyte-stimulating hormone
diurnal rhythm: response of the hypothalamus and then the pituitary and adrenals to wakefulness and sleeping
glands: organised groups of specialised cells that secrete hormones, or chemical messengers, directly into the bloodstream to communicate within the body
hormones: chemical messengers working within the endocrine system to communicate within the body
hypothalamic–pituitary axis (HPA): interconnection of the hypothalamus and pituitary to regulate the levels of certain endocrine hormones through a complex series of negative feedback systems
hypothalamus: 'master gland' of the neuroendocrine system; regulates both nervous and endocrine responses to internal and external stimuli
negative feedback system: control system in which increasing levels of a hormone lead to decreased levels of releasing and stimulating hormones, leading to decreased hormone levels, which stimulates the release of releasing and stimulating hormones; allows tight control of the endocrine system
neuroendocrine system: the combination of the nervous and endocrine systems, which work closely together to maintain regulatory control and homeostasis in the body
pituitary gland: gland found in the sella turcica of the brain; produces hormones, endorphins and encephalins and stores two hypothalamic hormones
posterior pituitary: lobe of the pituitary that receives antidiuretic hormone and oxytocin via nerve axons from the hypothalamus and stores them to be released when stimulated by the hypothalamus
releasing hormones or factors: chemicals released by the hypothalamus into the anterior pituitary to stimulate the release of anterior pituitary hormones

The endocrine system, in conjunction with the nervous system, works to maintain internal homeostasis and to integrate the body's response to the external environment. Their activities and functions are so closely related that it is probably more correct to refer to them as the **neuroendocrine system**. However, this section deals with drugs affecting the 'traditional' endocrine system, which includes **glands** – organised groups of specialised cells that produce and secrete chemical messengers called **hormones** directly into the bloodstream to communicate within the body.

Some organs function like endocrine glands, but they are not considered part of the traditional endocrine system. In addition, certain hormones that influence body functioning are not secreted by endocrine glands. For example, prostaglandins are tissue hormones produced in various tissues; they do not enter the bloodstream, but exert their effects just in the area where they are released. Moreover, neurotransmitters, such as noradrenaline and dopamine, can be classified as hormones because they are secreted directly into the bloodstream for dispersion throughout the body. There also are many gastrointestinal (GI) hormones that are produced in GI cells and act locally. All of these hormones are addressed in the chapters most related to their effects.*

STRUCTURE AND FUNCTION OF THE ENDOCRINE SYSTEM

The endocrine system provides communication within the body and helps to regulate growth and development, reproduction, energy use and electrolyte balance. The endocrine system is closely interconnected with the nervous system, and the two systems work to maintain homeostasis within the body to ensure maximum function and adequate response to various internal and external stressors.

Glands

The endocrine glands are collections of specialised cells that produce hormones that cause an effect at hormone-receptor sites. These glands do not have ducts, so they secrete their hormones directly into the bloodstream. There are many endocrine glands in the body. Table 34.1 lists the endocrine glands, the hormones that they produce and the clinical effects that the hormones cause.

Hormones

Hormones are chemicals that are produced in the body and that meet specific criteria. All hormones:

- are produced in very small amounts.
- are secreted directly into the bloodstream.
- travel through the blood to specific receptor sites throughout the body.
- act to increase or decrease the normal metabolic cellular processes when they react with their specific receptor sites.
- are immediately broken down.

Hormones may act in two different ways. Some hormones react with specific receptor sites on a cell membrane to stimulate the nucleotide cyclic adenosine monophosphate (cAMP) within the cell to cause an effect. For example, when insulin interacts with an insulin-receptor site, it activates intracellular enzymes that cause many effects, including changing the cell membrane's permeability to glucose. Hormones such as insulin that do not enter the cell but react with specific receptor sites on the cell membrane act very quickly – often within seconds – to produce an effect.

Other hormones, such as oestrogen, actually enter the cell and interact with a receptor site inside the cell to change messenger RNA, which enters the cell nucleus to affect cellular DNA and thereby alters the cell's function. These hormones that enter the cell before they can cause an effect take quite a while to produce an effect. The full effects of oestrogen may not be seen for months to years, as evidenced by the changes that occur at puberty. Because the neuroendocrine system tightly regulates the body's processes within a narrow range of normal limits, overproduction or underproduction of any hormone can affect the body's activities and other hormones within the system.

KEY POINTS

- The endocrine system and the nervous system regulate body functions and maintain homeostasis largely with the help of hormones. Hormones are chemicals produced within the body that increase or decrease cellular activity.
- The endocrine system regulates growth and development, reproduction, energy use in the body and electrolyte balance.
- Hormones can react with receptors on the cell membrane to cause an immediate effect on a cell by altering enzyme systems near the cell membrane, or they may enter the cell and react with receptor sites on messenger RNA, which then enters the nucleus and alters cell function.

*Gastrointestinal hormones are discussed in Part 11: Drugs acting on the gastrointestinal system. Neurotransmitters acting like hormones are discussed in Chapter 29: Introduction to the autonomic nervous system. The reproductive hormones are discussed in Chapter 39: Introduction to the reproductive system. Hormones active in the inflammatory and immune response are discussed in Part 3: Drugs acting on the immune system. Specific traditional endocrine glands and hormones are discussed in Chapter 35 (hypothalamic and pituitary hormones), Chapter 36 (adrenocortical hormones), Chapter 37 (thyroid and parathyroid hormones) and Chapter 38 (pancreatic hormones).

TABLE 34.1 Endocrine glands with associated hormones and clinical effects

Gland	Hormones produced	Principal effects
Adrenal cortex	Cortisol	Increases glucose levels, suppresses inflammatory and immune reactions
	Aldosterone	Sodium retention, potassium excretion
Intestine	Secretin, cholecystokinin	Decreases gastric movement, stimulates bile and pancreatic juice secretion
Kidney (juxtaglomerular cells)	Erythropoietin	Increases red blood cell production
	Renin	Stimulates increase in blood pressure and vascular volume
Ovaries	Oestrogen, progesterone	Promotes secondary sex characteristics, prepares the female body for pregnancy
Pancreas	Insulin, glucagon, somatostatin	Regulation of glucose, fat metabolism (islets of Langerhans)
Parathyroid glands	Parathyroid hormone	Increases serum calcium levels
Pineal gland	Melatonin	Affects secretion of hypothalamic hormones, particularly gonadotropin-releasing hormone
Placenta	Oestrogens, progesterones	Maintains fetal growth and development, prepares the body for birth
Stomach	Gastrin	Stimulates stomach acid production
Testes	Testosterone	Stimulates secondary sex characteristics in males
Thyroid	Thyroid hormone	Stimulates basal metabolic rate (how the body uses energy)
	Calcitonin	Decreases serum calcium levels

THE HYPOTHALAMUS

The **hypothalamus** is the coordinating centre for the nervous and endocrine responses to internal and external stimuli. The hypothalamus constantly monitors the body's homeostasis by analysing input from the periphery and the central nervous system (CNS) and coordinating responses through the autonomic, endocrine and nervous systems. In effect, it is the 'master gland' of the neuroendocrine system. This title was once given to the pituitary gland because of its many functions and well-protected location (see later discussion).

The hypothalamus has various neurocentres – areas specifically sensitive to certain stimuli – that regulate a number of body functions, including body temperature, thirst, hunger, water retention, blood pressure, respiration, reproduction and emotional reactions. Situated at the base of the forebrain, the hypothalamus receives input from virtually all other areas of the brain, including the limbic system and the cerebral cortex. Because of its positioning, the hypothalamus is able to influence, and be influenced by, emotions and thoughts. The hypothalamus is also located in an area of the brain that is poorly protected by the blood–brain barrier, so it is able to act as a sensor to various electrolytes, chemicals and hormones that are in circulation and do not affect other areas of the brain.

The hypothalamus maintains internal homeostasis by sensing blood chemistries and by stimulating or suppressing endocrine, autonomic and CNS activity. In essence, it can turn the autonomic nervous system and its effects on or off. The hypothalamus also produces and secretes a number of **releasing hormones or factors** that stimulate the pituitary gland, which in turn stimulates or inhibits various endocrine glands throughout the body (see Figure 34.1). These releasing hormones include growth hormone–releasing hormone (GHRH), thyrotropin-releasing hormone (TRH), gonadotropin-releasing hormone (GnRH), corticotropin-releasing hormone (CRH) and prolactin-releasing hormone (PRH). The hypothalamus also produces two inhibiting factors that act as regulators to shut off the production of hormones when levels become too high: growth hormone release–inhibiting factor (somatostatin) and prolactin-inhibiting factor (PIF). Recent research has indicated that PIF may actually be dopamine, a neurotransmitter. People who are taking dopamine-blocking drugs often develop galactorrhoea (inappropriate milk production) and breast enlargement, theoretically because PIF is also blocked and prolactin levels continue to rise, stimulating breast tissue and milk production. Research is ongoing about the chemical structure of several of the releasing factors.

The hypothalamus is connected to the pituitary gland by two networks: a vascular network carries the hypothalamic releasing factors directly into the anterior pituitary, and a neurological network delivers two other hypothalamic hormones – antidiuretic hormone (ADH) and oxytocin – to the posterior pituitary to be stored. These hormones are released as needed by the body when stimulated by the hypothalamus.

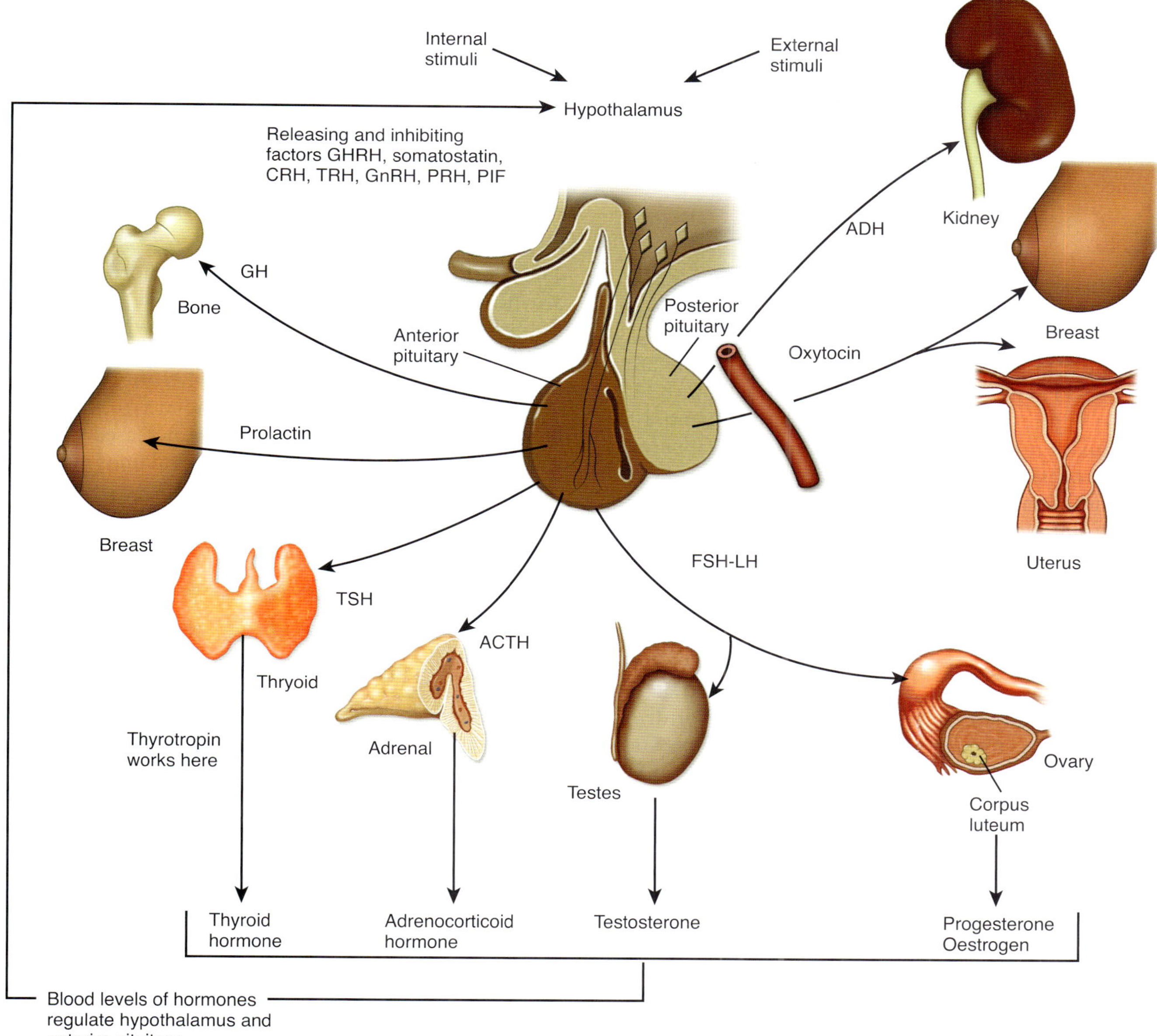

FIGURE 34.1 The traditional endocrine system. The hypothalamus secretes releasing factors to stimulate the parathyroid gland to produce stimulating factors that enter the circulation and react with specific target glands, which produce endocrine hormones.

KEY POINTS

- As the 'master gland' of the neuroendocrine system, the hypothalamus helps to regulate the central and autonomic nervous systems and the endocrine system to maintain homeostasis.
- The hypothalamus produces stimulating and inhibiting factors that travel to the anterior pituitary to stimulate the release of pituitary hormones or block the production of certain pituitary hormones when levels of target hormones get too high.
- The hypothalamus is connected to the posterior pituitary by a nerve network that delivers the hypothalamic hormones ADH and oxytocin to be stored in the posterior pituitary until the hypothalamus stimulates their release.

THE PITUITARY GLAND

The **pituitary gland** is located in the skull in the bony sella turcica under a layer of dura mater. It is divided into three lobes: an anterior lobe, a posterior lobe and an intermediate lobe. Traditionally, the anterior pituitary was known as the body's master gland because it has so many important functions and, through feedback mechanisms, regulates the function of many other endocrine glands. In addition, its unique and protected position in the brain led early scientists to believe that it must be the chief control gland. However, as knowledge of the endocrine system has grown, scientists now designate the hypothalamus as the master gland because it has even greater direct regulatory effects over the neuroendocrine system, including stimulation of the pituitary gland to produce its hormones.

The anterior pituitary

The **anterior pituitary** produces six major hormones: growth hormone (GH), adrenocorticotropic hormone (ACTH), follicle-stimulating hormone (FSH), luteinising hormone (LH), prolactin (PRL) and thyroid-stimulating hormone (TSH, also called thyrotropin) (Table 34.2; see also Figure 34.1). These hormones are essential for the regulation of growth, reproduction and some metabolic processes. Deficiency or overproduction of these hormones disrupts this regulation.

The anterior pituitary hormones are released in a rhythmic manner into the bloodstream. Their secretion varies with time of day (often referred to as **diurnal rhythm**) or with physiological conditions such as exercise or sleep. Their release is affected by activity in the CNS; by hypothalamic hormones; by hormones of the peripheral endocrine glands; by certain diseases that can alter endocrine functioning; and by a variety of drugs, which can directly or indirectly upset the homeostasis in the body and cause an endocrine response. Normally, diurnal rhythm occurs when the hypothalamus begins secretion of corticotropin-releasing factor (CRF) in the evening, peaking at about midnight; adrenocortical peak response is between 6 and 9 a.m.; levels fall during the day until evening, when the low level is picked up by the hypothalamus and CRF secretion begins again.

The anterior pituitary also produces melanocyte-stimulating hormone (MSH) and various lipotropins. MSH plays an important role in animals that use skin colour changes as an adaptive mechanism. It might also be important for nerve growth and development in humans. Lipotropins stimulate fat mobilisation but have not been clearly isolated in humans.

The posterior pituitary

The **posterior pituitary** stores two hormones that are produced by the hypothalamus and deposited in the posterior lobe via the nerve axons where they are produced. These two hormones are ADH, also referred to as vasopressin and oxytocin. ADH is directly released in response to increased plasma osmolarity or decreased blood volume (which often results in increased osmolarity). The osmoreceptors in the hypothalamus stimulate the release of ADH. Oxytocin stimulates uterine smooth muscle contraction in late phases of pregnancy and also causes milk release or 'let down' reflex in breastfeeding women. Its release is stimulated by various hormones and neurological stimuli associated with labour and with breastfeeding.

The intermediate lobe

The intermediate lobe of the pituitary produces endorphins and encephalins, which are released in response to severe pain or stress and occupy specific endorphin-receptor sites in the brainstem to block the perception of pain. These hormones are also produced in peripheral tissues and in other areas of the brain. They are released in response to overactivity of pain nerves, sympathetic stimulation, transcutaneous stimulation, guided imagery and vigorous exercise.

TABLE 34.2 Hypothalamic hormones, associated anterior pituitary hormones and target organ response

Hypothalamus hormones	Anterior pituitary hormones	Target organ response
Stimulating hormones		
CRH (corticotropin-releasing hormone)	ACTH (adrenocorticotropic hormone)	Production of adrenal corticosteroid hormones
TRH (thyroid-releasing hormone)	TSH (thyroid-stimulating hormone)	Production of thyroid hormone
GHRH (growth hormone–releasing hormone)	GH (growth hormone)	Cell growth
GnRH (gonadotropin-releasing hormone)	LH and FSH (luteinising hormone, follicle-stimulating hormone)	Production of oestrogen and progesterone (females) and testosterone (males)
PRH (prolactin-releasing hormone)	Prolactin	Milk production
	MSH (melanocyte-stimulating hormone)	Melanin stimulation (colour change in animals, nerve growth in humans)
Inhibiting hormones		
Somatostatin (growth hormone-inhibiting factor)		Stops release of GH
PIF (prolactin-inhibiting factors)		Stops release of prolactin

KEY POINTS

- The pituitary gland has three lobes: the anterior lobe produces stimulating hormones in response to hypothalamic stimulation.
- The posterior lobe of the pituitary stores ADH and oxytocin, which are two hormones produced by the hypothalamus.
- The intermediate lobe of the pituitary produces endorphins and encephalins to modulate pain perception.

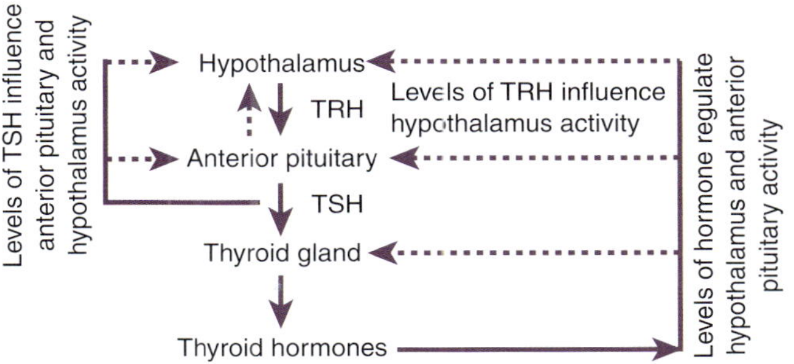

FIGURE 34.2 Negative feedback system. Thyroid hormone levels are regulated by a series of negative feedback systems influencing thyrotropin-releasing hormone (TRH), thyrotropin (TSH) and thyroid hormone levels.

ENDOCRINE REGULATION

The production and release of hormones needs to be tightly regulated within the body. Hormones are released in small amounts to accomplish what needs to be done to maintain homeostasis within the body. The fine tuning and regulation of hormone release through the hypothalamus is often regulated by a series of negative feedback systems. Other hormones are not controlled in this fashion but respond to other direct stimuli.

Hypothalamic–pituitary axis

Because of its position in the brain, the hypothalamus is stimulated by many things, such as light, emotion, cerebral cortex activity and a variety of chemical and hormonal stimuli. Together, the hypothalamus and the pituitary function closely to maintain endocrine activity along what is called the **hypothalamic–pituitary axis (HPA)** using a series of negative feedback systems.

A **negative feedback system** works much like the law of supply and demand in business. In business, when there is an adequate supply of a product, production of that product will slow down because there is an adequate supply and no current demand for it. When the supply is used up, demand will increase, and so production will pick up. Production continues until the supply is adequate and demand is reduced. When the hypothalamus senses a need for a particular hormone, for example, thyroid hormone, it secretes the releasing factor TRH directly into the anterior pituitary. In response to the TRH, the anterior pituitary secretes TSH, which in turn stimulates the thyroid gland to produce thyroid hormone. When the hypothalamus senses the rising levels of thyroid hormone, it stops secreting TRH, resulting in decreased TSH production and subsequent reduced thyroid hormone levels. The hypothalamus, sensing the falling thyroid hormone levels, secretes TRH again. The negative feedback system continues in this fashion, maintaining the levels of thyroid hormone within a relatively narrow range of normal (see Figure 34.2).

It is thought that this feedback system is more complex than once believed. The hypothalamus probably also senses TRH and TSH levels and regulates TRH secretion within a narrow range, even if thyroid hormone is not produced. The anterior pituitary may also be sensitive to TSH levels and thyroid hormone, regulating its own production of TSH. This complex system provides backup controls and regulation if any part of the HPA fails. This system can also create complications, especially when there is a need to override or interact with the total system, as is the case with hormone replacement therapy or the treatment of endocrine disorders. Supplying an exogenous hormone, for example, may increase the hormone levels in the body, but then may affect the HPA to stop production of releasing and stimulating hormones, leading to a decrease in the body's normal production of the hormone.

Two of the anterior pituitary hormones (i.e. growth hormone and prolactin) do not have a target organ to produce hormones and so cannot be regulated by the same type of feedback mechanism. The hypothalamus in this case responds directly to rising levels of growth hormone and prolactin. When levels rise, the hypothalamus releases the inhibiting factors somatostatin and PIF directly to inhibit the pituitary's release of growth hormone and prolactin, respectively. The HPA functions through negative feedback loops or the direct use of inhibiting factors to constantly keep these hormones regulated.

Other forms of regulation

Hormones other than stimulating hormones are also released in response to stimuli. For example, the pancreas produces and releases insulin, glucagon and somatostatin from different cells in response to varying blood glucose levels. The parathyroid glands release parathyroid hormone, or parathormone, in response to local calcium levels. The juxtaglomerular cells in the kidney release erythropoietin and renin in response to decreased pressure or decreased oxygenation of the blood flowing into the glomerulus. GI hormones are released in response to local stimuli in areas of the GI tract, such as acid, proteins or calcium. The thyroid gland produces and secretes another hormone, called calcitonin, in direct response to serum calcium levels. Many different prostaglandins are released throughout the body in response to local stimuli in the tissues that produce them. Activation of the sympathetic nervous system directly causes release of ACTH and the adrenocorticoid hormones to prepare the body for fight or flight. Aldosterone, an adrenocorticoid hormone, is released in response to ACTH but is also released directly in response to high potassium levels.

As more is learned about the interactions of the nervous and endocrine systems, new ideas are being formed about how the body controls its intricate homeostasis. When administering any drug that affects the endocrine or nervous systems, it is important for the nurse and midwife to remember how closely related all of these activities are. Expected or unexpected adverse effects involving areas of the endocrine and nervous systems often occur.

KEY POINTS

- The hypothalamus and pituitary operate by a series of negative feedback mechanisms called the hypothalamic–pituitary axis (HPA). The hypothalamus secretes releasing factors to cause the anterior pituitary to release stimulating hormones, which act with specific endocrine glands to cause the release of hormones.
- Growth hormone and prolactin are released by the anterior pituitary and directly influence cell activity. These hormones are regulated by the release of the hypothalamic inhibiting factors somatostatin and PIF in response to the levels of the pituitary hormones growth hormone and prolactin.
- Some hormones are not influenced by the HPA and are released in response to direct local stimulation.

CHAPTER SUMMARY

- The endocrine system is a regulatory system that communicates through the use of hormones.
- Because the endocrine and nervous systems are tightly intertwined in the regulation of body homeostasis, they are often referred to as the neuroendocrine system.
- A hormone is a chemical that is produced within the body, is needed in only small amounts, travels to specific receptor sites to cause an increase or decrease in cellular activity and is broken down immediately.
- As the 'master gland' of the neuroendocrine system, the hypothalamus helps to regulate the central and autonomic nervous systems and the endocrine system to maintain homeostasis.
- The pituitary is made up of three lobes: anterior, posterior and intermediate. The anterior lobe produces stimulating hormones in response to hypothalamic stimulation. The posterior lobe stores two hormones produced by the hypothalamus – ADH and oxytocin. The intermediate lobe produces endorphins and encephalins to modulate pain perception.
- The hypothalamus and pituitary operate by a series of negative feedback mechanisms called the hypothalamic–pituitary axis (HPA). The hypothalamus secretes releasing factors to cause the anterior pituitary to release stimulating hormones, which act with specific endocrine glands to cause the release of hormones or, in the case of growth hormone and prolactin, to stimulate cells directly. This stimulation shuts down the production of releasing factors, which leads to decreased stimulating factors and, subsequently, decreased hormone release.
- Growth hormone and prolactin are released by the anterior pituitary and directly influence cell activity. These hormones are regulated by the release of hypothalamic inhibiting factors in response to hormone levels or a cellular mediator.
- Some hormones are not influenced by the HPA and are released in response to direct local stimulation.
- When any drug that affects either the endocrine or the nervous system is given, adverse effects may occur throughout both systems because they are closely interrelated.

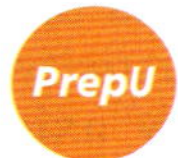

Knowing your strengths and weaknesses helps you to study more effectively. Take a PrepU Practice Quiz to find out how you measure up!

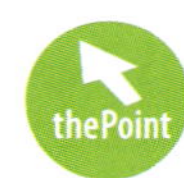

ONLINE RESOURCES

An extensive range of additional resources to enhance teaching and learning and to facilitate understanding of this chapter may be found online at the text's accompanying website, located on thePoint at http://thepoint.lww.com. These include Watch and Learn videos, Concepts in Action animations, journal articles, review questions, case studies, discussion topics and quizzes.

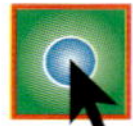

WEB LINKS

Students may want to explore up-to-date information from the following web resources:

www.innerbody.com/image/endoov.html
Travel through the virtual endocrine system.

www.vivo.colostate.edu/hbooks/pathphys/endocrine
Interactive review of the endocrine system and hormones.

BIBLIOGRAPHY

Finlayson, A. & Sanders, S. (2007). (Eds.). *Endocrine and Reproductive Systems* (3rd edn). Edinburgh: Mosby.

Gardner, D. G., Greenspan, F. S. & Shoback, D. M. (Eds.). (2011). *Basic and Clinical Endocrinology* (9th edn). New York: McGraw-Hill.

Goldman, L. & Shafer, A. I. (Eds.). (2012). *Goldman's Cecil's Medicine* (24th edn). Philadelphia: Saunders.

Goodman, L. S., Brunton, L. L., Chabner, B. & Knollmann, B.C. (2011). *Goodman and Gilman's Pharmacological Basis of Therapeutics* (12th edn). New York: McGraw-Hill.

Guyton, A. & Hall, J. (2011). *Textbook of Medical Physiology* (12th edn). Philadelphia: Saunders Elsevier.

Longo, D. L., Facui, A. S., Kasper, D. L., Hauser, S. L., Jameson, J. L. & Loscalzo, J. (2012). *Harrison's Principles of Internal Medicine* (18th edn). New York: McGraw-Hill.

McKenna, L. & Mirkov, S. (2019). *McKenna's Drug Handbook for Nursing and Midwifery* (8th edn). Sydney: Wolters Kluwer Health Australia.

Porth, C. M. (2011). *Essentials of Pathophysiology: Concepts of Altered Health States* (3rd edn). Philadelphia: Lippincott Williams & Wilkins.

Porth, C. M. (2009). *Pathophysiology: Concepts of Altered Health States* (8th edn). Philadelphia: Lippincott Williams & Wilkins.

Williams, R. H. & Melmed, S. (Eds.). (2011). *Williams Textbook of Endocrinology* (12th edn). Philadelphia: Elsevier Saunders.

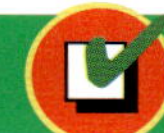

CHECK YOUR UNDERSTANDING

Answers to the questions in this chapter can be found in Appendix A at the back of this book.

MULTIPLE CHOICE

Select the best answer to the following.

1. Which of the following best describes aldosterone?
   a. It causes the loss of sodium and water from the renal tubules.
   b. It is under direct hormonal control from the hypothalamus.
   c. It is released into the bloodstream in response to angiotensin I.
   d. It is released into the bloodstream in response to high potassium levels.

2. When explaining the role of antidiuretic hormone (ADH) to a group of students, which of the following would the instructor include?
   a. It is produced by the anterior pituitary.
   b. It causes the retention of water by the kidneys.
   c. It is released by the hypothalamus.
   d. It causes the retention of sodium by the kidneys.

3. The endocrine glands:
   a. form part of the communication system of the body.
   b. cannot be stimulated by hormones circulating in the blood.
   c. cannot be viewed as integrating centres of reflex arcs.
   d. are only controlled by the hypothalamus.

4. The hypothalamus maintains internal homeostasis and could be considered the master endocrine gland because:
   a. it releases stimulating hormones that cause endocrine glands to produce their hormones.
   b. no hormone-releasing gland responds unless stimulated by the hypothalamus.
   c. it secretes releasing hormones that are an important part of the hypothalamic–pituitary axis.
   d. it regulates temperature control and arousal, as well as hormone release.

5. The posterior lobe of the pituitary gland:
   a. secretes a number of stimulating hormones.
   b. produces endorphins to modulate pain perception.
   c. has no function that has yet been identified.
   d. stores ADH and oxytocin, which are produced in the hypothalamus.

6. After teaching a group of students about the negative feedback system, identification of which of the following as an example would indicate that the students have understood the teaching?
   a. growth hormone control
   b. prolactin control
   c. melanocyte-stimulating hormone control
   d. thyroid hormone control

7. Internal body homeostasis and communication are regulated by:
   a. the cardiovascular and respiratory systems.
   b. the nervous and cardiovascular systems.
   c. the endocrine and nervous systems.
   d. the endocrine and cardiovascular systems.

MULTIPLE RESPONSE

Select all that apply.

1. Hormones exert their influence on human cells by influencing which of the following?
   a. enzyme-controlled reactions
   b. messenger RNA
   c. lysosome activity
   d. transcription RNA
   e. cellular DNA
   f. cyclic AMP activity

2. The specific criteria that define a hormone would include which of the following?
   a. It is produced in very small amounts.
   b. It is secreted directly into the bloodstream.
   c. It is slowly metabolised in the liver and lungs.
   d. It reacts with a very specific receptor set on a target cell.
   e. A mechanism is always available to immediately destroy it.
   f. It can change a cell's basic function.

3. Some endocrine glands do not respond to the hypothalamic–pituitary axis. These glands include the:
   a. thyroid gland.
   b. ovaries.
   c. parathyroid glands.
   d. adrenal cortex.
   e. endocrine pancreas.
   f. GI gastrin-secreting cells.

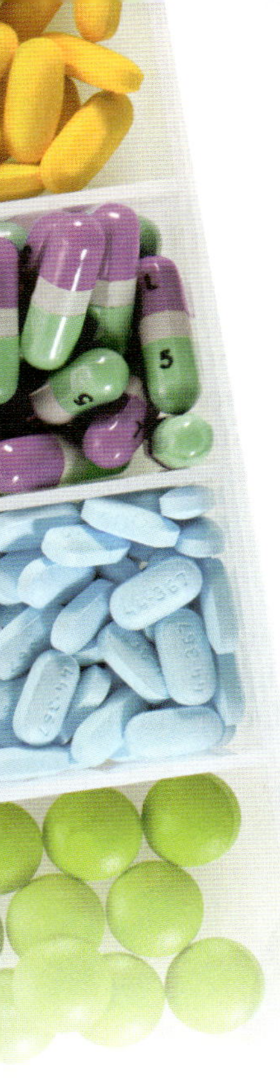

Hypothalamic and pituitary agents

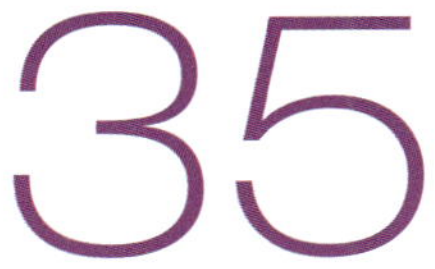

Learning objectives

On completing this chapter you should be able to:

1. Describe the anatomical and physiological relationship between the hypothalamus and the pituitary gland and list the hormones produced by each.
2. Describe the therapeutic actions, indications, pharmacokinetics, contraindications, most common adverse reactions and important drug–drug interactions associated with the hypothalamic and pituitary agents.
3. Discuss the use of hypothalamic and pituitary agents across the lifespan.
4. Compare and contrast the prototype drugs leuprorelin, somatropin, bromocriptine mesilate and desmopressin with other hypothalamic and pituitary agents.
5. Outline the care considerations, including important teaching points, for people receiving a hypothalamic or pituitary agent.

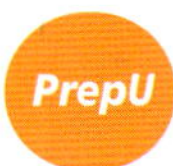

Test your current knowledge of hypothalamic and pituitary agents with a PrepU Practice Quiz!

Glossary of key terms

acromegaly: thickening of bony surfaces in response to excess growth hormone after the epiphyseal plates have closed
diabetes insipidus: condition resulting from a lack of antidiuretic hormone, which results in the production of copious amounts of glucose-free urine
dwarfism: small stature, resulting from lack of growth hormone in children
gigantism: response to excess levels of growth hormone before the epiphyseal plates close; heights of over 2 metres are not uncommon
hypopituitarism: lack of adequate function of the pituitary; reflected in many endocrine disorders

DRUGS AFFECTING HYPOTHALAMIC HORMONES

Agonists
goserelin
tetracosactide (tetracosactrin)

Antagonists
cetrorelix
ganirelix
(P) leuprorelin
nafarelin

DRUGS AFFECTING ANTERIOR PITUITARY HORMONES

Growth hormone agonist
(P) somatropin

Growth hormone antagonists
(P) bromocriptine mesilate
lanreotide
octreotide acetate
pegvisomant

Drugs affecting other anterior pituitary hormones
cabergoline
choriogonadotropin alfa
chorionic gonadotropin
quinagolide
thyrotropin alfa

DRUGS AFFECTING POSTERIOR PITUITARY HORMONES
argipressin (vasopressin)
(P) desmopressin

As described in Chapter 34, the endocrine system's main function is to maintain homeostasis. This is achieved through a complex balance of glandular activities that either stimulate or suppress hormone release. Too much or too little glandular activity disrupts the body's homeostasis, leading to various disorders and interfering with the normal functioning of other endocrine glands. The drugs presented in this chapter are those used to either replace or interact with the hormones or factors produced by the hypothalamus and pituitary. See Figure 35.1 for sites of action of hypothalamic and pituitary agents. Box 35.1 discusses the use of these drugs in various age groups.

DRUGS AFFECTING HYPOTHALAMIC HORMONES

The hypothalamus uses a number of hormones or factors to either stimulate or inhibit the release of hormones from the anterior pituitary. Factors that stimulate the release of hormones are growth hormone–releasing hormone (GHRH), thyrotropin-releasing hormone (TRH), gonadotropin-releasing hormone (GnRH), corticotropin-releasing hormone (CRH) and prolactin-releasing hormone (PRH). Factors that inhibit the release of hormones are somatostatin (growth hormone–inhibiting factor) and prolactin-inhibiting factor (PIF).

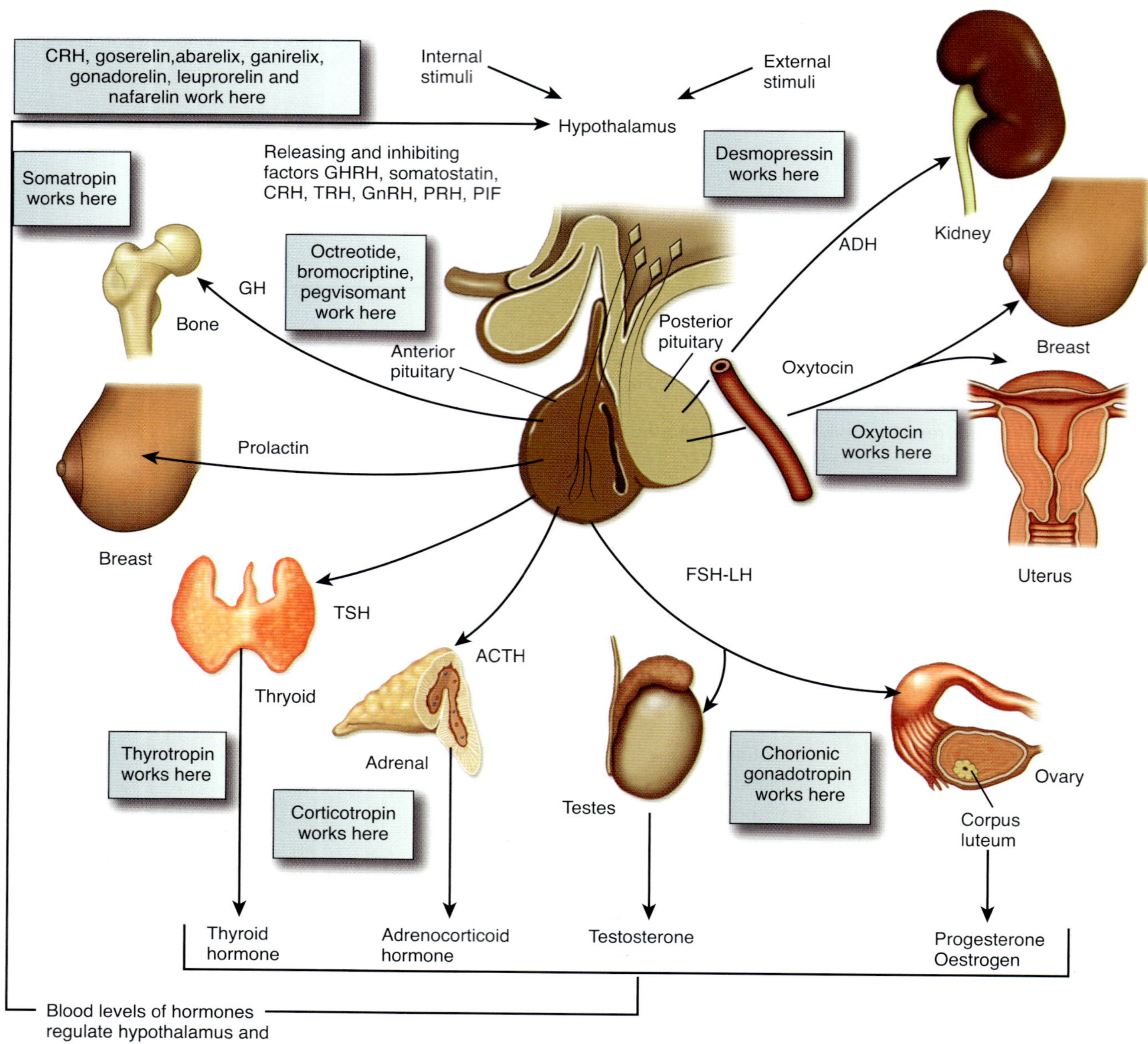

FIGURE 35.1 Sites of action of hypothalamic/pituitary agents.

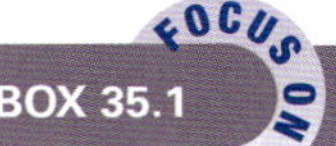

BOX 35.1 Drug therapy across the lifespan

Hypothalamic and pituitary agents

CHILDREN

Children who receive any of the hypothalamic or pituitary agents need to be monitored closely for adverse effects associated with changes in overall endocrine function, particularly growth, development and metabolism. Periodic radiograph of the long bones, as well as monitoring of blood sugar levels and electrolytes, should be a standard part of the treatment plan. Children receiving growth hormone pose many challenges (see Box 35.2). Children who are using desmopressin for diabetes insipidus need to have the administration technique monitored and should have an adult responsible for the overall treatment protocol.

ADULTS

Adults also need frequent monitoring of electrolytes and blood sugar levels when receiving any of these agents. Adults using nasal forms of drugs to control diabetes insipidus should review the proper administration of the drug with the primary care provider periodically; inappropriate administration can lead to complications and lack of therapeutic effect. Adults receiving regular injections of these drugs should learn the proper storage, preparation and administration of the drug, including rotation of injection sites.

PREGNANCY AND BREASTFEEDING

These drugs should not be used during pregnancy or breastfeeding unless the benefit to the mother clearly outweighs any risk to the fetus or neonate because of the potential for severe adverse effects associated with the use of these drugs.

OLDER ADULTS

Older adults may be more susceptible to the imbalances associated with alterations in the endocrine system. They should be evaluated periodically during treatment for hydration and nutrition, as well as for electrolyte balance. Proper administration technique should be reviewed and nasal mucous membranes should be evaluated regularly because older people are more apt to develop dehydrated membranes and possibly ulcerations, leading to improper dosing of drugs delivered nasally.

Not all of these hormones are available for pharmacological use (see Table 34.1 in Chapter 34).

Available hypothalamic releasing hormones include corticotropin-releasing hormone (CRH) (generic), and goserelin (*Zoladex*) (synthetic GnRH). Available antagonists that block the effects of hypothalamic releasing hormones include cetrorelix (*Cetrotide*) (blocks GnRH), ganirelix (*Orgalutran*) (blocks GnRH), leuprorelin (*Eligard*, *Lucrin*) (blocks GnRH effects) and nafarelin (*Synarel*) (blocks GnRH) (not available in New Zealand). See Table 35.1 for a complete list of these drugs.

Therapeutic actions and indications

The hypothalamic hormones are found in such minute quantities that the actual chemical structures of all of

TABLE 35.1 DRUGS IN FOCUS Drugs affecting hypothalamic hormones

Drug name	Dosage/route	Usual indications
Agonists		
tetracosactide (tetracosactrin) (*Synacten, Synacten Depot*)	*Synacten* test: 250 micrograms IM, IV; measure plasma cortisol immediately before and exactly 30 minutes after injection *Synacten Depot*, adult: initially 1 mg IM daily to q 12 hours in acute cases and in oncological indications; usual dosage is 1 mg IM q 2–3 days, reduced to 0.5 mg IM q 2–3 days or 1 mg IM weekly	Diagnosis of Cushing disease; being studied for treatment of peritumoral brain oedema Oncology: as adjuvant therapy to improve the tolerability of chemotherapy
goserelin (*Zoladex*)	Implant inserted SC into lower anterior abdominal wall: 3.6 mg implant q 28 days or 10.8 mg q 3 months	Antineoplastic agent for treatment of specific hormone-stimulated cancers Controlled ovarian hyperstimulation for in-vitro fertilisation Palliative treatment of advanced prostate cancer and high-risk localised or locally advanced hormone-dependent prostate cancer (with adjuvant radiotherapy)
Antagonists		
cetrorelix (*Cetrotide*)	250 micrograms/day SC lower abdominal wall, starting day 5 or 6 of ovarian stimulation; continue until day of ovulation induction	Prevention of ovulation in women undergoing assisted reproductive techniques

Continued on following page

TABLE 35.1 DRUGS IN FOCUS Drugs affecting hypothalamic hormones *(continued)*

Drug name	Dosage/route	Usual indications
Antagonists *(continued)*		
ganirelix (*Orgalutran*)	250 micrograms SC on day 6 of FSH administration	Inhibition of premature luteinising hormone surge in women undergoing controlled ovarian stimulation as part of a fertility program
(P) leuprorelin (*Eligard, Lucrin, Lucrin Depot*)	Prostate cancer: 1 mg/day SC or various depot preparations Endometriosis 3.75 mg IM once a month Ovarian hyperstimulation: 1 mg (0.2 mL) SCI at the beginning of the follicular phase (approximately day 1 of the cycle) until the administration of hCG hormone. Duration of treatment is 12–14 days, depending on the ovarian response to exogenous gonadotrophin stimulus Depot preparations: 7.5 mg SCI once a month or 22.5 mg SCI once q 3 months	Used as antineoplastic agent for treatment of specific cancers; treatment of endometriosis
nafarelin (*Synarel*)	400 micrograms/day divided as one spray in left nostril a.m. or p.m.; one spray in right nostril a.m. or p.m. May increase to 800 micrograms/day	Treatment of endometriosis

these hormones have not been clearly identified. Not all of the hypothalamic hormones are used as pharmacological agents. A number of the hypothalamic releasing hormones described here are used for diagnostic purposes only, and others are used primarily as antineoplastic agents.

Agonists

CRH stimulates the release of adrenocorticotropic hormone (ACTH) from the anterior pituitary and is used to diagnose Cushing disease (a condition characterised by hypersecretion of adrenocortical hormones in response to excessive ACTH release). Goserelin is an analogue of GnRH. After an initial burst of follicle-stimulating hormone (FSH) and luteinising hormone (LH) release, this drug inhibits pituitary gonadotropin secretion, with a resultant drop in the production of the sex hormones. See Table 35.1 for usual indications for each of these agents.

Antagonists

Cetrorelix, ganirelix, leuprorelin and nafarelin are antagonists of GnRH. Leuprorelin occupies pituitary GnRH receptor sites so that they no longer respond to GnRH; as a result, there is no stimulation for release of LH and FSH. Nafarelin, a potent agonist of GnRH, is used to decrease the production of gonadal hormones through repeated stimulation of their receptor sites. After about 4 weeks of therapy, gonadal hormone levels fall, and the cells they normally stimulate are quiet. See Table 35.1 for usual indications for each of these agents.

Pharmacokinetics

For the most part, these drugs are absorbed slowly when given intramuscularly (IM), subcutaneously (SC) or in depot form. Nafarelin is given in a nasal form. They tend to have very long half-lives of days to weeks. Metabolism is not understood, but it is thought that they are metabolised by endogenous hormonal pathways. Because they are hormones or similar to hormones, they cross the placenta and cross into breast milk. Most of them are excreted in the urine.

Contraindications and cautions

These drugs are contraindicated with known hypersensitivity to any component of the drug *because of the risk of hypersensitivity reactions*, and during pregnancy and breastfeeding *because of the potential adverse effects to the fetus or baby.* Caution should be used with renal impairment, *which could interfere with excretion of the drug*; with peripheral vascular disorders, *which could alter the absorption of injected drug*; and with rhinitis when using nafarelin, *which could alter the absorption of the nasal spray.*

Adverse effects

Adverse effects associated with these drugs are related to the stimulation or blocking of regular hormone control. Agonists can lead to increased cortisol and aldosterone levels, causing fluid retention, electrolyte imbalance, impaired healing and elevated glucose levels, or to increased release of sex hormones, leading

Prototype summary: leuprorelin

Indications: treatment of advanced prostatic cancer, endometriosis, uterine leiomyomata.

Actions: LHRH agonist that occupies pituitary gonadotropin-releasing hormone receptors and desensitises them; causes an initial increase and then profound decrease in LH and FSH levels.

Pharmacokinetics:

Route	Onset	Peak	Duration
IM depot	4 hours	Variable	1, 2, 3 or 4 months

$T_{1/2}$: 3 hours; metabolism and excretion are unknown.

Adverse effects: dizziness, headache, pain, peripheral oedema, myocardial infarction, nausea, vomiting, anorexia, constipation, urinary frequency, haematuria, hot flushes, increased sweating.

Care considerations for people receiving drugs affecting hypothalamic hormones

The specific care of the person who is receiving a hypothalamic releasing factor is related to the hormone (or hormones) that the drug is affecting (see Chapter 36 for adrenocorticoid hormones and Chapters 40 and 41 for sex hormones). Drugs used for diagnostic purposes are short lived; information about these agents should be included in any teaching about the diagnostic procedure. Guidelines for other agents can be found with the therapeutic drug class to which they belong (eg, antineoplastic agents, Chapter 14).

to ovarian overstimulation, flushing, increased temperature and appetite and fluid retention. Antagonists can lead to a decrease in testosterone levels, leading to loss of energy, decreased sperm count and activity and potential alterations in secondary sex characteristics, or to a decrease in female sex hormones, leading to lack of menstruation, fluid and electrolyte changes, insomnia and irritability.

KEY POINTS

- The hypothalamus releases hormones that act as releasing factors, stimulating the anterior pituitary to release specific stimulating factors and inhibiting factors that act to stop the production of specific anterior pituitary hormones.
- The hypothalamic hormones are not all available for pharmacological use; those that are available are used mostly for diagnostic testing, for treating some forms of cancer or as adjuncts in fertility programs.

DRUGS AFFECTING ANTERIOR PITUITARY HORMONES

Agents that affect pituitary function are used mainly to mimic or antagonise the effects of specific pituitary hormones. They may be used either as replacement therapy for conditions resulting from a hypoactive pituitary or for diagnostic purposes. Antagonists are also available that may be used to block the effects of the anterior pituitary hormones (Table 35.2).

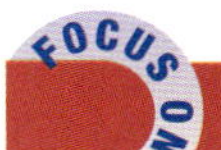

Safe medication administration

When receiving GH, the child's family will need instructions on storage, preparation and administration (see implementation in Care considerations). They must also be advised to report any lack of growth, as well as signs of glucose intolerance (thirst, hunger, voiding pattern changes) or thyroid dysfunction (fatigue, thinning hair, slow pulse, puffy skin, intolerance to the cold).

The use of GH involves an interrelationship among many subspecialists and expensive and regular medical evaluation and care. The key to the success of this therapy may be the attitude and cooperation of the young person.

GROWTH HORMONE AGONISTS

The anterior pituitary hormone that is most commonly used pharmacologically is growth hormone. GH is responsible for linear skeletal growth, the growth of internal organs, protein synthesis and the stimulation of many other processes that are required for normal growth. **Hypopituitarism** is often seen as GH deficiency before any other signs and symptoms occur. Hypopituitarism may occur as a result of developmental abnormalities or congenital defects of the pituitary, circulatory disturbances (eg, haemorrhage, infarction), acute or chronic inflammation of the pituitary and pituitary tumours. GH deficiency in children results in short stature (**dwarfism**). Adults with somatropin deficiency syndrome (SDS) may have hypopituitarism as a result of pituitary tumours or trauma, or they may have been treated for GH deficiency as children, resulting in a shutdown of the pituitary production of somatotropin.

TABLE 35.2 DRUGS IN FOCUS Drug affecting anterior pituitary hormones

Drug name	Dosage/route	Usual indications
Growth hormone agonists		
(P) somatropin (*Genotropin, Humatrope, Omnitrope, Zomacton*)	Dose varies with each product, check manufacturer's instructions; must be given SC or IM	Treatment of children with growth failure due to lack of growth hormone (GH) or to chronic renal failure replacement of GH in people with GH deficiency; long-term treatment of growth failure in children born small for gestational age who do not achieve catch-up growth by 2 years of age; treatment of short stature associated with Turner syndrome or Prader-Willi syndrome; also approved to increase protein production and growth in various AIDS-related states
Growth hormone antagonists		
(P) bromocriptine mesilate (generic, *Parlodel*)	Acromegaly: 1.25 PO bd–tid; may increase slowly to 10–20 mg/day Parkinson disease: initially 1.25 mg PO daily at bedtime, increasing gradually every 5–7 days as required. Usual range: 10–40 mg/day in divided doses, with food Inhibition of lactation: day 1: 1.25 mg morning and night with food, increasing on day 2–2.5 mg bd. Therapy should be continued for 14 days to prevent rebound lactation	Treatment of acromegaly in people who are not candidates for or cannot tolerate other therapy; not recommended for children < 15 years Treatment of Parkinson disease as monotherapy or as an adjunct to levodopa therapy Inhibition of lactation
lanreotide (*Somatuline Autogel, Somatuline LA*)	*Somatuline Autogel* Acromegaly: 60 mg SC q 28 days or 120 mg q 42–56 days Carcinoid syndrome: 60–120 mg SC q 28 days GEP-NETs: 120 mg SC q 28 days *Somatuline LA:* prolonged-release microparticles 30 mg IM q 14 days	Treatment of acromegaly, carcinoid syndrome associated with carcinoid tumours, and gastroenteropancreatic neuroendocrine tumours (GEP-NETs)
octreotide (*Sandostatin, Sandostatin LAR*)	Solution: SC 0.05–0.1 mg q 8–12 hours increasing to a maximum of 1.5 mg/day Modified-release injection: initially 20 mg IM q 4 weeks	Treatment of acromegaly in adults who are not candidates for or cannot tolerate other therapy Treatment of GEP-NETs
pegvisomant	80 mg SC as a loading dose, then 10 mg/day SC; maximum 30 mg/day	Treatment of acromegaly in adults who are not candidates for or who cannot tolerate other therapy
Drugs affecting other anterior pituitary hormones		
cabergoline (*Cabaser, Dostinex*)	2–3 mg PO daily	Treatment of signs and symptoms of Parkinson's disease
chorionic gonadotropin (*Pregnyl*)	Males, hypogonadism: 1000–2000 IU 2–3 times a week Females, sterility: 5000–10,000 IU + FSH preparation Cryptorchism, infants < 2 years: 250 IU twice weekly for 6 weeks; < 6 years: 500–1000 IU twice weekly for 6 weeks; > 6 years: 1500 IU twice weekly for 6 weeks	Treatment of male hypogonadism, to induce ovulation in females with functioning ovaries, for treatment of prepubertal cryptorchidism when there is no anatomical obstruction to testicular movement
choriogonadotropin alfa (*Ovidrel*)	250 micrograms SC given 1 day after last dose of a follicle-stimulating hormone (FSH) stimulator	Induction of ovulation in infertile females who have been pretreated with FSH
quinagolide (*Norprolac*)	25 micrograms/day PO for 3 days, then 50 micrograms/day for further 3 days then 75–125 micrograms/day PO	Treatment of hyperprolactinaemia
thyrotropin alfa (*Thyrogen*)	0.9 mg IM, followed by 0.9 mg IM in 24 hours	Adjunctive treatment for post-radioiodine ablation of thyroid tissue in people with near-total thyroidectomy and well-differentiated thyroid cancer without metastasis

BOX 35.2 Growth hormone therapy

In the past, growth hormone (GH) therapy was expensive and unsafe. The use of cadaver pituitaries resulted in unreliable hormone levels and, in many cases, hypersensitivity reactions to the proteins found in the drug. With the advent of genetic engineering and the development of safer, more reliable forms of growth hormone, there has been a surge in the use of the drug to treat children with short stature. Even so, the drug is still costly and not without adverse effects.

Growth hormone can be used to treat growth failure caused either by lack of growth hormone or by renal failure. It also can help children with normal growth hormone levels who are just genetically small. Before the drug is prescribed, the child must undergo screening procedures and specific testing (including radiographs and blood tests) and must display a willingness to have regular injections. The child taking this drug will need to have pretherapy and periodic tests of thyroid function, blood glucose levels, glucose tolerance tests, and tests for growth hormone antibodies (a risk that increases with the length of therapy). In addition, radiographs of the long bones will be taken to monitor for closure of the epiphyses, a sign that the drug must be stopped. Because the child who is taking growth hormone may experience sudden growth, they will need to be monitored for nutritional needs, as well as psychological trauma that may occur with the sudden change in body image. Insulin therapy and replacement thyroid therapy may be needed, depending on the child's response to the drug. (See also Focus on safe medication administration related to growth hormone therapy.)

GH deficiency was once treated with GH injections extracted from the pituitary glands of cadavers. The supply of GH was therefore rather limited and costly (Box 35.2). Synthetic human GH is now available from recombinant DNA sources, using genetic engineering. Synthetic GH is expensive, but it is thought to be safer than cadaver GH and is being used increasingly to treat GH deficiencies. Somatropin (*Genotropin*, *Omnitrope*, *Saizen*, *Zomacton* and others) are used for GH replacement today.

Therapeutic actions and indications

In clinical practice, the agents that are used purely as a replacement for anterior pituitary hormones are those acting as GH (somatropin). These drugs are produced with the use of recombinant DNA technology. See Table 35.2 for indications.

Pharmacokinetics

Somatropin is injected and reaches peak levels within 7 hours. Box 35.3 discusses a new delivery system for this drug. It is widely distributed in the body and localises in highly perfused tissues, particularly the liver and kidney. Excretion occurs through the urine and faeces. Individuals with liver or renal dysfunction may experience reduced clearance and increased concentrations of the drug.

BOX 35.3 New delivery system for growth hormone

Somatropin is a preparation of recombinant DNA–produced human growth hormone that is used to treat children with growth failure due to lack of growth hormone. The drug must be given by injection six or seven times a week. A new delivery form is now available to ease the discomfort and trauma of the frequent injections. For example, Genotropin is dispensed in a special glass ampoule, a so-called two-chamber cartridge, with the active substance in one chamber and solvent in the other. Genotropin cartridges are supplied as a reusable injection device (*Genotropin Pen*), or sealed in a disposable pre-filled pen (*Genotropin GoQuick*). Tests have shown a bioequivalency of this method with standard injection techniques, and the young people who must use this drug are much less resistant to the dosing. Various drug companies anticipate similar delivery systems, which will provide a therapeutic dose of drugs without the associated discomfort of IM or SC injection.

Contraindications and cautions

Somatropin is contraindicated with any known allergy to the drug or ingredients in the drug *to avoid hypersensitivity reactions*. It is also contraindicated in the presence of closed epiphyses or with underlying cranial lesions *because of the risk of serious complications*, and with abdominal surgery and acute illness secondary to complications of open-heart surgery *because of potential problems with healing*. It should be used with caution in pregnancy and breastfeeding *because of the potential for adverse effects on the fetus*.

Adverse effects

The adverse effects that most often occur when using GH include the development of antibodies to GH and subsequent signs of inflammation and autoimmune-type reactions, such as swelling and joint pain, and the endocrine reactions of hypothyroidism and insulin resistance.

Clinically important drug–drug interactions

Caution should be used when these agents are combined with any drugs using the cytochrome P450 liver enzyme system because of a risk for change in metabolism of the combined drugs.

Prototype summary: somatropin

Indications: long-term treatment of children with growth failure associated with various deficiencies, girls with Turner syndrome, AIDS wasting and cachexia, growth hormone deficiency in adults, and treatment of growth failure in children of small gestational age who do not achieve catch-up growth by 2 years of age.

Actions: replaces human growth hormone; stimulates skeletal growth, growth of internal organs, and protein synthesis.

Pharmacokinetics:

Route	Onset	Peak
IM, SC	Varies	5–7.5 hours

$T_{1/2}$: 15–50 minutes; metabolised in the liver and excreted in the urine and faeces.

Adverse effects: development of antibodies to growth hormone, insulin resistance, swelling, joint pain, headache, injection-site pain.

Care considerations for people receiving drugs affecting growth hormone agonists

Assessment: history and examination

- Assess history of allergy to any GH or binder, presence of closed epiphyses or underlying cranial lesions, serious infection after open-heart surgery, abdominal surgery and pregnancy or breastfeeding status *to determine contraindications to the use of the drug.*
- Assess height, weight, thyroid function tests, glucose tolerance tests and GH levels *to determine baseline status before beginning therapy and for any potential adverse effects.*

Implementation with rationale

- Reconstitute the drug following the manufacturer's directions *because individual products vary*; administer IM or SC *for appropriate delivery of drug.*
- Monitor response carefully when beginning therapy *to allow appropriate dose adjustments as needed.*
- Monitor thyroid function, glucose tolerance and GH levels periodically *to monitor endocrine changes and to institute treatment as needed.*
- Provide thorough teaching, including measures to take to avoid adverse effects, warning signs of problems and the need for regular evaluation (including blood tests) *to enhance knowledge about drug therapy and promote compliance.* Instruct a family member or carer in:
  - storage of the drug (refrigeration is required).
  - preparation of the drug (the reconstitution procedure varies depending on the brand name product used).
  - administration techniques: aseptic no-touch technique, need to rotate injection sites and need to monitor injection sites for atrophy or extravasation.

Evaluation

- Monitor response to the drug (return of GH levels to normal; growth and development).
- Monitor for adverse effects (hypothyroidism, glucose intolerance, nutritional imbalance).
- Evaluate the effectiveness of the teaching plan (person can name drug, dosage, adverse effects to watch for and specific measures to avoid them; family member can demonstrate proper technique for preparation and administration of the drug).
- Monitor the effectiveness of comfort measures and compliance with the regimen.

GROWTH HORMONE ANTAGONISTS

GH hypersecretion is usually caused by pituitary tumours and can occur at any time of life. This is often referred to as hyperpituitarism. If it occurs before the epiphyseal plates of the long bones fuse, it causes an acceleration in linear skeletal growth, producing **gigantism** of over 2 metres in height with fairly normal body proportions. In adults, after epiphyseal closure, linear growth is impossible. Instead, hypersecretion of GH causes enlargement in the peripheral parts of the body, such as the hands and feet, and the internal organs, especially the heart. **Acromegaly** is the term used to describe the onset of excessive GH secretion that occurs after puberty and epiphyseal plate closure.

Most conditions of GH hypersecretion are treated by radiation therapy or surgery. Drug therapy for GH excess can be used for those people who are not candidates for surgery or radiation therapy. The drugs include a dopamine agonist (the prototype drug bromocriptine mesilate [*Parlodel*]); somatostatin analogue (lanreotide [*Somatuline*]) and octreotide [*Sandostatin*]); and a GH analogue (pegvisomant).

Therapeutic actions and indications

Somatostatin is an inhibitory factor released from the hypothalamus. It is not used to decrease GH levels, although it does do that very effectively. Because it has multiple effects on many secretory systems (eg, it inhibits release of gastrin, glucagon and insulin) and a short duration of action, it is not desirable as a therapeutic agent. Analogues of somatostatin, lanreotide and octreotide, are considerably more potent in inhibiting GH release with less of an inhibitory effect on insulin release. Consequently, they are used instead of somatostatin.

Bromocriptine, a semisynthetic ergot alkaloid, is a dopamine agonist frequently used to treat acromegaly. It may be used alone or as an adjunct to irradiation. Dopamine agonists inhibit GH secretion in some individuals with acromegaly; the opposite effect occurs in normal individuals. Bromocriptine's GH-inhibiting effect may be explained by the fact that dopamine increases somatostatin release from the hypothalamus.

Pegvisomant is a GH analogue that was approved in late 2003 for the treatment of acromegaly in individuals who do not respond to other therapies. It binds to GH receptors on cells, inhibiting GH effects. It must be given by daily SC injection. Table 35.2 shows usual indications for each of these agents.

Pharmacokinetics

Octreotide must be administered SC. The drug is rapidly absorbed and widely distributed throughout the body, and it is metabolised in the tissues with about 30% excreted unchanged in the urine.

Lanreotide is administered by either deep SC or IM injection, peaking between 10 and 16 hours after administration.

Bromocriptine is administered orally and effectively absorbed from the gastrointestinal (GI) tract. The drug undergoes extensive first-pass metabolism in the liver and is primarily excreted in the bile.

Pegvisomant is given by SC injection and is slowly absorbed, reaching peak effects in 33–77 hours. It also clears from the body at a slow rate, with a half-life of 6 days. The drug is excreted in the urine.

Contraindications and cautions

Bromocriptine should not be used during pregnancy or breastfeeding *because of effects on the fetus and because it blocks breastfeeding*. There are no adequate studies of effects of octreotide and pegvisomant in pregnancy and during breastfeeding; use of these drugs should be reserved for situations in which the benefits to the mother clearly outweigh any potential risks to the fetus or neonate. Growth hormone antagonists are contraindicated in the presence of any known allergy to the drug *to prevent hypersensitivity reactions*. They should be used cautiously in the presence of any other endocrine disorder (eg, diabetes, thyroid dysfunction) *that could be exacerbated by the blocking of GH*.

Adverse effects

People with renal dysfunction may accumulate higher levels of octreotide. GI complaints (eg, constipation or diarrhoea, flatulence and nausea) are not uncommon because of the drug's effects on the GI tract. Octreotide and lanreotide have also been associated with the development of acute cholecystitis, cholestatic jaundice, biliary tract obstruction and pancreatitis. People must be assessed for the possible development of any of these problems. Other, less common adverse effects include headache, sinus bradycardia or other cardiac arrhythmias and decreased glucose tolerance. Because octreotide and lanreotide are administered SC, they can be associated with discomfort and/or inflammation at injection sites.

Bromocriptine is also associated with GI disturbances. Because of its dopamine-blocking effects, it may cause drowsiness and postural hypotension. It blocks breastfeeding and should not be used by breastfeeding women.

Pegvisomant may cause pain and inflammation at the injection site (common). Increased incidence of infection, nausea and diarrhoea and changes in liver function may also occur.

Clinically important drug–drug interactions

Increased serum bromocriptine levels and increased toxicity occur if bromocriptine is combined with erythromycin. This combination should be avoided.

The effectiveness of bromocriptine may decrease if it is combined with phenothiazines. If this combination is used, the person should be monitored carefully.

People receiving pegvisomant may require higher doses to receive adequate GH suppression if they are also taking opioids. The mechanism of action of this interaction is not understood.

Prototype summary: bromocriptine mesilate

Indications: treatment of Parkinson disease, hyperprolactinaemia associated with pituitary adenomas, female infertility associated with hyperprolactinaemia and acromegaly; short-term treatment of amenorrhoea or galactorrhoea.

Actions: acts directly on postsynaptic dopamine receptors in the brain.

Pharmacokinetics:

Route	Onset	Peak	Duration
PO	Varies	1–3 hours	14 hours

$T_{1/2}$: 3 hours, then 45–50 hours; metabolised in the liver and excreted in the bile.

Adverse effects: dizziness, fatigue, light-headedness, nasal congestion, drowsiness, nausea, vomiting, abdominal cramps, constipation, diarrhoea, headache.

Care considerations for people receiving growth hormone antagonists

Assessment: history and examination

- Assess for history of allergy to any GH antagonist or binder *to prevent hypersensitivity reactions*; other endocrine disturbances, *which could be exacerbated when blocking GH*; and pregnancy and breastfeeding *because of the potential for adverse effects to the fetus and the blocking of breastfeeding.*
- Assess orientation, affect and reflexes; blood pressure, pulse and orthostatic blood pressure; abdominal examination; glucose tolerance tests and GH levels, *to determine baseline status before beginning therapy and for any potential adverse effects.*

Implementation with rationale

- Reconstitute octreotide and pegvisomant following manufacturer's directions; administer these drugs SC and rotate injection sites regularly *to prevent skin breakdown and to ensure proper delivery of the drug.*
- Monitor thyroid function, glucose tolerance and GH levels periodically *to detect problems and to institute treatment as needed.*
- Arrange for baseline and periodic ultrasound evaluation of the gallbladder if using octreotide *to detect any gallstone development and to arrange for appropriate treatment.*
- Provide thorough teaching, including measures to avoid adverse effects, warning signs of problems and need for regular evaluation (including blood tests), *to enhance knowledge about drug therapy and promote compliance.* Instruct a family member in proper preparation and administration techniques to ensure that there is another responsible person to administer the drug if needed.

Evaluation

- Monitor response to the drug (return of GH levels to normal, growth and development).
- Monitor for adverse effects (hypothyroidism, glucose intolerance, nutritional imbalance, GI disturbances, headache, dizziness, cholecystitis).
- Evaluate the effectiveness of the teaching plan (person can name drug, dosage, adverse effects to watch for and specific measures to avoid them; family member can demonstrate proper technique for preparation and administration of drug).
- Monitor the effectiveness of comfort measures and compliance with the regimen.

DRUGS AFFECTING OTHER ANTERIOR PITUITARY HORMONES

Drugs that affect growth hormone are the most commonly used drugs affecting anterior pituitary hormones. There are several other anterior pituitary hormones that can now be affected by drugs. The other anterior pituitary hormones that are available for pharmacological use include chorionic gonadotropin (*Pregnyl*), choriogonadotropin alfa (*Ovidrel*) and thyrotropin alfa (*Thyrogen*) (not available in New Zealand).

Chorionic gonadotropin acts like LH and stimulates the production of testosterone and progesterone. Usual indications are presented in Table 35.2. (See Chapters 40 and 41 for nursing implications.) Choriogonadotropin alfa is used as a fertility drug to induce ovulation in women treated with FSH (see Chapters 40 and 41).

Thyrotropin alfa is used as adjunctive treatment for radioiodine ablation of thyroid tissue remnants in people who have undergone a near-total to total thyroidectomy for well-differentiated thyroid cancer and who do not have evidence of metastatic thyroid cancer.

Cabergoline (*Cabaser, Dostinex*) acts on dopamine receptors located on pituitary lactotrophic cells to decrease prolactin secretion and inhibit central dopaminergic effect.

KEY POINTS

- Hypothalamic releasing factors stimulate the anterior pituitary to release hormones, which in turn stimulate endocrine glands or cell metabolism. The anterior pituitary hormones are mostly used for diagnostic testing, for treating some cancers or in fertility programs.
- In children, deficiency of GH may be responsible for dwarfism; in adults it is associated with somatropin deficiency syndrome.
- GH may be replaced by substances produced by recombinant DNA processes, which are safer than replacement drugs used in the past.
- In cases of GH excess, drugs are used to block the effects of GH. Care must be taken to monitor these individuals because of the systemic effects of the drugs.

DRUGS AFFECTING POSTERIOR PITUITARY HORMONES

The posterior pituitary stores two hormones produced in the hypothalamus: antidiuretic hormone (ADH, also known as argipressin or vasopressin) and oxytocin. Oxytocin stimulates milk ejection or 'let down' in breastfeeding women. In pharmacological doses, it can

TABLE 35.3 DRUGS IN FOCUS Drugs affecting posterior pituitary hormones

Drug name	Dosage/route	Usual indications
Argipressin (vasopressin) (*Pitressin*)	Adult: 0.25 mL IM or SC. Can be increased to 0.5 mL if required and repeated at 3–4-hour intervals	Treatment of postoperative abdominal distension and diabetes insipidus
 desmopressin (*Minirin, Octostim*)	*Nasal spray* Adults, diabetes insipidus: 10–40 micrograms/day Children, nocturnal enuresis: 10–40 micrograms at bedtime *Nasal drops* Adults, diabetes insipidus: 10–40 micrograms/day *Injection* Control of bleeding or bleeding prophylaxis before an invasive operation in patients with prolonged bleeding time: 0.3 micrograms/kg in 50–100 mL normal saline IV over 15–30 minutes Adults, von Willebrand disease: 1–4 micrograms/day Children, von Willebrand disease: 0.4 micrograms/kg *Tablets* Adults, diabetes insipidus: 100–200 micrograms tid Children, nocturnal enuresis: 200 micrograms at bedtime; may increase to 400 micrograms at bedtime *Sublingual* Adults, diabetes insipidus: 60–120 micrograms tid Children, nocturnal enuresis: 120 micrograms at bedtime	Treatment of neurogenic diabetes insipidus, von Willebrand's disease, haemophilia; being studiec for the treatment of chronic autonomic failure

CRITICAL THINKING SCENARIO

Diabetes insipidus and posterior pituitary hormones (desmopressin)

THE SITUATION

B.T. is a 56-year-old teacher with diabetes insipidus. Her condition was eventually regulated on desmopressin nasal spray, one or two sprays per nostril four times a day. B.T. seemed highly interested in her disease and therapy and learned to control her dose by symptom control. For several years, her symptoms were well controlled. Then, at her last clinical visit, it was noted that she had postnasal ulcerations and nasal rhinitis. She also complained of several GI symptoms, including upset stomach, abdominal cramps and diarrhoea.

CRITICAL THINKING

Think about the pathophysiology of diabetes insipidus. What are the effects of desmopressin on the body, and what adverse effects might occur if the drug was being absorbed inappropriately?

Because B.T. has used the drug for so many years, she may have forgotten some of the teaching points about her disease and drug administration. Outline a care plan for B.T. that includes necessary teaching points and takes into consideration her long experience with her disease and her drug therapy. Think about specific warning signs that should be highlighted for B.T. and ways to involve her in the teaching program that might make it more pertinent to her and her needs.

DISCUSSION

An essential aspect of the ongoing care process is continual evaluation of the effectiveness of the drug therapy. An evaluation of this situation shows that B.T.'s postnasal mucosa was ulcerated, possibly as a result of overexposure to the vasoconstrictive properties of the drug. B.T.'s GI tract also seemed to show evidence of increased antidiuretic hormone effects. These factors suggest that perhaps the drug was being administered incorrectly, resulting in excessive exposure of the nasal mucosa to the drug, increased absorption and increased levels of the drug reaching the systemic circulation.

The care provider should watch B.T. administer a dose of the drug to herself, then discuss the signs and symptoms of problems that B.T. should watch for. In this case, B.T. remembered most of the details of her drug teaching. But when administering the drug, she tilted her head back, tipped the bottle upside down and then squirted the drug into each nostril. When questioned about her technique, she explained that she had seen an advertisement on TV about nasal sprays and realised that she had been doing it wrong all these years. The difference in the types of nasal sprays was explained and the entire care plan was reviewed with B.T. The drug was discontinued and B.T. was placed on SC antidiuretic hormone until the nasal ulcerations healed.

As a person becomes more familiar with drug therapy, the details about the drug may be forgotten. It is important to remember that an individual's teaching needs regular updating and evaluation. This point is often forgotten when dealing with people who have been taking a drug for years. However, remembering to assess the person's knowledge about the drug can prevent problems such as B.T.'s from developing. Because B.T. is a teacher, she might be interested in developing a teaching protocol that will meet her needs and serve as an appropriate reminder about the disease and drug therapy. If B.T. is actively involved in preparing such a plan, it will be more effective and might be remembered much longer.

CARE GUIDE FOR B.T.: DIABETES INSIPIDUS AND POSTERIOR PITUITARY HORMONES

Assessment: history and examination

Assess for allergies to any anticholinergic agent and other drugs. Also assess for a history of chronic obstructive pulmonary disease, narrow-angle glaucoma, myasthenia gravis, bowel or urinary obstruction, pregnancy or breastfeeding, tachycardia, and recent GI or urinary tract surgery.

Focus the physical assessment on the following:

CV: blood pressure, pulse rate, peripheral perfusion, electrocardiogram

CNS: orientation, affect, reflexes, vision

Skin: colour, lesions, texture, sweating

GU: urinary output, bladder tone

GI: abdominal examination

Respiratory: respiratory rate, adventitious sounds

Implementation

Ensure safe and appropriate administration of the drug.

Provide comfort and safety measures, such as physical assistance or raised side rails if B.T. is hospitalised; temperature control; dark eyeglasses; small, frequent meals; artificial saliva, fluids; sugarless lozenges, mouth care; and bowel program.

Provide support and reassurance to deal with drug effects, discomfort and GI effects.

Teach person about drug therapy, including drug name, dosage, adverse effects, precautions and warning signs of serious adverse effects to report.

Monitor blood pressure and pulse rate and adjust dosage as needed.

Evaluation

Evaluate drug effects, including decrease in signs and symptoms being treated.

Monitor for adverse effects: CV effects – tachycardia, heart failure; CNS – confusion, dreams; urinary retention; GI effects – constipation; visual blurring, photophobia.

Monitor for drug–drug interactions as indicated for each drug.

Evaluate the effectiveness of teaching program and comfort and safety measures.

TEACHING FOR B.T.

- The anterior pituitary hormone desmopressin, or antidiuretic hormone, acts to promote the resorption of water in your kidneys, replacing the action of antidiuretic hormone that you are missing in your body. This lack of antidiuretic hormone is the cause of your diabetes insipidus. This drug will replace the missing hormone. This drug also causes your blood vessels to contract and may increase the activity of your GI tract. Some of the following adverse effects may occur:
    - *Tremor, dizziness, vision changes:* if these occur, you should avoid driving a car, operating dangerous machinery or performing any other tasks that require alertness.
    - *GI cramping, passing of gas:* eating small, frequent meals may help.
    - *Nasal irritation, development of lesions:* proper administration of the drug will decrease this effect.
- Use caution to administer the nasal solution correctly. Sit upright and press a finger over one nostril to close it. Hold the spray bottle upright and place the tip of the bottle about 1.5 cm) into the open nostril. A firm squeeze on the bottle will deliver the drug. Do not use excessive force when squeezing the bottle. Do not tip your head back during administration.
- Tell any doctor, nurse or other health care provider involved in your care that you are taking this drug.
- Watch for any signs of water intoxication (drowsiness, light-headedness, headache, seizures, coma) and report this to your health care provider immediately.
- Report any nasal pain or runny nose, which might indicate that you are not administering the drug correctly.
- Keep this drug, and all medications, out of the reach of children. Do not share this drug with other people.

be used to initiate or improve uterine contractions in labour. Oxytocin is discussed in Chapter 40.

ADH possesses antidiuretic, haemostatic and vasopressor properties. Posterior pituitary disorders can occur secondary to metastatic cancer, lymphoma, disseminated intravascular coagulation (discussed in Chapter 48) or septicaemia. Posterior pituitary disorders that are seen clinically involve ADH release and include **diabetes insipidus**, which results from insufficient secretion, and syndrome of inappropriate antidiuretic hormone secretion (SIADH), which occurs with excessive secretion of ADH. Diabetes insipidus can be treated pharmacologically. (*See the Critical thinking scenario related to diabetes insipidus and posterior pituitary hormones.*)

Diabetes insipidus is characterised by the production of a large amount of dilute urine containing no glucose. Blood glucose levels are higher than normal, and the body responds with polyuria (excessive urine), polydipsia (excessive thirst) and dehydration. With this rare metabolic disorder, individuals produce large quantities of dilute urine and are constantly thirsty. Diabetes insipidus is caused by a deficiency in the amount of posterior pituitary ADH and may result from pituitary disease or injury (eg, head trauma, surgery, tumour). The condition can be acute and short in duration or it can be a chronic, lifelong problem.

ADH itself is never used as therapy for diabetes insipidus. Instead, synthetic preparations of ADH, which are purer and have fewer adverse effects, are used. The ADH preparations currently available are desmopressin (*Minirin, Octostim*) and argipressin (*Pitressin*) (see Table 35.3).

Therapeutic actions and indications

ADH is released in response to increases in plasma osmolarity or decreases in blood volume. It produces its antidiuretic activity in the kidneys, causing the cortical and medullary parts of the collecting duct to become permeable to water, thereby increasing water reabsorption and decreasing urine formation. These activities reduce plasma osmolarity and increase blood volume. See Table 35.3 for usual indications for desmopressin and argipressin.

Pharmacokinetics

Desmopressin and argipressin are rapidly absorbed and metabolised; they are excreted in the liver and kidneys. Desmopressin is available for oral, IV, SC and nasal administration. Argipressin is administered by SC or IM injection.

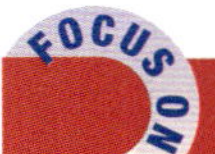

Safe medication administration

Administering a nasal spray

Instruct the person to sit upright and press a finger over one nostril to close it. Then, with the spray bottle held upright, have the person place the tip of the bottle about 1.5 cm into the open nostril. A firm squeeze should deliver the drug to the desired mucosal area for absorption. Caution the person not to use excessive force and not to tip the head back because these actions could result in ineffective administration.

Contraindications and cautions

Desmopressin and argipressin are contraindicated with any known allergy to the drugs or their components *to avoid potential hypersensitivity reactions* or with severe renal dysfunction, *which could alter the effects of the drug.* Caution should be used with any known vascular disease *because of its effects on vascular smooth muscle;* epilepsy; asthma; and with hyponatraemia, *which could be exacerbated by the effects of the drug.* This drug should not be used during pregnancy *because of the risk of uterine contractions that would harm the fetus* or breastfeeding *because of the potential for adverse effects to the fetus or baby.*

The drugs should be stopped during acute illnesses that might lead to fluid and/or electrolyte imbalance, and caution should be used in individuals who consume large amounts of fluid *because of the increased risk of electrolyte dilution and hyponatraemia.*

Adverse effects

The adverse effects associated with the use of these drugs include water intoxication (drowsiness, lightheadedness, headache, coma, convulsions) related to the shift to water retention and resulting electrolyte imbalance; tremor, sweating, vertigo and headache related to water retention (a 'hangover' effect); abdominal cramps, flatulence, nausea and vomiting related to stimulation of GI motility; and local nasal irritation related to nasal administration. Local reaction at injection sites is fairly common. Hypersensitivity reactions have also been reported, ranging from rash to bronchial constriction.

Clinically important drug–drug interactions

There is an increased risk of antidiuretic effects if the drugs are combined with carbamazepine; use caution if combinations are used.

Prototype summary: desmopressin

Indications: treatment of neurogenic diabetes insipidus, haemophilia A.

Actions: has pressor and antidiuretic effects; increases levels of clotting factor VIII.

Pharmacokinetics:

Route	Onset	Peak	Duration
Oral	1 hour	60–90 min	7 hours
IV, SC	30 min	90–120 min	Varies
Nasal	15–60 min	1–5 hours	5–21 hours

$T_{1/2}$: 7.8 minutes, then 75.5 minutes (IV); 1.5–2.5 hours (oral); 3.3–3.5 hours (nasal); metabolised in the tissues, excretion is unknown.

Adverse effects: headache, facial flushing, nausea, fluid retention, slight increase in blood pressure, local reaction at injection site, water intoxication at high doses.

Care considerations for people receiving drugs affecting posterior pituitary hormones

Assessment: history and examination

- Assess for history of allergy to any ADH preparation or components *to avoid hypersensitivity reactions*; vascular diseases; epilepsy; renal dysfunction; pregnancy; and breastfeeding, *which could be cautions or contraindications to use of the drug.*
- Assess for skin lesions; orientation, affect and reflexes; blood pressure and pulse; respiration and adventitious sounds; abdominal examination; renal function tests; and serum electrolytes, *to determine baseline status before beginning therapy and for any potential adverse effects.*

Implementation with rationale

- Monitor fluid volume *to watch for signs of water intoxication and fluid excess*; arrange to decrease dose as needed.
- Monitor individuals with vascular disease for any sign of exacerbation *to provide for immediate treatment.*
- Monitor condition of nasal passages if given intranasally *to observe for nasal ulceration, which can occur and could affect absorption of the drug.*
- Provide thorough teaching, including measures to avoid adverse effects, warning signs of problems, and the need for regular evaluation, including blood tests, *to enhance knowledge about drug therapy and promote compliance.*

Evaluation

- Monitor response to the drug (maintenance of fluid balance).
- Monitor for adverse effects (GI problems, water intoxication, headache, skin rash).
- Evaluate the effectiveness of the teaching plan (person can name drug, dosage, adverse effects to watch for and specific measures to avoid them; person can demonstrate proper administration of nasal preparations).
- Monitor the effectiveness of comfort measures and compliance with the regimen.

KEY POINTS

- Posterior pituitary hormones are produced in the hypothalamus and stored in the posterior pituitary. They include oxytocin and antidiuretic hormone (ADH).
- Lack of antidiuretic hormone produces diabetes insipidus, which is characterised by large amounts of dilute urine and excessive thirst.
- ADH replacement uses an analogue of ADH, desmopressin, and can be administered parenterally or intranasally.
- Fluid balance needs to be monitored when individuals are taking desmopressin.

CHAPTER SUMMARY

- Hypothalamic releasing factors stimulate the anterior pituitary to release hormones.
- The hypothalamic releasing factors are used mostly for diagnostic testing and for treating some forms of cancer.
- Anterior pituitary hormones stimulate endocrine glands or cell metabolism.
- Growth hormone (GH) deficiency can cause dwarfism in children and somatropin deficiency syndrome in adults.
- GH replacement is done with drugs produced by recombinant DNA processes; these agents are more reliable and cause fewer problems than drugs used in the past.
- GH excess causes gigantism in people whose epiphyseal plates have not closed and acromegaly in people with closed epiphyseal plates.
- GH antagonists include octreotide and bromocriptine. Blockage of other endocrine activity may occur when these drugs are used.
- Posterior pituitary hormones are produced in the hypothalamus and stored in the posterior pituitary. They include oxytocin and antidiuretic hormone (ADH).
- Lack of ADH produces diabetes insipidus, which is characterised by large amounts of dilute urine and excessive thirst.

- ADH replacement uses desmopressin, an analogue of ADH, which can be administered parenterally or intranasally.
- Fluid balance needs to be monitored when individuals are taking desmopressin or argipressin (vasopressin).

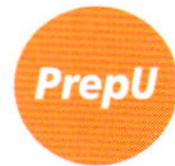

Knowing your strengths and weaknesses helps you to study more effectively. Take a PrepU Practice Quiz to find out how you measure up!

ONLINE RESOURCES

An extensive range of additional resources to enhance teaching and learning and to facilitate understanding of this chapter may be found online at the text's accompanying website, located on thePoint at http://thepoint.lww.com. These include Watch and Learn videos, Concepts in Action animations, journal articles, review questions, case studies, discussion topics and quizzes.

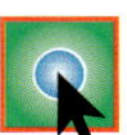

WEB LINKS

Patients, health care providers, and students may want to consult the following web resources:

www.acromegaly.org
Information on acromegaly – diagnosis, treatment and support.

http://pituitary.asn.au
The Australian Pituitary Foundation Ltd. Information and support for people with pituitary conditions.

www.rch.org.au/clinicalguide/cpg.cfm?doc_id=9745
Royal Children's Hospital, Melbourne, Clinical Practice Guidelines – Diabetes Insipidus.

BIBLIOGRAPHY

Barrett, K . E. & Ganong, W. F. (2010). *Ganong's Review of Medical Physiology* (23rd edn). New York: McGraw-Hill.

Farrell, M. & Dempsey, J. (2014). *Smeltzer & Bare's Textbook of Medical-Surgical Nursing* (3rd edn). Sydney: Lippincott Williams & Wilkins.

Finlayson, A. & Sanders, S. (2007). (Eds.). *Endocrine and Reproductive Systems* (3rd edn). Edinburgh: Mosby.

Gardner, D. G., Greenspan, F. S. & Shoback, D. M. (Eds.). (2011). *Basic and Clinical Endocrinology* (9th edn). New York: McGraw-Hill.

Goodman, L. S., Brunton, L. L., Chabner, B. & Knollmann, B. C. (2011). *Goodman and Gilman's Pharmacological Basis of Therapeutics* (12th edn). New York: McGraw-Hill.

Gordon, B. M (2007). Pharmacological management of secreting pituitary tumors. *Journal of Neuroscience Nursing, 39(1)*, 52–57.

Guyton, A. & Hall, J. (2011). *Textbook of Medical Physiology* (12th edn). Philadelphia: Saunders Elsevier.

Hanberg, A. (2005). Common disorders of the pituitary gland: Hyposecretion versus hypersecretion. *Journal of Infusion Nursing, 28*, 36–44.

Lim, E. M. (2009). Drug treatment of pituitary tumours. *Australian Prescriber, 32*, 19–21.

McKenna, L. & Mirkov, S. (2019). *McKenna's Drug Handbook for Nursing and Midwifery* (8th edn). Sydney: Wolters Kluwer Health Australia.

Porth, C. M. (2011). *Essentials of Pathophysiology: Concepts of Altered Health States* (3rd edn). Philadelphia: Lippincott Williams & Wilkins.

Porth, C. M. (2009). *Pathophysiology: Concepts of Altered Health States* (8th edn). Philadelphia: Lippincott Williams & Wilkins.

CHECK YOUR UNDERSTANDING

Answers to the questions in this chapter can be found in Appendix A at the back of this book.

MULTIPLE CHOICE

Select the best answer to the following.

1. Hypothalamic hormones are normally present in very small amounts. When used therapeutically, their main indication is:
   a. diagnosis of endocrine disorders and treatment of specific cancers.
   b. treatment of multiple endocrine disorders.
   c. treatment of CNS-related abnormalities.
   d. treatment of autoimmune-related problems.
2. Somatropin (*Genotropin* and others) is a genetically engineered growth hormone that is used:
   a. to diagnose hypothalamic failure.
   b. to treat precocious puberty.
   c. in the treatment of children with growth failure.
   d. to stimulate pituitary response.
3. Growth hormone deficiencies:
   a. occur only in children.
   b. always result in dwarfism.
   c. are treated only in children because GH is usually produced only until puberty.
   d. can occur in adults as well as children.

4. People who are receiving growth hormone replacement therapy must be monitored very closely. Routine follow-up examinations would include:
   a. a bowel program to deal with constipation.
   b. tests for thyroid function and glucose tolerance.
   c. a kilojoule check to control weight gain.
   d. tests of adrenal hormone levels.
5. Acromegaly and gigantism are both conditions related to excessive secretion of:
   a. thyroid hormone.
   b. melanin-stimulating hormone.
   c. growth hormone.
   d. oxytocin.
6. Diabetes insipidus is a relatively rare disease characterised by:
   a. excessive secretion of ADH.
   b. renal damage.
   c. the production of large amounts of dilute urine containing no glucose.
   d. insufficient pancreatic activity.
7. Treatment with ADH preparations is associated with adverse effects, including:
   a. constipation and paralytic ileus.
   b. cholecystitis and bile obstruction.
   c. nocturia and bed wetting.
   d. 'hangover' symptoms, including headache, sweating and tremors.
8. A person who is receiving an ADH preparation for diabetes insipidus may need instruction in administering the drug:
   a. orally or intramuscularly.
   b. orally or intranasally.
   c. rectally or orally.
   d. intranasally or by dermal patch.

MULTIPLE RESPONSE

Select all that apply.

1. Octreotide (*Sandostatin*) would be the drug of choice in the treatment of acromegaly in a person with which of the following conditions?
   a. diabetes
   b. gallbladder disease
   c. adrenal insufficiency
   d. hypothalamic lesions
   e. intolerance to other therapies
   f. acromegaly in a person older than the age of 18 years
2. A father brought his 15-year-old son to the endocrine clinic because the boy was only 152 centimetres tall. He wanted his son to receive growth hormone therapy because short stature would be a detriment to his success as an adult. The boy would be considered for this therapy under which of the following circumstances?
   a. If he were against the use of cadaver parts.
   b. If his epiphyses were closed.
   c. If his GH levels were very low.
   d. If he were also diabetic.
   e. If he had chronic renal failure.
   f. If he had hypothyroidism.

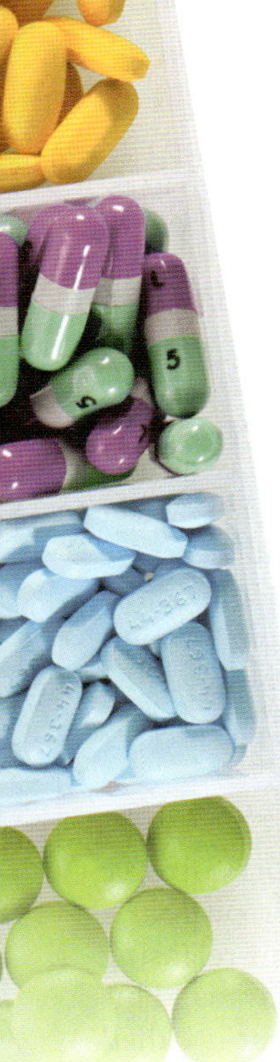

36 Adrenocortical agents

Learning objectives

On completing this chapter you should be able to:

1. Explain the control of the synthesis and secretion, and physiological effects of the adrenocortical agents.
2. Describe the therapeutic actions, indications, pharmacokinetics, contraindications, most common adverse reactions and important drug–drug interactions associated with the adrenocortical agents.
3. Discuss the use of adrenocortical agents across the lifespan.
4. Compare and contrast the prototype drugs prednisone and fludrocortisone with other adrenocortical agents.
5. Outline the care considerations, including important teaching points, for people receiving an adrenocortical agent.

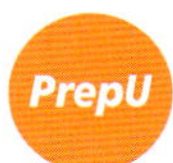

Test your current knowledge of adrenocortical agents with a PrepU Practice Quiz!

Glossary of key terms

adrenal cortex: outer layer of the adrenal gland; produces glucocorticoids and mineralocorticoids in response to adrenocorticotropic hormone (ACTH) stimulation; also responds to sympathetic stimulation

adrenal medulla: inner layer of the adrenal gland; a sympathetic ganglion, it releases noradrenaline and adrenaline into circulation in response to sympathetic stimulation

corticosteroids: steroid hormones produced by the adrenal cortex; include androgens, glucocorticoids and mineralocorticoids

diurnal rhythm: response of the hypothalamus and then the pituitary and adrenals to wakefulness and sleeping; normally, the hypothalamus begins secretion of corticotropin-releasing factor (CRF) in the evening, peaking at about midnight; adrenocortical peak response is between 6 and 9 a.m.; levels fall during the day until evening, when the low level is picked up by the hypothalamus and CRF secretion begins again

glucocorticoids: steroid hormones released from the adrenal cortex; they increase blood glucose levels, fat deposits and protein breakdown for energy

mineralocorticoids: steroid hormones released by the adrenal cortex; they cause sodium and water retention and potassium excretion

ADRENOCORTICAL AGENTS

Glucocorticoids

beclomethasone
betamethasone
budesonide
cortisone
dexamethasone
fluticasone
fluoromethalone
hydrocortisone
methylprednisolone
prednisolone
 prednisone
triamcinolone

Mineralocorticoids

cortisone
(P) fludrocortisone
hydrocortisone

Topical steroids

See Appendix C

Adrenocortical agents are widely used to suppress the immune system. These drugs do not, however, cure any inflammatory disorders. Once widely used to treat a number of chronic problems, adrenocortical agents are now reserved for short-term use to relieve inflammation during acute stages of illness or for replacement therapy to maintain hormone levels when the adrenal glands are not functioning adequately.

THE ADRENAL GLANDS

The two adrenal glands are flattened bodies that sit on top of each kidney. Each gland is made up of an inner core called the **adrenal medulla** and an outer shell called the **adrenal cortex.**

The adrenal medulla is actually part of the sympathetic nervous system (SNS). It is a ganglion of neurons that releases the neurotransmitters noradrenaline and adrenaline into circulation when the SNS is stimulated. (See Chapter 29 for a review of the sympathetic nervous system.) The secretion of these neurotransmitters directly into the bloodstream allows them to act as hormones, travelling from the adrenal medulla to react with specific receptor sites throughout the body. This is thought to be a backup system for the sympathetic system, adding an extra stimulus to the stress ('fight-or-flight') response.

The adrenal cortex surrounds the medulla and consists of three layers of cells, each of which synthesises chemically different types of steroid hormones that exert physiological effects throughout the body. The adrenal cortex produces hormones called **corticosteroids.** There are three types of corticosteroids: androgens, glucocorticoids and mineralocorticoids. Androgens are a form of the male sex hormone testosterone. They affect electrolytes, stimulate protein production and decrease protein breakdown. They are used pharmacologically to treat hypogonadism or to increase protein growth and red blood cell production. These hormones are discussed in Chapter 41.

Controls

The adrenal cortex responds to adrenocorticotropic hormone (ACTH) released from the anterior pituitary. ACTH, in turn, responds to corticotropin-releasing hormone (CRH) released from the hypothalamus. This happens regularly during a normal day in what is called **diurnal rhythm** (Box 36.1). A person who has a regular cycle of sleep and wakefulness will produce high levels of CRH during sleep, usually around midnight. A resulting peak response of increased ACTH and adrenocortical hormones occurs sometime early in the morning, around 6–9 a.m. This high level of hormones then suppresses any further CRH or ACTH release. The corticosteroids are metabolised and excreted slowly throughout the day

BOX 36.1 FOCUS ON **The evidence**

Diurnal rhythm

Research over the years has shown that the adrenocortical hormones are released in a pattern called the diurnal rhythm. The secretion of CRH, ACTH and cortisol are high in the morning in day-oriented people (those who have a regular cycle of wakefulness during the day and sleep during the night). In such individuals, the peak levels of cortisol usually come between 6 and 8 a.m. The levels then fall off slowly (with periodic spurts) and reach a low in the late evening, with lowest levels around midnight. It is thought that this cycle is related to the effects of sleeping on the hypothalamus, and that the hypothalamus is regulating its stimulation of the anterior pituitary in relation to sleep and activity. The cycle may also be connected to the hypothalamic response to light. This is important to keep in mind when treating people with corticosteroids. In order to mimic the normal diurnal pattern, corticosteroids should be taken immediately on waking in the morning.

Complications to this pattern arise, however, when people work shifts or change their sleeping patterns (eg, university students). In response, the hypothalamus shifts its release of CRH to correspond to the new cycle. For example, if a person works all night and goes to bed at 8 a.m., arising at 3 p.m. to carry on the day's activities before going to work at 11 p.m., the hypothalamus will release CRH at about 3 p.m. in accordance with the new sleep–wake cycle. It usually takes 2 or 3 days for the hypothalamus to readjust. A person on this schedule who is taking replacement corticosteroids would then need to take them at 3 p.m., or on rising. People who work several different shifts in a single week may not have time to reregulate their hypothalamus, and the corticosteroid cycle may be thrown off. People who have to change their sleep patterns repeatedly often complain about feeling weak, getting sick more easily, or having trouble concentrating. University students frequently develop a pattern of sleeping all day, then staying up all night – a cycle that becomes hard to break as their bodies and endocrine systems try to readjust.

It is a challenge to help people understand how the body works and to offer ways to decrease the stress of changing sleep patterns – especially if the health professional is also working several different shifts. Many employers are willing to have employees work several days of the same shift before switching back, mainly because they have noticed an increase in productivity and a decrease in absences when employees have enough time to allow their bodies to adjust to the new shift.

and fall to low levels by evening. At this point, the hypothalamus and pituitary sense low levels of the hormones and begin the production and release of CRH and ACTH again. This peaks around midnight and the cycle starts again.

Activation of the stress reaction through the SNS bypasses the usual diurnal rhythm and causes release of ACTH and secretion of the adrenocortical hormones – an important aspect of the stress response. The stress response is activated with cellular injury or when a person perceives fear or feels anxious. These hormones have many actions, including:

- increasing the blood volume (aldosterone effect)
- causing the release of glucose for energy
- slowing the rate of protein production (which preserves energy)
- blocking the activities of the inflammatory and immune systems (which preserves a great deal of energy).

These actions are important during an acute stress situation, but they can cause adverse reactions in periods of extreme or prolonged stress. For example, a person who is very fearful and stressed postoperatively may not heal well because protein building is blocked; infections may be hard to treat in such an individual because the inflammatory and immune systems are not functioning adequately.

Aldosterone is also released without ACTH stimulation when the blood surrounding the adrenal gland is high in potassium, a direct stimulus for aldosterone release. Aldosterone causes the kidneys to excrete potassium to restore homeostasis.

Adrenal Insufficiency

Some individuals can experience a shortage of adrenocortical hormones and develop signs of adrenal insufficiency (Table 36.1). This can occur when a person does not produce enough ACTH, when the adrenal glands are not able to respond to ACTH, when an adrenal gland is damaged and cannot produce enough hormones (as in Addison disease) or secondary to surgical removal of the glands.

A more common cause of adrenal insufficiency is prolonged use of corticosteroid hormones. When exogenous corticosteroids are used, they act to negate the regular feedback systems (Figure 36.1). The adrenal glands begin to atrophy because ACTH release is suppressed by the exogenous hormones, so the glands are no longer stimulated to produce or secrete hormones. It takes several weeks to recover from the atrophy caused by this lack of stimulation. To prevent this from happening, people should receive only short-term steroid therapy and should be weaned slowly from the hormones so that the adrenals have time to recover and start producing hormones again.

Adrenal crisis

Individuals who have an adrenal insufficiency may do quite well until they experience a period of extreme stress, such as a motor vehicle accident, a surgical procedure or a massive infection. Because they are not able to supplement the energy-consuming effects of the sympathetic reaction, they enter an adrenal crisis, which can include physiological exhaustion, hypotension, fluid shift, shock and even death. Individuals in adrenal crisis are treated with a massive infusion of replacement steroids, constant monitoring and life support procedures.

KEY POINTS

- There are two adrenal glands, one on top of each kidney.
- Each adrenal gland is composed of the adrenal medulla and the adrenal cortex.
- Corticosteroids help the body to conserve energy for the stress response.
- Prolonged use of corticosteroids suppresses the normal hypothalamic–pituitary axis and leads to adrenal atrophy from lack of stimulation.

TABLE 36.1 Signs and symptoms of adrenal dysfunction

Clinical effects	Hypoadrenal function (Addison disease)	Hyperadrenal function (Cushing disease)
Central nervous system	Confusion, disorientation	Emotional disturbances
Cardiovascular system	Hypotension, arrhythmias, cardiovascular collapse, loss of extracellular fluid	Cardiac hypertrophy, hypertension
Skin, hair, nails	Hyperpigmentation, sparse axillary and pubic hair; bluish-black oral mucosa	Thin, wrinkled skin; purpura; purple abdominal striae; hirsutism
Metabolic rate	Hyponatraemia, hyperkalaemia, hypoglycaemia, lethargy, fatigue, weakness	Hypernatraemia, hypokalaemia, hyperglycaemia, osteoporosis; renal calculi; amenorrhoea
General	Dehydration, fatigue, poor response to stress, limited ability to respond to infection	Moon face, buffalo hump, obesity, immune and inflammatory suppression, risk of gastric ulcers and bleeding

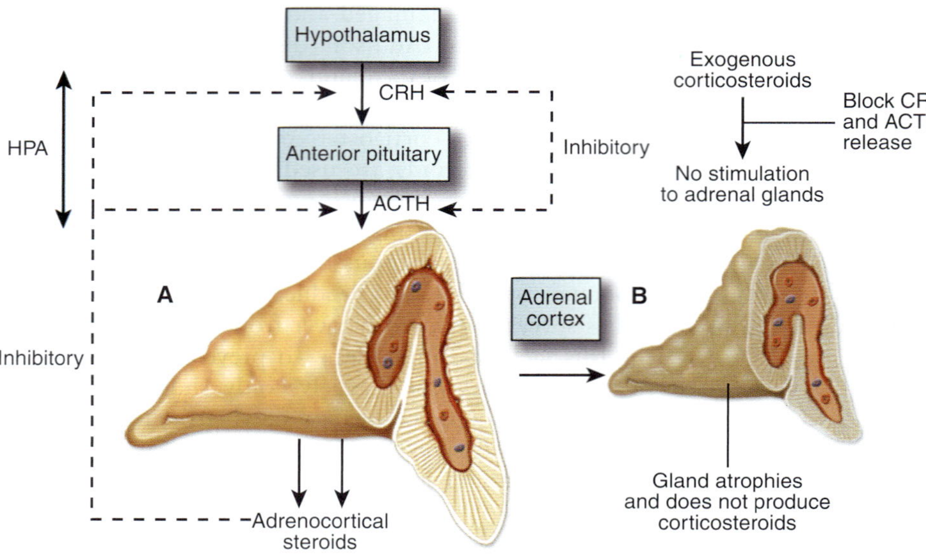

FIGURE 36.1 **A.** Normal controls of adrenal glands. The hypothalamus releases corticotropin-releasing hormone (CRH), which causes release of corticotropin (ACTH) from the anterior pituitary. ACTH stimulates the adrenal cortex to produce and release corticosteroids. Increasing levels of corticosteroids inhibit the release of CRH and ACTH. **B.** Exogenous corticosteroids act to inhibit CRH and ACTH release; the adrenal cortex is no longer stimulated and atrophies. Sudden stopping of steroids results in a crisis of adrenal hypofunction until hypothalamic–pituitary axis (HPA) controls stimulate the adrenal gland again.

ADRENOCORTICAL AGENTS

There are three types of corticosteroids: androgens (discussed in Chapter 41), glucocorticoids and mineralocorticoids. Not all adrenocortical agents are classified as only glucocorticoids or mineralocorticoids. Hydrocortisone, cortisone and prednisone also have glucocorticoid and some mineralocorticoid activity and affect potassium, sodium and water levels in the body when present in high levels (Table 36.2). Box 36.2 discusses their use in different age groups. Figure 36.2 displays the sites of action of the glucocorticoids and the mineralocorticoids.

Glucocorticoids

Glucocorticoids (Table 36.3) are so named because they stimulate an increase in glucose levels for energy. They also increase the rate of protein breakdown and decrease the rate of protein formation from amino acids, another way of preserving energy. Glucocorticoids also cause lipogenesis, or the formation and storage of fat in the body. This stored fat will then be available to be broken down for energy when needed.

Several glucocorticoids are available for pharmacological use. They differ mainly by route of administration and duration of action. Glucocorticoids include beclomethasone (*Beconase, Qvar*), betamethasone (*Celestone*, *Diprosone* and others), budesonide (*Entocort*, *Pulmicort*, *Rhinocort*, *Symbicort* and others), cortisone (*Cortate*), dexamethasone (*Dexmethsone* and others), hydrocortisone (*Sigmacort, Solu-Cortef*, and others), methylprednisolone (*Advantan*, *Depo-Medrol*, *Depo-Nisolone*), prednisolone (*Panafcortelone*, *Predsol*, *Redipred* and others), prednisone (*Panafcort*, *Sone*) and triamcinolone (*Aristocort*, *Kenacomb*, *Tricortone* and others).

TABLE 36.2 Selected corticosteroids: equivalent strength, glucocorticoid and mineralocorticoid effects and duration of effects

Drug	Equivalent dose (mg)	Glucocorticoid effects	Mineralocorticoid effects	Duration of effects (hours)
Short-acting corticosteroids				
cortisone	25	+	++++	8–12
hydrocortisone	20	+	++++	8–12
Intermediate-acting corticosteroids				
prednisone	5	++++	++	18–36
prednisolone	5	++++	++	18–36
triamcinolone	4	+++++	—	18–36
methylprednisolone	4	+++++	—	18–36
Long-acting corticosteroids				
dexamethasone	0.75	+++++++++	—	36–54
betamethasone	0.75	+++++++++	—	35–54

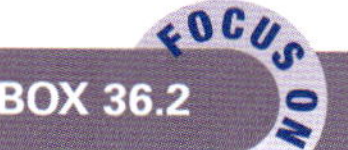

BOX 36.2 Drug therapy across the lifespan

Corticosteroids

CHILDREN

Corticosteroids are used in children for the same indications as in adults. The dose for children is determined by the severity of the condition being treated and the response to the drug, not on a weight or age formula.

Children need to be monitored closely for any effects on growth and development, and dose adjustments should be made or drug discontinued if growth is severely retarded.

Topical use of corticosteroids should be limited in children; because their body surface area is comparatively large, the amount of the drug absorbed in relation to weight is greater than in an adult. Apply sparingly and do not use in the presence of open lesions. Do not occlude treated areas with dressings or nappies, which may increase the risk of systemic absorption.

Children need to be supervised when using nasal sprays or respiratory inhalants to ensure that proper technique is being used.

Children receiving long-term therapy should be protected from exposure to infection, and special precautions should be instituted to avoid injury. If injuries or infections do occur, the child should be seen by a primary care provider as soon as possible.

ADULTS

Adults should be reminded of the importance of taking these drugs in the morning to approximate diurnal rhythm.

They should also be cautioned about the importance of tapering the drug rather than stopping abruptly.

Several over-the-counter topical preparations contain corticosteroids, and adults should be cautioned to avoid combining these preparations with prescription topical corticosteroids. They also should be cautioned to apply any of these sparingly and to avoid applying them to open lesions or excoriated areas.

With long-term therapy, the importance of avoiding exposure to infection – crowded areas, people with colds or the flu, activities associated with injury – should be stressed. If an injury or infection should occur, the person should be encouraged to seek medical care. Monitoring blood glucose levels should be done regularly.

PREGNANCY AND BREASTFEEDING

These drugs should not be used during pregnancy because they cross the placenta and could cause adverse effects on the fetus. If the benefit to the mother clearly outweighs the potential risk to the fetus, they should be used with caution. Breastfeeding women should find another method of feeding the baby if corticosteroids are needed because of the potential for serious adverse effects on the baby.

OLDER ADULTS

Older adults are more likely to experience the adverse effects associated with these drugs, and the dose should be reduced and the person monitored very closely. Older adults are more likely to have hepatic and/or renal impairment, which could lead to accumulation of the drug and resultant toxic effects. They are also more likely to have medical conditions that could be imbalanced by changes in fluid and electrolytes, metabolism changes, and other drug effects. Such conditions include diabetes, heart failure, osteoporosis, coronary artery disease and immune suppression. Careful monitoring of drug dose and response to the drug should be done on a regular basis.

Therapeutic actions and indications

Glucocorticoids enter target cells and bind to cytoplasmic receptors, initiating many complex reactions that are responsible for anti-inflammatory and immunosuppressive effects. Hydrocortisone, cortisone and prednisone also have some mineralocorticoid activity and affect potassium, sodium and water levels in the body.

Glucocorticoids are indicated for the short-term treatment of many inflammatory disorders, to relieve discomfort and to give the body a chance to heal from the effects of inflammation. They block the actions of arachidonic acid, which leads to a decrease in the formation of prostaglandins and leukotrienes. Without these chemicals, the normal inflammatory reaction is blocked. They also impair the ability of phagocytes to leave the bloodstream and move to injured tissues, and they inhibit the ability of lymphocytes to act within the immune system, including a blocking of the production of antibodies. They can be used to treat local inflammation as topical agents, intranasal or inhaled agents, intra-articular injections and ophthalmic agents. Systemic use is indicated for the treatment of some cancers, hypocalcaemia associated with cancer, haematological disorders and some neurological infections. When combined with mineralocorticoids, some of these drugs can be used in replacement therapy for adrenal insufficiency. See Table 36.3 for information on each type of glucocorticoid agent.

Pharmacokinetics

These drugs are absorbed well from many sites. They are metabolised by natural systems, mostly within the liver, and are excreted in the urine. The glucocorticoids are known to cross the placenta and to enter breast milk; they should be used during pregnancy and breastfeeding only if the benefits to the mother clearly outweigh the potential risks to the fetus or neonate.

Beclomethasone is available in the form of a respiratory inhalant and nasal spray.

Betamethasone is a long-acting steroid available for systemic, parenteral use in acute situations, as well as orally and as a topical application.

Budesonide is a relatively new steroid for intranasal use.

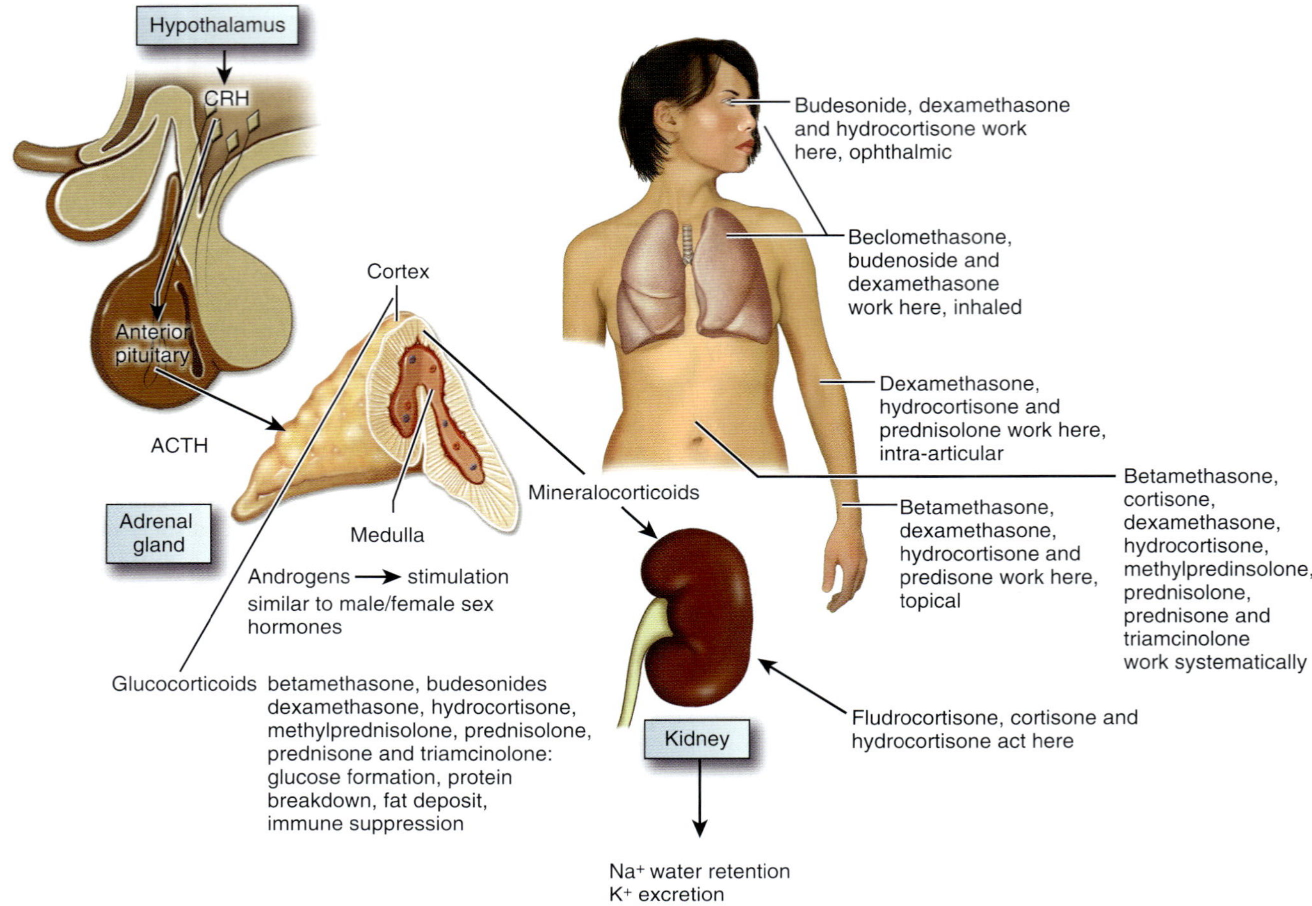

FIGURE 36.2 Sites of action of the adrenocortical agents.

Cortisone is used orally and parenterally.

Dexamethasone and triamcinolone are available in multiple forms for dermatological, ophthalmological, intra-articular, parenteral and inhalational uses. They peak quickly and effects can last for 2–3 days.

Hydrocortisone has largely been replaced for other uses (eg, intra-articular, intravenous) by other steroid hormones with less mineralocorticoid effect. It may be preferred for use as a topical or ophthalmic agent.

Methylprednisolone is available in multiple forms, including oral, parenteral, intra-articular and retention enema preparations.

Prednisolone is an intermediate-acting corticosteroid with effects lasting only a day or so. It is used

TABLE 36.3 DRUGS IN FOCUS Adrenocortical agents

Drug name	Dosage/route	Usual indications
Glucocorticoids		
beclomethasone (*Beconase, Qvar*)	*Asthma prophylaxis* Adults: 50–200 micrograms bd, up to 400 micrograms bd (maximum 800 micrograms/day) Children > 5 years: 50 micrograms bd *Allergic rhinitis* Adults and children > 12 years: 2 sprays in each nostril bd; maximum 8 sprays/day	Blocking inflammation in the respiratory tract
betamethasone (*Celestone, Diprosone*)	Adult, intra-articular: 1 mL (5.7 mg/mL) repeat in 1–2 weeks; intramuscular: 1 mL (5.7 mg/mL) weekly; not given IV or SC Paediatric: individualise dose based on severity and response, and monitor closely	Management of allergic intra-articular, topical and inflammatory disorders

TABLE 36.3 DRUGS IN FOCUS Adrenocortical agents *(continued)*

Drug name	Dosage/route	Usual indications
Glucocorticoids *(continued)*		
budesonide (*Butacort, Rhinocort, Entocort, Pulmicort, Rhinocort, Symbicort*)	Oral: 9 mg in the morning for 12 weeks (Crohn disease) Nasal, adults, *Butacort 50:* initially 1–2 sprays into each nostril morning and night, then after 2–3 days, 1 spray into each nostril bd; *Butacort 100:* initially 1–2 sprays into each nostril in the morning, then after 2–3 days, 1 spray into each nostril in the morning Nasal, children > 6 years: Rhinocort 32–64 micrograms in each nostril in the morning Foam enema: 1.2 g foam (1 application) daily morning or night for up to 6–8 weeks Inhaler, adults: 400–2400 micrograms/day in 2–4 divided doses, depending on severity Inhaler, children: 200–400 micrograms/day in 2–4 divided doses; maximum 800 micrograms/day Pulmicort respule for nebulisation, adults: 1–2 mg bd via nebuliser; children: 0.5–1 mg bd via nebuliser	Relief of symptoms of seasonal and allergic rhinitis with few side effects; approved in 2001 as an oral agent for the treatment of mild-to-moderate active Crohn disease
cortisone (*Cortate*)	Adult: 25 mg PO q 6 hours until remission, then reduced by 10–20 mg every few days Paediatric: base dose on response, monitor closely	Replacement therapy in adrenal insufficiency; allergic and inflammatory disorders treatment
dexamethasone (*Dexmethsone*)	*Adult* Oral: initially 0.5–10 mg daily in divided doses; then gradually reduce to 0.5–1 mg daily. No children's dose given IM or IV: 0.5–24 mg/day depending on condition and severity Eye drops: 1–2 drops 4–6 times daily Also available as an intravitreal implant	Management of allergic and inflammatory disorders, adrenal hypofunction
hydrocortisone (*Sigmacort, Solu-Cortef*)	*Adult* Tablets: usually 30 mg/day PO in divided doses Topical: apply 2–4 times daily Rectal foam: one application once or twice daily IM, IV: 100–500 mg q 2–6 hours Ophthalmic: apply ointment bd–qid Rectal foam: 1 applicator-full (ie, 90–100 mg) rectally 1–2 times daily for 2–3 weeks, then reduce	Replacement therapy, treatment of allergic and inflammatory disorders
methylprednisolone (*Advantan, Depo-Medrol, Depo-Nisolone*)	Oral, IV, IM, intra-articular Adult: 40–120 mg/day PO or IM; 10–40 mg IV slowly Paediatric: base dose on severity and response	Treatment of allergic and inflammatory disorders
prednisolone (*Panafcortelone, Predsol, Redipred*)	Tablets, oral liquid, adults: 5–20 mg/day; maximum 80 mg/day Oral tablets, oral liquid, paediatric: 0.5–1.5 mg/kg/day; maintenance dosage: 0.125–0.25 mg/kg/day Suppository: one (5 mg) bd Rectal enema: one at night for 2–4 weeks Eye drops: 1 drop as required for non-infected inflammatory eye condition	Treatment of allergic and inflammatory disorders

Continued on following page

TABLE 36.3 DRUGS IN FOCUS Adrenocortical agents (continued)

Drug name	Dosage/route	Usual indications
Glucocorticoids *(continued)*		
(P) prednisone (*Panafcort, Sone*)	Adult: 5–80 mg in divided dose (initial dose); 5–20 mg daily (maintenance dose). Dose individualised according to severity of the disease and individual's response rather than age or body weight Paediatric: base dose on severity and response	Replacement therapy for adrenal insufficiency; treatment of allergic and inflammatory disorders; severe bronchial asthma, status asthmaticus, acquired haemolytic anaemia, nephrotic syndrome
triamcinolone (*Aristocort, Kenacomb, Tricortone*)	Intra-articular: 2.5–15 mg depending on joint size Deep IM: 20–80 mg; usual dose 60 mg Topical: apply tid–qid Nasal spray, adults, children > 12 years: 2 sprays each nostril once a day Oral paste: apply at bedtime up to bid–tid	Treatment of allergic and inflammatory disorders, management of asthma; treatment of adrenal insufficiency when combined with a mineralocorticoid
Mineralocorticoids		
cortisone (*Cortate*)	Adult: 25 mg PO q 6 hours until remission, then reduced by 10–20 mg every few days Paediatric: base dose on severity and response	Used for replacement therapy in adrenal insufficiency, treatment of allergic and inflammatory disorders
(P) fludrocortisone (*Florinef*)	Adult: 0.1–0.2 mg/day PO	Used for replacement therapy and treatment of salt-losing adrenogenital syndrome with a glucocorticoid; not recommended for children; being tried for treatment of severe orthostatic hypotension because sodium and water retention effects can lead to increased blood pressure
hydrocortisone (*Solu-Cortef*)	Topical: apply bd–qid as necessary. Oral tablets, adults: usually 30 mg/day in divided doses; no children's dose Rectal foam: one application once or twice daily IM, IV: 100–500 mg q 2–6 hours Ophthalmic: bd–qid Paediatric: base dose on response and severity; 0.56–8 mg/kg/day (20–240 mg/m^2/day) IM/IV in 3–4 divided doses	Used for replacement therapy, treatment of allergic and inflammatory disorders

for intralesional and intra-articular injection and is also available in oral and topical forms.

Prednisone is available only as an oral agent.

Contraindications and cautions

These drugs are contraindicated in the presence of any known allergy to any steroid preparation *to avoid hypersensitivity reactions*; in the presence of an acute infection, *which could become serious or even fatal if the immune and inflammatory responses are blocked*; and with breastfeeding *because the anti-inflammatory and immunosuppressive actions could be passed to the baby.*

Caution should be used in people with diabetes *because the glucose-elevating effects disrupt glucose control*; with acute peptic ulcers *because steroid use is associated with the development of ulcers*; with other endocrine disorders, *which could be sent into imbalance*; and in pregnancy.

Use in children

Corticosteroids cause growth retardation in infancy, childhood and adolescence, which may be irreversible and therefore long-term administration of pharmacological doses should be avoided. If prolonged therapy is necessary, treatment should be limited to the minimum suppression of the hypothalamic–pituitary–adrenal axis, and the growth and development of infants and children should be closely monitored. Treatment should be administered where possible as a single dose on alternate days.

Children and adolescents should also be closely monitored for osteoporosis, avascular necrosis of the femoral heads, glaucoma or cataracts during prolonged

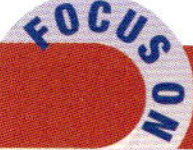

Safe medication administration

Adverse effects of corticosteroid use associated with various routes of administration

Systemic: *systemic effects are most likely to occur when the corticosteroid is given by the oral, intravenous, intramuscular or subcutaneous route. Systemic absorption is possible, however, if other routes of administration are not used correctly or if tissue breakdown or injury allows direct absorption.*

Central nervous system: vertigo, headache, paraesthesias, insomnia, convulsions, psychosis.

Gastrointestinal: peptic or oesophageal ulcers, pancreatitis, abdominal distension, nausea, vomiting, increased appetite, weight gain.

Cardiovascular: hypotension, shock, heart failure secondary to fluid retention, thromboembolism, thrombophlebitis, fat embolism, arrhythmias secondary to electrolyte disturbances.

Haematological: sodium and fluid retention, hypokalaemia, hypocalcaemia, increased blood sugar, increased serum cholesterol, decreased thyroid hormone levels.

Musculoskeletal: muscle weakness, steroid myopathy, loss of muscle mass, osteoporosis, spontaneous fractures.

Eyes, ears, nose and throat: cataracts, glaucoma.

Dermatological: frail skin, petechiae, ecchymoses, purpura, striae, subcutaneous fat atrophy.

Endocrine: amenorrhoea, irregular menses, growth retardation, decreased carbohydrate tolerance, glucose dysregulation and/or diabetes.

Other: immunosuppression, aggravation or masking of infections, impaired wound healing, suppression of hypothalamic–pituitary axis.

Intramuscular repository injections: *atrophy at the injection site.*

Retention enema: *local pain, burning; rectal bleeding.*

Intra-articular injection: *osteonecrosis, tendon rupture, infection.*

Intraspinal: *meningitis, adhesive arachnoiditis, conus medullaris syndrome.*

Intrathecal administration: *arachnoiditis.*

Topical: *local burning, irritation, acneiform lesions, striae, skin atrophy.*

Respiratory inhalant: *oral, laryngeal and pharyngeal irritation; fungal infections.*

Intranasal: *headache, nausea, nasal irritation, fungal infections, epistaxis, rebound congestion, perforation of the nasal septum, anosmia (lack of ability to perceive odours), urticaria.*

Ophthalmic: *infections, glaucoma, cataracts.*

Intralesional: *blindness when used on the face and head (rare).*

therapy. Children are at special risk from raised intracranial pressure.

Use in the elderly

Long-term use in the elderly should be planned bearing in mind the more serious consequences of the common side-effects of prednisone in old age, especially osteoporosis, diabetes, hypertension, hypokalaemia, susceptibility to infection and thinning of the skin. Close medical supervision is required to avoid life threatening reactions.

Adverse effects

Children are at risk of growth retardation associated with suppression of the hypothalamic–pituitary system. Additional adverse effects associated with the glucocorticoids are related to the route of administration that is used. Local use is associated with local inflammations and infections, as well as burning and stinging sensations.

Clinically important drug–drug interactions

Therapeutic and toxic effects increase if corticosteroids are given with erythromycin. Serum levels and effectiveness may decrease if corticosteroids are combined with salicylates, barbiturates, phenytoin or rifampicin.

 **Prototype summary: prednisone**

Indications: replacement therapy in adrenal cortical insufficiency, short-term management of various inflammatory and allergic disorders, hypercalcaemia associated with cancer, haematological disorders, ulcerative colitis, acute exacerbations of multiple sclerosis, palliation in some leukaemias, trichinosis with systemic involvement.

Actions: enters target cells and binds to intracellular corticosteroid receptors, initiating many complex reactions responsible for its anti-inflammatory and immunosuppressive effects.

Pharmacokinetics:

Route	Onset	Peak	Duration
PO	Varies	1–2 hours	1–1.5 days

$T_{1/2}$: 2–3 hours; metabolised in the liver to the active metabolite prednisolone and excreted in the urine.

Adverse effects: vertigo, headache, hypotension, shock, sodium and fluid retention, amenorrhoea, increased appetite, weight gain, immunosuppression, aggravation or masking of infections, impaired wound healing.

Care considerations for people receiving glucocorticoids

Assessment: history and examination

- Assess for history of allergy to any steroid preparations, acute infections, peptic ulcer disease, pregnancy, breastfeeding, endocrine disturbances and renal dysfunction, *which could be cautions or contraindications to use of the drug.*
- Assess weight; temperature; orientation and affect; grip strength; eye examination; blood pressure, pulse, peripheral perfusion and vessel evaluation; respiration and adventitious breath sounds; glucose tolerance, renal function, serum electrolytes and endocrine function tests as appropriate, *to determine baseline status before beginning therapy and for any potential adverse effects.*

Refer to the Critical thinking scenario for a full discussion of care for a person who is receiving glucocorticoids.

Implementation with rationale

- Administer drug daily at 8–9 a.m. *to mimic normal peak diurnal concentration levels and thereby minimise suppression of the hypothalamic–pituitary axis.*
- Space multiple doses evenly throughout the day *to try to achieve homeostasis.*
- Use the minimal dose for the minimal amount of time *to minimise adverse effects.*
- Taper doses when discontinuing from high doses or from long-term therapy *to give the adrenal glands a chance to recover and produce adrenocorticoids.*
- Arrange for increased dose when the person is under stress *to supply the increased demand for corticosteroids associated with the stress reaction.*
- Use alternate-day maintenance therapy with short-acting drugs whenever possible *to decrease the risk of adrenal suppression.*
- Do not give live virus vaccines when the person is immunosuppressed *because there is an increased risk of infection.*
- Protect the person from unnecessary exposure to infection and invasive procedures *because the steroids suppress the immune system and the person is at increased risk for infection.*
- Assess the person carefully for any potential drug–drug interactions *to avoid adverse effects.*
- Provide thorough teaching, including measures to avoid adverse effects, warning signs of problems and the need for regular evaluation, including blood tests, *to enhance knowledge of drug therapy and promote compliance.* Explain the need to protect from exposure to infections *to prevent serious adverse effects.*

Evaluation

- Monitor response to the drug (relief of signs and symptoms of inflammation, return of adrenal function to within normal limits).
- Monitor for adverse effects (increased susceptibility to infections, skin changes, endocrine dysfunctions, fatigue, fluid retention, peptic ulcer, psychological changes).
- Evaluate the effectiveness of the teaching plan (person can name drug, dosage, adverse effects to watch for and specific measures to avoid them).

KEY POINTS

- The glucocorticoids increase glucose production, stimulate fat deposition and protein breakdown and inhibit protein formation. They are used clinically to block inflammation and the immune response and in conjunction with mineralocorticoids to treat adrenal insufficiency.
- Individuals receiving glucocorticoids need to be protected from exposure to infection, have their blood glucose monitored regularly and dietary changes made as needed. They will also not heal well because of the inhibition of protein formation.

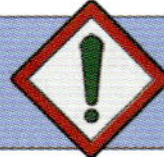

CRITICAL THINKING SCENARIO

Adrenocortical agents

THE SITUATION

M.W., a 48-year-old woman, was diagnosed with severe rheumatoid arthritis 7 years ago. She has been retired, on disability, from her job as an art teacher in the local high school. Her pain is no longer controlled by aspirin, and her doctor ordered 5 mg prednisone three times a day. Over the next 4 weeks, M.W.'s symptoms were markedly relieved; she was able to start painting again, and she became much more mobile. She also noted that for the first time in years she felt 'really good'. Her appetite increased, she was no longer fatigued and her outlook on life was markedly improved. At her follow-up visit, M.W. had gained 4 kilograms; she had slight oedema in both ankles, and her blood pressure was 150/92 mmHg. An inflamed, oozing lesion was found on her right hand, which she stated became infected a few weeks ago after she cut her hand while peeling potatoes. Her range of motion and joints were markedly improved. The doctor decided that M.W. was past her crisis and that the prednisone should be tapered to 5 mg/day over a 4-week period.

CRITICAL THINKING

Think about the pathophysiology of rheumatoid arthritis. What effects did the prednisone have on the process at work in M.W.'s joints?

What effects does the adrenocorticoid steroid have on the rest of M.W.'s body?

What can be expected to occur when a person is on prednisone for a month?

What precautions should be taken?

What care interventions are appropriate for M.W. at this visit?

DISCUSSION

The most urgent problem for M.W. at this time is the infected lesion on her hand.

Because steroids interfere with the normal inflammatory and immune response to infection, the lesion could progress to a very serious problem. The lesion should be cultured, cleansed and dressed. M.W. should be instructed in how to care for her hand and how to protect it from water or further injury. An antibiotic might be prescribed and then evaluated for its appropriateness when the culture report comes back.

The real challenge with M.W. will be helping her to cope with and understand the need to taper her prednisone. The drug-teaching information for prednisone should be thoroughly reviewed with M.W., pointing out the side effects of drug therapy that she is already experiencing and explaining, again, the effect that prednisone has on her body. A calendar should be prepared for M.W. to help her schedule the tapering of the drug. It usually progresses from 5 mg twice daily for 2 weeks to 5 mg/day. M.W. will need a great deal of encouragement and support to cope with the decrease in therapeutic benefit caused by the need to reduce the prednisone dose. She has felt so good and done so much better while receiving the drug that she may have a real dread of losing those benefits. She should be encouraged to discuss her feelings and to call in for support if she needs it. M.W. should be given an appointment for a return visit in 2 weeks to evaluate the lesion on her hand and to check her progress in the tapering of the drug. She should be urged to call if the lesion looks worse to her or if she has any difficulties with her drug therapy.

Patients with rheumatoid arthritis should start treatment with a disease modifying-anti-rheumatic drug (DMARD) as soon as possible, as early treatment has been shown to improve outcomes (see Chapter 16: Anti-inflammatory, antiarthritis and related agents).

M.W.'s case is a common example of the clinical problems that are encountered with a chronic inflammatory condition requiring steroid therapy. These people require strong support and continual teaching.

CARE GUIDE FOR M.W.: ADRENOCORTICAL AGENTS

Assessment: history and examination

Assess for allergies to any steroids and for heart failure, pregnancy, hypertension, acute infection, peptic ulcer, vaccination with a live virus, or endocrine disorders.

Also assess for concurrent use of azole antifungals, oestrogens, barbiturates, phenytoin, rifampicin or salicylates.

Focus the physical examination on the following:

Neurological: orientation, reflexes, affect

General: temperature, weight, site of hand infection

CV: pulse, cardiac auscultation, blood pressure, oedema

Respiratory: respiratory rate, adventitious sounds

Laboratory tests: urinalysis, blood glucose level, stool guaiac test, renal function tests, culture and sensitivity of wound specimen

Implementation

Administer around 9 a.m. to mimic normal diurnal rhythm.

Use the minimal dose for the minimal period of time that the dose is needed.

Arrange for increased doses during times of stress.

Taper gradually to allow adrenal glands to recover and produce their own steroids.

Protect the person from unnecessary exposure to infection.

Provide support and reassurance to deal with drug therapy.

Provide teaching regarding drug name, dosage, adverse effects, precautions and warning signs to report.

Evaluation

Evaluate drug effects: relief of signs and symptoms of inflammation.

Monitor for adverse effects: infection, peptic ulcer, fluid retention, hypertension, electrolyte imbalance or endocrine changes.

Monitor for drug–drug interactions as listed.

Evaluate the effectiveness of the teaching program.

Evaluate the effectiveness of comfort and safety measures and support offered.

TEACHING FOR M.W.

- The drug that has been prescribed for you is called prednisone. Prednisone is from a class of drugs called corticosteroids, which are similar to steroids produced naturally in your body. They affect a number of bodily functions, including your body's glucose levels, blocking your body's inflammatory and immune responses and slowing the healing process.

- You should never stop taking your drug suddenly. If your prescription is low or you are unable to take the medication for any reason, notify your health care provider.
- Some of the following adverse effects may occur:
  - *Increased appetite:* this may be a welcome change, but if you notice a continual weight gain, you may want to watch your kilojoules.
  - *Restlessness, trouble sleeping:* some people experience elation and a feeling of new energy; take frequent rest periods.
  - *Increased susceptibility to infection:* because your body's normal defenses will be decreased, you should avoid crowded places and people with known infections. If you notice any signs of illness or infection, notify your health care provider at once.
  - (Report any of the following to your health care provider): *sudden weight gain; fever or sore throat; black, tarry stools; swelling of the hands or feet; any signs of infection; or easy bruising.*
- If you are taking this drug for a prolonged period, limit your intake of salt and salted products and add proteins to your diet.
- Avoid the use of any over-the-counter medication without first checking with your health care provider. Several of these medications can interfere with the effectiveness of this drug.
- Tell any doctor, nurse or other health care provider involved in your care that you are taking this drug.
- Because this drug affects your body's natural defences, you will need special care during any stressful situations. You may want to wear or carry medical identification showing that you are taking this medication. This identification alerts any medical personnel taking care of you in an emergency to the fact that you are taking this drug.
- It is important to have regular medical follow-up. If your drug dose is being tapered, notify your health care provider if any of the following occurs: fatigue, nausea, vomiting, diarrhoea, weight loss, weakness or dizziness.
- Keep this drug out of the reach of children. Do not give this medication to anyone else or take any similar medication that has not been prescribed for you.

Mineralocorticoids

Mineralocorticoids (Table 36.3) affect electrolyte levels and homeostasis. These steroid hormones, such as aldosterone, directly affect the levels of electrolytes in the system. The classic mineralocorticoid is aldosterone. Aldosterone holds sodium – and with it, water – in the body and causes the excretion of potassium by acting on the renal tubule. Aldosterone is no longer available for pharmacological use. Mineralocorticoids that are available include cortisone (*Cortate*), fludrocortisone (*Florinef*) and hydrocortisone (*Solu-Cortef*).

Therapeutic actions and indications

The mineralocorticoids increase sodium reabsorption in renal tubules, leading to sodium and water retention, and increase potassium excretion (see Figure 36.2). Fludrocortisone is a powerful mineralocorticoid and is preferred for replacement therapy over cortisone and hydrocortisone; it is used in combination with a glucocorticoid. Hydrocortisone and cortisone also exert mineralocorticoid effects at high doses; however, this effect is not usually enough to maintain electrolyte balance in adrenal insufficiency. These drugs are indicated (in combination with a glucocorticoid) for replacement therapy in primary and secondary adrenal insufficiency. They are also indicated for the treatment of salt-wasting adrenogenital syndrome when taken with appropriate glucocorticoids. See Table 36.3 for usual indications for each mineralocorticoid.

Pharmacokinetics

These drugs are absorbed slowly and distributed throughout the body. They undergo hepatic metabolism to inactive forms. They are known to cross the placenta and to enter breast milk. They should be avoided during pregnancy and breastfeeding because of the potential for adverse effects in the fetus or baby.

Contraindications and cautions

These drugs are contraindicated in the presence of any known allergy to the drug *to avoid hypersensitivity reactions*; with severe hypertension, heart failure or cardiac disease *because of the resultant increased blood pressure*; and with breastfeeding *due to potential adverse effects on the baby*. Caution should be used in pregnancy *because of the potential for adverse effects on the fetus*, in the presence of any infection, *which will alter adrenal response*, and with high sodium intake *because severe hypernatraemia could occur.*

Adverse effects

Adverse effects commonly associated with the use of mineralocorticoids are related to the increased fluid volume seen with sodium and water retention (eg, headache, oedema, hypertension, heart failure, arrhythmias, weakness) and possible hypokalaemia. Allergic reactions, ranging from skin rash to anaphylaxis, have also been reported.

Clinically important drug–drug interactions

Decreased effectiveness of salicylates, barbiturates, phenytoin, rifampicin and anticholinesterases has been reported when these drugs are combined with mineralocorticoids. Such combinations should be avoided if possible, but if they are necessary, the person should be monitored closely and the dose increased as needed.

Prototype summary: fludrocortisone

Indications: partial replacement therapy in cortical insufficiency conditions, treatment of salt-losing adrenogenital syndrome; off-label use: treatment of hypotension.

Actions: increases sodium reabsorption in the renal tubules and increases potassium and hydrogen excretion, leading to water and sodium retention.

Pharmacokinetics:

Route	Onset	Peak	Duration
PO	Gradual	1.7 hours	18–36 hours

$T_{1/2}$: 3.5 hours; metabolised in the liver and excreted in the urine.

Adverse effects: frontal and occipital headaches, arthralgia, weakness, increased blood volume, oedema, hypertension, heart failure, rash, anaphylaxis.

Care considerations for people receiving mineralocorticoids

Assessment: history and examination

- Assess for allergy to these drugs *to avoid hypersensitivity reactions*; history of heart failure, hypertension or infections; high sodium intake; breastfeeding; and pregnancy, *which could be cautions or contraindications to use of the drug.*
- Assess blood pressure, pulse and adventitious breath sounds, weight and temperature, tissue turgor, reflexes, bilateral grip strength and serum electrolyte levels, *to determine baseline status before beginning therapy and for any potential adverse effects.*

Implementation with rationale

- Use only in conjunction with appropriate glucocorticoids *to maintain control of electrolyte balance.*
- Increase dose in times of stress *to prevent adrenal insufficiency and to meet increased demands for corticosteroids under stress.*
- Monitor for hypokalaemia (weakness, serum electrolytes) *to detect the loss early and treat appropriately.*
- Discontinue if signs of overdose (excessive weight gain, oedema, hypertension, cardiomegaly) occur *to prevent the development of more severe toxicity.*
- Provide thorough teaching, including drug name, dosage and administration; measures to avoid adverse effects; warning signs of problems; and the need for regular evaluation, including blood tests, *to enhance knowledge about drug therapy and promote compliance.*

Evaluation

- Monitor response to the drug (maintenance of electrolyte balance).
- Monitor for adverse effects (fluid retention, oedema, hypokalaemia, headache).
- Evaluate the effectiveness of the teaching plan (person can name drug, dosage, adverse effects to watch for and specific measures to avoid them).
- Monitor effectiveness of comfort measures and compliance with the regimen.

KEY POINTS

- The mineralocorticoids stimulate retention of sodium and water and excretion of potassium. These drugs are used therapeutically in conjunction with glucocorticoids to treat adrenal insufficiency.
- Individuals receiving mineralocorticoids need to be evaluated for possible hypokalaemia and its associated cardiac effects and for fluid retention that could exacerbate heart failure and cause electrolyte abnormalities.

CHAPTER SUMMARY

- The adrenal medulla is basically a sympathetic nerve ganglion that releases noradrenaline and adrenaline into the bloodstream in response to sympathetic stimulation.
- The adrenal cortex produces three types of corticosteroids: androgens (male and female sex hormones), glucocorticoids and mineralocorticoids.
- The corticosteroids are released normally in a diurnal rhythm, with the hypothalamus producing peak levels of corticotropin-releasing hormone (CRH) around midnight; peak adrenal response occurs around 9 a.m. The steroid levels drop slowly

during the day to reach low levels in the evening, when the hypothalamus begins CRH secretion, with peak levels again occurring around midnight. Corticosteroids are also released as part of the sympathetic stress reaction to help the body conserve energy for the fight-or-flight response.

- Prolonged use of corticosteroids suppresses the normal hypothalamic–pituitary axis and leads to adrenal atrophy from lack of stimulation. Corticosteroids need to be tapered slowly after prolonged use to allow the adrenals to resume steroid production.
- The glucocorticoids increase glucose production, stimulate fat deposition and protein breakdown and inhibit protein formation. They are used clinically to block inflammation and the immune response and in conjunction with mineralocorticoids to treat adrenal insufficiency.
- The mineralocorticoids stimulate retention of sodium and water and excretion of potassium. They are used therapeutically in conjunction with glucocorticoids to treat adrenal insufficiency.
- Adverse effects of corticosteroids are related to exaggeration of the physiological effects; they include immunosuppression, peptic ulcer formation, fluid retention and oedema.
- Corticosteroids are used topically and locally to achieve the desired anti-inflammatory effects at a particular site without the systemic adverse effects that limit the usefulness of these drugs.

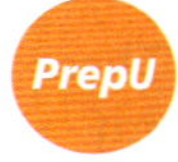

Knowing your strengths and weaknesses helps you to study more effectively. Take a PrepU Practice Quiz to find out how you measure up!

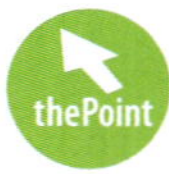

ONLINE RESOURCES

An extensive range of additional resources to enhance teaching and learning and to facilitate understanding of this chapter may be found online at the text's accompanying website, located on thePoint at http://thepoint.lww.com. These include Watch and Learn videos, Concepts in Action animations, journal articles, review questions, case studies, discussion topics and quizzes.

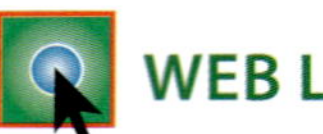

WEB LINKS

Health care providers and students may want to consult the following web resources:

www.arthritisaustralia.com.au
Information on rheumatoid and inflammatory diseases.

www.arthritis.org.nz
Information on arthritis – treatment, processes and support.

BIBLIOGRAPHY

Bennett, S. (2008). Corticosteroids: Uses and prescribing rationale. *Nurse Prescribing, 6(6)*, 259–265.

Carlos, G., Uribe, P. & Fernandez-Penas, P. (2013). Rational use of topical corticosteroids. *Australian Prescriber, 36(5)*, 159–161.

Chakera, A. J. & Valdya, B. (2010). Addison disease in adults: Diagnosis and management. *American Journal of Medicine, 123(5)*, 409–413.

Crawford, A. & Harris, H. (2012). Adrenal cortex disorders: Hormones out of kilter. *Nursing, 42(10)*, 32–39.

Farrell, M. & Dempsey, J. (2014). *Smeltzer & Bare's Textbook of Medical-Surgical Nursing* (3rd edn). Sydney: Lippincott Williams & Wilkins.

Goodman, L. S., Brunton, L. L., Chabner, B. & Knollmann, B. C. (2011). *Goodman and Gilman's Pharmacological Basis of Therapeutics* (12th edn). New York: McGraw-Hill.

Guyton, A. & Hall, J. (2011). *Textbook of Medical Physiology* (12th edn). Philadelphia: Saunders Elsevier.

Jenkins, C. (2006). Starting steroids for asthma. *Australian Prescriber, 29*, 63–66.

Lim, A., Hussainy, S. Y. & Abramson, M. J. (2013). Asthma drugs in pregnancy and lactation. *Australian Prescriber, 36(5)*, 150–153.

McKenna, L. & Mirkov, S. (2019). *McKenna's Drug Handbook for Nursing and Midwifery* (8th edn). Sydney: Wolters Kluwer Health Australia.

Porth, C. M. (2011). *Essentials of Pathophysiology: Concepts of Altered Health States* (3rd edn). Philadelphia: Lippincott Williams & Wilkins.

Porth, C. M. (2009). *Pathophysiology: Concepts of Altered Health States* (8th edn). Philadelphia: Lippincott Williams & Wilkins.

Prague, J. K., May, S. & Cameron Whitelaw, B. (2013). Cushing's syndrome. *British Medical Journal, 346(7901)*, 33–35.

Rhen, T. & Cidlowski, J. A. (2005). Antiinflammatory actions of glucocorticoids. *New England Journal of Medicine, 353*, 1711–1723.

CHECK YOUR UNDERSTANDING

Answers to the questions in this chapter can be found in Appendix A at the back of this book.

MULTIPLE CHOICE

Select the best answer to the following.

1. Adrenocortical agents are widely used:
   a. to cure chronic inflammatory disorders.
   b. for short-term treatment to relieve inflammation.
   c. for long-term treatment of chronic disorders.
   d. to relieve minor aches and pains and to make people feel better.
2. If a health care professional was asked to explain the adrenal medulla to a person, it would be appropriate for her to tell that person that it:
   a. is the outer core of the adrenal gland.
   b. is the site of production of aldosterone and corticosteroids.
   c. is actually a neural ganglion of the sympathetic nervous system.
   d. consists of three layers of cells that produce different hormones.
3. Glucocorticoids are hormones that:
   a. are released in response to high glucose levels.
   b. help to regulate electrolyte levels.
   c. help to regulate water balance in the body.
   d. promote the preservation of energy through increased glucose levels, protein breakdown and fat formation.
4. Diurnal rhythm in a person with a regular sleep cycle would show:
   a. high levels of ACTH during the night while sleeping.
   b. rising levels of corticosteroids throughout the day.
   c. peak levels of ACTH and corticosteroids early in the morning.
   d. hypothalamic stimulation to release CRH around noon.
5. People who have been receiving corticosteroid therapy for a prolonged period and suddenly stop the drug will experience an adrenal crisis because their adrenal glands will not be producing any adrenal hormones. Your assessment of a person for the possibility of adrenal crisis may include:
   a. physiological exhaustion, shock and fluid shift.
   b. acne development and hypertension.
   c. water retention and increased speed of healing.
   d. hyperglycaemia and water retention.
6. A person is started on a regimen of prednisone because of a crisis in her ulcerative colitis. Care of this person would need to include:
   a. immunisations to prevent infections.
   b. increased kilojoules to deal with metabolic changes.
   c. fluid restriction to decrease water retention.
   d. administration of the drug around 8 or 9 a.m. to mimic normal diurnal rhythm.
7. A person who is taking corticosteroids is at increased risk for infection and should:
   a. be protected from exposure to infections and invasive procedures.
   b. take anti-inflammatory agents regularly throughout the day.
   c. receive live virus vaccine to protect themselves from infection.
   d. be at no risk if elective surgery is needed.
8. Mineralocorticoids are used to maintain electrolyte balance in situations of adrenal insufficiency. Mineralocorticoids:
   a. are usually given alone.
   b. can be given only intravenously.
   c. are always given in conjunction with appropriate glucocorticoids.
   d. are separate in their function from the glucocorticoids.

MULTIPLE RESPONSE

Select all that apply.

1. People who are taking corticosteroids would be expected to report which of the following?
   a. weight gain
   b. round or 'moon face' appearance
   c. feeling of wellbeing
   d. weight loss
   e. excessive hair growth
   f. fragile skin
2. Corticosteroid hormones are released during a sympathetic stress reaction. They would act to do which of the following?
   a. increase blood volume
   b. cause the release of glucose for energy
   c. increase the rate of protein production
   d. block the effects of the inflammatory and immune systems
   e. store glucose to preserve energy
   f. block protein production to save energy

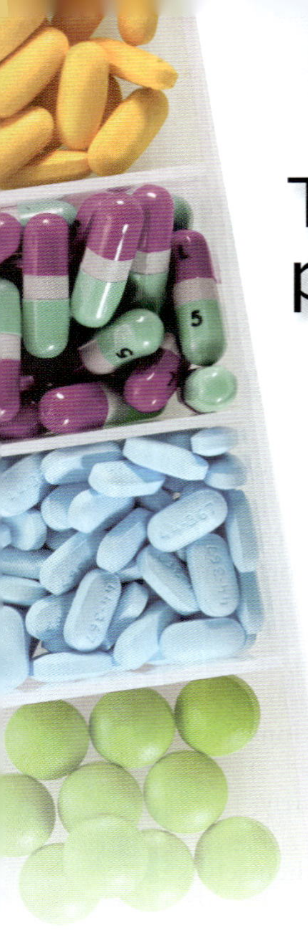

37 Thyroid and parathyroid agents

Learning objectives

On completing this chapter you should be able to:

1. Explain the control of the synthesis and secretion of thyroid hormones and parathyroid hormones, applying this to alterations in the control process (eg, using thyroid hormones to treat obesity, Paget disease, etc.).
2. Describe the therapeutic actions, indications, pharmacokinetics, contraindications, most common adverse reactions, and important drug–drug interactions associated with thyroid and parathyroid agents.
3. Discuss the use of thyroid and parathyroid drugs across the lifespan.
4. Compare and contrast thyroid and parathyroid prototype drugs with agents in their class.
5. Outline care considerations, including important teaching points, for people receiving drugs used to affect thyroid or parathyroid function.

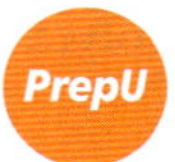

Test your current knowledge of thyroid and parathyroid agents with a PrepU Practice Quiz!

Glossary of key terms

bisphosphonates: drugs used to block bone resorption (the process by which osteoclasts break down bone) and lower serum calcium levels in several conditions

calcitonin: hormone produced by the parafollicular cells of the thyroid; counteracts the effects of parathyroid hormone to maintain calcium levels

cretinism: lack of thyroid hormone in an infant; if untreated, leads to mental retardation

follicles: structural unit of the thyroid gland; cells arranged in a circle

hypercalcaemia: excessive calcium levels in the blood

hyperparathyroidism: excessive parathormone

hyperthyroidism: excessive levels of thyroid hormone

hypocalcaemia: calcium deficiency

hypoparathyroidism: rare condition of absence of parathormone; may be seen after thyroidectomy

hypothyroidism: lack of sufficient thyroid hormone to maintain metabolism

iodine: important dietary element used by the thyroid gland to produce thyroid hormone

levothyroxine (L-thyroxine)**:** a synthetic salt of thyroxine (T_4), a thyroid hormone; the most frequently used replacement hormone for treating hypothyroidism

liothyronine: the L-isomer of triiodothyronine (T_3), and the most potent thyroid hormone, with a short half-life of 12 hours

metabolism: rate at which the cells burn energy

myxoedema: severe lack of thyroid hormone in adults

Paget disease: a genetically linked disorder of overactive osteoclasts that are eventually replaced by enlarged and softened bony structures

parathormone: hormone produced by the parathyroid glands; responsible for maintaining calcium levels in conjunction with calcitonin

postmenopausal osteoporosis: condition in which dropping levels of oestrogen allow calcium to be pulled out of the bone, resulting in a weakened and honeycombed bone structure

thioamides: drugs used to prevent the formation of thyroid hormone in the thyroid cells, lowering thyroid hormone levels

thyroxine: one of the hormones produced by the thyroid gland

THYROID AGENTS	**Iodine solution**	**Antihypercalcaemic agents**	**Calcitonin**
Thyroid hormones	sodium iodide ^{131}I	**Bisphosphonates**	(P) calcitonin salmon (salcatonin)
levothyroxine		(P) alendronate	
liothyronine	**PARATHYROID AGENTS**	clodronate	**Calcimimetic**
	Antihypocalcaemic agents	etidronate	cinacalcet
Antithyroid agents	(P) calcitriol	ibandronate	
Thioamides	teriparatide	pamidronate	
carbimazole		risedronate	
(P) propylthiouracil		zoledronic acid	

This chapter reviews drugs that are used to affect the function of the thyroid and parathyroid glands. These two glands are closely situated in the middle of the neck and share a common goal of calcium homeostasis. Serum calcium levels need to be maintained within a narrow range to promote effective blood coagulation, as well as nerve and muscle function. In most respects, however, these glands are very different in structure and function.

THE THYROID GLAND

The thyroid gland is located in the middle of the neck, where it surrounds the trachea like a shield (Figure 37.1). Its name comes from the Greek words *thyros* (shield) and *eidos* (gland). It produces two hormones – thyroid hormone and calcitonin.

Structure and function

The thyroid is a vascular gland with two lobes – one on each side of the trachea – and a small isthmus connecting the lobes. The gland is made up of cells arranged in circular **follicles**. The centre of each follicle is composed of colloid tissue, in which the thyroid hormones produced by the gland are stored. Cells found around the follicle of the thyroid gland are called parafollicular cells (see Figure 37.1). These cells produce another hormone, **calcitonin**, which affects calcium levels and

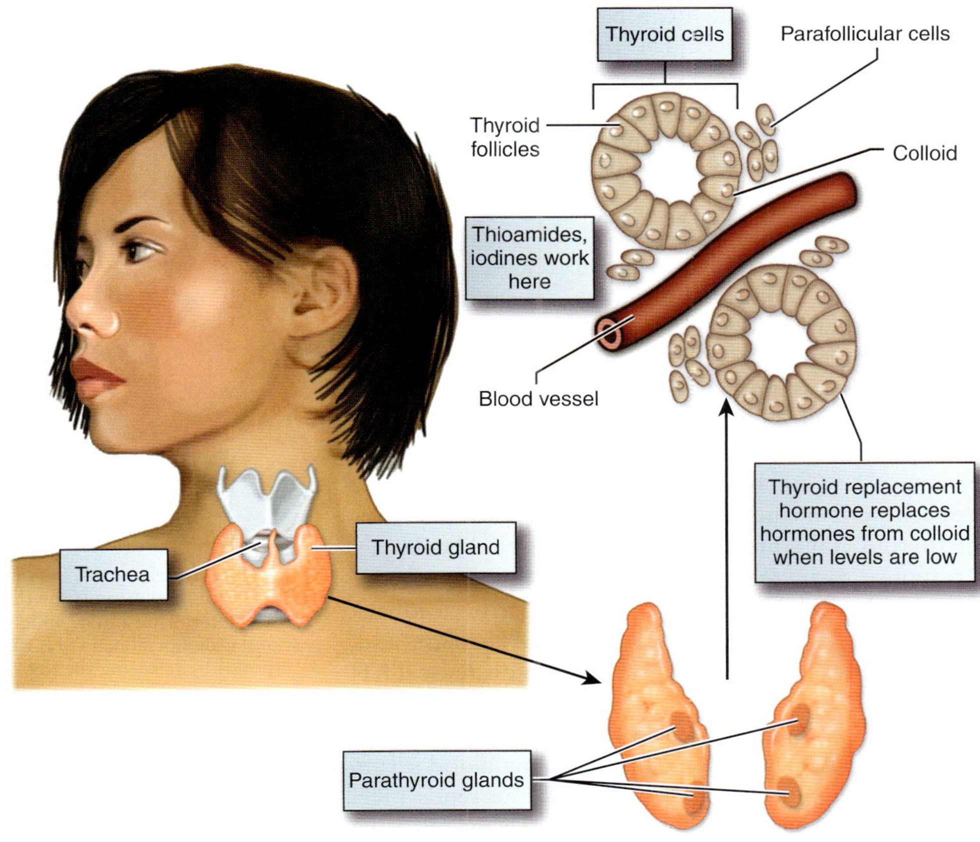

FIGURE 37.1 The thyroid and parathyroid glands. The basic unit of the thyroid gland is the follicle.

acts to balance the effects of the parathyroid hormone (PTH), **parathormone**. Calcitonin will be discussed later in connection with the parathyroid glands.

The thyroid gland produces two slightly different thyroid hormones, using **iodine** that is found in the diet: thyroxine, or tetraiodothyronine (T_4), so named because it contains four iodine atoms, which is given therapeutically in the synthetic form **levothyroxine** (L-thyroxine), and triiodothyronine (T_3), so named because it contains three iodine atoms, which is given in the synthetic form **liothyronine**. The thyroid cells remove iodine from the blood, concentrate it and prepare it for attachment to tyrosine, an amino acid. A person must obtain sufficient amounts of dietary iodine to produce thyroid hormones. The thyroid hormone regulates the rate of **metabolism** – that is, the rate at which energy is burned – in almost all the cells of the body. The thyroid hormones affect heat production and body temperature; oxygen consumption and cardiac output; blood volume; enzyme system activity; and metabolism of carbohydrates, fats and proteins. Thyroid hormone is also an important regulator of growth and development, especially within the reproductive and nervous systems. Because the thyroid has such widespread effects throughout the body, any dysfunction of the thyroid gland will have numerous systemic effects.

When thyroid hormone is needed in the body, the stored thyroid hormone molecule is absorbed into the thyroid cells, where the T_3 and T_4 are broken off and released into circulation. These hormones are carried on plasma proteins, which can be measured as protein-bound iodine (PBI) levels. The thyroid gland produces more T_4 than T_3. More T_4 is released into circulation, but T_3 is approximately four times more active than T_4. Most T_4 (with a half-life of about 12 hours) is converted to T_3 (with a half-life of about 1 week) at the tissue level.

Control

Thyroid hormone production and release are regulated by the anterior pituitary hormone called thyroid-stimulating hormone (TSH). The secretion of TSH is regulated by thyrotropin-releasing hormone (TRH), a hypothalamic regulating factor. A delicate balance exists among the thyroid, the pituitary and the hypothalamus in regulating the levels of thyroid hormone. See Chapter 36 for a review of the negative feedback system and the hypothalamic–pituitary axis. The thyroid gland produces increased thyroid hormones in response to increased levels of TSH. The increased levels of thyroid hormones send a negative feedback message to the pituitary to decrease TSH release and, at the same time, to the hypothalamus to decrease TRH release. A drop in TRH levels subsequently results in a drop in TSH levels, which in turn leads to a drop in thyroid hormone levels. In response to low blood serum levels of thyroid hormone, the hypothalamus sends TRH to the anterior pituitary, which responds by releasing TSH, which in turn stimulates the thyroid gland to again produce and release thyroid hormone. The rising levels of thyroid hormone are sensed by the hypothalamus and the cycle begins again. This intricate series of negative feedback mechanisms keeps the level of thyroid hormone within a narrow range of normal (Figure 37.2).

Thyroid dysfunction

Thyroid dysfunction involves either underactivity (hypothyroidism) or overactivity (hyperthyroidism). This dysfunction can affect any age group. Box 37.1 explains use of thyroid agents across the lifespan.

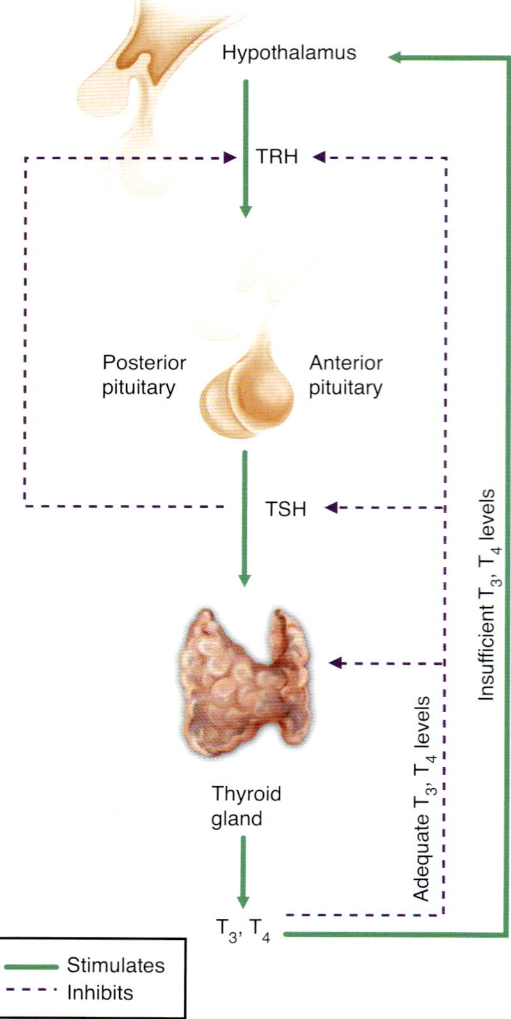

FIGURE 37.2 In response to low blood serum levels of thyroid hormone, the hypothalamus sends the thyrotropin-releasing hormone (TRH) to the anterior pituitary, which responds by releasing the thyroid-stimulating hormone (TSH) to the thyroid gland; it, in turn, responds by releasing the thyroid hormone (T_3 and T_4) into the bloodstream. The anterior pituitary is also sensitive to the increase in blood serum levels of the thyroid hormone and responds by decreasing production and release of TSH. As thyroid hormone production and release subside, the hypothalamus senses the lower serum levels and the process is repeated by the release of TRH again. This intricate series of negative feedback mechanisms keeps the level of thyroid hormone within normal limits.

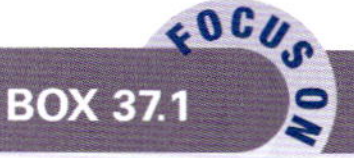

BOX 37.1 Drug therapy across the lifespan

Thyroid and parathyroid agents

CHILDREN

Thyroid replacement therapy is required when a child is hypothyroid. Levothyroxine is the drug of choice in children. Dose is determined based on serum thyroid hormone levels and the response of the child, including growth and development. Dose in children tends to be higher than in adults because of the higher metabolic rate of the growing child. Usually, the starting dose to consider is 10–15 micrograms/kg per day.

Regular monitoring, including growth records, is necessary to determine the accurate dose as the child grows. Maintenance levels at the adult dose usually occurs after puberty and when active growing stops.

If an antithyroid agent is needed, propylthiouracil (PTU) is the drug of choice because it is less toxic. Unless other agents are ineffective, radioactive agents are not used in children because of the effects of radiation on chromosomes and developing cells.

Hypercalcaemia is relatively rare in children, although it may be seen with certain malignancies. If a child develops a malignancy-related hypercalcaemia, the bisphosphonates may be used, with dose adjustments based on age and weight. Serum calcium levels should be monitored very closely in the child and dose adjustments made as necessary.

ADULTS

Adults who require thyroid replacement therapy need to understand that this will be a lifelong replacement need. An established routine of taking the tablet first thing in the morning may help the person to comply with the drug regimen. Levothyroxine is the drug of choice for replacement, but in some cases other agents may be needed. Periodic monitoring of thyroid hormone levels is necessary to ensure that dose needs have not changed.

If antithyroid drugs are needed, the person's underlying problems should be considered. Sodium iodide ^{131}I should not be used in adults in their reproductive years unless they are aware of the possibility of adverse effects on fertility.

Alendronate and risedronate are commonly used drugs for osteoporosis and calcium lowering. Serum calcium levels need to be monitored carefully with any of the drugs that affect calcium levels. People should be encouraged to take calcium and vitamin D in their diet or as supplements in cases of hypocalcaemia, and also for prevention and treatment of osteoporosis.

PREGNANCY AND BREASTFEEDING

Thyroid replacement therapy is necessary during pregnancy for women who have been maintained on this regimen. It is not uncommon for hypothyroidism to develop during pregnancy. Levothyroxine is again the drug of choice.

If an antithyroid drug is essential during pregnancy, PTU is the drug of choice because it is less likely to cross the placenta and cause problems for the fetus. Radioactive agents should not be used. Bisphosphonates should be used during pregnancy only if the benefit to the mother clearly outweighs the potential risk to the fetus. Breastfeeding women who need thyroid replacement therapy should continue with their prescribed regimen and report any adverse reactions in the baby. Bisphosphonates and antithyroid drugs should not be used during breastfeeding because of the potential for adverse reactions in the baby; another method of feeding the baby should be used.

OLDER ADULTS

Because the signs and symptoms of thyroid disease mimic many other problems that are common to older adults – hair loss, slurred speech, fluid retention, heart failure and so on – it is important to screen older adults for thyroid disease carefully before beginning any therapy. The dose should be started at a very low level and increased based on the response. Levothyroxine is the drug of choice for hypothyroidism. Periodic monitoring of thyroid hormone levels, as well as cardiac and other responses, is essential with this age group.

If antithyroid agents are needed, sodium iodide ^{131}I may be the drug of choice because it has fewer adverse effects than the other agents. The person should be monitored closely for the development of hypothyroidism, which usually occurs within a year after starting antithyroid therapy.

Older adults may have dietary deficiencies related to calcium and vitamin D. They should be encouraged to eat dairy products and foods high in calcium and to supplement their diet if necessary. Postmenopausal women, who are prone to develop osteoporosis, may want to consider hormone replacement therapy and calcium supplements to prevent osteoporosis. Many postmenopausal women, and some older men, respond well to the effect of bisphosphonates in moving calcium back into the bone. They need specific instructions on the proper way to take these drugs and may not be able to comply with the restrictions about staying upright and swallowing the tablet with a full glass of water.

Older adults have a greater incidence of renal impairment and kidney function should be evaluated before starting any of these drugs. Bisphosphonates should be used in lower doses in people with moderate renal impairment and are not recommended for those who have severe renal impairment. With any of these drugs, regular monitoring of calcium levels is important to ensure that therapeutic effects are achieved with a minimum of adverse effects.

Hypothyroidism

Hypothyroidism is a lack of sufficient levels of thyroid hormones to maintain a normal metabolism. This condition occurs in a number of pathophysiological states:

- Absence of the thyroid gland
- Lack of sufficient iodine in the diet to produce the needed level of thyroid hormone
- Lack of sufficient functioning thyroid tissue due to tumour or autoimmune disorders

- Lack of TSH due to pituitary disease
- Lack of TRH related to a tumour or disorder of the hypothalamus.

Hypothyroidism is the most common type of thyroid dysfunction. It is estimated that approximately 5%–10% of women older than 50 years of age are hypothyroidic. Hypothyroidism is also a common finding in elderly men. The symptoms of hypothyroidism can be varied and vague, such as obesity and fatigue (Box 37.2), and are frequently overlooked or mistaken for signs of normal ageing (Table 37.1).

Children who are born without a thyroid gland or who have a non-functioning gland develop a condition called **cretinism**. If untreated, these children will have

BOX 37.2 FOCUS ON The evidence

Thyroid hormones for obesity

Treatment trends for obesity have changed over the years. Not long ago, one of the suggested treatments was the use of thyroid hormone. The thinking was that obese people had slower metabolisms and therefore would benefit from a boost in metabolism from extra thyroid hormone.

If an obese person is truly hypothyroid, this might be a good idea. Unfortunately, many of the people who received thyroid hormone for weight loss were not tested for thyroid activity and ended up with excessive thyroid hormone in their systems. This situation triggered a cascade of events. The exogenous thyroid hormone disrupted the hypothalamic–pituitary–thyroid control system, resulting in decreased production of thyrotropin-releasing hormone (TRH) and thyroid-stimulating hormone (TSH) as the hypothalamus and pituitary sensed the rising levels of thyroid hormone. Because the thyroid was no longer stimulated to produce and secrete thyroid hormone, thyroid levels would actually fall. Lacking stimulation by TSH, the thyroid gland would start to atrophy. If exogenous thyroid hormone were stopped, the atrophied thyroid would not be able to immediately respond to the TSH stimulation and produce thyroid hormone. Ultimately, these people experienced an endocrine imbalance. What's more, they did not lose weight – and in the long run may actually have gained weight as the body's compensatory mechanisms tried to deal with the imbalances.

Today, thyroid hormone is no longer considered a good choice for treating obesity. Many people, especially middle-aged people who may recall that thyroid hormone was once used for weight loss, ask for it as an answer to their weight problem. People have even been known to 'borrow' thyroid replacement hormones from others for a quick weight loss solution or to order the drug over the Internet without supervision or monitoring.

People with obesity need reassurance, understanding and education about the risks of borrowed thyroid hormone. Insistent people should undergo thyroid function tests. If the results are normal, they should receive teaching about the controls and actions of thyroid hormone in the body and an explanation of why taking these hormones can cause problems. Obesity is a chronic and frustrating problem that poses continual challenges for health care providers.

TABLE 37.1 Signs and symptoms of thyroid dysfunction

Clinical effects	Hypothyroidism	Hyperthyroidism
Central nervous system	Depressed: hypoactive reflexes, lethargy, sleepiness, slow speech, emotional dullness	Stimulated: hyperactive reflexes, anxiety, nervousness, insomnia, tremors, restlessness, increased basal temperature
Cardiovascular system	Depressed: bradycardia, hypotension, anaemia, oliguria, decreased sensitivity to catecholamines	Stimulated: tachycardia, palpitations, increased pulse pressure, systolic hypertension, increased sensitivity to catecholamines
Skin, hair and nails	Skin is pale, coarse, dry, thickened; puffy eyes and eyelids; hair is coarse and thin; hair loss; nails are thick and hard	Skin is flushed, warm, thin, moist, sweating; hair is fine and soft; nails are soft and thin
Metabolic rate	Decreased: lower body temperature, intolerance to cold, decreased appetite, higher levels of fat and cholesterol, weight gain, hypercholesterolaemia	Increased, overactive cellular metabolism: low-grade fever, intolerance to heat, increased appetite with weight loss, muscle wasting and weakness, thyroid myopathy
Generalised myxoedema	Accumulation of mucopolysaccharides in the heart, tongue and vocal cords; periorbital oedema, cardiomyopathy, hoarseness, and thickened speech	Localised with accumulation of mucopolysaccharides in eyeballs, ocular muscles; periorbital oedema, lid lag, exophthalmos; pretibial oedema
Ovaries	Decreased function: menorrhagia, habitual abortion, sterility, decreased sexual function	Altered tendency toward oligomenorrhoea, amenorrhoea
Goitre	Rare; simple non-toxic type may occur	Diffuse, highly vascular; very frequent

poor growth and development and mental retardation because of the lack of thyroid hormone stimulation. Severe adult hypothyroidism is called **myxoedema**. Myxoedema usually develops gradually as the thyroid slowly stops functioning. It can develop as a result of autoimmune thyroid disease (Hashimoto disease), viral infection or overtreatment with antithyroid drugs or because of surgical removal or irradiation of the thyroid gland. People with myxoedema exhibit many signs and symptoms. Hypothyroidism is treated with replacement thyroid hormone therapy.

Hyperthyroidism

Hyperthyroidism occurs when excessive amounts of thyroid hormones are produced and released into the circulation. Graves' disease, a poorly understood condition that is thought to be an autoimmune problem, is the most common cause of hyperthyroidism. Goitre (enlargement of the thyroid gland) is an effect of hyperthyroidism, which occurs when the thyroid is overstimulated by TSH. This can happen if the thyroid gland does not make sufficient thyroid hormones to turn off the hypothalamus and anterior pituitary; in the body's attempt to produce the needed amount of thyroid hormone, the thyroid is continually stimulated by increasing levels of TSH. Additional signs and symptoms of hyperthyroidism can be found in Table 37.1.

Hyperthyroidism may be treated by surgical removal of the gland or portions of the gland, treatment with radiation to destroy parts or all of the gland, or drug treatment to block the production of **thyroxine** in the thyroid gland or to destroy parts or the entire gland. The metabolism of these individuals must then be regulated with replacement thyroid hormone therapy.

KEY POINTS

- The thyroid gland uses iodine to produce the thyroid hormones that regulate body metabolism.
- Control of the thyroid gland involves an intricate balance among TRH, TSH and circulating levels of thyroid hormone.
- Hypothyroidism is treated with replacement thyroid hormone; hyperthyroidism is treated with thioamides or iodines.

THYROID AGENTS

When thyroid function is low, thyroid hormone needs to be replaced to ensure adequate metabolism and homeostasis in the body. When thyroid function is too high, the resultant systemic effects can be serious and the thyroid will need to be removed or destroyed pharmacologically. The hormone normally produced by the gland will then need to be replaced with thyroid hormone. Thyroid agents include thyroid hormones and antithyroid drugs, which are further classified as thioamides and iodine solutions. Table 37.2 includes a complete list of each type of thyroid agent.

THYROID HORMONES

Several replacement hormone products are available for treating hypothyroidism. These hormones replace the low or absent levels of natural thyroid hormone and suppress the overproduction of TSH by the pituitary. These products can contain both natural and synthetic thyroid hormone. Levothyroxine (*Eutroxsig, Oroxine*), a synthetic salt of T_4, is the most frequently used replacement hormone because of its predictable bioavailability and reliability. Another thyroid hormone, liothyronine (*Tertroxin*), is a synthetic salt of T_3.

Therapeutic actions and indications

The thyroid replacement hormones increase the metabolic rate of body tissues, increasing oxygen consumption, respiration, heart rate, growth and maturation, and the metabolism of fats, carbohydrates and proteins. They are indicated for replacement therapy in hypothyroid states, treatment of myxoedema coma, suppression of TSH in the treatment and prevention of goitres and management of thyroid cancer. In conjunction with antithyroid drugs, they also are indicated to treat thyroid toxicity, prevent goitre formation during thyroid overstimulation and treat thyroid overstimulation during pregnancy. See Table 37.2 for usual indications for each drug.

Pharmacokinetics

These drugs are well absorbed from the gastrointestinal (GI) tract and bound to serum proteins. Because liothyronine contains only T_3, it has a rapid onset and a long duration of action. De-iodination of the drugs occurs at several sites, including the liver, kidney and other body tissues. Elimination is primarily in the bile. Thyroid hormone does not cross the placenta and seems to have no effect on the fetus. Thyroid replacement therapy should not be discontinued during pregnancy, and the need for thyroid replacement often becomes apparent or increases during pregnancy. Thyroid hormone does enter breast milk in small amounts. Caution should be used during breastfeeding.

Contraindications and cautions

These drugs should not be used with any known allergy to the drugs or their binders *to prevent hypersensitivity reactions*, during acute thyrotoxicosis (unless used in conjunction with antithyroid drugs) or during acute myocardial infarction (unless complicated by

TABLE 37.2 DRUGS IN FOCUS Thyroid agents

Drug name	Dosage/route	Usual indications
Thyroid hormones		
(P) levothyroxine (*Eutroxsig, Oroxine*)	Adults: 50–200 micrograms/day Paediatric: initially 50 micrograms every other day, increased by increments of 25 micrograms (given as 50 micrograms on alternate days) q 2–4 weeks	Replacement therapy in hypothyroidism and congenital hypothyroidism in infants; suppression of TSH release; treatment of myxoedema coma and thyrotoxicosis
liothyronine (*Tertroxin*)	Adult: 10–20 micrograms PO q 8 hours up to maximum of 60 micrograms daily Paediatric: initially, 5 micrograms PO daily up to 10–40 micrograms PO daily	Replacement therapy in hypothyroidism; suppression of TSH release; treatment of thyrotoxicosis; synthetic hormone used in people allergic to desiccated thyroid **Special considerations:** not for use with cardiac or anxiety problems
Antithyroid agents		
Thionamides		
carbimazole (*Neo-Mercazole*)	Adult: initially 15–60 mg/day PO in divided doses; maintenance: 10–15 mg/day PO	Treatment of hyperthyroidism; before thyroidectomy
(P) propylthiouracil (*PTU*)	Adult: initially 100–1200 mg/day PO in divided doses; maintenance: 50–800 mg PO daily in 2–4 divided doses Paediatric: 50 mg/m² PO tds	Treatment of hyperthyroidism
Iodine solutions		
sodium iodide ^{131}I (generic, radioactive iodine)	Adult, hyperthyroidism: 148–370 MBq. Antithyroid drugs should be discontinued for 3–4 days before administration of the dose and withheld for 7–14 days afterwards Adult, thyroid imaging: 0.185–3.7 MBq	Treatment of hyperthyroidism; thyroid blocking in radiation emergencies; destruction of thyroid tissue in people who are not candidates for surgical removal of the gland

hypothyroidism) *because the thyroid hormones could exacerbate these conditions*. Caution should be used during breastfeeding *because the drug enters breast milk and could suppress the infant's thyroid production*, and with hypoadrenal conditions such as Addison disease. Liothyronine has a greater incidence of cardiac side effects and is not recommended for use in individuals with potential cardiac problems or those who are prone to anxiety reactions.

Adverse effects

When the correct dose of the replacement therapy is being used, few if any adverse effects are associated with these drugs. Skin reactions and loss of hair are sometimes seen, especially during the first few months of treatment in children. Symptoms of hyperthyroidism may occur as the drug dose is regulated. Some of the less predictable effects are associated with cardiac stimulation (arrhythmias, hypertension), central nervous system (CNS) effects (anxiety, sleeplessness, headache) and difficulty swallowing (taking the drug with a full glass of water may help).

Clinically important drug–drug interactions

Decreased absorption of the thyroid hormones occurs if they are taken concurrently with colestyramine. If this combination is needed, the drugs should be taken 2 hours apart.

The effectiveness of oral anticoagulants is increased if they are combined with thyroid hormone. Because this may lead to increased bleeding, the dose of the oral anticoagulant should be reduced and the bleeding time checked periodically.

Decreased effectiveness of digitalis glycosides can occur when these drugs are combined. Consequently, digitalis levels should be monitored and an increased dose may be required.

Theophylline clearance is decreased in hypothyroid states. As the person approaches normal thyroid function, theophylline dose may need to be adjusted frequently.

Prototype summary: levothyroxine

Indications: replacement therapy in hypothyroidism; pituitary TSH suppression in the treatment of euthyroid goitres and in the management of thyroid cancer; thyrotoxicosis in conjunction with other therapy; myxoedema coma.

Actions: increases the metabolic rate of body tissues, increasing oxygen consumption, respiration and heart rate; the rate of fat, protein and carbohydrate metabolism; and growth and maturation.

Pharmacokinetics:

Route	Onset	Peak	Duration
PO	Slow	1–3 weeks	1–3 weeks
IV	6–8 hours	24–48 hours	unknown

$T_{1/2}$: 6–7 days; metabolised in the liver and excreted in the bile.

Adverse effects: tremors, headache, nervousness, palpitations, tachycardia, allergic skin reactions, loss of hair in the first few months of therapy in children, diarrhoea, nausea, vomiting.

Care considerations for people receiving thyroid hormones

Assessment: history and examination

- Assess for history of allergy to any thyroid hormone or binder, breastfeeding, Addison disease, acute myocardial infarction not complicated by hypothyroidism and thyrotoxicosis, *which could be contraindications or cautions to use of the drug.*
- Assess for the presence of any skin lesions; orientation and affect; baseline pulse, blood pressure and electrocardiogram (ECG); respiration and adventitious sounds; and thyroid function tests, *to determine baseline status before beginning therapy and for any potential adverse effects.*

Refer to the Critical thinking scenario for a full discussion of care for a person who is receiving a thyroid hormone.

Implementation with rationale

- Administer a single daily dose before breakfast each day *to ensure consistent therapeutic levels.*
- Administer with a full glass of water *to help prevent difficulty swallowing.*
- Monitor response carefully when beginning therapy *to adjust dose according to individual response.*
- Monitor cardiac response *to detect cardiac adverse effects.*
- Assess the person carefully *to detect any potential drug–drug interactions if giving thyroid hormone in combination with other drugs.*
- Arrange for periodic blood tests of thyroid function *to monitor the effectiveness of the therapy.*
- Provide thorough teaching, including drug name, dosage and administration, measures to avoid adverse effects, warning signs of problems and the need for regular evaluation if used for longer than recommended, *to enhance knowledge of drug therapy and promote compliance.*

Evaluation

- Monitor person's response to the drug (return of metabolism to normal, prevention of goitre).
- Monitor for adverse effects (tachycardia, hypertension, anxiety, skin rash).
- Evaluate the effectiveness of the teaching plan (person can name drug, dosage, adverse effects to watch for and specific measures to avoid them).

CRITICAL THINKING SCENARIO

Hypothyroidism

THE SITUATION

H.R., a 38-year-old Caucasian woman, complains of 'exhaustion, lethargy and sleepiness'. Her past history is sketchy, her speech seems slurred and her attention span is limited. Mr R., her husband, reports feeling frustrated with H.R., stating that she has become increasingly lethargic, disorganised and uninvolved at home. He also notes that she has gained weight and lost interest in her appearance.

Physical examination reveals the following remarkable findings: pulse rate, 52/minute; blood pressure, 90/62 mmHg; temperature, 36°C (oral); pale, dry and thick skin; periorbital oedema; thick and asymmetric tongue; height, 165 cm; weight, 75 kg. The immediate impression is that of hypothyroidism. Laboratory tests confirm this, revealing elevated TSH and very low levels of triiodothyronine (T_3) and thyroxine (T_4). Levothyroxine 200 micrograms mg daily PO, is prescribed.

CRITICAL THINKING

What teaching plans should be developed for this woman?
What interventions would be appropriate in helping Mr and Mrs R. accept the diagnosis and the pathophysiological basis for Mrs R's complaints and problems?
What body image changes will H.R. experience as her body adjusts to the thyroid therapy?
How can H.R. be helped to adjust to these changes and re-establish her body image and self-concept?

DISCUSSION

Hypothyroidism develops slowly. With it comes fatigue, lethargy and lack of emotional affect – conditions that result in the person's losing interest in appearance, activities and responsibilities. In this case, the woman's husband, not knowing that there was a physical reason for the problem, became increasingly frustrated and even angry. Mr R. should be involved in the teaching program so that his feelings can be taken into consideration. Any teaching content should be written down for later reference. (When H.R. starts to return to normal, her attention span and interest should return; anything that was missed or forgotten can be referred to in the written teaching program.)

H.R. may be encouraged to bring a picture of herself from a year or so ago to help her to understand and appreciate the changes that have occurred. Many people are totally unaware of changes in their appearance and activity level because the disease progresses so slowly and brings on lethargy and lack of emotional affect.

The teaching plan should include information about the function of the thyroid gland and the anticipated changes that will be occurring to H.R. over the next week and beyond. The importance of taking the medication daily should be emphasised. The need to return for follow-up to evaluate the effectiveness of the medication and the effects on her body should also be stressed. Both H.R. and her husband will need support and encouragement to deal with past frustrations and the return to normal. Lifelong therapy will probably be needed, so further teaching will be important once things have stabilised.

CARE GUIDE FOR H.R.: THYROID HORMONE

Assessment: history and examination

Review the person's history for allergies to any of these drugs, Addison disease, acute myocardial infarction not complicated by hypothyroidism, breastfeeding and thyrotoxicosis.

Focus the physical examination on the following:
Neurological: orientation and affect
Skin: colour and lesions
CV: pulse, cardiac auscultation, blood pressure and electrocardiogram findings
Respiratory: respirations, adventitious sounds
Haematological: thyroid function tests

Implementation

Administer the drug once a day before breakfast with a full glass of water.
Provide comfort, safety measures (eg, temperature control, rest as needed, safety precautions).
Provide support and reassurance to deal with drug effects and lifetime need.
Provide teaching regarding drug name, dosage, adverse effects, precautions and warning signs to report.

Evaluation

Evaluate drug effects: return of metabolism to normal; prevention of goitre.
Monitor for adverse effects: anxiety, tachycardia, hypertension, skin reaction.
Monitor for drug–drug interactions as indicated for each drug.
Evaluate the effectiveness of the teaching program and comfort and safety measures.

TEACHING FOR H.R.

- This hormone is designed to replace the thyroid hormone that your body is not able to produce. The thyroid hormone is responsible for regulating your body's metabolism, or the speed with which your body's cells burn energy. Thyroid hormone actions affect many body systems, so it is very important that you take this medication only as prescribed.
- Never stop taking this drug without consulting with your health care provider. The drug is used to replace a very important hormone and will probably have to be taken for life. Stopping the medication can lead to serious problems.
- Take this drug before breakfast each day with a full glass of water.
- Thyroid hormone usually causes no adverse effects. You may notice a slight skin rash or hair loss in the first few months of therapy. You should notice the signs and symptoms of your thyroid deficiency subsiding, and you will feel 'back to normal'.
- Report any of the following to your health care provider: chest pain, difficulty breathing, sore throat, fever, chills,

weight gain, sleeplessness, nervousness, unusual sweating or intolerance to heat.

- Avoid taking any over-the-counter medication without first checking with your health care provider because several of these medications can interfere with the effectiveness of this drug.
- Tell any doctor, nurse, midwife or other health care provider involved in your care that you are taking this drug. You may also want to wear or carry medical identification showing that you are taking this medication. This would alert any health care personnel taking care of you in an emergency to the fact that you are taking this drug.
- While you are taking this drug, you will need regular medical follow-up, including blood tests to check the activity of your thyroid gland, to evaluate your response to the drug and any possible underlying problems.
- Keep this drug, and all medications, out of the reach of children. Do not give this medication to anyone else or take any similar medication that has not been prescribed for you.

ANTITHYROID AGENTS

Drugs used to block the production of thyroid hormone and to treat hyperthyroidism include the thioamides and iodide solutions (Table 37.2). Although these groups of drugs are not chemically related, they both block the formation of thyroid hormones within the thyroid gland (see Therapeutic actions and indications).

Therapeutic actions and indications

Thioamides

Thioamides lower thyroid hormone levels by preventing the formation of thyroid hormone in the thyroid cells, which lowers the serum levels of thyroid hormone. They also partially inhibit the conversion of T_4 to T_3 at the cellular level. These drugs are indicated for the treatment of hyperthyroidism. Thioamides include carbimazole (*Neo-Mercazole*) and propylthiouracil (PTU). Carbimazole is the most commonly used drug in New Zealand. PTU is an unapproved medicine in New Zealand reserved for people who are intolerant of carbimazole.

Iodine solutions

Low doses of iodine are needed in the body for the formation of thyroid hormone. High doses, however, block thyroid function. Therefore, iodine preparations are sometimes used to treat hyperthyroidism but are not used as often as they once were in the clinical setting (see Pharmacokinetics). The iodine solutions cause the thyroid cells to become oversaturated with iodine and stop producing thyroid hormone. In some cases, the thyroid cells are actually destroyed. Radioactive iodine (sodium iodide ^{131}I) (not available in New Zealand) is taken up into the thyroid cells, which are then destroyed by the beta-radiation given off by the radioactive iodine. Except during radiation emergencies, the use of sodium iodide is reserved for individuals who are not candidates for surgery, women who cannot become pregnant and elderly people with such severe, complicating conditions that immediate thyroid destruction is needed. See Table 37.2 for usual indications.

Pharmacokinetics

Thioamides

These drugs are well absorbed from the GI tract and are then concentrated in the thyroid gland. The onset and duration vary with each person. PTU has a low potential for crossing the placenta and for entering breast milk (see Contraindications and cautions).

Iodine solutions

These drugs are rapidly absorbed from the GI tract and widely distributed throughout the body fluids. Excretion occurs through the urine. Strong iodine products, potassium iodide and sodium iodide are taken orally and have a rapid onset of action, with effects seen within 24 hours and peak effects seen in 10–15 days. The effects are short lived and may even precipitate further thyroid enlargement and dysfunction (see Adverse effects). For this reason, the drugs are not used as often as they once were in the clinical setting.

The strong iodine products cross the placenta and are known to enter breast milk, but the effects on the neonate are not known. Sodium iodide ^{131}I enters breast milk and is rated pregnancy category X (see Contraindications and cautions).

Contraindications and cautions

Antithyroid agents are contraindicated in the presence of any known allergy to antithyroid drugs *to prevent hypersensitivity reactions* and during pregnancy *because of the risk of adverse effects on the fetus and the development of cretinism.* (If an antithyroid drug is absolutely essential and the woman has been informed about the risk of cretinism in the infant, PTU is the drug of choice, but caution should still be used.) Another method of feeding the baby should be chosen if an

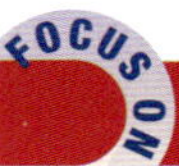

Safe medication administration

Name confusion has been reported between propylthiouracil (PTU) and Puri-Nethol *(mercaptopurine), an antineoplastic agent. Serious adverse effects could occur. Use extreme caution when using these drugs.*

antithyroid drug is needed during breastfeeding *because of the risk of antithyroid activity in the infant, including the development of a neonatal goitre.* (Again, if an antithyroid drug is needed, PTU is the drug of choice.)

Use of strong iodine products is also contraindicated with pulmonary oedema or pulmonary tuberculosis.

Adverse effects

Thioamides

The adverse effects most commonly seen with thioamides are the effects of thyroid suppression: drowsiness, lethargy, bradycardia, nausea, skin rash and so on. They are also associated with nausea, vomiting and GI complaints.

Iodine solutions

The most common adverse effect of iodine solutions is hypothyroidism; the person will need to be started on replacement thyroid hormone to maintain homeostasis. Other adverse effects include iodism (metallic taste and burning in the mouth, sore teeth and gums, diarrhoea, cold symptoms and stomach upset), staining of teeth, skin rash and the development of goitre.

Sodium iodide (radioactive ^{131}I) is usually reserved for use in individuals who are older than 30 years of age because of the adverse effects associated with the radioactivity.

Clinically important drug–drug interactions

Thioamides

An increased risk for bleeding exists when PTU or carbimazole are administered with oral anticoagulants. Changes in serum levels of theophylline, metoprolol, propranolol and digoxin may lead to changes in the effects of the antithyroid agent as the person moves from the hyperthyroid to the euthyroid state.

Iodine solutions

Because the use of drugs to destroy thyroid function moves the person from hyperthyroidism to hypothyroidism, individuals who are taking drugs that are metabolised differently in hypothyroid and hyperthyroid states or drugs that have a small margin of safety that could be altered by the change in thyroid function should be monitored closely. These drugs include anticoagulants, theophylline, digoxin, metoprolol and propranolol.

Prototype summary: propylthiouracil

Indications: treatment of hyperthyroidism.

Actions: inhibits the synthesis of thyroid hormones, partially inhibits the peripheral conversion of T_4 to T_3.

Pharmacokinetics:

Route	Onset
PO	Varies

$T_{1/2}$: 1–2 hours; metabolised in the liver and excreted in the urine.

Adverse effects: paraesthesias, neuritis, vertigo, drowsiness, skin rash, urticaria, skin pigmentation, nausea, vomiting, epigastric distress, nephritis, bone marrow suppression, arthralgia, myalgia, oedema.

Prototype summary: strong iodine products

Indications: adjunct therapy for hyperthyroidism; thyroid blocking in a radiation emergency.

Actions: inhibit the synthesis of thyroid hormones and inhibit the release of these hormones into the circulation.

Pharmacokinetics:

Route	Onset	Peak	Duration
PO	24 hours	10–15 days	6 weeks

$T_{1/2}$: unknown; metabolised in the liver and excreted in the urine.

Adverse effects: rash, hypothyroidism, goitre, swelling of the salivary glands, iodism (metallic taste, burning mouth and throat, sore teeth and gums, head cold symptoms, stomach upset, diarrhoea), allergic reactions.

Care considerations for people receiving antithyroid agents

Assessment: history and examination

- Assess for history of allergy to any antithyroid drug; pregnancy and breastfeeding status; and pulmonary oedema or pulmonary tuberculosis if using strong iodine solution, *which could be cautions or contraindications to use of the drug.*
- Assess for skin lesions; orientation and affect; baseline pulse, blood pressure and ECG; respiration and adventitious sounds; and thyroid function tests, *to determine baseline status before beginning therapy and for any potential adverse effects.*

Implementation with rationale

- Administer propylthiouracil three times a day, around the clock, *to ensure consistent therapeutic levels.*
- Give iodine solution through a straw *to decrease staining of teeth;* tablets can be crushed.
- Monitor response carefully and arrange for periodic blood tests *to assess response and to monitor for adverse effects.*
- Monitor people receiving iodine solution for any sign of iodism *so the drug can be stopped immediately if such signs appear.*
- Provide thorough teaching, including measures to avoid adverse effects, warning signs of problems and the need for regular evaluation if used for longer than recommended, *to enhance knowledge of drug therapy and promote compliance.*

Evaluation

- Monitor response to the drug (lowering of thyroid hormone levels).
- Monitor for adverse effects (bradycardia, anxiety, blood dyscrasias, skin rash).
- Evaluate the effectiveness of the teaching plan (person can name drug, dosage, adverse effects to watch for and specific measures to avoid them).
- Monitor the effectiveness of comfort measures and adherence to the regimen.

KEY POINTS

- Hypothyroidism, or lower-than-normal levels of thyroid hormone, is treated with replacement thyroid hormone.
- Hyperthyroidism, or higher-than-normal levels of thyroid hormone, is treated with thioamides, which block the thyroid from producing thyroid hormone, or with iodines, which prevent thyroid hormone production, or by surgery or radioactive iodine, which destroy parts of the gland.

THE PARATHYROID GLANDS

The parathyroid glands are four very small groups of glandular tissue located on the back of the thyroid gland (Figure 37.3). The parathyroid glands produce parathyroid hormone, an important regulator of serum calcium levels.

Structure and function

As mentioned earlier, the parafollicular cells of the thyroid gland produce the hormone calcitonin. Calcitonin responds to high calcium levels to cause lower serum calcium levels and acts to balance the effects of the PTH, which works to elevate calcium levels. PTH is the most important regulator of serum calcium levels

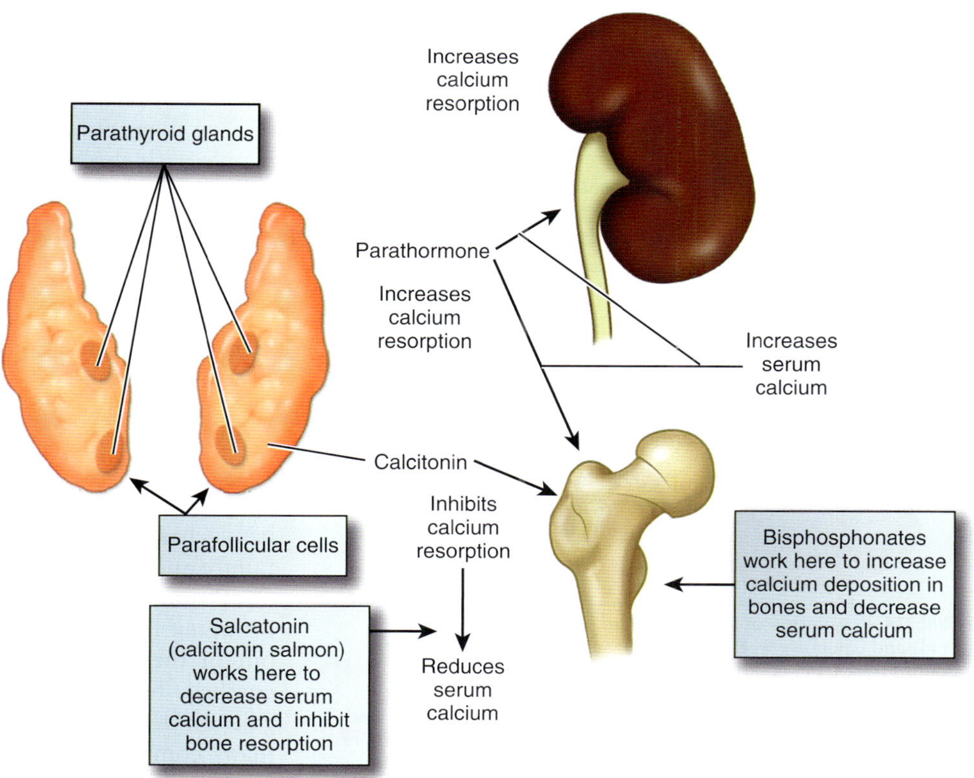

FIGURE 37.3 Calcium control. Parathormone and calcitonin work to maintain calcium homeostasis in the body.

in the body. PTH has many actions, including the following:

- Stimulation of osteoclasts or bone cells to release calcium from the bone
- Increased intestinal absorption of calcium
- Increased calcium resorption from the kidneys
- Stimulation of cells in the kidney to produce calcitriol, the active form of vitamin D, which stimulates intestinal transport of calcium into the blood.

Control

Calcium is an electrolyte that is used in many of the body's metabolic processes. These processes include membrane transport systems, conduction of nerve impulses, muscle contraction and blood clotting. To achieve all of these effects, serum levels of calcium must be maintained between 2.1 and 2.6 mmol/L. This is achieved through regulation of serum calcium by PTH and calcitonin (Figure 37.4).

The release of calcitonin is not controlled by the hypothalamic–pituitary axis but is regulated locally at the cellular level. Calcitonin is released when serum calcium levels rise. Calcitonin works to reduce calcium levels by blocking bone resorption and enhancing bone formation. This action pulls calcium out of the serum for depositing into the bone. When serum calcium levels are low, PTH release is stimulated. When serum calcium levels are high, PTH release is blocked.

Another electrolyte – magnesium – also affects PTH secretion by mobilising calcium and inhibiting the release of PTH when concentrations rise above or fall below normal. An increased serum phosphate level indirectly stimulates parathyroid activity. Renal tubular phosphate reabsorption is balanced by calcium secretion into the urine, which causes a drop in serum calcium, stimulating PTH secretion. The hormones PTH and calcitonin work together to maintain the delicate balance of serum calcium levels in the body and to keep serum calcium levels within the normal range.

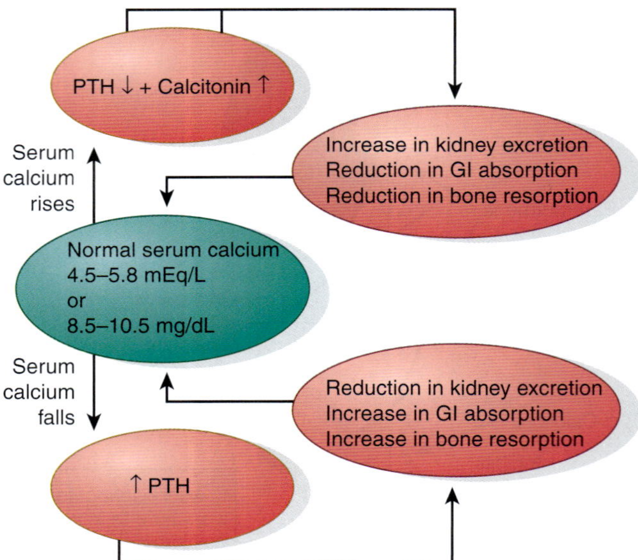

FIGURE 37.4 Regulation of serum calcium. Parathyroid hormone (PTH) and calcitonin regulate normal serum calcium. As serum calcium rises, PTH is inhibited by calcitonin. The kidney then excretes more calcium, the GI system absorbs less and a reduction in bone resorption occurs. As serum calcium falls, PTH is secreted and raises the calcium level by decreasing the amount of calcium lost in the kidney, increasing the amount absorbed in the GI tract and increasing bone resorption.

Parathyroid dysfunction and related disorders

Parathyroid dysfunction involves either absence of PTH (hypoparathyroidism) or overproduction of PTH (hyperparathyroidism). This dysfunction can affect any age group. Box 37.1 explains the use of parathyroid agents across the lifespan.

Hypoparathyroidism

The absence of PTH results in a low calcium level (**hypocalcaemia**) and a relatively rare condition called **hypoparathyroidism**. This is most likely to occur with the accidental removal of the parathyroid glands during thyroid surgery. Treatment consists in calcium and vitamin D therapy to increase serum calcium levels (see section on antihypocalcaemic agents).

Hyperparathyroidism

The excessive production of PTH leads to an elevated calcium level (**hypercalcaemia**) and a condition called **hyperparathyroidism**. This can occur as a result of parathyroid tumour or certain genetic disorders. The person presents with signs of high calcium levels (see Table 37.3). Primary hyperparathyroidism occurs more often in women between 60 and 70 years of age. Secondary hyperparathyroidism occurs most frequently in people with chronic renal failure (see Box 37.3 for more information). When plasma concentrations of calcium are elevated secondary to high PTH levels, inorganic phosphate levels are usually decreased. Pseudorickets (renal fibrocystic osteosis or renal rickets) may occur as a result of this phosphorus retention (hyperphosphataemia), which results from increased stimulation of the parathyroid glands and increased PTH secretion.

The genetically linked disorder **Paget disease** is a condition of overactive osteoclasts that are eventually replaced by enlarged and softened bony structures. People with this disease complain of deep bone pain, headaches and hearing loss, and usually have cardiac failure and bone malformation.

Postmenopausal osteoporosis can occur when dropping levels of oestrogen allow calcium to be pulled out of the bone, resulting in a weakened and honeycombed bone structure. Oestrogen normally causes calcium deposits in the bone; osteoporosis is one of the many complications that accompany the loss of oestrogen at menopause (Box 37.4).

TABLE 37.3 Signs and symptoms of calcium imbalance

System	Hypocalcaemia	Hypercalcaemia
Central nervous system	Hyperactive reflexes, paraesthesias, positive Chvostek and Trousseau signs	Lethargy, personality and behaviour changes, polydipsia, stupor, coma
Cardiovascular	Hypotension, prolonged QT interval, oedema and signs of cardiac insufficiency	Hypertension, shortening of the QT interval, atrioventricular block
Gastrointestinal	Abdominal spasms and cramps	Anorexia, nausea, vomiting, constipation
Muscular	Tetany, skeletal muscle cramps, carpopedal spasm, laryngeal spasm, tetany	Muscle weakness, muscle atrophy, ataxia, loss of muscle tone
Renal		Polyuria, flank pain, kidney stones, acute and/or chronic renal insufficiency
Skeletal	Bone pain, osteomalacia, bone deformities, fractures	Osteopenia, osteoporosis

BOX 37.3 Treatments for secondary hyperparathyroidism

In 2004, a new drug in a new class of calcimimetic agents, cinacalcet hydrochloride (*Sensipar*), was approved for treatment of secondary hyperparathyroidism in people undergoing dialysis for chronic kidney disease and for treatment of hypercalcaemia in people with parathyroid carcinoma. Cinacalcet is a calcimimetic drug that increases the sensitivity of the calcium-sensing receptor to activation by extracellular calcium. In increasing the receptors' sensitivity, cinacalcet lowers parathyroid hormone (PTH) levels, causing a concomitant decrease in serum calcium levels.

The usual initial adult doses for secondary hyperparathyroidism are 30 mg/day PO, after which PTH, serum calcium and serum phosphorus levels are monitored to achieve the desired therapeutic effect. The usual dose range is 60–180 mg/day. The drug must be used in combination with vitamin D and/or phosphate binders.

For parathyroid carcinoma, the initial dose is 30 mg PO twice a day titrated every 2–4 weeks to maintain serum calcium levels within a normal range; 30–90 mg twice a day up to 90 mg three to four times daily may be needed. Side effects that the person may experience include nausea, vomiting, diarrhoea and dizziness.

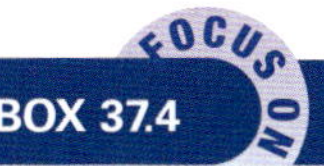

BOX 37.4 Gender considerations

Osteoporosis

Osteoporosis is the most common bone disease found in adults. It results from a lack of bone-building cell (osteoclast) activity and a decrease in bone matrix and mass, with less calcium and phosphorus being deposited in the bone. This can occur with advancing age, when the endocrine system is slowing down and the stimulation to build bone is absent; with menopause, when the calcium-depositing effects of oestrogen are lost; with malnutrition states, when vitamin C and proteins essential for bone production are absent from the diet; and with a lack of physical stress on the bones from lack of activity, which promotes calcium removal and does not stimulate osteoclast activity. The inactive, elderly, postmenopausal woman with a poor diet is a prime candidate for osteoporosis. Fractured hips and wrists, shrinking size, and curvature of the spine are all evidence of osteoporosis in this age group. Besides the use of bisphosphonates to encourage calcium deposition in the bone, several other interventions can help prevent severe osteoporosis in this group or in any other people with similar risk factors.

- *Aerobic exercise:* walking, even 10 minutes a day, has been shown to help increase osteoclast activity. Encourage people to walk around the block or to park their car far from the door and walk. Exercise does not have to involve vigorous gym activity to be beneficial.
- *Proper diet:* calcium and proteins are essential for bone growth. The person who eats only pasta and avoids milk products could benefit from calcium supplements and encouragement to eat protein at least two or three times a week. Weight loss can also help to improve activity and decrease pressure on bones at rest.
- *Hormone replacement therapy (HRT):* for women, HRT has been very successful in decreasing the progression of osteoporosis. Results of the Women's Health Study showed an increase in cardiovascular events with long-term HRT, making it a less desirable treatment. Women who are at high risk for breast cancer or who do not elect to take HRT may be good candidates for bisphosphonates.

The risk of osteoporosis should be taken into consideration as part of the health care regimen for all people as they age. Prevention can save a great deal of pain and debilitation in the long run.

KEY POINTS

- Parathyroid glands produce PTH, which, together with calcitonin, maintains the body's calcium balance.
- A low calcium level (hypocalcaemia) is treated with vitamin D and calcium replacement therapy.
- Hypercalcaemia and hypercalcaemic states are associated with postmenopausal osteoporosis, Paget disease and malignancies.

PARATHYROID AGENTS

The drugs used to treat disorders associated with parathyroid function are drugs that affect serum calcium levels. There is one parathyroid replacement hormone available and one form of calcitonin; the other drugs affect calcium levels in other ways.

ANTIHYPOCALCAEMIC AGENTS

Deficient levels of PTH result in hypocalcaemia (calcium deficiency). Vitamin D stimulates calcium absorption from the intestine and restores the serum calcium to a normal level. Hypoparathyroidism is treated primarily with vitamin D and, if necessary, dietary supplements of calcium. However, there is one parathyroid hormone available for therapeutic use, teriparatide (*Forteo*), a parathyroid hormone genetically engineered from *Escherichia coli* bacteria using recombinant DNA technology. The drug was approved in 2002 to increase bone mass in postmenopausal women and men with primary or hypogonadal osteoporosis who are at high risk for fracture. Additional hypocalcaemic agents include calcitriol (*Kosteo, Rocaltrol and others*) which is the most commonly used form of vitamin D (see Table 37.4).

Therapeutic actions and indications

Vitamin D compounds regulate the absorption of calcium and phosphate from the small intestine, mineral resorption in bone and reabsorption of phosphate from the renal tubules. Working along with PTH and calcitonin to regulate calcium homeostasis, vitamin D actually functions as a hormone. With the once-daily administration, teriparatide stimulates new bone formation, leading to an increase in skeletal mass. It increases serum calcium and decreases serum phosphorus.

Use of these agents is indicated for the management of hypocalcaemia in people undergoing chronic renal dialysis and for the treatment of hypoparathyroidism; teriparatide is used for the treatment of postmenopausal or hypogonadal osteoporosis (see Table 37.4).

Pharmacokinetics

Calcitriol is well absorbed from the GI tract and widely distributed through the body. It is stored in the liver, fat, muscle, skin and bones. Calcitriol has a half-life of approximately 5–8 hours and a duration of action of 3–5 days. After being metabolised in the liver, it is primarily excreted in the bile, with some found in the urine (see Contraindications and cautions for use of this drug during pregnancy and breastfeeding).

Teriparatide is given by subcutaneous injection every day. It is rapidly absorbed from the subcutaneous tissues, reaching peak concentration within 3 hours. The half-life of teriparatide is about 1 hour. Serum calcium levels will begin to decline after about 6 hours and return to baseline 16–24 hours after dosing. Parathyroid hormone is believed to be metabolised in the liver and excreted through the kidneys.

Contraindications and cautions

These drugs should not be used in the presence of any known allergy to any component of the drug, *to avoid hypersensitivity reactions*, or hypercalcaemia or vitamin D toxicity, *which would be exacerbated by these drugs*. At therapeutic levels, these drugs should be used during pregnancy only if the benefit to the mother clearly outweighs the potential for adverse effects on the fetus. Calcitriol has been associated with hypocalcaemia (excessive calcium levels in the blood) in the baby when used by breastfeeding women. Another method of feeding the baby should be used if these drugs are needed during breastfeeding. Caution should be used with a history of renal stones or during breastfeeding, *when high calcium levels could cause problems*.

Teriparatide is associated with osteosarcoma – a bone cancer – in animal studies, so its use is limited to postmenopausal women who have osteoporosis, are at high risk for fractures and are intolerant of standard therapies, and to men with primary or hypogonadal osteoporosis who are at high risk for fracture and are intolerant of standard therapies. Individuals should be informed of the risk of osteosarcoma. These people should also take supplemental calcium and vitamin D, increase weight-bearing exercise and decrease risk factors such as smoking and alcohol consumption.

Adverse effects

The adverse effects most commonly seen with these drugs are related to GI effects: metallic taste, nausea, vomiting, dry mouth, constipation and anorexia. CNS effects such as weakness, headache, somnolence and irritability may also occur. These are possibly related to the changes in electrolytes that occur with these drugs. People with liver or renal dysfunction may experience increased levels of the drugs and/or toxic effects.

TABLE 37.4 DRUGS IN FOCUS Parathyroid agents

Drug name	Dosage/route	Usual indications
Antihypocalcaemic agents		
(P) calcitriol (*Kosteo, Rocaltrol*)	Osteoporosis: 0.25 microgram PO bd. Uraemic osteodystrophy: 0.5–1 microgram/day PO in the morning	Management of hypocalcaemia and reduction of parathormone levels
teriparatide (*Forteo*)	20 micrograms SC daily	Management of osteoporosis in postmenopausal women and men with primary hypogonadal osteoporosis who do not respond to standard therapy
Antihypercalcaemic agents		
Bisphosphonates		
alendronate (generic)	Males and for postmenopausal osteoporosis: 10 mg daily or 70 mg weekly Paget disease: 40 mg/day for up to 6 months	Treatment of Paget disease, postmenopausal osteoporosis treatment and prevention, treatment of glucocorticoid-induced osteoporosis, osteoporosis in men
clodronate (*Bonefos*)	Initially, 2400–3200 mg PO daily in divided doses Maintenance: 1600 mg PO daily	Treatment of hypercalcaemia in malignancy; treatment of osteolytic metastases
etidronate (generic)	5–10 mg/kg/day PO for 14 days followed by a 76-day period of calcium (minimum recommended supplement is 500 mg/day of elemental calcium)	Treatment of Paget disease, postmenopausal osteoporosis, hypercalcaemia of malignancy, osteolytic bone lesions in people with cancer
ibandronate (*Bondronat*)	50 mg PO daily or 6 mg IV q 4 weeks	Treatment of metatstic bone disease in breast cancer and tumour induced hypercalcaemia
pamidronate (*Pamisol*)	Bone metastases from breast cancer and advanced multiple myeloma: 90 mg IV infusion q 4 weeks Paget disease: 60 mg IV infusion	Treatment of Paget disease, postmenopausal osteoporosis in women, hypercalcaemia of malignancy, osteolytic bone lesions in people with cancer
risedronate (*Acris, Actonel*)	35 mg PO once weekly or 150 mg PO once monthly	Treatment of osteoporosis and preservation of bone mineral density in patients receiving corticosteroids long term
zoledronic acid (*Aclasta, Zometa*)	*Aclasta:* 5 mg once yearly IV infusion *Zometa:* prevention of skeletal-related events in advanced malignancies: 4 mg IV infusion over 15 minutes q 3–4 weeks	Treatment of Paget disease, postmenopausal osteoporosis in women, hypercalcaemia of malignancy, osteolytic bone lesions in certain people with cancer
Calcitonins (salcatonin)		
(P) calcitonin salmon (salcatonin) (*Miacalcic*)	Paget disease: 50–100 International Units/day SC or IM Hypercalcaemia: 5–10 IU/kg/day by slow IV infusion, or IM or SC undiluted for volumes > 2 mL. IM is preferred and multiple sites of injection should be used	Treatment of Paget disease, postmenopausal osteoporosis in conjunction with vitamin D and calcium supplements; emergency treatment of hypercalcaemia

Clinically important drug–drug interactions

The risk of hypermagnesaemia increases if these drugs are taken with magnesium-containing antacids. This combination should be avoided.

Reduced absorption of these compounds may occur if they are taken with colestyramine or mineral oil because they are fat-soluble vitamins. If this combination is used, the drugs should be separated by at least 2 hours.

Prototype summary: calcitriol

Indications: management of hypocalcaemia in people on chronic renal dialysis, management of hypocalcaemia associated with hypoparathyroidism.

Actions: a vitamin D compound that regulates the absorption of calcium and phosphate from the small intestine, mineral resorption in bone, and reabsorption of phosphate from the renal tubules, increasing the serum calcium level.

Pharmacokinetics:

Route	Onset	Peak	Duration
PO	Slow	4 hours	3–5 days

$T_{1/2}$: 5–8 hours; metabolised in the liver and excreted in the bile.

Adverse effects: weakness, headache, nausea, vomiting, dry mouth, constipation, muscle pain, bone pain, metallic taste.

Care considerations for people receiving antihypocalcaemic agents

Assessment: history and examination

- Assess for history of allergy to any component of the drugs, hypercalcaemia, vitamin toxicity, renal stone and pregnancy or breastfeeding, *which could be cautions or contraindications to use of the drug.*
- Assess for the presence of any skin lesions; orientation and affect; liver evaluation; serum calcium, magnesium and alkaline phosphate levels; and radiographs of bones as appropriate, *to determine baseline status before beginning therapy and any potential adverse effects.*

Implementation with rationale

- Monitor serum calcium concentration before and periodically during treatment *to allow for adjustment of dose to maintain calcium levels within normal limits.*
- Provide supportive measures *to help the person deal with GI and CNS effects of the drug* (analgesics, small and frequent meals, help with activities of daily living).
- Arrange for a nutritional consultation if GI effects are severe *to ensure nutritional balance.*
- Provide thorough teaching, including measures to avoid adverse effects, warning signs of problems and the need for regular evaluation, *to enhance their knowledge about drug therapy and promote compliance.*

Evaluation

- Monitor response to the drug (return of serum calcium levels to normal).
- Monitor for adverse effects (weakness, headache, GI effects).
- Evaluate the effectiveness of the teaching plan (person can name drug, dosage, adverse effects to watch for and specific measures to avoid them).
- Monitor the effectiveness of comfort measures and compliance with the regimen.

Antihypercalcaemic agents

Drugs used to treat PTH excess or hypocalcaemia include the bisphosphonates and calcitonin salmon. These drugs act on the serum levels of calcium and do not suppress the parathyroid gland or PTH (see Table 37.4).

Therapeutic actions and indications

Bisphosphonates

The **bisphosphonates** act to slow or block bone resorption; by doing this, they help to lower serum calcium levels, but they do not inhibit normal bone formation and mineralisation. Bisphosphonates include alendronate (generic), clodronate (*Bonefos*), etidronate (generic), ibandronate (*Bondronat*), pamidronate (*Pamisol*), risedronate (*Acris*, *Actonel*), and zoledronic acid (*Aclasta, Zometa*). These drugs are used in the treatment of Paget disease and of postmenopausal osteoporosis in women, and alendronate is also used to treat osteoporosis in men. See Table 37.4 for usual indications for each drug.

Calcitonins

The calcitonins are hormones secreted by the thyroid gland to balance the effects of PTH. Currently the only calcitonin readily available is calcitonin salmon (salcatonin) (synthetic calcitonin salmon) (*Miacalcic*). This hormone inhibits bone resorption, lowers serum calcium levels in children and in people with Paget disease and increases the excretion of phosphate, calcium and sodium from the kidney. See Table 37.4 for usual indications for this drug.

Pharmacokinetics

Bisphosphonates

These drugs are well absorbed from the small intestine and do not undergo metabolism. They are excreted relatively unchanged in the urine. The onset of action is slow, and the duration of action is days to weeks. Individuals with renal dysfunction may experience toxic levels of the drug and should be evaluated for a dose reduction. See

Contraindications and cautions for use of these drugs during pregnancy and breastfeeding.

Calcitonins

These drugs are metabolised in the body tissues to inactive fragments, which are excreted by the kidney. Calcitonins cross the placenta and have been associated with adverse effects on the fetus in animal studies. These drugs inhibit breastfeeding in animals; it is not known whether they are excreted in breast milk (see Contraindications and cautions). Calcitonin salmon (salcatonin) can be given by injection. Peak effects are seen within 40 minutes, and the duration of effect is 8–24 hours.

Contraindications and cautions

Bisphosphonates

These drugs should not be used in the presence of hypocalcaemia, *which could be made worse by lowering calcium levels*, or with a history of any allergy to bisphosphonates *to avoid hypersensitivity reactions*. Fetal abnormalities have been associated with these drugs in animal trials, and they should not be used during pregnancy unless the benefit to the mother clearly outweighs the potential risk to the fetus or neonate. Extreme caution should be used when breastfeeding *because of the potential for adverse effects on the baby*.

Alendronate should not be used by breastfeeding mothers. Caution should be used in people with renal dysfunction, *which could interfere with excretion of the drug*, or with upper GI disease, *which could be aggravated by the drug*.

Alendronate and risedronate need to be taken on rising in the morning, with a full glass of water, fully 30 minutes before any other food or beverage, and the person must then remain upright for at least 30 minutes; *taking the drug with a full glass of water and remaining upright for at least 30 minutes facilitates delivery of the drug to the stomach*. These drugs should not be given to anyone who is unable to remain upright for 30 minutes after taking the drug *because serious oesophageal erosion can occur*.

Zoledronic acid should be used cautiously in people with asthma who are aspirin sensitive. Alendronate and risedronate are now available in a once-a-week formulation *to decrease the number of times the person must take the drug*, which should increase compliance with the drug regimen.

Calcitonins

These drugs should be used in pregnancy only if the benefit to the mother clearly outweighs the potential risk to the fetus. They should not be used during breastfeeding *because the calcium-lowering effects could cause problems for the baby*. These drugs should be used with caution in people with renal dysfunction or pernicious anaemia, *which could be exacerbated by these drugs*.

Adverse effects

Bisphosphonates

The most common adverse effects seen with bisphosphonates are headache, nausea and diarrhoea. There is also an increase in bone pain in individuals with Paget disease, but this effect usually passes after a few days to a few weeks. Oesophageal erosion has been associated with alendronate if the person has not remained upright for at least 30 minutes after taking the tablets.

Calcitonins

The most common adverse effects seen with these drugs are flushing of the face and hands, skin rash, nausea and vomiting, urinary frequency and local inflammation at the site of injection. Many of these side effects lessen with time, the time varying with each individual person.

Clinically important drug–drug interactions

Bisphosphonates

Oral absorption of bisphosphonates is decreased if they are taken concurrently with antacids, calcium products, iron or multiple vitamins. If these drugs need to be taken, they should be separated by at least 30 minutes.

GI distress may increase if bisphosphonates are combined with aspirin; this combination should be avoided if possible.

Calcitonins

There have been no clinically important drug–drug interactions reported with the use of calcitonins.

Prototype summary: alendronate

Indications: treatment and prevention of osteoporosis in postmenopausal women and in men; treatment of glucocorticoid-induced osteoporosis; treatment of Paget disease in certain people.

Actions: slows normal and abnormal bone resorption without inhibiting bone formation and mineralisation.

Pharmacokinetics:

Route	Onset	Duration
PO	Slow	Days

$T_{1/2}$: greater than 10 days; not metabolised, but excreted in the urine.

Adverse effects: headache, nausea, diarrhoea, increased or recurrent bone pain, oesophageal erosion.

 **Prototype summary: calcitonin salmon (salcatonin)**

Indications: Paget disease, postmenopausal osteoporosis, emergency treatment of hypercalcaemia.

Actions: inhibits bone resorption; lowers elevated serum calcium in children and people with Paget disease; increases the excretion of filtered phosphate, calcium and sodium by the kidney.

Pharmacokinetics:

Route	Onset	Peak	Duration
IM, SC	15 min	3–4 hours	8–24 hours
Nasal	Rapid	31–39 min	8–24 hours

$T_{1/2}$: 1.43 hours; metabolised in the kidneys and excreted in urine.

Adverse effects: flushing of face and hands, nausea, vomiting, local inflammatory reactions at injection site, nasal irritation if nasal form is used.

Care considerations for people receiving antihypercalcaemic agents

Assessment: history and examination

- Assess for history of allergy to any of these products *to avoid hypersensitivity reaction*; pregnancy or breastfeeding; hypocalcaemia; and renal dysfunction, *which could be cautions or contraindications to use of the drug.*
- Assess for the presence of any skin lesions; orientation and affect; abdominal examination; serum electrolytes; and renal function tests, *to determine baseline status before beginning therapy and for any potential adverse effects.*

Implementation with rationale

- Ensure adequate hydration with any of these agents *to reduce the risk of renal complications.*
- Arrange for concomitant vitamin D, calcium supplements and hormone replacement therapy *if used to treat postmenopausal osteoporosis.*
- Rotate injection sites and monitor for inflammation if using calcitonin salmon (salcatonin) *to prevent tissue breakdown and irritation.*
- Monitor serum calcium regularly *to allow for dose adjustment as needed.*
- Assess the person carefully for any potential drug–drug interactions if giving in combination with other drugs *to prevent serious effects.*
- Arrange for periodic blood tests of renal function if using gallium *to monitor for renal dysfunction.*
- Provide comfort measures and analgesics *to relieve bone pain if it returns as treatment begins.*
- Provide thorough teaching, including measures to avoid adverse effects, warning signs of problems, the need for regular evaluation if used for longer than recommended and proper administration of nasal spray, *to enhance knowledge about drug therapy and promote compliance.*

Evaluation

- Monitor the person's response to the drug (return of calcium levels to normal; prevention of complications of osteoporosis; control of Paget disease).
- Monitor for adverse effects (skin rash; nausea and vomiting; hypocalcaemia; renal dysfunction).
- Evaluate the effectiveness of the teaching plan (person can name drug, dosage, adverse effects to watch for and specific measures to avoid them).
- Monitor the effectiveness of comfort measures and compliance with the regimen.

KEY POINTS

- The parathyroid glands are located behind the thyroid gland and produce PTH, which works with calcitonin, produced by thyroid cells, to maintain the calcium balance in the body.
- Hypocalcaemia, or low levels of calcium, is treated with vitamin D products and calcium replacement therapy.
- Hypercalcaemia can occur in postmenopausal osteoporosis and Paget disease, as well as hypercalcaemia related to malignancy.
- Hypercalcaemia is treated with bisphosphonates, which slow or block bone resorption to lower serum calcium levels, or calcitonin, which inhibits bone resorption, lowers serum calcium levels in children and people with Paget disease and increases the excretion of phosphate, calcium and sodium from the kidney.

CHAPTER SUMMARY

- The thyroid gland uses iodine to produce thyroid hormones. Thyroid hormones control the rate at which most body cells use energy (metabolism).
- Control of the thyroid gland is an intricate balancing process between TRH, released by the hypothalamus; TSH, released by the anterior pituitary; and circulating levels of thyroid hormone.
- Hypothyroidism, or lower-than-normal levels of thyroid hormone, is treated with replacement thyroid hormone.

- Hyperthyroidism, or higher-than-normal levels of thyroid hormone, is treated with thioamides, which block the thyroid from producing thyroid hormone, or with iodines, which prevent thyroid hormone production or destroy parts of the gland.
- The parathyroid glands are located behind the thyroid gland and produce PTH, which works with calcitonin, produced by thyroid cells, to maintain the calcium balance in the body.
- Hypocalcaemia, or low levels of calcium, is treated with vitamin D products and calcium replacement therapy.
- Hypercalcaemia and hypercalcaemic states include postmenopausal osteoporosis and Paget disease, as well as hypercalcaemia related to malignancy.
- Hypercalcaemia is treated with bisphosphonates or calcitonin. Bisphosphonates slow or block bone resorption, which lowers serum calcium levels. Calcitonin inhibits bone resorption, lowers serum calcium levels in children and in people with Paget disease, and increases the excretion of phosphate, calcium and sodium from the kidney.

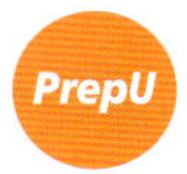

Knowing your strengths and weaknesses helps you to study more effectively. Take a PrepU Practice Quiz to find out how you measure up!

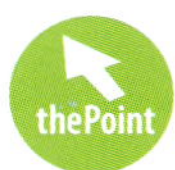

ONLINE RESOURCES

An extensive range of additional resources to enhance teaching and learning and to facilitate understanding of this chapter may be found online at the text's accompanying website, located on thePoint at http://thepoint.lww.com. These include Watch and Learn videos, Concepts in Action animations, journal articles, review questions, case studies, discussion topics and quizzes.

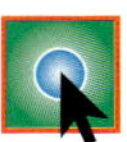

WEB LINKS

Health care providers and students may want to consult the following web resource:

www.osteoporosis.org.au
Information on osteoporosis – support groups, screening, treatment and research.

BIBLIOGRAPHY

Brown, E. & Lambert, K. (2008). Bisphosphonate infusions for hypercalcaemia of malignancy. *European Journal of Palliative Care, 15(5)*, 217–220.

Burton, J. E. (2011). Hyperthyroidism. *MEDSURG Nursing, 20(3)*, 152–153.

Crowley, R. & Gittoes, N. (2013). How to approach hypercalcaemia. *Clinical Medicine, 13(3)*, 287–290.

Davoren, P. (2008). Modern management of thyroid replacement therapy. *Australian Prescriber, 31*, 159–161.

Farrell, M. & Dempsey, J. (2014). *Smeltzer & Bare's Textbook of Medical-Surgical Nursing* (3rd edn). Sydney: Lippincott Williams & Wilkins.

Goodman, L. S., Brunton, L. L., Chabner, B. & Knollmann, B. C. (2011). *Goodman and Gilman's Pharmacological Basis of Therapeutics* (12th edn). New York: McGraw-Hill.

Granjean, C. K. & McMullen, P. C. (2010). Hypercalcaemia: What constitutes reasonable follow-up? *Journal for Nurse Practitioners, 6(9)*, 691–693.

Joshi, D., Center, J. R. & Eisman, J. A. (2010). Vitamin D deficiency in adults. *Australian Prescriber, 33*, 103–106.

LabPlus Auckland (2011). Test Guide. Auckland. Author.

McKenna, L. & Mirkov, S. (2019). *McKenna's Drug Handbook for Nursing and Midwifery* (8th edn). Sydney: Wolters Kluwer Health Australia.

Pettifer, A. & Grant, S. (2013). The management of hypercalcaemia in advanced cancer. *International Journal of Palliative Nursing, 19(7)*, 327–331.

Porth, C. M. (2011). *Essentials of Pathophysiology: Concepts of Altered Health States* (3rd edn) Philadelphia: Lippincott Williams & Wilkins.

Porth, C. M. (2009). *Pathophysiology: Concepts of Altered Health States* (8th edn). Philadelphia: Lippincott Williams & Wilkins.

Roberts, D. M. (2010). Management of renal bone disease. *Australian Prescriber, 33*, 34–37.

Sabry, N. A. & Habib, E. E. (2011). Zoledronic acid and clodronate in the treatment of malignant bone metastases with hypercalcaemia: Efficacy and safety comparative study. *Medical Oncology, 28(2)*, 584–590.

Schenk, D., Donaldson, M. & Cheetham, T. (2012). Which antithyroid drug regimen in paediatric Grave's disease? *Clinical Endocrinology, 77(6)*, 806–807.

Weetman, A. (2013). Current choice of treatment for hypo- and hyperthyroidism. *Prescriber, 24(13–16)*, 23–33.

CHECK YOUR UNDERSTANDING

Answers to the questions in this chapter can be found in Appendix A at the back of this book.

MULTIPLE CHOICE

Select the best answer to the following.

1. The thyroid gland produces the thyroid hormones T_3 and T_4, which are dependent on the availability of:
   a. iodine produced in the liver.
   b. iodine found in the diet.
   c. iron absorbed from the gastrointestinal tract.
   d. parathyroid hormone to promote iodine binding.
2. The thyroid gland is dependent on the hypothalamic–pituitary axis for regulation. Increasing the levels of thyroid hormone (by taking replacement thyroid hormone) would:
   a. increase hypothalamic release of TRH.
   b. increase pituitary release of TSH.
   c. suppress hypothalamic release of TRH.
   d. stimulate the thyroid gland to produce more T_3 and T_4.
3. Goitre, or enlargement of the thyroid gland, is usually associated with:
   a. hypothyroidism.
   b. iodine deficiency.
   c. hyperthyroidism.
   d. underactive thyroid tissue.
4. Thyroid replacement therapy is indicated for the treatment of:
   a. obesity.
   b. myxoedema.
   c. Graves' disease.
   d. acute thyrotoxicosis.
5. Assessing a person's knowledge of their thyroid replacement therapy would show good understanding if the person stated:
   a. 'My wife may use some of my drug, since she wants to lose weight.'
   b. 'I should only need this drug for about 3 months.'
   c. 'I can stop taking this drug as soon as I feel like my old self.'
   d. 'I should call if I experience unusual sweating, weight gain, or chills and fever.'
6. Administration of propylthiouracil (PTU) would include giving the drug:
   a. once a day in the morning.
   b. around the clock to assure therapeutic levels.
   c. once a day at bedtime to decrease adverse effects.
   d. if the person is experiencing slow heart rate, skin rash or excessive bleeding.
7. The parathyroid glands produce PTH, which is important in the body as:
   a. a modulator of thyroid hormone.
   b. a regulator of potassium.
   c. a regulator of calcium.
   d. an activator of vitamin D.
8. A drug of choice for the treatment of postmenopausal osteoporosis would be:
   a. paracetamol.
   b. alendronate.
   c. calcitonin salmon (salcatonin).
   d. calcitriol.

MULTIPLE RESPONSE

Select all that apply.

1. A person who is receiving a bisphosphonate for the treatment of postmenopausal osteoporosis should be taught:
   a. to also take vitamin D, calcium, and hormone replacement.
   b. to restrict fluids as much as possible.
   c. to take the drug before any food for the day, with a full glass of water.
   d. to stay upright for at least 30 minutes after taking the drug.
   e. to take the drug with meals to avoid GI upset.
   f. to avoid exercise to prevent bone fractures.
2. Hypothyroidism is a very common and often missed disorder. Signs and symptoms of hypothyroidism include:
   a. increased body temperature.
   b. thickening of the tongue.
   c. bradycardia.
   d. loss of hair.
   e. excessive weight loss.
   f. oily skin.

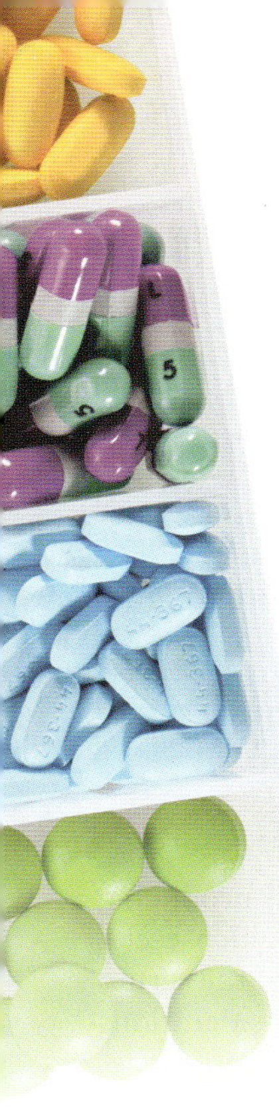

Agents to control blood glucose levels

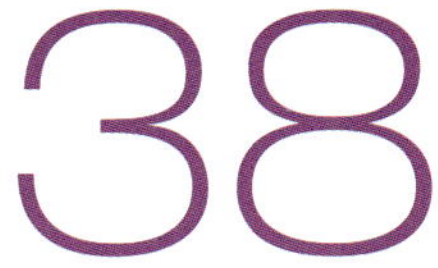

Learning objectives

On completing this chapter you should be able to:

1. Describe the pathophysiology of diabetes mellitus, including alterations in metabolic pathways and changes to basement membranes.
2. Describe the therapeutic actions, indications, pharmacokinetics, contraindications, most common adverse reactions, and important drug–drug interactions associated with insulin and other hypoglycaemic agents and glucose-elevating agents.
3. Discuss the use of hypoglycaemic agents and glucose-elevating agents across the lifespan.
4. Compare and contrast the prototype drugs insulin, glibenclamide and metformin with other hypoglycaemic agents in their class.
5. Outline the care considerations, including important teaching points, for people receiving a hypoglycaemic or glucose-elevating agent.

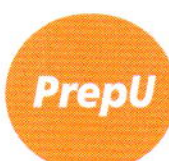

Test your current knowledge of agents to control blood glucose levels with a PrepU Practice Quiz!

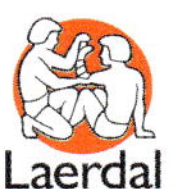

Simulation-based learning
On completion of the chapter, explore the scenario of Skyler Hanson (Part 1) who has been taken to the emergency department with diabetic ketoacidosis. Continue onto the second scenario (Part 2) where Skyler is brought at a different time to the emergency department by his friends. Consider the medication management of Skyler's condition throughout his episode of care. What learning from the chapter can be applied to the case?

Glossary of key terms

adiponectin: hormone produced by adipocytes that acts to increase insulin sensitivity, decrease the release of glucose from the liver and protect the blood vessels from inflammatory changes

diabetes mellitus: a metabolic disorder characterised by high blood glucose levels and altered metabolism of proteins and fats; associated with thickening of the basement membrane, leading to numerous complications

dipeptidyl peptidase-4 (DPP-4): enzyme that quickly metabolises glucagon-like polypeptide-1

endocannabinoid receptors: receptors found in the adipose tissue, muscles, liver, satiety centre in the hypothalamus and GI tract that are part of a signalling system within the body to keep the body in a state of energy gain

glucagon-like polypeptide-1 (GLP-1): a peptide produced in the GI tract in response to carbohydrates that increases insulin release, decreases glucagon release, slows GI emptying and stimulates the satiety centre in the hypothalamus

glycogen: storage form of glucose; can be broken down for rapid glucose level increases during times of stress

glycosuria: presence of glucose in the urine

glycated haemoglobin: a blood glucose marker that provides a 3-month average of blood glucose levels

hyperglycaemia: elevated fasting plasma glucose levels > 7.0 mmol/L (126 mg/dL) leading to multiple signs and symptoms and abnormal metabolic pathways

hypoglycaemia: lower-than-normal blood sugar < 4.4 mmol/L (40 mg/dL); often results from imbalance between insulin or oral agents and person's eating, activity and stress

incretins: peptides that are produced in the GI tract in response to food that help to modulate insulin and glucagon activity

insulin: hormone produced by the beta cells in the pancreas; stimulates insulin receptor sites to move glucose into the cells; promotes storage of fat and glucose in the body

ketosis: breakdown of fats for energy, resulting in an increase in ketones to be excreted from the body

polydipsia: increased thirst; seen in diabetes when loss of fluid and increased tonicity of the blood lead the hypothalamic thirst centre to make the person feel thirsty

polyphagia: increased hunger; sign of diabetes when cells cannot use glucose for energy and sense they are starving, causing hunger

sodium–glucose co-transporter 2 (SGLT2): protein that promotes reabsorption of glucose in the proximal tubule of the nephron
sulfonylureas: oral hypoglycaemia agents used to stimulate the pancreas to release more insulin

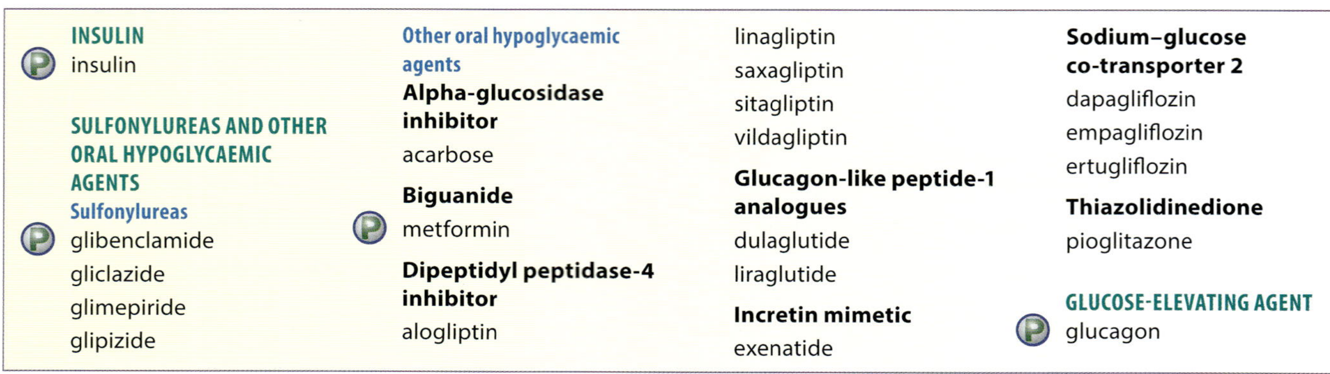

INSULIN
(P) insulin

SULFONYLUREAS AND OTHER ORAL HYPOGLYCAEMIC AGENTS
Sulfonylureas
(P) glibenclamide
gliclazide
glimepiride
glipizide

Other oral hypoglycaemic agents
Alpha-glucosidase inhibitor
acarbose

Biguanide
(P) metformin

Dipeptidyl peptidase-4 inhibitor
alogliptin
linagliptin
saxagliptin
sitagliptin
vildagliptin

Glucagon-like peptide-1 analogues
dulaglutide
liraglutide

Incretin mimetic
exenatide

Sodium–glucose co-transporter 2
dapagliflozin
empagliflozin
ertugliflozin

Thiazolidinedione
pioglitazone

GLUCOSE-ELEVATING AGENT
(P) glucagon

Hypoglycaemic agents, as the name implies, are used to treat **diabetes mellitus**, the most common of all metabolic disorders. It is estimated that almost 1 million people in Australia have been diagnosed with diabetes mellitus, and there are many others not yet diagnosed. Furthermore, diabetes mellitus has been reported as three times more common in the Indigenous Australian population than the non-Indigenous (AIHW, 2013). As a major problem that significantly impacts on the health of Australians, diabetes mellitus is one of the nine National Health Priority Areas identified by the Australian government. For more information on diabetes mellitus in Australia, see www.aihw.gov.au/diabetes. In New Zealand, the Ministry of Health has a big focus on diabetes prevention and active diabetes management, especially of type 2 diabetes, resulting in increased funding for diabetes services over the last few years (www.diabetes.org.nz).

Diabetes mellitus is a complicated disorder that alters the metabolism of glucose, fats and proteins, affecting many end organs and causing numerous clinical complications. The World Health Organization diagnostic criteria for diabetes are fasting plasma glucose level ≥ 7.0 mmol/L (126 mg/dL) or 2-hour plasma glucose level (venous plasma glucose level 2 hours after ingestion of a 75 g oral glucose load) ≥ 11.1 mmol/L (200 mg/dL). Diabetes mellitus is part of the 'metabolic syndrome', a collection of conditions that predispose to cardiovascular disease (Chapter 46).

Treatment of diabetes is aimed at tightly regulating the blood glucose level through diet and the use of insulin or other glucose-lowering drugs. Maintaining serum glucose within a therapeutic range is very important to the nervous system. The nerves in the central nervous system (CNS) receive glucose by diffusion. The presence of too much glucose, which is a large molecule, takes water into the CNS and can cause swelling and nerve instability. The presence of too little glucose results in less energy for the nerves to use to function and loss of cell membrane integrity. Maintaining a therapeutic glucose level is a complicated process that involves diet, exercise and drug management. At times, the blood glucose level is lowered too much, producing a state of hypoglycaemia. When this occurs, glucose-elevating agents need to be used to quickly return the serum glucose levels to a therapeutic range. Considerations related to the use of insulin and other oral hypoglycaemic agents based on age are highlighted in Box 38.1. Nurses, midwives and diabetes educators play a major role in education and management for individuals with diabetes and their families.

GLUCOSE REGULATION

Glucose is the leading energy source for the human body. Glucose is stored in the body for rapid release in times of stress. As a result, blood glucose levels can be readily maintained so that the neurons always receive a constant supply of glucose to function. The body's control of glucose is intricately related to fat and protein metabolism, balancing energy conservation with energy consumption to maintain homeostasis in a variety of situations. Many factors have an impact on this balance and the body's ability to adapt and to maintain metabolism.

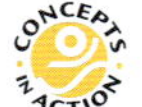

Endocrine: Hormonal control of blood glucose

The pancreas

The pancreas is both an endocrine gland, producing hormones, and an exocrine gland, releasing sodium bicarbonate and pancreatic enzymes directly into the common bile duct to be released into the small intestine, where they neutralise the acid chyme from the stomach and aid digestion. The endocrine part of the pancreas produces hormones in collections of tissue called the islets of Langerhans. These islets contain endocrine cells that produce specific hormones. The alpha cells release glucagon in direct response to low blood glucose levels. The beta cells release insulin in direct response to high blood glucose levels. Delta cells produce somatostatin in response to very low blood glucose levels; somatostatin

BOX 38.1 FOCUS ON **Drug therapy across the lifespan**

Hypoglycaemic agents

CHILDREN

Treatment of diabetes in children is a difficult challenge of balancing diet, activity, growth, stressors and insulin requirements. Children need to be carefully monitored for any sign of hypoglycaemia or hyperglycaemia and treated quickly because their fast metabolism and lack of body reserves can push them into a severe state quickly.

Insulin dose, especially in infants, may be so small that it is difficult to calibrate. Insulin often needs to be diluted to a volume that can be detected on the syringe. A second person should always check the calculations and dose of insulin being given to small children.

Teenagers often present a real challenge for diabetes management. The desire to be 'normal' often leads to a resistance to dietary restrictions and insulin injections. The metabolism of the teenager is also in flux, leading to complications in regulating insulin dose. A team approach, including the child, family members, teachers, coaches, and even friends, may be the best way to help the child deal with the disease and the required therapy. New delivery methods for insulin may help this age group cope with the drug therapy in the future.

Metformin is the only oral hypoglycaemic drug approved for children. It has established dosing for children 10 years of age and older. With the increasing number of children being diagnosed with type 2 diabetes, the use of other agents in children is being tested.

ADULTS

Adults need extensive education about the disease, as well as about the drug therapy. Warning signs and symptoms should be stressed repeatedly as the adult learns to juggle insulin needs with exercise, stressors, other drug effects and diet. Adults maintained on oral agents need to be monitored for changes in response to the drugs. Often additional drugs are added or doses are changed as the disease progresses over time.

Exercise and diet should always be emphasised as the mainstay of dealing with diabetes. Adults need to be cautioned about the use of over-the-counter and herbal or alternative therapies. Many of these products contain agents that alter blood glucose levels and will change insulin or oral agent requirements. Adults should always be asked specifically whether they use any of these agents and adjustments should be made accordingly.

PREGNANCY AND BREASTFEEDING

Insulin therapy is the best choice for women with diabetes mellitus during pregnancy and breastfeeding, which are times of high stress and metabolic demands. Needs may change on a daily basis, and the mother should have ready support and extensive teaching about what to do if hypoglycaemia or hyperglycaemia occurs. The period of labour and birth is often a critical time in diabetes management because of the stress and sudden changes in body fluid volume and hormone levels. The obstetrician and the endocrinologist or primary care provider should consult frequently about the best way to support the woman through this period.

OLDER ADULTS

Older adults can have many underlying problems that complicate diabetes management. Poor vision and/or coordination may make it difficult to prepare a syringe. A week's supply of syringes can be prepared and refrigerated for the usual dose of insulin.

Dietary deficiencies related to changes in taste, absorption or attitude may lead to wide fluctuations in blood sugar levels, making it difficult to control diabetes. Many areas have nutritional assistance programs for older adults (eg, Meals on Wheels) or have places that can refer people to appropriate agencies that might be able to offer assistance.

Older adults have a greater incidence of renal or hepatic impairment, and kidney and liver function should be evaluated before starting any of these drugs. Combinations of oral agents may not be feasible with severe dysfunction and the person may need to use insulin to control blood glucose levels.

Older adults should receive periodic educational reminders about diet, the need for exercise, skin and foot care, and warning signs to report to the health care provider.

The older person is also more likely to experience end organ damage related to the diabetes – loss of vision, kidney problems, coronary artery disease, infections – and the drug regimen of these people can become quite complex. Careful screening for drug interactions is an important aspect of the assessment of these people.

blocks the secretion of both insulin and glucagon. These hormones work together to maintain the blood glucose level within normal limits.

Insulin

Insulin is the hormone produced by the pancreatic beta cells of the islets of Langerhans. The hormone is released into circulation when the levels of glucose around these cells rise. It is also released in response to **incretins**, peptides that are produced in the gastrointestinal (GI) tract in response to food. One of these incretins, **glucagon-like polypeptide-1 (GLP-1)**, increases insulin release and decreases glucagon release (in preparation for the nutrients that will soon be absorbed). GLP-1 also slows GI emptying to allow more absorption of nutrients and stimulates the satiety centre in the hypothalamus to decrease the desire to eat because food is already in the GI tract. GLP-1 has a very short half-life and is metabolised by the enzyme **dipeptidyl-peptidase-4 (DPP-4)**.

Insulin circulates through the body and reacts with specific insulin receptor sites to stimulate the transport of glucose into the cells to be used for energy, a process called facilitated diffusion. Insulin also stimulates the synthesis of **glycogen** (glucose stored for immediate release during times of stress or low glucose), the conversion of lipids into fat stored in the form of adipose tissue and the synthesis of needed proteins from amino acids.

Insulin is released after a meal, when the blood glucose levels rise. It circulates and affects metabolism, allowing the body to either store or use the nutrients from the meal effectively. As a result of the insulin release, blood glucose levels fall and insulin release drops off. Sometimes, an insufficient amount of insulin is released. This may occur because the pancreas cannot produce enough insulin, the insulin receptor sites have lost their sensitivity to insulin and they require more insulin to lower glucose effectively or the person does not have enough receptor sites to support his or her body size, as in obesity.

Glucagon

Glucagon is released from the alpha cells in the islets of Langerhans located in the pancreas in response to low blood glucose levels. Glucagon causes an immediate mobilisation of glycogen stored in the liver and raises blood glucose levels.

Other factors affecting glucose control

Other factors in the body have been found to have an impact on glucose, fat and protein metabolism. These factors play a role in the overall energy balance in the body.

Adipocytes, or fat cells, were once thought to just store fat for energy. However, they have been found to have a major impact on glucose and fat metabolism throughout the body through the secretion of **adiponectin**. This hormone acts to increase insulin sensitivity, decrease the release of glucose from the liver and protect the blood vessels from inflammatory changes. When adiponectin levels are high, it exerts a protective effect on the body. When adiponectin levels are low, as in cases of intra-abdominal fat accumulation, glucose levels rise and blood vessel injury increases.

Endocannabinoid receptors have been identified in the adipose tissue, muscles, liver, the satiety centre and the GI tract. These receptors seem to be part of a signalling system within the body to keep the body in a state of energy gain, to prepare for stressful situations. When stimulated, these receptors promote food intake, decrease adiponectin release, increase fat breakdown, decrease insulin sensitivity, increase fat storage and alter gastric emptying to promote greater nutrient absorption. People who are obese have been shown to have increased stimulation of these receptors.

The sympathetic nervous system, through noradrenaline and adrenaline effects, directly causes a decrease in insulin release, an increase in the release of stored glucose and an increase in fat breakdown. A person under stress will have increased glucose levels and increased free fatty acid (FFA) levels, which will provide the energy needed for the immediate 'fight or flight' associated with a stress reaction. Prolonged stress can alter the control of metabolism that regulates the body's energy balance.

Corticosteroids, which are released diurnally but also during a stress reaction, decrease insulin sensitivity, increase glucose release and decrease protein building. All of these actions conserve energy and provide immediate glucose for any stressful situation.

Growth hormone causes decreased insulin sensitivity, increased FFA levels and increase in protein building. Fluctuating levels of growth hormone can upset the metabolic homeostasis. Box 38.2 summarises effects of various factors on blood glucose levels.

Loss of blood glucose control

When an insufficient amount of insulin is released or insulin receptors are no longer responding, several metabolic changes occur, beginning with hyperglycaemia, or increased blood sugar. Hyperglycaemia results in **glycosuria**: sugar is excreted into the urine because the concentration of glucose in the blood is too high for complete reabsorption. Because this sugar-rich urine is an ideal environment for bacteria, cystitis is a common finding. The person experiences fatigue because the body's cells cannot use the glucose that is there; they need insulin to facilitate transport of the glucose into the cells. **Polyphagia** (increased hunger) occurs because the hypothalamic centres cannot take in glucose; thus

BOX 38.2 Glucose control mechanisms

Insulin	Decreases blood glucose; glycogen storage; adipose tissue deposit; synthesis of proteins to form amino acids
Glucagon	Increases blood glucose
Somatostatin	Decreases insulin release; decreases glucagon release; slows GI emptying
Growth hormone	Decreases insulin sensitivity; increases protein building; increases free fatty acid formation
Incretins	Increase insulin release; decrease glucagon release; stimulate satiety centre; slows GI emptying
Adiponectin	Increases insulin sensitivity; decreases glucose output from liver; protects vessels from inflammatory reactions
Catecholamines	Decrease insulin release; increase glucose output from liver and muscles; increase breakdown of fat to free fatty acids
Corticosteroids	Increase glucose output; decrease insulin sensitivity
Endocannabinoid system	Increases food intake by blocking satiety signals; decreases adiponectin release; decreases insulin sensitivity; increases fat synthesis; alters gastric motility

the cells sense that they are requiring glucose. **Polydipsia** (increased thirst) occurs because the tonicity of the blood is increased owing to the increased glucose and waste products in the blood and the loss of fluid with glucose in the urine. The hypothalamic cells that are sensitive to fluid levels sense a need to increase fluid in the system, which in turn causes the person to feel thirsty.

Lipolysis, or fat breakdown, occurs when the body breaks down stored fat into FFAs for energy because glucose is not usable. The person experiences **ketosis** as metabolism shifts to the use of fat for energy. Ketones are produced that cannot be removed effectively. Acidosis also occurs because the liver cannot remove all of the waste products (acid being a primary waste product) that result from the breakdown of glucose, fat and proteins. Muscles break down because proteins are being broken down for their essential amino acids. The breakdown of proteins results in an increase in nitrogen wastes, which is manifested by an elevated blood urea nitrogen (BUN) concentration and sometimes by protein in the urine. People with hyperglycaemia do not heal quickly because of this protein breakdown, as well as the lack of a stimulus to initiate protein building. All of these actions eventually contribute to development of the complications associated with chronic hyperglycaemia or diabetes.

DIABETES MELLITUS

Diabetes mellitus (literally, 'honey urine') is characterised by complex disturbances in metabolism. Diabetes affects carbohydrate, protein and fat metabolism. The most frequently recognised clinical signs of diabetes are hyperglycaemia (fasting plasma glucose level greater than 7.0 mmol/L [126 mg/dL]) and glycosuria (the presence of sugar in the urine). The alteration in the body's ability to effectively deal with carbohydrate, fat and protein metabolism over the long term results in a thickening of the basement membrane (a thin layer of collagen filament that lies just below the endothelial lining of blood vessels) in large and small blood vessels. This thickening leads to changes in oxygenation of the vessel lining; damage to the vessel lining, which leads to narrowing, vessel remodelling and decreased blood flow through the vessel; and an inability of oxygen to rapidly diffuse across the membrane to the tissues. These changes result in an increased incidence of a number of disorders, including the following:

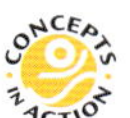

Endocrine: Diabetes

- *Atherosclerosis*: heart attacks and strokes related to the development of atherosclerotic plaques in the vessel lining
- *Retinopathy*: resultant loss of vision as tiny vessels in the eye are narrowed and closed
- *Neuropathies*: motor and sensory changes in the feet and legs and progressive changes in other nerves as the oxygen supply to these nerves is slowly cut off
- *Nephropathy*: renal dysfunction related to changes in the basement membrane of the glomerulus

The overall metabolic disturbances associated with diabetes are thought to be caused by a mosaic of problems, including low insulin and loss of insulin receptor sensitivity.

The diagnosis of diabetes mellitus has involved monitoring of fasting blood glucose levels and sometimes challenging the system with glucose for a glucose tolerance test. However, recent research indicates that the body's response to food may be a more important indicator of impending diabetes. Current thinking is that a fasting blood glucose level may not be as important as a postprandial (after a meal) blood glucose level, which reveals the body's ability to respond to a glucose challenge. The importance of looking at a variety of different glucose markers is being stressed. Box 38.3 highlights some cultural variations in blood glucose levels.

Glycated haemoglobin levels, or an HbA_{1c} test, provide a 3-month average of glucose levels. Red blood cells are freely permeable to glucose, and this test gives

BOX 38.3 FOCUS ON **Cultural considerations**

Diabetes and blood glucose variations

Certain ethnic groups tend to have a genetically predetermined variation in blood glucose levels, possibly caused by a variation in metabolism. In New Zealand, certain ethnic groups (particularly Māori, Pacific Islanders and people from South Asia) are at a higher risk of developing diabetes, and data suggest that the incidence of diabetes for Māori and Pacific Islander peoples are more than three times higher than the European rates, with Māori and Pacific Islander peoples are more than five times as likely to die from type 2 diabetes. Similarly, it has been estimated that Indigenous Australians have a three times higher incidence of type 2 diabetes than the non-Indigenous population, and are twice as likely to die from a diabetes-related condition. People in these groups should be screened regularly for type 2 diabetes. They can also benefit from teaching about warning signs of diabetes. Beyond Australia and New Zealand, similar problems exist for many cultural groups including First Nation people in Canada, and African and Native Americans.

The clinical importance of this relates to proper screening of individuals for hypoglycaemia and diabetes mellitus. Individuals in these groups who have fasting glucose tolerance tests need to have the standard readjusted before a diagnosis is made. Such people also require an understanding of potential differences in normal levels on home blood glucose monitoring units when they are regulating insulin at home.

Sources: Dissanayake, A. (2008). *About Diabetes*. New Zealand Society for the Study of Diabetes (NZSSD). www.nzssd.org.nz/education/diabetes.html; Australian Institute of Health and Welfare (AIHW). (2013). *Diabetes*. www.aihw.gov.au/diabetes.

an average range of glucose exposure over the life of the red blood cell (about 120 days). This test does not require fasting before blood is drawn or the oral intake of glucose before testing. Elevations above 6% may be an early indicator of a prediabetic state, before changes are noted in the fasting blood sugar level. Once a baseline is established, the goal of therapy for a person with diabetes is an HbA_{1c} level less than 7%. Researchers believe that very early intervention – diet, exercise and lifestyle changes – may delay the onset of diabetes and the complications, including coronary artery disease, that come with it.

Diabetes mellitus is classified as either type 1, formerly known as insulin-dependent diabetes mellitus (IDDM), or type 2, formerly non–insulin-dependent diabetes mellitus (NIDDM) or adult-onset diabetes. Type 1 diabetes is usually associated with rapid onset, mostly in younger people, and is connected in many cases to viral destruction of the beta cells of the pancreas. Type 1 diabetes always requires insulin replacement because the beta cells are no longer functioning.

Type 2 diabetes was once thought to be a disease of mature adults with a slow and progressive onset. However, studies released in 2001 reported that the incidence of type 2 diabetes in teenagers and young adults is increasing markedly. People with type 2 diabetes are able to produce insulin, but perhaps not enough to maintain glucose control, or perhaps their insulin receptors are not sensitive enough to insulin, leading to increased serum glucose levels.

Questions are being raised about the impact of early diet and lack of exercise in contributing to this new increase in type 2 diabetes in young people. The treatment of Type 2 diabetes usually begins with changes in diet and exercise. Dieting controls the amount and timing of glucose introduction into the body, and weight loss decreases the number of insulin receptor sites that need to be stimulated, as well as the intra-abdominal fat that blocks adiponectin release. Exercise increases the movement of glucose into the cells by sympathetic nervous system (SNS) activation and by the increased potassium in the blood that occurs directly after exercising. Potassium acts as part of a polarising system during exercise that pushes glucose into the cells. Clinical studies have shown that controlling serum glucose levels can decrease the risk of complications by up to 40% (ADA, 2008).

When diet and exercise no longer work, other agents (discussed later) are used to stimulate the production of insulin in the pancreas, increase the sensitivity of the insulin receptor sites, or control the entry of glucose into the system. Injection of insulin may eventually be needed. This concept is often confusing for people who are learning about diabetes. Type 2 diabetes often evolves until insulin is needed. Timing of the injections of insulin is correlated with food intake and anticipated increases in blood glucose levels, as well as exercise levels and anticipated stress (ADA, 2008). See Box 38.4

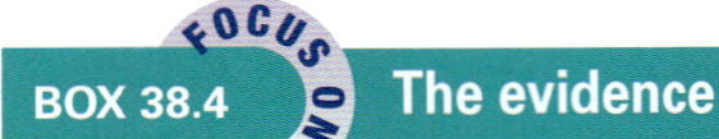

BOX 38.4 The evidence

Managing glucose levels during stress

The body has many compensatory mechanisms for ensuring that blood glucose levels stay within a safe range. The sympathetic stress reaction elevates blood glucose levels to provide ready energy for fight or flight (see Chapter 29). The stress reaction causes the breakdown of glycogen to release glucose and the breakdown of fat and proteins to release other energy.

STRESS REACTIONS

The stress reaction elevates the blood glucose concentration above the normal range. In severe stress situations – such as an acute myocardial infarction or a car crash – the blood glucose level can be very high (above 8.0 mmol/L). The body uses that energy to fight the insult or flee from the stressor.

Nurses and midwives in acute care situations need to be aware of this reflex elevation in glucose when caring for people in acute stress, especially people in emergency situations whose medical history is unknown. The usual medical response to a blood glucose concentration of above 8.8 mmol/L would be the administration of insulin. In many situations, that is exactly what is done, especially if the person's history is not known and the effects of such a high glucose level could cause severe systemic reactions. Insulin administration causes a drop in the blood glucose level as glucose enters cells to be either used for energy or converted to glycogen for storage.

However, a problem may arise in the acute care setting, particularly in a non-diabetic person. Relieving the stress reaction can also drop glucose levels as the stimulus to increase these levels is lost and the glucose that was there is used for energy. A person in this situation who has been treated with insulin is at risk for development of potentially severe hypoglycaemia. The body's response to low glucose levels is a sympathetic stress reaction, which again elevates the blood glucose concentration. If treated, the person potentially can enter a cycle of high and low glucose levels.

BEST CARE PRACTICE

Nurses and midwives are often the ones in closest contact with the highly stressed person – in the emergency room, the intensive care unit, the post-anaesthesia room – and should be constantly aware of the normal and reflex changes in blood glucose that accompany stress. Careful monitoring, with awareness of stress and the relief of stress, can prevent a prolonged treatment program to maintain blood glucose levels within the range of normal, a situation that is not 'normal' during a stress reaction.

People with diabetes who are in severe stress situations require changes in their insulin doses. They should be allowed some elevation of blood glucose, even though their inability to produce sufficient insulin will make it difficult for their cells to make effective use of the increased glucose levels. It is a clinical challenge to balance glucose levels with the needs of the person because so many factors can affect the glucose level.

Source: American Diabetes Association (ADA). (2008). Standards of medical care for patients with diabetes mellitus. *Diabetes Care, 38,* S14–S36.

for more information about managing glucose levels during stress.

Hyperglycaemia

Hyperglycaemia, or high blood sugar, results when there is an increase in glucose in the blood. Clinical signs and symptoms include fatigue, lethargy, irritation, glycosuria, polyphagia, polydipsia and itchy skin (from accumulation of wastes that the liver cannot clear). If the hyperglycaemia goes unchecked, the person will experience ketoacidosis and CNS changes that can progress to coma. Signs of impending dangerous complications of hyperglycaemia include:

- fruity breath as the ketones build up in the system and are excreted through the lungs
- dehydration as fluid and important electrolytes are lost through the kidneys
- slow, deep respirations (Kussmaul respirations) as the body tries to rid itself of high acid levels
- loss of orientation and coma.

This level of hyperglycaemia needs to be treated immediately with insulin. Where available, intravenous (IV) insulin will most rapidly reduce blood glucose levels.

Hypoglycaemia

Hypoglycaemia, or a blood glucose concentration lower than 4.4 mmol/L (40 mg/dL), occurs in a number of clinical situations, including starvation, and if treatment of hyperglycaemia with insulin or oral agents lowers the blood glucose level too far. The body immediately reacts to lowered blood glucose because the cells require glucose to survive, the neurons being among the cells most sensitive to the lack of glucose. The initial reaction to falling blood glucose level is parasympathetic stimulation – increased GI activity to increase digestion and absorption. Rather rapidly, the SNS responds with a 'fight-or-flight' reaction that increases blood glucose levels by initiating the breakdown of fat and glycogen to release glucose for rapid energy. The pancreas releases glucagon, a hormone that counters the effects of insulin and works to increase glucose levels, and somatostatin, which help the body to conserve energy. In many cases, the response to the hypoglycaemic state causes a hyperglycaemic state. Balancing the body's responses to glucose is sometimes difficult when one is trying to treat and control diabetes. Table 38.1 offers a comparison of the signs and symptoms of hyperglycaemia and hypoglycaemia.

INSULIN

Insulin is the only parenteral hypoglycaemic agent available for exogenous replacement (Table 38.2). It is used to treat type 1 diabetes and to treat type 2 diabetes in adults who have no response to diet, exercise and other agents. (See Box 38.1 for considerations related to the use of insulin based on age.) The types of insulin that are available include insulin analogue or lispro (*Humalog*), insulin aspart (*NovoRapid*), insulin glargine (*Lantus*), insulin glulisine (*Apidra*), insulin detemir (*Levemir*), regular (neutral) insulin (*Actrapid, Humulin R*) and isophane insulin (*Humulin NPH*).

Originally, insulin was prepared from pork and beef pancreas. Today, virtually all insulin is prepared by recombinant DNA technology and is human insulin produced by genetically altered bacteria. This purer form of insulin is not associated with the sensitivity problems that many people developed when using the animal products. Animal insulins may still be obtained for people most responsive to them, but they are not generally used. Box 38.5 describes the various forms

TABLE 38.1 Signs and symptoms of hypoglycaemia and hyperglycaemia

Clinical effects	Hypoglycaemia	Hyperglycaemia
Central nervous system	Headache, blurred vision, diplopia; drowsiness progressing to coma; ataxia; hyperactive reflexes	Decreased level of consciousness, sluggishness progressing to coma; hypoactive reflexes
Neuromuscular	Paraesthesias; weakness; muscle spasms; twitching progressing to seizures	Weakness, lethargy
Cardiovascular	Tachycardia; palpitations; normal to high blood pressure	Tachycardia; hypotension
Respiratory	Rapid, shallow respirations	Rapid, deep respirations (Kussmaul); acetone-like or fruity breath
Gastrointestinal	Hunger, nausea	Nausea; vomiting; thirst
Other	Diaphoresis; cool and clammy skin; normal eyeballs	Dry, warm, flushed skin; soft eyeballs
Laboratory tests	Urine glucose negative; blood glucose low	Urine glucose strongly positive; urine ketone levels positive; blood glucose levels high
Onset	Sudden; person appears anxious, drunk; associated with overdose of insulin, missing a meal, increased stress	Gradual; person is slow and sluggish; associated with lack of insulin, increased stress

TABLE 38.2 DRUGS IN FOCUS Insulin

Drug name	Dosage/route	Usual indications
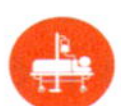 insulin (various types)	Varies based on response, diet, and activity level	Treatment of type 1 diabetes mellitus; treatment of type 2 diabetes mellitus in people whose diabetes cannot be controlled by diet or other agents; treatment of severe ketoacidosis or diabetic coma; treatment of hyperkalaemia (in conjunction with a glucose infusion to produce a shift of potassium into the cells [polarising solution]); also used for short courses of therapy during periods of stress (eg, surgery, disease) in people with type 2 diabetes, for newly diagnosed people being stabilised, for people with poor control of glucose levels, and for people with gestational diabetes

of insulin delivery that are available or under study for future use.

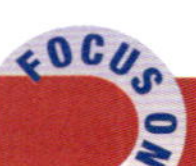 **Hyperglycaemic crisis**

Therapeutic actions and indications

Insulin is a hormone that promotes the storage of the body's fuels, facilitates the transport of various metabolites and ions across cell membranes and stimulates the synthesis of glycogen from glucose, fats from lipids, and proteins from amino acids. Insulin does these things by reacting with specific receptor sites on the cell. Figure 38.3 shows the sites of action of replacement insulin and other drugs used to treat diabetic conditions. See Table 38.2 for indications.

FOCUS ON Safe medication administration

In 2009, lente insulin was removed from the market, as name confusion had occurred between Lantus *insulin and lente insulin. The pharmacokinetics and dose of insulins vary greatly. Use caution to make sure you know which insulin is intended for the individual person.* Lantus *and* Levemir *insulin cannot be mixed in a syringe with any other insulin or any other drug. Use particular caution when working with these two insulins.*

The DHBNZ Safe and Quality Use of Medicines has released an alert informing health care professionals to take extra care when giving insulin Humalog preparation. There are three Humalog preparations available in Australia and New Zealand: Humalog, Humalog Mix25 and Humalog Mix50. Potential harm can result if a person is given Humalog rapid release as opposed to Humalog intermediate release.

The Australian Commission on Safety and Quality in Health Care (ACSQHC) has developed 10 National Safety and Quality Health Service Standards. These Standards aim to improve the quality of health service provision across Australia and provide a national statement of the level of care consumers should be able to expect from health services. Awareness and knowledge of Standard 4 on Medication Safety is an important part of the nurse's and midwife's clinical repertoire. For more information, see www.safetyandquality.gov.au/our-work/accreditation/nsqhss.

Pharmacokinetics

Various preparations of insulin are available to provide short- and long-term coverage. These preparations are processed within the body like endogenous insulin. However, the peak, onset and duration of each vary because of the placement or addition of glycine and/or arginine chains. Maintenance doses are given by the subcutaneous (SC) route only, and injection sites need to be rotated regularly to avoid damage to muscles and to prevent SC atrophy. Regular insulin is given intramuscularly (IM) or IV in emergency situations.

Insulin is available in various preparations with a wide range of peaks and durations of action. A person may receive a combination of regular and isophane insulin in the morning to cover the glucose peak from breakfast (regular onset, 30–60 minutes) and the lunch and dinner glucose peaks. The person may then require another injection before bed. The types of insulin used are determined by the anticipated eating and exercise activities of any particular individual. It is very important to make sure that one is using the correct insulin preparation when administering the drug. Insulin glargine (*Lantus*) and insulin detemir (*Levemir*) cannot be mixed in solution with any other drug, including other insulins.

Contraindications and cautions

Because insulin is used as a replacement hormone, there are no contraindications. Care should be taken during pregnancy and breastfeeding to monitor glucose levels

BOX 38.5 Insulin delivery: past, present and future

Past

Subcutaneous insulin injection. The delivery of insulin by SC injection was introduced in the 1920s and changed the way that people with diabetes were managed clinically, giving them a chance for a normal lifestyle. Research is ongoing to find more efficient and acceptable ways to deliver insulin to people with diabetes.

Present

Subcutaneous insulin injection. This remains the primary delivery system.

Insulin jet injector. This cylindrical device shoots a fine spray of insulin through the skin under very high pressure. Although it is appealing for people who do not like needles or have problems disposing of needles properly, it can be very expensive.

Insulin pen. This syringe-like device looks like a pen. It has a small needle at the tip and a barrel that holds insulin (Figure 38.1). The person 'dials' the amount of insulin to be given and injects the insulin SC by pressing on the top of the pen. This is advantageous for people who need insulin two or three times during the day but cannot easily transport syringes and needles. It is a subtle way to give insulin, and is popular with students and business people on the go. It is important to rotate the syringe 15–20 times before injecting the insulin to disperse it. People often forget this point after using the pens for a while, and as a result, may inject far too much or too little insulin when it is needed. Periodic reinforcement of the administration instructions is important.

External insulin pump. This battery-operated pump device can be worn on a belt or hidden in a pocket and is attached to a small tube inserted into the SC tissue of the abdomen. The device slowly leaks a base rate of insulin into the abdomen all day; the person can pump or inject booster doses throughout the day to correspond with meals and activity. Only fast-acting insulin is used in the pump. The device does have several disadvantages. For example, it is awkward, the tubing poses an increased risk of infection and requires frequent changing, and the person has to frequently check blood glucose levels throughout the day to monitor response.

Future

Implantable insulin pump. This pump is surgically implanted into the abdomen and delivers base insulin as well as insulin boluses as needed directly into the abdomen to be absorbed by the liver, just as pancreatic insulin is (Figure 38.2). The disadvantages are risk of infection, mechanical problems with the pump and lack of long-term data on its effectiveness. This method is not yet available for general use.

Insulin patch. The patch is placed on the skin and delivers a constant low dose of insulin. When the person eats a meal, tabs are pulled on the patch to release more insulin. The problem with this delivery method is that insulin does not readily pass through the skin, so there is tremendous variability in its effects. This route is not yet commercially available.

Inhaled insulin. The lung tissue is one of the best sites for insulin absorption. An aerosol delivery system has been developed that delivers a powdered insulin formulation directly into the lung tissue. Research has been very promising, suggesting that this may be a more reliable method of delivering insulin in the future.

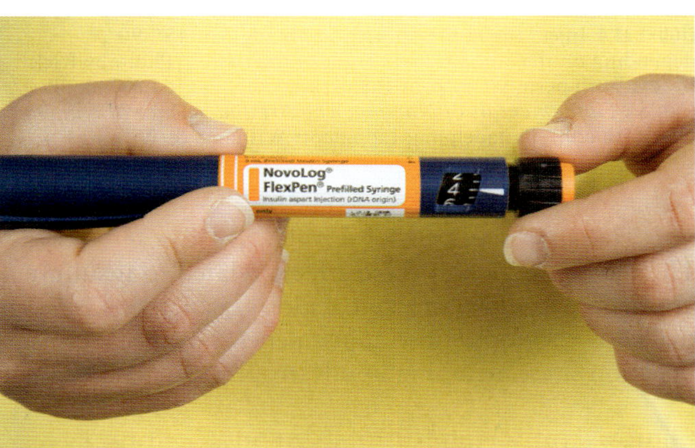

FIGURE 38.1 Pre-filled insulin syringe. (From Farrell, M. & Dempsey, J. (2014). *Smeltzer & Bare's Textbook of Medical-Surgical Nursing* (3rd edn). Sydney: Lippincott Williams & Wilkins.)

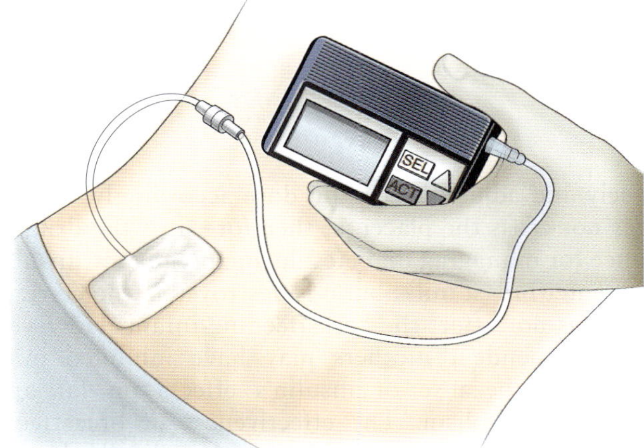

FIGURE 38.2 Person wearing an insulin pump. (From Dempsey, J., Hillege, S. & Hill, R. (2014). *Fundamentals of Nursing and Midwifery* (2nd edn). Sydney: Lippincott Williams & Wilkins.)

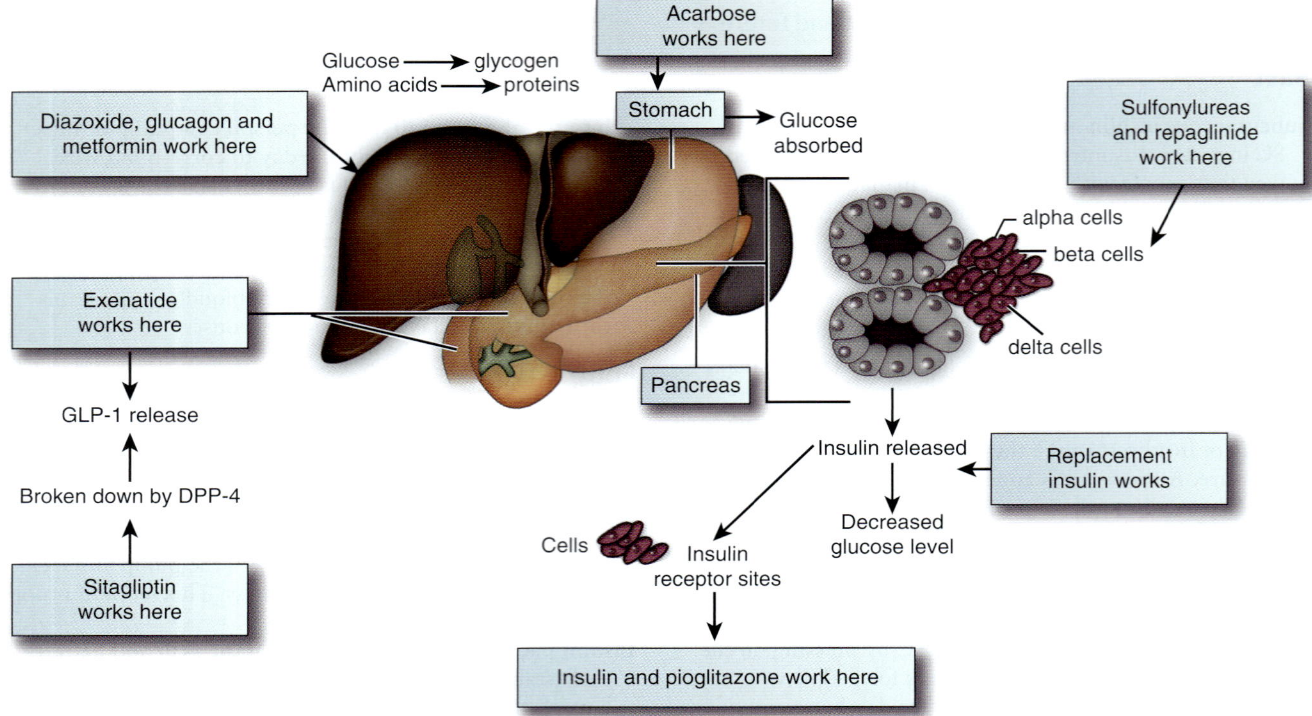

FIGURE 38.3 Sites of action of drugs used to treat diabetic conditions.

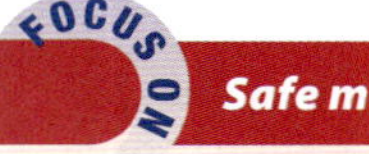

Safe medication administration

Insulin is usually given by SC injection. Using an insulin syringe with a 25-gauge, ½" needle, inject the insulin into the loose connective tissue underneath the skin (Figure 38.4). The areas of the body that are best able to be pinched up to access this tissue are the abdomen, the upper thigh and the upper arm. Inject the needle quickly at an angle of 45–90°, depending on the amount and turgor of the tissue. Inject the insulin. Remove the needle and syringe and apply gentle pressure at the injection site. Rotate sites regularly to prevent tissue damage.

Insulins should only be drawn up into insulin-specific syringes due to potential for drug errors with regular syringes.

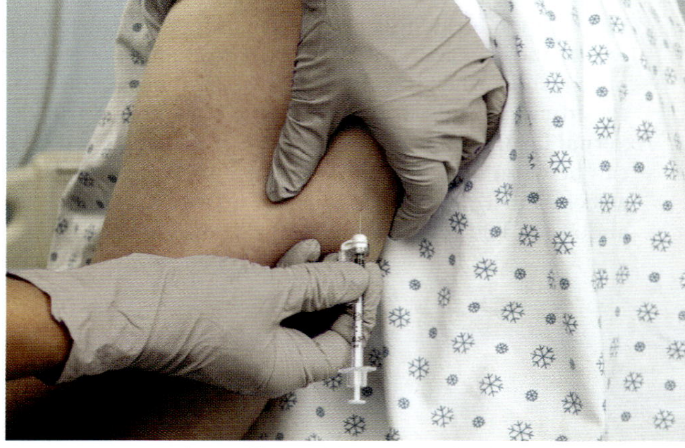

FIGURE 38.4 Inject the needle quickly at an angle of 45°–90°, depending on the amount and turgor of the tissue. [Photo by Rick Brady. With permission from Taylor, C., Lillis, C. & LeMone, P. (2005). *Fundamentals of Nursing: The Art and Science of Nursing Care* (5th edn). Philadelphia: Lippincott Williams & Wilkins.]

closely and adjust the insulin dose accordingly. Insulin does not cross the placenta; therefore, it is the drug of choice for managing diabetes during pregnancy. Insulin does enter breast milk, but it is destroyed in the GI tract and does not affect the breastfeeding infant. However, insulin-dependent mothers may have inhibited milk production because of insulin's effects on fat and protein metabolism. The effectiveness of breastfeeding the infant should be evaluated periodically. People with allergies to beef or pork products should use only human insulins.

Adverse effects

The most common adverse effects related to insulin use are hypoglycaemia and ketoacidosis, which can be controlled with proper dose adjustments. Local reactions at injection sites, including lipodystrophy, can also occur.

Clinically important drug–drug interactions

Caution should be used when giving a person stabilised on insulin any drug that decreases glucose levels (eg, monoamine oxidase inhibitors, beta blockers, salicylates, alcohol). Dose adjustments are needed when any of these drugs are added or removed. Care should also be taken when combining insulin with any beta blocker. The blocking of the SNS also blocks many of the signs and symptoms of hypoglycaemia, hindering the person's ability to recognise problems. People taking beta blockers need to learn other ways to recognise hypoglycaemia. Individuals should also be warned about possible interactions with various herbal and complementary therapies and over-the-counter preparations (Box 38.6).

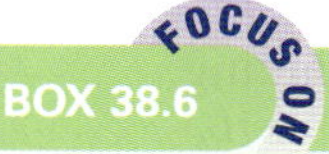

BOX 38.6 FOCUS ON Herbal and alternative therapies

People being treated with hypoglycaemic therapies are at an increased risk of developing hypoglycaemia if they use juniper berries, ginseng, garlic, fenugreek, coriander, dandelion root or celery. If a person uses these therapies, blood glucose levels should be monitored closely and appropriate dose adjustment made in the prescribed drug.

Care considerations for people taking insulin

Assessment: history and examination

- Assess for contraindications or cautions: any known allergy to any insulin and current status of pregnancy or breastfeeding *so that appropriate monitoring and dose adjustments can be completed, including possible need to use animal-source insulin.*
- Perform a physical assessment *to establish a baseline before beginning therapy*, and during therapy *to evaluate the effectiveness of therapy and for any potential adverse effects.*
- Assess for presence of any skin lesions; orientation and reflexes; baseline pulse and blood pressure; respiration or adventitious breath sounds, *which could indicate response to high or low glucose levels and potential risk factors in giving insulin.*
- Assess body systems *for changes suggesting possible complications associated with poor blood glucose control.*
- Investigate nutritional intake, *noting any problems with intake and adherence to prescribed diet that could alter the anticipated response to insulin therapy.*

Prototype summary: insulin

Indications: treatment of type 1 diabetes; treatment of type 2 diabetes when other agents have failed; short-term treatment of type 2 diabetes during periods of stress; management of diabetic ketoacidosis, hyperkalaemia and marked insulin resistance.

Actions: replacement of endogenous insulin.

Pharmacokinetics:

Generic (*brand*)	Onset	Peak	Duration
regular (neutral)	30–60 min	2–4 hours	8–12 hours
semilente isophane	1–1.5 hours	5–10 hours	12–16 hours
isophane (*Humulin NPH*)	1–1.5 hours	4–12 hours	24 hours
lispro (*Humalog*)	< 15 min	30–90 min	2–5 hours
aspart (*NovoRapid*)	15 min	1–3 hours	3–5 hours
glargine (*Lantus*)	60–70 min	None	24 hours
glulisine (*Apidra*)	2–5 min	30–90 min	1–2.5 hours
detemir (*Levemir*)	1–2 hours	6–8 hours	24 hours
Combination insulins			
neutral and isophane (*Humulin 70/30, Mixtard 70/30*)	30–60 min, then 1–2 hours	2–4 hours, then 6–12 hours	6–8 hours, then 18–24 hours

$T_{1/2}$: varies with each preparation; metabolised at the cellular level.

Adverse effects: hypersensitivity reaction, local reactions at injection site, hypoglycaemia, ketoacidosis.

- Assess activity level, including amount and degree of exercise, *which could alter anticipated response to insulin therapy.*
- Inspect skin areas that will be used for injection of insulin; note any areas that are bruised, thickened or scarred, *which could interfere with insulin absorption and alter anticipated response to insulin therapy.*
- Obtain blood glucose levels as ordered *to monitor response to insulin and need to adjust dose as needed.*
- Monitor the results of laboratory tests, including urinalysis, *for evidence of glucosuria.*
- Assess level of cognitive ability and dexterity in planning for education related to the condition.

Refer to the Critical thinking scenario for a full discussion of care for a person with type 1 diabetes mellitus.

Implementation with rationale

- Ensure the person is following a dietary and exercise regimen and using good hygiene practices *to improve the effectiveness of the insulin and decrease adverse effects of the disease.*
- Gently rotate the vial containing the agent and avoid vigorous shaking *to ensure uniform suspension of insulin.*
- Select a site that is free of bruising and scarring *to ensure good absorption of the insulin.*
- Give maintenance doses by the SC route only (see Focus on safe medication administration under Pharmacokinetics for insulin), and rotate injection sites regularly *to avoid damage to muscles and to prevent SC atrophy.* Give regular insulin IM or IV in emergency situations.
- Monitor response carefully *to avoid adverse effects*; blood glucose monitoring is the most effective way to evaluate insulin dose.
- Monitor the person for signs and symptoms of hypoglycaemia, especially during peak insulin times, when these signs and symptoms would be most likely to appear, *to assess the response to insulin and the need for dose adjustment or medical intervention.*
- Always verify the name of the insulin being given *because each insulin has a different peak and duration, and the names can be confused.*
- Use caution when mixing types of insulin; administer mixtures of regular and isophane or regular and lente insulins within 15 minutes after combining them *to ensure appropriate suspension and therapeutic effect.*
- Store insulin in a cool place away from direct sunlight *to ensure effectiveness.* Pre-drawn syringes are stable for 1 week if refrigerated; *they offer a good way to ensure the proper dose for people who have limited vision.*
- Monitor during times of trauma or severe stress *for potential dose adjustment needs.*
- Monitor food intake; ensure that the person eats when using insulin *to ensure therapeutic effect and avoid hypoglycaemia.*
- Monitor exercise and activities; ensure that the person considers the effects of exercise in relationship to eating and insulin dose *to ensure therapeutic effect and avoid hypoglycaemia.*
- Protect the person from infection, including good skin care and foot care, *to prevent the development of serious infections and changes in therapeutic insulin doses.*
- Monitor the person's sensory losses *to incorporate his or her needs into safety issues, as well as potential problems in drawing up and administering insulin.*
- Help the person to deal with necessary lifestyle changes, including diet and exercise needs, sensory loss and the impact of a drug regimen that includes giving injections, *to help encourage compliance with the treatment regimen.*
- Instruct people receiving beta blockers about ways to monitor glucose levels and signs and symptoms of glucose abnormalities *to prevent hypoglycaemic and hyperglycaemic episodes when SNS and warning signs are blocked.*
- Provide thorough teaching, including diet and exercise needs; measures to avoid adverse effects, including proper food care and screening for injuries; warning signs of problems, including signs and symptoms of hypoglycaemia and hyperglycaemia; the importance of increased screening when ill or unable to eat properly; proper administration techniques and proper disposal of needles and syringes; and the need to monitor disease status, *to enhance knowledge about drug therapy and promote compliance.*

Evaluation

- Monitor the person's response to the drug (stabilisation of blood glucose levels).
- Monitor for adverse effects (hypoglycaemia, ketoacidosis, injection-site irritation).
- Evaluate the effectiveness of the teaching plan (person can name drug, dosage, adverse effects to watch for, specific measures to avoid them and proper administration technique).
- Monitor the effectiveness of comfort measures and compliance with the regimen.

KEY POINTS

- Insulin replaces the endogenous hormone when the body does not produce enough insulin or when there are not enough insulin receptor sites to provide adequate glucose control.
- Blood glucose levels vary with food intake, exercise and stress levels, possibly necessitating a change in insulin dose.
- Individuals need to learn to recognise the signs of hypoglycaemia and hyperglycaemia to effectively manage their drug therapy.

CRITICAL THINKING SCENARIO

Type 1 diabetes mellitus

THE SITUATION

M.J. is a 22-year-old woman who has newly diagnosed type 1 diabetes mellitus. She was stabilised on insulin while hospitalised for diagnosis and management. One week after discharge, M.J. experienced nausea and anorexia. She was unable to eat, but she took her insulin as usual in the morning. That afternoon, she experienced profuse sweating and was tremulous and apprehensive, so she went to the hospital emergency room. The initial diagnosis was insulin reaction from taking insulin and not eating, combined with the stress of her gastrointestinal upset. M.J. was treated at the emergency room with IV glucose. After she had rested and her glucose levels had returned to normal, she was discharged to home.

CRITICAL THINKING

What instructions should M.J. receive before she leaves?
Think about the ways that stress can alter the blood glucose levels. Then consider the stress that a person with newly diagnosed type 1 diabetes undergoes while trying to cope with the diagnosis, learn self-injection, and think about complications of the disease that may arise in the future.

What teaching approaches could help M.J. to decrease her stress and to effectively plan her medical regimen? What sort of support would be useful for M.J. as she adjusts to her new life?

DISCUSSION

The diagnosis of type 1 diabetes is a life-changing event. M.J. had to learn about the disease and how to test her blood and give herself injections, manage a new diet and exercise program, and cope with the knowledge that the long-term complications of diabetes can be devastating. Many people who are regulated on insulin in the hospital experience a change in insulin demand after discharge. The stress of being in hospital may increase the activity of the SNS, and one of the effects of increased SNS activity is increased glucose level – preparing the body for fight or flight. For some people, returning home eases the stress that activated the SNS and glucose levels fall. If the person continues to use the same insulin dose, hypoglycaemia can occur. Other people may feel protected in the hospital and experience stress when they are sent home. They may feel anxious about taking care of themselves while coping with everyday problems and tensions. These people need an increased insulin dose because their stress reaction intensifies when they get home, driving their blood glucose level up.

People are taught how to measure their blood glucose levels before they leave the hospital. After they get used to doing this and regulating their insulin based on glucose concentrations, they usually manage well. The first few days to weeks are often the hardest. The health care professional should review with M.J. how to test her glucose, draw up her insulin and regulate the dose. The health care professional should also give M.J. written information that she can refer to later.

In addition, the health care professional should give M.J. a chance to talk and to vent her feelings about her diagnosis and her future. To help decrease M.J.'s stress and to avoid problems during this adjustment period, the health care professional can give M.J. a telephone number to call if she has problems or questions. M.J. should return in a few days to review her progress and have any questions answered. In the meantime, the health care professional should encourage M.J. to write down any questions or problems that arise so that they can be addressed during the follow-up visit. Support and encouragement will be crucial to helping M.J. adjust to her disease and her drug therapy. She can also be referred to a diabetes association in her community that offers support services to help diabetics.

CARE GUIDE FOR M.J.: TYPE 1 DIABETES MELLITUS

Assessment: history and examination

Review the person's history for allergies to drug products, pregnancy, breastfeeding and other drugs in current use. M.J. denies allergies, pregnancy and breastfeeding. She is taking no other medications.

Focus the physical examination on the following:

Neurological: orientation, reflexes; M.J. appears shaky and her pupils are dilated.

Skin: colouration and/or lesions; M.J.'s appearance (pale, sweaty) is consistent with diaphoresis.
Cardiovascular: pulse, 110 beats/minute; blood pressure, 155/92 mmHg.
Respiratory: respiratory rate, 24/minute; lungs clear on auscultation; rapid respiratory rate is indicative of acidosis.
Laboratory tests: urinalysis – negative for glucose, positive for ketones; blood glucose level, 72 mg/dL.

Implementation

Provide teaching regarding drug name, dosage, adverse effects, precautions, warning signs to report and proper administration technique.
Assist M.J. to restore blood glucose to normal levels by using insulin and constantly monitoring blood glucose levels during normal times and during times of stress and trauma so that insulin dose can be adjusted to needed amount.
Review proper SC injection technique and site rotation.
Provide support and reassurance to help M.J. deal with drug injections, this hypoglycaemic episode and her lifetime need for insulin.
Teach M.J. how to store insulin in a cool place away from light and to use caution when mixing insulin types.
Review with M.J. the name and type of insulin, dosage, adverse effects, precautions, warning signs of adverse effects to report and proper administration technique.

Evaluation

Evaluate drug effects: return of glucose levels to normal.
Monitor for adverse effects: hypoglycaemia and/or injection-site reaction.
Monitor for drug–drug interactions as indicated for insulin.
Evaluate the effectiveness of teaching program and comfort and safety measures.

TEACHING FOR M.J.

- Diet modifications and increased exercise are very important aspects of your diabetes management. You should also practise good skin care and hygiene measures. Check for any injury or sign of infection regularly.
- Insulin is a hormone that is normally produced by your pancreas. It helps to regulate your energy balance by affecting the way the body uses sugar and fats. The lack of insulin produces a disease called diabetes mellitus. By injecting insulin each day, you can help your body use the sugars and fats in your food effectively.
- Check the expiration date on your insulin. Store the insulin at room temperature, and avoid extremes of heat and light. Gently rotate the vial between your palms before use to dispense any crystals that may have formed. Do not shake the vial because vigorous shaking can inactivate the drug.
- A prescription is required to get the syringes that you will need to administer your insulin. Keep the syringes sealed until ready to use and dispose of them appropriately. Rotate your injection sites regularly to prevent tissue damage and to ensure that the proper amount of insulin is absorbed.
- You should be aware of the signs and symptoms of hypoglycaemia (too much insulin). If any of these occur, eat or drink something high in sugar, such as a lolly, orange juice, honey or sugar. The signs and symptoms to watch for include the following: nervousness, anxiety, sweating, pale and cool skin, headache, nausea, hunger and shakiness. These may happen if you skip a meal, exercise too much or experience extreme stress. If these symptoms happen very often, notify your health care provider. If you cannot eat because of illness or other problems, do not take your usual insulin dose. Contact your health care provider for assistance.
- Avoid the use of any over-the-counter medications or herbal therapies without first checking with your health care provider. Several of these medications and many commonly used herbs can interfere with the effectiveness of insulin. Avoid the use of alcohol because it increases the chances of having hypoglycaemic attacks.
- Tell any doctor, nurse or other health care provider involved in your care that you are taking this drug. You may want to wear or carry a MedicAlert tag showing that you are on this medication. This would alert any medical personnel taking care of you in an emergency to the fact that you are taking this drug.
- Report any of the following to your health care provider: loss of appetite, blurred vision, fruity odour to your breath, increased urination, increased thirst, nausea or vomiting.
- While you are taking this drug, it is important to have regular medical follow-up, including blood tests to monitor your blood glucose levels, to evaluate you for any adverse effects of your diabetes.
- Keep this drug and your syringes out of the reach of children. Use proper disposal techniques for your needles and syringes. Do not give this medication to anyone else or take any similar medication that has not been prescribed for you.

SULFONYLUREAS AND OTHER HYPOGLYCAEMIC AGENTS

Other hypoglycaemic agents may be used in individuals who still have a functioning pancreas. These agents include the sulfonylureas and other agents that do not fit into a specific classification (see Table 38.3). The sulfonylureas were the first oral agents introduced to treat type 2 diabetes. They stimulate the pancreas to release insulin. Other agents discussed in this section

TABLE 38.3 DRUGS IN FOCUS Other oral hypoglycaemic agents

Drug name	Dosage/route	Usual indications
Sulfonylureas		
(P) glibenclamide (*Daonil*)	2.5 mg PO increased by 2.5 mg/week to maximum of 20 mg/day	Adjunct to diet for the management of type 2 diabetes; adjunct to insulin for management in certain people with type 2 diabetes, reducing the insulin dose and decreasing the risk of hypoglycaemia
gliclazide (*Diamicron, Diamicron MR, Glyade, Glyade MR*)	Adults, immediate-release tablets: initially 40 mg daily; may increase to a maximum of 320 mg/day Adults, modified-release tablets: initially 30 mg/day; may increase to a maximum of 120 mg/day	Adjunct to diet for the management of type 2 diabetes
glimepiride (*Amaryl*)	1–4 mg/day PO; lower doses with elderly people	Adjunct to diet for the management of type 2 diabetes; adjunct to insulin for management in certain people with type 2 diabetes, reducing the insulin dose and decreasing the risk of hypoglycaemia
glipizide (*Melizide, Minidiab*)	Initially 2.5–5 mg before breakfast; may increase by 2.5–5 mg at intervals of several days; divide doses > 15 mg; maximum 40 mg/day	Adjunct to diet for the management of type 2 diabetes; adjunct to insulin for management in certain people with type 2 diabetes, reducing the insulin dose and decreasing the risk of hypoglycaemia
Other oral hypoglycaemic agents		
Alpha-glucosidase inhibitor		
acarbose (*Glucobay*)	50–100 mg PO tid at the start of each meal; may increase to 200 mg tid	Adjunct to diet to lower blood glucose level in people with type 2 diabetes; in combination with sulfonylureas to control blood sugar in people whose diabetes cannot be controlled with either drug alone
Biguanide		
(P) metformin (*Diaformin, Diaformin XR, Glucophage*)	*Immediate-release tablets* Adults: 500 mg 1–2 times daily; may increase dose gradually to a maximum of 3000 mg/day in divided doses Paediatric: > 10 years: 500–850 mg/day; may increase to a maximum of 2000 mg/day in divided doses *Extended-release tablets* Adults: 500 mg 1–2 times daily; may increase dose gradually to a maximum of 2000 mg/day in divided doses Paediatric: not recommended *Note: metformin XR tablets cannot be divided*	Adjunct to diet to lower blood glucose level in type 2 diabetes
Dipeptidyl peptidase-4 (DPP-4) inhibitors		
alogliptin (*Nesina*)	25 mg/day PO in combination with mefromin, a thiazolidinedione, sulfonylurea, or insulin	Adjunct to diet and exercise to improve glucose control in people with type 2 diabetes
linagliptin (*Trajenta*)	5 mg/day PO	Adjunct to diet and exercise to improve glucose control in people with type 2 diabetes as monotherapy or combined with metformin, pioglitazone or other agents

Continued on following page

TABLE 38.3 **DRUGS IN FOCUS** **Other oral hypoglycaemic agents *(continued)***

Drug name	Dosage/route	Usual indications
Other oral hypoglycaemic agents *(continued)*		
saxagliptin (*Onglyza*)	5 mg/day PO in combination with metformin, a thiazolidinedione, sulfonylurea, or insulin	Adjunct to metformin, a thiazolidinedione or sulfonylurea
sitagliptin (*Januvia*)	100 mg/day PO	Adjunct to diet and exercise to improve glucose control in people with type 2 diabetes, as monotherapy or combined with metformin, pioglitazone or other agents
vildagliptin (*Galvus*)	Individualised up to 100 mg/day in 2 divided doses	Adjunct to diet and exercise to improve glucose control in individuals with type 2 diabetes, as monotherapy or combined
Glucagon-like peptide-1 analogue		
liraglutide (*Victoza*)	0.6–1.8 mg/day by SC injection	Adjunct to diet and exercise to improve glucose control in people with type 2 diabetes, as monotherapy or combined with other agents
Incretin mimetic		
exenatide (*Byetta*, *Bydureon*)	*Byetta:* 5 micrograms by SC injection within 60 minutes before morning and evening meals; may be increased to 10 micrograms bd after 1 month *Bydureon:* adults: 2 mg once weekly SC	Adjunct to diet and oral agents to improve glycaemic control in people with type 2 diabetes
Sodium–glucose co-transporter inhibitors		
dapagliflozin (*Forxiga*)	10 mg/day PO	Adjunct to diet and exercise to improve glucose control in people with type 2 diabetes, as monotherapy or combined with other agents
empagliflozin (*Jardiance*)	Adult: 10 mg PO once daily up to 25 mg once daily	Treatment of type 2 diabetes mellitus as monotherapy in patients for whom use of metformin is considered inappropriate due to intolerance of, or in combination with, other glucose-lowering medications, including insulin To reduce the risk of cardiovascular death in patients with type 2 diabetes mellitus and established cardiovascular disease
ertugliflozin (*Steglatro*)	Adult: 5 mg once daily up to 15 mg once daily	Adjunct to diet and exercise to improve glycaemic control in adults with type 2 diabetes mellitus; as monotherapy when metformin is considered inappropriate because of intolerance or in combination with other antihyperglycaemic agents
Thiazolidinedione		
pioglitazone (*Actos*)	15–30 mg/day PO as a single dose; maximum 45 mg/day use caution with hepatic impairment	Adjunct to diet to lower blood glucose in type 2 diabetes; in combination with insulin or sulfonylureas to control blood sugar in people whose diabetes cannot be controlled with either drug alone

have been introduced more recently for use in people with type 1 and type 2 diabetes. These agents interact with the body's glucose controls in a number of ways, including affecting insulin release, decreasing insulin resistance or altering glucose absorption from the GI tract and release of glucose by the liver. They often are combined with a sulfonylurea to increase glycaemic control.

SULFONYLUREAS

The **sulfonylureas** bind to potassium channels on pancreatic beta cells. They may improve insulin binding to insulin receptors and increase the number of insulin receptors. They are also known to increase the effect of antidiuretic hormone on renal cells. They are effective only in people who have functioning beta cells. They are not effective for all people with diabetes and may lose their effectiveness over time with others. Sulfonylureas are further classified as first-generation or second-generation sulfonylureas. All of the sulfonylureas can cause hypoglycaemia.

First-generation sulfonylureas

The first-generation sulfonylureas included chlorpropamide and tolbutamide. However, these drugs are no longer used in Australia and New Zealand.

The first-generation sulfonylureas were associated with an increased risk of cardiovascular disease and death in a somewhat controversial study. They are now thought to possibly cause an increase in cardiovascular deaths.

Second-generation sulfonylureas

The second-generation drugs include glibenclamide (*Daonil*, *Gliben*, *Glimel* and others), gliclazide (*Diamicron*, *Glyade*), glimepiride (*Amaryl*) and glipizide (*Melizide*, *Minidiab*). See Table 38.3 for usual indications for each drug. Second-generation sulfonylureas have several advantages over the first-generation drugs, including the following:

- They are excreted in urine and bile, making them safer for individuals with renal dysfunction.
- They do not interact with as many protein-bound drugs as the first-generation drugs.
- They have a longer duration of action, making it possible to take them only once or twice a day, thus increasing compliance.

Prescribers may try different agents (first- or second-generation drugs) before finding the one that is most effective for a given person.

Therapeutic actions and indications

The sulfonylureas stimulate insulin release from the beta cells in the pancreas (see Figure 38.3). They improve insulin binding to insulin receptors and may actually increase the number of insulin receptors. They are indicated as an adjunct to diet and exercise to lower blood glucose levels in type 2 diabetes mellitus. They have the off-label use of being an adjunct to insulin to improve glucose control in people with type 2 diabetes.

Pharmacokinetics

These drugs are rapidly absorbed from the GI tract and undergo hepatic metabolism. They are excreted in the urine. The peak effects and duration of effects differ because of the activity of various metabolites of the different drugs.

Contraindications and cautions

Sulfonylureas are contraindicated in the presence of known allergy to any sulfonylureas *to avoid hypersensitivity reactions* and in diabetes complicated by fever, severe infection, severe trauma, major surgery, ketoacidosis, severe renal or hepatic disease, pregnancy or breastfeeding, *which require tighter control of glucose levels using insulin.* These drugs are also contraindicated for use in people with type 1 diabetes mellitus, *who do not have functioning beta cells and would have no benefit from the drug.*

These drugs are not for use during pregnancy. Insulin should be used if a hypoglycaemic agent is needed during pregnancy. Some of these drugs cross into breast milk, and adequate studies are not available on others. *Because of the risk of hypoglycaemic effects in the baby*, these drugs should not be used during breastfeeding. Another method of feeding the baby should be used. The safety and efficacy of these drugs for use in children have not been established.

Adverse effects

The most common adverse effects related to the sulfonylureas are hypoglycaemia (caused by an imbalance in levels of glucose and insulin) and GI distress, including nausea, vomiting, epigastric discomfort, heartburn and anorexia. (Anorexia should be monitored because affected individuals may not eat after taking the sulfonylurea, which could lead to hypoglycaemia.) Allergic skin reactions have been reported with some of these drugs and, as mentioned earlier, there may be an increased risk of cardiovascular mortality, particularly with the first-generation agents.

Clinically important drug–drug interactions

Care should be taken with any drug that acidifies the urine because excretion of the sulfonylurea may be decreased. Caution should also be used with beta blockers, which may mask the signs of hypoglycaemia, and with alcohol, which can lead to altered glucose levels when combined with sulfonylureas. Caution must also be used with many herbal therapies that could alter blood glucose levels.

Prototype summary: glibenclamide

Indications: adjunct to diet and exercise in the management of type 2 diabetes; with metformin or insulin for stabilisation of people with diabetes.

Actions: stimulates insulin release from functioning beta cells in the pancreas; may improve insulin binding to insulin receptor sites or increase the number of insulin receptor sites.

Pharmacokinetics:

Route	Onset	Duration
Oral	1 hour	24 hours

$T_{1/2}$: 4 hours; metabolised in the liver and excreted in bile and urine.

Adverse effects: GI discomfort, anorexia, nausea, vomiting, heartburn, diarrhoea, allergic skin reactions, hypoglycaemia.

OTHER ORAL HYPOGLYCAEMIC AGENTS

Several other oral hypoglycaemic agents are available. Although these drugs are structurally unrelated to the sulfonylureas, they are frequently effective when used in combination with sulfonylureas or insulin. These drugs include the alpha-glucosidase inhibitor acarbose (*Glucobay*); the biguanide metformin (*Diaformin*, *Glucophage*); the DPP-4 inhibitors alogliptin (*Nesina*), linagliptin (*Trajenta*), saxagliptin (*Onglyza*), sitagliptin (*Januvia*) and vildagliptin (*Galvumet*, *Galvus*); the GLP-1 analogue liraglutide (*Victoza*) (not available in New Zealand); the incretin mimetic exenatide (*Byetta*); the sodium–glucose co-transporters dapagliflozin (*Forxiga*), empagliflozin (*Jardiance*) and ertugliflozin (*Steglatro*); and the thiazolidinedione pioglitazone (*Actos*) (see Table 38.3).

Acarbose is an inhibitor of alpha-glucosidase (an enzyme that breaks down glucose for absorption); it delays the absorption of glucose. It has only a mild effect on glucose levels and has been associated with severe hepatic toxicity. It does not enhance insulin secretion, so its effects are additive to those of the sulfonylureas in controlling blood glucose. Alpha-glucosidase inhibitors are used in combination with sulfonylureas, metformin and insulin for individuals whose glucose levels cannot be controlled with a single agent or diet and exercise alone.

Metformin decreases the production and increases the cellular uptake of glucose. It is effective in lowering blood glucose levels and does not cause hypoglycaemia, as the sulfonylureas do. It has been associated with the development of lactic acidosis. Both acarbose and metformin can cause GI distress. Metformin is approved for use in children 10 years of age and older. It is also being used in the treatment of women with polycystic ovary syndrome (see Box 38.7).

The thiazolidinediones (*Actos* and others) are drugs that decrease insulin resistance; they are used in combination with sulfonylureas, insulin or metformin to treat individuals with insulin resistance. The first drug of this class, troglitazone, was withdrawn from the market after reports of serious hepatotoxicity. The sole drug available now, pioglitazone, is not associated with the same severe liver toxicity, although in late 2007 reports were published linking this drug and another thiazolidinedione, rosiglitazone, to an increase in cardiovascular events. Rosiglitazone was withdrawn from the New Zealand market in April 2011, and from the Australian market (except in fixed-dose combinations with metformin) in February 2017, due to safety concerns related to increased cardiovasular risk. People should still be monitored for any change in liver function while they are taking pioglitazone. This drug is also being studied for use in increasing ovulation frequency in woman who have polycystic ovary syndrome (Box 38.7). Box 38.8 describes some of the new fixed-dose combination oral agents, which provide two different agents in one tablet to make it easier for the person to be compliant.

Therapeutic actions and indications, pharmacokinetics, contraindications and cautions, adverse effects and clinically important drug–drug interactions for these drugs are basically the same as for the

BOX 38.7 Polycystic ovary syndrome and oral hypoglycaemic drugs

Polycystic ovary syndrome is an ovarian function disorder associated with obesity, infrequent or absent menses and infertility. Women who have this disorder have elevated insulin levels with normal fasting blood glucose levels, elevated luteinising hormone (LH) levels, and normal oestrogen and follicle-stimulating hormone levels. Because of the alterations in hormone activity, follicles develop on the ovaries, but ovulation does not occur, and the developed follicles turn into cysts. The high LH levels tend to cause an increase in androgen production, which is associated with insulin resistance.

Treatment is aimed at altering the metabolic changes to allow ovulation (if pregnancy is desired) or stop the follicle development (if pregnancy is not desired). Weight loss is very important and may correct the alterations in metabolism and allow ovulation to occur without medical treatment. Metformin and pioglitazone have proven effective in increasing insulin sensitivity and decreasing androgen and LH levels to break the cycle and allow ovulation to occur if pregnancy is desired. A fertility drug is often used with the oral hypoglycaemic agent. Hormonal contraceptives are used if pregnancy is not desired, to halt the development of the follicles and stop the cyst production.

BOX 38.8 Available fixed-dose combination oral agents

Several fixed-dose combination oral hypoglycaemic agents have become available in the last 5 years. These combination products are intended to decrease the number of tablets the person needs to take each day and thereby increase compliance with the drug regimen. The person should be stabilised on the individual products first and then switched to the combination product after the correct dose combination for that person has been established. The person should be reminded that diet and exercise are still the key parts of the diabetes management regimen. Some examples* of the fixed-dose combination oral hypoglycaemic agents are:

- *Avandamet,* a combination of rosiglitazone and metformin and is available in four dose sizes:
  2 mg rosiglitazone with 1000 mg metformin,
  2 mg rosiglitazone with 500 mg metformin,
  4 mg rosiglitazone with 1000 mg metformin,
  4 mg rosiglitazone with 500 mg metformin.
- *Galvumet,* a combination of vildagliptin and metformin and is available in three dose sizes:
  50 mg vildagliptin with 1000 mg metformin,
  50 mg vildagliptin with 500 mg metformin,
  50 mg vildagliptin with 850 mg metformin.
- *Glucovance,* a combination of metformin and glibenclamide and is available in three dose sizes:
  250 mg metformin with 1.25 mg glibenclamide,
  500 mg metformin with 2.5 mg glibenclamide,
  500 mg metformin with 5 mg glibenclamide.
- *Janumet,* a combination of sitagliptin and metformin and is available in three dose sizes:
  50 mg sitagliptin with 1000 mg metformin,
  50 mg sitagliptin with 500 mg metformin,
  50 mg sitagliptin with 850 mg metformin.

* There are many more: see *McKenna's Drug Handbook for Nursing and Midwifery* (8th edn, 2019).

sulfonylureas. The safety and efficacy of these drugs for use in children have not been established, except for the use of metformin in children 10 years of age and older. The newest of the oral hypoglycaemic agents include: exenatide, which was released in 2005; the GLP-1 analogue, liraglutide, released in 2005; the DPP-4 inhibitors, which first became available in 2007; and the sodium–glucose co-transporter (SGLT2) inhibitors, dapagliflozin and empagliflozin, released in 2013, later followed by ertugliflozin.

Exenatide and liraglutide mimic the effects of GLP-1, leading to enhancement of glucose-dependent insulin secretion by the beta cells in the pancreas, depression of elevated glucagon secretion and slowed gastric emptying to help moderate and lower blood glucose levels. Exenatide is given by SC injection twice a day, within 60 minutes before the morning and evening meals. It has a rapid onset of action and peaks within 2 hours; its effects last 8–10 hours. It is given in combination with oral agents to improve glycaemic control in people with type 2 diabetes who cannot achieve glycaemic control on oral agents alone. It should not be given if the person is unable to eat. Liraglutide is also given by SC injection once daily and independent of meals. It has a duration of action of 24 hours.

Sitagliptin is a DPP-4 inhibitor. It slows the breakdown of GLP-1 in the body, prolonging the effects of increased insulin secretion, decreased glucagon secretion and slowed GI emptying. It is an oral drug, taken once a day, often in combination with other agents. It is rapidly absorbed, with peak effects in 1–4 hours. It has a half-life of 12.4 hours and is excreted unchanged in the urine. Few adverse effects have been reported with this drug, and it also must be used in combination with an appropriate diet and exercise program.

SGLT2 inhibitors are among the newest oral hypoglycaemic agents on the market. These drugs lower glucose reabsorption by lowering the renal threshold for glucose. Hence, more glucose can be eliminated in the urine. Both drugs are rapidly absorbed and extensively metabolised. SGLT2 inhibitors have been associated with cases of diabetic ketoacidosis (DKA). Patients should be informed of the signs and symptoms of DKA and advised to seek immediate medical attention if they occur.

Prototype summary: metformin

Indications: either alone or in combination, or with insulin) initial therapy and mainstay in the oral treatment of hyperglycemia. Also an adjunct to diet and exercise for the treatment of type 2 diabetes in people older than 10 years of age; extended-release form for people older than 17 years of age; adjunctive treatment with polycystic ovary syndrome.

Actions: may increase the peripheral use of glucose, increase production of insulin, decrease hepatic glucose production and alter intestinal absorption of glucose.

Pharmacokinetics:

Route	Onset	Peak	Duration
Oral	Slow	2–2.5 hours	10–16 hours

$T_{1/2}$: 6.2 and then 17 hours; metabolised in the liver and excreted in the urine.

Adverse effects: hypoglycaemia, lactic acidosis, GI upset, nausea, anorexia, diarrhoea, heartburn, allergic skin reaction.

Care considerations for people taking other oral hypoglycaemic agents

Assessment: history and examination

- Assess for contraindications or cautions: history of allergy to any of these agents *to avoid hypersensitivity reactions*; severe renal or hepatic dysfunction, *which could interfere with metabolism and excretion of the drugs*; and status of pregnancy or breastfeeding, *which are contraindications to the use of these agents*.
- Perform a complete physical assessment to establish baseline status *before beginning therapy and to evaluate effectiveness and any potential adverse effects during therapy*.
- Assess for the presence of any skin lesions *for indication of possible infection and to establish appropriate sites for SC administration as appropriate*; orientation and reflexes; baseline pulse and blood pressure; adventitious breath sounds; abdominal sounds and function, *to monitor effects of altered glucose levels*.
- Assess body systems *for changes suggesting possible complications associated with poor blood glucose control*.
- Investigate nutritional intake, noting any problems with intake and adherence to prescribed diet.
- Assess activity level, including amount and degree of exercise.
- Monitor blood glucose levels as ordered.
- Monitor results of laboratory tests, including urinalysis, for evidence of glycosuria, and renal and liver function tests, especially with use of the thiazolidinediones, which can cause liver failure, *to determine the need for possible dose adjustment and evaluate for signs of toxicity*.

Implementation with rationale

- Administer the drug as prescribed in the appropriate relationship to meals *to ensure therapeutic effectiveness*.
- Ensure that the individual is following diet and exercise modifications *to improve effectiveness of the drug and decrease adverse effects*.
- Monitor nutritional status *to provide nutritional consultation as needed*.
- Monitor response carefully; blood glucose monitoring is the most effective way *to evaluate dose*. Obtain blood glucose levels as ordered.
- Monitor liver enzymes of people receiving pioglitazone very carefully *to avoid liver toxicity*; arrange to discontinue the drug *to avert serious liver damage if liver toxicity develops*.
- Monitor individuals during times of trauma, pregnancy or severe stress, *and arrange to switch to insulin coverage as needed*.
- Provide thorough teaching, including drug name, dosage and schedule for administration; administration technique if appropriate; need for food intake within specified time period; signs and symptoms of hypo- and hyperglycaemia; skin assessment, including daily inspection of feet; signs and symptoms to report immediately; measures to use when ill or unable to eat; proper diet and exercise program; hygiene measures; recommended schedule for follow-up and disease monitoring; and the need for follow-up lab testing *to enhance knowledge of drug therapy and to promote compliance*.

Evaluation

- Monitor the person's response to the drug (stabilisation of blood glucose levels).
- Monitor for adverse effects (hypoglycaemia, GI distress).
- Evaluate the effectiveness of the teaching plan (person can name drug, dosage, adverse effects to watch for and specific measures to avoid them).
- Monitor the effectiveness of comfort measures and compliance with the regimen.

KEY POINTS

- Sulfonylureas work only if the pancreas has functioning beta cells.
- Other oral hypoglycaemic agents work to slow GI absorption of glucose, increase release of insulin by beta cells, increase insulin-receptor-site sensitivity and/or block liver release of glucose.
- In times of severe stress, individuals regulated on other oral hypoglycaemic agents usually need to be switched to insulin to control blood glucose levels.
- Proper diet and exercise are the backbone of diabetes mellitus management; oral hypoglycaemic drugs are adjuncts to help control blood glucose levels.

GLUCOSE-ELEVATING AGENTS

Glucose-elevating agents, as the name implies, raise the blood level of glucose when severe hypoglycaemia occurs (less than 4.4 mmol/L [40 mg/dL]). Some adverse conditions are associated with hypoglycaemia, including pancreatic disorders, kidney disease, certain cancers, disorders of the anterior pituitary and unbalanced treatment of diabetes mellitus (which can occur if the person takes the wrong dose of insulin or oral hypoglycaemic agents or if something interferes with food intake or changes stress or exercise levels). One agent is used to elevate glucose in these conditions: glucagon (*GlucaGen*). Pure glucose can also be given orally or IV to increase glucose levels.

Therapeutic actions and indications

These agents increase the blood glucose level by decreasing insulin release and accelerating the breakdown of glycogen in the liver to release glucose. They are indicated for the treatment of hypoglycaemic reactions related to insulin or oral hypoglycaemic agents, for the treatment of hypoglycaemia related to pancreatic or other cancers and for short-term treatment of acute hypoglycaemia related to anterior pituitary dysfunction (Table 38.4).

Pharmacokinetics

Glucagon is given parenterally only and is the preferred agent for emergency situations. Glucagon is rapidly absorbed and widely distributed throughout the body. It is excreted in the urine.

Contraindications and cautions

There are no adequate studies on glucagon and pregnancy, so use should be reserved for those situations in which the benefits to the mother outweigh any potential risks to the fetus. Caution should be used during breastfeeding because the drug may cause hyperglycaemic effects in the baby. Caution should be used in individuals with renal or hepatic dysfunction or cardiovascular disease.

Prototype summary: glucagon

Indications: counteracts severe hypoglycaemic reactions in people with diabetes treated with insulin.

Actions: accelerates the breakdown of glycogen to glucose in the liver, causing an increase in blood glucose levels.

Pharmacokinetics:

Route	Onset	Peak	Duration
IV	1 min	15 min	9–20 min

$T_{1/2}$: 3–10 minutes; metabolised in the liver and excreted in the urine and bile.

Adverse effects: hypotension, hypertension, nausea, vomiting, respiratory distress with hypersensitivity reactions, hypokalaemia with overdose.

Adverse effects

Glucagon is associated with GI upset, nausea and vomiting.

Clinically important drug–drug interactions

Increased anticoagulation effects have been noted when glucagon is combined with oral anticoagulants. If this combination is needed, the dose should be adjusted.

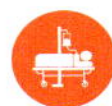

Patient with diabetes and hypertension

Care considerations for people taking glucose-elevating agents

Assessment: history and examination

- Perform a complete physical assessment *to establish a baseline before beginning therapy, monitor effectiveness of therapy and evaluate for any potential adverse effects during therapy.*
- Assess orientation and reflexes and baseline pulse, blood pressure and adventitious sounds *to monitor the effects of altered glucose levels*, and abdominal sounds and function, *which could be altered by these drugs.*
- Monitor blood glucose levels as ordered *to assess the effectiveness of the drug and response to treatment.*
- Monitor the results of laboratory tests, including urinalysis, *to evaluate for glycosuria*, serum glucose levels *to evaluate response to therapy*, and renal and liver function tests *to determine the need for possible dose adjustment or identify possible toxic effects.*

Implementation with rationale

- Monitor blood glucose levels *to evaluate the effectiveness of the drug.*
- Have insulin on standby during emergency use *to treat severe hyperglycaemia if it occurs as a result of overdose.*
- Monitor nutritional status *to provide nutritional consultation as needed.*
- Provide thorough teaching, including drug name, dosage and schedule for administration; signs and symptoms of hyperglycaemia; administration technique if indicated; signs and symptoms of

TABLE 38.4 DRUGS IN FOCUS Glucose-elevating agent

Drug name	Dosage/route	Usual indications
glucagon (*GlucaGen*)	Adults and children > 25 kg: 1 mg SC, IM or IV Children < 25 kg: 0.5 mg SC, IM or IV	To counteract severe hypoglycaemic reactions

adverse effects; need for follow-up monitoring and laboratory testing if indicated; nutritional measures; and blood glucose monitoring.

Evaluation

- Monitor response to the drug (stabilisation of blood glucose levels).
- Monitor for adverse effects (hyperglycaemia, GI distress).
- Evaluate the effectiveness of the teaching plan (person can name drug, dosage, adverse effects to watch for and specific measures to avoid them).
- Monitor the effectiveness of comfort measures and adherence to the regimen.

KEY POINTS

- Glucose-elevating agents are used to increase glucose when levels become dangerously low. Imbalance in glucose levels while taking insulin or oral agents is a common cause of hypoglycaemia.
- Individuals need to be carefully monitored to determine the effectiveness of therapy with these drugs and to prevent inadvertent overdose, which could lead to hyperglycaemia.

CHAPTER SUMMARY

- Diabetes mellitus is the most common metabolic disorder. It is characterised by high blood glucose levels and alterations in the metabolism of fats, proteins and glucose.
- Glucose control is a complicated process affected by various hormones, enzymes and receptor sites.
- Diabetes mellitus is complicated by many end-organ problems. These are related to thickening of basement membranes and the resultant decrease in blood flow to these areas.
- Treatment of diabetes involves tight control of blood glucose levels using diet and exercise, a combination of other agents to stimulate insulin release or alter glucose absorption, or the injection of replacement insulin.
- Replacement insulin was once obtained from beef and pork pancreas. Today, most replacement insulin is human, derived from genetically altered bacteria.
- The amount and type of insulin given must be regulated daily. People taking insulin must learn to inject the drug, to test their blood glucose levels and to recognise the signs of hypoglycaemia and hyperglycaemia.
- Insulin is used for type 1 diabetes and for type 2 diabetes in times of stress or when other therapies have failed.
- Other oral hypoglycaemic agents include first- and second-generation sulfonylureas, which stimulate the pancreas to release insulin, and other agents that alter glucose absorption, decrease insulin resistance, decrease the formation of glucose or increase the urinary excretion of glucose. These agents are often used in combination to achieve effectiveness.
- Glucose-elevating agents are used to increase glucose when levels become dangerously low. Imbalance in glucose levels while taking insulin or oral agents is a common cause of hypoglycaemia.
- Nurses and midwives play a major role in the health care team with regard to management of care and education for people with diabetes.

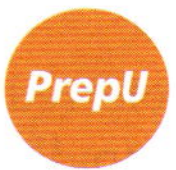

Knowing your strengths and weaknesses helps you to study more effectively. Take a PrepU Practice Quiz to find out how you measure up!

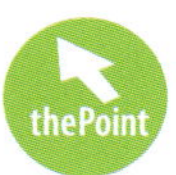

ONLINE RESOURCES

An extensive range of additional resources to enhance teaching and learning and to facilitate understanding of this chapter may be found online at the text's accompanying website, located on thePoint at http://thepoint.lww.com. These include Watch and Learn videos, Concepts in Action animations, journal articles, review questions, case studies, discussion topics and quizzes.

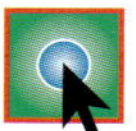

WEB LINKS

Health care providers and students may want to consult the following web resources:

www.aihw.gov.au/diabetes
Australian Institute of Health and Welfare information about diabetes mellitus in Australia.

www.diabetesaustralia.com.au
Australian information on diabetes research, management and support.

www.diabetesinfo.org.nz
New Zealand Information on diabetes.

www.clinicalguidelines.gov.au/portal/2438/new-blood-glucose-management-algorithm-type-2-diabetes-position-statement-australian
A new blood glucose management algorithm for type 2 diabetes. A position statement of the Australian Diabetes Society.

BIBLIOGRAPHY

American Diabetes Association (ADA). (2008). Standards of medical care for patients with diabetes mellitus. *Diabetes Care, 38*, S14–S36.

Australian Institute of Health and Welfare (AIHW). (2013). Diabetes. www.aihw.gov.au/diabetes.

Davis, T. (2014). Sodium–glucose co-transporter inhibitors: Clinical applications. *Australian Prescriber*, www.australianprescriber.com/online-first/27/sodium-glucose-co-transporter-inhibitors.

Derosa, G. & Maffioli, P. (2010). Effects of thiazolidinediones and sulfonylureas in patients with diabetes. *Diabetes Technology & Therapeutics, 12(6)*, 491–501.

Dissanayake, A. (2008). About Diabetes. New Zealand Society for the Study of Diabetes (NZSSD). www.nzssd.org.nz/education/diabetes.html.

Donovan, P. J. (2010). Drugs for gestational diabetes. *Australian Prescriber, 33*, 141–144.

Farrell, M. & Dempsey, J. (2014). *Smeltzer & Bare's Textbook of Medical-Surgical Nursing* (3rd edn). Sydney: Lippincott Williams & Wilkins.

Fleming, S. E. & Corbett, C. (2010). Promoting stringent glycemic control before and during pregnancy: Evidence- and theory-based strategies. *Nursing for Women's Health, 14*, 280–288.

Goodman, L. S., Brunton, L. L., Chabner, B. & Knollmann, B. C. (2011). *Goodman and Gilman's Pharmacological Basis of Therapeutics* (12th edn). New York: McGraw-Hill.

Hamilton, C. A. (2012). Pharmacological management of type 2 diabetes mellitus in patients with CKD. *Journal of Renal Care, 38(supp)*, 59–66.

Kellow, N. & Khalil, H. (2013). A review of the pharmacological management of type 2 diabetes in a rural Australian primary care cohort. *International Journal of Pharmacy Practice, 21(5)*, 297–304.

Lange, V. Z. (2010). Successful management of in-hospital hyperglycemia: The pivotal role of nurses in facilitating effective insulin use. *MEDSURG Nursing, 19*, 323–328.

McElduff, A. (2013). Non-type 1, non-type 2 diabetes: What's in a name? *Australian Prescriber, 36*, 196–198.

McKenna, L. & Mirkov, S. (2019). *McKenna's Drug Handbook for Nursing and Midwifery* (8th edn). Sydney: Wolters Kluwer Health Australia.

O'Dea, K., Rowley, K. G. & Brown, A. (2007). Diabetes in Indigenous Australians: Possible ways forward. *Medical Journal of Australia, 185*, 494–495.

Porth, C. M. (2011). *Essentials of Pathophysiology: Concepts of Altered Health States* (3rd edn). Philadelphia: Lippincott Williams & Wilkins.

Porth, C. M. (2009). *Pathophysiology: Concepts of Altered Health States* (8th edn). Philadelphia: Lippincott Williams & Wilkins.

Srinivasan, S. & Donaghue, K. C. (2007). Paediatric diabetes – which children can gain insulin independence? *Medical Journal of Australia 186*, 436–437.

Taylor, C., Lillis, C. & LeMone, P. (2005). *Fundamentals of Nursing: The Art and Science of Nursing Care* (5th edn). Philadelphia: Lippincott Williams & Wilkins

Thynne, T. & Doogue, M. (2014). Sodium–glucose co-transporter inhibitors: Mechanisms of action. *Australian Prescriber*, www.australianprescriber.com/online-first/26/sodium-glucose-co-transporter-inhibitors.

Wong, J. (2004). Starting insulin treatment in type 2 diabetes. *Australian Prescriber, 27*, 93–96.

CHECK YOUR UNDERSTANDING

Answers to the questions in this chapter can be found in Appendix A at the back of this book.

MULTIPLE CHOICE

Select the best answer to the following.

1. Currently, the medical management of diabetes mellitus is aimed at:
   a. controlling kilojoule intake.
   b. increasing exercise levels.
   c. regulating blood glucose levels.
   d. decreasing fluid loss.
2. The HbA_{1c} blood test is a good measure of overall glucose control because:
   a. it reflects the level of glucose after a meal.
   b. fasting for 8 hours before the test ensures accuracy.
   c. it reflects a 3-month average glucose level in the body.
   d. the test can be affected by the glucose challenge.
3. A person with hyperglycaemia will present with:
   a. polyuria, polydipsia and polyphagia.
   b. polycythaemia, polyuria and polyphagia.
   c. polyadenitis, polyuria and polydipsia.
   d. polydipsia, polycythaemia and polyarteritis.
4. The long-term alterations in fat, carbohydrate and protein metabolism associated with diabetes mellitus result in:
   a. obesity.
   b. thickening of the capillary basement membrane.
   c. chronic obstructive pulmonary disease.
   d. lactose intolerance.
5. Insulin is available in several forms or suspensions, which differ in their:
   a. effect on the pancreas.
   b. onset and duration of action.
   c. means of administration.
   d. tendency to cause adverse effects.
6. Acarbose differs from the sulfonylureas in that it:
   a. greatly stimulates pancreatic insulin release.
   b. greatly increases the sensitivity of insulin receptor sites.
   c. delays the absorption of glucose, leading to lower glucose levels.
   d. cannot be used in combination with other oral hypoglycaemic agents.

7. Teaching subjects for the person with diabetes should include:
   a. diet and exercise changes that are needed.
   b. the importance of avoiding exercise and eating one meal a day.
   c. protection from exposure to any infection and avoiding tiring activities.
   d. avoiding pregnancy and taking hygiene measures.

MULTIPLE RESPONSE

Select all that apply.

1. Treatment of diabetes may include which of the following?
   a. replacement therapy with insulin
   b. control of glucose absorption through the GI tract
   c. drugs that stimulate insulin release or increase sensitivity of insulin receptor sites
   d. surgical clearing of the capillary basement membranes
   e. slowing of gastric emptying
   f. diet and exercise programs
2. A person is recently diagnosed with diabetes. In reviewing his past history, which of the following would be early indicators of the problem?
   a. lethargy
   b. fruity-smelling breath
   c. boundless energy
   d. weight loss
   e. increased sweating
   f. getting up often at night to go to the bathroom

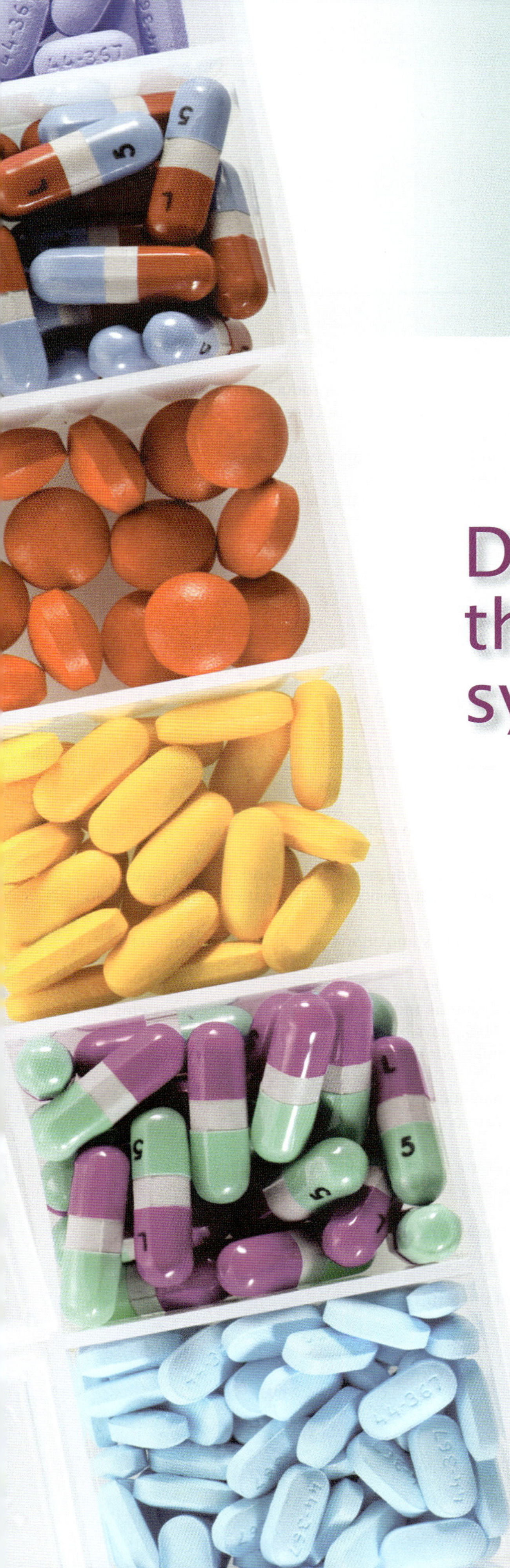

PART 7

Drugs acting on the reproductive system

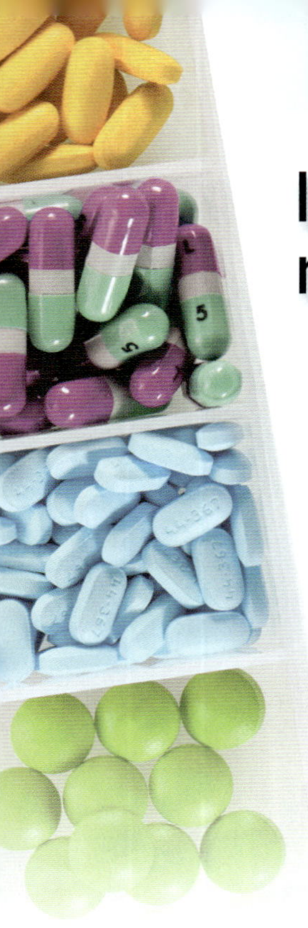

Introduction to the reproductive system

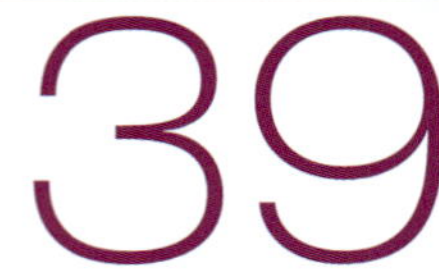

Learning objectives

On completing this chapter you should be able to:

1. Explain the functions of the female ovaries and male testes as part of the reproductive systems.
2. Outline the control mechanisms involved with the male and female reproductive systems, using this outline to explain the negative feedback systems involved with each system.
3. List five effects for each of the sex hormones: oestrogen, progesterone and testosterone.
4. Describe the changes that occur to the female body during pregnancy.
5. Describe the phases of the human sexual response and briefly describe the clinical presentation of each stage.

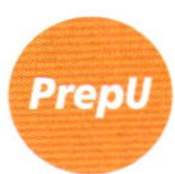

Test your current knowledge of the reproductive system with a PrepU Practice Quiz!

Glossary of key terms

corpus luteum: remains of a follicle that releases a mature ovum at ovulation; becomes an endocrine gland producing oestrogen and progesterone
follicle: storage site of each ovum in the ovary; allows the ovum to grow and develop; produces oestrogen and progesterone
inhibin: oestrogen-like substance produced by seminiferous tubules during sperm production; acts as a negative feedback stimulus to decrease release of follicle-stimulating hormone (FSH)
interstitial or Leydig cells: part of the testes that produce testosterone in response to stimulation by luteinising hormone (LH)
menarche: the onset of the menstrual cycle
menopause: depletion of the female ova; results in lack of oestrogen and progesterone
menstrual cycle: cycling of female sex hormones in interaction with the hypothalamus and anterior pituitary feedback systems
menstruation: expulsion of the uterine lining occurring approximately every 28–32 days
oestrogen: hormone produced by the ovary, placenta and adrenal gland; stimulates development of female characteristics and prepares the body for pregnancy
ova: eggs; the female gamete; contain half of the information needed in a human nucleus
ovaries: female sexual glands that store ova and produce oestrogen and progesterone
ovulation: release of the ovum from the follicle into the abdomen
progesterone: hormone produced by the ovary, placenta and adrenal gland; promotes maintenance of pregnancy
puberty: point at which the hypothalamus starts releasing gonadotropin-releasing factor (GnRF) to stimulate the release of FSH and LH and begin sexual development
seminiferous tubules: part of the testes that produce sperm in response to stimulation by FSH
sperm: male gamete; contains half of the information needed for a human cell nucleus
testes: male sexual glands that produce sperm and testosterone
testosterone: male sex hormone; produced by the interstitial or Leydig cells of the testes
uterus: the womb; site of growth and development of the embryo and fetus

The reproductive systems in males and females are composed of the structures that support conception and development of a fetus and the endocrine glands that produce the hormones necessary for the regulation and maintenance of these structures and that facilitate reproduction. Though anatomically the two systems appear to be very different, they have many underlying similarities. The same fetal cells in males and females give rise to the glands that produce sexual hormones (gonads). In the female, those cells remain in the abdomen and develop into the **ovaries**, the female sexual glands. In the male, the cells migrate out of the abdomen to form the **testes** (the male sexual glands), which are suspended from the body in the scrotum. Both male and female glands respond to follicle-stimulating hormone (FSH) and luteinising hormone (LH), which are released from the anterior pituitary in response to stimulation from gonadotropin-releasing hormone (GnRH) released from the hypothalamus.

FEMALE REPRODUCTIVE SYSTEM

The female reproductive system consists of two ovaries, two oviducts, the uterus and accessory structures, including the vagina, clitoris, labia and breast tissue. The hormones that stimulate and maintain these structures are oestrogen and progesterone. See Figure 39.1.

Structures

The ovaries are almond-shaped organs located on each side of the pelvic cavity. The ovaries store the **ova**, or eggs. Eggs contain half of the genetic material needed to produce a whole cell. At birth, a female's ovaries contain all of the ova that a woman will have. No new ova will ever be produced by the ovaries. The ova are released into the abdomen throughout a woman's life or slowly degenerate over time. Each ovum is contained in a storage site called a **follicle**; the follicles act as endocrine glands producing the hormones **oestrogen** and **progesterone**. The primary goal of these hormones is to prepare the body for pregnancy and to maintain the pregnancy until delivery.

Very near to each ovary is an oviduct. The oviduct is a muscular tube with a ciliated lining that is constantly moving. This movement propels the ovum released into the abdomen down the oviduct and into the **uterus**, or womb, for the developing embryo and fetus. The uterus is a muscular organ that can develop a blood-filled inner lining, or endometrium, which allows for implantation of the fertilised egg and supports the development of the placenta. The placenta provides nourishment for the developing fetus and acts as an endocrine gland producing the hormones needed to maintain the active metabolic state of the pregnancy. The muscular walls of the uterus are important for expelling the developed fetus through the vagina at delivery. The external genitalia – the clitoris,

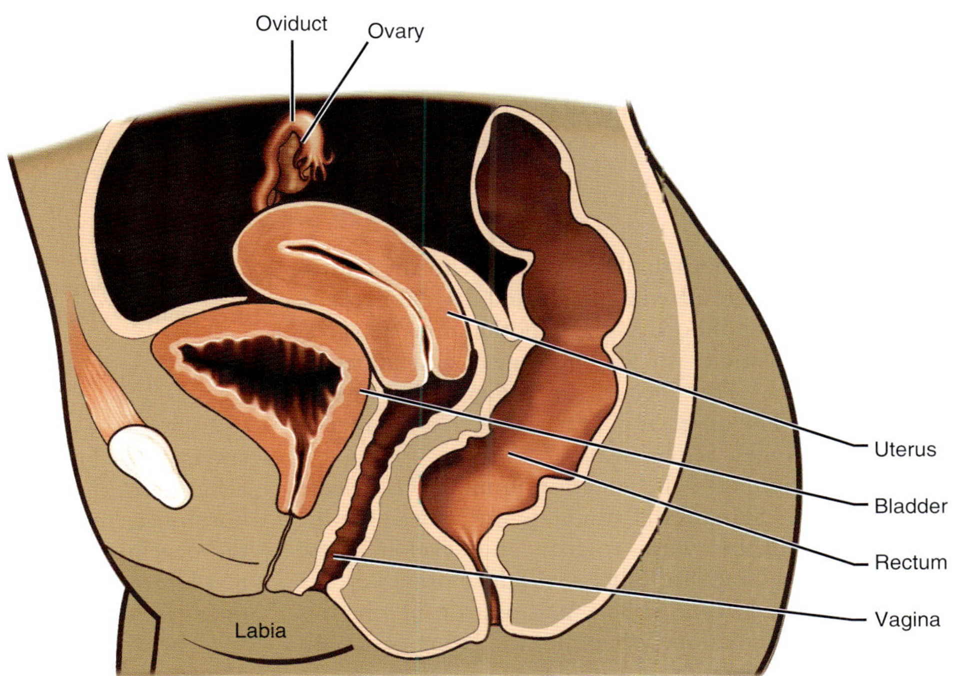

FIGURE 39.1 The female reproductive system.

labia and vagina – are sites of erogenous stimulation and the entry way for sperm to reach the uterus to allow conception and the exit path for the developed fetus at birth. Development of the breast tissue, also considered a secondary sex characteristic, is controlled by the female sex hormones and is necessary for producing milk for the nourishment of the baby when it has been expelled from the uterus and is no longer able to be dependent on the mother's blood supply for nourishment.

Hormones

The hormones produced in the ovaries are oestrogen and progesterone. These two hormones influence many other body systems while preparing the body for pregnancy or maintenance of pregnancy.

Oestrogen

The oestrogens produced by the ovaries include oestradiol, oestrone and oestriol. The oestrogens enter cells and bind to receptors within the cytoplasm to promote messenger RNA (mRNA) activity, which results in production of specific proteins for cell activity or structure. Many of these effects are first noticed at menarche (the onset of the menstrual cycle), when the hormones begin cycling for the first time. Female characteristics are associated with the effects of oestrogen on many of the body's systems – wider hips, soft skin, breast growth and so on. Box 39.1 summarises the effects of oestrogen on the body.

Progesterone

Progesterone is released into circulation after ovulation. Progesterone has many effects that support the early development of the fetus. Progesterone's effects on body temperature are monitored in the 'rhythm method' of birth control to indicate that ovulation has just occurred. Box 39.2 summarises the effects of progesterone on the body.

Control mechanisms

The developing hypothalamus is sensitive to the androgens released by the adrenal glands and does not release GnRH during childhood. As the hypothalamus matures, it loses its sensitivity to the androgens and starts to release GnRH. This occurs at **puberty**, or sexual development. The onset of puberty leads to a number of hormonal changes. See Figure 39.2.

GnRH stimulates the anterior pituitary to release FSH and LH. FSH and LH stimulate the follicles on the outer surface of the ovaries to grow and develop. These follicles, called Graafian follicles, produce progesterone, which is retained in the follicle, and oestrogen, which is released into circulation. When the circulating oestrogen level rises high enough, it stimulates a massive release of LH from the anterior pituitary. This is called the 'LH surge'. This burst of LH causes one of the developing follicles to burst and release the ovum, with its stored hormones, from the ovary. LH also causes the rest of the developing follicles to shrink in on themselves, or involute and eventually disappear. The release of an ovum from the follicle is called **ovulation.**

The ovum is released into the abdomen near the end of one of the oviducts, and the constant movement of cilia within the tube helps to propel the ovum into the

BOX 39.1 Effects of oestrogen

Growth of genitalia (in preparation for childbirth)
Growth of breast tissue (in preparation for pregnancy and breastfeeding)
Characteristic triangular female pubic hair distribution
Stimulation of protein building (important for the developing fetus)
Increased total blood cholesterol (for energy for the mother as well as the developing fetus) with an increase in high-density lipoprotein levels ('good' cholesterol, which serves to protect the female blood vessels against atherosclerosis)
Retention of sodium and water (to provide cooling for the heat generated by the developing fetus and to increase diffusion of sodium and water to the fetus through the placenta)
Inhibition of calcium resorption from the bones (helps to deposit calcium in the fetal bone structure; when this property is lost at menopause, osteoporosis, or loss of calcium from the bone, is common)
Alteration of pelvic bone structure to a wider and flaring pelvis (to promote easier delivery)
Closure of the epiphyses (to conserve energy for the fetus by halting growth of the mother)
Increased thyroid hormone globulin (metabolism needs to be increased greatly during pregnancy, and the increase in thyroid hormone facilitates this)
Increased elastic tissue of the skin (to allow for the tremendous stretch of the abdominal skin during pregnancy)
Increased vascularity of the skin (to allow for radiation loss of heat generated by the developing fetus)
Increased uterine motility (oestrogen is high when the ovum first leaves the ovary, and increased uterine motility helps to move the ovum towards the uterus and to propel the sperm towards the ovum)
Thin, clear cervical mucus (allows easy penetration of the sperm into the uterus as ovulation occurs; used in fertility programs as an indication that ovulation will soon occur)
Proliferative endometrium (to prepare the lining of the uterus for implantation with the fertilised egg)
Anti-insulin effect, with increased glucose levels (to allow increased diffusion of glucose to the developing fetus)
T-cell inhibition (to protect the non-self cells of the embryo from the immune surveillance of the mother)

■ BOX 39.2 Effects of progesterone

Decreased uterine motility (to provide increased chance that implantation can occur)
Development of a secretory endometrium (to provide glucose and a rich blood supply for the developing placenta and embryo)
Thickened cervical mucus (to protect the developing embryo and keep out bacteria and other pathogens; this is lost at the beginning of labour as the mucous plug)
Breast growth (to prepare for breastfeeding)
Increased body temperature (a direct hypothalamic response to progesterone, which stimulates metabolism and promotes activities for the developing embryo; this increase in temperature is monitored in the 'rhythm method' of birth control to indicate that ovulation has occurred)
Increased appetite (this is a direct effect on the satiety centres of the hypothalamus and results in increased nutrients for the developing embryo)
Depressed T-cell function (again, this protects the non-self cells of the developing embryo from the immune system)
Anti-insulin effect (to generate a higher blood glucose concentration to allow rapid diffusion of glucose to the developing embryo)

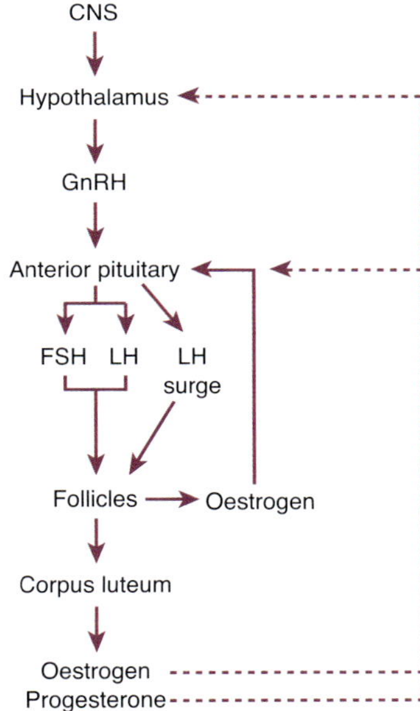

FIGURE 39.2 Interaction of the hypothalamic, pituitary and ovarian hormones that underlies the menstrual cycle. Dotted lines indicate negative feedback surge. CNS, central nervous system; FSH, follicle-stimulating hormone; GnRH, gonadotropin-releasing hormone; LH, luteinising hormone.

oviduct and then into the uterus. The ruptured follicle becomes a functioning endocrine gland called the **corpus luteum**. It will continue to produce oestrogen and progesterone for 10–14 days unless pregnancy occurs.

Fertilisation of the ovum and implantation in the uterine wall results in the production of human chorionic gonadotropin (HCG). This hormone stimulates the corpus luteum to continue to produce oestrogen and progesterone until the placenta develops and becomes functional, producing these hormones at a level high enough to sustain the pregnancy.

If pregnancy does not occur, the corpus luteum involutes and becomes a white scar on the ovary. This scar is called the corpus albicans. Initially, the rising levels of oestrogen and progesterone produced by the corpus luteum act as a negative feedback system to the hypothalamus and the pituitary, stopping the production and secretion of GnRH, FSH and LH. Later in the cycle, the corpus luteum atrophies, the falling levels of oestrogen and progesterone stimulate the hypothalamus to release GnRH and the cycle begins again.

Factors influencing control mechanisms

Because of its position in the brain, the hypothalamus is influenced by many internal and external factors. For example, high levels of stress can interrupt the reproductive cycle. Tremendous amounts of energy are expended in reproduction, and if the body needs energy for 'fight or flight', the hypothalamus shuts down the reproductive activities, stopping the release of GnRH, which results in no FSH or LH release and no stimulation of the follicles. This saves a tremendous amount of energy in the body, energy that the body will use for fight or flight. In addition to stress, starvation, extreme exercise and emotional problems are all associated with a decrease in reproductive capacity related to the controls of the hypothalamus.

The menstrual cycle

The cyclical nature of the female sex hormones on the body produces the **menstrual cycle**. The onset of the menstrual cycle at puberty is called the **menarche**. Each cycle starts with release of FSH and LH and stimulation of the ovarian follicles. For about the next 14 days, the developing follicles release oestrogen into the body. Thus the woman may notice the many effects of oestrogen, such as breast tenderness and water retention. In addition, oestrogen thins cervical mucosa and increases susceptibility to infections.

By about day 14, the oestrogen levels have caused the LH surge and ovulation occurs. The woman experiences increased body temperature, increased appetite, breast tenderness, bloating and abdominal fullness and constipation, among others – the effects associated with progesterone, which is released into the system when the follicle ruptures. The uterus becomes thicker and more vascular as the cycle progresses, and develops a proliferative endometrium. After ovulation, the lining of the uterus begins to produce glucose and other nutrients

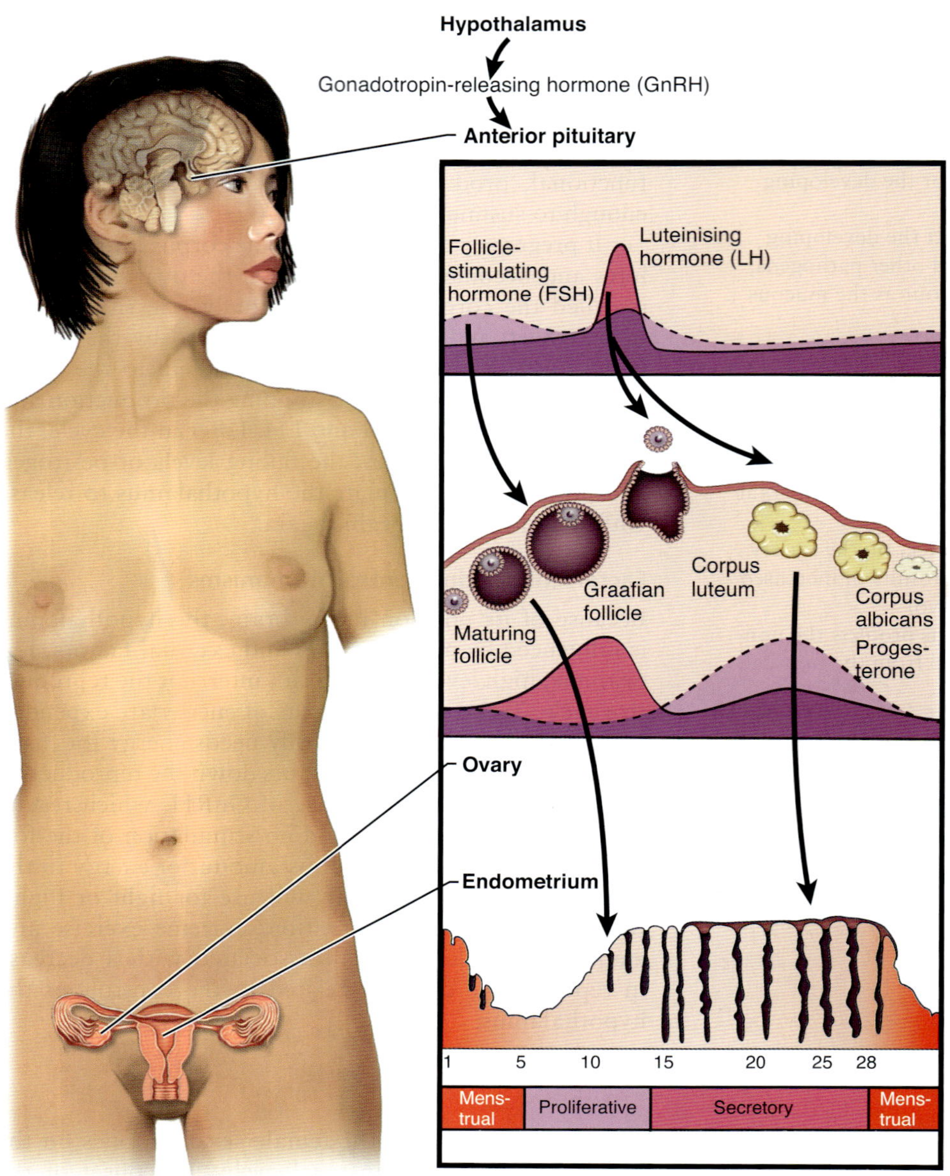

FIGURE 39.3 Relation of pituitary and ovarian hormone levels to the menstrual cycle and to ovarian and endometrial function.

which would nurture a growing embryo; this is called a secretory endometrium. If pregnancy does not occur, after about 14 days the corpus luteum involutes, and the levels of oestrogen and progesterone drop off (Figure 39.3).

The dropping levels of oestrogen and progesterone trigger the release of FSH and LH again, along with the start of another menstrual cycle. Lowered hormone levels also cause the inner lining of the uterus to slough off because it is no longer stimulated by the hormones. High levels of plasminogen in the uterus prevent clotting of the lining as the vessels shear off. Prostaglandins in the uterus stimulate uterine contraction to clamp off vessels as the lining sheds away. This causes menstrual cramps. This loss of the uterine lining, called **menstruation**, repeats approximately every 28–32 days. Figure 39.3 depicts the various phases of the menstrual cycle.

Pregnancy

When the ovum is fertilised by a sperm, a new cell is produced that rapidly divides to produce the embryo. The embryo implants in the wall of the uterus, and the interface between the fetal cells and the uterus produces the placenta, a large, vascular organ that serves as a massive endocrine gland and a transfer point for nutrients from the mother to the fetus. The placenta maintains high levels of oestrogens and progesterone to support the uterus and the developing fetus. When the placenta ages, the levels of progesterone and oestrogens fall off.

Eventually, the tendency to block uterine activity (an effect of progesterone) is overcome by the stimulation to increase uterine activity caused by oxytocin (a hypothalamic hormone stored in the posterior pituitary). At this point, local prostaglandins stimulate uterine contraction and the onset of labour. Once the fetus and the placenta have been expelled from the uterus, the hormone levels plummet towards the non-pregnant state. It often takes 6–8 weeks to reverse the effects of these hormones. This is a time of tremendous adjustment for the body as it tries to re-achieve homeostasis.

Menopause

The follicles contained in the ovary become depleted over time, the ovaries no longer produce oestrogen and progesterone, and **menopause** – the cessation of menses – occurs. The hypothalamus and pituitary produce increased levels of GnRH, FSH and LH for a while in an attempt to stimulate the ovaries to produce oestrogen and progesterone. If that does not happen, the levels of these hormones fall back within a normal range in response to their own negative feedback systems. Menopause is associated with loss of many of the effects of these two hormones on the body, including retention of calcium in the bones, lowered serum lipid levels and maintenance of secondary sex characteristics.

KEY POINTS

- The female ovary stores ova and produces the sex hormones oestrogen and progesterone.
- The hypothalamus releases GnRH at puberty to stimulate the anterior pituitary release of FSH and LH, thus stimulating the production and release of the sex hormones. Levels are controlled by a series of negative feedback systems.
- Female sex hormones prepare the body for pregnancy and the maintenance of the pregnancy. If pregnancy does not occur, the prepared inner lining of the uterus sloughs off as menstruation in the menstrual cycle.
- Menopause occurs when the supply of ova is exhausted and the woman's body no longer produces the hormones oestrogen and progesterone.

MALE REPRODUCTIVE SYSTEM

The male reproductive system consists of two testes, the vas deferens, the prostate gland, the penis and the urethra. The hormone that stimulates and maintains these structures is testosterone.

Structures

The male reproductive system originates from the same fetal cells as in the female. The major male reproductive system structure is the testes, the two endocrine glands that continually produce **sperm**, as well as the hormone **testosterone**. During fetal development, the two testes migrate down the abdomen and descend into the scrotum outside the body. There they are protected from the heat of the body to prevent injury to the sperm-producing cells. The testes are made up of two distinct parts: the **seminiferous tubules**, which produce the sperm, and the **interstitial** or **Leydig cells**, which produce the hormone testosterone. Other components include the vas deferens, which stores produced sperm and carries sperm from the testes to be ejaculated from the body; the prostate gland, which produces enzymes to stimulate sperm maturation, as well as lubricating fluid; the penis, which includes two corpora cavernosa and a corpus spongiosum, structures that allow massively increased blood flow and erection; the urethra, through which urine and the sperm and seminal fluid are delivered; and other glands and ducts that promote sperm and seminal fluid development (Figure 39.4).

Hormones

The primary hormone associated with the male reproductive system is testosterone. Testosterone is responsible for many sexual and metabolic effects in the male. Like oestrogen, testosterone enters the cell and reacts with a cytoplasmic receptor site to influence mRNA activity, resulting in the production of proteins for cell structure or function. Box 39.3 summarises the effects of testosterone on the body.

If the testes are lost before puberty occurs, there will be no development of the secondary male sex characteristics or the other effects seen when testosterone is released. Such a person would require testosterone replacement therapy to develop these characteristics. However, once puberty and the physical changes brought about by testosterone have occurred, the androgens released by the adrenal glands are sufficient to sustain the male characteristics. Androgens are very similar in structure to testosterone and are able to influence cells to maintain the changes caused by testosterone. This is important information for adults undergoing testicular surgery or chemical castration.

Control mechanisms

The activity of the male sex glands is not thought to be cyclical like that of the female. The hypothalamus in the male child is also sensitive to circulating levels of adrenal androgens and suppresses GnRH release. After the hypothalamus matures, this sensitivity is lost and the hypothalamus releases GnRH. This in turn stimulates the anterior pituitary to release FSH and LH, or what is sometimes called interstitial cell–stimulating hormone (ICSH) in males. FSH directly stimulates the seminiferous tubules to produce sperm, a process called spermatogenesis. FSH also stimulates the Sertoli cells in the seminiferous tubules to produce oestrogens, which provide negative feedback to the pituitary and hypothalamus to cause a decrease in the release of GnRH, FSH and LH.

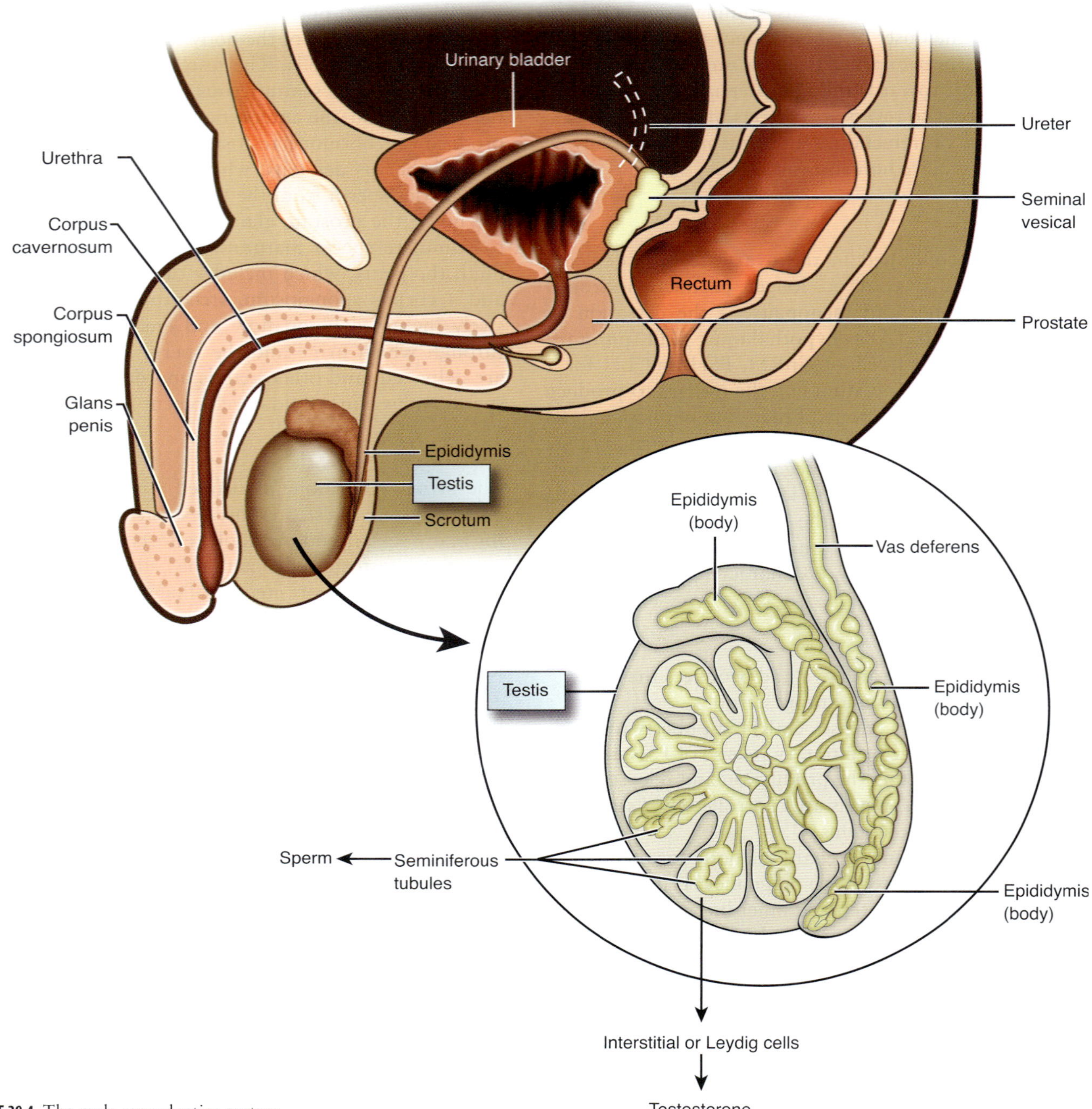

FIGURE 39.4 The male reproductive system.

The Sertoli cells also produce a substance called **inhibin**, an oestrogen-like molecule. On the sensing of inhibin by the hypothalamus and anterior pituitary, a negative feedback response occurs, decreasing the circulating level of FSH. When the FSH level falls low enough, the hypothalamus is stimulated to again release GnRH to stimulate FSH release. This feedback system prevents overproduction of sperm in the testes (Figure 39.5). Inhibin has been investigated for many years as a possible male birth control drug because it is thought to affect only sperm production.

The LH stimulates the interstitial (Leydig) cells to produce testosterone. The concentration of testosterone acts in a similar negative feedback system with the hypothalamus. When the concentration is high enough, the hypothalamus decreases GnRH release, leading to a subsequent decrease in FSH and LH release. The levels of testosterone are thought to remain within a fairly well-defined range of normal.

With age, the seminiferous tubules and interstitial cells atrophy and the male climacteric, a period of lessened sexual activity and loss of testosterone effects,

BOX 39.3 Effects of testosterone

Growth of male and sexual accessory organs (penis, prostate gland, seminal vesicles, vas deferens)
Growth of testes and scrotal sac
Thickening of vocal cords, producing the deep, male voice
Hair growth on the face, body, arms, legs and trunk
Male-pattern baldness
Increased protein anabolism and decreased protein catabolism (this causes larger and more powerful muscle development)
Increased bone growth in length and width, which ends when the testosterone stimulates closure of the epiphyses
Thickening of the cartilage and skin, leading to the male gait
Vascular thickening
Increased haematocrit

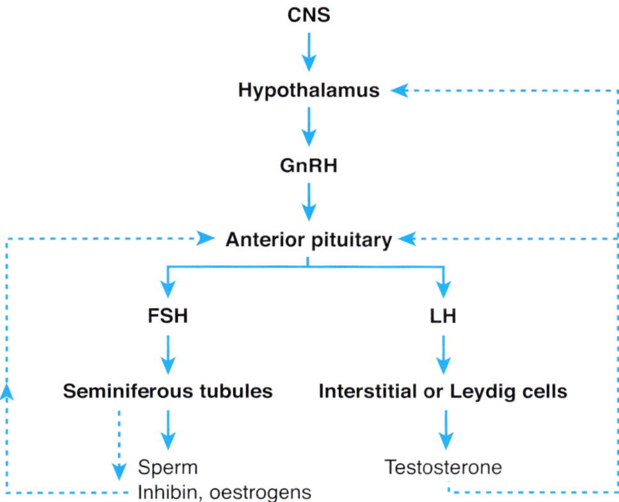

FIGURE 39.5 Interaction of the hypothalamic, pituitary, and testicular hormones that underlies the male sexual hormone system. CNS, central nervous system; FSH, follicle-stimulating hormone; GnRH, gonadotropin-releasing hormone; LH, luteinising hormone.

occurs. This is similar to female menopause. The hypothalamus and anterior pituitary put out larger amounts of GnRH, FSH and LH in an attempt to stimulate the gland. If no increase in testosterone or inhibin occurs, the levels of GnRH, FSH and LH eventually return to normal levels.

KEY POINTS

- The testes produce sperm in the seminiferous tubules in response to FSH stimulation, and testosterone in the interstitial cells in response to LH stimulation.
- Testosterone is responsible for the development of male sex characteristics. These characteristics can be maintained by the androgens from the adrenal gland once the body has undergone the changes of puberty.

THE HUMAN SEXUAL RESPONSE

Many animals require particular endocrine stimuli, called an oestrous cycle, for sexual response to occur. Humans and ferrets are the only animals known to be sexually stimulated and responsive at will. Humans can be sexually stimulated by thoughts, sights, touch or a variety of combined stimuli. The human sexual response consists of four phases:

- A period of stimulation with mild increases in sensitivity and beginning stimulation of the sympathetic nervous system
- A plateau stage when stimulation levels off
- A climax, which results from massive sympathetic stimulation of the body
- A period of recovery or resolution, when the effects of the sympathetic stimulation are resolved (Figure 39.6)

Previously, it was believed that male and female responses were very different. However, it is now thought that the physiology of the responses is quite similar. Sexual stimulation and activity are a normal response and, in healthy individuals, are probably necessary for complete health of the body's systems. The sympathetic stimulation causes increased heart rate, increased blood pressure, sweating, pupil dilation, glycogenolysis (breakdown of stored glycogen to glucose for energy) and other sympathetic responses. This stimulation could be dangerous in some cardiovascular conditions that could be exacerbated by the sympathetic effects. In the male, the increased blood flow to the penis causes erection, which is necessary for penetration of the female and deposition of the sperm. Any drug therapy or disease process that interferes with the sympathetic response or the innervation of the sexual organs will change the person's ability to experience the human sexual response. This is important to keep in mind when teaching and when evaluating the effects of a drug.

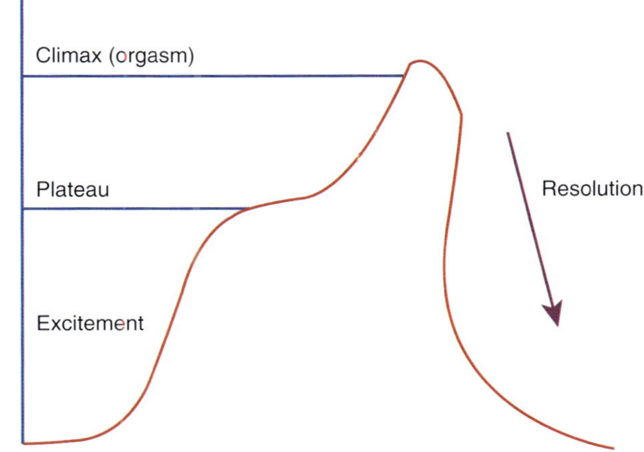

FIGURE 39.6 Human sexual response.

KEY POINTS

- The human sexual response involves activation of the sympathetic nervous system to allow a four-phase response: stimulation, plateau, climax and resolution.
- Sexual stimulation and activity are a normal response and, in healthy individuals, are probably necessary for complete health of the body's systems.
- Since activation of the sympathetic response is an integral part of the human sexual response, any disease process or drug therapy that interferes with the sympathetic response will alter the person's ability to experience a sexual response.

CHAPTER SUMMARY

- Male and female reproductive systems arise from the same fetal cells. The female ovaries store ova and produce the sex hormones oestrogen and progesterone; the male testes produce sperm and the sex hormone testosterone.
- The hypothalamus releases GnRH at puberty to stimulate the anterior pituitary release of FSH and LH, thus stimulating the production and release of the sex hormones. Levels are controlled by a series of negative feedback systems.
- Female sex hormones are released in a cyclical fashion. Release of an ovum for possible fertilisation is termed ovulation. The female hormones prepare the body for pregnancy, including maintenance of the pregnancy if fertilisation occurs.
- If pregnancy does not occur, the prepared inner lining of the uterus is sloughed off as menstruation in the menstrual cycle, so that the lining can be prepared again when ovulation recurs.
- Menopause in women and the male climacteric in men occur when the body no longer produces sex hormones; the hypothalamus and anterior pituitary respond by releasing increasing levels of GnRH, FSH and LH in an attempt to achieve higher levels of sex hormones.
- The testes produce sperm in the seminiferous tubules in response to FSH stimulation, and testosterone in the interstitial cells in response to LH stimulation.
- Testosterone is responsible for the development of male sex characteristics. These characteristics can be maintained by the androgens from the adrenal gland once the body has undergone the changes of puberty.
- The human sexual response involves activation of the sympathetic nervous system to allow a four-phase response: stimulation, plateau, climax and resolution.

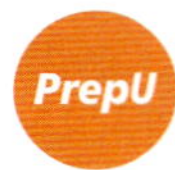

Knowing your strengths and weaknesses helps you to study more effectively. Take a PrepU Practice Quiz to find out how you measure up!

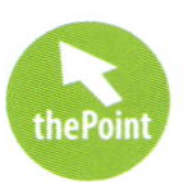

ONLINE RESOURCES

An extensive range of additional resources to enhance teaching and learning and to facilitate understanding of this chapter may be found online at the text's accompanying website, located on thePoint at http://thepoint.lww.com. These include Watch and Learn videos, Concepts in Action animations, journal articles, review questions, case studies, discussion topics and quizzes.

BIBLIOGRAPHY

Barrett, K. E. & Ganong, W. F. (2010). *Ganong's Review of Medical Physiology* (23rd edn). New York: McGraw-Hill.

Basson, R. (2007). Women's sexual function and dysfunction. *JAMA*, 297, 895–897.

Camacho, P. M., Gharib, H. & Sizemore, G. W. (Eds.). (2012) *Evidence-based Endocrinology* (3rd edn). Philadelphia: Lippincott Williams & Wilkins.

Finlayson, A. & Sanders, S. (2007). (Eds.). *Endocrine and Reproductive Systems* (3rd edn). Edinburgh: Mosby.

Fritz, M. A. & Speroff, L. (2010). *Clinical Gynecologic Endocrinology and Infertility* (8th edn). Philadelphia: Lippincott Williams & Wilkins.

Gardner, D. G., Greenspan, F. S. & Shoback, D. M. (Eds.). (2011). *Basic and Clinical Endocrinology* (9th edn). New York: McGraw-Hill.

Guyton, A. & Hall, J. (2011). *Textbook of Medical Physiology* (12th edn). Philadelphia: Saunders Elsevier.

Melmed, S., Polonsky, K. S., Larsen, P. R. & Kronenberg, H. M. (Eds.). (2011). *Williams Textbook of Endocrinology* (12th edn). Philadelphia: Elsevier Saunders.

White, B. A. & Porterfield, S. P. (2013). *Endocrine and Reproductive Physiology*. Philadelphia: Elsevier Mosby.

CHECK YOUR UNDERSTANDING

Answers to the questions in this chapter can be found in Appendix A at the back of this book.

MULTIPLE CHOICE

Select the best answer to the following.

1. In a non-pregnant woman, the levels of the sex hormones fluctuate in a cyclical fashion until:
   a. all of the ova are depleted.
   b. the FSH and LH are depleted.
   c. the hypothalamus no longer senses FSH and LH.
   d. the hypothalamus becomes more sensitive to androgens.
2. A woman develops ova (or eggs):
   a. continually until menopause.
   b. during fetal life.
   c. until menopause.
   d. starting with puberty
3. Control of the female sex hormones starts with the release of GnRH from the hypothalamus. Because of this, the cycling of these hormones may be influenced by:
   a. body temperature.
   b. stress or emotional problems.
   c. age.
   d. androgen release.
4. The rhythm method of birth control depends on the effects of progesterone:
   a. to increase uterine motility.
   b. to decrease and thicken cervical secretions.
   c. to elevate body temperature.
   d. to depress appetite.
5. The menstrual cycle:
   a. always repeats itself every 28 days.
   b. is associated with changing hormone levels.
   c. is necessary for a human sexual response.
   d. cannot occur if ovulation does not occur.
6. In the male reproductive system:
   a. the seminiferous tubules produce sperm and testosterone.
   b. the interstitial cells produce sperm.
   c. the seminiferous tubules produce sperm and the interstitial cells produce testosterone.
   d. the interstitial cells produce sperm and testosterone.
7. Spring fever occurs as a result of increased light. In males, this increase in light causes an increase in the production of:
   a. inhibin.
   b. adrenal androgens.
   c. oestrogen.
   d. testosterone.
8. The human sexual response depends on stimulation of:
   a. the sympathetic nervous system.
   b. the parasympathetic nervous system.
   c. the hypothalamic sex drive centre.
   d. adrenal androgens.

MULTIPLE RESPONSE

Select all that apply.

1. After teaching a group of students about the effects of the various sex hormones, the instructor determines that the teaching was successful when the group identifies which of the following as related to oestrogen?
   a. increased levels of high-density lipoproteins
   b. increased calcium density in the bone
   c. closing of the epiphyses
   d. development of a thick cervical plug
   e. increased body temperature
   f. triangle-shaped body hair distribution
2. A group of students are reviewing material in preparation for an examination on the sex hormones. Which of the following, if identified by the students as effects of testosterone, demonstrates understanding of the information?
   a. thickening of skin and vocal cords
   b. development of a wide and flat pelvis
   c. development of facial hair
   d. closure of the epiphyses
   e. increased haematocrit
   f. increased aggression

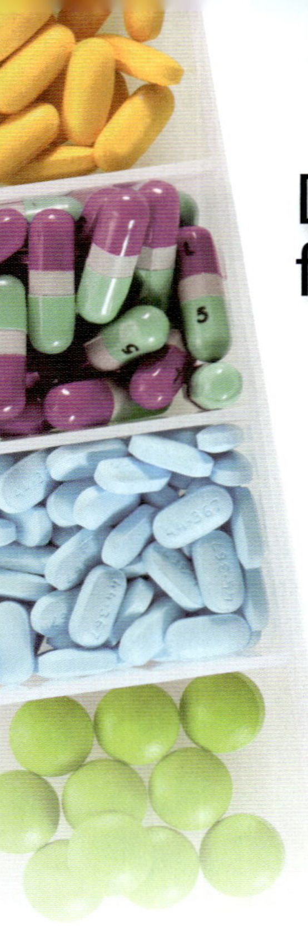

Drugs affecting the female reproductive system

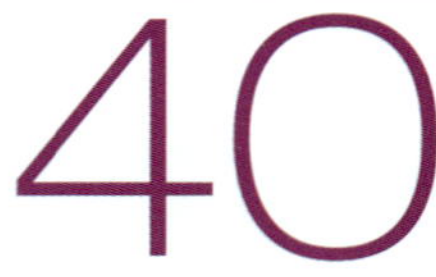

Learning objectives

On completing this chapter you should be able to:

1. Integrate knowledge of the effects of sex hormones on the female body to explain the therapeutic and adverse effects of these agents when used clinically.
2. Describe the therapeutic actions, indications, pharmacokinetics, contraindications, most common adverse reactions and important drug–drug interactions associated with drugs that affect the female reproductive system.
3. Discuss the use of drugs that affect the female reproductive system across the lifespan.
4. Compare and contrast the prototype drugs estradiol, raloxifene, norethisterone, clomifene, oxytocin and dinoprostone with other agents in their class.
5. Outline the nursing and midwifery considerations, including important teaching points to stress, for women receiving drugs that affect the reproductive system.

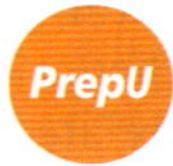

Test your current knowledge of drugs affecting the female reproductive system with a PrepU Practice Quiz!

Glossary of key terms

fertility drugs: drugs used to stimulate ovulation and pregnancy in women with functioning ovaries who are having trouble conceiving

oxytocics: drugs that act like the hypothalamic hormone oxytocin; they stimulate uterine contraction and contraction of the lacteal glands in the breast, promoting milk ejection

oestrogen: the endogenous female sex hormone, produced by the ovary, placenta, testes, and possibly the adrenal cortex

pessary: vaginal suppository

progestin: a synthetic progestogen

progestogens: the endogenous female hormone progesterone and its various derivatives, important in maintaining a pregnancy and supporting many secondary sex characteristics

SEX HORMONES AND OESTROGEN-RECEPTOR MODULATORS

Sex hormones

Ethinylestradiol

Estrogens

(P) estradiol

conjugated estrogens

Progestogens

desogestrel

drospirenone

etonogestrel

levonorgestrel

medroxyprogesterone

nomegestrol

(P) norethisterone

progesterone

Oestrogen-receptor modulators

bazedoxifene

(P) raloxifene

toremifene

FERTILITY DRUGS

cetrorelix

choriogonadotropin alfa

chorionic gonadotropin

(P) clomifene

follitropin alfa

follitropin beta

ganirelix

lutropin alfa

menopausal gonadotropin

UTERINE MOTILITY DRUGS

Oxytocics

carbetocin

ergometrine

(P) oxytocin

Prostaglandins

(P) dinoprostone

gemeprost

mifepristone

misoprostol

The female reproductive system functions in a cyclical fashion, not in the steady-state fashion seen with much of the rest of the endocrine system. Altering any component of this cycle or the system can have a wide variety of effects on the entire body. Drugs that affect the female reproductive system typically include hormones and hormonal-like agents. Figure 40.1 reviews the female reproductive system and sites of action of the drugs used to affect the system. Box 40.1 highlights considerations related to the use of drugs discussed in this chapter as they affect the female reproductive system throughout the lifespan.

SEX HORMONES AND OESTROGEN-RECEPTOR MODULATORS

The female sex hormones can be used to replace hormones that are missing or to act on the control mechanisms of the endocrine system to decrease the release of endogenous hormones. Drugs that act like oestrogen, particularly at specific oestrogen receptors, are also used to stimulate the effects of oestrogen in the body with fewer of the adverse effects. See Table 40.1 for information on these agents.

SEX HORMONES

Female sex hormones include oestrogens and the **progestogens** (the endogenous female hormone progesterone and its various derivatives). Exogenous estrogens that are available for use include estradiol (*Estraderm*, *Climara* and others) and conjugated estrogens (*Premarin*).

Progestogens include desogestrel (*Marvelon*), drospirenone (with ethinylestradiol as *Yasmin*, *YAZ*), etonogestrel (*Implanon*), levonorgestrel (*Microlut*, *Mirena*), medroxyprogesterone (*Provera*), and nomegestrol (with estradiol as *Zoely*), norethisterone (with ethinylestradiol as *Brevinor*) and progesterone (*Crinone, ProFeme*).

Estrogens

Therapeutic actions and indications

Estrogens are used in many clinical situations; for example, in small doses, they are used for hormone replacement

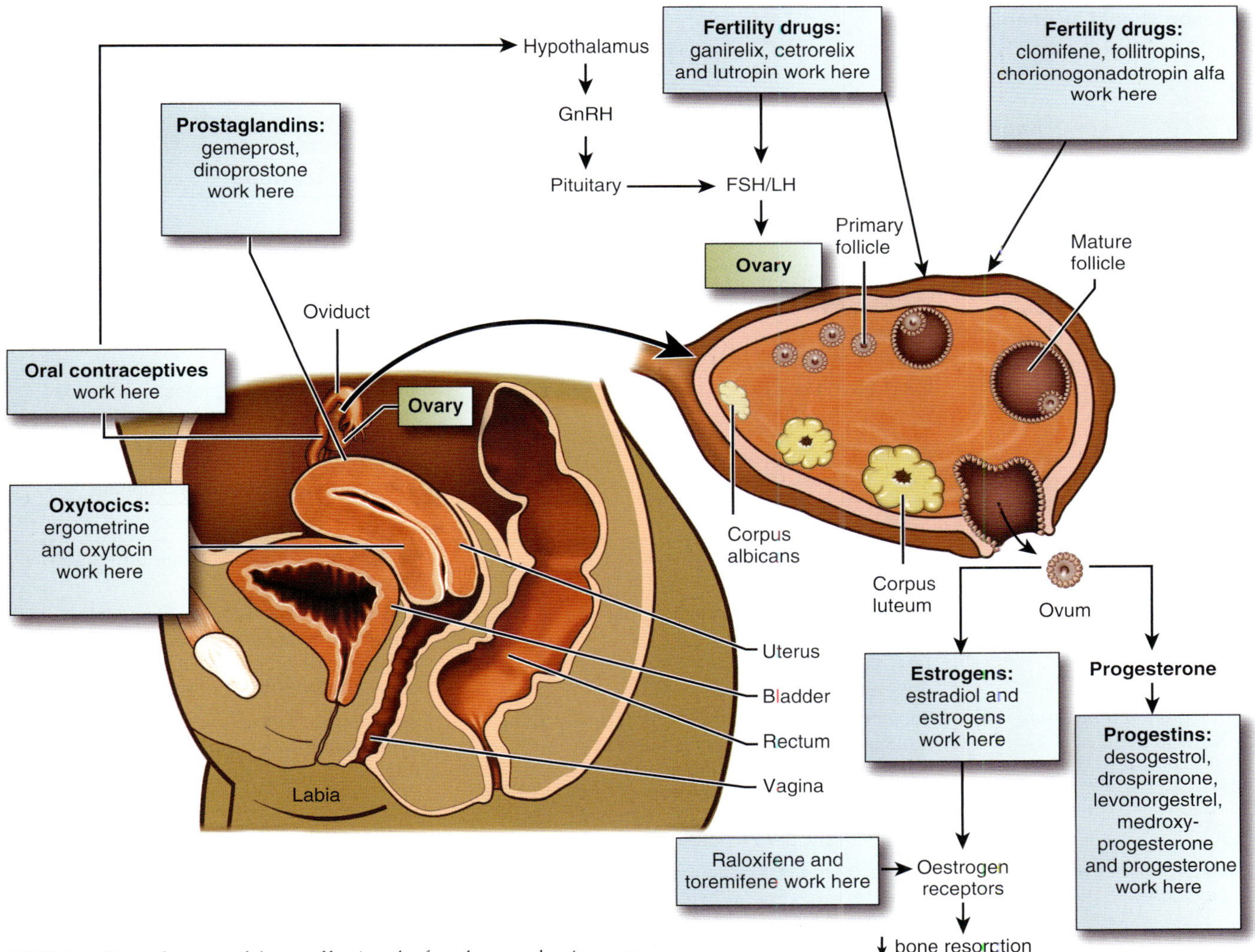

FIGURE 40.1 Sites of action of drugs affecting the female reproductive system.

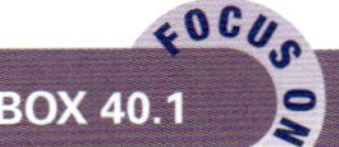

BOX 40.1 Drug therapy across the lifespan

Drugs affecting the female reproductive system

CHILDREN

The estrogens and progestins have undergone little testing in children. Because of their effects on closure of the epiphyses, they should be used only with great caution in growing children.

If oral contraceptives are prescribed for teenage girls, the smallest dose possible should be used and the child should be monitored carefully for metabolic and other effects.

ADULTS

Women who are receiving any of these drugs should receive an annual medical examination, including breast examination and Pap smear, to monitor for adverse effects and underlying medical conditions. The potential for adverse effects should be discussed and comfort measures provided. Women taking estrogen should be advised not to smoke because of the increased risk of thrombotic events.

If any of these drugs is used in males for the treatment of specific cancers, the person should be advised about the possibility of oestrogenic effects, and appropriate support should be offered.

PREGNANCY AND BREASTFEEDING

When combinations of these hormones are used as part of fertility programs, women need a great deal of psychological support and comfort measures to cope with the many adverse effects associated with these drugs. The risk of multiple births should be explained, as should the need for frequent monitoring.

When prostaglandins are used, people need a great deal of psychological support. Written lists of signs and symptoms to report and what to expect are more effective than just verbal lists in this time of potential stress.

These agents are not for use during pregnancy or breastfeeding because of the potential for adverse effects on the fetus or neonate.

OLDER ADULTS

Hormone replacement therapy (HRT) is no longer commonly used by postmenopausal women. Reports of benefits and risks are frequent and conflicting, and women need support and reliable information to make informed decisions about the use of these drugs.

If women are also using alternative therapies, their effects on the HRT and other possible prescription drugs need to be carefully evaluated.

TABLE 40.1 *DRUGS IN FOCUS* Sex hormones and oestrogen-receptor modulators

Drug name	Dosage/route	Usual indications
Sex hormones		
Estrogens		
(P) estradiol (*Climara, Estrofem, Estradot*)	Transdermal patch: 1 patch once weekly releasing 25–100 micrograms estradiol in 24 hours Tablet: 1–2 mg/day PO	Hormone replacement therapy; short-term management of oestrogen deficiency due to menopause
conjugated estrogens (*Premarin*)	0.3–1.25 mg/day PO	Oestrogen-deficiency states: menopause, female hypogonadism or castration, primary ovarian failure, postmenopausal osteoporosis prevention when non-estrogen alternatives inappropriate
Progestogens		
desogestrel (*Marvelon*)	desogestrel 150 micrograms daily with ethinylestradiol 30 micrograms PO daily	Available only in combination form, used as oral contraceptive
drospirenone (*Yasmin, YAZ*)	*Yasmin:* 3 mg with 30 micrograms ethinylestradiol *YAZ:* 3 mg with 20 micrograms estradiol	Used in combination contraceptives; treatment of acne and premenstrual dysphoric disorder (PMDD); relief of signs and symptoms of menopause
etonogestrel (*Implanon, NuvaRing*)	*Implanon:* 68 mg implanted subdermally for up to 3 years, may be replaced at that time *NuvaRing:* 11.7 mg etonogestrel and 2.7 mg ethinylestradiol as a vaginal ring releasing 120 micrograms and 15 micrograms, respectively, per 24 hours	Contraceptive for women; being investigated as a male contraceptive agent
levonorgestrel (*Mirena, Levonelle*)	*Mirena:* 52 mg inserted intrauterine for up to 5 years *Levonelle:* 1.5 mg PO taken within 72 hours of sexual intercourse	Intrauterine contraceptives; also used as 'morning after' pill; component in many combination contraceptives

TABLE 40.1 DRUGS IN FOCUS Sex hormones and oestrogen-receptor modulators *(continued)*

Drug name	Dosage/route	Usual indications
Progestogens *(continued)*		
medroxyprogesterone (*Provera*)	*Oral* Amenorrhoea: 2.5–10 mg /day for 10 days Carcinoma: 200–500 mg/day Endometriosis: 10 mg tid for 90 days *IM injection* Carcinoma: 600–1200 mg weekly Endometriosis: 50 mg/week or 100 mg/2 weeks Contraception: 150 mg every 90 days	Treatment of amenorrhoea (orally); palliation of certain cancers (injection)
nomegestrol (*Zoely*)	1 tablet (nomegestrol 2.5 mg daily with estradiol 1.5 mg) PO daily	Oral contraception
(P) norethisterone (*Noriday, Primolut*)	Dysfunctional bleeding: 5 mg tid Amenorrhoea: 5 mg once or twice daily Endometriosis: 5–10 mg bd Contraception: 350 micrograms/day Also in various combination contraceptives along with an estrogen	Used in combination contraceptives; used alone for treatment of amenorrhoea
progesterone (generic)	Intravaginally: 25–200 mg/day PV as vaginal cream 3.2% or 10%, vaginal gel 8%, or vaginal pessaries 100–200 mg Oral capsules: 200 mg daily at bedtime for 12 days beginning on day 15 of the cycle and ending on day 26; or 100 mg at bedtime from day 1 to day 25	Used as contraceptive and in fertility programs; treatment of amenorrhoea
Oestrogen-receptor modulators		
bazedoxifene (*Duavive*)	Adult: 1 tablet (bazedoxifene acetate 20 mg with conjugated estrogens 450 micrograms) PO daily. Tablets should be swallowed whole, not chewed, crushed or broken. Use for shortest duration consistent with treatment goals and risks. Not recommended in renal impairment; contraindicated in liver impairment; limited use in people > 65 years	Treatment of moderate to severe vasomotor symptoms associated with menopause in women with an intact uterus
(P) raloxifene (*Evista*)	60 mg/day PO	Used therapeutically to stimulate specific oestrogen-receptor sites, which results in an increase in bone mineral density without stimulating the endometrium in women; reduces risk of invasive breast cancer in postmenopausal women with osteoporosis who are at high risk for invasive breast cancer
toremifene (*Fareston*)	60 mg/day PO	Used as an antineoplastic agent because of its effects on oestrogen-receptor sites (see Chapter 14) for treatment of advanced breast cancer in postmenopausal women with oestrogen receptor–positive and oestrogen receptor–unknown tumours

therapy (HRT) when ovarian activity is blocked or absent. (Box 40.2 lists combination products used as HRT.) Estrogens are also used as palliation for discomforts of menopause when many of the beneficial effects of oestrogen are lost, or as part of combination oral contraceptives (OC), to promote calcium retention in osteoporosis and for palliation in certain cancers that have known receptor sensitivity (see Chapter 14). See Table 40.1 for usual indications for each type of estrogen. See also Box 40.4 for a discussion of the advantages and disadvantages of HRT.

Oestrogens are important for the development of the female reproductive system and secondary sex characteristics. They affect the release of pituitary follicle-stimulating hormone (FSH) and luteinising hormone (LH); cause capillary dilation, fluid retention, protein anabolism and thin the cervical mucus; conserve calcium and phosphorus, and

BOX 40.2 Combination drugs used for menopause

Many fixed-dose combination drugs containing estrogen and a progestin are available specifically for relieving the signs and symptoms associated with menopause in women who have an intact uterus. The benefits include reduction in the risk of osteoporosis and coronary artery disease with short-term use. These drugs are taken as one tablet, once a day. Women should receive regular medical follow-up and monitoring while taking these drugs:

ethinylestradiol/drospirenone (*Yasmin, Yaz*)
estradiol/drospirenone (*Angeliq*)
estradiol/norethisterone (*Kliogest, Kliovance*)
estradiol/dydrogesterone (*Femoston*)
medroxyprogesterone/conjugated estrogen (*Premia*)
norethisterone/estradiol (*Trisequens*)

Also available as a combination patch: estradiol/norethisterone (*Estalis, Kliogest, Kliovance*).

encourage bone formation; inhibit ovulation; and prevent postpartum breast discomfort. Oestrogens are also responsible for the proliferation of the endometrial lining (Figure 40.1). An absence or decrease in oestrogen produces the signs and symptoms of menopause in the uterus, vagina, breasts and cervix. Oestrogens are known to compete with androgens for receptor sites; this trait makes them beneficial in certain androgen-dependent prostate cancers. Oestrogens produce a wide variety of systemic effects, including protecting the heart from atherosclerosis, retaining calcium in the bones and maintaining the secondary female sex characteristics (see Box 39.1 in Chapter 39 for a complete list of estrogen effects).

Pharmacokinetics

Oral estrogens are well absorbed through the gastrointestinal (GI) tract and undergo extensive hepatic metabolism. They are excreted in the urine. Estrogens cross the placenta and enter breast milk.

Contraindications and cautions

Estrogens are contraindicated in the presence of any known allergies to estrogens and in people with idiopathic vaginal bleeding, breast cancer, any oestrogen-dependent cancer or with a history of thromboembolic disorders, including cerebrovascular accident. Heavy smokers are at *increased risk of thrombus and embolus development.*

Estrogens are contraindicated during pregnancy *because of the risk of serious fetal defects* and should be avoided during breastfeeding *because of possible effects on the neonate.* Estrogens should be used cautiously in people with metabolic bone disease *because of the bone-conserving effect of oestrogen, which could exacerbate the disease*; with renal insufficiency, *which could interfere with the renal excretion of the drug and increase the risk for potential adverse effects on fluid and electrolyte balance*; and with hepatic impairment, *which could alter the metabolism of the drug and increase the risk for the adverse effects, including those on the liver and GI tract.*

Adverse effects

Many of the most common adverse effects associated with estrogens involve the genitourinary (GU) tract. They include breakthrough bleeding, menstrual irregularities, dysmenorrhoea, amenorrhoea and changes in libido. Other effects can result from the systemic effects of estrogens, including fluid retention, electrolyte disturbances, headache, dizziness, mental changes, weight changes and oedema. GI effects are also fairly common and include nausea, vomiting, abdominal cramps and bloating and colitis. Potentially serious GI effects, including acute pancreatitis, cholestatic jaundice and hepatic adenoma, have been reported with the use of estrogens.

Clinically important drug–drug interactions

If estrogens are given in combination with drugs that enhance their hepatic metabolism (eg, barbiturates, rifampicin, tetracyclines, phenytoin), serum estrogen levels may decrease. Whenever a drug is added to or removed from a drug regimen that contains estrogens, the health professional should evaluate that drug for possible interactions and consult with the prescriber for appropriate dose adjustments.

Estrogens have been associated with increased therapeutic and toxic effects of corticosteroids, so people taking both drugs should be monitored very closely.

Smoking while taking estrogens should be strongly discouraged because the combination with nicotine increases the risk for development of thrombi and emboli.

Grapefruit juice can inhibit the metabolism of estradiols, leading to increased serum levels. People should be discouraged from drinking large quantities of grapefruit juice if they are taking estrogens. St John's wort can affect the metabolism of estrogens and can make estrogen-containing contraceptives less effective. This combination should be discouraged. Other herbal and alternative therapies used for menopausal symptoms may interact with estrogens.

Progestogens

Progestogens are used as contraceptives, most effectively in combination with estrogens (Box 40.3 lists available contraceptives). They are used to treat primary and secondary amenorrhoea and functional uterine bleeding and as part of fertility programs. Like the estrogens, some progestogens are useful in treating specific cancers with specific receptor-site sensitivity (see Chapter 14). See Table 40.1 for usual indications for each type of progestogen.

The progestogens transform the proliferative endometrium into a secretory endometrium, inhibit the secretion of FSH and LH, prevent follicle maturation and ovulation, inhibit uterine contractions and may have some anabolic and oestrogenic effects. When they are used

BOX 40.3 Contraceptives: forms and dosing

Oral contraceptives are available as monophasic, triphasic and quadriphasic. Active tablets generally begin on the fifth day of the cycle (day 1 of the cycle is the first day of menstrual bleeding).

Missed doses. If 1 tablet is missed, it should be taken as soon as possible, or 2 tablets taken the next day.

Postcoital or emergency contraception ('morning after'). Tablet must be taken within 72 hours after unprotected intercourse. This can be taken as 750 micrograms levonorgestrel followed by a second dose 12 hours after the first, or as a 1.5 mg dose. Available emergency contraception includes:

Levonelle-1	1.5 mg levonorgestrel
NorLevo-1	1.5 mg levonorgestrel
Postinor-1	1.5 mg levonorgestrel

Monophasic oral contraceptives

Brenda-35 ED	2 mg cyproterone acetate, 35 micrograms ethinylestradiol
Brevinor	500 micrograms norethisterone, 35 micrograms ethinylestradiol
Brevinor-1	1 mg norethisterone, 35 micrograms ethinylestradiol
Diane-35 ED	2 mg cyproterone acetate, 35 micrograms ethinylestradiol
Estelle-35 ED	2 mg cyproterone acetate, 35 micrograms ethinylestradiol
Juliet-35 ED	2 mg cyproterone acetate, 35 micrograms ethinylestradiol
Laila-35 ED	2 mg cyproterone acetate, 35 micrograms ethinylestradiol
Levlen ED	150 micrograms levonorgestrel, 30 micrograms ethinylestradiol
Loette	100 micrograms levonorgestrel, 20 micrograms ethinylestradiol
Marvelon 28	150 micrograms desogestrel, 30 micrograms ethinylestradiol
Microgynon 20 ED	100 micrograms levonorgestrel, 20 micrograms ethinylestradiol
Microgynon 30 ED	150 micrograms levonorgestrel, 30 micrograms ethinylestradiol
Microgynon 50 ED	125 micrograms levonorgestrel, 50 micrograms ethinylestradiol
Microlevlen ED	100 micrograms levonorgestrel, 20 micrograms ethinylestradiol
Minulet	75 micrograms gestodene, 30 micrograms ethinylestradiol
Monofeme	30 micrograms ethinylestradiol, 150 micrograms levonorgestrel
Nordette	30 micrograms ethinylestradiol, 150 micrograms levonorgestrel
Norimin	500 micrograms norethisterone, 35 micrograms ethinylestradiol
Norimin-1	1 mg norethisterone, 35 micrograms ethinylestradiol
Norinyl-1	1 mg norethisterone, 50 micrograms mestranol
Valette	30 micrograms ethinylestradiol, 2 mg dienogest
Yasmin	30 micrograms ethinylestradiol, 3 mg drospirenone
Yaz	20 micrograms ethinylestradiol, 3 mg drospirenone
Zoely	2.5 mg nomegestrol, 1.5 mg estradiol

Triphasic oral contraceptives

Logynon ED	Phase 1, 6 tablets: 50 micrograms levonorgestrel, 30 micrograms ethinylestradiol; phase 2, 5 tablets: 75 micrograms levonorgestrel, 40 micrograms ethinylestradiol; phase 3, 10 tablets: 125 micrograms levonorgestrel, 30 micrograms ethinylestradiol
Trifeme	Phase 1, 6 tablets: 50 micrograms levonorgestrel, 30 micrograms ethinylestradiol; phase 2, 5 tablets: 75 micrograms levonorgestrel, 40 micrograms ethinylestradiol; phase 3, 10 tablets
Triphasil	Phase 1, 6 tablets: 50 micrograms levonorgestrel, 30 micrograms ethinylestradiol; phase 2, 5 tablets: 75 micrograms levonorgestrel, 40 micrograms ethinylestradiol; phase 3, 10 tablets: 125 micrograms levonorgestrel, 30 micrograms ethinylestradiol
Triquilar ED	Phase 1, 6 tablets: 50 micrograms levonorgestrel, 30 micrograms ethinylestradiol; phase 2, 5 tablets: 75 micrograms levonorgestrel, 40 micrograms ethinylestradiol; phase 3, 10 tablets: 125 micrograms levonorgestrel, 30 micrograms ethinylestradiol

Quadriphasic oral contraceptives

Qlaira	Phase 1, 2 tablets: 3 mg estradiol valerate; phase 2: 5 tablets: 2 mg estradiol valerate, 2 mg dienogest; phase 3, 17 tablets: 2 mg estradiol valerate, 3 mg dienogest; phase 4, 2 tablets: 1 mg estradiol valerate

Progestogen-only oral contraceptives

Microlut	30 micrograms levonorgestrel
Micronor	350 micrograms norethisterone
Noriday 28	350 micrograms norethisterone

Injectables

Depo-Provera	150 mg medroxyprogesterone, given by deep IM injection q 3 months
Depo-Ralovera	150 mg medroxyprogesterone, given by deep IM injection q 3 months

Continued on following page

BOX 40.3 Contraceptives: forms and dosing *(continued)*

Intrauterine device

Mirena	52 mg levonorgestrel: inserted into the uterus; releases low-dose levonorgestrel over a 5-year period

Vaginal ring

NuvaRing	11.7 mg etonogestrel, 2.7 mg ethinylestradiol; NuvaRing releases an average of 120 micrograms etonogestrel and 15 micrograms ethinylestradiol per 24 hours over 3 weeks. *NuvaRing* is inserted vaginally once a month and kept in place for 3 weeks; after 1 week rest, a new ring is inserted

Subdermal implant

Implanon NXT	68 mg etonogestrel implanted subdermally, effective up to 3 years, may be replaced at that time if desired

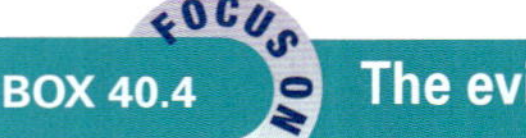

BOX 40.4 The evidence

Menopause and hormone replacement therapy (HRT) – The Women's Health Initiative

Women experience the menarche (onset of the menstrual cycle) in adolescence and menopause (cessation of the menstrual cycle) in midlife. The age at which a woman experiences menopause or 'the change' of life varies. The family history of onset of menopause is a good guide for when the effects can be expected. Just as the physical changes associated with puberty can take a few years to be accomplished, so too can the changes associated with menopause. The signs and symptoms of menopause (vaginal dryness, hot flushes, moodiness, loss of bone density, increased risk of cardiovascular (CV) disease, somnolence) are related to the loss of oestrogen and progesterone effects on the body.

HORMONE REPLACEMENT THERAPY OR NOT?

For centuries, women have proceeded through this time in their lives without pharmacological intervention, although many herbal and alternative therapies may help to ease the transition through menopause (see Box 40.5). Women who rely on these therapies need to be cautioned about potential drug–drug interactions and advised to always report the use of these agents to their health care providers. Today, with more research and safer drugs available to counteract some of the effects of menopause, many women choose to use HRT if the adverse effects of menopause become too uncomfortable or difficult to tolerate. The use of HRT can decrease the discomforts associated with menopause, although various forms of HRT have been associated with increased risks of breast and cervical cancer. Many women are reluctant to consider HRT because of these effects.

The newer drugs used in HRT have been shown to be associated with only a possible increase in risk of breast and cervical cancer, but with long-term use, they are associated with an increased risk of CV events. Women with many risk factors for developing these cancers are at greater risk than women with no risk factors. Other drugs – the oestrogen-receptor modulators – have anti-oestrogen effects on the breast and may remove the cancer risk. However, these drugs may be less reliable in their management of the signs and symptoms of menopause and have not been correlated with a reduction in the risk of coronary artery disease.

EARLY RESEARCH

The Women's Health Initiative was a long-term, multi-site study of the effects of hormones on menopausal women. When the initial reports were published, after the third and fourth years of the study, it seemed that the use of HRT was protective in many ways. It seemed that women using HRT had decreased coronary artery disease and CV events, decreased osteoporosis and bone fractures, decreased breast and colon cancer, and improved memory. HRT was then being prescribed to prevent a number of these chronic conditions.

LATER RESEARCH

In 2002, however, the study was stopped when it was found that women using HRT for 5 or more years had an increased incidence for CV disease and stroke, as well as blood clots, gallstones and ovarian cancer. The news headlines were confusing at best; many women simply stopped HRT, and women new to menopause would not even consider it.

APPLYING THE EVIDENCE

The woman who is entering menopause should have all of the information available before deciding whether HRT is for her. This can be a very difficult decision for many women, because the risks involved may outweigh the benefits or vice versa. The nurse and midwife are often in the best position to provide information, listen to concerns and help the woman to decide what is best for her.

A complete family and personal history of cancer and coronary artery disease risk factors should be completed to help the woman balance the benefits versus the risks of this therapy. If the decision is made to use HRT, the woman may need support in dealing with the effects of the drugs and may have to try several different preparations before the one best suited to her is found. This can be a very frustrating time, so the woman will need a consistent, reliable person to turn to with questions and for support. As researchers continue to study women's health issues, better therapies may be developed to help women through this transition in life. Keeping up with the research as it is reported can be a difficult task, but for anyone who works with women in clinical practice it is a necessity.

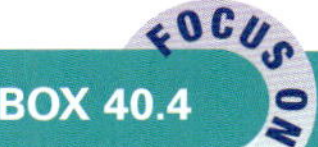

BOX 40.4 The evidence *(continued)*

The current recommendation of the US Preventative Services Task Force is that women should feel comfortable taking HRT to reduce the symptoms of menopause for short-term therapy (fewer than 5 years). The task force summarised all of the studies and noted that long-term use of HRT provides a decreased risk of osteoporosis and related fractures, possibly a reduced risk of dementia and a reduction in risk of colon cancer. The negative aspects of this therapy include a definite but small increased risk for heart disease, stroke and breast cancer. The harms of long-term use outweigh the benefits for most women. The benefits of short-term use, however, must be considered if a woman is having a difficult time getting through menopause (US Preventative Services Task Force, 2002).

Critics of the study also point out that the women in the study were much older than most early postmenopausal groups who could benefit from HRT; they concluded that more research is needed on this issue (Neves-e-Castro, 2003). Follow-up research using this study has found no correlation between use of HRT and the prevention of Alzheimer disease, and no drop in bone fractures in women using HRT.

BOX 40.5 Herbal and alternative therapies

black cohosh: 40 mg/day active ingredient, should not be used for longer than 60 days; monitor for dizziness, nausea, vomiting, visual disturbances; contains alcohol – do not combine with disulfiram, metronidazole.

borage: 90–500 mg/day PO in soft gel capsules, not for long-term use; use caution with seizure disorders or liver impairment.

chaste tree: 150–325 mg PO once or twice daily; may cause increased blood pressure – avoid use with antihypertensives or beta blockers; may cause rash and itching.

clary: 8 drops (gtt) in 30 mL of water daily as an atomiser or dissolved in bath water; may cause sedation – avoid use with alcohol; not for internal use.

devil's claw: 1.5–6 g/day PO depending on preparation; increases stomach acid and may interfere with many prescription drugs; use with caution.

dong quai: 500 mg/day PO; causes photosensitivity – avoid exposure to the sun; do not use with warfarin – increased bleeding can occur.

false unicorn root: 1–2 mL PO three times a day; do not use with estrogen or progestins – may alter uterine effects.

red clover: 4 g PO three times a day as tea; 30–60 gtt PO three times a day of liquid extract; do not use with heparin or warfarin because of increased bleeding effects; do not combine with hormone replacement therapy because of risk of increased oestrogenic effects.

soy: 25 g/day PO; do not use with calcium, iron or zinc products; may decrease effects of estrogen, raloxifene, tamoxifen – alert health care provider if combining these drugs.

wild yam: 1–6 g/day PO; contains progesterone – do not use with hormone replacement therapy; may cause increased blood glucose and other toxic effects; do not combine with disulfiram or metronidazole – severe reaction may occur.

as contraceptives, the exact mechanism of action is not known, but it is thought that circulating progestogens and estrogens 'trick' the hypothalamus and pituitary, and prevent the release of gonadotropin-releasing hormone (GnRH), FSH and LH, thus preventing follicle development and ovulation. The low levels of these hormones do not produce a lush endometrium that is receptive to implantation, and if ovulation and fertilisation were to occur, the chances of implantation would be remote.

Pharmacokinetics

The progestogens are well absorbed, undergo hepatic metabolism and are excreted in the urine. They are known to cross the placenta and to enter breast milk. Like estrogens, progestogens are available in several forms. Etonogestrel, in addition to being available with ethinylestradiol as a vaginal ring (*NuvaRing)*, is available as a subdermal implant (*Implanon NXT*) that may be left in place for up to 3 years and then must be removed. Another implant could be placed at that time. Levonorgestrel is available in combination-form oral contraceptives or as an intrauterine device (*Mirena*). It is also used for emergency contraception as the 'morning after' pill (*Levonelle, Postinor*).

Contraindications and cautions

Contraindications and cautions for progestogens are similar to those for estrogens. Progestogens are also contraindicated in the presence of pelvic inflammatory disease (PID), sexually transmitted infections, endometriosis or pelvic surgery *because of the effects of progestogens on the vasculature of the uterus.* Drospirenone is contraindicated in people who are at risk of hyperkalaemia due to renal disorders, liver disease, adrenal dysfunction or the use of other drugs that can affect potassium levels *because of its antimineralocorticoid effects and the risk of hyperkalaemia.*

Progestogens should be used with caution in people with epilepsy, migraine headaches, asthma or cardiac or renal dysfunction *because of the potential exacerbation of these conditions.*

Adverse effects

Adverse effects associated with progestogens vary with the administration route used. Systemic effects are very similar to the adverse effects of estrogens. Dermal patch contraceptives are associated with the same systemic

Prototype summary: estradiol

Indications: palliation of moderate to severe vasomotor symptoms associated with menopause; prevention of postmenopausal osteoporosis; treatment of female hypogonadism, female castration, female ovarian failure; palliation of inoperable and progressing breast cancer and inoperable prostatic cancer.

Actions: the most potent endogenous female sex hormone, responsible for oestrogenic effects on the body.

Pharmacokinetics:

Route	Onset	Peak	Duration
PO	Slow	Days	Unknown

Topical preparations are not generally absorbed systemically.

$T_{1/2}$: not known; with hepatic metabolism and excretion in the urine.

Adverse effects: corneal changes, photosensitivity, peripheral oedema, chloasma, hepatic adenoma, nausea, vomiting, abdominal cramps, bloating, breakthrough bleeding, change in menstrual flow, dysmenorrhoea, premenstrual-like syndrome.

Prototype summary: norethisterone

Indications: treatment of amenorrhoea, abnormal uterine bleeding due to hormonal imbalance; treatment of endometriosis; component of some hormonal contraceptives.

Actions: progesterone derivative that transforms the proliferative endometrium into a secretory endometrium; inhibits the secretion of pituitary FSH and LH, which prevents ovulation; inhibits uterine contractions.

Pharmacokinetics:

Route	Onset	Peak	Duration
PO	Varies	Unknown	Unknown

$T_{1/2}$: unknown, with hepatic metabolism and excretion in the faeces and urine.

Adverse effects: venous thromboembolism, loss of vision, diplopia, migraine headache, rash, acne, chloasma, alopecia, breakthrough bleeding, spotting, amenorrhoea, fluid retention, oedema, increase in weight.

effects, as well as local skin irritation. Vaginal gel use is associated with headache, nervousness, constipation, breast enlargement and perineal pain. Intrauterine systems are associated with abdominal pain, endometriosis, abortion, PID and expulsion of the intrauterine device. Vaginal use is associated with local irritation and swelling. Drospirenone, used in combination contraceptives, has anti-mineralocorticoid activity and can block aldosterone, leading to increased potassium levels.

Clinically important drug–drug interactions

Interaction with barbiturates, carbamazepine, phenytoin, griseofulvin, penicillins, tetracyclines or rifampicin may reduce the effectiveness of progestogens. People using any of these drugs should use another method of contraception if birth control is needed. St John's wort can affect the metabolism of progestogens and can make progestogen-containing contraceptives less effective. This combination should be discouraged.

OESTROGEN-RECEPTOR MODULATORS

Three available oestrogen-receptor modulators are bazedoxifene (*Duavive*), raloxifene (*Evista*) and toremifene (*Fareston*). The long-term effects of these two drugs are not yet known.

Therapeutic actions and indications

Oestrogen-receptor modulators are not hormones but affect specific oestrogen-receptor sites, stimulating some and blocking others. They were developed to produce some of the positive effects of oestrogen replacement while limiting the adverse effects. See Table 40.1 for usual indications for these drugs. Toremifene is discussed in greater detail in Chapter 14, which discusses antineoplastic agents.

Pharmacokinetics

Administered orally, raloxifene is well absorbed from the GI tract and is metabolised in the liver. Excretion occurs through the faeces. It is known to cross the placenta and enter into breast milk.

Contraindications and cautions

Raloxifene is contraindicated in the presence of any known allergy to raloxifene *to avoid hypersensitivity reactions* and during pregnancy and breastfeeding *because of potential effects on the fetus or neonate.* Caution should be used in people with a history of venous thrombosis or smoking *because of an increased risk of blood clot formation if smoking and estrogen are combined.*

Adverse effects

Raloxifene has been associated with GI upset, nausea and vomiting. Changes in fluid balance may also cause headache, dizziness, visual changes and mental changes. Hot flushes, skin rash, oedema and vaginal bleeding may occur secondary to specific oestrogen-receptor stimulation. Venous thromboembolism is a potentially dangerous side effect that has been reported.

Clinically important drug–drug interactions

Colestyramine reduces the absorption of raloxifene. Highly protein-bound drugs, such as diazepam (*Valium*), ibuprofen (*Brufen*), indometacin (*Indocid*) and naproxen (*Naprosyn*), may interfere with binding sites. Warfarin taken with raloxifene may decrease the prothrombin time (PT); people using this combination must be monitored closely.

 **Prototype summary: raloxifene**

Indications: prevention and treatment of osteoporosis in postmenopausal women.

Actions: increases bone mineral density without stimulating the endometrium; modulates effects of endogenous oestrogen at specific receptor sites.

Pharmacokinetics:

Route	Onset	Peak	Duration
PO	Varies	4–7 hours	24 hours

$T_{1/2}$: 27.7 hours, with hepatic metabolism and excretion in the faeces.

Adverse effects: venous thromboembolism, hot flushes, skin rash, nausea, vomiting, vaginal bleeding, depression, light-headedness.

Care considerations for people receiving sex hormones or oestrogen-receptor modulators

Assessment: history and examination

- Assess for contraindications or cautions: history of allergy to any sex hormone or component of the drug product *to avoid hypersensitivity reactions*; current status related to pregnancy and breastfeeding *due to adverse effects on the fetus and neonate*; hepatic dysfunction *that might interfere with drug metabolism*; cardiovascular disease, breast or genital cancer, renal disease or metabolic bone disease, *which could be exacerbated by estrogen use*; history of thromboembolism or smoking, *which may increase the person's risk for embolic conditions*; idiopathic vaginal bleeding or pelvic disease, *which could represent an underlying problem that could be exacerbated with the use of these drugs*; and history of asthma or epilepsy, *which could be exacerbated by progestogen use.*
- Perform a physical assessment to establish a baseline status before beginning therapy and during therapy *to determine the effectiveness of therapy and evaluate for any potential adverse effects.*
- Assess the abdomen, including auscultation of bowel sounds and palpation of the liver, *to identify abnormalities.* Measure abdominal girth as indicated *to evaluate for bloating.*
- Assess skin colour, lesions and texture; affect, orientation, mental status and reflexes; and blood pressure, pulse, cardiac auscultation, oedema and perfusion, *which will reflect circulatory status and show any changes associated with thromboembolism.*
- Complete or assist with pelvic and breast examinations. Ensure specimen collection for Pap smear; obtain a history of the woman's menstrual cycle *to provide baseline data and to monitor for any adverse effects that could occur.*
- Arrange for ophthalmic examination (particularly if the person wears contact lenses) *because hormonal changes can alter the fluid in the eye and curvature of the cornea, which can change the fit of contact lenses and alter visual acuity.*
- Monitor the results of laboratory tests, including urinalysis and renal and/or liver function tests, *to determine the need for possible dose adjustment and identify early indications of dysfunction.*

See the Critical thinking scenario for additional information related to a person who is taking contraceptives.

Implementation with rationale

- Administer drug as prescribed *to prevent adverse effects*; administer with food if GI upset is severe *to relieve GI distress.*
- Provide analgesics *for relief of headache as appropriate.*
- Strongly urge the woman to stop smoking *to reduce the risk of thromboembolism.*
- Encourage taking of small, frequent meals *to assist with nausea and vomiting.*
- Monitor for swelling and changes in vision or fit of contact lenses *to monitor for fluid retention and fluid changes.*
- Arrange for at least an annual physical examination, including pelvic examination, Pap smear and breast examination, *to reduce the risk of adverse effects and to monitor drug effects.*

- Assess the woman periodically for changes in perfusion or signs of vessel occlusion *because of the risk of thromboembolism.*
- Monitor liver function periodically for the person on long-term therapy *to evaluate liver function and ensure discontinuation of the drug at any sign of hepatic dysfunction.*
- Offer support and reassurance *to deal with the drug and drug effects.*
- Provide thorough teaching, including steps to take if a dose is missed or lost, measures to avoid adverse effects, and signs and symptoms that may indicate a problem and the need for regular evaluation, *to enhance knowledge about drug therapy and to promote compliance.*

Evaluation

- Monitor response to the drug (palliation of signs and symptoms of menopause, prevention of pregnancy, decreased risk factors for coronary artery disease, palliation of certain cancers).
- Monitor for adverse effects (liver changes, GI upset, oedema, changes in secondary sex characteristics, headaches, thromboembolic episodes, breakthrough bleeding).
- Monitor for potential drug–drug interactions as indicated.
- Evaluate the effectiveness of the teaching plan: person can name drug, dosage, adverse effects to watch for, specific measures to avoid them and warning signs and symptoms.
- Monitor the effectiveness of comfort measures and compliance with the regimen.

KEY POINTS

- Oestrogens are hormones associated with the development of the female reproductive system and secondary sex characteristics; pharmacologically, estrogens are used to prevent conception, to stimulate ovulation in women with hypogonadism and, to a lesser extent, to replace hormones after menopause.
- Progestogens maintain pregnancy and are also involved with development of secondary sex characteristics. Progestogens are used as part of combination contraceptives, to treat amenorrhoea and functional uterine bleeding and as part of fertility programs.
- Oestrogen-receptor modulators are used to stimulate specific oestrogen receptors to achieve therapeutic effects of increased bone mass without stimulating the endometrium and causing other, less desirable oestrogenic effects.

CRITICAL THINKING SCENARIO

Birth control

THE SITUATION

J.M. is a 25-year-old woman who is being seen in her gynaecologist's office for a routine annual physical examination and Pap test. J.M. reports that she has just become sexually active and would like to start using contraceptives. She has some concerns about stories she has heard about 'the pill' and would like to know the safest and most effective birth control to use. She is interested in what other methods are available and what the advantages and disadvantages of each form might be.

CRITICAL THINKING

What teaching and counselling issues will be important for J.M. at this time?

What important issues should be discussed when explaining the benefits and drawbacks of various contraceptive measures?

What teaching information needs to be stressed with J.M. if she elects to use oral contraceptives?

DISCUSSION

This appointment presents a good opportunity for the health care provider to allow J.M. to discuss this new aspect of her life. She may have questions about the experience and about things she should be doing or should be questioning. The risk of sexually transmitted infections, as well as pregnancy, can be discussed. J.M. needs full information about the various forms of birth control that are available for use. Non-pharmacological measures such as condoms and the rhythm method and their reliability can be discussed.

The use of hormones for birth control should then be explained, including the 96%–98% reliability of these methods when used correctly. The numerous delivery methods for these hormones should be outlined. A variety of possibilities exists, ranging from the transdermal patch, to injection, to the vaginal ring, to the traditional tablet, and the use of the subdermal implant and intrauterine devices.

J.M. elects to go with an oral contraceptive (OC). She states that she has a good memory, and taking them every day won't be a problem. She swims regularly and thinks that the patch might be an issue if it comes off, and she is not comfortable with anything being injected or inserted into her body. J.M. will need teaching about drug and herbal interactions with the OC and will need to have written instructions on what to do if a dose is missed. The action that should be taken if a dose is missed can be very complicated and involves knowing on which day in the cycle the dose was missed.

It is also important to stress that the OC will not protect J.M. from sexually transmitted infections and that precautions will need to be taken to avoid exposure to these diseases. She should also be advised not to smoke because smoking combined with OC use increases the risk for emboli. The adverse effects that she might experience should be reviewed and the importance of an annual pelvic examination and Pap test should be stressed. A trusting relationship is important at this time so that J.M. can feel free to call with questions or problems in the future.

CARE GUIDE FOR J.M.: ORAL CONTRACEPTIVES

Assessment: history and examination

Assess the woman's health history for allergies to any estrogens, pregnancy or breastfeeding status, breast or genital cancer, hepatic dysfunction, coronary artery disease, thromboembolic disease, renal disease, idiopathic vaginal bleeding, metabolic bone disease, diabetes, and smoking history.

Focus the physical examination on the following:

Neurological: orientation, reflexes, affect, mental status

Skin: colour, lesions

CV: pulse, cardiac auscultation, blood pressure, oedema, perfusion

GI: abdominal examination, liver examination

GU: pelvic examination, Pap smear, urinalysis

Eye: ophthalmological examination

Implementation

Administer medication as prescribed.

Administer with meals if upset stomach is a problem.

Provide analgesics for headache if appropriate.

Advise the woman that if she wears contact lenses, the shape of her cornea may change and she may need a new prescription or may no longer be able to wear them.

Provide at least an annual physical examination, including Pap smear and breast examination.

Monitor perfusion and complaints of pain, tingling or numbness.

Provide support and reassurance to deal with drug therapy.

Provide teaching regarding drug name, dosage, what to do if a dose is missed, adverse effects, precautions, warnings to report and safe administration.

Evaluation

Evaluate drug effects: prevention of pregnancy.

Monitor for adverse effects: signs of liver dysfunction; GI upset; oedema; changes in secondary sex characteristics; headaches; thromboembolic episodes; breakthrough bleeding.

Evaluate the effectiveness of the teaching program and comfort and safety measures.

TEACHING FOR J.M.

- An oral contraceptive (OC), or birth control pill, contains specific amounts of female sex hormones that work to make the body unreceptive to pregnancy and to prevent ovulation (the release of the egg from the ovary). Because these hormones affect many systems in your body, it is important to have regular physical checkups while you are taking this drug.
- Many drugs affect the way that OCs work. To be safe, avoid the use of over-the-counter drugs and other drugs unless you first check with your health care provider.
- Some of the following adverse effects may occur:
  - *Headache, nervousness.* Check with your health care provider about the use of an analgesic; this effect usually passes after a few months on the drug.
  - *Nausea, loss of appetite.* This usually passes with time; consult your health care provider if it is a problem.
  - *Swelling, weight gain.* Water retention is a normal effect of these hormones. Limiting salt intake may help. You may have trouble with contact lenses if you wear them because the body often retains fluid, which may change the shape of your eye. This usually adjusts over time.
  - *Blood clots in women who smoke cigarettes.* Cigarette smoking can aggravate serious side effects of OCs, such as the formation of blood clots. When taking OCs, it is advisable to cut down, or preferably to stop, cigarette smoking.
- Tell any doctor, nurse or other health care provider that you are taking this drug.
- Report any of the following to your health care provider: pain in the calves or groin; chest pain or difficulty breathing; lump in the breast; severe headache, dizziness, visual changes; severe abdominal pain; yellowing of the skin; pregnancy.
- Bleeding (a false menstrual period) should occur during the time that the drug is withdrawn. Report bleeding at *any* other time to your health care provider.
- It is important to have regular medical checkups, including Pap tests, while you are taking this drug. If you decide to stop the drug to become pregnant, consult with your health care provider.
- A package insert is included with the drug. Read this information and feel free to ask any questions that you might have.
- Keep this drug and all medications out of the reach of children.

TABLE 40.2 DRUGS IN FOCUS Fertility drugs

Drug name	Dosage/route	Usual indications
cetrorelix (*Cetrotide*)	250 micrograms SC once daily in lower abdominal wall Morning administration: start day 5–6 of ovarian stimulation, continue until day of ovulation induction Evening administration: start day 5 of ovarian stimulation, continue until evening before ovulation induction	Inhibition of premature LH surges in women undergoing controlled ovarian stimulation
choriogonadotropin alfa (*Ovidrel*)	250 micrograms SC, timing depending on indication	Induction of final follicular maturation and ovulation induction in infertile women
chorionic gonadotropin (*Pregnyl*)	500–10,000 International Units SC depending on timing and indication	Stimulation of ovulation, hypogonadism, prepubertal cryptorchidism
(P) clomifene (*Clomid* and others)	50–100 mg/day PO, with length of therapy and timing dependent on the particular situation	Treatment of infertility; also found to be effective in the treatment of male infertility
follitropin alfa (*Gonal-F*)	75–150 International Units/day SC, dose increases based on response; do not exceed 450 International Units/day	Stimulation of follicular development in the treatment of infertility and for harvesting of ova for in vitro fertilisation
follitropin beta (*Puregon*)	75–225 International Units/day SC, dose increases based on response; do not exceed 300 International Units/day	Stimulation of follicular development in the treatment of infertility and for harvesting of ova for in vitro fertilisation
ganirelix (*Orgalutran*)	250 micrograms/day SC during early follicular phase	Inhibition of premature LH surges in women undergoing controlled ovarian hyperstimulation as part of a fertility program
lutropin alfa (*Luveris*)	37.5–225 units SC with follitropin alfa	Used in combination with follitropin alfa to stimulate follicle development and help to prepare the uterus for implantation
menopausal gonadotropin (*Menopur*)	75–150 International Units/day SC for at least 7 days, dose increased based on response; do not exceed 225 International Units/day	Treatment of anovulatory fertility and controlled ovarian hyperstimulation to induce multiple follicle development

FERTILITY DRUGS

Fertility drugs stimulate the female reproductive system. The following fertility drugs are in use: cetrorelix (*Cetrotide*), chorionic gonadotropin (*Pregnyl*), choriogonadotropin alfa (*Ovidrel*), clomifene (*Clomid* and others), follitropin alfa (*Gonal-F*), follitropin beta (*Puregon*), ganirelix (*Orgalutran*), lutropin alfa (*Luveris*) and menopausal gonadotropin (*Menopur*). Table 40.2 gives more information on these agents.

Therapeutic actions and indications

Women without primary ovarian failure who cannot get pregnant after 1 year of trying may be candidates for the use of fertility drugs. Fertility drugs work either directly to stimulate follicles and ovulation or stimulate the hypothalamus to increase FSH and LH levels, leading to ovarian follicular development and maturation of ova. Given in sequence with human chorionic gonadotropin (HCG) to maintain the follicle and hormone production, these drugs are used to treat infertility in women with functioning ovaries whose partners are fertile. Fertility drugs also may be used to stimulate multiple follicle development for the harvesting of ova for in vitro fertilisation.

Cetrorelix inhibits premature LH surges in women undergoing controlled ovarian stimulation by acting as a GnRH antagonist. Chorionic gonadotropin is used to stimulate ovulation by acting like GnRH and affecting FSH and LH release. Follitropin alfa and follitropin beta are FSH molecules; they are injected to stimulate follicular development in the treatment of infertility and for harvesting of ova for in vitro fertilisation. See Table 40.2 for usual indications for each fertility drug.

Pharmacokinetics

These drugs are well absorbed and are treated like endogenous hormones within the body, undergoing hepatic metabolism and renal excretion. Drugs that are available in injectable form include cetrorelix, chorionic gonadotropin, choriogonadotropin alpha, follitropin alfa, follitropin beta, lutropin alfa and ganirelix. Clomifene is available as an oral agent.

Contraindications and cautions

These drugs are contraindicated in the presence of primary ovarian failure (*they only work to stimulate functioning ovaries*); thyroid or adrenal dysfunction *because of the effects on the hypothalamic–pituitary axis*; ovarian cysts, *which could be stimulated and become larger due to the effects of the drugs*; pregnancy *due to the potential for serious fetal effects*; idiopathic uterine bleeding, *which could represent an underlying problem that could be exacerbated by the stimulatory effects of these drugs*; and known allergy to any fertility drug *to avoid hypersensitivity reactions*.

Caution should be used in women who are breast-feeding *because of the risk of adverse effects on the baby*, in those with thromboembolic disease *because of the risk of increased thrombus formation*, as well as in women with respiratory diseases *because of alterations in fluid volume and blood flow that could overtax the respiratory system*.

Adverse effects

Adverse effects associated with fertility drugs include a greatly increased risk of multiple births and birth defects; ovarian overstimulation (abdominal pain, distension, ascites, pleural effusion); and headache, fluid retention, nausea, bloating, uterine bleeding, ovarian enlargement, gynaecomastia and febrile reactions (possibly due to stimulation of progesterone release).

Prototype summary: clomifene

Indications: treatment of ovarian failure in women with normal liver function and normal endogenous oestrogens; off-label use: treatment of male sterility.

Actions: binds to oestrogen receptors, decreasing the number of available oestrogen receptors, which gives the hypothalamus the false signal to increase FSH and LH secretion, leading to ovarian stimulation.

Pharmacokinetics:

Route	Onset	Peak	Duration
PO	5–8 days	Unknown	6 weeks

$T_{1/2}$: 5 days, with hepatic metabolism and excretion in the faeces.

Adverse effects: vasomotor flushing, visual changes, abdominal discomfort, distension and bloating, nausea, vomiting, ovarian enlargement, breast tenderness, ovarian overstimulation, multiple pregnancies.

Care considerations for people receiving fertility drugs

Assessment: history and examination

- Assess for contraindications or cautions: history of allergy to any fertility drug *to avoid hypersensitivity reactions*; current status of pregnancy and breastfeeding, *which are contraindications or cautions to the use of the drug*; primary ovarian failure, *which would not respond to these agents*; thyroid or adrenal dysfunction *due to effects on hypothalamic–pituitary axis*; ovarian cysts, *which could be stimulated and become larger as a result of the drug's stimulatory effects*; idiopathic uterine bleeding, *which could reflect an underlying medical problem that could be exacerbated by the stimulatory effects of the drug*; thromboembolic diseases, *which could increase the woman's risk for thrombus formation*; and respiratory diseases, *which would be exacerbated by the effects of the drug*.
- Perform a complete physical assessment *to establish baseline status before beginning therapy and during therapy to monitor for any potential adverse effects*.
- Assess skin and lesions; orientation, affect and reflexes; and blood pressure, pulse, respiration and adventitious sounds *to determine cardiac function and perfusion and to detect changes in blood flow or thromboembolism*.
- Complete, or assist with, pelvic and breast examinations and ensure collection of specimen for Pap smear *to establish a baseline of GU health and detect early changes as a result of drug therapy*.
- Monitor the results of laboratory tests, such as renal and hepatic function studies, *to evaluate for possible dysfunction that might interfere with metabolism and excretion of the drug*; and check hormonal levels as indicated *to determine the effectiveness of therapy and reduce the risk of ovarian hyperstimulation*.

Implementation with rationale

- Assess the cause of dysfunction before beginning therapy *to ensure appropriate use of the drug*.
- Complete a pelvic examination before each use of the drug *to rule out ovarian enlargement, pregnancy or uterine problems*.
- Check urine oestrogen and oestradiol levels before beginning therapy *to verify ovarian function*.
- Administer with an appropriate dose of HCG as indicated *to ensure beneficial effects*.

- Discontinue the drug at any sign of ovarian overstimulation and arrange for hospitalisation *to monitor and support the person* if this occurs.
- Provide women with a calendar of treatment days, explanations of adverse effects to anticipate, and instructions on when intercourse should occur *to increase the therapeutic effectiveness of the drug.*
- Provide warnings about the risk and hazards of multiple births *so the person can make informed decisions about drug therapy.*
- Offer support and encouragement *to deal with low self-esteem issues associated with infertility.*
- Provide teaching about proper administration technique, appropriate disposal of needles and syringes, measures to avoid adverse effects, warning signs of problems and the need for regular evaluation *to enhance the person's knowledge about drug therapy and to promote compliance.*

Evaluation

- Monitor woman's response to the drug (ovulation).
- Monitor for adverse effects (abdominal bloating, weight gain, ovarian hyperstimulation, multiple births).
- Evaluate the effectiveness of the teaching plan (woman can name drug, dosage, adverse effects to watch for and specific measures to avoid them).
- Monitor effectiveness of comfort measures and compliance with the regimen.

KEY POINTS

- In women with functioning ovaries, fertility drugs increase follicle development by stimulating FSH and LH to increase the chances for pregnancy.
- Women receiving fertility drugs need to be monitored for ovarian hyperstimulation, need to be aware of the possibility of multiple births and need support and encouragement to deal with the self-esteem issues associated with infertility.

UTERINE MOTILITY DRUGS

Uterine motility drugs stimulate uterine contractions to assist labour or induce termination. Salbutamol, a beta$_2$-selective adrenergic agonist, has been used as a uterine motility agent to relax the gravid uterus to prolong pregnancy. This drug is administered if uterine contractions become strong before term to prevent

TABLE 40.3 ***DRUGS IN FOCUS*** **Uterine motility drugs**

Drug name	Dosage/route	Usual indications
Oxytocics		
carbetocin (*Duratocin*)	100 micrograms by bolus IV injection over 1 minute following birth of baby; given as single dose only	Prevention and treatment of postpartum uterine atony and excessive bleeding following caesarean section under epidural or spinal anaesthesia
ergometrine (generic)	0.2 mg IM	Prevention and treatment of postpartum and postabortion uterine atony; management of third stage of labour
(P) oxytocin (*Syntocinon*)	Induction or enhancement of labour: 5 IU of oxytocin in 500 mL normal saline given at 1–4 milliunits/min IV through an infusion pump; increase as needed, do not exceed 20 milliunits/min; 10 units IM after delivery of the placenta	Induction of labour; promotion of uterine contractions postpartum; management of third stage of labour
Prostaglandins		
(P) dinoprostone (*Cervidil, Prostin E2*)	20 mg vaginal pessary, may repeat q 3–5 hours as needed Vaginal gel: 1 mg intravaginally, additional 1–2 mg may be administered after 6 hours to a maximum of 3 mg	A prostaglandin used for evacuation of the uterus; stimulation of cervical ripening before labour
gemeprost (*Cervagem*)	Pre-operatively: 1 mg pessary into posterior vaginal fornix. Termination: one pessary q 3 hours to maximum of five pessaries	Preoperative cervical softening; first or second trimester pregnancy termination
misoprostol (*GyMiso*)	800 micrograms PO as a single dose, or 2 doses of 400 micrograms within 2 hours Must be administered 36–48 hours after oral mifepristone	Medical termination of pregnancy up to 49 days' gestation

premature labour and delivery, which could result in detrimental effects on the neonate, including death. Salbutamol is usually reserved for use after 20 weeks of gestation, when the fetus has a chance of survival outside of the uterus. If this drug is administered, the person will need to be monitored for sympathetic stimulation in the rest of the body (see Chapter 55, which deals with drugs used to treat obstructive pulmonary diseases, for a full discussion of salbutamol). However, nifedipine (a calcium channel blocker) is now commonly preferred in place of salbutamol. Prostaglandins are often used to 'ripen' the cervix to promote the onset of labour or termination of pregnancy. Oxytocics and prostaglandins are discussed in detail in this section and in Table 40.3.

Oxytocics

Oxytocics stimulate contraction of the uterus, much like the action of the hypothalamic hormone oxytocin, which is stored in the posterior pituitary. These drugs include ergometrine and oxytocin (*Syntocinon*) as well as combined ergometrine and oxytocin (*Syntometrine*).

Therapeutic actions and indications

The oxytocics directly affect neuroreceptor sites to stimulate contraction of the uterus. They are especially effective in the gravid uterus. Oxytocin, a synthetic form of the hypothalamic hormone, also stimulates the lacteal glands in the breast to contract, promoting milk ejection in breastfeeding women. Oxytocics are indicated for the prevention and treatment of uterine atony after birth. This is important to prevent postpartum haemorrhage. See Table 40.3 for usual indications for each of these drugs.

Pharmacokinetics

The oxytocics are rapidly absorbed after parenteral or oral administration, metabolised in the liver and excreted in urine and faeces. They cross the placenta and enter breast milk.

The oxytocics are administered intramuscularly or intravenously.

Contraindications and cautions

Oxytocics are contraindicated in the presence of any known allergy to oxytocics *to avoid hypersensitivity reactions* and with cephalopelvic disproportion, unfavourable fetal position, complete uterine atony or early pregnancy, *which could be compromised by uterine stimulation*. Caution should be used in women with coronary disease and hypertension *due to the effect of causing arterial contraction, which could raise blood pressure or compromise coronary blood flow*, or in women who have had previous caesarean births *because of the effects on uterine contraction, which could compromise scars from previous procedures*. Caution should be used in hepatic or renal impairment, *which could alter the metabolism or excretion of the drug.*

Adverse effects

The adverse effects most often associated with the oxytocics are related to excessive effects (eg, uterine hypertonicity and spasm, uterine rupture, postpartum haemorrhage, decreased fetal heart rate). GI upset, nausea, headache and dizziness are also common. Ergometrine can produce ergotism, manifested by nausea, blood pressure changes, weak pulse, dyspnoea, chest pain, numbness and coldness in extremities, confusion, excitement, delirium, convulsions and even coma. Oxytocin has caused severe water intoxication with coma and even maternal death when used for a prolonged period. This is thought to occur because of related effects of antidiuretic hormone (ADH), which is also stored in the posterior pituitary and may be released in response to oxytocin activity, causing water retention by the kidney.

Prototype summary: oxytocin

Indications: to initiate or improve uterine contractions for early vaginal delivery; to stimulate or reinforce labour in selected cases of uterine inertia; to manage inevitable or incomplete abortion; for second-trimester abortion; to control postpartum bleeding or haemorrhage; to treat breastfeeding deficiency.

Actions: synthetic form stimulates the uterus, especially the gravid uterus; causes myoepithelium of the lacteal glands to contract, resulting in milk ejection in breastfeeding women.

Pharmacokinetics:

Route	Onset	Peak	Duration
IV	Immediate	Unknown	60 min
IM	3–5 min	Unknown	2–3 hours

$T_{1/2}$: 1–6 minutes, with tissue metabolism and excretion in the urine.

Adverse effects: cardiac arrhythmias, hypertension, fetal bradycardia, nausea, vomiting, uterine rupture, pelvic haematoma, uterine hypertonicity, severe water intoxication, anaphylactic reaction.

Care considerations for women receiving oxytocics

Assessment: history and examination

- Assess for contraindications or cautions: history of allergy to oxytocics *to avoid hypersensitivity reactions*; early status of pregnancy, *which might lead to early onset of labour*; current status of breastfeeding; uterine atony, undesirable fetal position and cephalopelvic disproportion, *which could be compromised by the stimulatory effects of the drug*; hypertension, *which could be exacerbated due to the drug's effect on arteries*; and history of caesarean birth, *which could lead to uterine rupture or damage to previous surgical sites due to the drug's stimulatory effect on uterine contraction.*

- Perform a complete physical assessment *to establish a baseline before beginning therapy and during therapy to evaluate drug effectiveness and to determine potential adverse effects.*
- Assess the woman's neurological status, including level of orientation, affect, reflexes and papillary response.
- Monitor vital signs, including pulse and blood pressure; auscultate lungs for evidence of adventitious sounds.
- Assess labour pattern, including uterine contractions, cervical dilation and effacement, and fetal status, including fetal heart rate, rhythm and position. Institute electronic fetal monitoring as appropriate.
- Evaluate uterine tone, noting any indications of atony; assess fundal height and uterine involution, and amount and characteristics of vaginal bleeding.
- Monitor the results of laboratory tests, including coagulation studies and full blood count *to evaluate haematological status.*

Implementation with rationale

- Ensure fetal position (if appropriate) and cephalopelvic proportions *to prevent serious complications of delivery.*
- Regulate oxytocin delivery using an infusion pump between contractions if it is being given to stimulate labour *to regulate dose appropriately.*
- Monitor blood pressure and fetal heart rate frequently during and after administration *to monitor for adverse effects.* Discontinue the drug if blood pressure rises dramatically.
- Monitor uterine tone and involution and amount of bleeding *to ensure safe and therapeutic drug use.*
- Discontinue the drug at any sign of uterine hypertonicity *to avoid potentially life-threatening effects*; provide life support as needed.
- Monitor fetal heart rate and rhythm if given during labour *to ensure safety of the fetus.*

Evaluation

- Monitor woman's response to the drug (uterine contraction, prevention of haemorrhage, milk 'let down').
- Monitor for adverse effects (blood pressure changes, uterine hypertonicity, water intoxication, ergotism).
- Evaluate the effectiveness of the teaching plan (woman can name drug, dosage, adverse effects to watch for and specific measures to avoid them).
- Monitor the effectiveness of comfort measures and compliance with the regimen.

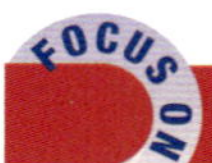

Safe medication administration

Name confusion has been reported among Prostin VR *(alprostadil) and* Prostin E2 *(dinoprostone). Use extreme caution to make sure that the person is receiving the correct drug. Serious adverse effects and lack of therapeutic effects can occur if the wrong drug is given to the person.*

PROSTAGLANDINS

Prostglandins are used to stimulate labour or termination of a pregnancy via intense uterine contractions. The available forms include gemeprost and dinoprostone. Gemeprost (*Cervagem*) is administered via vaginal **pessary** usually for termination of pregnancy. Dinoprostone (*Prostin E2, Cervidil*) assists with ripening the cervix in preparation for induction of labour and stimulates uterine contractions. It is available as a gel or pessary.

Therapeutic actions and indications

Prostaglandins stimulate uterine activity, dislodging any implanted trophoblasts and preventing implantation of any fertilised egg. Gemeprost is approved for use to terminate pregnancy in the second trimester of pregnancy. See Table 40.3 for usual indications for each of these agents.

Pharmacokinetics

These drugs are well absorbed when administered. They are metabolised in the liver and excreted in the urine. Because of their effects on the uterus, they are used during pregnancy only to end the pregnancy. They are not recommended for use during breastfeeding.

Contraindications and cautions

Prostaglandins should not be used with any known allergy to prostaglandins *to avoid hypersensitivity reactions*; after 20 weeks from the last menstrual period, *which would be too late into the pregnancy for a termination*; or with active PID or acute cardiovascular, hepatic, renal or pulmonary disease, *which could be exacerbated by the effects of these drugs*. They are not recommended for use during breastfeeding *because of the potential for serious effects on the neonate*. If these drugs are to be used by a breastfeeding mother, another method of feeding the baby should be used.

Caution should be used with any history of asthma, hypertension or adrenal disease, *which could be exacerbated by the drug effects*, and with acute vaginitis (inflammation of the vagina) or scarred uterus, *which could be aggravated by the uterine contractions*.

Adverse effects

Adverse effects associated with prostaglandins include abdominal cramping, heavy uterine bleeding, perforated uterus and uterine rupture, all of which are related to exaggeration of the desired effects of the drug. Other adverse effects include headache, nausea and vomiting, diarrhoea, diaphoresis (sweating), backache and rash.

Prototype summary: dinoprostone

Indications: evacuation of the uterus in the management of missed abortion or intrauterine fetal death; management of non-metastatic gestational trophoblastic disease; initiation of cervical ripening.

Actions: stimulates the myometrium of the pregnant uterus to contract, evacuating the contents of the uterus.

Pharmacokinetics:

Route	Onset	Peak	Duration
Intravaginal	10 min	15 min	2–3 hours

$T_{1/2}$: 5–10 hours, with tissue metabolism and excretion in the urine.

Adverse effects: headache, paraesthesias, hypotension, vomiting, diarrhoea, nausea, uterine rupture, uterine or vaginal pain, chills, diaphoresis, backache, fever.

Care considerations for women receiving prostaglandins

Assessment: history and examination

- Assess for contraindications or cautions: history of allergy to any prostaglandin preparation *to avoid hypersensitivity reactions*; active PID, *which could be exacerbated by the increased uterine activity*; cardiac, hepatic, pulmonary or renal disease problems, *which could be exacerbated by the effects of the drug*; history of asthma, *which predisposes the woman to hypersensitivity reactions*; hypotension, hypertension and epilepsy, *which require cautious use of the drug*; and scarred uterus or acute vaginitis, *which could be exacerbated by the strong uterine contractions*.
- Perform a complete physical assessment before beginning therapy *to establish baseline status* and during therapy *to determine drug effectiveness and evaluate for any potential adverse effects*.
- Confirm date of last menstrual period and estimated duration of pregnancy *to ensure appropriate use of the drug*.
- Assess vital signs, including skin and lesions; orientation and affect; and blood pressure, pulse and respiration; and auscultate lung sounds, *to monitor for vascular effects, including bleeding and hypersensitivity reactions*.
- Assist with, or complete, a pelvic examination, observe for vaginal discharge and evaluate uterine tone to *monitor effectiveness of the drug and the occurrence of adverse effects*.
- Monitor the results of laboratory tests, including complete blood count, leucocyte count, haemoglobin and haematocrit, *to monitor for excess bleeding*, and urinalysis *to monitor for potential infection or reaction to the procedure*.

Implementation with rationale

- Administer via route indicated, following the manufacturer's directions for storage and preparation, *to ensure safe and therapeutic use of the drug*.
- Confirm the pregnancy gestation before administering the drug *to ensure appropriate use of the drug*.
- Confirm that termination or uterine evacuation is complete by assessing vaginal bleeding and passing of tissue in the vaginal blood *to avoid potential bleeding problems;* prepare for dilation and curettage if necessary *to stop excessive blood loss*.
- Monitor blood pressure frequently during and after administration *to assess for adverse effects*; discontinue the drug if blood pressure rises dramatically.
- Monitor uterine tone and involution and the amount of bleeding during, and for several days after, use of the drug *to ensure appropriate response to and recovery from the drug*.
- Provide support and appropriate referrals *to help the woman deal with the termination or fetal death*.
- Provide teaching, including monitoring necessary during drug administration, comfort measures, signs and symptoms of adverse effects, measures to

minimise or prevent adverse effects, danger signs and symptoms to report immediately, need for follow-up monitoring and evaluation and sources for support and referrals *to enhance the person's knowledge about drug therapy and to promote compliance.*

Evaluation

- Monitor woman's response to the drug (evacuation of uterus).
- Monitor for adverse effects (GI upset, nausea, blood pressure changes, haemorrhage, uterine rupture).
- Evaluate the effectiveness of the teaching plan (woman can name drug, dosage, adverse effects to watch for and specific measures to avoid them).
- Monitor the effectiveness of comfort measures and compliance with the regimen.

KEY POINTS

- Oxytocic drugs act like the hypothalamic hormone oxytocin to stimulate uterine contractions and induce or speed up labour and to control bleeding and promote postpartum involution of the uterus.
- Prostaglandins are drugs that stimulate uterine activity to cause uterine evacuation. These drugs can be used to induce termination in early pregnancy or to promote uterine evacuation after intrauterine fetal death.
- Tocolytics are drugs that relax the uterine smooth muscle; they are used to stop premature labour in women after 20 weeks of gestation.

CHAPTER SUMMARY

- Estrogens are primarily used pharmacologically: to replace hormones lost at menopause to reduce the signs and symptoms associated with menopause, to stimulate ovulation in women with hypogonadism and in combination with progestogens for oral contraceptives.
- Progestogens, which include progesterone and all of its derivatives, are female sex hormones that are responsible for the maintenance of a pregnancy and for the development of some secondary sex characteristics.
- Progestogens are used in combination with estrogens for contraception, to treat uterine bleeding and for palliation in certain cancers with sensitive receptor sites.
- Fertility drugs stimulate FSH and LH in women with functioning ovaries to increase follicle development and improve the chances for pregnancy.
- A major adverse effect of fertility drugs is multiple births and birth defects.
- Oxytocic drugs act like the hypothalamic hormone oxytocin to stimulate uterine contractions and induce or speed up labour and to control bleeding and promote postpartum involution of the uterus.
- Prostaglandins are drugs that stimulate uterine activity to cause uterine evacuation. These drugs can be used to induce labour at term, induce termination in early pregnancy or to promote uterine evacuation after intrauterine fetal death.
- Tocolytics are drugs that relax the uterine smooth muscle; they are used to stop premature labour in women after 20 weeks of gestation.

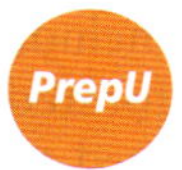

Knowing your strengths and weaknesses helps you to study more effectively. Take a PrepU Practice Quiz to find out how you measure up!

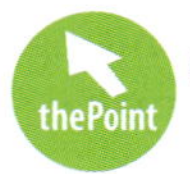

ONLINE RESOURCES

An extensive range of additional resources to enhance teaching and learning and to facilitate understanding of this chapter may be found online at the text's accompanying website, located on thePoint at http://thepoint.lww.com. These include Watch and Learn videos, Concepts in Action animations, journal articles, review questions, case studies, discussion topics and quizzes.

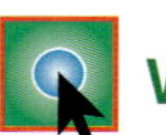

WEB LINKS

Health care providers and students may want to explore the following web resources:

www1.health.gov.au/internet/main/publishing.nsf/Content/national-womens-health-strategy-2020-2030
National Women's Health Strategy: 2020–2030.

www.menopause.org.au/
Australasian Menopause Society.

www.jeanhailes.org.au/
The Jean Hailes Foundation for Women's Health.

www.thewomens.org.au/health-professionals/clinical-resources/clinical-guidelines-gps
The Royal Women's Hospital. Clinical Practice Guidelines.

BIBLIOGRAPHY

Campbell, P. & Pickard, S. (2007). Prescribing and advising on oral contraception. *Nurse Prescribing, 5(1)*, 8–14.

Farrell, M. & Dempsey, J. (2014). *Smeltzer & Bare's Textbook of Medical-Surgical Nursing* (3rd edn). Sydney: Lippincott Williams & Wilkins.

Fehring, R. (2004). The future of professional education in natural family planning. *Journal of Obstetric, Gynecologic, and Neonatal Nursing, 33*, 34–43.

Goodman, L. S., Brunton, L. L., Chabner, B. & Knollmann, B. C. (2011). *Goodman and Gilman's Pharmacological Basis of Therapeutics* (12th edn). New York: McGraw-Hill.

Heiss, G., Wallace, R., Anderson, G. L., Aragaki, A., Beresford, S. A., Brzyski, R., et al.; WHI Investigators. (2008). Health risks and benefits 3 years after stopping randomized treatment with estrogen and progestin. *JAMA, 299*, 1036–1045.
Kass-Wolff, J. H. & Fisher, J. E. (2011). Menopause and the hormone controversy: Clarification or confusion? *Nurse Practitioner, 36(7)*, 22–30.
McKenna, L. & Mirkov, S. (2019). *McKenna's Drug Handbook for Nursing and Midwifery* (8th edn). Sydney: Wolters Kluwer Health Australia
Neves-e-Castro, M. (2003). Menopause in crisis post-Women's Health Initiative? A view based on personal clinical experience. *Human Reproduction, 18*, 2512–2518.
Parke, A. & Abernethy, K. (2008). Hormone replacement therapy: Risks and benefits. *Nurse Prescribing, 6(10)*, 433–439.
Porth, C. M. (2011). *Essentials of Pathophysiology: Concepts of Altered Health States* (3rd edn). Philadelphia: Lippincott Williams & Wilkins.
Porth, C. M. (2009). *Pathophysiology: Concepts of Altered Health States* (8th edn). Philadelphia: Lippincott Williams & Wilkins.
Robinson, G. (2012). Oral contraception for women: A brief overview. *Nurse Prescribing, 10(3)*, 124–145.
U.S. Preventative Services Task Force. (2002). Post-menopausal hormone replacement therapy to prevent chronic conditions: Recommendations. *Annals of Internal Medicine, 127*, 1–4.

CHECK YOUR UNDERSTANDING

Answers to the questions in this chapter can be found in Appendix A in the back of this book.

MULTIPLE CHOICE

Select the best answer to the following.

1. A postmenopausal woman is to receive short-term hormonal replacement therapy to control her menopausal symptoms. Which of the following would the nurse include when teaching the woman about possible adverse effects of this therapy?
   a. constipation
   b. breakthrough bleeding
   c. weight loss
   d. persistently elevated body temperature

2. An oestrogen-receptor modulator might be the drug of choice in the treatment of postmenopausal osteoporosis in a woman with a family history of breast or uterine cancer. The nurse would instruct the woman that she might experience which of the following?
   a. constipation and dry, itchy skin
   b. flushing and dry vaginal mucosa
   c. hot flushes and vaginal bleeding
   d. diarrhoea and weight loss

3. Combination estrogens and progestins are commonly used as oral contraceptives. It is thought that this combination has its effect by:
   a. acting to block the release of FSH and LH, preventing follicle development.
   b. directly suppressing the ovaries and preventing ovulation.
   c. keeping the endometrium constantly lush and blood filled.
   d. preventing menstruation, which prevents pregnancy.

4. Any person who is taking estrogens, progestins or combination products should be cautioned to avoid smoking because:
   a. nicotine increases the metabolism of the hormones, making them less effective.
   b. the risk for potentially dangerous thromboembolic episodes increases.
   c. nicotine amplifies the adverse effects of the hormones.
   d. nicotine blocks hormone receptor sites, and they may no longer be effective.

5. Oxytocin, a synthetic form of the hypothalamic hormone, is used to:
   a. induce labour by stimulating uterine contraction.
   b. stimulate milk production in the breastfeeding woman.
   c. increase fertility and the chance of conception.
   d. relax the gravid uterus to prevent preterm labour.

6. The use of a prostaglandin drug is contraindicated in a woman:
   a. who is 15 weeks pregnant.
   b. who is older than 50 years of age.
   c. who has a history of four previous caesarean births.
   d. who is 10 weeks pregnant.

7. A young woman chooses oral contraceptives because she feels that it is not the right time for her to get pregnant. You would evaluate her teaching about the drug to be effective if she tells you which of the following?
   a. 'I shouldn't smoke for the first month to make sure I don't react severely to the pills.'
   b. 'If I forget to take a pill, I'll just start over the next day with a new series of pills.'
   c. 'I may not be able to wear my contact lenses while taking these pills, or I might have to be fitted for a new pair.'
   d. 'If I have to take an antibiotic while I am using these pills, I should take double pills on those days that I am using the antibiotic.'

MULTIPLE RESPONSE

Select all that apply.

1. Oestrogens produce a wide variety of systemic effects. Effects attributed to oestrogen include:
   a. protecting the heart from atherosclerosis.
   b. retaining calcium in the bones.
   c. maintaining the secondary female sex characteristics.
   d. relaxing the gravid uterus to prolong pregnancy.
   e. stimulating the uterus to increase the chances of conception.
   f. relaxing blood vessels.
2. A woman is taking clomifene after 6 years of inability to conceive a child. The woman will need to be informed about which of the following?
   a. the need for a complete physical and pelvic examination before each course of drug therapy
   b. the risks and hazards of multiple births
   c. the importance of scheduling treatments and intercourse to increase the chance of conception
   d. the need to use oral contraceptives during drug therapy
   e. the need to report blurred vision
   f. common adverse effects include light-headedness, dizziness, and drowsiness
3. A woman is receiving an oxytocic drug to stimulate labour. The care of this woman would include which of the following?
   a. monitoring of fetal heart rate during labour
   b. regulation of drug delivery between contractions
   c. administration of blood pressure–lowering drugs to balance hypertensive effects
   d. monitoring of maternal blood pressure periodically during and after administration
   e. close monitoring of maternal blood loss following delivery
   f. isolation of mother and newborn to prevent infection

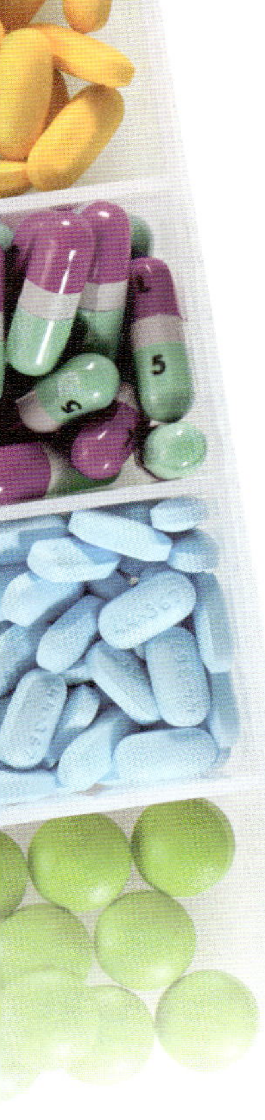

Drugs affecting the male reproductive system

41

Learning objectives

On completing this chapter you should be able to:

1. Discuss the effects of testosterone and other androgens on the male body and use this information to explain the therapeutic and adverse effects of these agents when used clinically.
2. Describe the therapeutic actions, indications, pharmacokinetics, contraindications, most common adverse reactions and important drug–drug interactions associated with drugs affecting the male reproductive system.
3. Discuss the use of drugs that affect the male reproductive system across the lifespan.
4. Compare and contrast the prototype drugs testosterone and sildenafil with other agents in their class.
5. Outline the nursing considerations, including important teaching points, for men receiving drugs used to affect the reproductive system.

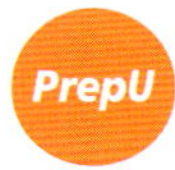

Test your current knowledge of drugs affecting the male reproductive system with a PrepU Practice Quiz!

Glossary of key terms

anabolic steroids: androgens developed with more anabolic or protein-building effects than androgenic effects
androgenic effects: effects associated with development of male sexual characteristics and secondary characteristics (eg, deepening of voice, hair distribution, genital development, acne)
androgens: male sex hormones, primarily testosterone; produced in the testes and adrenal glands
hirsutism: hair distribution associated with male secondary sex characteristics (eg, increased hair on trunk, arms, legs, face)
hypogonadism: underdevelopment of the gonads (testes in the male)
penile erectile dysfunction: condition in which the corpus cavernosum does not fill with blood to allow for penile erection; can be related to ageing or to neurological or vascular conditions

ANDROGENS
danazol
mesterolone
(P) testosterone

ANABOLIC STEROIDS
nandrolone

DRUGS FOR TREATING PENILE ERECTILE DYSFUNCTION
alprostadil
avanafil
 sildenafil
tadalafil
vardenafil

Drugs that are used to affect the male reproductive system include androgens (male steroid hormones), anabolic steroids and drugs that act to improve penile dysfunction. The male steroids are produced in the testes and affect the entire male reproductive system (Figure 41.1). Box 41.1 describes the effect of these drugs across the lifespan.

ANDROGENS

Androgens are male sex hormones and include testosterone, which is produced in the testes, and the androgens, which are produced in the adrenal glands. Testosterone, the primary natural androgen, is the classic androgen in use today. It is used for replacement therapy in cases

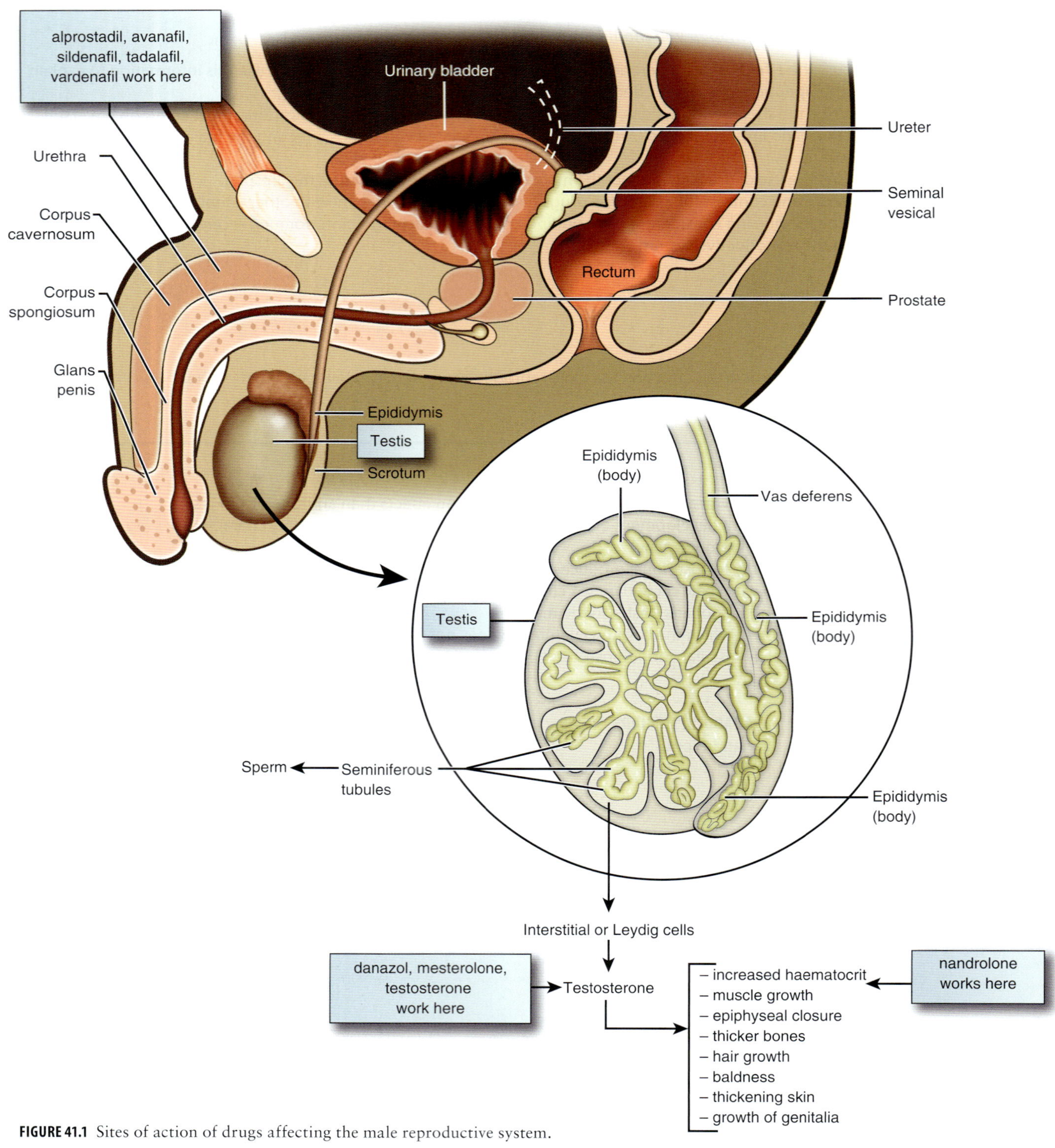

FIGURE 41.1 Sites of action of drugs affecting the male reproductive system.

BOX 41.1 FOCUS ON Drug therapy across the lifespan

Drugs affecting the male reproductive system

CHILDREN

These drugs are used in children as replacement therapy and to increase red blood cell production in renal failure. Because of the effects of these hormones on epiphyseal closure, children should be closely monitored with hand and wrist radiographs pretreatment and every 6 months. If precocious puberty occurs, the drug should be stopped.

Adolescents who are prescribed androgens should be alerted to the potential for increased acne and other effects.

Adolescent athletes need constant education about the risks associated with the use of anabolic steroids to improve athletic prowess and the lack of scientific evidence of beneficial effect.

ADULTS

Adults also need reinforcement of the information about anabolic steroid use and athletics.

Women who are prescribed these drugs may experience masculinising effects and may need support in coping with these body changes. Men who are receiving these drugs for replacement therapy may need to learn self-injection techniques and may benefit from information on depot forms or dermal systems. Periodic liver function tests are important in monitoring the effects of these drugs on the liver.

PREGNANCY AND BREASTFEEDING

These drugs are not indicated for use in pregnancy or breastfeeding because of the potential for serious effects on the male fetus or neonate.

OLDER ADULTS

Older adults may have problems with androgen therapy because of underlying conditions that are aggravated by the drug effects. Hypertension, heart failure and coronary artery disease may be aggravated by the fluid retention associated with these drugs. Benign prostatic hypertrophy, a common problem in older men, may be aggravated by androgenic effects that may enlarge the prostate further, leading to urinary difficulties and increased risk of prostate cancer.

Many older adults have hepatic dysfunction and these drugs can be hepatotoxic. Older people should be monitored very carefully and dose should be reduced. If signs of liver failure or hepatitis occur, the drug should be stopped immediately.

of **hypogonadism** (underdeveloped testes) and to treat certain breast cancers. The usual dosages and indications can be found in Table 41.1.

Therapeutic actions and indications

The androgens are forms of testosterone. They are responsible for the growth and development of male sex organs and the maintenance of secondary sex characteristics. They act to increase the retention of nitrogen, sodium, potassium and phosphorus and to decrease the urinary excretion of calcium. Testosterones increase protein anabolism and decrease protein catabolism (breakdown). They also increase the production of red blood cells. Hence, they can also be used for delayed male puberty or hypogonadism. Testosterone is long acting and is available in several forms, including depot (deep, slow-release) injections and a dermal patch. Mesterolone (*Proviron*) is an

TABLE 41.1 DRUGS IN FOCUS Androgens

Drug name	Dosage/route	Usual indications
danazol (*Azol*)	200–800 mg daily in 2–4 divided doses, depending on condition	Blockade of follicle-stimulating hormone and luteinising hormone release in women to prevent ovulation for treatment of endometriosis; prevention of hereditary angioedema
mesterolone (*Proviron*)	Initially 25–50 mg PO tid; maintenance 25 mg bd–tid	Replacement therapy in male hypogonadism
(P) testosterone (*Androderm, Testogel*), testosterone cypionate (*Depo Testosterone*), testosterone esters (*Sustanon*), testosterone enantate (*Primoteston Depot*), testosterone undecanoate (*Andriol Testocaps, Reandron 1000*)	Transdermal patch: 2.5–7.5 mg/day Cream 1% 2% or 5%: apply once daily Transdermal solution: 30 mg (1.5 mL)/day; maximum 120 mg/day Transdermal gel: 50 mg (5 g of gel) daily IM injection: 250 mg/1 mL every 3 weeks or 1000 mg every 10–14 weeks PO capsules: 40–160 mg/day	Replacement therapy in hypogonadism; treatment of delayed puberty in males and certain breast cancers in postmenopausal women; prevention of postpartum breast engorgement

androgen derivative available in oral form. Danazol, a synthetic androgen, is also long-acting but is available only in oral form.

Pharmacokinetics

The androgens are well absorbed and widely distributed throughout the body. They are metabolised in the liver and excreted in the urine. It is not known whether androgens enter breast milk (see Contraindications and cautions).

Contraindications and cautions

These drugs are contraindicated with any known allergy to the drug or ingredients in the drug; during pregnancy and breastfeeding *because of potential adverse effects on the male neonate* (another method of feeding the baby should be used if these drugs are needed during breastfeeding); and in the presence of prostate or breast cancer in men, *which could be aggravated by the testosterone effects of the drugs.* They should be used cautiously in the presence of any liver dysfunction or cardiovascular disease *because these disorders could be exacerbated by the effects of the hormones.*

Adverse effects

Androgenic effects include acne, oedema, **hirsutism** (increased hair distribution), deepening of the voice, oily skin and hair, weight gain, decrease in breast size and testicular atrophy. Anti-oestrogen effects – flushing, sweating, vaginitis, nervousness and emotional lability – can be anticipated when these drugs are used with women. Other common effects include headache (possibly related to fluid and electrolyte changes), dizziness, sleep disorders and fatigue, rash and altered serum electrolytes. A potentially life-threatening effect that has been documented is hepatocellular cancer. This may occur because of the effect of testosterone on hepatic cells. People on long-term therapy should have liver function tests monitored regularly – before beginning therapy and every 6 months during therapy.

Clinically significant drug–laboratory test interferences

While a person is taking androgens, there may be decreased thyroid function, as well as increased creatinine clearance, results that are not associated with disease states. These effects can last up to 2 weeks after the discontinuation of therapy.

 **Prototype summary: testosterone**

Indications: replacement therapy in hypogonadism, inoperable breast cancer.

Actions: primary natural androgen, responsible for growth and development of male sex organs and maintenance of secondary sex characteristics; increases the retention of nitrogen, sodium, potassium and phosphorus; decreases urinary excretion of calcium; increases protein anabolism; stimulates red blood cell production.

Pharmacokinetics:

Route	Onset	Peak
IM	Slow	1–3 days
IM cypionate	Slow	2–4 weeks
IM esters	Slow	2–4 weeks
Dermal	Rapid	24 hours

$T_{1/2}$: 10–100 minutes, with hepatic metabolism and excretion in the urine and faeces.

Adverse effects: dizziness, headache, sleep disorders, fatigue, rash, androgenic effects (acne, deepening voice, oily skin), hypo-oestrogenic effects (flushing, sweating, vaginitis), polycythaemia, nausea, hepatocellular carcinoma.

Care considerations for people receiving androgens

Assessment: history and examination

- Assess for contraindications or cautions to the use of the drug, including history of allergy to any testosterone or androgen *to avoid hypersensitivity reactions*; pregnancy or breastfeeding *to avoid potential adverse effects on the male fetus or baby*; hepatic dysfunction *to avoid the risk of hepatocellular disorders*; and cardiovascular disease and breast or prostate cancer in men, *which could be aggravated by the drug.*
- Perform a physical assessment *to determine baseline status before beginning therapy and for any potential adverse effects.*
- Assess skin colour, lesions, texture and hair distribution *to monitor for drug effects on the body and potential adverse effects.*
- Monitor affect, orientation and peripheral sensation *to assess central nervous system (CNS) effects related to drug use.*
- Perform abdominal examination and serum electrolytes, serum cholesterol and liver function tests *to monitor for potential effects on liver function.*
- Arrange for radiography of the long bones in children *to assess for testosterone effects on growth.*

Implementation with rationale

- Reconstitute the drug according to the manufacturer's directions *to ensure proper reconstitution and to administer as prescribed.*
- Remove any old dermal system before applying a new system to clean, dry, intact skin *to ensure accurate administration and decrease risk of toxic levels.*

- Monitor response carefully when beginning therapy *so that the dose can be adjusted accordingly.*
- Monitor liver function periodically with long-term therapy, and *arrange to discontinue the drug at any sign of hepatic dysfunction.*
- Provide thorough teaching, including measures to avoid adverse effects, warning signs of problems and the need for regular evaluation, including blood tests. Instruct a family member or carer in proper preparation and administration techniques as appropriate *to enhance knowledge about drug therapy and to promote compliance with the drug regimen.*

Evaluation

- Monitor response to the drug.
- Monitor for adverse effects (androgenic effects, cardiac effects, serum electrolyte imbalance, headache, sleep disturbances, rash, hepatocellular carcinoma).
- Evaluate the effectiveness of the teaching plan (person can name drug, dosage, adverse effects to watch for and specific measures to avoid them; family member or carer can demonstrate proper technique for preparation and administration of the drug as appropriate).
- Monitor the effectiveness of comfort measures and compliance with the regimen.

KEY POINTS

- Androgens are the male sex hormones that are responsible for the development and maintenance of male sex characteristics and secondary sex characteristics or androgenic effects.
- Androgens are used for replacement therapy or to block other hormonal effects.

ANABOLIC STEROIDS

The **anabolic steroids** are analogues of testosterone that have been developed to produce the tissue-building effects of testosterone with less androgenic effect. Nandrolone is an available form for the management of acute and chronic renal failure and associated anaemia.

Therapeutic actions and indications

Anabolic steroids promote body tissue-building processes, reverse catabolic or tissue-destroying processes and increase haemoglobin and red blood cell mass. Indications for particular anabolic steroids vary with the drug (see Table 41.2). They can be used to treat anaemias, certain cancers and angioedema, to promote weight gain and tissue repair in debilitated people, and protein anabolism in individuals who are receiving long-term corticosteroid therapy.

Anabolic steroids are also known to be used illegally for the enhancement of athletic performance by promoting increased muscle mass, increased haematocrit and, theoretically, an increase in strength and endurance. The adverse effects of these drugs can be deadly when they are used in the amounts needed for enhanced athletic performance (see Adverse effects).

Pharmacokinetics

Like the androgens, the anabolic steroids are well absorbed and widely distributed throughout the body. They are metabolised in the liver and excreted in the urine. Anabolic steroids are contraindicated for use in pregnancy because of adverse effects on the male fetus. It is not known whether anabolic steroids enter breast milk, but because of the potential for adverse effects, another method of feeding the baby should be used if these drugs are needed during breastfeeding.

Contraindications and cautions

These drugs are contraindicated in the presence of any known allergy to anabolic steroids; during pregnancy and breastfeeding *because of potential masculinisation in the neonate*; and in the presence of liver dysfunction *because these drugs are metabolised in the liver and are known to cause liver toxicity*, and coronary disease *because of cholesterol-raising effects through effects on the liver* or prostate or breast cancer in males.

Adverse effects

In prepubertal males, adverse effects include virilisation (eg, phallic enlargement, hirsutism, increased skin pigmentation). Postpubertal males may experience inhibition of testicular function, gynaecomastia, testicular

TABLE 41.2 DRUGS IN FOCUS Anabolic steroids

Drug name	Dosage/route	Usual indications
Nitrates		
nandrolone (*Deca-Decabolin*)	25–150 mg/week to q 2–3 weeks, depending on condition, by deep IM injection	Treatment of acute renal failure, chronic renal insufficiency or associated anaemia, management of inoperative breast cancer, osteoporosis, aplastic anaemia; promotion of catabolism with prolonged corticosteroid use

atrophy, priapism (a painful and continual erection of the penis), baldness and change in libido (increased or decreased). Women may experience hirsutism, hoarseness, deepening of the voice, clitoral enlargement, baldness and menstrual irregularities. As with the androgens, serum electrolyte changes, liver dysfunction (including life-threatening hepatitis), insomnia and weight gain may occur. These drugs all have black box warnings as alerts to the potentially serious effects of liver tumours, hepatitis and blood lipid level changes that might be associated with increased risk of coronary artery disease. There is an increased risk of prostate problems, especially in older people.

See the Critical thinking scenario for additional information about treating a person experiencing adverse effects of anabolic steroids.

Clinically important drug–drug interactions

Because the anabolic steroids affect the liver, there is a potential for interaction with oral anticoagulants and a potentially decreased need for hypoglycaemic agents, which may not be metabolised normally. They may alter lipid metabolism and cause a lack of effectiveness for lipid-lowering agents. People should be monitored closely and appropriate dose adjustments made. People who are taking a prescribed androgen or anabolic steroid for a medical condition should check with their health care provider before taking any complementary and alternative therapies because of a risk of adverse effects (see Box 41.2).

Care considerations for people receiving anabolic steroids

Assessment: history and examination

- Assess for the following conditions, *which could be cautions or contraindications to use of the drug*: history of allergy to any androgens or anabolic steroids; pregnancy or breastfeeding *because of masculinisation of the neonate*; prostrate or breast cancer; coronary disease; and hepatic dysfunction.
- Perform a physical assessment *to determine baseline status before beginning therapy and for any potential adverse effects.*
- Assess skin colour, lesions, texture and hair distribution *to monitor for drug effects on the body and potential adverse effects.*
- Monitor affect, orientation and peripheral sensation *to assess CNS effects related to drug use.*
- Perform abdominal examination and serum electrolytes, serum cholesterol and liver function tests *to monitor for potential effects on liver function.*
- Arrange for radiography of the long bones in children *to assess for testosterone effects on growth.*

Implementation with rationale

- Administer with food if GI effects are severe *to relieve GI distress.*

BOX 41.2 FOCUS ON Herbal and alternative therapies

With an increasing awareness of the risks associated with anabolic steroid use and increasing pressures to make it difficult to get these drugs even illegally, there is an increased push in advertising of alternative or 'natural' products that are reported to enhance athletic performance.

Bee pollen – reported to contain amino acids and other minerals and enzymes.There are no scientific studies regarding its effectiveness. Serious allergic reactions have been reported with the use of this product. Random studies have found a wide variety of ingredients in each product, depending on the season, growing conditions and geographical area.

Creatine – contains a substance that is found in muscle and naturally occurs in red meats and other dietary sources. No scientific data are available on its actual effects on energy or athletic performance. It interacts with many other drugs, including non-steroidal anti-inflammatory drugs, cimetidine, probenecid and trimethoprim, and can cause serious effects on kidney functioning. Users should be advised to drink plenty of fluids while taking this drug and to monitor for swelling, muscle cramps and dizziness. Suggested only for short-term use.

Damiana – used to increase muscle strength, as an aphrodisiac and to boost mental health. It can cause liver toxicity. It interferes with antidiabetic agents and causes elevated blood sugar concentrations. Users should report muscle spasms or hallucinations.

Spirulina – used to increase energy and boost metabolism. It may contain toxic metals and can cause serious reactions in children and pets. It interferes with vitamin B12 absorption. No scientific studies validate the claims of its effectiveness.

Wild yam – found to have many oestrogen-like effects, this herb is used to increase athletic performance because it may contain a constituent of dehydroepiandrosterone (DHEA) used to slow the ageing process and to improve energy and stamina. Preparations interact with disulfiram and metronidazole because they contain alcohol. It is known to be toxic to the liver. Users may experience oestrogen-like effects, including breast pain. Users should be monitored closely and urged to report any adverse effects.

- Monitor endocrine function, hepatic function and serum electrolytes before and periodically during therapy *so that dose can be adjusted appropriately and severe adverse effects can be avoided.*
- Arrange for radiography of the long bones of children every 3–6 months *so that the drug can be discontinued if bone growth reaches the norm for the child's age.*
- Provide thorough teaching, including measures to avoid adverse effects and warning signs of problems, as well as the need for regular evaluation, including blood tests, *to enhance knowledge about drug therapy and to promote compliance with the drug regimen.*

Evaluation

- Monitor response to the drug (increase in haematocrit, protein anabolism).
- Monitor for adverse effects (androgenic effects, serum electrolyte disturbances, epiphyseal closure, hepatic dysfunction, personality changes, cardiac effects).
- Evaluate the effectiveness of the teaching plan (person can name drug, dosage, adverse effects to watch for and specific measures to avoid them).
- Monitor the effectiveness of comfort measures and compliance with the regimen.

KEY POINTS

- Anabolic steroids are testosterone analogues with more anabolic or protein-building effects than androgenic effects.
- Deadly effects may result from the abuse of anabolic steroids by athletes trying to build muscle mass and improve performance.

CRITICAL THINKING SCENARIO

Adverse effects of anabolic steroids

THE SITUATION

Senior nursing student K.S. recently became engaged. Her fiancé is a university senior who is training as a javelin thrower in hopes of competing in the Olympics. K.S. noticed that her fiancé had been suffering from GI upset for the last 3 weeks and more recently had developed tremors and muscle cramps. K.S. first suspected that he was suffering from a viral infection, but when the symptoms did not resolve, she became concerned. K.S. tried to get her fiancé to see a doctor, but he refused. Eventually, he admitted that he had begun using anabolic steroids to develop his muscles and improve his athletic prowess. He said that the friend who gave him the drugs told him that stomach upset was normal. He refuses to see a doctor because he knows that the use of these drugs is illegal. He believes that using the anabolic steroids for a while will put him closer to his goal. K.S. accepts his explanation but is upset about the use of anabolic steroids. She consults with her clinical instructor about the effects of these drugs.

CRITICAL THINKING

What does K.S. need to know? *Think about the systemic effects of anabolic steroids and the possible long-term effects from their abuse.*

What implications do these effects have for the athlete? *Consider the concern that K.S. must be experiencing. Suggest ways for K.S. to share the information about the actual effects of anabolic steroids with her fiancé and still cope with her own feelings and concerns.*

What are the ethical and legal issues involved when a heathcare provider knows about illegal drug use and abuse? *Outline a plan for helping K.S. and her fiancé cope with this issue and its implications for their futures.*

DISCUSSION

Use of anabolic steroids is illegal in almost all organised athletic contests. Random drug testing is done to rule out use of these and other drugs. Not surprisingly, K.S. feels insecure about her fiancé's decision. She needs to know that her discussion will be confidential and that she will receive support for her concerns and her fears. K.S. needs to review the effects of anabolic steroids. Although they do promote muscle development, there has never been any evidence that they actually improve athletic performance. The potential adverse effects of these drugs can be deadly, especially if K.S.'s fiancé is receiving the drugs from a friend and has no medical evaluation or dosage guidance to reduce the risk. Personality changes, cardiomyopathy, liver cancer and impotence are just a few of the possible adverse effects.

K.S. is in a precarious position. She does not want to interfere with her fiancé's dreams or cause problems in their relationship. She should be encouraged to explain the adverse effects of the drugs to her fiancé, pointing out that he is already experiencing some of them. Adverse effects associated with the drugs can ultimately interfere with, not enhance, his athletic performance. She might be encouraged to practise what she will tell her fiancé and to seek other support as needed.

The sale or distribution of anabolic steroids without a prescription is illegal, and this fact further complicates the situation for K.S. Because she is planning to become a health care provider, she may be obliged by law to report this information to the authorities. K.S. should research these issues and discuss them further with her clinical instructor and other resource people.

CARE GUIDE FOR K.S.: ANDROGENS, ANABOLIC STEROIDS

A person receiving an anabolic steroid for a medical condition would have the following care plan:

Assessment: history and examination

Assess the person's health history for allergies to any steroids, breast cancer or prostate cancer in men, hepatic dysfunction, coronary artery disease, pregnancy or breastfeeding in women, or concurrent use of insulin or oral anticoagulants.

Focus the physical examination on the following:

Neurological: orientation, reflexes, affect

Skin: colour, lesions, hair

CV: pulse, cardiac auscultation, blood pressure, oedema

GI: abdominal examination, liver examination

Laboratory tests: serum electrolytes, liver function tests, long-bone X-ray studies

Implementation

Administer as prescribed.

Monitor liver function before and periodically during therapy.

Monitor response and adjust dose as appropriate.

Provide support and reassurance to deal with drug therapy.

Provide teaching regarding drug name, dosage, adverse effects, precautions, warnings to report and safe administration.

Evaluation

Evaluate drug effects: maintenance of male sex characteristics, suppression of breastfeeding in women.

Monitor for adverse effects: androgenic effects, hypo-oestrogenic effects, hepatic dysfunction, electrolyte imbalance, endocrine changes.

Monitor for drug–drug interactions: decreased need for insulin, increased bleeding with oral anticoagulants.

Evaluate the effectiveness of the teaching program and comfort and safety measures.

TEACHING FOR K.S.

If the person is taking these drugs to increase body mass after severe weight loss due to trauma, you would teach about the following. Sharing this information with those considering the unprescribed use of the drugs might be helpful.

- Androgens or anabolic steroids have properties similar to those of the male sex hormones. Because the formulations have widespread effects, there are often many adverse effects associated with their use.
- These drugs are controlled substances because the tendency for people, and athletes in particular, to abuse them can cause serious medical problems. When the drug is used as prescribed, it is safe, but you will need to be monitored.
- Some of the following adverse effects may occur:
  - *GI upset, nausea, vomiting:* taking the drug with food usually helps to relieve these effects.
  - *Acne:* this is a hormonal effect; washing your face regularly and avoiding oily foods may help.
  - *Increased facial hair, decreased head hair:* these are hormonal effects; if they become bothersome, consult with your health care provider.
  - *Menstrual irregularities (women):* this is a normal effect of the androgens; if you suspect that you might be pregnant, consult with your health care provider immediately.
  - *Weight gain, increased muscle development:* these are common hormonal effects.
  - *Change in sex drive:* this can be distressing and difficult to deal with; consult with your health care provider if this is a serious concern.
  - (Report any of the following to your health care provider): swelling in fingers or legs; continual erection; uncontrollable sex drive; yellowing skin; fever, chills or rash; chest pain or difficulty breathing; hoarseness, loss of hair or growth of facial hair (women).
- Tell any doctor, nurse or other health care provider involved in your care that you are taking this drug.
- Take this medicine only as directed. In addition schedule regular medical follow-up, including blood tests, to monitor your response to this drug.
- Keep this drug and all medications out of the reach of children. Do not give this medication to anyone else or take any similar medication that has not been prescribed for you.

DRUGS FOR TREATING PENILE ERECTILE DYSFUNCTION

Penile erectile dysfunction is a condition in which the corpus cavernosum does not fill with blood to allow for penile erection. This can result from the ageing process and in vascular and neurological conditions. Two very different types of drugs are approved for the treatment of this condition. These include the prostaglandin alprostadil (*Caverject*) and the phosphodiesterase type 5 (PDE5) receptor inhibitors avanafil (*Spedra*) and sildenafil (*Viagra*, also available as *Revatio* for the treatment of pulmonary

BOX 41.3 FOCUS ON The evidence

Viagra – wonder drug?

The release of the drug sildenafil (*Viagra*) to treat penile erectile dysfunction caused a tremendous stir in society. This was the first oral drug developed to treat a disorder that was common in ageing men but was seldom mentioned or discussed. *Viagra*, which facilitates penile erection approximately 1 hour after it is taken, returned sexual function to many of these men.

For many months after its release, the drug was the centre of controversy, news coverage and debate. Stand-up comedians, television situation comedies and Internet joke networks were buzzing with the latest *Viagra* jokes. Insurance companies debated covering the cost of this drug. Was it like cosmetic surgery, and not a necessary treatment, or was it a necessary aid to human physiology? Most insurance companies ended up covering the cost of *Viagra*.

Women's rights groups voiced concern that no drug was approved and covered to help facilitate a woman's sexual response. *Viagra* is in trial stages for the treatment of sexual dysfunction in women; early reports seem to indicate that it is not effective. However, *Viagra* has proven to be very effective at increasing sexual functioning for many men. Its success has led to the development of three other drugs in the same class of phosphodiesterase type 5 (PDE5) inhibitors, avanafil (*Spedra*), tadalafil (*Cialis*) and vardenafil (*Levitra*).

The use of these drugs is not without risks. Deaths have occurred when these drugs were combined with nitrates (eg, glyceryl trinitrate) or alpha-adrenergic blockers. Headache, flushing, stomach upset and urinary tract infections often occur. There have been reports of sudden loss of vision and hearing. These drugs can be used only once daily, and they do not work without sexual stimulation. Absorption is delayed if they are taken with a high-fat meal, and people need to plan accordingly. People also should be reminded that they need to use protection against sexually transmitted infections.

When *Viagra* was the hot, new drug, there was tremendous demand for it from the public. This demand put health care providers in the position of ensuring that the drug was right for the person's actual needs. The cause of penile erectile dysfunction should be determined, if at all possible. If this is a problem that the person has never before discussed with the health care provider, there could be an underlying medical condition that should be addressed. The adverse effects, timing of administration and drug combinations to avoid should be discussed with the person before the drug is prescribed.

With pharmaceutical companies now advertising in magazines, on television and over the Internet, health care providers are often asked for specific prescription drugs based on media advertising. This relatively new phenomenon in health care presents new challenges to the health care provider to ensure quality teaching to help the person understand the actual uses, effects and rationales for a specific drug therapy.

hypertension), tadalafil (*Cialis*) and vardenafil (*Levitra*). Box 41.3 contains more information about *Viagra*.

Therapeutic actions and indications

When injected directly into the cavernosum, alprostadil acts locally to relax the vascular smooth muscle and allow filling of the corpus cavernosum, causing penile erection. The PDE5 inhibitors avanafil, sildenafil, tadalafil and vardenafil are selective inhibitors of cyclic guanosine monophosphate (cGMP). The PDE5 inhibitors are taken orally and act to increase nitrous oxide levels in the corpus cavernosum. Nitrous oxide activates the enzyme cGMP, which causes smooth muscle relaxation, allowing the flow of blood into the corpus cavernosum. They prevent the breakdown of cGMP by phosphodiesterase, leading to increased cGMP levels and prolonged smooth muscle relaxation, thus promoting the flow of blood into the corpus cavernosum, resulting in penile erection.

The prostaglandin alprostadil and the PDE5 inhibitors are indicated for the treatment of penile erectile dysfunction. The PDE5 inhibitors have the advantage of being oral drugs that can be timed in coordination with sexual activity, based on the drug's onset. Sildenafil (*Revatio*) is also approved for the treatment of pulmonary arterial hypertension. By relaxing smooth muscle, the pulmonary artery relaxes and there is less resistance and pressure in the pulmonary bed. Tadalafil is also approved for daily use in men who are very active sexually. A person might select this drug if the timing of sexual stimulation is not known and may be several hours away. See Table 41.3 for usual indications for all four of these drugs.

Pharmacokinetics

After injection, alprostadil is metabolised to inactive compounds in the lungs and excreted in the urine. The PDE5 inhibitors are well absorbed from the GI tract, undergo metabolism in the liver and are excreted in the faeces. The differences among the three PDE5 inhibitors lie in their onset and duration of action. Sildenafil has a median onset of 27 minutes and duration of 4 hours. People are encouraged to take the drug 1 hour before anticipated sexual stimulation. Vardenafil has a mean onset of action of 26 minutes and duration of 4 hours; it is also intended to be taken 1 hour before sexual stimulation. Tadalafil has an onset of action of 45 minutes and duration of 36 hours.

None of these drugs is indicated for use in women, so no adequate studies have been done during pregnancy and breastfeeding. Because the effects on pregnancy are not known, if alprostadil is being used, condoms should be used during intercourse with a pregnant woman.

TABLE 41.3 DRUGS IN FOCUS Drugs used to treat penile erectile dysfunction

Drug name	Dosage/route	Usual indications
alprostadil (*Caverject*)	2.5 micrograms injected intracavernously, titrate the dose to one that will allow a satisfactory erection that is maintained no longer than 1 hour; usual dose 10–20 micrograms; maximum 60 micrograms. Maximum of once in 24 hours, maximum of 3 times a week	Treatment of penile erectile dysfunction
avanafil (*Spedra*)	50–200 mg PO prn 15–30 minutes before sexual stimulation	Treatment of penile erectile dysfunction
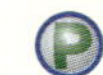 sildenafil (*Viagra, Revatio*)	*Viagra:* 25–100 mg PO taken 1 hour before sexual stimulation *Revatio:* 20 mg PO tds, at least 4–6 hours apart	Treatment of penile erectile dysfunction Treatment of pulmonary arterial hypertension in men and women
tadalafil (*Cialis*)	10 mg PO taken before sexual activity; range 5–20 mg PO; limit use to once a day; 2.5–5 mg/day PO for very sexually active males	Treatment of penile erectile dysfunction
vardenafil (*Levitra*)	5–10 mg PO taken 1 hour before sexual stimulation; range 5–20 mg; limit use to once a day	Treatment of penile erectile dysfunction

Contraindications and cautions

These drugs are contraindicated in the presence of any anatomical obstruction or condition that might predispose to priapism. They cannot be used with penile implants, and they are not indicated for use in women. However, sildenafil is used in women for the treatment of pulmonary arterial hypertension.

Caution should be used in people with bleeding disorders. The PDE5 inhibitors should also be used cautiously in people with coronary artery disease, active peptic ulcer, retinitis pigmentosa, optic neuropathy, hypotension or severe hypertension, congenital prolonged QT interval or severe hepatic or renal disorders *because of the risk of exacerbating these diseases.*

Adverse effects

Adverse effects associated with alprostadil are local effects such as pain at the injection site, infection, priapism, fibrosis and rash. The PDE5 inhibitors are associated with more systemic effects, including headache, flushing (related to relaxation of vascular smooth muscle), dyspepsia, urinary tract infection, diarrhoea, dizziness, possible optic neuropathy, possible eighth cranial nerve toxicity, loss of hearing and rash.

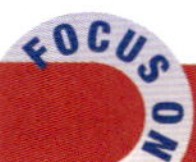

Safe medication administration

People who are using PDE5 inhibitors need to be advised to avoid drinking grapefruit juice while using the drug. Grapefruit juice can cause a decrease in the metabolism of the PDE5 inhibitor, leading to increased serum levels and a risk of toxicity. They should also be advised to avoid taking the drug with or just after a high-fat meal. The presence of fat in the GI tract will delay the absorption and onset of action of the drug, which could cause problems for individuals who are timing onset of action with their sexual activity.

These drugs can have serious cardiovascular effects. Deaths have been reported in people combining use of such drugs with other cardiovascular medications. People need to be aware of the potential risks in taking the drugs alongside other medications.

Prototype summary: sildenafil

Indications: treatment of erectile dysfunction in the presence of sexual stimulation; treatment of pulmonary arterial hypertension.

Actions: inhibits PDE5 receptors, leading to a release of nitrous oxide, which activates cGMP to cause a prolonged smooth muscle relaxation, allowing the flow of blood into the corpus cavernosum and facilitating erection.

Pharmacokinetics:

Route	Onset	Peak	Duration
PO	15–30 min	30–120 min	4 hours

$T_{1/2}$: 4 hours, with hepatic metabolism and excretion in the faeces and urine.

Adverse effects: headache, abnormal vision, flushing, dyspepsia, urinary tract infection, rash.

Clinically important drug–drug interactions

The PDE5 inhibitors cannot be taken in combination with any organic nitrates or alpha-adrenergic blockers; serious cardiovascular effects, including death, have occurred. There is also a possibility of increased vardenafil or tadalafil levels and effects if PDE5 inhibitors are taken with itraconazole or erythromycin; monitor the person and reduce dose as needed.

Vardenafil and tadalafil serum levels can increase if these drugs are combined with indinavir or ritonavir. If these drugs are being used, limit the dose of the PDE5 inhibitor.

Care considerations for people receiving drugs to treat penile erectile dysfunction

Assessment: history and examination

- Assess for the following conditions, *which could be cautions or contraindications to the use of the drug:* history of allergy to any of the preparations, penile structural abnormalities, penile implants, bleeding disorders, active peptic ulcer, coronary artery disease, hypotension or severe hypertension, congenital prolonged QT interval or severe hepatic or renal disorders.
- Assess baseline status before beginning therapy *to determine any potential adverse effects.*
- Assess skin and lesions *to monitor for adverse reactions to the drug and cardiovascular perfusion.*
- Monitor orientation, affect and reflexes *to evaluate CNS changes that might be related to changes in blood pressure and blood flow.*
- Assess blood pressure, pulse, respiration and adventitious sounds *to evaluate blood flow and potential changes in cardiovascular function.*
- When using alprostadil, perform a local inspection of the penis *to assess local reaction to injection and to monitor for potential infection.*
- Evaluate laboratory tests for bleeding time and liver function *to monitor potential adverse effects on the liver.*

Implementation with rationale

- Assess the cause of dysfunction before beginning therapy *to ensure appropriate use of these drugs.*
- Monitor people with vascular disease for any sign of exacerbation *so that the drug can be discontinued before severe adverse effects occur.*
- Instruct the person in the injection of alprostadil, storage of the drug, filling of the syringe, sterile technique, site rotation and proper disposal of needles *to ensure safe and proper administration of the drug.*
- Monitor people who are taking PDE5 inhibitors for use of nitrates or alpha-blockers *to avert potentially serious cardiovascular drug–drug interactions.*
- Provide thorough teaching, including measures to avoid adverse effects and warning signs of problems, as well as the need for regular evaluation, *to enhance knowledge about drug therapy and to promote compliance with the drug regimen.*

Evaluation

- Monitor response to the drug (improvement in penile erection).
- Monitor for adverse effects (dizziness, flushing, local inflammation or infection, fibrosis, diarrhoea, dyspepsia).
- Evaluate the effectiveness of the teaching plan (person can name drug, dosage, adverse effects to watch for and specific measures to avoid them; person can demonstrate proper administration of injected drug).
- Monitor the effectiveness of comfort measures and compliance with the regimen.

KEY POINTS

- Penile erectile dysfunction can inhibit erection and male sexual function.
- Alprostadil, a prostaglandin, can be injected into the penis to stimulate erection.
- The PDE5 inhibitors are oral agents that act quickly to promote vascular filling of the corpus cavernosum and promote penile erection. They differ in duration and time of onset. They are effective only in the presence of sexual stimulation.

CHAPTER SUMMARY

- Androgens are male sex hormones – specifically testosterone or testosterone-like compounds.
- Androgens are responsible for the development and maintenance of male sex characteristics and secondary sex characteristics or androgenic effects.
- Side effects related to androgen use involve excess of the desired effects, as well as potentially deadly hepatocellular carcinoma.
- Androgens can be used for replacement therapy or to block other hormone effects, as is seen with their use in the treatment of specific breast cancers.
- Anabolic steroids are analogues of testosterone that have been developed to have more anabolic or protein-building effects and fewer androgenic effects.

- Anabolic steroids have been abused to enhance muscle development and athletic performance, often with deadly effects.
- Anabolic steroids are used to increase haematocrit and improve protein anabolism in certain depleted states.
- Penile erectile dysfunction can inhibit erection and male sexual function.
- Alprostadil, a prostaglandin, can be injected into the penis to stimulate erection.
- The PDE5 inhibitors are oral agents that act quickly to promote vascular filling of the corpus cavernosum and promote penile erection. They differ in duration and time of onset. They are effective only in the presence of sexual stimulation.
- Dangerous cardiovascular effects, including death, have occurred when the PDE5 inhibitors are combined with organic nitrates or alpha blockers. Careful teaching is very important to avoid this drug–drug interaction.

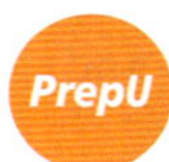

Knowing your strengths and weaknesses helps you to study more effectively. Take a PrepU Practice Quiz to find out how you measure up!

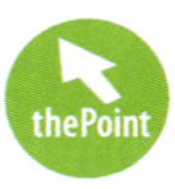

ONLINE RESOURCES

An extensive range of additional resources to enhance teaching and learning and to facilitate understanding of this chapter may be found online at the text's accompanying website, located on thePoint at http://thepoint.lww.com. These include Watch and Learn videos, Concepts in Action animations, journal articles, review questions, case studies, discussion topics and quizzes.

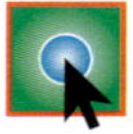

WEB LINKS

Health care providers and students may want to consult the following web resources:

www.andrologyaustralia.org
Andrology Australia.

www.health.gov.au/internet/main/publishing.nsf/Content/national+mens+health-1
Department of Health, Australia. National Male Health Policy.

BIBLIOGRAPHY

Cawley, M. A. (2009). Testosterone replacement therapy: What to look for, when to treat. *Nurse Practitioner, 34(9)*, 47–52.

Conaglen, H. M. & Conaglen, J. V. (2013). Drug-induced sexual dysfunction in men and women. *Australian Prescriber, 36(2)*, 42–45.

Farrell, M. & Dempsey, J. (2014). *Smeltzer & Bare's Textbook of Medical-Surgical Nursing* (3rd edn). Sydney: Lippincott Williams & Wilkins.

Goodman, L. S., Brunton, L. L., Chabner, B. & Knollmann, B. C. (2011). *Goodman and Gilman's Pharmacological Basis of Therapeutics* (12th edn). New York: McGraw-Hill.

Kirby, M. (2012). In the balance: Testosterone deficiency and cardiovascular health. *British Journal of Primary Care Nursing, 9(3)*, 107–109.

McKenna, L. & Mirkov, S. (2019). *McKenna's Drug Handbook for Nursing and Midwifery* (8th edn). Sydney: Wolters Kluwer Health Australia.

Peale, I. (2012). Breaking the silence: Helping men with erectile dysfunction. *British Journal of Community Nursing, 17(7)*, 310–317.

Porth, C. M. (2011). *Essentials of Pathophysiology: Concepts of Altered Health States* (3rd edn). Philadelphia: Lippincott Williams & Wilkins.

Porth, C. M. (2009). *Pathophysiology: Concepts of Altered Health States* (8th edn). Philadelphia: Lippincott Williams & Wilkins.

Steggall, M. J. (2011). Clinical management of erectile dysfunction. *International Journal of Urological Nursing, 5(2)*, 52–58.

Turkoski, B. B. (2008). Drugs used to treat erectile dysfunction. *Orthopaedic Nursing, 27(3)*, 201–206.

CHECK YOUR UNDERSTANDING

Answers to the questions in this chapter can be found in Appendix A at the back of this book.

MULTIPLE CHOICE

Select the best answer to the following.

1. Testosterone is approved for use in:
   a. treatment of breast cancers.
   b. increasing muscle strength in athletes.
   c. oral contraceptives.
   d. increasing hair distribution in male-pattern baldness.
2. Illegal use of large quantities of unprescribed anabolic steroids to enhance athletic performance has been associated with:
   a. increased sexual prowess.
   b. muscle rupture from overexpansion.
   c. development of chronic obstructive pulmonary disease (COPD).
   d. cardiomyopathy and liver cancers.
3. Anabolic steroids would be indicated for the treatment of:
   a. hair loss
   b. angioedema.
   c. debilitation and severe weight loss.
   d. breast cancers in males.
4. Erectile penile dysfunction is a condition in which:
   a. problems with childhood authority figures prevent a male erection.
   b. the corpus cavernosum does not fill with blood to allow for penile erection.
   c. the sympathetic nervous system fails to function.
   d. past exposure to sexually transmitted infections causes physical damage within the penis.
5. A potentially deadly drug–drug interaction can occur if a PDE5 inhibitor (sildenafil, tadalafil or vardenafil) is combined with:
   a. corticosteroids.
   b. oral contraceptives.
   c. organic nitrates.
   d. halothane anaesthetics.
6. To achieve erection, a person taking sildenafil (*Viagra*) would require:
   a. sexual stimulation of the penis.
   b. no additional stimulation.
   c. privacy.
   d. 10–15 minutes after taking the oral drug.
7. Men taking alprostadil for treatment of erectile dysfunction must:
   a. take the drug orally about 1 hour before anticipated intercourse.
   b. arrange for sexual stimulation to promote erection.
   c. learn to inject the drug directly into the penis.
   d. avoid the use of nitrates for cardiovascular disorders.
8. Sildenafil is known to:
   a. cause unexpected and enlarged erections.
   b. make a person young and agile.
   c. promote interpersonal relationships between partners.
   d. increase nitrous oxide levels in the corpus cavernosum, causing vascular relaxation and promoting blood flow into the corpus cavernosum.

MULTIPLE RESPONSE

Select all that apply.

1. In assessing a person for androgenic effects, you would expect to find which of the following?
   a. hirsutism
   b. deepening of the voice
   c. testicular enlargement
   d. acne
   e. elevated body temperature
   f. sudden growth
2. A child treated with anabolic steroids because of anaemia associated with renal disease will need:
   a. early sex education classes because of the effects of the drug.
   b. X-rays of the long bones every 3–6 months so the drug can be stopped when the bone size is appropriate to the child's age.
   c. to learn to shave.
   d. to learn to cope with an altered body image.
   e. regular monitoring of liver function tests.
   f. monitoring for the development of oedema.

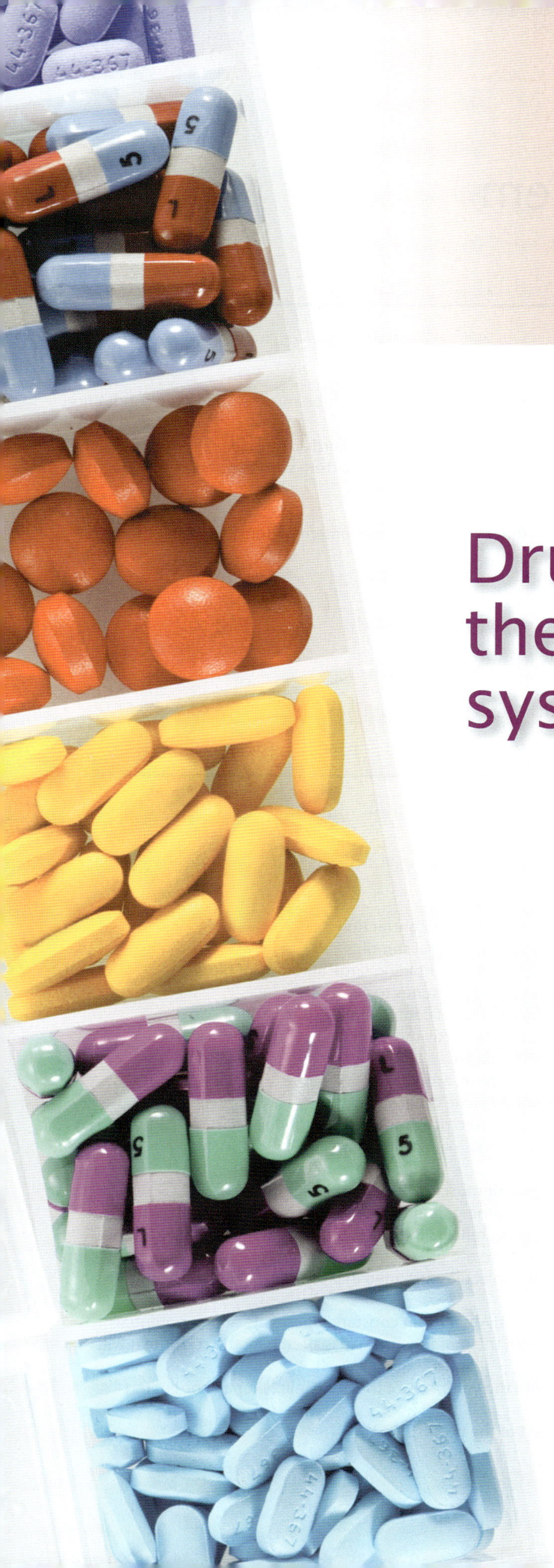

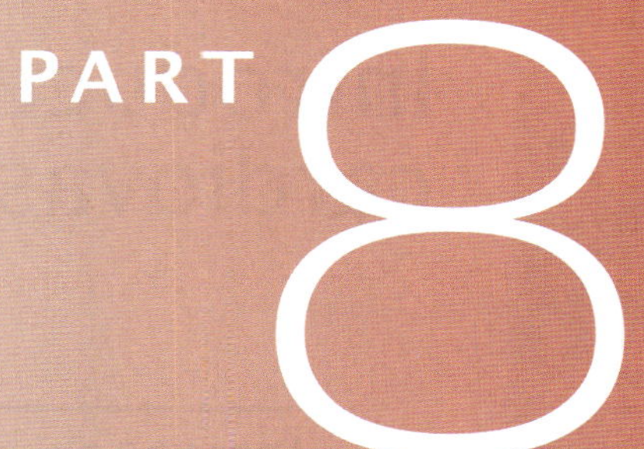

PART 8

Drugs acting on the cardiovascular system

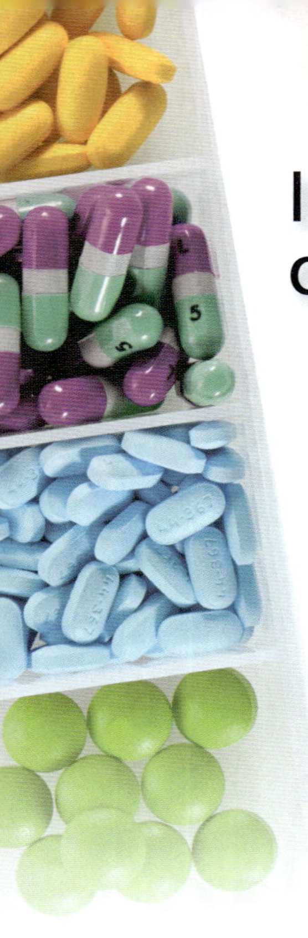

Introduction to the cardiovascular system

42

Learning objectives

On completing this chapter you should be able to:

1. Label a diagram of the heart, including all chambers, valves, great vessels, coronary vessels and the conduction system.
2. Describe the flow of blood during the cardiac cycle, including flow to the cardiac muscle.
3. Outline the conduction system of the heart, correlating the normal ECG pattern with the underlying electrical activity in the heart.
4. Discuss four normal controls of blood pressure.
5. Describe the capillary fluid shift, including factors that influence the movement of fluid in clinical situations.

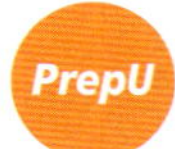

PrepU Test your current knowledge of the cardiovascular system with a PrepU Practice Quiz!

Glossary of key terms

actin: thin muscle filament, a component of a sarcomere or muscle unit
arrhythmia: a disruption in cardiac rate or rhythm
arteries: vessels that take blood away from the heart; muscular, resistance vessels
atrium: top chamber of the heart, receives blood from veins
auricle: appendage on the atria of the heart, holds blood to be pumped out with atrial contraction
automaticity: property of heart cells to generate an action potential without an external stimulus
capacitance system: the venous system; distensible, flexible veins that are capable of holding large amounts of blood
capillary: small vessel made up of loosely connected endothelial cells that connect arteries to veins
cardiac cycle: a period of cardiac muscle relaxation (diastole) followed by a period of contraction (systole) in the heart
conductivity: property of heart cells to rapidly conduct an action potential of electrical impulse
diastole: resting phase of the heart; blood is returned to the heart during this phase
dysrhythmia: another term for disruption in cardiac rate or rhythm; preferred term: arrhythmia
ectopic focus: a shift in the pacemaker of the heart from the sinoatrial node to some other site
electrocardiogram (ECG): an electrical tracing reflecting the conduction of an electrical impulse through the heart muscle; does not reflect mechanical activity
myocardium: the muscle of the heart
myosin: thick muscle filament with projections, a component of a sarcomere or muscle unit
oncotic pressure: the pulling pressure of plasma proteins, responsible for returning fluid to the vascular system at the capillary level
pulse pressure: the systolic blood pressure minus the diastolic blood pressure; reflects the filling pressure of the coronary arteries
resistance system: the arteries; the muscles of the arteries provide resistance to the flow of blood, leading to control of blood pressure
sarcomere: functional unit of a muscle cell, composed of actin and myosin molecules arranged in layers to give the unit a striped or striated appearance
sinoatrial (SA) node: the normal pacemaker of the heart; composed of primitive cells that constantly generate action potentials
Starling's law of the heart: addresses the contractile properties of the heart; the more the muscle is stretched, the stronger it will react, until it is stretched to a point at which it will not react at all
syncytia: intertwining networks of muscle fibres that make up the atria and the ventricles of the heart; allow for a coordinated pumping contraction
systole: contracting phase of the heart, during which blood is pumped out of the heart

troponin: chemical in heart muscle that prevents the reaction between actin and myosin, leading to muscle relaxation; it is inactivated by calcium during muscle stimulation to allow actin and myosin to react, causing muscle contraction
veins: vessels that return blood to the heart; distensible tubes
ventricle: bottom chamber of the heart, which contracts to pump blood out of the heart

The cardiovascular system is responsible for delivering oxygen and nutrients to all of the cells of the body and for removing waste products for excretion. The cardiovascular system consists of a pump – the heart – and an interconnected series of vessels that continually move blood throughout the body.

STRUCTURE AND FUNCTION OF THE HEART

The heart is a hollow, muscular organ that is divided into four chambers. The heart may actually be viewed as two joined hearts: a right heart and a left heart, each of which is divided into two parts, an upper part called the **atrium** (literally 'porch' or entryway) and a lower part called the **ventricle**.

Attached to each atrium is an appendage called the **auricle**, which collects blood that is then pumped into the ventricles by atrial contraction. The right auricle is quite large; the left auricle is very small. The ventricles pump blood out of the heart to the lungs (right ventricle) or the body (left ventricle). Between the atria and ventricles are two cardiac valves – thin tissues that are anchored to an annulus, or fibrous ring, which also gives the hollow organ some structure and helps to keep the organ open and divided into distinct chambers.

A partition called a septum separates the right half of the heart from the left half. The right half receives deoxygenated blood from everywhere in the body through the **veins** (vessels that carry blood towards the heart) and directs that blood into the lungs. The left half receives the now-oxygenated blood from the lungs and directs it into the aorta. The aorta delivers blood into the systemic circulation by way of **arteries** (vessels that carry blood away from the heart) (Figure 42.1). The circulatory system is composed of about 96,500 kilometres of interconnecting blood vessels that carry the needed oxygen and nutrients to the cells and carry away the metabolic waste products from the tissues.

Cardiac cycle

The heart, a muscle that contracts thousands of millions of times in a lifetime, possesses structural and functional properties that are different from those of other muscles. The fibres of the cardiac muscle, or **myocardium**, form two intertwining networks called the atrial and ventricular **syncytia**. These interlacing structures

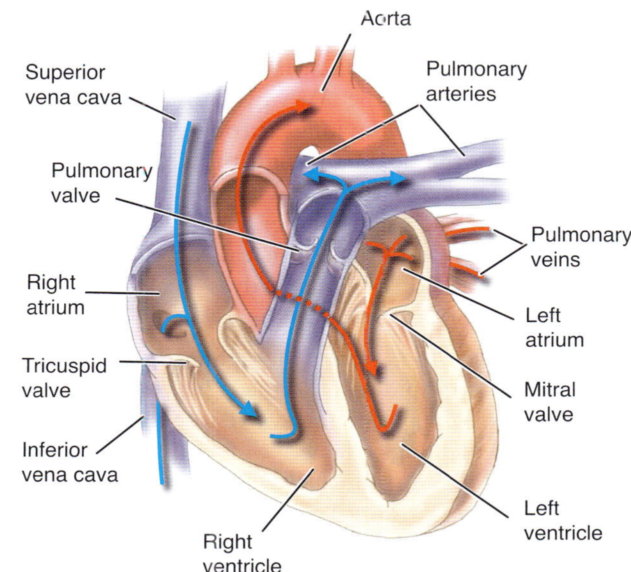

FIGURE 42.1 Blood flow into and out of the heart. Deoxygenated blood enters the right atrium from the great cardiac vein and the superior and inferior venae cavae and flows through the tricuspid valve into the right ventricle, which contracts and sends the blood through the pulmonary valve into the pulmonary artery and to the lungs. Oxygenated blood from the lungs enters the left atrium through the pulmonary veins and passes through the mitral valve into the left ventricle, which contracts and ejects the blood through the aortic valve into the aorta and out to the systemic circulation.

enable the atria and then the ventricles to contract synchronously when excited by the same stimulus.

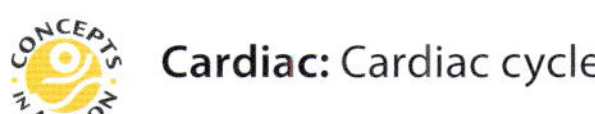

Cardiac: Cardiac cycle

Simultaneous contraction is a necessary property for a muscle that acts as a pump. A hollow pumping mechanism must also pause long enough in the pumping cycle to allow the chambers to fill with fluid. The heart muscle relaxes long enough to ensure adequate filling; the more completely it fills, the stronger is the subsequent contraction. This occurs because the muscle fibres of the heart, stretched by the increased volume of blood that has returned to them, spring back to normal size. This is similar to the stretching of a rubber band, which returns to its normal size after it is stretched – the further it is stretched, the stronger is the spring back to normal. This property is defined through **Starling's law of the heart.**

During **diastole** – the period of cardiac muscle relaxation – blood returns to the heart from the systemic and pulmonary veins, flowing into the right and left atria, respectively. When the pressure generated by the blood volume in the atria is greater than the pressure in the ventricles, blood flows through the atrioventricular (AV) valves into the ventricles. The valve on the right side of the heart is called the tricuspid valve because it is composed of three leaflets or cusps. The valve on the left side of the heart, called the mitral or bicuspid valve, is composed of two leaflets or cusps (see Figure 42.1). Just before the ventricles are stimulated to contract, the atria contract, pushing about one more tablespoon of blood into each ventricle. The much more powerful ventricles then contract, forcing the AV valves to snap shut, and pumping blood out to the lungs through the pulmonary valve or out to the aorta through the aortic valve and into the systemic circulation. The contraction of the ventricles is referred to as **systole**. Each period of systole followed by a period of diastole is called a **cardiac cycle**. The heart's series of one-way valves keeps the blood flowing in the correct direction:

- *Deoxygenated blood enters* the right atrium, flows through the tricuspid valve to the right ventricle, and flows through the pulmonary valve to pulmonary arteries and the lungs.
- *Oxygenated blood from the lungs returns* through the pulmonary veins to the left atrium, flows through the mitral valve into the left ventricle, and then flows through the aortic valve to the aorta and the rest of the body.

The AV valves close very tightly when the ventricles contract, preventing blood from flowing backwards into the atria, thereby keeping blood moving forwards through the system. The pulmonary and aortic valves open with the pressure of ventricular contraction and close tightly during diastole, keeping blood from flowing backwards into the ventricles. These valves operate much like one-way automatic doors: you can go through in the intended direction, but if you try to go the wrong way, the doors close and stop your movement. The proper functioning of the cardiac valves is important in maintaining the functioning of the cardiovascular system.

Cardiac conduction

Each cycle of cardiac contraction and relaxation is controlled by impulses that arise spontaneously in certain pacemaker cells of the **sinoatrial (SA) node** of the heart. These impulses are conducted from the pacemaker cells by a specialised conducting system that activates all of the parts of the heart muscle almost simultaneously. These continuous, rhythmic contractions are controlled by the heart itself; the brain does not stimulate the heart to beat. This safety feature allows the heart to beat as long as it has enough nutrients and oxygen to survive, regardless of the status of the rest of the body. This property protects the vital cardiovascular function in many disease states; it is the same property that allows the heart to continue functioning in a person who is 'brain dead'.

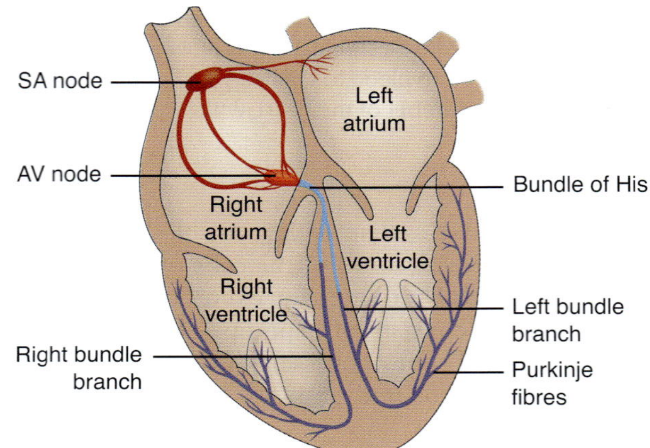

FIGURE 42.2 The conducting system of the heart. Impulses originating in the sinoatrial (SA) node are transmitted through the atrial bundles to the atrioventricular (AV) node and down the bundle of His and the bundle branches by way of the Purkinje fibres through the ventricles.

The conduction system of the heart consists of the SA node, atrial bundles, AV node, bundle of His, bundle branches and Purkinje fibres (Figure 42.2). The SA node, which is located near the top of the right atrium, acts as the pacemaker of the heart. Atrial bundles conduct the impulse through the atrial muscle. The AV node, which is located near the bottom of the right atrium, slows the impulse and allows the delay needed for ventricular filling. The AV node then sends the impulse from the atria into the ventricles by way of the bundle of His, which enters the septum and then divides into three bundle branches. These bundle branches, which conduct the impulses through the ventricles, break into a fine network of conducting fibres called the Purkinje fibres, which deliver the impulse to the ventricular cells.

Automaticity

The cells of the impulse-forming and conducting system are rather primitive, uncomplicated cells called pale or P cells. Because of their simple cell membrane, these cells possess a special property that differentiates them from other cells: they can generate action potentials or electrical impulses without being excited to do so by external stimuli. This property is called **automaticity**.

All cardiac cells possess some degree of automaticity. During diastole or rest, these cells undergo a spontaneous depolarisation because they decrease the flow of potassium ions out of the cell and probably leak sodium into the cell, causing an action potential. This action potential is basically the same as the action potential of the neuron (see Chapter 19). The action potential of the cardiac muscle cell consists of five phases:

- Phase 0 occurs when the cell reaches a point of stimulation. The sodium gates open along the cell membrane and sodium rushes into the cell, resulting in a positive flow of electrons into the cell – an electrical potential. This is called depolarisation.

- Phase 1 is the very short period when the sodium ion concentrations are equal inside and outside the cell.
- Phase 2, or the plateau stage, occurs as the cell membrane becomes less permeable to sodium. Calcium slowly enters the cell and potassium begins to leave the cell. The cell membrane is trying to return to its resting state, a process called repolarisation.
- Phase 3 is a period of rapid repolarisation as the gates are closed and potassium rapidly moves out of the cell.
- Phase 4 occurs when the cell comes to rest as the sodium–potassium pump returns the membrane to its previous state, with sodium outside and potassium inside the cell. Spontaneous depolarisation begins again.

Each area of the heart has an action potential that appears slightly different from the other action potentials, reflecting the complexity of the cells in that particular area. Because of these differences in the action potential, each area of the heart has a slightly different rate or rhythm. The SA node generates an impulse about 90–100 times a minute, the AV node about 40–50 times a minute and the complex ventricular muscle cells only about 10–20 times a minute (Figure 42.3).

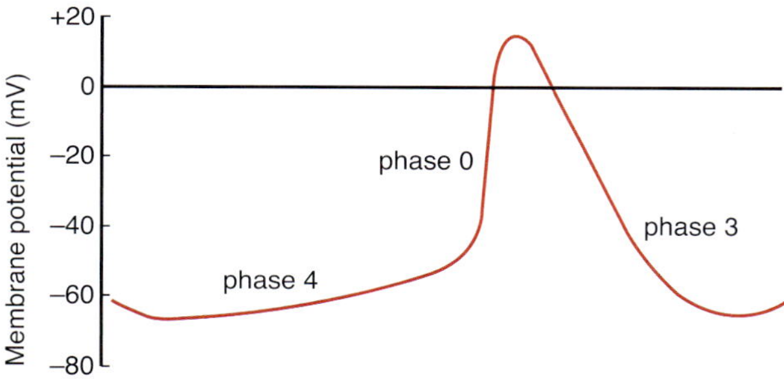

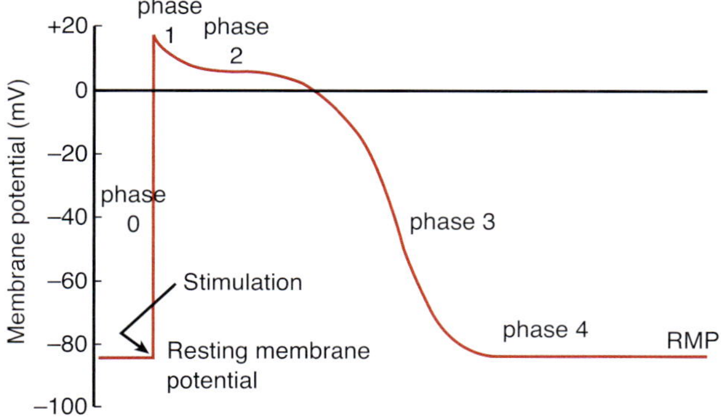

FIGURE 42.3 Action potentials recorded from a cell in the sinoatrial (SA) node (**A**) showing diastolic depolarisation in phase 4 and recorded from a ventricular muscle cell (**B**). In phase 0, the cell is stimulated, sodium rushes into the cell, and the cell is depolarised. In phase 1, sodium levels equalise. In phase 2, the plateau phase, calcium enters the cell (the slow current), and potassium and sodium leave. In phase 3, the slow current stops, and sodium and potassium leave the cell. In phase 4, the resting membrane potential (RMP) returns and the pacemaker potential begins in the SA node cell.

Conductivity

Normally, the SA node sets the pace for the heart rate because it depolarises faster than any cell in the heart. However, the other cells in the heart are capable of generating an impulse if anything happens to the SA node, which is another protective feature of the heart. As mentioned earlier, the SA node is said to be the pacemaker of the heart because it acts to stimulate the rest of the cells to depolarise at its rate. When the SA node sets the pace for the heart rate, the person is said to be in sinus rhythm.

The specialised cells of the heart can conduct an impulse rapidly through the system so that the muscle cells of the heart are stimulated at approximately the same time. This property of cardiac cells is called **conductivity**. The conduction velocity, or the speed at which the cells can pass on the impulse, is slowest in the AV node and fastest in the Purkinje fibres.

A delay in conduction at the AV node, between the atria and the ventricles, accounts for the fact that the atria contract a fraction of a second before the ventricles contract. This allows extra time for the ventricles to fill completely before they contract. The almost simultaneous spread of the impulse through the Purkinje fibres permits a simultaneous and powerful contraction of the ventricle muscles, making them an effective pump.

After a cell membrane has conducted an action potential, there is a span of time, called the absolute refractory period, in which it is impossible to stimulate that area of membrane. The absolute refractory period is the minimal amount of time that must elapse between two stimuli applied at one site in the heart for each of these stimuli to cause an action potential. This time reflects the responsiveness of the heart cells to stimuli. Cardiac drugs may affect the refractory period of the cells to make the heart more or less responsive.

Autonomic influences

The heart can generate action potentials on its own and could function without connection to the rest of the body. However, the autonomic nervous system (see Chapter 29) can influence the heart rate and rhythm and the strength of contraction. The parasympathetic nerves – primarily the vagus nerve, or 10th cranial nerve – can slow the heart rate and decrease the speed of conduction through the AV node. This allows the heart to rest and conserve its strength. In addition, the parasympathetic influence on the SA node is the dominant influence most of the time, keeping the resting heart rate at 70–80 beats per minute.

The sympathetic nervous system stimulates the heart to beat faster, speeds conduction through the AV node and causes the heart muscle to contract harder. This action is important during exercise or stress, when the body's cells need to have more oxygen delivered.

These two branches of the autonomic nervous system work together to help the heart meet the body's demands. Drugs that influence either branch can exert autonomic effects on the heart.

Myocardial contraction

The end result of the electrical stimulation of the heart cells is the unified contraction of the atria and ventricles, which moves the blood throughout the vascular system. The basic unit of the cardiac muscle is the **sarcomere** (Figure 42.4). A sarcomere is made up of two contractile proteins: **actin**, a thin filament, and **myosin**, a thick filament with small projections on it. These proteins are anchored at the Z bands, the outer edges of each sarcomere. These proteins readily react with each other, but are at rest they are kept apart by the protein **troponin.**

When a cardiac muscle cell is stimulated, calcium enters the cell though channels in the cell membrane and also from storage sites within the cell. This occurs during phase 3 of the action potential, when the cell is starting to repolarise. The calcium reacts with the troponin and inactivates it. This action allows the actin and myosin proteins to react with each other, forming actomyosin bridges. These bridges then break quickly, and the myosin slides along to form new bridges.

As long as calcium is present, the actomyosin bridges continue to form. This action slides the proteins together, shortening or contracting the sarcomere. Cardiac muscle cells are linked together: when one cell is stimulated to contract, they are all stimulated to contract.

The shortening of numerous sarcomeres causes the contraction and pumping action of the heart muscle. As the cell reaches its repolarised state, calcium is removed from the cell by a sodium–calcium pump, and calcium released from storage sites within the cell returns to the storage sites. The contraction process requires energy and oxygen for the chemical reaction that allows the formation of the actomyosin bridges, and calcium to allow the bridge formation to occur.

The degree of shortening (the strength of contraction) is determined by the amount of calcium present – the more calcium present, the more bridges will be formed – and by the stretch of the sarcomere before contraction begins. The further apart the actin and myosin proteins are before the cell is stimulated, the more bridges will be formed and the stronger the contraction will be. This correlates with Starling's law of the heart. The more the cardiac muscle is stretched, the greater is the contraction. The more blood that enters the heart, the greater is the contraction that is needed to empty the heart, up to a point; however, if the actin and myosin molecules are stretched too far apart, they will not be able to reach each other to form the actomyosin bridges, and no contraction will occur.

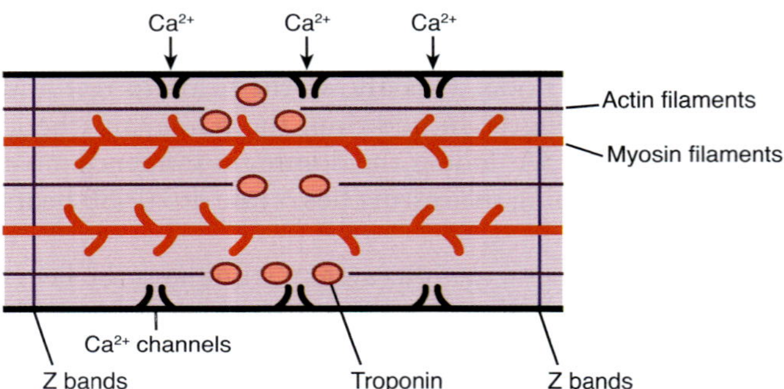

FIGURE 42.4 A sarcomere, the functioning unit of cardiac muscle.

KEY POINTS

- The heart, a hollow muscle with four chambers comprising two upper atria and two lower ventricles, pumps oxygenated blood to the body's cells and also collects waste products from the tissues.
- The two-step process known as the cardiac cycle includes diastole (resting period when the veins carry blood back to the heart) and systole (contraction period when the heart pumps blood out to the arteries for distribution to the body).
- Impulses generated in the heart – not the brain – stimulate contraction of the heart muscle.
- The heart's conduction (or stimulatory) system consists of the sinoatrial (SA) node, the atrial bundles, the AV node, the bundle of His, the bundle branches and the Purkinje fibres.

ELECTROCARDIOGRAPHY

Electrocardiography is a process of recording the patterns of electrical impulses as they move through the heart. It is an important diagnostic tool in the care of the person experiencing cardiac problems. The electrocardiography machine detects the patterns of electrical impulse generation and conduction through the heart and translates that information into a recorded pattern, which is displayed as a waveform on a cardiac monitor or printout on calibrated paper. An **electrocardiogram (ECG)** is a measure of electrical activity; it provides no information about the mechanical activity of the heart. The important aspect of cardiac output – the degree to which the heart is doing its job of pumping blood out to all of the tissues – needs to be carefully assessed by looking at and evaluating the person.

The normal ECG waveform is made up of five main waves: the P wave, which is formed as impulses originating in the SA node or pacemaker pass through the atrial tissues; the QRS complex, which represents depolarisation of the bundle of His (Q) and the ventricles (RS); and the T wave, which represents repolarisation of the ventricles (Figure 42.5).

The P wave immediately precedes the contraction of the atria. The QRS complex immediately precedes the contraction of the ventricles and then relaxation of the ventricles during the T wave. The repolarisation of the atria (the Ta wave) occurs during the QRS complex and usually is not seen on an ECG. In certain conditions of atrial hypertrophy, the Ta wave may appear around the QRS complex.

In addition to the five waves, several areas represent critical points on the ECG. These include the following:

PR interval: reflects the normal delay of conduction at the AV node

QT interval: reflects the critical timing of repolarisation of the ventricles

ST segment: reflects important information about the repolarisation of the ventricles

A person with a normal ECG pattern and a heart rate within the normal range for that person's age group is said to be in normal sinus rhythm. However, abnormalities in the shape or timing of each part of an ECG tracing help to reveal the presence of particular cardiac disorders.

Arrhythmias

A disruption in cardiac rate or rhythm is called an **arrhythmia** (formerly dysrhythmia). Various factors, such as drugs, acidosis, decreased oxygen levels, changes in the electrolytes in the area and build-up of waste products, can change the cardiac rate and rhythm. Arrhythmias can arise because of changes in the automaticity or conductivity of the heart cells. They are significant because they interfere with the work of the heart and can disrupt the cardiac output, which eventually will affect every cell in the body. Several different types of arrhythmias may occur.

Sinus arrhythmias

The SA node is influenced by the autonomic nervous system to change the rate of firing to meet the body's

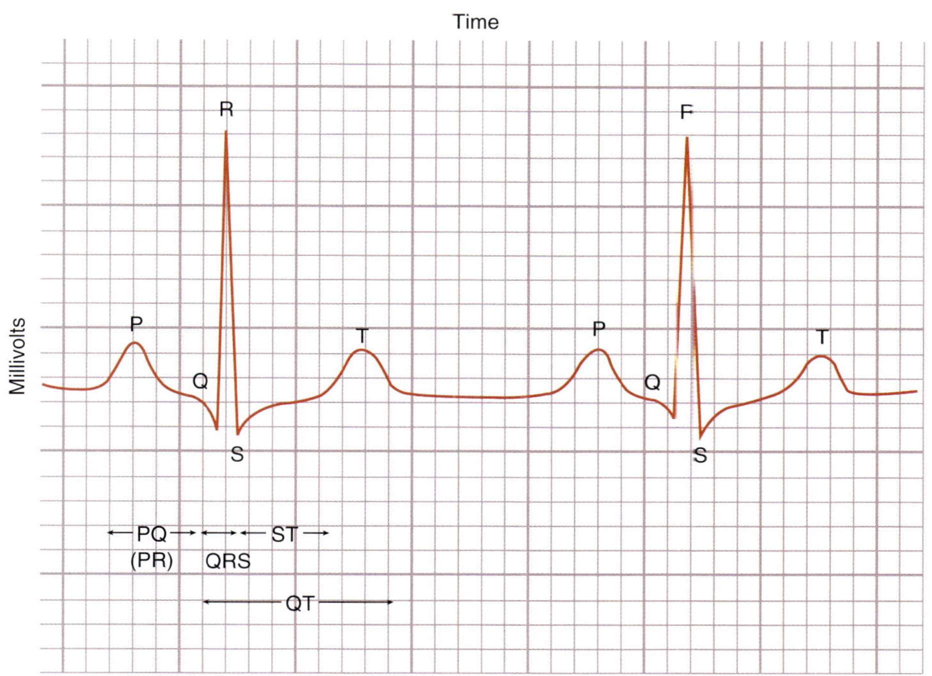

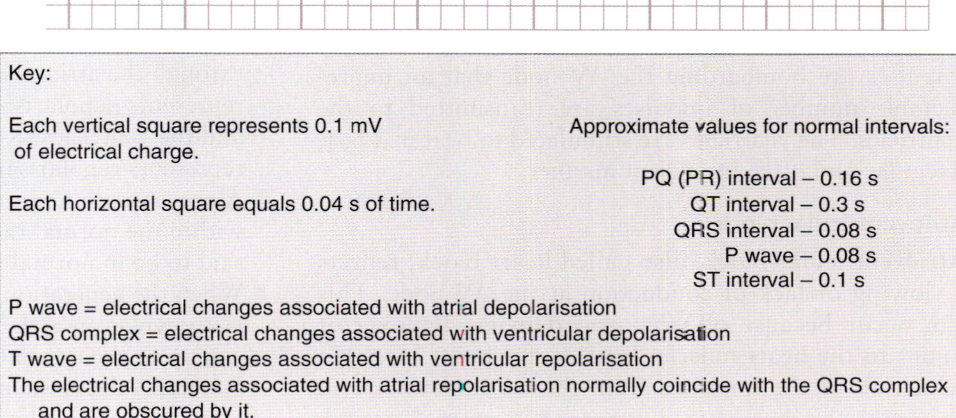

FIGURE 42.5 The normal electrocardiogram waveform.

demands for oxygen. A faster-than-normal heart rate – usually anything faster than 100 beats/min in an adult – with a normal-appearing ECG pattern is called sinus tachycardia. If sinus tachycardia becomes too fast, it can lead to a decreased time for cardiac filling and a decrease in cardiac output. Many activities or conditions can cause a sinus tachycardia, such as exercise, fear or stress. The underlying physical condition of the person will determine whether this fast heart rate is problematic. Sinus bradycardia is a slower-than-normal heart rate (usually less than 60 beats/min) with a normal-appearing ECG pattern. Sinus bradycardia allows increased time for ventricular filling and an increased cardiac output. This is often seen with athletes who have a slow heart rate. In other people, this rate might be too slow to adequately perfuse all of the tissues.

Supraventricular arrhythmias

Arrhythmias that originate above the ventricles but not in the SA node are called supraventricular arrhythmias. These arrhythmias feature an abnormally-shaped P wave because the site of origin is not the sinus node. However, they show normal QRS complexes because the ventricles are still conducting impulses normally. Supraventricular arrhythmias include the following:

- *Premature atrial contractions (PACs)*, which reflect an **ectopic focus** (a shift in the pacemaker of the heart from the SA node to some other site) in the atria that is generating an impulse out of the normal rhythm.
- *Paroxysmal atrial tachycardia (PAT)*, sporadically occurring runs of rapid heart rate originating in the atria.
- *Atrial flutter*, characterised by sawtooth-shaped P waves reflecting a single ectopic focus that is generating a regular, fast atrial depolarisation.
- *Atrial fibrillation*, with irregular P waves representing many ectopic foci firing in an uncoordinated manner through the atria.

With atrial flutter, often one of every two or one of every three impulses is transmitted to the ventricles. The person may have a 2:1 or 3:1 ratio of P waves to QRS complexes. The ventricles beat faster than normal, losing some efficiency. With atrial fibrillation, so many impulses are bombarding the AV node that an unpredictable number of impulses are transmitted to the ventricles. The ventricles are stimulated to beat in a fast, irregular and often inefficient manner.

Atrioventricular block

Atrioventricular block, also called heart block, reflects a slowing or lack of conduction at the AV node. This can occur because of structural damage, hypoxia or injury to the heart muscle. First-degree heart block, in which all of the impulses from the SA node arrive in the ventricles but after a longer-than-normal period, is characterised by a lengthening of the P–R interval beyond the normal 0.16–0.20 seconds. Each P wave is followed by a QRS complex. In second-degree heart block, some of the impulses are lost and do not get through, resulting in a slow rate of ventricular contraction. With this arrhythmia, a QRS complex may follow one, two, three or four P waves. In third-degree heart block, or complete heart block, no impulses from the SA node get through to the ventricles, and the much slower ventricular automaticity takes over. The waveform shows a total dissociation of P waves from QRS complexes and T waves. Because the P waves can come at any time, the P–R interval is not constant. The QRS complexes appear at a very slow rate and may not be sufficient to meet the body's needs.

Ventricular arrhythmias

Impulses that originate below the AV node originate from ectopic foci that do not use the normal conduction pathways. The QRS complexes appear wide and prolonged, and the T waves are inverted, reflecting the slower conduction across cardiac tissue that is not part of the rapid conduction system. Premature ventricular contractions (PVCs) can arise from a single ectopic focus in the ventricles, with all of them having the same shape, or from many ectopic foci, which produces PVCs with different shapes. Runs or bursts of PVCs from many different foci are more ominous because they can reflect extensive damage or hypoxia in the myocardium. Runs of several PVCs at a rapid rate are called ventricular tachycardia. Ventricular fibrillation is seen as a bizarre, irregular, distorted wave. It is potentially fatal because it reflects a lack of any coordinated stimulation of the ventricles. The ventricles' inability to contract in a coordinated fashion results in no blood being pumped to the body or the brain. Thus there is a total loss of cardiac output.

KEY POINTS

- The normal ECG waveform is made up of five main waves: the P wave, which is formed as impulses originating in the SA node or pacemaker pass through the atrial tissues; the QRS complex, which represents depolarisation of the bundle of His (Q) and the ventricles (RS); and the T wave, which represents repolarisation of the ventricles.
- A person with a normal ECG pattern and a heart rate within the normal range for that person's age group is said to be in normal sinus rhythm.
- When the generation of impulses is altered, the result is known as an arrhythmia (or dysrhythmia) that can upset the normal balance in the cardiovascular system. A decrease in cardiac output, which affects all of the cells of the body, follows.

CIRCULATION

The purpose of the heart's continual pumping action is to keep blood flowing to and from all of the body's tissues and cells. Blood delivers oxygen and much-needed nutrients to the cells for producing energy, and it carries away carbon dioxide and other waste products of metabolism. The steady circulation of blood is essential for the proper functioning of all of the body's organs, including the heart.

The circulation of the blood follows two courses:

- *Heart–lung or pulmonary circulation*: the right side of the heart sends blood to the lungs, where carbon dioxide and some waste products are removed from the blood and oxygen is picked up by the red blood cells.
- *Systemic circulation*: the left side of the heart sends oxygenated blood out to all of the cells in the body.

In addition, the heart muscle, like any other muscle, requires adequate oxygen and nutrients to function. This is accomplished via coronary circulation.

The blood moves from areas of high pressure to areas of lower pressure. The system is a 'closed' system; that is, it has no openings or holes that would allow blood to leak out. The closed nature of the system is what keeps the pressure differences in the proper relationship so that blood always flows in the direction in which it is intended to flow (Figure 42.6).

Pulmonary circulation

The right atrium is a very low pressure area in the cardiovascular system. All of the deoxygenated blood from the body flows into the right atrium from the inferior and superior venae cavae (see Figure 42.1) and from the great cardiac vein, which returns deoxygenated blood from the heart muscle. As the blood flows into the atrium, the pressure increases. When the pressure becomes greater than the pressure in the right ventricle, most of the blood flows into the right ventricle; this is called the rapid-filling phase. At this point in the cardiac cycle, the atrium is stimulated to contract and pushes the remaining blood into the right ventricle. The ventricle is then stimulated to contract; it generates pressure that opens the pulmonary valve (see Figure 42.1) and sends blood into the pulmonary artery, which takes the blood into the lungs, a very low pressure area. The

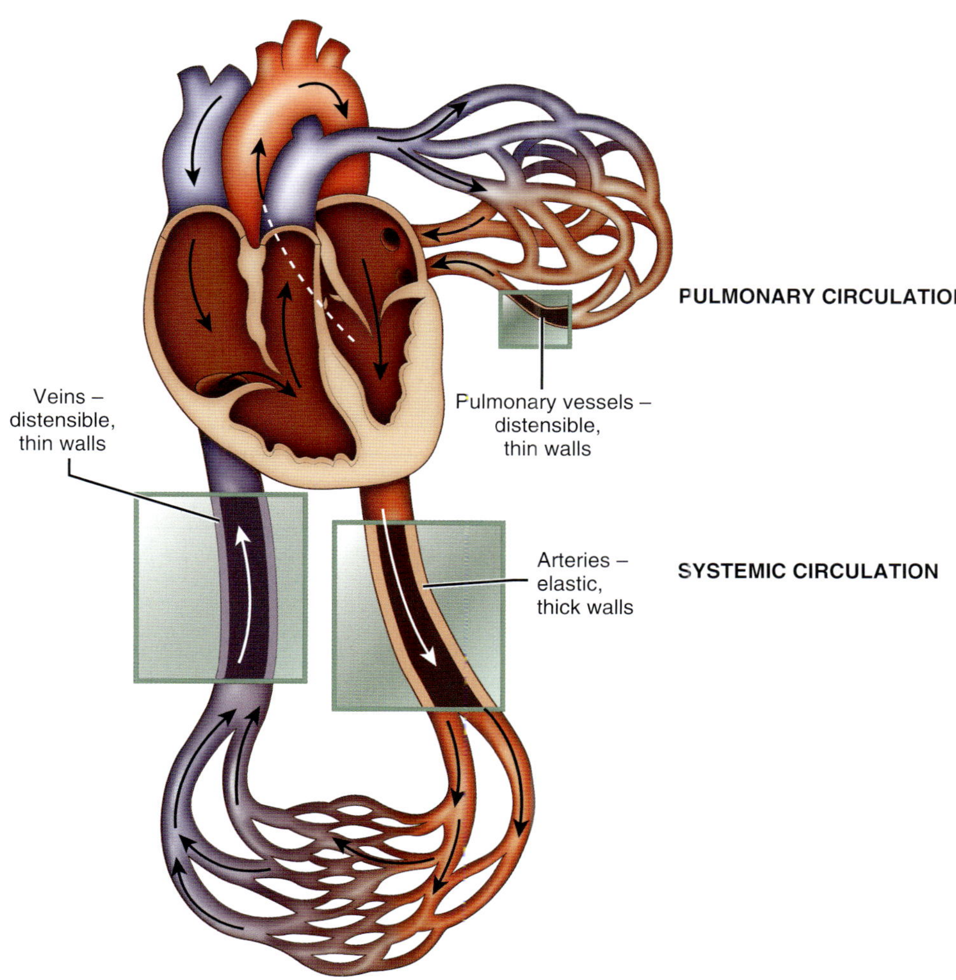

FIGURE 42.6 Blood flow through the systemic and pulmonary vasculature circuits.

blood then circulates around the alveoli of the lungs, picking up oxygen and getting rid of carbon dioxide; flows through pulmonary capillaries (the tiny blood vessels that connect arteries and veins) into the pulmonary veins; and then returns to the left atrium.

Systemic circulation

When the pressure of blood volume in the left atrium is greater than the pressure in the large left ventricle, this oxygenated blood flows into the left ventricle. The left atrium contracts and pushes any remaining blood into the left ventricle, which is stimulated to contract and generates tremendous pressure to push the blood into the aorta, carrying it throughout the body. The aorta and other large arteries have thick, muscular walls. The entire arterial system contains muscles in the walls of the vessels all the way to the terminal branches or arterioles, which consist of fragments of muscle and endothelial cells. These muscles offer resistance to the blood that is sent pumping into the arterial system by the left ventricle, generating pressure. The arterial system is referred to as a **resistance system**. The vessels can either constrict or dilate, increasing or decreasing resistance, respectively, based on the needs of the body. The arterioles are able to completely shut off blood flow to some areas of the body; that is, they can shunt blood to another area where it is needed more. The arterioles, because of their ability to increase or decrease resistance in the system, are one of the main regulators of blood pressure.

Blood from the tiny arterioles flows into the **capillary** system, which connects the arterial and venous systems. These microscopic vessels are composed of loosely connected endothelial cells. Oxygen, fluid and nutrients are able to pass through the arterial end of the capillaries and enter the interstitial area between tissue cells. Fluid at the venous end of the capillary, which contains carbon dioxide and other waste products, is drawn back into the vessel. This shifting of fluid in the capillaries, called the capillary fluid shift, is carefully regulated by a balance between hydrostatic (fluid pressure) forces on the arterial end of the capillary and **oncotic pressure** (the pulling pressure of the large, vascular proteins) on the venous end of the capillary. In a normal situation, the higher pressure at the arterial end of a capillary forces fluid out of the vessel and into the tissue, and the now-concentrated proteins (which are too large to leave the capillary) exert a pull on the fluid at the venous end of the capillary to pull it back in. A disruption in the hydrostatic pressure or in the concentration of proteins in the capillary can lead to fluid being left in the tissue, a condition referred to as oedema. The capillaries merge into venules, which merge into veins, the vessels responsible for returning the blood to the heart (Figure 42.7).

The veins are thin-walled, very elastic, low-pressure vessels that can hold large quantities of blood if necessary. The venous system is referred to as a **capacitance system** because the veins have the capacity to hold large quantities of fluid as they distend with fluid volume. These capacitance vessels have a great deal of influence on the venous return to the heart – the amount of blood that is delivered to the right atrium.

Coronary circulation

The heart muscle requires a constant supply of oxygenated blood to keep contracting. The myocardium receives its blood through two main coronary arteries that branch off the base of the aorta from an area called the sinuses of Valsalva. These arteries encircle the heart

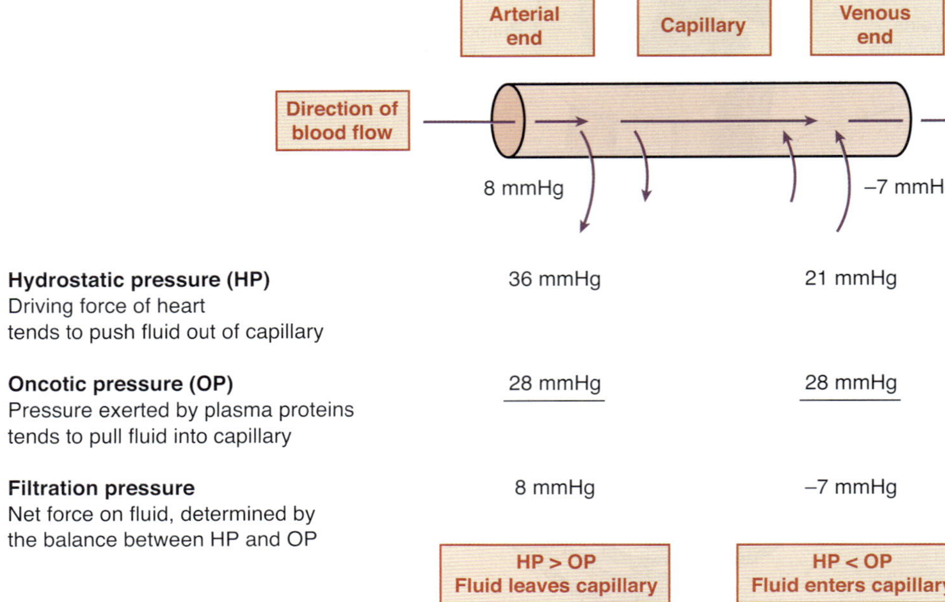

FIGURE 42.7 The net shift of fluid out of and into the capillary is determined by the balance between the hydrostatic pressure (HP) and the oncotic pressure (OP). The HP tends to push fluid out of the capillary and the OP tends to pull it back into the capillary. At the arterial end of the capillary bed, the blood pressure is higher than at the venous end. At the arterial end, HP exceeds OP and fluid filters out. At the venous end, HP has fallen, and HP is less than OP; fluid is pulled back into the capillary from the surrounding tissue. The lymphatic system also returns fluids and substances from the tissues to the circulation.

in a pattern resembling a crown, which is why they are called 'coronary' arteries.

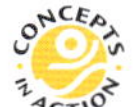

Cardiac: Myocardial blood flow

The left coronary artery arises from the left side of the aorta and bifurcates, or divides, into two large vessels called the left circumflex artery (which travels down the left side of the heart and feeds most of the left ventricle) and the left anterior descending coronary artery (which travels down the front of the heart and feeds the septum and anterior areas, including much of the conduction system). The artery arising from the right side of the aorta, called the right coronary artery, supplies most of the right side of the heart, including the SA node.

The coronary arteries receive blood during diastole, when the muscle is at rest and relaxed so that blood can flow freely into the muscle. When the ventricle contracts, it forces the aortic valve open, which in turn causes the leaflets of the valve to cover the openings of the coronary arteries. When the ventricles relax, the blood is no longer pumped forwards and starts to flow back towards the ventricle. The blood flowing down the sides of the aorta closes the aortic valve and fills the coronary arteries. The pressure that fills the coronary arteries is the difference between the systolic (ejection) pressure and the diastolic (resting) pressure. This is called the **pulse pressure** (systolic minus diastolic blood pressure readings). The pulse pressure is monitored clinically to evaluate the filling pressure of the coronary arteries. The oxygenated blood that is fed into the heart by the coronary circulation reaches every cardiac muscle fibre as the vessels divide and subdivide throughout the myocardium (Figure 42.8).

The heart has a pattern of circulation called end-artery circulation. The arteries go into the muscle and end without a great deal of backup or collateral circulation. Normally this is an efficient system and is able to meet the needs of the heart muscle. The heart's supply of and demand for oxygen are met by changes in the delivery of oxygen through the coronary artery system. Problems can arise, however, when an imbalance develops between the supply of oxygen delivered to the heart muscle and the myocardial demand for oxygen.

The main forces that determine the heart's use of oxygen or oxygen consumption include the following:

- *Heart rate*: the more the heart has to pump, the more oxygen it requires.
- *Preload (amount of blood that is brought back to the heart to be pumped throughout the body)*: the more blood that is returned to the heart, the harder it will have to work to pump the blood around. The volume of blood in the system is a determinant of preload.
- *Afterload (resistance against which the heart has to beat)*: the higher the resistance in the system, the harder the heart will have to contract to force open the valves and pump the blood along. Blood pressure is a measure of afterload.
- *Stretch on the ventricles*: if the ventricular muscle is stretched before it is stimulated to contract, more actomyosin bridges will be formed, which will take more energy; alternatively, if the muscle is stimulated to contract harder than usual (which happens with sympathetic stimulation), more bridges will be formed, which also will require more energy.

The muscle can be stretched, as in ventricular hypertrophy related to chronic hypertension or cardiac muscle damage, or in heart failure when the ventricle does not empty completely and blood backs up in the system.

The supply of blood to the myocardium can be altered if the heart fails to pump effectively and cannot deliver blood to the coronary arteries. This happens in

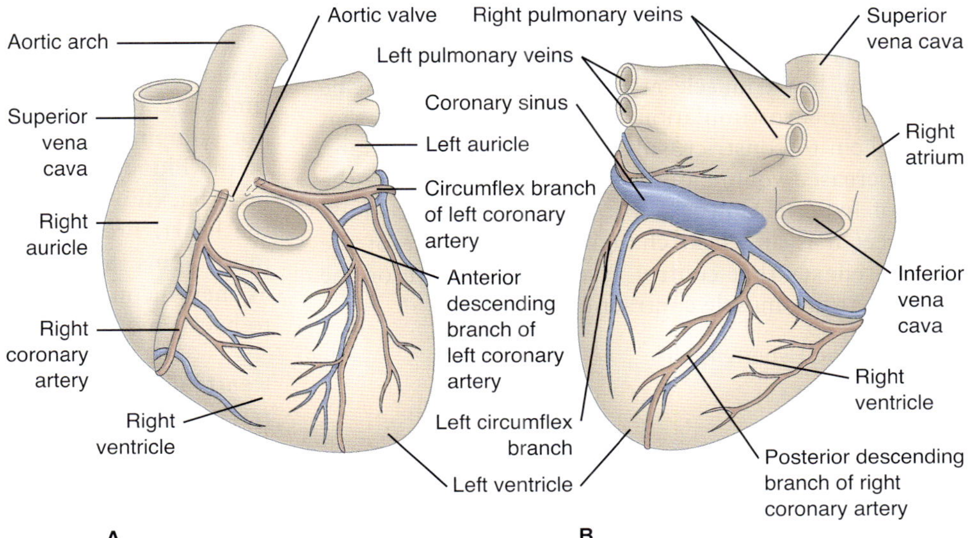

FIGURE 42.8 Coronary arteries and veins. **A.** Anterior view. **B.** Posterior view.

heart failure and cases of hypotension. The supply is most frequently altered, however, when the coronary vessels become narrowed and unresponsive to stimuli to dilate and deliver more blood. This happens in atherosclerosis or coronary artery disease. The end result of this narrowing can be total blockage of a coronary artery, leading to hypoxia and eventual death of the cells that depend on that vessel for oxygen. This is called a myocardial infarction (MI), and it is one of the leading causes of death in Australia and New Zealand.

Systemic arterial pressure

The contraction of the left ventricle, which sends blood surging out into the aorta, creates a pressure that continues to force blood into all of the branches of the aorta. This pressure against arterial walls is greatest during systole (cardiac contraction) and falls to its lowest level during diastole. Measurement of both the systolic and the diastolic pressure indicates both the pumping pressure of the ventricle and the generalised pressure in the system, or the pressure the ventricle has to overcome to pump blood out of the heart.

Hypotension

The pressure of the blood in the arteries needs to remain relatively high to ensure that blood is delivered to every cell in the body and to keep the blood flowing from high-pressure to low-pressure areas. The pressure can fall dramatically – termed hypotension – from loss of blood volume or from failure of the heart muscle to pump effectively. Severe hypotension can progress to shock and even death as cells are cut off from their oxygen supply.

Hypertension

Constant, excessive high blood pressure – called hypertension – can damage the fragile inner lining of blood vessels and cause a disruption of blood flow to the tissues. It also puts a tremendous strain on the heart muscle, increasing myocardial oxygen consumption and putting the heart muscle at risk. Hypertension can be caused by neurostimulation of the blood vessels that causes them to constrict, subsequently raising pressure, or by increased volume in the system. In most cases, the cause of hypertension is not known and drug therapy to correct it is aimed at changing one or more of the normal reflexes that control vascular resistance or the force of cardiac muscle contraction.

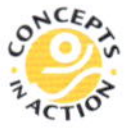

Cardiac: Hypertension

Vasomotor tone

The smooth muscles in the walls of the arteries receive constant input from nerve fibres of the sympathetic nervous system. These impulses work to dilate the vessels if more blood flow is needed in an area, to constrict vessels if increased pressure is needed in the system, and to maintain muscle tone so that the vessel remains patent and responsive.

The coordination of these impulses is regulated through the medulla in an area called the cardiovascular centre. If increased pressure is needed, this centre increases sympathetic flow to the vessels. If pressure rises too high, this is sensed by baroreceptors or pressure receptors and the sympathetic flow is decreased. Chapter 43 discusses the drugs that are used to influence the stimulation of vessels to alter blood pressure.

Renin–angiotensin–aldosterone system

Another determinant of blood pressure is the renin–angiotensin–aldosterone system. This system is activated when blood flow to the kidneys is decreased. Cells in the kidney release an enzyme called renin. Renin is transported to the liver, where it converts angiotensinogen (produced in the liver) to angiotensin I. Angiotensin I travels to the lungs, where it is converted by angiotensin-converting enzyme (ACE) to angiotensin II. Angiotensin II travels through the body and reacts with angiotensin II–receptor sites on blood vessels to cause a severe vasoconstriction. This increases blood pressure and should increase blood flow to the kidneys to decrease the release of renin. Angiotensin II also causes the release of aldosterone from the adrenal cortex, which causes retention of sodium and water, leading to the release of antidiuretic hormone (ADH) to retain water and increase blood volume. Increasing blood volume increases blood flow to the kidney. This system works constantly, whenever a position change alters flow to the kidney or blood volume or pressure changes, to help maintain the blood pressure within a range that ensures perfusion (delivery of blood to all of the tissues) (Figure 42.9).

Venous pressure

Blood in the veins also exerts a pressure that may sometimes rise above normal. This can happen if the heart is not pumping effectively and is unable to pump out all of the blood that is trying to return to it. This results in a backup or congestion of blood waiting to enter the heart. Pressure rises in the right atrium and then in the veins that are trying to return blood to the heart as they encounter resistance. The venous system begins to back up or become congested with blood.

Heart failure

If the heart muscle fails to do its job of effectively pumping blood through the system, blood backs up and the system becomes congested. This is called heart failure (HF). The rise in venous pressure that results from this backup of blood increases the hydrostatic

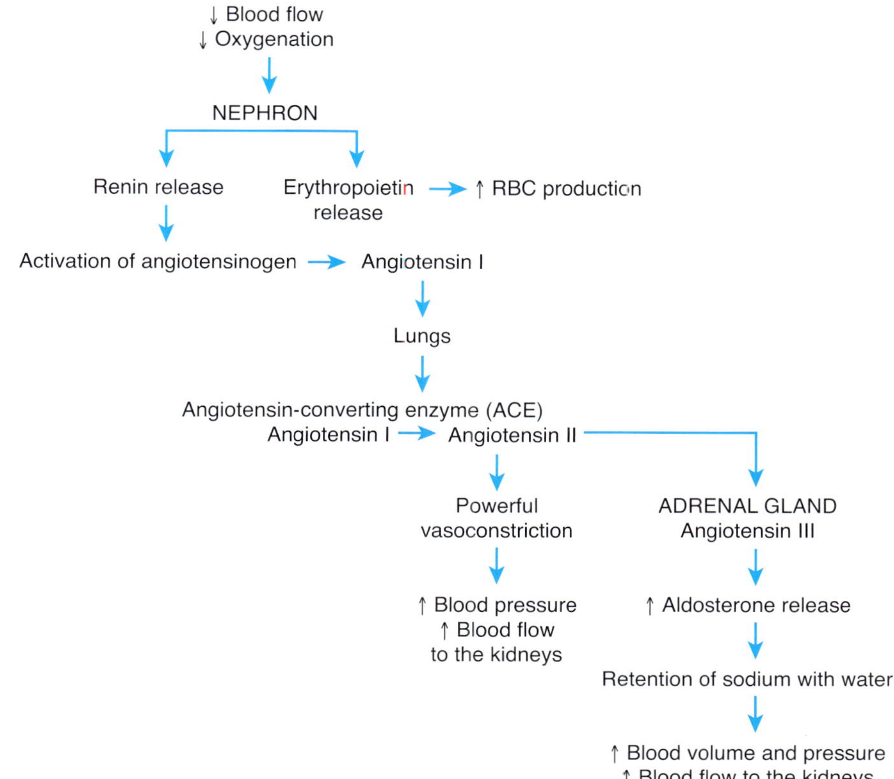

FIGURE 42.9 The renin–angiotensin–aldosterone system for reflex maintenance of blood pressure control.

pressure on the venous end of the capillaries. The hydrostatic pressure pushing fluid out of the capillary is soon higher than the oncotic pressure that is trying to pull the fluid back into the vessel, causing fluid to be lost into the tissues. This shift of fluid accounts for the oedema seen with HF. Pulmonary oedema results when the left side of the heart fails; peripheral, abdominal and liver oedema occur when the right side of the heart fails.

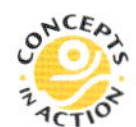

Cardiac: Congestive heart failure

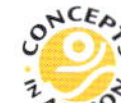

Cardiac: Oedema

Other factors can contribute to a loss of fluid in the tissues, including protein loss and fluid retention. Protein loss can lead to a fall in oncotic pressure and an inability to pull fluid back into the vascular system. Protein levels fall in renal failure, when protein is lost in the urine, and in liver failure, when the liver is no longer able to produce plasma proteins. Fluid retention, which is often stimulated by aldosterone and ADH as described earlier, can increase the hydrostatic pressure so much that fluid is pushed out under higher pressure and the balancing pressure to pull it back into the vessel is not sufficient. Drugs that are used to treat HF may affect the vascular system at any of these areas in an attempt to return a balance to the pressures in the system.

KEY POINTS

- Blood pressure is maintained by stimulus from the sympathetic system and reflex control of blood volume and pressure by the renin–angiotensin system and the aldosterone–ADH system. Alterations in blood pressure (hypotension or hypertension) can upset the balance of the cardiovascular system and lead to problems in blood delivery.
- Fluid shifts out of the blood at the arterial ends of capillaries to deliver oxygen and nutrients to the tissues. It moves out due to the hydrostatic or fluid pressure of the arterial side of the system. Fluid returns to the system at the venous end of the capillaries because of the oncotic pull of proteins in the vessels. Disruptions in these pressures can lead to oedema or loss of fluid in the tissues.

CHAPTER SUMMARY

- The heart is a hollow muscle that is divided into a right and a left side by a thick septum and into four chambers – the two upper atria and the two lower ventricles. The right side of the heart receives all of the deoxygenated blood from the body through the veins and directs it into the lungs. The left side of the heart receives oxygenated blood from the lungs and pumps it out to every cell in the body through the arteries.
- The heart is responsible for pumping oxygenated blood to every cell in the body and for picking up waste products from the tissues.
- The cardiac cycle consists of a period of rest, or diastole, when blood is returned to the heart by veins, and a period of contraction, or systole, when the blood is pumped out of the heart.
- The heart muscle possesses the properties of automaticity (the ability to generate an action potential in the absence of stimulation) and conductivity (the ability to rapidly transmit an action potential).
- The heart muscle is stimulated to contract by impulses generated in the heart, not by stimuli from the brain. The autonomic nervous system can affect the heart to increase (sympathetic) or decrease (parasympathetic) activity.
- In normal sinus rhythm, cells in the SA node generate an impulse that is transmitted through the atrial bundles and delayed slightly at the AV node before being sent down the bundle of His into the ventricles. When cardiac muscle cells are stimulated, they contract.
- Alterations in the generation of conduction of impulses in the heart cause arrhythmias (dysrhythmias), which can upset the normal balance in the cardiovascular system and lead to a decrease in cardiac output, affecting all of the cells of the body.
- Heart muscle contracts by the sliding of actin and myosin filaments in a functioning unit called a sarcomere. Contraction requires energy and calcium to allow the filaments to react with each other and slide together.
- The heart muscle needs a constant supply of blood, which is furnished by the coronary arteries. Increase in demand for oxygen can occur with changes in heart rate, preload, afterload or stretch on the muscle.
- The cardiovascular system is a closed pressure system that uses arteries (muscular, pressure or resistance vessels) to carry blood from the heart, veins (flexible, distensible capacitance vessels) to return blood to the heart and capillaries (which connect arteries to veins) to keep blood flowing from areas of high pressure to areas of low pressure.
- Blood pressure is maintained by stimulus from the sympathetic system and reflex control of blood volume and pressure by the renin–angiotensin system and the aldosterone–ADH system. Alterations in blood pressure (hypotension or hypertension) can upset the balance of the cardiovascular system and lead to problems in blood delivery.
- Fluid shifts out of the blood at the arterial ends of capillaries to deliver oxygen and nutrients to the tissues. It moves out due to the hydrostatic or fluid pressure of the arterial side of the system. Fluid returns to the system at the venous end of the capillaries because of the oncotic pull of proteins in the vessels. Disruptions in these pressures can lead to oedema or loss of fluid in the tissues.

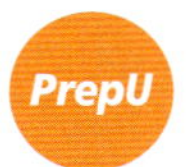

Knowing your strengths and weaknesses helps you to study more effectively. Take a PrepU Practice Quiz to find out how you measure up!

ONLINE RESOURCES

An extensive range of additional resources to enhance teaching and learning and to facilitate understanding of this chapter may be found online at the text's accompanying website, located on thePoint at http://thepoint.lww.com. These include Watch and Learn videos, Concepts in Action animations, journal articles, review questions, case studies, discussion topics and quizzes.

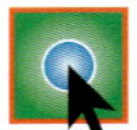

WEB LINK

To explore the virtual cardiovascular system, consult the following web resource:

www.InnerBody.com

BIBLIOGRAPHY

Barrett, K. E. & Ganong, W. F. (2010). *Ganong's Review of Medical Physiology* (23rd edn). New York: McGraw-Hill.

Braunwald, E., Bonow, R. O., Mann, D. L., Zipes, D. P. & Libby, P. (2012). *Braunwald's Heart Disease: A Textbook of Cardiovascular Medicine* (9th edn). Philadelphia: Elsevier Saunders.

Goodman, L. S., Brunton, L. L., Chabner, B. & Knollmann, B. C. (2011). *Goodman and Gilman's Pharmacological Basis of Therapeutics* (12th edn). New York: McGraw-Hill.

Guyton, A. & Hall, J. (2011). *Textbook of Medical Physiology* (12th edn). Philadelphia: Saunders Elsevier.

Hurst, J. W., Fuster, V., Walsh, R. A. & Harrington, R. A. (Eds.). (2011). *Hurst's the Heart* (13th edn). New York: McGraw-Hill.

Porth, C. M. (2011). *Essentials of Pathophysiology: Concepts of Altered Health States* (3rd edn). Philadelphia: Lippincott Williams & Wilkins.

Porth, C. M. (2009). *Pathophysiology: Concepts of Altered Health States* (8th edn). Philadelphia: Lippincott Williams & Wilkins.

CHECK YOUR UNDERSTANDING

Answers to the questions in this chapter can be found in Appendix A at the back of this book.

MULTIPLE CHOICE

Select the best answer to the following.

1. When describing heart valves to a group of students, which of the following would the instructor include?
   a. The closing of the AV valves is what is responsible for heart sounds.
   b. Small muscles attached to the AV valves are responsible for opening and closing the valves.
   c. The aortic valve opens when the pressure in the left ventricle becomes greater than the aortic pressure.
   d. The valves leading to the great vessels are called the cuspid valves.
2. In the heart:
   a. the ventricles will not contract unless they are stimulated by action potentials arising from the SA node.
   b. fibrillation of the atria will cause blood pressure to fall to zero.
   c. spontaneous depolarisation of the muscle membrane can occur in the absence of nerve stimulation.
   d. the muscle can continue to contract for a long period of time in the absence of oxygen.
3. The activity of the heart depends on both the inherent properties of the cardiac muscle cells and the activity of the autonomic nerves to the heart. Therefore:
   a. cutting all of the autonomic nerves to the heart produces a decrease in heart rate.
   b. blocking the parasympathetic nerves to the heart decreases the heart rate.
   c. stimulating the sympathetic nerves to the heart increases the time available to fill the ventricles during diastole.
   d. the heart rate will increase in cases of dehydration, which leads to low cardiac output.
4. A person with a transplanted heart has no nerve connections to the transplanted heart. In such an individual, one would expect to find:
   a. a slower-than-normal resting heart rate.
   b. atria that contract at a different rate than ventricles.
   c. an increase in heart rate during emotional stress.
   d. inability to exercise because there is no way to increase heart rate.
5. The baroreceptors in the carotid sinus and aortic arch:
   a. are in appropriate position to protect the brain.
   b. decrease the frequency of impulses sent to the cardiovascular centre when arterial blood pressure is increased.
   c. monitor the magnitude of concentration of oxygen in the vessels.
   d. react to high levels of carbon dioxide in the aorta or carotid.
6. Cardiac cells differ from skeletal muscle cells in that:
   a. they contain actin and myosin.
   b. they possess automaticity and conductivity.
   c. calcium must be present for muscle contraction to occur.
   d. they do not require oxygen to survive.
7. Clinically, arrhythmias (or dysrhythmias) cause:
   a. altered cardiac output that could affect all cells.
   b. changes in capillary filling pressures.
   c. alterations in osmotic pressure.
   d. valvular dysfunction.
8. A person is brought to the emergency room with a suspected myocardial infarction. The person is very upset because he had just had an ECG in his doctor's office and it was fine. The explanation of this common phenomenon would include the fact that:
   a. the ECG only reflects changes in cardiac output.
   b. the ECG is not a very accurate test.
   c. the ECG only measures the flow of electrical current through the heart.
   d. the ECG is not related to the heart problems.
9. Blood flow to the myocardium differs from blood flow to the rest of the cells of the body in that:
   a. blood perfuses the myocardium during systole.
   b. blood flow is determined by many local factors, including buildup of acid.
   c. blood perfuses the myocardium during diastole.
   d. oxygenated blood flows to the myocardium via veins.

MULTIPLE RESPONSE

Select all that apply.

1. During diastole, which of the following would occur?
   a. opening of the atrioventricular valves
   b. relaxation of the myocardial muscle
   c. flow of blood from the atria to the ventricles
   d. contraction of the ventricles
   e. closing of the semilunar valves
   f. filling of the coronary arteries

2. The sympathetic nervous system would be expected to have which of the following effects?
   a. stimulate the heart to beat faster
   b. speed conduction through the AV node
   c. cause the heart muscle to contract harder
   d. slow conduction through the AV node
   e. decrease overall vascular volume
   f. increase total peripheral resistance

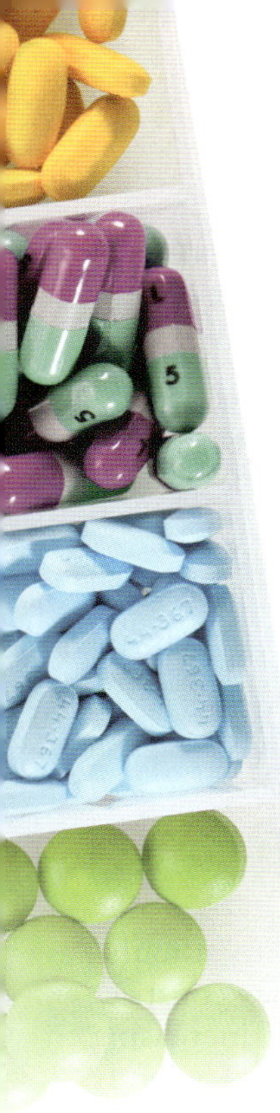

Drugs affecting blood pressure

43

Learning objectives

On completing this chapter you should be able to:

1. Outline the normal controls of blood pressure and explain how the various drugs used to treat hypertension or hypotension affect these controls.
2. Describe the therapeutic actions, indications, pharmacokinetics, contraindications, most common adverse reactions and important drug–drug interactions associated with drugs affecting blood pressure.
3. Discuss the use of drugs that affect blood pressure across the lifespan.
4. Compare and contrast the drugs captopril, losartan, diltiazem, nitroprusside and midodrine with other agents in their class and with other agents used to affect blood pressure.
5. Outline the care considerations, including important teaching points, for people receiving drugs used to affect blood pressure.

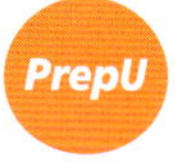

Test your current knowledge of drugs affecting blood pressure with a PrepU Practice Quiz!

Glossary of key terms

angiotensin-converting enzyme (ACE) inhibitor: drug that blocks ACE, the enzyme responsible for converting angiotensin I to angiotensin II in the lungs; this blockage prevents the vasoconstriction and aldosterone release related to angiotensin II

angiotensin II receptors: specific receptors found in blood vessels and in the adrenal gland that react with angiotensin II to cause vasoconstriction and release of aldosterone

baroreceptor: pressure receptor; located in the arch of the aorta and in the carotid artery; responds to changes in pressure and influences the medulla to stimulate the sympathetic system to increase or decrease blood pressure

cardiovascular centre: area of the medulla at which stimulation will activate the sympathetic nervous system to increase blood pressure, heart rate and so forth

essential hypertension: sustained blood pressure above normal limits with no discernible underlying cause

hypotension: sustained blood pressure that is lower than that required to adequately perfuse all of the body's tissues

peripheral resistance: force that resists the flow of blood through the vessels, mostly determined by the arterioles, which contract to increase resistance; important in determining overall blood pressure

renin–angiotensin–aldosterone system: compensatory process that leads to increased blood pressure and blood volume to ensure perfusion of the kidneys; important in the continual regulation of blood pressure

shock: severe hypotension that can lead to accumulation of waste products and cell death

stroke volume: the amount of blood pumped out of the ventricle with each beat; important in determining blood pressure

ANTIHYPERTENSIVE AGENTS

Angiotensin-converting-enzyme inhibitors
- (P) captopril
- enalapril
- fosinopril
- lisinopril
- perindopril
- quinapril
- ramipril
- trandolapril

Angiotensin II–receptor blockers
- candesartan
- eprosartan
- irbesartan
- (P) losartan
- olmesartan
- telmisartan
- valsartan

Calcium channel blockers
- amlodipine
- (P) diltiazem
- felodipine
- isradipine
- lercanidipine
- nifedipine
- verapamil

Vasodilators
- diazoxide
- hydralazine
- minoxidil
- (P) sodium nitroprusside

Other antihypertensive agents

Diuretic agents

Thiazide and thiazide-like diuretics

bendroflumethiazide (bendrofluazide)

chlortalidone

hydrochlorothiazide

indapamide

Loop diuretics

bumetanide

furosemide (frusemide)

Potassium-sparing diuretics / aldosterone antagonists

amiloride

eplerenone

spironolactone

triamterene

Sympathetic nervous system drugs

Beta blockers

atenolol

metoprolol

nadolol

nebivolol

pindolol

propranolol

Alpha and beta blockers

carvedilol

labetalol

Alpha blockers

phenoxybenzamine

Alpha-1 blockers

doxazosin

prazosin

terazosin

Alpha-2 blockers

clonidine

methyldopa

moxonidine

ANTIHYPOTENSIVE AGENTS

Alpha-specific adrenergic agent

midodrine

Sympathetic adrenergic agonists or vasopressors

adrenaline (epinephrine)

dobutamine

dopamine

ephedrine

isoprenaline

metaraminol

noradrenaline (norepinephrine)

phenylephrine

The cardiovascular system is a closed system of blood vessels that is responsible for delivering oxygenated blood to the tissues and removing waste products from the tissues. The blood in this system flows from areas of higher pressure to areas of lower pressure. The area of highest pressure in the system is always the left ventricle during systole. The pressure in this area propels the blood out of the aorta and into the system. The lowest pressure is in the right atrium, which collects all of the deoxygenated blood from the body. The maintenance of this pressure system is controlled by specific areas of the brain and various hormones. If the pressure becomes too high, the person is said to be hypertensive. If the pressure becomes too low and blood cannot be delivered effectively, the person is said to be hypotensive. Helping the person to maintain the blood pressure within normal limits is the goal of drug therapy. Cardiovascular health is one of the Australian government's nine National Health Priority Areas (AIHW, 2013).

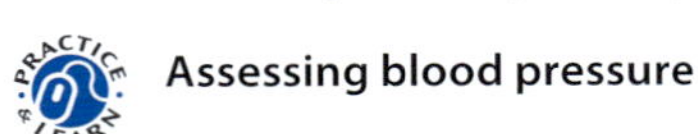

REVIEW OF BLOOD PRESSURE CONTROL

The pressure in the cardiovascular system is determined by three elements:

- Heart rate
- **Stroke volume**, or the amount of blood that is pumped out of the ventricle with each heartbeat (primarily determined by the volume of blood in the system)
- Total **peripheral resistance**, or the resistance of the muscular arteries to the blood being pumped through.

The small arterioles are thought to be the most important factors in determining peripheral resistance. Because they have the smallest diameter, they are able to almost stop blood flow into capillary beds when they constrict, building up tremendous pressure in the arteries behind them as they prevent the blood from flowing through. The arterioles are very responsive to stimulation from the sympathetic nervous system; they constrict when the sympathetic system is stimulated, increasing total peripheral resistance and blood pressure. The body uses this responsiveness to regulate blood pressure on a constant basis, to ensure that there is enough pressure in the system to deliver sufficient blood to the brain.

Baroreceptors

As the blood leaves the left ventricle through the aorta, it influences specialised cells in the arch of the aorta called **baroreceptors** (pressure receptors). Similar cells are located in the carotid arteries, which deliver blood to the brain. If there is sufficient pressure in these vessels, the baroreceptors are stimulated, sending that information to the brain. If the pressure falls, the stimulation of the baroreceptors falls off. That information is also sent to the brain.

The sensory input from the baroreceptors is received in the medulla in an area called the **cardiovascular centre** or vasomotor centre. If the pressure is high, the medulla stimulates vasodilation and a decrease in cardiac rate and output, causing the pressure in the system to drop. If the pressure is low, the medulla directly stimulates an increase in cardiac rate and output, and vasoconstriction; this increases total peripheral resistance and raises the blood pressure. The medulla mediates these effects through the autonomic nervous system (see Chapter 29).

The baroreceptor reflex functions continually to maintain blood pressure within a predetermined range of normal. For example, if you have been lying down flat and suddenly stand up, the blood will rush to your feet (an effect of gravity). You may even feel light-headed or dizzy for a short time. When you stand and the blood flow drops, the baroreceptors are not stretched. The medulla senses this drop in stimulation of the baroreceptors and stimulates a rise in heart rate and cardiac output, and a generalised vasoconstriction, which increases total peripheral resistance and blood pressure. These increases should raise pressure in the system, which restores blood flow to the brain and stimulates the baroreceptors. The stimulation of the baroreceptors leads to a decrease in stimulatory impulses from the medulla, and the blood pressure falls back within normal limits (Figure 43.1).

Renin–angiotensin–aldosterone system

Another compensatory system is activated when the blood pressure within the kidneys falls. Because the kidneys require a constant perfusion to function properly, they have a compensatory mechanism to help ensure that blood flow is maintained. This mechanism is called the **renin–angiotensin–aldosterone system.**

Low blood pressure or poor oxygenation of a nephron causes the release of renin from the juxtaglomerular cells, a group of cells that monitor blood pressure and flow into the glomerulus. Renin is released into the bloodstream and arrives in the liver to convert the compound

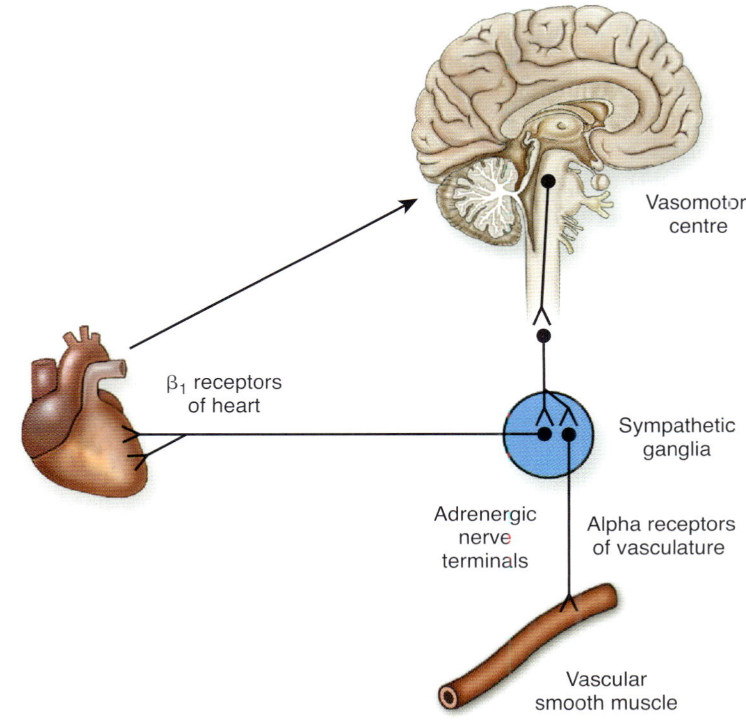

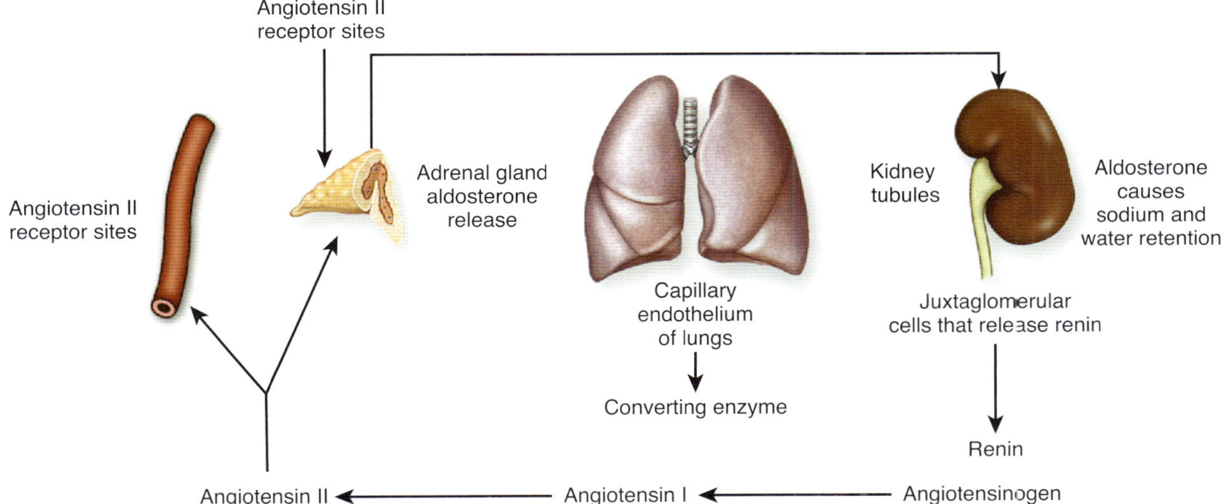

FIGURE 43.1 Control of blood pressure. The vasomotor centre in the medulla responds to stimuli from aortic and carotid baroreceptors to cause sympathetic stimulation. The kidneys release renin to activate the renin–angiotensin system, causing vasoconstriction and increased blood volume.

angiotensinogen (produced in the liver) to angiotensin I. Angiotensin I travels in the bloodstream to the lungs, where the metabolic cells of the alveoli use angiotensin-converting enzyme (ACE) to convert angiotensin I to angiotensin II. Angiotensin II reacts with specific angiotensin II–receptor sites on blood vessels to cause intense vasoconstriction. This effect raises the total peripheral resistance and the blood pressure, restoring blood flow to the kidneys and decreasing the release of renin.

Angiotensin II, probably after conversion to angiotensin III, also stimulates the adrenal cortex to release aldosterone. Aldosterone acts on the nephrons to cause the retention of sodium and water. This effect increases blood volume, which should also contribute to increasing blood pressure. The sodium-rich blood stimulates the osmoreceptors in the hypothalamus to cause the release of antidiuretic hormone (ADH), which in turn causes retention of water in the nephrons, further increasing the blood volume. This increase in blood volume increases the blood pressure, which should increase blood flow to the kidneys. This should lead to a decrease in the release of renin, thus causing the compensatory mechanisms to stop (Figure 43.2).

Hypertension

When a person's blood pressure is above normal limits for a sustained period, a diagnosis of hypertension is made (Table 43.1). High blood pressure can damage the heart and kidneys. It can also lead to ischaemic heart disease, stroke and kidney (renal) failure. In New Zealand, high blood pressure accounted for about 8% of illness, disability and premature mortality in 2013. One in six adults (17%) reported taking medication for high blood pressure in 2015/16; however, just over half (53%) of them had their blood pressure under control when measured in the survey. Māori people were the main ethnic group highly represented for cardiovascular death. Ischaemic heart disease was the leading cause of death for Māori men and both non-Māori men and women, and the second leading cause of death for Māori women. In Australia, the Australian Bureau of Statistics (2014) reported in 2012–13 that 20% of the Indigenous population over the age of 55 years had hypertension.

Ninety per cent of the people with hypertension have what is called **essential hypertension**, or hypertension with no known cause. People with essential hypertension usually have elevated total peripheral resistance. Their organs are being perfused effectively, and they usually display no symptoms. A few people develop secondary hypertension, or high blood pressure resulting from a known cause. For example, a tumour in the adrenal medulla called a phaeochromocytoma can cause hypertension related to the release of large amounts of noradrenaline from tumour cells, which resolves after the tumour is removed.

The underlying danger of hypertension of any type is the prolonged force on the vessels of the vascular system. The muscles in the arterial system eventually thicken, leading to a loss of responsiveness in the system. The left ventricle thickens because the muscle must constantly work hard to expel blood at a greater force. The thickening of the heart muscle and the increased pressure that the muscle has to generate every time it contracts increase the workload of the heart and the risk of coronary artery disease (CAD) as well. The force of the blood being propelled against them damages the inner linings of the arteries, making these vessels susceptible

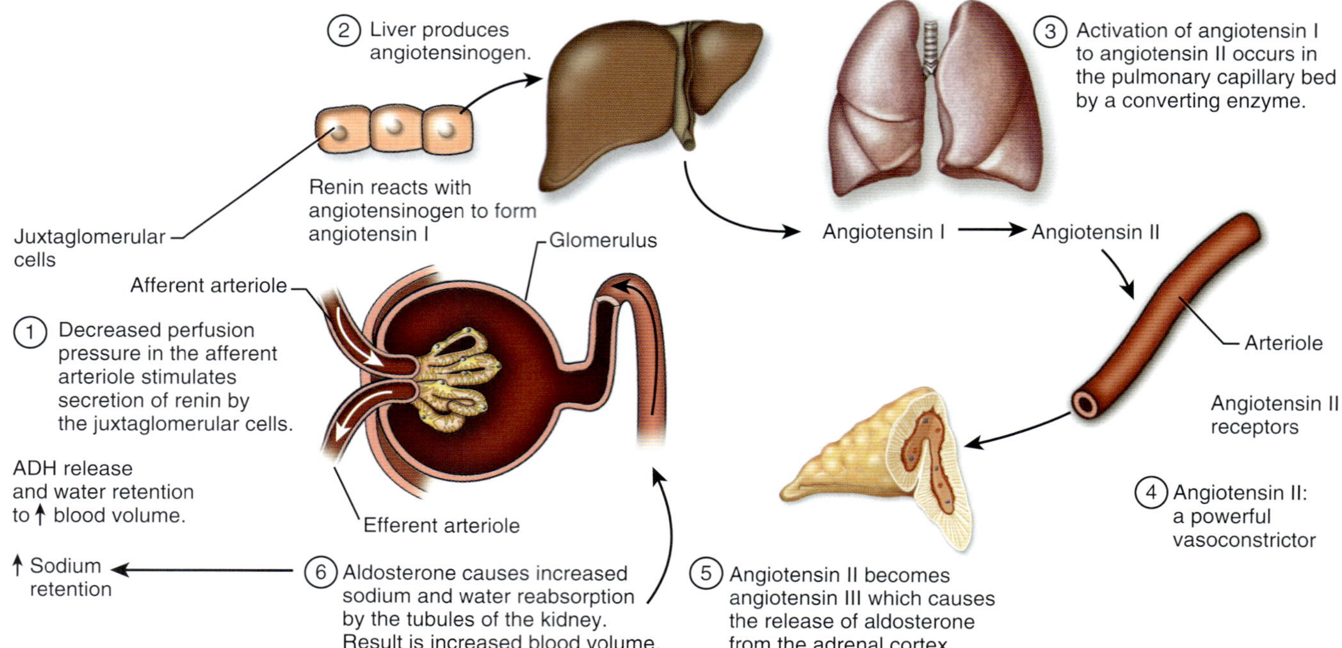

FIGURE 43.2 The renin–angiotensin–aldosterone system.

BOX 43.1 FOCUS ON The evidence

'White coat' hypertension

The diagnosis of hypertension is accompanied by the impact of serious ramifications, such as increased risk of numerous diseases and cardiovascular death, as well as the potential need for significant lifestyle changes and also drug therapy, which may include many unpleasant adverse effects. Consequently, it is important that a person be correctly diagnosed before being labelled hypertensive.

Researchers in the 1990s discovered that some people were hypertensive only when they were in their doctor's office having their blood pressure measured. This was correlated to a sympathetic stress reaction (which elevates systolic blood pressure) and a tendency to tighten the muscles (isometric exercise, which elevates diastolic blood pressure) while waiting to be seen and during the blood pressure measurement. The researchers labelled this phenomenon 'white coat' hypertension.

The Heart Foundation has published new guidelines for the diagnosis of hypertension. A person should have multiple consecutive blood pressure readings above normal. These guidelines point out the importance of using the correct technique when taking a person's blood pressure, especially because the results can have such a tremendous impact on a person. It is good practice to periodically review the process for performing this routine task. For example, the nurse should:

- select a cuff that is the correct size for the person's arm (a cuff that is too small may give a high reading; a cuff that is too large may give a lower reading)
- try to put the person at ease; remember that waiting alone in a cold room can be stressful to the body and mind and can increase the blood pressure
- ensure that the arm that will be used for the cuff is supported
- make sure the rest of the person's muscles are not tensed while the blood pressure is being taken
- place both the cuff and the stethoscope directly on the person instead of on clothing
- listen carefully and record the first sound heard, the muffling of sounds, and the absence of sound (the actual diastolic pressure is thought to be between these two sounds).

Blood pressure machines found in grocery stores and pharmacies often give higher readings than the actual blood pressure, so people should not be encouraged to use these machines for follow-up readings. The Heart Foundation offers many guidelines for accurate blood pressure measurement. Nurses and midwives are often the health care providers most likely to be taking and recording blood pressure, so it is important to always use proper technique and to make accurate records.

TABLE 43.1 Categories rating the severity of hypertension

Diagnostic category	Systolic (mmHg)	Diastolic (mmHg)
Optimal	< 120	< 80
Normal	120–129	80–84
High-normal	130–139	85–89
Grade 1 (mild) hypertension	140–159	90–99
Grade 2 (moderate) hypertension	160–179	100–109
Grade 3 (severe) hypertension	≥ 180	≥ 110
Isolated systolic hypertension	≥ 140	< 90

Source: National Heart Foundation of Australia, 2016. *Guideline for the diagnosis and management of hypertension in adults – 2016.* www.heartfoundation.org.au/images/uploads/publications/PRO-167_Hypertension-guideline-2016_WEB.pdf

to atherosclerosis and to narrowing of the lumen of the vessels (see Chapter 46). Tiny vessels can be damaged and destroyed, leading to loss of vision (if the vessels are in the retina), loss of kidney function (if the vessels include the glomeruli in the nephrons) or loss of cerebral function (if the vessels are small and fragile vessels in the brain).

Untreated hypertension increases a person's risk for CAD and cardiac death, stroke, renal failure and loss of vision. Because hypertension has no symptoms, it is difficult to diagnose and treat, and it is often called the 'silent killer'. All of the drugs used to treat hypertension have adverse effects, many of which are seen as unacceptable by otherwise healthy people. Health professionals face a difficult challenge trying to convince people to comply with their drug regimens when they experience adverse effects and do not see any positive effects on their bodies. Research into the cause of hypertension is ongoing. Many theories have been proposed for the cause of the disorder, and it may well be due to a mosaic of factors. Factors that are known to increase blood pressure in some people include high levels of psychological stress, exposure to high-frequency noise, a high-salt diet, lack of rest and genetic predisposition.

Hypotension

If blood pressure becomes too low, the vital centres in the brain, as well as the rest of the tissues of the body, may not receive enough oxygenated blood to continue functioning. **Hypotension** can progress to **shock**, in which the body is in serious jeopardy as waste products accumulate and cells die from lack of oxygen. Hypotensive states can occur:

- when the heart muscle is damaged and unable to pump effectively
- with severe blood loss, when volume drops dramatically
- when there is extreme stress and the body's levels of noradrenaline are depleted, leaving the body unable to respond to stimuli to raise blood pressure.

KEY POINTS

- The cardiovascular system depends on pressure changes to circulate blood to the tissues and back to the heart.
- Heart rate, stroke volume and peripheral vascular resistance are factors that determine blood pressure.
- Constriction and relaxation of the arterioles result in peripheral resistance.
- The baroreceptors stimulate the medulla, which stimulates the sympathetic nervous system to constrict the blood vessels and increase fluid retention if pressure is low in the aorta and the carotid arteries. If pressure is too high, vasodilation and loss of fluid result.
- A decrease in blood flow to the kidneys triggers the renin–angiotensin–aldosterone system, by which the blood vessels constrict and water is retained. This activity increases blood pressure and restores blood flow to the kidney.
- Hypertension is a sustained state of higher-than-normal blood pressure that can lead to blood vessel damage, atherosclerosis and damage to small vessels in end organs.
- The cause of essential hypertension is unknown; treatment varies among individuals.

ANTIHYPERTENSIVE AGENTS

Because an underlying cause of hypertension is usually unknown, altering the body's regulatory mechanisms is the best treatment currently available. Drugs used to treat hypertension work to alter the normal reflexes that control blood pressure. See Figure 43.3 for a review of the sites of action of drugs used to treat hypertension. Treatment for essential hypertension does not cure the disease but is aimed at maintaining the blood pressure within normal limits to prevent the damage that hypertension can cause. Not all people respond in the same way to antihypertensive drugs because different factors may contribute to each person's hypertension. Individuals may have complicating conditions, such as diabetes or acute myocardial infarction (AMI), that make it unwise to use certain drugs.

Several different types of drugs that affect different areas of blood pressure control may need to be used in combination to maintain a person's blood pressure within normal limits. Trials of drugs and combinations of drugs are often needed to develop an individual regimen that is effective without producing adverse effects that are unacceptable to the person (Box 43.2). Research is ongoing into the treatment of more specific hypertensions (eg, pulmonary hypertension). The development of drugs that target specific blood vessel sites and chemicals could lead to a new approach to the treatment of essential hypertension (Box 43.3).

Antihypertensive agents include angiotensin-converting enzyme inhibitors, angiotensin II–receptor blockers, calcium channel blockers, vasodilators and other antihypertensive agents, including diuretic agents, ganglionic receptors, renin inhibitors and sympathetic nervous system drugs (see Chapter 31). See Table 43.2 for a complete list of antihypertensive agents. See Box 43.4 for use of these agents across the lifespan.

Treating hypertension

The importance of treating hypertension has been proven in numerous research studies. If hypertension is controlled, the person's risk of cardiovascular death and disease is reduced. The risk of developing cardiovascular complications is directly related to the person's degree of hypertension (see Table 43.1). Lowering the degree of hypertension lowers the risk.

Hypertensive treatment is further complicated by the presence of other chronic conditions. The Heart Foundation has published an algorithm for the treatment of hypertension to help prescribers select an antihypertensive agent in the light of complicating conditions (Figure 43.4). A person's response to a given antihypertensive agent is very individual, so the drug of choice for one person may have little to no effect on another person.

ANGIOTENSIN-CONVERTING-ENZYME INHIBITORS

The **angiotensin-converting-enzyme (ACE) inhibitors** include the following agents: captopril (*Capoten*, *Zedace*, others), enalapril (*Acetec*, *Renitec*, others), fosinopril (*Monace*), lisinopril (*Fibsol*, *Zestril*, others), perindopril (*Coversyl*, *Indopril*, *Perindo*), quinapril (*Accupril*, *Acquin*, *Qpril*), ramipril (*Prilace*, *Ramace*) and trandolapril (*Dolapril*, *Gopten*).

Therapeutic actions and indications

ACE inhibitors act in the lungs to prevent ACE from converting angiotensin I to angiotensin II, a powerful vasoconstrictor and stimulator of aldosterone release (see Figure 43.3). This action leads to a decrease in blood pressure and in aldosterone secretion, with a resultant slight increase in serum potassium and a loss of serum sodium and fluid.

These drugs are indicated for the treatment of hypertension, alone or in combination with other drugs. They are also used in conjunction with digoxin and diuretics for the treatment of heart failure and left ventricular dysfunction. Their therapeutic effect in these cases is thought to be related to a decrease in cardiac workload associated with the decrease in peripheral resistance and blood volume. See Table 43.2 for usual indications for each of these drugs.

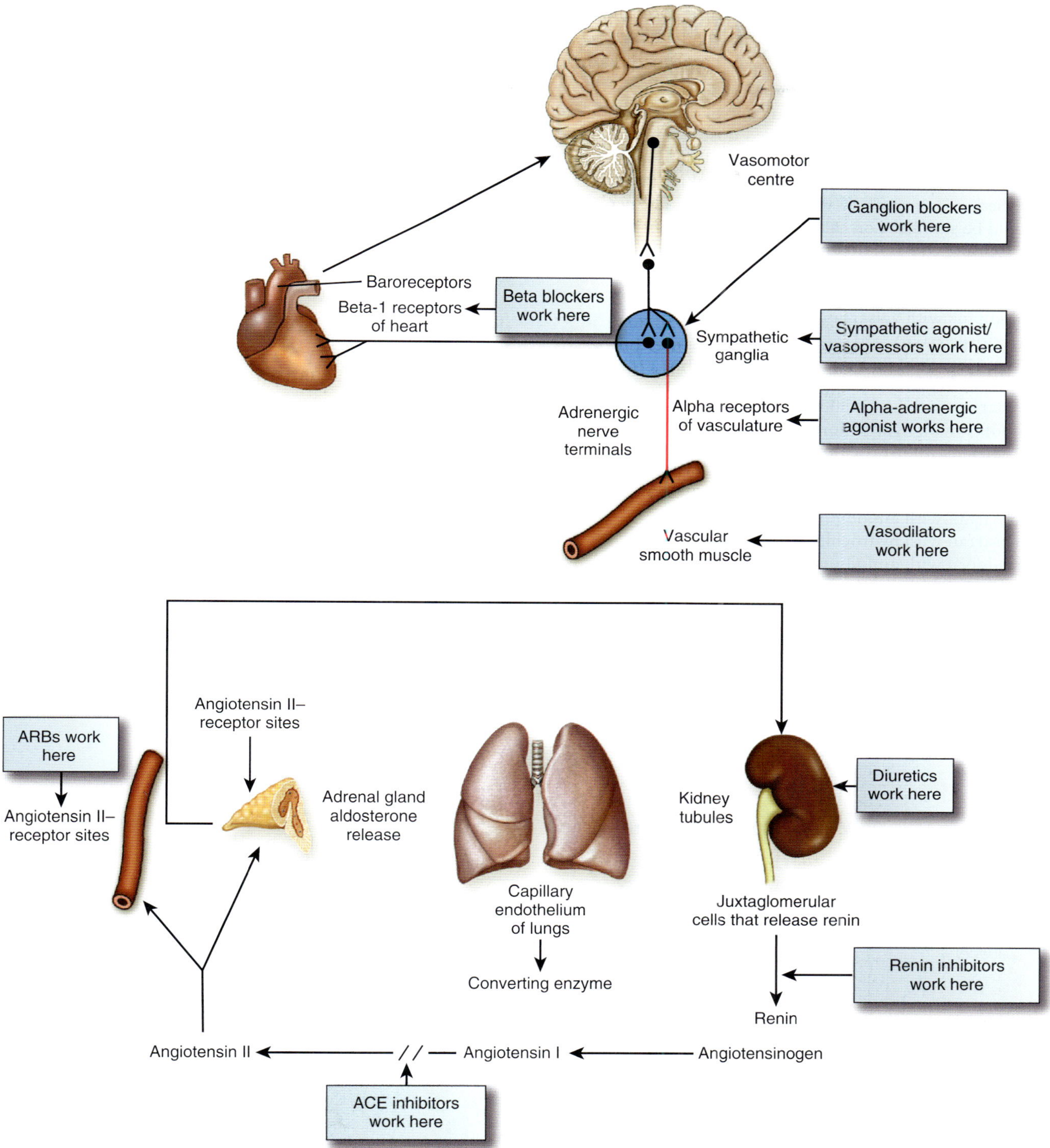

FIGURE 43.3 Sites of action of antihypertensive drugs.

Pharmacokinetics

All of the ACE inhibitors are administered orally. These drugs are well absorbed, widely distributed, metabolised in the liver and excreted in the urine and faeces. They have been detected in breast milk, are known to cross the placenta and have been associated with serious fetal abnormalities, so they should not be used during pregnancy.

Contraindications and cautions

ACE inhibitors are contraindicated in the presence of allergy to any of the ACE inhibitors and with impaired

BOX 43.2 Fixed-dose combination drugs for the treatment of hypertension

Many people require more than one type of antihypertensive to achieve good control of their blood pressure. There are now many fixed-dose combination drugs available for treating hypertension. This allows for fewer tablets or capsules each day, making it easier for the person to comply with drug therapy. The person should be stabilised on each drug first, and then an appropriate combination product can be used.

amlodipine with valsartan (*Exforge*)
amlodipine with valsartan and hydrochlorothiazide (*Exforge HCT*)
candesartan with hydrochlorothiazide (*Adesan HCT*, *Atacand Plus*)
eprosartan with hydrochlorothiazide (*Teveten Plus*)
fosinopril with hydrochlorothiazide (*Fosetic*, *Hyforil*)
irbesartan with hydrochlorothiazide (*Avapro HCT*, *Karvezide*, *KSART HCT*)
lercanidipine with enalapril (*Zan-Extra*)
olmesartan with amlodipine (*Sevikar*)
olmesartan with hydrochlorothiazide (*Olmetec Plus*)
perindopril with amlodipine (*Coveram*, *Reaptan*)
perindopril with indapamide (*Coversyl Plus*, *Perindo Combo*, *Indosyl Combi*)
quinapril with hydrochlorothiazide (*Accuretic*)
telmisartan with amlodipine (*Twynsta*)
telmisartan with hydrochlorothiazide (*Micardis Plus*)
trandolapril with verapamil (*Tarka*)
valsartan with hydrochlorothiazide (*Co-Diovan*)

BOX 43.3 Treatment of pulmonary arterial hypertension

In late 2001, bosentan (*Tracleer*, *Bosleer*) became the first endothelin receptor antagonist to be approved for use in the treatment of pulmonary arterial hypertension. This drug specifically blocks receptor sites for endothelin (ET_A and ET_B) in the endothelium and vascular smooth muscles; these endothelins are chemicals that are elevated in the plasma and lung tissues of people with pulmonary arterial hypertension. Blockade of these receptor sites allows the vessels to relax and dilate, relieving the pressure in the arteries.

Bosentan is an oral drug that is given to adults, initially as 62.5 mg PO bd for 4 weeks, and then increased to 125 mg PO bd if the person's exercise tolerance improves on the drug. People need to be monitored closely for any change in their respiratory function, signs of liver toxicity, or signs of peripheral vasodilation, including flushing, headache, hypotension and palpitations. The drug is pregnancy category X and is known to interact with other drugs, including the statins, glibenclamide and oral contraceptives.

In 2005, sildenafil, a drug known for the treatment of erectile dysfunction, was approved for the treatment of pulmonary arterial hypertension. *Revatio* is an oral drug, with 20 mg given three times a day. The doses should be at least 4–6 hours apart. *Revatio* inhibits cGMP; this allows nitrous oxide in the blood vessel to cause smooth muscle relaxation and decreases vessel pressure (see Chapter 41).

TABLE 43.2 *DRUGS IN FOCUS* Antihypertensive agents

Drug name	Dosage/route	Usual indications
Angiotensin-converting-enzyme (ACE) inhibitors		
(P) captopril (*Capoten*, *Zedace*)	Heart failure: initially 6.25–12.5 mg bd–tid under medical supervision, increased gradually at intervals of at least 2 weeks up to a target dose of 50 mg tid; maximum 150 mg/day Hypertension: 12.5–25 mg bd; maximum 150 mg/day Diabetic nephropathy: 25–50 mg PO tid Ventricular dysfunction after MI: initially 6.25 mg once daily, then 12.5 mg tid, increasing over several days; maximum 150 mg/day Reduce dose for kidney disease and elderly patients	Treatment of left ventricular dysfunction after myocardial infarction (MI) in clinically stable individuals; diabetic nephropathy; for use in adults
enalapril (*Acetec*, *Renitec*)	10–40 mg/day PO; reduce dose in elderly people and people with renal impairment; 2.5 mg PO bd increasing to maintenance dose of 10–20 mg/day for HF or left ventricular dysfunction	Treatment of hypertension, HF, left ventricular dysfunction in adults
fosinopril (*Monace*)	10–40 mg/day PO; reduce dose in elderly people and people with renal impairment	Treatment of hypertension; adjunct therapy for HF; for use in adults

TABLE 43.2 **DRUGS IN FOCUS** **Antihypertensive agents *(continued)***

Drug name	Dosage/route	Usual indications
Angiotensin-converting-enzyme (ACE) inhibitors *(continued)*		
lisinopril (*Fibsol, Zestril*)	Hypertension, usual maintenance: 10–20 mg/day; may require up to 80 mg/day Heart failure: initially 2.5 mg once daily, increased to 10–20 mg/day After MI: 5–10 mg/day Diabetic nephropathy: 10–20 mg once daily; titrate up to a maximum of 80 mg daily. Reduce dose in elderly people and people with renal impairment	Treatment of hypertension, HF; treatment of stable people within 24 hours after acute MI to increase survival; for use in adults
perindopril arginine (*Coversyl*) perindopril erbumine (*Indopril, Perindo*)	Perindopril arginine: 5 mg/day, maximum 10 mg/day Perindopril erbumine: 4 mg/day, maximum 8 mg/day Reduce dose in elderly people and people with renal impairment reduce dose in elderly people and people with renal impairment	Treatment of hypertension; may be used alone or as combination drug to control blood pressure; for use in adults
quinapril (*Accupril, Acquin, Qpril*)	Hypertension: 10 mg once daily, usual maintenance 20–40 mg daily in 1–2 divided doses, maximum 80 mg/day Heart failure: 2.5 mg bd, increased q 2 weeks up to 10 mg bd, maximum 40 mg/day Reduce dose in elderly people and people with renal impairment	Treatment of hypertension; adjunctive treatment of HF; for use in adults
ramipril (*Prilace, Ramace*)	Hypertension: initially 2.5 mg once daily, increased up to 10 mg/day Heart failure after MI: 2.5 mg PO bd increased gradually up to a maximum of 10 mg/day Reduce dose in elderly people and people with renal impairment	Treatment of hypertension; adjunctive treatment of HF for use in adults
trandolapril (*Dolapril, Gopten*)	Hypertension: initially 1–2 mg/day; maximum 4 mg/day Heart failure: 0.5 mg/day increasing slowly to a maximum of 4 mg/day Reduce dose in elderly people and people with renal impairment	Treatment of hypertension, HF, and after MI; for use in adults
Angiotensin II–receptor blockers		
candesartan (*Atacand*)	Initially 8–16 mg/day, to a maximum of 32 mg/day	Used alone or as part of combination therapy for treatment of hypertension in adults
eprosartan (*Teveten*)	Usual dose: 600 mg/day PO Elderly: 400 mg/day PO	Used alone or as part of combination therapy for treatment of hypertension in adults
irbesartan (*Abisart, Avapro*)	150–300 mg/day PO	Used alone or as part of combination therapy for treatment of tension in adults; slowing progression of diabetic nephropathy in people with hypertension and type 2 diabetes
(P) losartan (*Cozaar, Cozavan*)	Hypertension: 25 mg bd or 50 mg once daily; maximum 100 mg/day Heart failure: initially 12.5 mg once daily, increased at weekly intervals to a maximum of 150 mg/day	Used alone or as part of combination therapy for treatment of hypertension in adults; slowing progression of diabetic nephropathy with elevated serum creatinine level and proteinuria in people with hypertension and type 2 diabetes
olmesartan (*Olmetec*)	20–40 mg/day PO	Used alone or as part of combination therapy to treat hypertension in adults (newest angiotensin II–receptor blocker)

Continued on following page

TABLE 43.2 DRUGS IN FOCUS Antihypertensive agents (continued)

Drug name	Dosage/route	Usual indications
Angiotensin II–receptor blockers *(continued)*		
telmisartan (*Micardis*)	40–80 mg/day PO	Used alone or as part of combination therapy for treatment of hypertension in adults
valsartan (*Diovan*)	Usually 80–160 mg/day; maximum 320 mg/day	Used alone or as part of combination therapy for treatment of hypertension in adults; treatment of heart failure in people who are intolerant of ACE inhibitors
Calcium channel blockers		
amlodipine (*Norvasc*)	Usually 2.5–5 mg once daily; maximum 10 mg/day Reduce dose in elderly people and people with renal impairment	Used alone or in combination with other agents for treatment of hypertension and angina in adults
(P) diltiazem (*Cardizem CD, Dilzem*)	Immediate release: 30 mg qid; maximum 360 mg/day in divided doses Sustained release: 180–240 mg/day; maximum 360 mg/day	Extended-release preparation used to treat hypertension in adults; other preparations are used for angina
felodipine (*Felodil ZR, Felodur ER, Fendex ER, Plendil ER*)	10–15 mg/day PO; initially 5 mg daily, usual maintenance 5–10 mg once daily; maximum 20 mg/day Elderly or people with hepatic impairment: initially 2.5 mg daily; maximum 10 mg/day	Used alone or in combination with other agents for treatment of hypertension in adults
isradipine (*DynaCirc*)	5 mg once daily; maintenance dose 2.5 mg or 5 mg once daily Elderly, people with renal or hepatic impairment: initially 2.5 mg once daily	Used alone or in combination with thiazide diuretics for treatment of hypertension in adults
lercanidipine (*Lercan, Zanidip, Zircol*)	10–20 mg/day PO	Used alone or in combination with other agents for treatment of hypertension in adults
nifedipine: immediate release (*Adalat*); sustained-release twice-daily preparation (*Adalat Modified Release, Nyefax Retard*); sustained-release once-daily preparation (*Adalat OROS, Adefin XL*)	Immediate release: 5 mg tid Sustained-release twice-daily preparation: 10–20 mg bd; maximum 30 mg bd Sustained-release once-daily preparation: 30 mg once daily, increased if necessary, to 60 mg once daily; maximum 120 mg/day (hypertension) or 90 mg/day (angina)	Extended-release preparations only for the treatment of hypertension in adults; other preparations are used for angina
verapamil (*Anpec, Cordilox SR, Isoptin, Isoptin SR, Verapamil, Verapamil SR*)	Immediate release: 80–160 mg bd; maximum 160 mg tid Sustained release: 180–240 mg in the morning; maximum 240 mg bd	Extended-release formulations for the treatment of essential hypertension; other preparations are used for angina and treating various arrhythmias in adults
Vasodilators		
diazoxide (generic)	IV: traditionally 300 mg IV or 5 mg/kg over 30 seconds, whichever is the least Mini-bolus 1–3 mg/kg, maximum 150 mg, over 30 seconds every 5–15 minutes Oral: initially 5 mg/kg daily in 2–3 divided doses; usual maintenance dose 3–8 mg/kg daily in 2–3 divided doses	Treatment of severe hypertension in hospitalised adults
hydralazine (*Alphapress, Apresoline*)	Oral: 25 mg bd, maximum 50 mg bd IV: 5–10 mg by slow IV, or continuous infusion 200–300 micrograms/minutes; maintenance usually 50–150 micrograms/min	Treatment of severe hypertension
minoxidil (*Loniten*)	Adults usually 5–40 mg/day increasing slowly to a maximum of 100 mg/day Child > 12 years: 5 mg/day increasing slowly to a maximum of 100 mg/day	Treatment of severe hypertension unresponsive to other therapy

TABLE 43.2 DRUGS IN FOCUS Antihypertensive agents *(continued)*

Drug name	Dosage/route	Usual indications
Vasodilators *(continued)*		
(P) sodium nitroprusside (generic)	Adult and paediatric: 3 micrograms/kg per minute, do not exceed 10 micrograms/kg per minute	Treatment of hypertensive crisis; also used to maintain controlled hypotension during surgery
Other antihypertensive agents		
Diuretic agents		
See Chapter 51	See Chapter 51	Treatment of mild hypertension; often first agents used; often used in combination with other agents
Sympathetic nervous system blockers		
See Chapter 31	See Chapter 31	

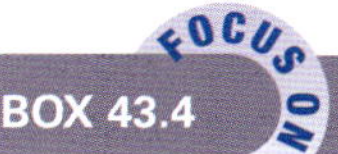

BOX 43.4 Drug therapy across the lifespan

Drugs affecting blood pressure

CHILDREN

National standards for determining normal levels of blood pressure in children are quite new. It has been determined that hypertension may start as a childhood disease, and more screening studies are being done to establish normal values for each age group.

Children are thought to be more likely to have secondary hypertension, caused by renal disease or congenital problems such as coarctation of the aorta.

Treatment of childhood hypertension should be done very cautiously because the long-term effects of the antihypertensive agents are not known. Lifestyle changes should be instituted before drug therapy if at all possible. Weight loss and increased activity may bring elevated blood pressure back to normal in many children.

If drug therapy is used, a mild diuretic may be tried first, with monitoring of blood glucose and electrolyte levels on a regular basis. Beta blockers have been used with success in some children; adverse effects may limit their usefulness in others. The safety and efficacy of the ACE inhibitors and the angiotensin II–receptor blockers (ARBs) have not been established in children. Calcium channel blockers have been used to treat hypertension in children and may be a first consideration if drug therapy is needed. Careful follow-up of the growing child is essential to monitor for changes in blood pressure, as well as for adverse effects.

ADULTS

Adults receiving any of these drugs need to be instructed about adverse reactions that should be reported immediately. They need to be reminded of safety precautions that may be needed in hot weather or with conditions that cause fluid depletion (eg, diarrhoea, vomiting). If they are taking any other drugs, the interacting effects of the various drugs should be evaluated. The importance of other measures to help lower blood pressure – weight loss, smoking cessation, increased activity – should be stressed.

PREGNANCY AND BREASTFEEDING

The safety for the use of these drugs during pregnancy has not been established. ACE inhibitors, ARBs and renin inhibitors should not be used during pregnancy. Women of childbearing age should be advised to use barrier contraceptives to prevent pregnancy while taking these drugs. Calcium channel blockers and vasodilators should not be used in pregnancy unless the benefit to the mother clearly outweighs the potential risk to the fetus. The drugs do enter breast milk and can cause serious adverse effects in the baby. Caution should be used or another method of feeding the baby should be used if one of these drugs is needed during breastfeeding.

OLDER ADULTS

Older adults frequently are prescribed one of these drugs. They are more susceptible to the toxic effects of the drugs and are more likely to have underlying conditions that could interfere with drug metabolism and excretion. Renal or hepatic impairment can lead to accumulation of the drugs in the body. If renal or hepatic dysfunction is present, the dose should be reduced and the person monitored very closely.

The total drug regimen of the older person should be coordinated, with careful attention to interactions among drugs and alternative therapies.

Older adults need to use special caution in any situation that could lead to a fall in blood pressure, such as loss of fluids from diarrhoea or vomiting, lack of fluid intake, or excessive heat with decreased sweating that comes with age. Dizziness, falls or syncope can occur if the blood pressure falls too far in these situations. The blood pressure should always be taken immediately before an antihypertensive is administered to an older adult in an institutional setting to avoid excessive lowering of blood pressure.

Older people should be especially cautioned about sustained-release antihypertensives that cannot be cut, crushed or chewed to avoid the potential for excessive dosing if these drugs are inappropriately cut.

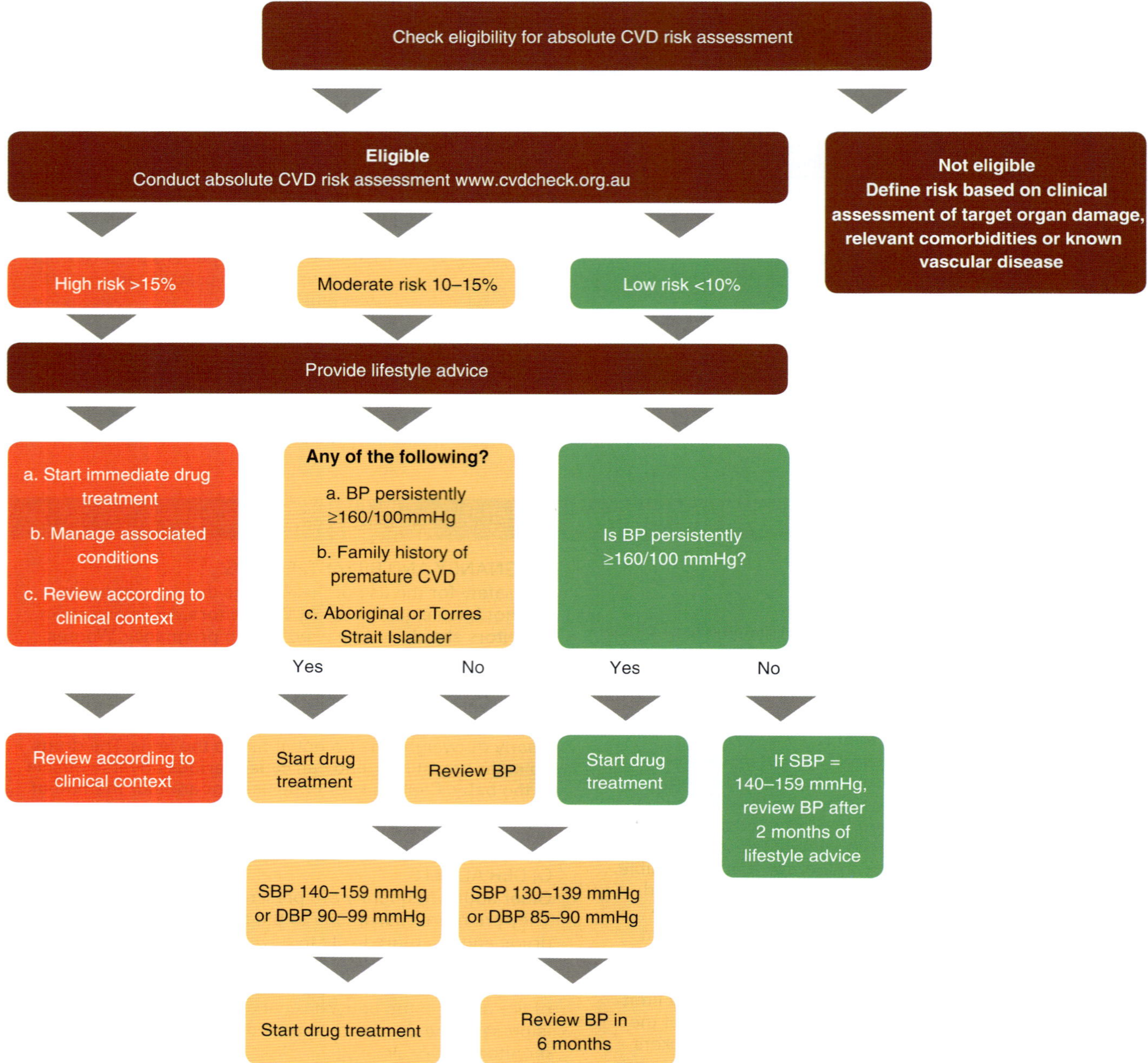

FIGURE 43.4 Treatment strategy for patients with newly diagnosed hypertension. In National Heart Foundation of Australia, 2016. *Guideline for the diagnosis and management of hypertension in adults – 2016*. Source: www.heartfoundation.org.au/images/uploads/publications/PRO-167_Hypertension-guideline-2016_WEB.pdf.

renal function, *which could be exacerbated by the effects of this drug in decreasing renal blood flow.* Caution should be used in individuals with heart failure *because the change in haemodynamics could be detrimental in some cases* and in those with salt/volume depletion, *which could be exacerbated by the drug effects.* Women of childbearing age who choose to use one of these drugs should be encouraged to use barrier contraceptives to avoid pregnancy while taking the drug. Use is contraindicated during pregnancy *because of the potential for serious adverse effects on the fetus* and during breastfeeding *because of potential decrease in milk production and effects on the neonate.*

Adverse effects

The adverse effects most commonly associated with the ACE inhibitors are related to the effects of vasodilation and alterations in blood flow. Such effects include reflex tachycardia, chest pain, angina, heart failure and cardiac arrhythmias; gastrointestinal (GI) irritation, ulcers, constipation and liver injury; renal insufficiency, renal failure and proteinuria; and rash, alopecia, dermatitis and photosensitivity. Quinapril, ramipril and trandolapril are fairly well tolerated and not associated with as many adverse effects as some of the other agents are. Enalapril and fosinopril are generally well tolerated but cause an unrelenting cough, possibly related to effects in the lungs, where the ACE is inhibited, that may lead people to discontinue the drug.

Captopril and perindopril are associated with more-serious adverse effects. Captopril has been associated with a sometimes-fatal pancytopenia, cough and unpleasant GI distress. Pancytopenia is a condition in which a person has low levels of red blood cells, white blood cells and platelets. Perindopril and lisinopril are associated with a sometimes fatal pancytopenia, as well as serious to fatal airway obstruction.

Clinically important drug–drug interactions

The risk of hypersensitivity reactions increases if these drugs are taken with allopurinol. There is a risk of decreased antihypertensive effects if taken with non-steroidal anti-inflammatory drugs; people should be monitored.

Clinically important drug–food interactions

Absorption of oral ACE inhibitors decreases if they are taken with food. They should be taken on an empty stomach 1 hour before or 2 hours after meals.

Prototype summary: captopril

Indications: treatment of hypertension, heart failure, diabetic nephropathy, and left ventricular dysfunction after an MI.

Actions: blocks ACE from converting angiotensin I to angiotensin II, leading to a decrease in blood pressure, a decrease in aldosterone production, and a small increase in serum potassium levels, along with sodium and fluid loss.

Pharmacokinetics:

Route	Onset	Peak
Oral	15 min	30–90 min

$T_{1/2}$: 2 hours; excreted in urine.

Adverse effects: tachycardia, MI, rash, pruritus, gastric irritation, aphthous ulcers, peptic ulcers, dysgeusia, proteinuria, bone marrow suppression, cough.

Care considerations for people receiving ACE inhibitors

Assessment: history and examination

- Assess for the following conditions, *which could be cautions or contraindications to use of the drug*: any known allergies to these drugs; impaired kidney function, *which could be exacerbated by these drugs*; pregnancy or breastfeeding *because of the potential adverse effects on the fetus or neonate*; salt/volume depletion and heart failure, *which could be exacerbated by these drugs.*
- Assess baseline status before beginning therapy to determine *any potential adverse effects*. This includes body temperature and weight; skin colour, lesions and temperature; pulse, blood pressure, baseline electrocardiogram (ECG) and perfusion; respirations and adventitious breath sounds; bowel sounds and abdominal examination; and renal function tests, full blood count with differential and serum electrolytes.

Implementation with rationale

- Encourage the person to implement lifestyle changes, including weight loss, smoking cessation, decreased alcohol and salt in the diet, and increased exercise, *to increase the effectiveness of antihypertensive therapy.*
- Administer on an empty stomach 1 hour before or 2 hours after meals *to ensure proper absorption of the drug.*
- Alert the surgeon and mark the person's chart prominently if the person is to undergo surgery *to alert medical personnel that the blockage of compensatory angiotensin II could result in hypotension after surgery that would need to be reversed with volume expansion.*
- Consult with the prescriber to reduce the dose in individuals with renal failure *to account for their decreased production of renin and lower-than-normal levels of angiotensin II.*
- Monitor the person carefully in any situation that might lead to a drop in fluid volume (eg, excessive sweating, vomiting, diarrhoea, dehydration) *to detect and treat excessive hypotension that may occur.*
- Provide comfort measures *to help the person tolerate drug effects*. These include small, frequent meals; access to bathroom facilities; bowel program as needed; environmental controls; safety precautions; and appropriate skin care as needed.
- Provide thorough teaching, including the name of the drug, dosage prescribed, measures to avoid adverse effects, warning signs of problems and the need for periodic monitoring and evaluation, *to enhance knowledge about drug therapy and to promote compliance.*
- Offer support and encouragement *to help the person deal with the diagnosis and the drug regimen.*

Evaluation

- Monitor response to the drug (maintenance of blood pressure within normal limits).

- Monitor for adverse effects (hypotension, cardiac arrhythmias, renal dysfunction, skin reactions, cough, pancytopenia, heart failure).
- Evaluate the effectiveness of the teaching plan (person can name drug, dosage, adverse effects to watch for, specific measures to avoid them and the importance of continued follow-up).
- Monitor the effectiveness of comfort measures and compliance with the treatment regimen.

ANGIOTENSIN II–RECEPTOR BLOCKERS

The angiotensin II–receptor blockers (ARBs) include the following drugs: candesartan (*Atacand*), eprosartan (*Teveten*), irbesartan (*Abisart, Avapro*), losartan (*Cozaar, Cozavan*), olmesartan (*Olmetec* [not available in New Zealand]), telmisartan (*Micardis* [not available in New Zealand]) and valsartan (*Diovan* [not available in New Zealand]).

Therapeutic actions and indications

The ARBs selectively bind with the **angiotensin II receptors** in vascular smooth muscle and in the adrenal cortex to block vasoconstriction and the release of aldosterone. These actions block the blood pressure–raising effects of the renin–angiotensin system and lower blood pressure. They are indicated to be used alone or in combination therapy for the treatment of hypertension and for the treatment of heart failure in individuals who are intolerant to ACE inhibitors. Recently, they were also found to slow the progression of renal disease in people with hypertension and type 2 diabetes. This action is thought to be related to the effects of blocking angiotensin receptors in the vascular endothelium. See Table 43.2 for indications for each drug.

Pharmacokinetics

These agents are all given orally. They are well absorbed and undergo metabolism in the liver by the cytochrome P450 system. They are excreted in faeces and in urine. The ARBs cross the placenta. It is not known whether they enter breast milk during breastfeeding (see Contraindications and cautions).

Contraindications and cautions

The ARBs are contraindicated in the presence of allergy to any of these drugs *to prevent hypersensitivity reactions*. Caution should be used in the presence of hepatic or renal dysfunction, *which could alter the metabolism and excretion of these drugs*, and with hypovolaemia, *because of the blocking of potentially life-saving compensatory mechanisms*. These drugs are also contraindicated during pregnancy: candesartan, eprosartan, irbesartan, olmesartan and telmisartan should not be used during the second or third trimester of pregnancy *because of association with serious fetal abnormalities and even death when given in the second or third trimester*; losartan and valsartan should not be used at any time during pregnancy. Although it is not known whether the ARBs enter breast milk during breastfeeding, these drugs should not be used during breastfeeding *because of the potential for serious adverse effects in the neonate*. Women of childbearing age should be advised to use barrier contraceptives to avoid pregnancy; if a pregnancy does occur, the ARB should be discontinued immediately.

Adverse effects

The adverse effects most commonly associated with ARBs include the following: headache, dizziness, syncope and weakness, which could be associated with drops in blood pressure; hypotension; GI complaints, including diarrhoea, abdominal pain, nausea, dry mouth and tooth pain; symptoms of upper respiratory tract infections and cough; and rash, dry skin and alopecia. In preclinical trials, these drugs have been associated with the development of various cancers.

Clinically important drug–drug interactions

The risk of decreased serum levels and loss of effectiveness increases if the ARB is taken in combination with phenobarbital (phenobarbitone), indometacin or a rifamycin. If this combination is used, the person should be monitored closely and dose adjustments made. There may be a decrease in anticipated antihypertensive effects if the drug is combined with fluconazole or diltiazem. Monitor the person closely and adjust dose as needed.

Prototype summary: losartan

Indications: alone or as part of combination therapy for the treatment of hypertension; treatment of diabetic nephropathy with an elevated serum creatinine level and proteinuria in people with type 2 diabetes and hypertension.

Actions: selectively blocks the binding of angiotensin II to specific tissue receptors found in the vascular smooth muscle and adrenal glands; blocks the vasoconstriction and release of aldosterone associated with the renin–angiotensin–aldosterone system.

Pharmacokinetics:

Route	Onset	Peak	Duration
Oral	Varies	1–3 hours	24 hours

$T_{1/2}$: 2 hours, then 6–9 hours; metabolised in the liver and excreted in urine and faeces.

Adverse effects: dizziness, headache, diarrhoea, abdominal pain, symptoms of upper respiratory tract infection, cough, back pain, fever, muscle weakness, hypotension.

Care considerations for people receiving angiotensin II–receptor blockers

Assessment: history and examination

- Assess for the following conditions, *which could be cautions or contraindications to use of the drug*: any known allergies to these drugs *to prevent hypersensitivity reactions*; impaired kidney or liver function, *which could be exacerbated by these drugs*; pregnancy and breastfeeding *because of the potential adverse effects on the fetus and neonate*; and hypovolaemia, *which could potentiate the blood pressure–lowering effects.*
- Assess baseline status before beginning therapy *to determine any potential adverse effects*; this includes body temperature and weight; skin colour, lesions and temperature; pulse, blood pressure, baseline ECG and perfusion; respirations and adventitious breath sounds; bowel sounds and abdominal examination; and renal and liver function tests.

Implementation with rationale

- Encourage the person to implement lifestyle changes, including weight loss, smoking cessation, decreased alcohol and salt in the diet, and increased exercise *to increase the effectiveness of antihypertensive therapy.*
- Administer without regard to meals; give with food *to decrease GI distress if needed.*
- Alert the surgeon and mark the person's chart prominently if undergoing surgery *to notify medical personnel that the blockage of compensatory angiotensin II could result in hypotension after surgery that would need to be reversed with volume expansion.*
- Ensure that women are not pregnant before beginning therapy, and suggest the use of barrier contraceptives while taking these drugs, *to avert potential fetal abnormalities and fetal death, which have been associated with these drugs.*
- Find an alternative method of feeding the baby if the woman is breastfeeding *to prevent the potentially dangerous blockade of the renin–angiotensin–aldosterone system in the neonate.*
- Monitor the person carefully in any situation that might lead to a drop in fluid volume (eg, excessive sweating, vomiting, diarrhoea, dehydration) *to detect and treat excessive hypotension that may occur.*
- Provide comfort measures *to help the person tolerate drug effects*, including small, frequent meals; access to bathroom facilities; safety precautions if central nervous system (CNS) effects occur; environmental controls; appropriate skin care as needed; and analgesics as needed.
- Provide thorough teaching, including the name of the drug, dosage prescribed, measures to avoid adverse effects, warning signs of problems and the need for periodic monitoring and evaluation, *to enhance knowledge about drug therapy and to promote compliance.*
- Offer support and encouragement *to help the person deal with the diagnosis and the drug regimen.*

Evaluation

- Monitor response to the drug (maintenance of blood pressure within normal limits).
- Monitor for adverse effects (hypotension, GI distress, skin reactions, cough, headache, dizziness).
- Evaluate the effectiveness of the teaching plan (person can name drug, dosage, adverse effects to watch for, measures to avoid them and the importance of continued follow-up).
- Monitor the effectiveness of comfort measures and compliance with the regimen.

CALCIUM CHANNEL BLOCKERS

Calcium channel blockers decrease blood pressure, cardiac workload and myocardial oxygen consumption. The effects of these drugs on cardiac workload also make them very effective in the treatment of angina (see Chapter 46). The calcium channel blockers available in immediate-release and sustained-release forms that are used in treating hypertension are amlodipine (*Norvasc*), felodipine (*Fendex ER*, *Plendil ER*) and isradipine (*DynaCirc SRO* [not available in Australia]). Other calcium channel blockers are safe and effective for this use only if they are given as sustained-release or extended-release preparations. These include diltiazem (*Cardizem*, *Dilzem*), lercanidipine (*Lercan*, *Zanidip*, *Zircol*), nifedipine (*Adalat*, *Adefin*) and verapamil (*Anpec*, *Isoptin*, *Cordilox SR*). See Contraindications and cautions for important safety information regarding use of controlled-release products.

Therapeutic actions and indications

Calcium channel blockers inhibit the movement of calcium ions across the membranes of myocardial and arterial muscle cells, altering the action potential and blocking muscle cell contraction. This effect depresses myocardial contractility, slows cardiac impulse formation in the conductive tissues and relaxes and dilates arteries, causing a fall in blood pressure and a decrease in venous return. See Table 43.2 for indications for each of these drugs.

Pharmacokinetics

Calcium channel blockers are given orally and are generally well absorbed, metabolised in the liver and excreted in the urine. These drugs cross the placenta and enter breast milk (see Contraindications and cautions).

Contraindications and cautions

These drugs are contraindicated in the presence of allergy to any of these drugs *to prevent hypersensitivity reactions*; with heart block or sick sinus syndrome, *which could be exacerbated by the conduction-slowing effects of these drugs*; and with renal or hepatic dysfunction, *which could alter the metabolism and excretion of these drugs*. Although there are no well-defined studies about effects during pregnancy, fetal toxicity has been reported in animal studies; therefore, these drugs should not be used during pregnancy unless the benefit to the mother clearly outweighs any potential risk to the fetus *because of the potential for adverse effects on the fetus or neonate. Because of the potential for serious adverse effects on the baby*, another method of feeding the infant should be used if these drugs are required during breastfeeding.

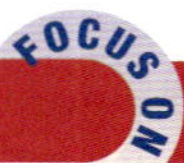

Safe medication administration

Several drugs that are used to treat hypertension cannot be cut, crushed or chewed. This is very important information to share with people on antihypertensive drugs. Sometimes individuals cut tablets in half to facilitate swallowing or to get twice the number of days for any given prescription. Most drugs formulated for extended release or sustained release are delivered in a matrix system that slowly dispenses the drug into the system. If the coating of the matrix is cut, all of the drug is released at once, leading to the release of too much drug at one time and, consequently, toxic levels of the drug when first taking it. Then the person receives no drug as the day goes on. Some antihypertensives to be aware of are diltiazem, nifedipine and verapamil.

Adverse effects

The adverse effects associated with these drugs relate to their effects on cardiac output and on smooth muscle. CNS effects include dizziness, light-headedness, headache and fatigue. GI problems include nausea and hepatic injury related to direct toxic effects on hepatic cells. Cardiovascular effects include hypotension, bradycardia, peripheral oedema and heart block. Skin flushing and rash may also occur.

Clinically important drug–drug interactions

Drug–drug interactions vary with each of the calcium channel blockers used to treat hypertension. A potentially serious effect to note is an increase in serum levels and toxicity of ciclosporin if taken with diltiazem.

Clinically important drug–food interactions

The calcium channel blockers are a class of drugs that interact with grapefruit juice. When grapefruit juice is present in the body, the concentrations of calcium channel blockers increase, sometimes to toxic levels. Advise people to avoid the use of grapefruit juice if they are taking a calcium channel blocker. If a person on a calcium channel blocker reports toxic effects, ask whether they are drinking grapefruit juice and if so advise them to stop drinking the juice.

Prototype summary: diltiazem

Indications: treatment of essential hypertension in the extended-release form.

Actions: inhibits the movement of calcium ions across the membranes of cardiac and arterial muscle cells, depressing the impulse and leading to slowed conduction, decreased myocardial contractility and dilation of arterioles, which lowers blood pressure and decreases myocardial oxygen consumption.

Pharmacokinetics:

Route	Onset	Peak	Duration
Oral, ext. release	30–60 min	6–11 hours	12 hours

$T_{1/2}$: 5–7 hours; metabolised in the liver and excreted in urine.

Adverse effects: dizziness, light-headedness, headache, peripheral oedema, bradycardia, atrioventricular block, flushing, nausea.

Care considerations for people receiving calcium channel blockers

The main use of calcium channel blockers is for the treatment of angina. See Chapter 46 for the care considerations of calcium channel blockers. *See the Critical thinking scenario for the initiation of antihypertensive therapy using calcium channel blockers.*

CRITICAL THINKING SCENARIO

Starting antihypertensive therapy

THE SITUATION

B.R., a 46-year-old Indigenous Australian male business executive, was seen for a routine insurance physical. His examination was normal except for a blood pressure reading of 164/102 mmHg. He also was approximately 10 kg overweight. Urinalysis and blood work results were all within normal limits. He was given a 5000 kilojoule/day diet to follow and was encouraged to reduce his salt and alcohol intake, start exercising and stop smoking. He was asked to return in 3 weeks for a follow-up appointment. Three weeks later, B.R. returned with a 3.5 kg weight loss and an average blood pressure reading (of three readings) of 145/92 mmHg. Discussion was held about starting B.R. on a diuretic in addition to the lifestyle changes that B.R. was undertaking. B.R. was reluctant to take a diuretic and, after much discussion, was prescribed a calcium channel blocker. B.R. asked for a couple more weeks to try to bring his blood pressure down with lifestyle changes before starting the drug.

CRITICAL THINKING

What care interventions should be done at this point?
Consider the risk factors that B.R. has for hypertension and the damage that hypertension can cause.
What are the chances that B.R. can bring his blood pressure within a normal range with lifestyle changes alone?
What additional teaching points should be covered with B.R. before a treatment decision is made?
What implication does the diagnosis of hypertension have for B.R.'s insurance and job security?
What effects could diuretic therapy have on B.R.'s busy business day?

DISCUSSION

B.R. was asked to change many things in his life over the last 3 weeks. These changes themselves can be stressful and can increase a person's blood pressure. B.R.'s reluctance to take a diuretic is understandable for a business executive who might not want his day interrupted by many bathroom stops.

B.R. should receive a complete teaching program outlining what is known about hypertension and all of the risk factors involved with the disease. The good effects of weight loss, exercise and other lifestyle changes should be stressed, and B.R. should be praised for his success over the last 3 weeks.

B.R. may benefit from trying for a couple more weeks to make lifestyle changes that will help bring his blood pressure into normal range. He will then feel that he has some control and input into the situation, and if drug therapy is needed, he may be more willing to comply with the prescribed treatment. The diagnosis of hypertension may be delayed for these 2 weeks while B.R. changes his lifestyle. Such a diagnosis should be made only after three consecutive blood pressure readings in the high range are recorded. B.R. may be able to have his blood pressure checked at work in a comfortable environment, which will improve the accuracy of the reading.

In the past, many insurance companies and some employers, viewed hypertension as a hiring and insurability risk. As a business executive, B.R. may be well aware of this increased risk category – another reason to give him a little more time. He may wish to look into biofeedback for relaxation, a fitness program, smoking-cessation programs (if appropriate) and stress reduction. As long as B.R. receives regular follow-up and frequent blood pressure checks, it may be a good idea to allow him to take some control and continue lifestyle changes. If at the end of the 2 weeks no further progress has been made or B.R.'s blood pressure has risen, drug therapy should be considered. Teaching should be aimed at helping B.R. to incorporate the drug effects into his lifestyle, to improve his compliance and tolerance of the therapy.

CARE GUIDE FOR B.R.: CALCIUM CHANNEL BLOCKERS

Assessment: history and examination

Concentrate the health history on allergies to any calcium channel blocker, renal dysfunction, salt/volume depletion, or heart failure and concurrent use of barbiturates, phenytoin, erythromycin, cimetidine, ranitidine, antifungal agents and/or grapefruit juice.
Focus the physical examination on the following:
Cardiovascular: blood pressure, pulse, perfusion, baseline ECG
CNS: orientation, affect
Skin: colour, lesions, texture, temperature
Respiratory system: respiration, adventitious sounds
GI: abdominal examination, bowel sounds
Laboratory tests: renal function tests, FBC, electrolyte levels

Implementation

Encourage lifestyle changes to increase drug effectiveness.
Do not cut, crush or chew this tablet. Give with food if GI upset occurs.
Provide comfort and safety measures.
Reduce dosage if person has renal failure.
Monitor for any situation that might lead to a drop in blood pressure.

Provide support and reassurance to deal with drug effects.
Provide teaching regarding drug, dosage, adverse effects, signs and symptoms of problems to report, and safety precautions.

Evaluation

Evaluate drug effects: maintenance of blood pressure within normal limits.
Monitor for adverse effects: nausea, dizziness; hypotension, congestive heart failure, skin reactions.
Monitor for drug–drug interactions as listed.
Evaluate effectiveness of teaching program and comfort and safety measures.

TEACHING FOR B.R.

- The drug that has been prescribed to treat your hypertension is called a calcium channel blocker. When used to treat high blood pressure, this drug is called an antihypertensive. High blood pressure is a disorder that may have no symptoms but that can cause serious problems, such as heart attack, stroke or kidney problems, if left untreated.
- It is very important to take your medication every day, as prescribed, even if you feel perfectly well without the medication. It is possible that you may feel worse because of the adverse effects associated with the medication when you take it. Even if this happens, it is crucial that you take your medication.
- If you find that the adverse effects of this drug are too uncomfortable, discuss the possibility of taking a different antihypertensive medication with your health care provider.
- This drug should be taken on an empty stomach, 1 hour before or 2 hours after meals.
- Common effects of these drugs include:
  - *Dizziness, drowsiness, light-headedness:* these effects often pass after the first few days. Until they do, avoid driving or performing hazardous or delicate tasks that require concentration. If these effects occur, change positions slowly to decrease the light-headedness.
  - *Nausea, vomiting, change in taste perception:* small, frequent meals may help ease these effects, which may pass with time. If they persist and become too uncomfortable, consult with your health care provider.
  - *Skin rash, mouth sores:* frequent mouth care may help. Keep the skin dry and use prescribed skin care (lotions, coverings, medication) if needed.
  - Report any of the following to your health care provider: *difficulty breathing; mouth sores; swelling of the feet, hands, or face; chest pain; palpitations; sore throat; fever or chills.*
- Do not stop taking this drug for any reason. Consult with your health care provider if you have problems taking this medication.
- You should avoid the use of grapefruit juice while you are taking this drug, because the combination of grapefruit juice and a calcium channel blocker may case toxic effects.
- Tell any doctor, nurse or others involved in your health care that you are taking this drug.
- Avoid taking over-the-counter medications while you are taking this drug. If you feel that you need one of these, consult with your health care provider for the best choice. Many of these drugs may interfere with the antihypertensive effect that usually occurs with this drug.
- Be extremely careful in any situation that might lead to a drop in blood pressure (eg, excessive sweating, vomiting, diarrhoea, dehydration). If you experience light-headedness or dizziness in any of these situations, consult your health care provider immediately.
- Keep this drug, and all medications, out of the reach of children.

VASODILATORS

If other drug therapies do not achieve the desired reduction in blood pressure, it is sometimes necessary to use a direct vasodilator. Most of the vasodilators are reserved for use in severe hypertension or hypertensive emergencies. These include diazoxide (generic), hydralazine (*Alphapress, Apresoline*), minoxidil (*Loniten*) and sodium nitroprusside (generic).

Therapeutic actions and indications

The vasodilators act directly on vascular smooth muscle to cause muscle relaxation, leading to vasodilation and drop in blood pressure. They do not block the reflex tachycardia that occurs when blood pressure drops. They are indicated for the treatment of severe hypertension that has not responded to other therapy (see Table 43.2).

Pharmacokinetics

Diazoxide and sodium nitroprusside are used intravenously; hydralazine is available for oral and intravenous use; and minoxidil is available as an oral agent only. These drugs are rapidly absorbed and widely distributed. They are metabolised in the liver and primarily excreted in urine. They cross the placenta and enter breast milk (see Contraindications and cautions).

Contraindications and cautions

The vasodilators are contraindicated in the presence of known allergy to the drug *to prevent hypersensitivity reactions* and with any condition *that could be exacerbated by a sudden fall in blood pressure*, such as cerebral insufficiency. Caution should be used in people with peripheral vascular disease, CAD, heart failure or tachycardia, *all of which could be exacerbated by the fall in blood pressure*. Diazoxide must be used with extreme caution in people with functional hypoglycaemia *because this drug increases blood glucose levels by blocking insulin release*.

These drugs are also contraindicated with pregnancy unless the benefit to the mother clearly outweighs the potential risk *because of the potential for adverse effects on the fetus or neonate*. If they are needed by a breastfeeding woman, another method of feeding the baby should be selected, *because of the potential for adverse effects on the baby*.

Adverse effects

The adverse effects most frequently seen with these drugs are related to the changes in blood pressure. These include dizziness, anxiety and headache; reflex tachycardia, heart failure, chest pain, oedema; skin rash and lesions (abnormal hair growth with minoxidil); and GI upset, nausea and vomiting. Cyanide toxicity (dyspnoea, headache, vomiting, dizziness, ataxia, loss of consciousness, imperceptible pulse, absent reflexes, dilated pupils, pink colour, distant heart sounds and shallow breathing) may occur with nitroprusside, which is metabolised to cyanide and also suppresses iodine uptake and can cause hypothyroidism.

Clinically important drug–drug interactions

Each of these drugs works differently in the body, so each drug should be checked for potential drug–drug interactions before use.

Prototype summary: sodium nitroprusside

Indications: severe hypertension, maintenance of controlled hypotension during anaesthesia, acute heart failure.

Actions: acts directly on vascular smooth muscle to cause vasodilation and drop of blood pressure; does not inhibit cardiovascular reflexes and tachycardia; renin release will occur.

Pharmacokinetics:

Route	Onset	Peak	Duration
IV	1–2 min	Rapid	1–10 min

$T_{1/2}$: 2 min; metabolised in the liver and excreted in urine.

Adverse effects: apprehension, headache, retrosternal pressure, palpitations, cyanide toxicity, diaphoresis, nausea, vomiting, abdominal pain, irritation at the injection site.

Care considerations for people receiving vasodilators

Assessment: history and examination

- Assess for the following conditions, *which could be cautions or contraindications to use of the drug*: any known allergies to these drugs; impaired kidney or liver function; pregnancy or breastfeeding *because of the potential adverse effects on the fetus or neonate*; and cardiovascular dysfunction, *which could be exacerbated by a fall in blood pressure*.
- Assess baseline status before beginning therapy *to determine any potential adverse effects*; this includes body temperature and weight; skin colour, lesions and temperature; pulse, blood pressure, baseline ECG and perfusion; respirations and adventitious breath sounds; bowel sounds and abdominal examination; renal and liver function tests; and blood glucose.

Implementation with rationale

- Encourage the person to implement lifestyle changes, including weight loss, smoking cessation, decreased alcohol and salt in the diet and increased exercise, *to increase the effectiveness of antihypertensive therapy*.
- Monitor blood pressure closely during administration *to evaluate for effectiveness and to ensure quick response if blood pressure falls rapidly or too much*.
- Monitor blood glucose and serum electrolytes *to avoid potentially serious adverse effects*.
- Monitor the person carefully in any situation that might lead to a drop in fluid volume (eg, excessive sweating, vomiting, diarrhoea, dehydration) *to detect and treat excessive hypotension that may occur*.
- Provide comfort measures *to help the person tolerate drug effects*, including small, frequent meals; access to bathroom facilities; safety precautions if CNS effects occur; environmental controls; appropriate skin care as needed; and analgesics as needed.
- Provide thorough teaching, including the name of the drug, dosage prescribed, measures to avoid adverse effects, warning signs of problems and the need for periodic monitoring and evaluation, *to enhance knowledge about drug therapy and to promote compliance*.
- Offer support and encouragement *to help the person deal with the diagnosis and the drug regimen*.

Evaluation

- Monitor response to the drug (maintenance of blood pressure within normal limits).
- Monitor for adverse effects (hypotension, GI distress, skin reactions, tachycardia, headache, dizziness).
- Evaluate the effectiveness of the teaching plan (person can name drug, dosage, adverse effects to watch for, specific measures to avoid them and the importance of continued follow-up).
- Monitor the effectiveness of comfort measures and compliance with the regimen.

OTHER ANTIHYPERTENSIVE AGENTS

Diuretic agents

Diuretics are drugs that increase the excretion of sodium and water from the kidney (Figure 43.3). See Chapter 51 for a detailed discussion of these agents. Diuretics are very important for the treatment of hypertension. These drugs are often the first agents tried in mild hypertension; they affect blood sodium levels and blood volume. A somewhat controversial study, the Antihypertensive and Lipid-Lowering Treatment to Prevent Heart Attack Trial (ALLHAT), reported in 2002 that people taking the less expensive, less toxic diuretics did better and had better blood pressure control than people using other antihypertensive agents. Replications of this study have supported its findings and the use of a thiazide diuretic as the first drug used in the management of hypertension. Although these drugs increase urination and can disturb electrolyte and acid–base balances, they are usually tolerated well by most people. Diuretic agents used to treat hypertension include the following:

- *Thiazide and thiazide-like diuretics*: hydrochlorothiazide (*Dithiazide*), chlortalidone (*Hygroton*) and indapamide (*Natrilix, Dapa-Tabs*).
- *Loop diuretics*: bumetanide (*Burinex*) and furosemide (*frusemide*) (*Diurin, Lasix, Uremide, Urex, Urex M, Urex Forte*).
- *Potassium-sparing diuretics / aldosterone antagonists*: amiloride (*Amizide, Kaluril*), eplerenone (*Espler, Inpler, Inspra*), spironolactone (*Aldactone, Spiractin*) and hydrochlorothiazide with triamterene (*Hydrene*).

Sympathetic nervous system blockers

Drugs that block the effects of the sympathetic nervous system are useful in blocking the compensatory effects of the sympathetic nervous system that lead to increased blood pressure (see Figure 43.3). See Chapters 30 and 31 for a detailed discussion of these drugs.

- Beta blockers block vasoconstriction, decrease heart rate, decrease cardiac muscle contraction and tend to increase blood flow to the kidneys, leading to a decrease in the release of renin. These drugs have many adverse effects and are not recommended for all people. They are often used as monotherapy, and in some people they control blood pressure adequately. Beta blockers used to treat hypertension include the following agents: atenolol (*Tenormin*), metoprolol (*Betaloc, Lopresor*), nadolol (*Apo-Nadol, Apo-Nadolol* [not available in Australia]), nebivolol (*Nebilet* [not available in New Zealand]), pindolol (*Barbloc, Visken*) and propranolol (*Deralin, Inderal*).
- Alpha and beta blockers are useful in conjunction with other agents and tend to be somewhat more powerful, blocking all of the receptors in the sympathetic system. People often complain of fatigue, loss of libido, inability to sleep, and GI and genitourinary disturbances. As a result, they may be unwilling to continue taking these drugs. Alpha and beta blockers used to treat hypertension include the following agents: carvedilol (*Dilatrend, Dicarz*) and labetalol (*Presolol, Trandate*).
- Alpha-adrenergic blockers inhibit the postsynaptic alpha-1-adrenergic receptors, decreasing sympathetic tone in the vasculature and causing vasodilation, which leads to a lowering of blood pressure. However, these drugs also block presynaptic alpha-2 receptors, preventing the feedback control of noradrenaline release. The result is an increase in the reflex tachycardia that occurs when blood pressure decreases. These drugs are used to diagnose and manage episodes of phaeochromocytoma, but they have limited usefulness in essential hypertension because of the associated adverse effects. The alpha-adrenergic blocker phenoxybenzamine (*Dibenyline*) (not currently registered) is indicated for hypertensive episodes in phaeochromocytoma.
- Alpha-1 blockers are used to treat hypertension because of their ability to block the postsynaptic alpha-1-receptor sites. This decreases vascular tone and promotes vasodilation, leading to a fall in blood pressure. These drugs do not block the presynaptic alpha-2-receptor sites, and therefore the reflex tachycardia that accompanies a fall in blood pressure does not occur. Alpha-1 blockers used to treat hypertension include the following agents: doxazosin (*Dosan* [not available in Australia]), prazosin (*Minipress*) and terazosin (*Hytrin*).
- Alpha-2 agonists (see Chapter 30) stimulate the alpha-2 receptors in the CNS and inhibit the cardiovascular centres, leading to a decrease in sympathetic outflow from the CNS and a resultant drop in blood pressure. These drugs are associated with many adverse CNS and GI effects, as well as cardiac arrhythmias. Alpha-2 blockers used to

treat hypertension include clonidine (*Catapres*) and methyldopa (*Aldomet*, *Hydopa*). Moxonidine (*Physiotens* [not available in New Zealand]) binds to both I_1-imidazoline receptors and alpha-2 adrenoreceptors, reducing sympathetic nervous system activity, and thus lowering blood pressure.

KEY POINTS

- Hypertension is a sustained state of higher-than-normal blood pressure that can lead to blood vessel damage, atherosclerosis and damage to small vessels in end organs.
- The cause of essential hypertension is unknown; treatment varies among individuals.
- Drug treatment of hypertension aims to change one or more of the normal reflexes that control blood pressure.
- Sodium levels and fluid volume are decreased by diuretic agents.
- ACE inhibitors prevent the conversion of angiotensin I to angiotensin II, leading to a fall in blood pressure.
- ARBs prevent the body from responding to angiotensin II, causing a loss of effectiveness of the renin–angiotensin system.
- Calcium channel blockers interfere with the ability of muscles to contract, which leads to vasodilation, which in turn reduces blood pressure.
- Other drugs used to treat hypertension include diuretics, which decrease the sodium content in the body, and various sympathetic blockers, which block the blood pressure–raising effects of the sympathetic system.

ANTIHYPOTENSIVE AGENTS

As mentioned earlier, if blood pressure becomes too low (hypotension), the vital centres in the brain and the rest of the tissues of the body may not receive sufficient oxygenated blood to continue functioning. Severe hypotension or shock puts the body in serious jeopardy; it is often an acute emergency situation, with treatment required to save the person's life. The first-choice drug for treating shock is usually a sympathomimetic drug. See Figure 43.3 for sites of action of drugs used to treat hypotension. Antihypotensive agents are also discussed in Table 43.3.

SYMPATHETIC ADRENERGIC AGONISTS, OR VASOPRESSORS

Sympathomimetic drugs are the first choice for treating severe hypotension or shock. The sympathomimetic drugs are discussed in detail in Chapter 30. Sympathomimetic drugs used to treat shock include adrenaline (epinephrine) (*Adrenaline*, *EpiPen*), dobutamine (*Dobutrex*), dopamine (generic), ephedrine (generic), isoprenaline (*Isuprel*), metaraminol (generic), noradrenaline (norepinephrine) (*Levophed*) and phenylephrine (*Neo-Synephrine*).

Therapeutic actions and indications

Sympathomimetic drugs react with sympathetic adrenergic receptors to cause the effects of a sympathetic stress response: increased blood pressure, increased blood volume and increased strength of cardiac muscle contraction. These actions increase blood pressure and may restore balance to the cardiovascular system while the underlying cause of the shock (eg, volume depletion, blood loss) is treated.

Adverse effects

The adverse effects related to these drugs are the effects of stimulation of the sympathetic system; decreased GI activity with nausea and constipation; increased respiratory rate and changes in blood pressure; headache; and changes in peripheral blood flow with numbness, tingling and even gangrene in extreme cases. These drugs should be used with caution with any disease that limits blood flow, with tachycardia or with hypertension.

ALPHA-SPECIFIC ADRENERGIC AGENTS

Midodrine (*Gutron*) is an alpha-specific adrenergic agent used to treat orthostatic hypotension – hypotension that occurs with position change – that interferes with

TABLE 43.3 *DRUGS IN FOCUS* Antihypotensive agents

Drug name	Dosage/route	Usual indications
Alpha-specific adrenergic agent		
midodrine (*Gutron*)	2.5–10 mg PO tds; maximum 30 mg/day	Treatment of orthostatic hypotension in adults
Sympathetic adrenergic agonists or vasopressors		
See Chapter 30	See Chapter 30	First-choice drugs for treatment of hypotension or shock

a person's ability to function and has not responded to any other therapy (Table 43.3). It is currently available in New Zealand but not Australia.

Therapeutic actions and indications

Midodrine activates alpha receptors in arteries and veins to produce an increase in vascular tone and an increase in blood pressure. It is indicated for the symptomatic treatment of orthostatic hypotension in individuals whose lives are impaired by the disorder and who have not had a response to any other therapy.

Pharmacokinetics

Midodrine is rapidly absorbed from the GI tract, reaching peak levels within 1–2 hours. It is metabolised in the liver and excreted in the urine with a half-life of 3–4 hours. It should be reserved in pregnancy for cases in which the benefit to the mother clearly outweighs the potential risk to the fetus. It is not known whether midodrine enters breast milk, so caution should be used during breastfeeding.

Contraindications and cautions

Midodrine is contraindicated in the presence of supine hypertension, CAD or phaeochromocytoma *because of the risk of precipitating a hypertensive emergency*; with acute renal disease, *which might interfere with excretion of the drug*; with urinary retention *because the stimulation of alpha receptors can exacerbate this problem*; and with thyrotoxicosis, *which could further increase blood pressure*. Caution should be used with pregnancy and breastfeeding *because of the potential for adverse effects on the fetus or neonate*; with visual problems, *which could be exacerbated by vasoconstriction*; and with renal or hepatic impairment, *which could alter the metabolism and excretion of the drug*.

Adverse effects

The most common adverse effects associated with this drug are related to the stimulation of alpha receptors and include piloerection, chills and rash; hypertension and bradycardia; dizziness, vision changes, vertigo and headache; and problems with urination.

Clinically important drug–drug interactions

There is a risk of increased effects and toxicity of cardiac glycosides, beta blockers, alpha-adrenergic agents and corticosteroids if they are taken with midodrine. People who are receiving any of these combinations should be monitored carefully for the need for a dose adjustment.

Care considerations for people receiving alpha-specific adrenergic agents

Assessment: history and examination

- Assess for the following conditions, *which could be contraindications or cautions*: any known allergy to midodrine *to prevent hypersensitivity reactions*; impaired kidney or liver function, *which could interfere with metabolism and excretion of the drugs*; pregnancy or breastfeeding *because of the potential adverse effects on the fetus or neonate*; cardiovascular dysfunction; visual problems; urinary retention; and phaeochromocytoma, *which could be exacerbated by the effects of the drugs.*
- Assess baseline status before beginning therapy *to determine any potential adverse effects*; this includes body temperature and weight; skin colour, lesions and temperature; pulse, blood pressure, orthostatic blood pressure and perfusion; respiration and adventitious sounds; bowel sounds and abdominal examination; and renal and liver function tests.

Implementation with rationale

- Monitor blood pressure carefully *to monitor effectiveness and blood pressure changes.*
- Do not administer the drug to people who are bedridden, but only to people who are up and mobile, *to ensure therapeutic effects and decrease the risk of severe hypertension.*
- Monitor heart rate regularly when beginning therapy *to monitor for bradycardia, which commonly occurs at the beginning of therapy; if bradycardia persists, it may indicate a need to discontinue the drug.*
- Monitor the person with known visual problems carefully *to ensure that the drug is discontinued if visual fields change.*
- Encourage the person to void before taking a dose of the drug *to decrease the risk of urinary retention problems.*
- Provide comfort measures *to help the person tolerate drug effects,* including small, frequent meals; access to bathroom facilities; safety precautions if CNS effects occur; environmental controls; appropriate skin care as needed; and analgesics as needed.
- Provide thorough teaching, including the name of the drug, dosage prescribed, measures to avoid adverse effects, warning signs of problems and the need for periodic monitoring and evaluation, *to enhance knowledge about drug therapy and to promote compliance.*
- Offer support and encouragement *to help the person deal with the diagnosis and the drug regimen.*

Evaluation

- Monitor response to the drug (maintenance of blood pressure within normal limits).
- Monitor for adverse effects (hypertension, dizziness, visual changes, piloerection, chills, urinary problems).
- Evaluate the effectiveness of the teaching plan (person can name drug, dosage, adverse effects to watch for, specific measures to avoid them and the importance of continued follow-up).
- Monitor the effectiveness of comfort measures and compliance with the regimen.

KEY POINTS

- Severe hypotension, or shock, is treated with sympathomimetic drugs that stimulate the sympathetic system to increase blood pressure.
- Midodrine, an alpha-specific adrenergic stimulant, is an oral drug used to treat people with orthostatic hypotension whose lives are considerably impaired by the fall in blood pressure when they stand.

CHAPTER SUMMARY

- The cardiovascular system is a closed system that depends on pressure differences to ensure the delivery of blood to the tissues and the return of that blood to the heart.
- Blood pressure is related to heart rate, stroke volume and the total peripheral resistance against which the heart has to push the blood.
- Peripheral resistance is primarily controlled by constriction or relaxation of the arterioles. Constricted arterioles raise pressure; dilated arterioles lower pressure.
- Control of blood pressure involves baroreceptor (pressure receptor) stimulation of the medulla to activate the sympathetic nervous system, which causes vasoconstriction and increased fluid retention when pressure is low in the aorta and carotid arteries, and vasodilation and loss of fluid when pressure is too high.
- The kidneys activate the renin–angiotensin–aldosterone system when blood flow to the kidneys is decreased.
- Renin activates the conversion of angiotensinogen to angiotensin I in the liver; angiotensin I is converted by angiotensin-converting enzyme (ACE) to angiotensin II in the lungs; angiotensin II then reacts with specific receptor sites on blood vessels to cause vasoconstriction to raise blood pressure and in the adrenal gland to cause the release of aldosterone, which leads to the retention of fluid and increased blood volume.
- Hypertension is a sustained state of higher-than-normal blood pressure that can lead to damage to blood vessels, increased risk of atherosclerosis and damage to small vessels in end organs. Because hypertension often has no signs or symptoms, it is called the silent killer.
- Essential hypertension has no underlying cause, and treatment can vary widely from individual to individual. Treatment approaches include lifestyle changes first, followed by careful addition and adjustment of various antihypertensive drugs.
- Drug treatment of hypertension is aimed at altering one or more of the normal reflexes that control blood pressure: diuretics decrease sodium levels and volume; sympathetic nervous system drugs alter the sympathetic response and lead to vascular dilation and decreased pumping power of the heart; ACE inhibitors prevent the conversion of angiotensin I to angiotensin II; ARBs prevent the body from responding to angiotensin II; renin inhibitors directly block the effects of renin; calcium channel blockers interfere with the ability of muscles to contract and lead to vasodilation; and vasodilators directly cause the relaxation of vascular smooth muscle.
- Hypotension is a state of lower-than-normal blood pressure that can result in decreased oxygenation of the tissues, cell death, tissue damage and even death.
- Hypotension is most often treated with sympathomimetic drugs, which stimulate the sympathetic receptor sites to cause vasoconstriction, fluid retention and return of normal pressure.

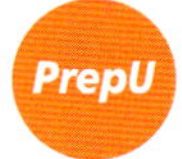

Knowing your strengths and weaknesses helps you to study more effectively. Take a PrepU Practice Quiz to find out how you measure up!

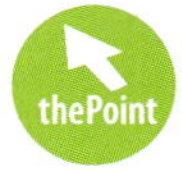

ONLINE RESOURCES

An extensive range of additional resources to enhance teaching and learning and to facilitate understanding of this chapter may be found online at the text's accompanying website, located on thePoint at http://thepoint.lww.com. These include Watch and Learn videos, Concepts in Action animations, journal articles, review questions, case studies, discussion topics and quizzes.

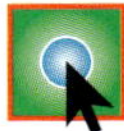

WEB LINKS

Health care providers and students may want to consult the following web resources:

https://www1.health.gov.au/internet/main/publishing.nsf/Content/hist-chronic-cardio-heartstr
National strategy for heart, stroke and vascular health in Australia.

www.heartfoundation.org.au
Information on research, alternative methods of therapy and pharmacology.

www.heartfoundation.org.nz
Information on research, alternative methods of therapy and pharmacology.

BIBLIOGRAPHY

Australian Bureau of Statistics. (2014). *4727.055.001 Australian Aboriginal and Torres Strait Islander Health Survey: First Results, Australia, 2012–13*. ABS: Canberra.

Australian Institute of Health and Welfare (AIHW). (2013). Cardiovascular health, www.aihw.gov.au/cardiovascular-health.

Ayer, J. G. & Sholler, G. F. (2012). Cardiovascular risk factors in Australian children: Hypertension and lipid abnormalities. *Australian Prescriber, 35(2)*, 51–55.

Bostock-Cox, B. (2013). Nurse prescribing for the management of hypertension. *British Journal of Cardiac Nursing, 8(11)*, 531–536.

Braunwald, E. & Bonow, R. O., MD Consult LLC. (2012). *Braunwald's Heart Disease: A Textbook of Cardiovascular Medicine* (9th edn). Philadelphia: Elsevier Saunders.

Davis, L. L. (2013). Using the latest evidence to manage hypertension. *Journal for Nurse Practitioners, 9(10)*, 621–628.

Elsik, M. & Krum, H. (2007). Should beta blockers remain first-line drugs for hypertension? *Australian Prescriber, 30*, 5–7.

Farrell, M. & Dempsey, J. (2014). *Smeltzer & Bare's Textbook of Medical-Surgical Nursing* (3rd edn). Sydney: Lippincott Williams & Wilkins.

Goodman, L. S., Brunton, L. L., Chabner, B. & Knollmann, B. C. (2011). *Goodman and Gilman's Pharmacological Basis of Therapeutics* (12th edn). New York: McGraw-Hill.

Hardy, S. (2009). Encouraging effective use of antihypertensives. *Practice Nursing, 20(7)*, 342–346.

Heart Foundation. (2010). *Guide to Management of Hypertension: Assessing and Managing Raised Blood Pressure in Adults*. www.heartfoundation.org.au/SiteCollectionDocuments/HypertensionGuidelines2008to2010Update.pdf.

Huang, N. & Duggan, K. (2008). Lifestyle management of hypertension. *Australian Prescriber, 31*, 150–153.

Matchar, D. B., McCrory, D. C., Orlando, L. A., Patel, M. R., Patel, U. D., Patwardhan, M. B., et al. (2008). Systematic review: Comparative effectiveness of angiotensin-converting enzyme inhibitors and angiotensin II receptor blockers for treating essential hypertension. *Annals of Internal Medicine, 148*, 16–29.

McKenna, L. & Mirkov, S. (2019). *McKenna's Drug Handbook for Nursing and Midwifery* (8th edn). Sydney: Wolters Kluwer Health Australia.

Parfrey, P. S. (2008). Inhibitors of the renin angiotensin system: Proven benefits, unproven safety. *Annals of Internal Medicine, 48*, 76–77.

Porth, C. M. (2011). *Essentials of Pathophysiology: Concepts of Altered Health States* (3rd edn). Philadelphia: Lippincott Williams & Wilkins.

Porth, C. M. (2009). *Pathophysiology: Concepts of Altered Health States* (8th edn). Philadelphia: Lippincott Williams & Wilkins.

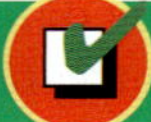

CHECK YOUR UNDERSTANDING

Answers to the questions in this chapter can be found in Appendix A at the back of this book.

MULTIPLE CHOICE

Select the best answer to the following.

1. The baroreceptors are the most important factor in continual control of blood pressure. The baroreceptors:
   a. are evenly distributed throughout the body to maintain pressure in the system.
   b. sense pressure and immediately send that information to the medulla in the brain.
   c. are directly connected to the sympathetic nervous system.
   d. are as sensitive to oxygen levels as to pressure changes.
2. Essential hypertension is the most commonly diagnosed form of high blood pressure. Essential hypertension is:
   a. caused by a tumour in the adrenal gland.
   b. associated with no known cause.
   c. related to renal disease.
   d. caused by liver dysfunction.
3. Hypertension is associated with:
   a. loss of vision.
   b. strokes.
   c. atherosclerosis.
   d. all of the above.
4. ACE inhibitors work on the renin–angiotensin system to prevent the conversion of angiotensin I to angiotensin II. Because this blocking occurs in the cells in the lung, which is usually the site of this conversion, use of ACE inhibitors often results in:
   a. spontaneous pneumothorax.
   b. pneumonia.
   c. unrelenting cough.
   d. respiratory depression.
5. A person taking an ACE inhibitor is scheduled for surgery. The nurse or midwife should:
   a. stop the drug.
   b. alert the surgeon and mark the person's chart prominently.
   c. cancel the surgery and consult with the prescriber.
   d. monitor fluid levels and make sure the fluids are restricted before surgery.

6. A woman who is hypertensive becomes pregnant. The drug of choice for this woman is:
   a. an angiotensin II–receptor blocker.
   b. an ACE inhibitor.
   c. a diuretic.
   d. a calcium channel blocker.

7. Midodrine, an antihypotensive drug, should be used:
   a. only with people who are confined to bed.
   b. in the treatment of acute shock.
   c. in people with known phaeochromocytoma.
   d. to treat orthostatic hypotension in people whose lives are impaired by the disorder.

MULTIPLE RESPONSE

Select all that apply.

1. Pressure within the vascular system is determined by which of the following?
   a. peripheral resistance
   b. stroke volume
   c. sodium load
   d. heart rate
   e. total intravascular volume
   f. rate of erythropoietin release

2. The renin–angiotensin system is associated with which of the following?
   a. intense vasoconstriction and blood pressure elevation
   b. blood flow through the kidneys
   c. production of surfactant in the lungs
   d. release of aldosterone from the adrenal cortex
   e. retention of sodium and water in the kidneys
   f. liver production of fibrinogen

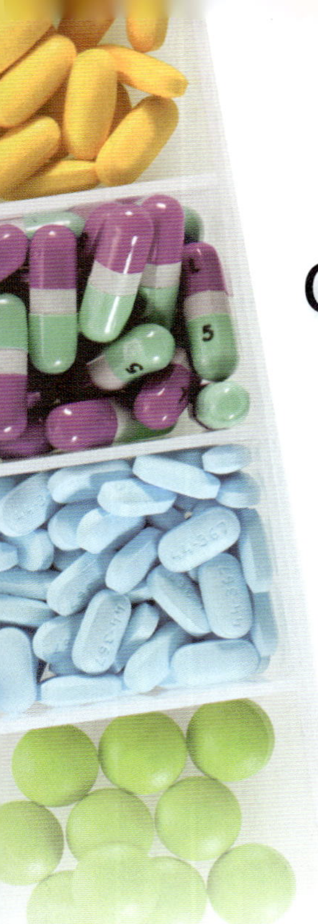

44

Cardiotonic agents

Learning objectives

On completing this chapter you should be able to:

1. Describe the pathophysiological process of heart failure and the resultant clinical signs.
2. Explain the body's compensatory mechanisms that occur in response to heart failure.
3. Describe the therapeutic actions, indications, pharmacokinetics, contraindications and cautions, most common adverse reactions and important drug–drug interactions associated with the cardiotonic agents.
4. Discuss the use of cardiotonic agents across the lifespan.
5. Compare and contrast the drugs digoxin and digoxin immune Fab.
6. Outline the care considerations, including important teaching points, for people receiving cardiotonic agents.

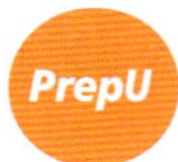

Test your current knowledge of cardiotonic agents with a PrepU Practice Quiz!

Glossary of key terms

cardiomegaly: enlargement of the heart, commonly seen with chronic hypertension, valvular disease and heart failure

cardiomyopathy: a disease of the heart muscle that leads to an enlarged heart and eventually to complete heart muscle failure and death

dyspnoea: discomfort with breathing, often with a feeling of anxiety and inability to breathe, seen with left-sided heart failure

haemoptysis: blood-tinged sputum, seen in left-sided heart failure when blood backs up into the lungs and fluid leaks out into the lung tissue

heart failure (HF): a condition in which the heart muscle fails to adequately pump blood around the cardiovascular system, leading to a backup or congestion of blood in the system

nocturia: getting up to void at night, reflecting increased renal perfusion with fluid shifts in the supine position when a person has gravity-dependent oedema related to heart failure; other medical conditions, including urinary tract infection, increase the need to get up and void

orthopnoea: difficulty breathing when lying down, often referred to by the number of pillows required to allow a person to breath comfortably

positive inotropic effect: results in an increased force of contraction

pulmonary oedema: severe left-sided heart failure with backup of blood into the lungs, leading to loss of fluid into the lung tissue

tachypnoea: rapid and shallow respirations, seen with left-sided heart failure

CARDIOTONIC AGENTS Cardiac glycoside	Phosphodiesterase type 3 inhibitor	Phosphodiesterase type 5 inhibitor	DIGOXIN ANTIDOTE
Ⓟ digoxin	milrinone	sildenafil	digoxin immune Fab

Cardiotonic agents are drugs used to increase the contractility of the heart muscle of people experiencing heart failure. **Heart failure (HF)** is a condition in which the heart fails to pump blood around the body effectively. Because the cardiac cycle normally involves a tight balance between the pumping of the right and left sides of the heart, any failure of the muscle to pump blood out of either side of the heart can result in a backup of blood. If this happens, the blood vessels become congested; eventually, the body's cells are deprived of oxygen and nutrients, and waste products build up in the tissues. The primary treatment for HF involves helping the heart muscle to contract more efficiently to restore system balance.

HEART FAILURE

HF, a condition that was once called 'dropsy', or decompensation, is a syndrome that usually involves dysfunction of the cardiac muscle, of which the sarcomere is the basic unit. The sarcomere contains two contractile proteins, actin and myosin, which are highly reactive with each other but at rest are kept apart by the chemical troponin. When a cardiac muscle cell is stimulated, calcium enters the cell and inactivates the troponin, allowing the actin and myosin to form actomyosin bridges. The formation of these bridges allows the muscle fibres to slide together or contract (Figure 44.1). The formation of these bridges and subsequent contraction require a constant supply of oxygen, glucose and calcium. (See Chapter 42 for a review of heart muscle contraction processes.)

Heart failure can occur with any of the disorders that damage or overwork the heart muscle:

- Coronary artery disease (CAD) is the leading cause of HF, accounting for approximately 95% of the cases diagnosed (see Chapter 47 for a discussion of CAD). CAD results in an insufficient supply of blood to meet the oxygen demands of the myocardium. Consequently, the muscles become hypoxic and can no longer function efficiently. When CAD evolves into a myocardial infarction (MI), muscle cells die or are damaged, leading to an inefficient pumping effort.
- **Cardiomyopathy** is a disease of the heart muscle that leads to an enlarged heart and eventually to complete muscle failure and death. It can occur as a result of a viral infection, alcoholism, anabolic steroid abuse or a collagen disorder. It causes muscle alterations and ineffective contraction and pumping.
- Hypertension eventually leads to an enlarged cardiac muscle because the heart must work harder than normal to pump against the high pressure in the arteries. Hypertension puts constant, increased demands for oxygen on the system because the heart is pumping so forcibly.
- Valvular heart disease leads to an overload of the ventricles because the valves do not close tightly, which allows blood to leak backwards into the ventricles. This overloading leads to muscle stretching

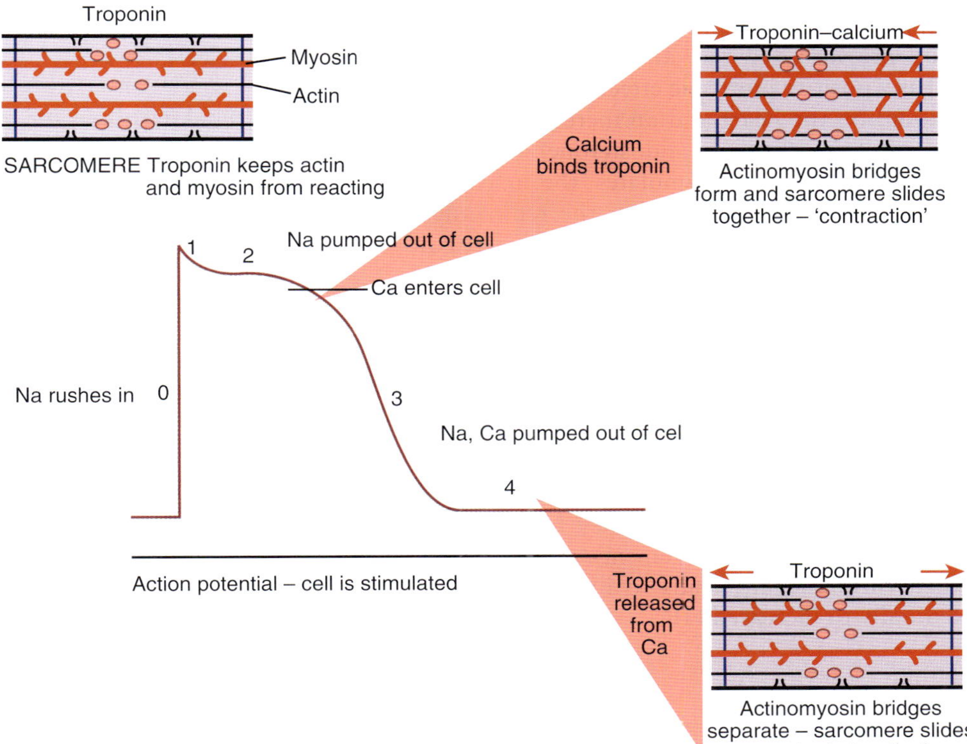

FIGURE 44.1 The sliding filaments of myocardial muscles. Calcium entering the cell deactivates troponin and allows actin and myosin to react, causing contraction. Calcium pumped out of the cell frees troponin to separate actin and myosin; the sarcomere filament slides apart, and the cell relaxes.

and increased demand for oxygen and energy as the heart muscle must constantly contract harder. (Valvular heart disease is seen less often today owing to the success of cardiac surgery and effective treatment for rheumatic fever.)

The end result of all of these conditions is that the heart muscle cannot pump blood effectively throughout the vascular system. If the left ventricle pumps inefficiently, blood backs up into the lungs, causing pulmonary vessel congestion and fluid leakage into the alveoli and lung tissue. In severe cases, **pulmonary oedema** (manifested by rales, wheezes, blood-tinged sputum, low oxygenation and development of a third heart sound [S_3]) can occur. If the right side of the heart is the primary problem, blood backs up in the venous system leading to the right side of the heart. Liver congestion and oedema of the legs and feet reflect right-sided failure. Because the cardiovascular system works as a closed system, one-sided failure, if left untreated, eventually leads to failure of both sides, and the signs and symptoms of total HF occur.

Clinincal management of a person with heart failure

Compensatory mechanisms

Because effective pumping of blood to the cells is essential for life, the body has several compensatory mechanisms that function if the heart muscle begins to fail (Figure 44.2). Decreased cardiac output stimulates the baroreceptors in the aortic arch and the carotid arteries, causing increased sympathetic activity (see Chapter 29). This stimulates an increase in heart rate, blood pressure and rate and depth of respirations, as well as a **positive inotropic effect** (increased force of contraction) on the heart and an increase in blood volume (through the release of aldosterone). The decrease in cardiac output also stimulates the release of renin from the kidneys and activates the renin–angiotensin–aldosterone system, which further increases blood pressure and blood volume.

If these mechanisms work effectively, compensation is occurring and the person may show no signs or symptoms of HF. Over time, however, all of these effects increase the workload of the heart, contributing to further development of HF. Eventually, the heart muscle overstretches from the increased workload, and the chambers of the heart dilate secondary to the increased blood volume that they have had to handle. This hypertrophy (enlargement) of the heart muscle, called **cardiomegaly**, leads to inefficient pumping and eventually to increased HF.

Cellular changes

The myocardial cells are changed with prolonged HF. Unlike healthy heart cells, the cells of the failing heart seem to lack the ability to produce the energy needed for effective contractions. Movement of calcium ions into and out of the cell is no longer effective, leading to further deterioration because the muscle contracts inefficiently and is unable to deliver blood to the cardiac muscle.

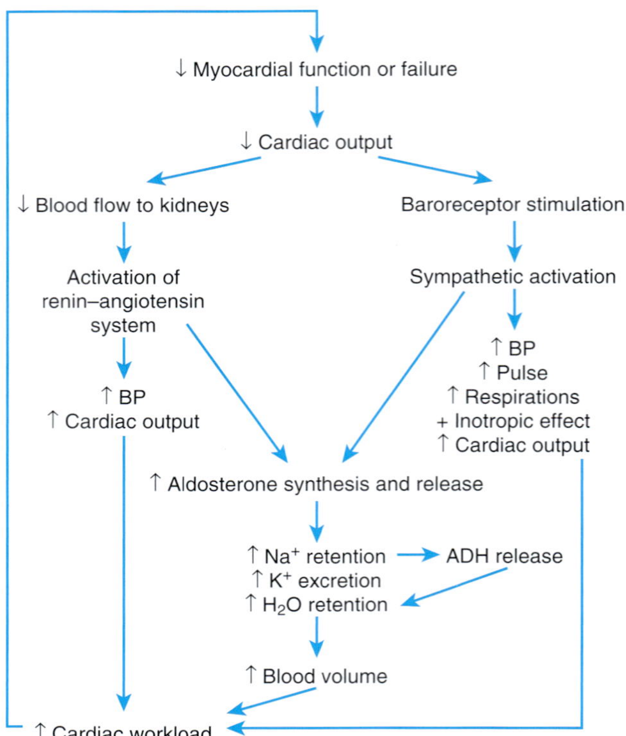

FIGURE 44.2 Compensatory mechanisms in heart failure (HF), which lead to increased cardiac workload and further HF. ADH, antidiuretic hormone; BP, blood pressure.

Clinical manifestations

The person with HF presents a predictable clinical picture that reflects not only the problems with heart pumping, but also the compensatory mechanisms that are working to balance the problem. Radiography, electrocardiography (ECG) and direct percussion and palpation help to detect changes in the heart muscle and function. The heart rate will be rapid secondary to sympathetic stimulation, and the person may develop atrial flutter or fibrillation as atrial cells are stretched and damaged. Anxiety often occurs as the body stimulates the sympathetic stress reaction. Heart murmurs may develop when the muscle is no longer able to support the papillary muscles that support the valve leaflets or the annuli that anchor the heart valves.

Peripheral congestion and oedema occur as the organs and vessels become engorged waiting for blood to be pumped through the heart as a result of pump failure. With right-sided failure, there is enlarged liver (hepatomegaly); enlarged spleen (splenomegaly); decreased blood flow to the gastrointestinal (GI) tract causing feelings of nausea and abdominal pain; swollen legs and feet; and dependent oedema in the coccyx or other dependent areas, with decreased peripheral pulses and hypoxia of those tissues. In addition, with left-sided failure, oedema of the lungs reflected in engorged vessels, and increased hydrostatic pressure throughout the cardiovascular system is also seen (Figure 44.3).

Left-sided heart failure

Left-sided HF reflects engorgement of the pulmonary veins, which eventually leads to difficulty in breathing. The person complains of **tachypnoea** (rapid, shallow respirations), **dyspnoea** (discomfort with breathing, often accompanied by a panicked feeling of being unable to breathe), and **orthopnoea** (increased difficulty breathing when lying down). Orthopnoea occurs in the supine position when the pattern of blood flow changes because of the effects of gravity, which increases pressure and perfusion in the lungs. Orthopnoea is usually relieved when the person sits up, thereby reducing the blood flow through the lungs. The degree of HF is often calculated by the number of pillows required to get relief (eg, one-pillow, two-pillow, or three-pillow orthopnoea).

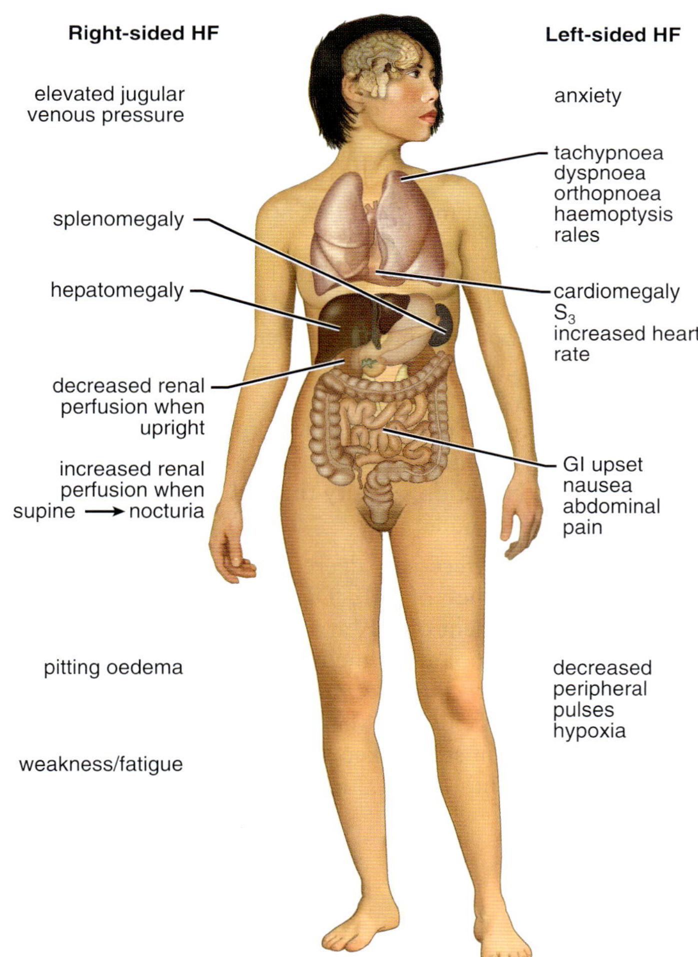

FIGURE 44.3 Signs and symptoms of heart failure (HF).

The person with left-sided HF may also experience coughing and **haemoptysis** (coughing up of blood). Rales may be present, signalling the presence of fluid in the lung tissue. In severe cases, the person may develop pulmonary oedema; this can be life-threatening because, as the spaces in the lungs fill up with fluid, there is no place for gas exchange to occur.

Right-sided heart failure

Right-sided HF usually occurs as a result of chronic obstructive pulmonary disease (COPD) or other lung diseases that elevate the pulmonary pressure. It often results when the right side of the heart, normally a very low-pressure system, must generate more and more force to move the blood into the lungs. It also commonly occurs with ageing, when the venous system fails to deliver blood to the heart effectively and the hydrostatic pressure in the venous end of the capillary increases, leading to a loss of fluid in the tissues and changes in the overall efficiency of the vascular system.

In right-sided HF, venous return to the heart is decreased because of the increased pressure in the right side of the heart. This causes congestion and a backup of blood in the systemic system. Jugular venous pressure (JVP) rises and can be seen in distended neck veins, reflecting increased central venous pressure (CVP). The liver enlarges and becomes congested with blood, which leads initially to pain and tenderness and eventually to liver dysfunction and jaundice.

Dependent (lower) areas develop oedema or swelling of the tissues as fluid leaves the congested blood vessels and pools in the tissues. Pitting oedema in the legs is a common finding, reflecting fluid pooling in the tissues. For example, when the person with right-sided HF changes position and the legs are no longer dependent, the fluid moves back into circulation to be returned to the heart. This increase in cardiovascular volume increases blood flow to the kidneys, causing increased urine output. This is often seen as **nocturia** (excessive voiding during the night) in a person who is up and around during the day and supine at night. The person may need to get up during the night to eliminate all of the urine that has been produced as a result of the fluid shift.

Treatments

Several different approaches are used to treat HF. This chapter focuses on the cardiotonic drugs (also called inotropic drugs) that work to directly increase the force of cardiac muscle contraction. Other drug therapies used to treat HF include the following:

- Vasodilators, such as angiotensin-converting-enzyme (ACE) inhibitors and nitrates, decrease cardiac workload, relax vascular smooth muscle to decrease afterload and allow pooling in the veins, thereby decreasing preload of the heart and helping to improve function (see Chapter 43 for a discussion of ACE inhibitors and Chapter 46 for a discussion of nitrates). Diuretics decrease blood volume, which decreases venous return and blood pressure, resulting in decreased afterload, preload and cardiac workload. (See Chapter 51 for additional information.)

- Beta-adrenergic agonists stimulate the beta receptors in the sympathetic nervous system, increasing calcium flow into the myocardial cells and causing increased contraction, a positive inotropic effect. Other sympathetic stimulation effects can cause increased HF because the heart's workload is increased by most sympathetic activity. (See Chapter 30 for additional information.)
- Human B-type natriuretic peptides are normally produced by myocardial cells as a compensatory response to increased cardiac workload and increased stimulation by the stress hormones. They bind to endothelial cells, leading to dilation and resulting in decreased venous return, peripheral resistance and cardiac workload. They also suppress the body's response to the stress hormones, leading to increased fluid loss and further decrease in cardiac workload.

KEY POINTS

- In HF, the heart pumps blood so ineffectively that blood builds up, causing congestion in the cardiovascular system.
- HF can result from damage to the heart muscle combined with an increased workload related to CAD, hypertension, cardiomyopathy, valvular disease or congenital heart abnormalities. As the heart pump fails, the muscle cells can no longer work to move calcium into the cell, and cardiac contractions become weak and ineffective.
- Signs and symptoms of HF result from the backup of blood in the vascular system and the loss of fluid in the tissues. Right-sided HF is characterised by oedema, liver congestion, elevated jugular venous pressure and nocturia, whereas left-sided failure is marked by tachypnoea, dyspnoea, orthopnoea, haemoptysis, anxiety and poor oxygenation of the blood.
- Treatment agents include vasodilators (to lighten the heart's workload); diuretics (to reduce blood volume and workload); beta blockers (to decrease the heart's workload by activating sympathetic reaction); human B-type natriuretic peptides (to decrease the heart's workload by vasodilation and suppression of the response to the sympathetic reaction); and cardiotonic (inotropic) agents (to stimulate more effective muscle contractions).

CARDIOTONIC AGENTS

Cardiotonic (inotropic) drugs affect the intracellular calcium levels in the heart muscle, leading to increased contractility. This increase in contraction strength leads to increased cardiac output, which causes increased renal blood flow and increased urine production. Increased renal blood flow decreases renin release, and hence reduces the effects of the renin–angiotensin–aldosterone system, increasing urine output, and leading to decreased blood volume. The result is a decrease in the heart's workload and relief of HF. Two types of cardiotonic drugs are used: the classic cardiac glycosides, which have been used for hundreds of years, and the newer phosphodiesterase inhibitors. Table 44.1 presents a complete list of these agents. Box 44.1 summarises the use of cardiotonic drugs in different age groups.

CARDIAC GLYCOSIDES

The cardiac glycosides were originally derived from the foxglove or digitalis plant. These plants were once ground up to make digitalis leaf. Today, digoxin (*Lanoxin, Sigmaxin*) is used as a second-line treatment for HF.

Therapeutic actions and indications

Digoxin increases intracellular calcium level and allows more calcium to enter myocardial cells during depolarisation (Figure 44.4), causing:

- increased force of myocardial contraction (a positive inotropic effect)
- increased cardiac output and renal perfusion (which has a diuretic effect, increasing urine output and decreasing blood volume while decreasing renin release and activation of the renin–angiotensin–aldosterone system)
- slowed heart rate, owing to slowing of the rate of cellular repolarisation (a negative chronotropic effect)
- decreased conduction velocity through the atrioventricular node.

The overall effect is a decrease in the myocardial workload and relief of HF. Digoxin is indicated for second-line treatment of HF, atrial flutter, atrial fibrillation and paroxysmal atrial tachycardia (see Table 44.1). Digoxin has a very *narrow margin of safety* (meaning that the therapeutic dose is very close to the toxic dose), so extreme care must be taken when using this drug (see Adverse effects and Box 44.3 for information on digoxin antidote).

Pharmacokinetics

Digoxin is available for oral and parenteral administration. The drug has a rapid onset of action and rapid absorption (30–120 minutes when taken orally,

TABLE 44.1 DRUGS IN FOCUS Cardiotonic agents

Drug name	Dosage/route	Usual indications
Cardiac glycosides		
digoxin (*Lanoxin, Sigmaxin*)	Adult, tablets and oral solution: loading dose, 0.75–1.5 mg over 24 hours in divided doses; maintenance dose: AF: 62.5–250 micrograms daily; HF: 62.5–125 micrograms once daily; decrease for elderly people and people with renal disease Adult, IV infusion: loading dose (emergency), 0.75–1 mg over at least 2 hours then maintenance dose by mouth the next day Monitor serum digoxin concentration	Treatment of acute heart failure, atrial arrhythmias
Phosphodiesterase inhibitors		
milrinone (*Primacor*)	Loading dose: 50 micrograms/kg slow IVI over 10 minutes Maintenance: minimum 0.6 mg/kg/24 hours; usually 0.77 mg/kg/24 hours; maximum 1.13 mg/kg/24 hours Reduce dose in renal impairment	Short-term management of HF in adults receiving digoxin and diuretics
sildenafil (*Revatio, Silvasta, Vedafil, Viagra*)	Adult: 25 mg 3 tid 6–8 hours apart	Pulmonary arterial hypertension

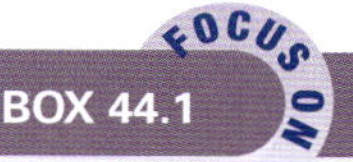

BOX 44.1 Drug therapy across the lifespan

Cardiotonic agents

CHILDREN

Digoxin is used widely in children with heart defects and related cardiac problems. The margin of safety for the dosage of this drug is very small with children. The dosage needs to be very carefully calculated and should be independently checked by another health care provider before administration.

Children should be monitored closely for any sign of impending digitalis toxicity and should have serum digoxin levels monitored.

The phosphodiesterase inhibitors are not recommended for use in children.

ADULTS

Adults receiving any of these drugs need to be instructed as to what adverse reactions to report immediately. They should learn to take their own pulse and should be encouraged to keep track of rate and regularity on a calendar. They may be asked to weigh themselves in the same clothing and at the same time of the day to monitor for fluid retention. Any changes in diet, GI activity, or medications should be reported to the health care provider because of the potential for altering serum levels and causing toxic reactions or ineffective dosing.

PREGNANCY AND BREASTFEEDING

Digoxin safety has been well established in pregnancy (Pregnancy Category A). There have been no reports linking digitalis or the various digitalis glycosides with congenital defects. Animal studies have not shown a teratogenic effect. Digoxin is not excreted in clinically significant amount in human milk and it is considered to be safe in breastfeeding.

Milrinone is classified as Pregnancy Category B3; there may or may not be human pregnancy experience, but the potential maternal benefit far outweighs the known or unknown embryo–fetal risk. Animal reproduction data are not relevant. There are no data on excretion in human milk.

OLDER ADULTS

Older adults frequently are prescribed one of these drugs. They, like children at the other end of the life spectrum, are more susceptible to the toxic effects of the drugs and are more likely to have underlying conditions that could interfere with their metabolism and excretion.

Renal impairment can lead to accumulation of digoxin in the body. If renal dysfunction is present, the dosage needs to be reduced and the person monitored very closely for signs of digoxin toxicity.

The total drug regimen of the older person should be coordinated, with careful attention to interacting drugs or alternative therapies.

For backup in situations of stress or illness, a significant other should be instructed in how to take the person's pulse and the adverse effects to watch for while the person is taking this drug.

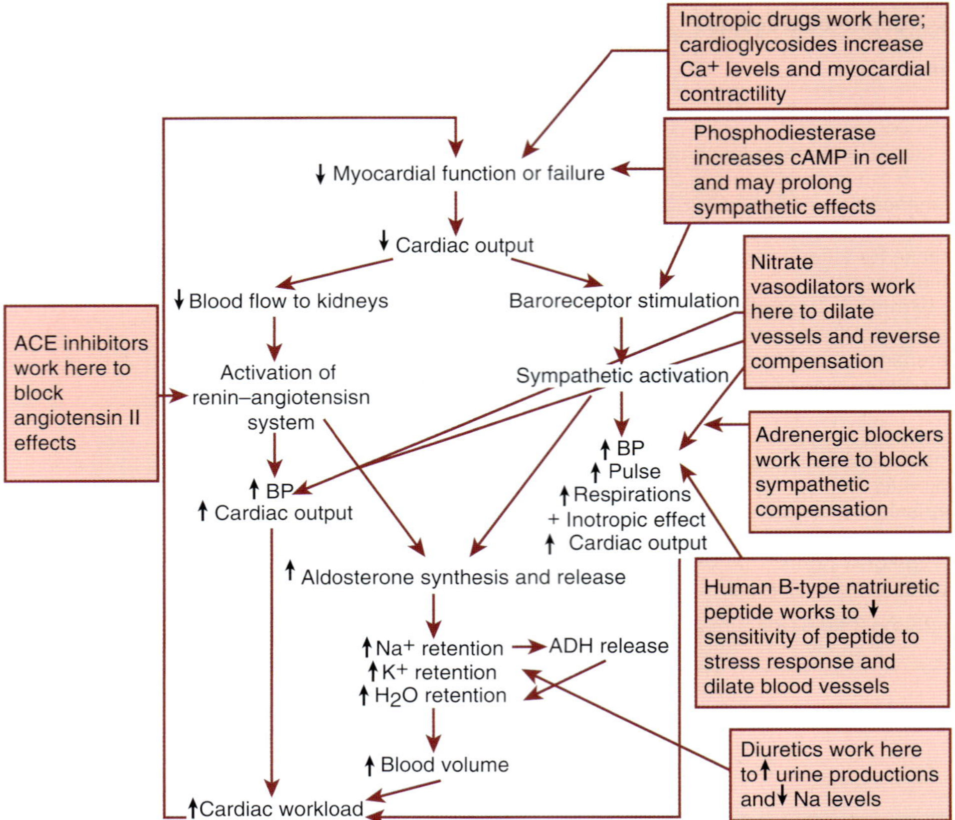

FIGURE 44.4 Sites of action of drugs used to treat heart failure (HF).

5–30 minutes when given intravenously [IV]). It is widely distributed throughout the body. Digoxin is primarily excreted unchanged in the urine. Because of this, caution should be used in the presence of renal impairment because the drug may not be excreted and could accumulate, causing toxicity.

Contraindications and cautions

Cardiac glycosides are contraindicated in the presence of allergy to any component of the digitalis preparation. Digoxin is contraindicated in the following conditions: ventricular tachycardia or fibrillation, *which are potentially fatal arrhythmias and should be treated with other drugs*; heart block or sick sinus syndrome, *which could be made worse by slowing of conduction through the atrioventricular node*; idiopathic hypertrophic subaortic stenosis (IHSS) *because the increase in force of contraction could obstruct the outflow tract to the aorta and cause severe problems*; acute MI *because the increase in force of contraction could cause more muscle damage and infarct*; renal insufficiency *because the drug is excreted through the kidneys and toxic levels could develop*; and electrolyte abnormalities (eg, increased calcium, decreased potassium, decreased magnesium levels), *which could alter the action potential and change the effects of the drug.*

Digoxin should be used cautiously in women who are pregnant or breastfeeding *because of the potential for adverse effects on the fetus or neonate*. It is not known whether digoxin causes fetal toxicity; it should be given during pregnancy only if the benefit to the mother clearly outweighs the risk to the fetus. Digoxin does enter breast milk, but it has not been shown to cause problems for the neonate. Caution should be used, however, during breastfeeding. Children and older people are also at higher risk (Box 44.2).

Adverse effects

The adverse effects most frequently seen with the cardiac glycosides include headache, weakness, drowsiness and vision changes (a yellow halo around objects is often reported). Gastrointestinal upset and anorexia also commonly occur. Arrhythmias may develop because the glycosides affect the action potential and conduction system of the heart. Digoxin toxicity is a serious syndrome that can occur when digoxin levels are too high. The person may present with anorexia, nausea, vomiting, malaise, depression, irregular heart rhythms including heart block, atrial arrhythmias and ventricular tachycardia. This can be a life-threatening situation. A digoxin antidote, **digoxin immune Fab**, has been developed to rapidly treat digoxin toxicity (Box 44.3). *See the Critical thinking scenario for additional information about inadequate digoxin absorption.*

BOX 44.2 FOCUS ON The evidence

Preventing digoxin toxicity in children and the elderly

Children and older adults are at increased risk for digoxin toxicity. Individuals in both of these groups have body masses that are smaller than the average adult body mass, and they may have immature or ageing kidneys. Digoxin is excreted unchanged in the kidneys, so any change in kidney function can result in increased serum digoxin levels and subsequent digoxin toxicity. Extreme care should be taken when administering digoxin to people in either of these age groups.

Paediatric findings

Many institutions require that paediatric digoxin doses be checked by a second health care professional before administration. This practice provides an extra check to help prevent the toxicity of this potentially dangerous drug. The child should then be assessed before the drug is given, including careful cardiac auscultation and apical pulse measurement to monitor heart rate and rhythm to detect any possible toxic effects.

Geriatric findings

Older adults may not receive the same kind of attention as a policy, but they should be monitored for any factor that might affect digoxin levels when the drug is administered. Such factors may include:

- renal function (Is the blood urea nitrogen concentration elevated?)
- low body mass (Is the person underweight, undernourished, taking laxatives?)
- current pulse, including quality and rhythm
- hydration (Is the skin loose? Are the mucous membranes dry? The presence of these conditions could signal potential electrolyte disturbances.)

Many elderly people eventually need a decrease in dose, from 0.25 mg once a day to 0.125 mg once a day or 0.25 mg every other day. The health care professional administering the drug is often in the best position to detect any changes in the person's condition that might indicate a need for further evaluation.

BOX 44.3 Digoxin antidote: digoxin immune Fab

Digoxin immune Fab (*Digibind*) [not available in New Zealand] is an antigen-binding fragment (Fab) derived from specific anti-digoxin antibodies. These antibodies bind molecules of digoxin, making them unavailable at their site of action. The digoxin antibody–antigen complexes accumulate in the blood and are excreted through the kidney. Digoxin immune Fab is used for the treatment of life-threatening digoxin intoxication (serum levels 0.10 ng/mL with serum potassium 0.5 mmol/L in a setting of digoxin intoxication) and potential life-threatening digoxin overdose.

The amount of digoxin immune Fab that is infused IV is determined by the amount of digoxin ingested or by the serum digoxin level if the ingested amount is unknown. The person's cardiac status should be monitored continually while the drug is given and for several hours after the infusion is finished. Because there is a risk of hypersensitivity reaction to the infused protein, life-support equipment should be on standby.

Serum digoxin levels will be very high and unreliable for about 3 days after the digoxin immune Fab infusion because of the high levels of digoxin in the blood. The person should not receive further digoxin for several days to 1 week after digoxin immune Fab has been used, because of the potential of remaining fragments in the blood.

Clinically important drug–drug interactions

There is a risk of increased therapeutic effects and toxic effects of digoxin if it is taken with verapamil, amiodarone, quinine, erythromycin or ciclosporin. If digoxin is combined with any of these drugs, it may be necessary to decrease the digoxin dose to prevent toxicity. If one of these drugs has been part of a medical regimen with digoxin and is discontinued, the digoxin dose may need to be increased. The risk of cardiac arrhythmias could increase if these drugs are taken with potassium-losing diuretics. If this combination is used, the person's potassium levels should be checked regularly and appropriate replacement done. Digoxin may be less effective if it is combined with thyroid hormones, metoclopramide

Prototype summary: digoxin

Indications: treatment of HF, atrial fibrillation.

Actions: increases intracellular calcium level and allows more calcium to enter the myocardial cell during depolarisation; this causes a positive inotropic effect (increased force of contraction), increased renal perfusion with a diuretic effect and decrease in renin release, a negative chronotropic effect (slower heart rate), and slowed conduction through the atrioventricular (AV) node.

Pharmacokinetics:

Route	Onset	Peak	Duration
Oral	30–120 min	2–6 hours	6–8 days
IV	5–30 min	1–5 hours	4–5 days

$T_{1/2}$: 30–40 hours; largely excreted unchanged in the urine.

Adverse effects: headache, weakness, drowsiness, visual disturbances, arrhythmias, GI upset.

or penicillamine, and increased digoxin dose may be needed. Absorption of oral digoxin may be decreased if it is taken with colestyramine, charcoal, colestipol, antacids, bleomycin, cyclophosphamide monohydrate or methotrexate. If it is used in combination with any of these agents, the drugs should not be taken at the same time but should be administered 2–4 hours apart. Box 44.4 highlights important information about the interactions between digoxin and common herbal remedies.

BOX 44.4 FOCUS ON Herbal and alternative therapies

St John's wort and psyllium have been shown to decrease the effectiveness of digoxin; this combination should be avoided. Increased digoxin toxicity has been reported with ginseng, hawthorn and licorice. People should be advised to avoid these combinations.

Care considerations for people receiving cardiac glycosides

Assessment: history and examination

- Assess for contraindications or cautions: known allergies to any digitalis product *to avoid hypersensitivity reactions*; impaired kidney function, *which could alter the excretion of the drug*; ventricular tachycardia or fibrillation, *which require treatment with other life-saving drugs*; heart block, sick sinus syndrome or IHSS, *which could be exacerbated by the drug*; acute MI, *which could lead to increased muscle damage and infarction*; electrolyte abnormalities (increased calcium, decreased potassium or decreased magnesium levels), *which could alter the action potential and drug effects*; and current status of pregnancy or breastfeeding.
- Perform a physical assessment *to establish baseline status before beginning therapy, determine the effectiveness of therapy and evaluate for any potential adverse effects*.
- Obtain the person's weight, noting any recent increases or decreases, *to determine the person's fluid status*.
- Assess cardiac status closely, including pulse and blood pressure, *to identify changes requiring a change in dosage of the drug or the presence of adverse effects*; and auscultate heart sounds, noting any evidence of abnormal sounds, *to identify conduction problems*.
- Inspect the skin and mucous membranes for colour, and check nail beds and capillary refill *for evidence of perfusion*.
- Monitor affect, orientation and reflexes *to evaluate central nervous system (CNS) effects of the drug*.
- Assess the person's respiratory rate and auscultate the lungs *for evidence of adventitious breath sounds to monitor for evidence of left-sided heart failure*.
- Examine the abdomen for distension; auscultate bowel sounds *to evaluate GI motility*.
- Assess voiding patterns and urinary output *to provide a gross indication of renal function*.
- Obtain a baseline electrocardiogram (ECG) *to identify rate and rhythm and evaluate for possible changes*.
- Monitor the results of laboratory tests, including serum electrolyte levels and renal function tests, *to determine the need for possible dose adjustment*.

Implementation with rationale

- Consult with the prescriber about the need for a loading dose when beginning therapy *to achieve desired results as soon as possible*.
- Monitor apical pulse for 1 full minute before administering the drug *to monitor for adverse effects*. Withhold the dose if the pulse is less than 60 beats/minute in an adult or less than 90 beats/minute in an infant; retake the pulse in 1 hour. If the pulse remains low, document it, withhold the drug and notify the prescriber *because the pulse rate could indicate digoxin toxicity* (see Table 44.2 for Signs and symptoms).
- Monitor the pulse for any change in quality or rhythm *to detect arrhythmias or early signs of toxicity*.
- Check the dose and preparation carefully *because digoxin has a very small margin of safety and inadvertent drug errors can cause serious problems*.
- Check paediatric dose with extreme care *because children are more apt to develop digoxin toxicity*. Have the dose double-checked by another nurse or midwife before administration.
- Follow dilution instructions carefully for IV use; use promptly *to avoid drug degradation*.
- Administer IV doses very slowly over at least 5 minutes *to avoid cardiac arrhythmias and adverse effects*.
- Avoid intramuscular administration, *which could be quite painful*.
- Arrange for the person to be weighed at the same time each day, in the same clothes, *to monitor for fluid retention and HF*. Assess dependent areas for oedema; note the amount and degree of pitting *to evaluate the severity of fluid retention*.
- Avoid administering the oral drug with food or antacids *to avoid delays in absorption*.

- Maintain emergency equipment on standby: potassium salts, lidocaine (lignocaine) (*for treatment of arrhythmias*), phenytoin (*for treatment of seizures*), atropine (*to increase heart rate*) and a cardiac monitor, *in case severe toxicity should occur.*
- Obtain digoxin level as ordered; monitor the person for therapeutic digoxin level (0.5–2 ng/mL) *to evaluate therapeutic dosing and to monitor for the development of toxicity.*
- Provide comfort measures *to help the person tolerate drug effects.* These include small, frequent meals *to help alleviate GI upset or nausea*; access to bathroom facilities if GI upset is severe and *to accommodate increased urination related to increased cardiac output*; safety precautions *to reduce the risk of injury secondary to weakness and drowsiness*; adequate lighting *to accommodate vision changes if they occur*; positioning for comfort; and frequent rest periods *to balance supply and demand of oxygen.*
- Offer support and encouragement *to help the person deal with the diagnosis and the drug regimen.*
- Provide thorough teaching, including the name of the drug, dosage prescribed, technique for monitoring pulse and acceptable pulse parameters, dietary measures if appropriate, measures to avoid adverse effects, warning signs of possible toxicity and need to notify health care provider and the need for periodic monitoring and evaluation, including ECGs and laboratory testing, *to enhance knowledge about drug therapy and to promote compliance.*

Evaluation

- Monitor response to the drug (improvement in signs and symptoms of HF, resolution of atrial arrhythmias, serum digoxin level of 0.5–2 ng/mL).
- Monitor for adverse effects (vision changes, arrhythmias, HF, headache, dizziness, drowsiness, GI upset, nausea).
- Monitor the effectiveness of comfort measures and compliance with the regimen.
- Evaluate the effectiveness of the teaching plan (person can name drug, dosage, proper administration, adverse effects to watch for, specific measures to avoid them and the importance of continued follow-up).

TABLE 44.2 Congestive heart failure and response to cardiac glycosides

	Response	
Signs and symptoms*	**During congestive heart failure**	**After treatment with digitalis+**
Heart rate, rhythm and size	Heart hypertrophied, dilated; rate rapid, irregular; 'palpitations'; auscultation – S_3	Dilatation decreased, hypertrophy remains; rate, 70–80 beats/minute, may be regular; auscultation – no S_3
Lungs	Dyspnoea on exertion; orthopnoea; tachypnoea; paroxysmal nocturnal dyspnoea; wheezing, rales, cough, haemoptysis (pulmonary oedema)	↓ Rate of respiration; wheezes, rales gone
Peripheral congestion	Pitting oedema of dependent parts; hepatomegaly; ↑ jugular venous pressure; cyanosis; oliguria; nocturia	↑ Cardiac output and renal blood flow leads to ↑ urine flow, ↓ oedema, ↓ signs and symptoms of poor perfusion
Other	Weakness, fatigue, anorexia, insomnia, nausea, vomiting, abdominal pain	↑ Appetite: ↑ strength, energy

*Because the clinical picture in heart failure varies with the stage and degree of severity, the signs and symptoms may vary considerably in different people.
+Treatment with digitalis will not overcome similar symptoms when they are caused by conditions other than heart failure. Overdosage may actually cause symptoms similar to those of heart failure (eg, anorexia, nausea, vomiting, cardiac arrhythmias, peripheral congestion).

CRITICAL THINKING SCENARIO

Inadequate digoxin absorption

THE SITUATION

G.J. is an 82-year-old Caucasian woman with a 50-year history of rheumatic mitral valve disease. She has been stabilised on digoxin for 10 years in a compensated state of heart failure (HF). G.J. recently moved into an extended-care facility because she was having difficulty caring for herself independently. She was examined by the admitting facility doctor and was found to be stable An irregular pulse of 76 beats/minute was noted with electrocardiographic documentation of her chronic atrial fibrillation.

Three weeks after her arrival at the nursing home, G.J. began to develop progressive weakness, dyspnoea on exertion, two-pillow orthopnoea and peripheral 2+ pitting oedema. These signs and symptoms became progressively worse, and 5 days after the first indication that her HF was returning, G.J. was admitted to the hospital with a diagnosis of HF. Physical examination revealed a heart rate of 96 beats/minute with atrial fibrillation, third heart sound, rales, wheezes, 2+ pitting oedema bilaterally up to the knees, elevated jugular venous pressure, cardiomegaly, weak pulses and poor peripheral perfusion. G.J.'s serum digoxin level was 0.12 ng/mL (therapeutic range, 0.5–2 ng/mL). G.J. was treated with diuretics and digitalis in the hospital, with close cardiac monitoring.

After her condition stabilised, G.J. reported that she knew she had been taking her digoxin every day because she recognised the pill. The only difference she could identify was that she was given the pill in the afternoon with a dish of ice cream, while at home she always took it on an empty stomach first thing in the morning. The nursing home staff confirmed that G.J. had received the drug daily in the afternoon and that it was the same brand name she had used at home.

CRITICAL THINKING

What care interventions should be made at this point? *Think about the signs and symptoms of HF and how they show its progression.*

How could the change in the timing of drug administration be related to the decreased serum digoxin levels noted on G.J.'s admission?

Consider the factors that affect absorption of a drug. What alterations in dosing could be suggested that would prevent this from happening to G.J. again?

What potential problems with trust could develop for G.J. on her return to the nursing home? Suggest an explanation for what happened to G.J. and possible ways that this problem could have been averted.

DISCUSSION

G.J.'s immediate needs involve trying to alleviate the alteration to her cardiac output that occurred when she lost the therapeutic effects of digoxin. Positioning, cool environment, small and frequent meals, and rest periods can help to decrease the workload on her heart. Digoxin has a narrow margin of safety and requires an adequate serum level to be therapeutic. G.J. was not absorbing enough digoxin to achieve a therapeutic serum level; consequently, her body began to go through the progression of HF, first right-sided and then left-sided.

CARE GUIDE FOR G.J.: DIGOXIN

Assessment: history and examination

Assess the person's health history for allergies to any digitalis product, renal dysfunction, idiopathic hypertrophic subaortic stenosis (IHSS), pregnancy, breastfeeding, arrhythmias, heart block and electrolyte abnormalities.

Focus the physical examination on the following areas:
Cardiovascular: blood pressure, pulse, perfusion, ECG
Neurological (CNS): orientation, affect, reflexes, vision
Skin: colour, lesions, texture, perfusion
Respiratory system: respiratory rate and character, adventitious sounds
GI: abdominal examination, bowel sounds
Laboratory tests: serum electrolytes, body weight

Implementation

Administer a loading dose to provide rapid therapeutic effects.

Monitor apical pulse for 1 full minute before administering to assess for adverse and therapeutic effects.

Check dose very carefully.

Provide comfort and safety measures: give small, frequent meals; ensure access to bathroom facilities; avoid intramuscular injection; administer IV over 5 minutes; keep emergency equipment on standby.

Provide support and reassurance to deal with drug effects.

Provide teaching regarding drug, dosage, adverse effects, what to report, safety precautions.

Evaluation

Evaluate drug effects: relief of signs and symptoms of HF, resolution of atrial arrhythmias, serum digoxin levels 0.5–2 ng/mL.

Monitor for adverse effects, including arrhythmias, vision changes (yellow halo), GI upset, headache, drowsiness.

Monitor for drug–drug interactions as indicated for each drug.

Evaluate the effectiveness of teaching program.

Evaluate the effectiveness of comfort and safety measures.

TEACHING FOR G.J.

- Digoxin is a digitalis preparation. Digitalis has many helpful effects on the heart; for example, it helps the heart to beat more slowly and efficiently. These effects promote better circulation and should help to reduce the swelling in your ankles or legs. It also should increase the amount of urine that you produce every day.
- Digoxin is a very powerful drug and must be taken exactly as prescribed. It is important to have regular medical checkups to ensure that the dose of the drug is correct for you and that it is having the desired effect on your heart.
- Do not stop taking this drug without consulting your health care provider. Never skip doses and never try to

'catch up' any missed doses, because serious adverse effects could occur.

- Learn to take your pulse. Take it each morning before engaging in any activity. Write your pulse rate on a calendar so you will be aware of any changes and can notify your health care provider if the rate or rhythm of your pulse shows a consistent change. Your normal pulse rate is __________.
- Try to monitor your weight fairly closely. Weigh yourself every other day, at the same time of the day and in the same amount of clothing. Record your weight on your calendar for easy reference. If you gain or lose 1.5 kg or more in 1 day, it may indicate a problem with your drug. Consult your health care provider.
- Some of the following adverse effects may occur:
  - *Dizziness, drowsiness, headache*: avoid driving or performing hazardous tasks or delicate tasks that require concentration if these occur. Consult your health care provider for an appropriate analgesic if the headache is a problem.
  - *Nausea, GI upset, loss of appetite*: small, frequent meals may help; monitor your weight loss; if it becomes severe, consult your health care provider.
  - *Vision changes, 'yellow' halos around objects*: these effects may pass with time. Take extra care in your activities for the first few days. If these reactions do not go away after 3–4 days, consult with your health care provider.
  - Report any of the following to your health care provider: *unusually slow or irregular pulse; rapid weight gain; 'yellow vision'; unusual tiredness or weakness; skin rash or hives; swelling of the ankles, legs or fingers; difficulty breathing.*
- Tell any doctor, nurse, dentist or other health care provider that you are taking this drug.
- Keep this drug, and all medications, out of the reach of children.
- Avoid the use of over-the-counter medications while you are taking this drug. If you think that you need one of these, consult with your health care provider for the best choice. Many of these drugs contain ingredients that could interfere with your digoxin.
- Consider wearing or carrying a medical identification to alert any medical personnel who might take care of you in an emergency that you are taking this drug.
- Schedule regular medical checkups to evaluate the actions of the drug and to adjust the dose if necessary.

PHOSPHODIESTERASE INHIBITORS

The phosphodiesterase inhibitors (Table 44.1) belong to a second class of drugs that act as cardiotonic (inotropic) agents. These include milrinone (*Primacor*) and sildenafil (*Revatio, Silvasta, Vedafil, Viagra*).

Therapeutic actions and indications

The phosphodiesterase inhibitors block the enzyme phosphodiesterase. This blocking effect leads to an increase in myocardial-cell cyclic adenosine monophosphate (cAMP) level, which increases calcium level in the cell (Figure 44.4). Increased cellular calcium level causes a stronger contraction and prolongs the effects of sympathetic stimulation, which can lead to vasodilation, increased oxygen consumption and arrhythmias. These drugs are indicated for the short-term treatment of HF that has not responded to digoxin or diuretics alone or that has had a poor response to digoxin, diuretics and vasodilators. See Table 44.1 for usual indications for each drug. Because these drugs have been associated with the development of potentially fatal ventricular arrhythmias, their use is limited to severe situations.

Pharmacokinetics

Milrinone is available only for IV use. It is widely distributed after injection, metabolised in the liver and excreted primarily in the urine.

Contraindications and cautions

Phosphodiesterase inhibitors are contraindicated in the presence of allergy to either of these drugs or to bisulfites. They also are contraindicated in the following conditions: severe aortic or pulmonary valvular disease, *which could be exacerbated by increased contraction*; acute MI, *which could be exacerbated by increased oxygen consumption and increased force of contraction*; fluid volume deficit, *which could be made worse by increased renal perfusion*; and ventricular arrhythmias, *which could be exacerbated by these drugs.*

Caution should be used in the elderly, *who are more likely to develop adverse effects.*

There are no adequate studies about the effects of these drugs during pregnancy, and their use should be reserved for situations in which the benefit to the mother clearly outweighs the potential risk to the fetus. *It is not known whether these drugs enter breast milk*, so caution should be used if the woman is breastfeeding.

Adverse effects

The adverse effects most frequently seen with these drugs are ventricular arrhythmias (which can progress to fatal ventricular fibrillation), hypotension and chest pain. GI effects include nausea, vomiting, anorexia and abdominal pain. Thrombocytopenia can occur with milrinone. Hypersensitivity reactions associated with these drugs include vasculitis, pericarditis, pleuritis and ascites. Burning at the IV injection site is also a frequent adverse effect.

Clinically important drug–drug interactions

Precipitates form when these drugs are given in solution with frusemide. Avoid this combination in solution. Use alternative lines if both of these drugs are being given IV.

Care considerations for people receiving phosphodiesterase inhibitors

Assessment: history and examination

- Assess for contraindications or cautions: any known allergies to these drugs or to bisulfites *to avoid hypersensitivity reactions*; acute aortic or pulmonary valvular disease, acute MI or fluid volume deficit and ventricular arrhythmias, *which could be exacerbated by these drugs*; and current status of pregnancy and breastfeeding *to prevent potential adverse effects to the fetus or baby.*
- Perform a physical assessment *to establish baseline status before beginning therapy, determine the effectiveness of therapy and evaluate for any potential adverse effects.*
- Assess cardiac status closely, including pulse and blood pressure, *to identify changes or the presence of adverse effects*; auscultate heart sounds, noting any evidence of abnormal sounds.
- Obtain the person's weight, noting any recent increases or decreases, *to determine the fluid status.*
- Inspect skin and mucous membranes for colour, and check nail beds and capillary refill *for evidence of perfusion.*
- Examine the abdomen for distension; auscultate bowel sounds *to evaluate GI motility.*
- Assess voiding patterns and urinary output *to provide a gross indication of renal function.*
- Obtain a baseline ECG *to identify rate and rhythm and evaluate for possible changes.*
- Monitor the results of laboratory tests, including serum electrolyte levels, full blood count, and renal and liver function tests, *to determine the need for possible dose adjustment.*

Implementation with rationale

- Protect the drug from light *to prevent drug degradation.*
- Ensure that the person has a patent IV access site available *to allow for IV administration of the drug.*
- Monitor pulse and blood pressure frequently during administration *to monitor for adverse effects so that the dose can be altered if needed to avoid toxicity.*
- Monitor input and output and record daily weight *to evaluate the resolution of HF.*
- Monitor platelet counts before and regularly during therapy *to ensure that the dose is appropriate*; inspect the skin for bruising or petechiae *to detect early signs of thrombocytopenia*; consult with the prescriber about the need to decrease the dose at the first sign of thrombocytopenia.
- Monitor IV injection sites and provide comfort measures *if infusion is causing irritation.*
- Provide life support equipment on standby *in case of severe reaction to the drug or development of ventricular arrhythmias.*
- Provide comfort measures *to help the person tolerate drug effects.* These include small, frequent meals *to alleviate GI upset and anorexia*; access to bathroom facilities to provide needed facilities if GI upset is severe and when increased urination occurs secondary to increased cardiac output; safety precautions *to protect the person if visual changes, dizziness or weakness occurs*; and orientation to surroundings *to support the person if CNS changes occur.*
- Offer support and encouragement *to help the person deal with the diagnosis and the drug regimen.*
- Provide thorough teaching, including the name of the drug, dosage prescribed, measures to avoid adverse effects, warning signs of problems and the need for periodic monitoring and evaluation, *to enhance knowledge about drug therapy and to promote compliance.*

Evaluation

- Monitor response to the drug (alleviation of signs and symptoms of HF).
- Monitor for adverse effects (hypotension, cardiac arrhythmias, GI upset, thrombocytopenia).
- Monitor the effectiveness of comfort measures and compliance with the regimen.
- Evaluate the effectiveness of the teaching plan (person can name drug, dosage, adverse effects to watch for, specific measures to avoid them and the importance of continued follow-up).

KEY POINTS

- The cardiac glycoside digoxin increases the movement of calcium into the heart muscle. This results in increased force of contraction, which increases blood flow to the kidneys (causing a diuretic effect), slows the heart rate and slows conduction through the atrioventricular node. All of these effects decrease the heart's workload.
- Phosphodiesterase inhibitors block the breakdown of cAMP in the cardiac muscle. This allows more calcium to enter the cell (leading to more intense contraction) and increases the effects of sympathetic stimulation (which can lead to vasodilation but also can increase pulse, blood pressure and workload on the heart).
- Phosphodiesterase inhibitors are associated with severe effects. They are reserved for use in extreme situations. They are only available for IV use.

CHAPTER SUMMARY

- HF, a condition in which the heart muscle fails to effectively pump blood through the cardiovascular system, can be the result of a damaged heart muscle and increased demand to work harder.
- The sarcomere – the functioning unit of the heart muscle – is made up of protein fibres: thin actin fibres and thick myosin fibres, which react with each other when calcium is present to inactivate troponin. The fibres slide together, resulting in contraction. Failing cardiac muscle cells lose the ability to effectively use energy to move calcium into the cell, and contractions become weak and ineffective.
- Cardiotonic (inotropic) agents are one class of drugs used in the treatment of heart failure. These agents directly stimulate the muscle to contract more effectively.
- Cardiac glycosides increase the movement of calcium into the heart muscle. This results in increased force of contraction, which increases blood flow to the kidneys (causing a diuretic effect), slows the heart rate and slows conduction through the atrioventricular node. All of these effects decrease the heart's workload. Digoxin is the cardiac glycoside most commonly used to treat HF.
- Phosphodiesterase inhibitors block the breakdown of cAMP in the cardiac muscle. This allows more calcium to enter the cell (leading to more forceful contraction) and enhances the effects of sympathetic stimulation (which can lead to vasodilation but also can increase pulse, blood pressure and workload on the heart). Because these drugs are associated with severe effects, they are reserved for use in extreme situations.

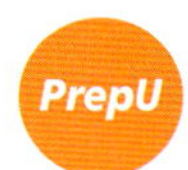

Knowing your strengths and weaknesses helps you to study more effectively. Take a PrepU Practice Quiz to find out how you measure up!

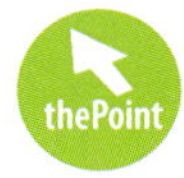

ONLINE RESOURCES

An extensive range of additional resources to enhance teaching and learning and to facilitate understanding of this chapter may be found online at the text's accompanying website, located on thePoint at http://thepoint.lww.com. These include Watch and Learn videos, Concepts in Action animations, journal articles, review questions, case studies, discussion topics and quizzes.

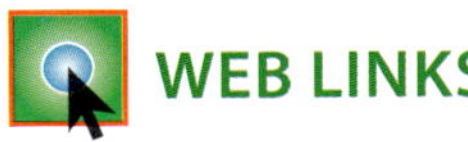

WEB LINKS

Health care providers and students may want to consult the following web resources:

www.aihw.gov.au/reports/heart-stroke-vascular-disease/cardiovascular-health-compendium/contents/how-many-australians-have-cardiovascular-disease
Cardiovascular disease snapshot 2018 – an Australian Institute of Health and Welfare publication.

www.heartfoundation.org.nz/resources/csanz-2018-heart-failure-guideline
National Heart Foundation of Australia and Cardiac Society of Australia and New Zealand. *Guidelines for the Prevention, Detection, and Management of Heart Failure in Australia 2018.*

BIBLIOGRAPHY

Aarnoudse, A. L. H. J., Dieleman, J. P. & Stricker, B. H. C. (2007). Age- and gender-specific incidence of hospitalisation for digoxin intoxication. *Drug Safety, 30(5)*, 431–436.

Albert, N. M. (2012). Fluid management strategies in heart failure. *Critical Care Nurse, 32(2)*, 20–33.

Bowers, M. T. (2013). Managing patients with heart failure. *Journal for Nurse Practitioners, 9(10)*, 634–642.

Braunwald, E. & Bonow, R. O., MD Consult LLC (2012). *Braunwald's Heart Disease: A Textbook of Cardiovascular Medicine* (9th edn). Philadelphia: Elsevier Saunders.

Chan, K. E., Lazarus, J. M. & Hakim, R. M. (2010). Digoxin associates with mortality in ESRD. *Journal of the American Society of Nephrology, 21*, 1550–1559.

Farrell, M. & Dempsey, J. (2014). *Smeltzer & Bare's Textbook of Medical-Surgical Nursing* (3rd edn). Sydney: Lippincott Williams & Wilkins.

Goodman, L. S., Brunton, L. L., Chabner, B. & Knollmann, B. C. (2011). *Goodman and Gilman's Pharmacological Basis of Therapeutics* (12th edn). New York: McGraw-Hill.

Gover, T. L. & Galvan, E. (2013). Diabetes and heart failure. *Critical Care Nursing Clinics of North America, 25(1)*, 93–99.

Graven, L. J. & Grant, J. (2013). The impact of social support on depressive symptoms in individuals with heart failure. *Journal Cardiovascular Nursing, 28(5)*, 429–443.

Hurst, J. W., Fuster, V., Walsh, R. A. & Harrington, R. A. (Eds.). (2011). *Hurst's the Heart* (13th edn). New York: McGraw-Hill.

McKenna, L. & Mirkov, S. (2019). *McKenna's Drug Handbook for Nursing and Midwifery* (8th edn). Sydney: Wolters Kluwer Health Australia.

Porth, C. M. (2011). *Essentials of Pathophysiology: Concepts of Altered Health States* (3rd edn). Philadelphia: Lippincott Williams & Wilkins.

Porth, C. M. (2009). *Pathophysiology: Concepts of Altered Health States* (8th edn). Philadelphia: Lippincott Williams & Wilkins.

Pressler, S. J., Gradus-Pizio, I., Chubinski, S. D., Smith, G., Wheeler, S., Sloan, R. & Jung, M. (2013). Family caregivers of patients with heart failure. *Journal of Cardiovascular Nursing, 28(5)*, 417–428.

Raja Rao, M. P., Panduranga, P., Sulaiman, K. & Al-Jufaili, M. (2013). Digoxin toxicity with normal digoxin and serum potassium levels: Beware of magnesium, the hidden malefactor. *Journal of Emergency Medicine, 45(2)*, e31–e34.

Scott, I. & Jackson, C. (2013) Chronic heart failure management in Australia: Time for general practice centred models of care? *Australian Family Physician, 42(5)*, 343–346.

Sykes, C. & Simpson, S. (2011). Managing the psychosocial aspects of heart failure: A case study. *British Journal of Nursing, 20(5)*, 272–279.

CHECK YOUR UNDERSTANDING

Answers to the questions in this chapter can be found in Appendix A at the back of this book.

MULTIPLE CHOICE

Select the best answer to the following.

1. A nurse or midwife assessing a person with HF would expect to find which of the following:
   a. cardiac arrest.
   b. congestion of blood vessels.
   c. a myocardial infarction.
   d. a pulmonary embolism.
2. Calcium is needed in the cardiac muscle:
   a. to break apart actin–myosin bridges.
   b. to activate troponin.
   c. to promote contraction via sliding.
   d. to maintain the electrical rhythm.
3. When assessing a person with right-sided HF, the nurse or midwife would expect to find oedema:
   a. in gravity-dependent areas.
   b. in the hands and fingers.
   c. around the eyes.
   d. when the person is lying down.
4. ACE inhibitors and other vasodilators are used in the early treatment of HF. They act to:
   a. cause loss of volume.
   b. increase arterial pressure and perfusion.
   c. cause pooling of the blood and decreased venous return to the heart.
   d. increase the release of aldosterone and improve fluid balance.
5. A nurse or midwife is preparing to administer a prescribed cardiotonic drug to a person based on the understanding that this group of drugs act in which way?
   a. They block the sympathetic nervous system.
   b. They block the renin–angiotensin system.
   c. They block the parasympathetic influence on the heart muscle.
   d. They affect intracellular calcium levels in the heart muscle.
6. A nurse or midwife would instruct a person taking digoxin (*Lanoxin*) for the treatment of HF to do which of the following?
   a. Make up any missed doses the next day.
   b. Report changes in heart rate.
   c. Avoid exposure to the sun.
   d. Switch to generic tablets if less expensive.
7. A nurse or midwife is about to administer *Lanoxin* to a person whose apical pulse is 48 beats/min. She should:
   a. give the drug and notify the prescriber that the heart rate is low.
   b. retake the pulse in 15 minutes and give the drug if the pulse has not changed.
   c. retake the pulse in 1 hour and withhold the drug if the pulse is still less than 60 beats/minute.
   d. withhold the drug and notify the prescriber that the heart rate is below 60 beats/minute.
8. Before giving digoxin to an infant, the health care professional should:
   a. notify the prescriber that the dose is about to be given and recheck the ordered dose.
   b. check the apical pulse and have another health care professional independently check the dose.
   c. make sure that the infant has eaten, has a full stomach and has been given an antacid.
   d. check the apical pulse and give the drug very slowly.

MULTIPLE RESPONSE

Select all that apply.

1. HF occurs when the heart fails to pump effectively. Which of the following could cause HF?
   a. coronary artery disease
   b. chronic hypertension
   c. cardiomyopathy
   d. fluid overload
   e. pneumonia
   f. cirrhosis
2. A person develops left-sided HF after an MI. Which of the following would the nurse expect to find during the person's assessment?
   a. orthopnoea
   b. polyuria
   c. tachypnoea
   d. dyspnoea
   e. blood-tinged sputum
   f. swollen ankles

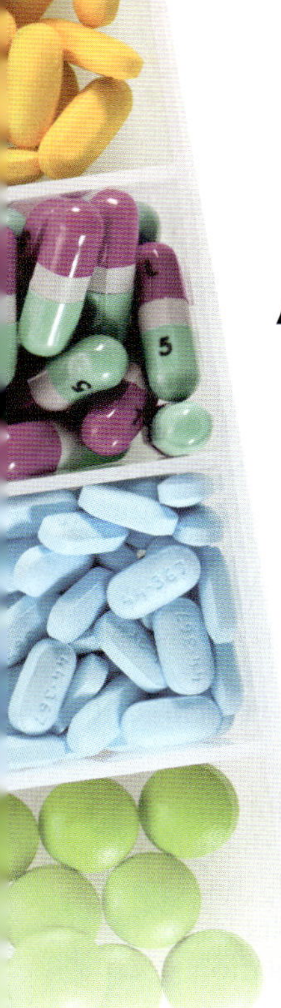

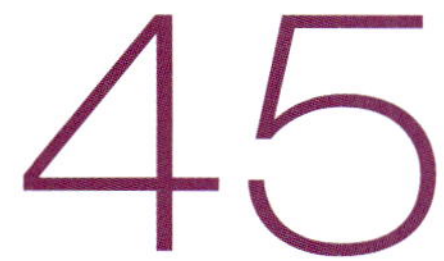

Antiarrhythmic agents

Learning objectives

On completing this chapter you should be able to:

1. Describe the cardiac action potential and its phases to explain the changes made by each class of antiarrhythmic agents.
2. Describe the therapeutic actions, indications, pharmacokinetics, contraindications and cautions, most common adverse reactions and important drug–drug interactions associated with antiarrhythmic agents.
3. Discuss the use of antiarrhythmic agents across the lifespan.
4. Compare and contrast the prototype antiarrhythmic drugs lidocaine (lignocaine), propranolol, amiodarone and diltiazem with other agents in their class and with other classes of antiarrhythmics.
5. Outline the care considerations, including important teaching points, for people receiving antiarrhythmic agents.

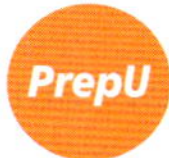

Test your current knowledge of antiarrhythmic agents with a PrepU Practice Quiz!

Glossary of key terms

antiarrhythmics: drugs that affect the action potential of cardiac cells and are used to treat arrhythmias and restore normal rate and rhythm

bradycardia: slower-than-normal heart rate (usually less than 60 beats/minute)

Cardiac Arrhythmia Suppression Trial (CAST): a large research study run by the US National Heart and Lung Institute, which found that long-term treatment of arrhythmias may have a questionable effect on mortality, and in some cases actually lead to increased cardiac death; basis for the current indication for antiarrhythmics (short-term use to treat life-threatening ventricular arrhythmias)

cardiac output: the amount of blood the heart can pump per beat; influenced by the coordination of cardiac muscle contraction, heart rate and blood return to the heart

haemodynamics: the study of the forces moving blood throughout the cardiovascular system

heart blocks: blocks to conduction of an impulse through the cardiac conduction system; can occur at the atrioventricular node, interrupting conduction from the atria into the ventricles, or in the bundle branches within the ventricles, preventing the normal conduction of the impulse

premature atrial contraction (PAC): caused by an ectopic focus in the atria that stimulates an atrial response

premature ventricular contraction (PVC): caused by an ectopic focus in the ventricles that stimulates the cells and causes an early contraction

proarrhythmic: tending to cause arrhythmias; many of the drugs used to treat arrhythmias have been found to generate them

tachycardia: faster-than-normal heart rate (usually greater than 100 beats/minute)

ANTIARRHYTHMIC AGENTS

Class I antiarrhythmics

Class Ia
disopyramide

Class Ib
(P) lidocaine (lignocaine)

Class Ic
flecainide
propafenone

Class II antiarrhythmics
esmolol
(P) propranolol

Class III antiarrhythmics
(P) amiodarone
sotalol

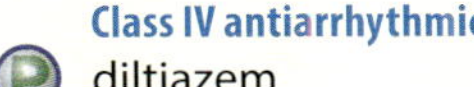
Class IV antiarrhythmics
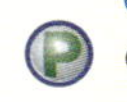
(P) diltiazem
verapamil

Other antiarrhythmics
adenosine
digoxin

As discussed in earlier chapters, disruptions in impulse formation and in the conduction of impulses through the myocardium are called arrhythmias. (They also are called dysrhythmias by some health care providers.) Arrhythmias occur in the heart because all of the cells of the heart possess the property of automaticity (discussed later in this chapter) and therefore can generate an excitatory impulse. Disruptions in the normal rhythm of the heart can interfere with myocardial contractions and affect the **cardiac output**, the amount of blood pumped with each beat. Arrhythmias that seriously disrupt cardiac output can be fatal. Drugs used to treat arrhythmias, called antiarrhythmics, suppress automaticity or alter the conductivity of the heart.

ARRHYTHMIAS

Arrhythmias involve changes to the automaticity or conductivity of the heart cells. These changes can result from several factors, including electrolyte imbalances that alter the action potential, decreased oxygen delivery to cells that changes their action potential, structural damage that changes the conduction pathway, or acidosis or waste product accumulation that alters the action potential. In some cases, changes to the heart's automaticity or conductivity may result from drugs that alter the action potential or cardiac conduction.

Conductivity

With normal heart function, each cycle of cardiac contraction and relaxation is controlled by impulses arising spontaneously in the sinoatrial (SA) node and transmitted via a specialised conducting system to activate all parts of the heart muscle almost simultaneously (see Chapter 42) (Figure 45.1). These continuous, rhythmic contractions are controlled by the heart itself. This property allows the heart to beat as long as it has enough nutrients and oxygen to survive, regardless of the status of the rest of the body.

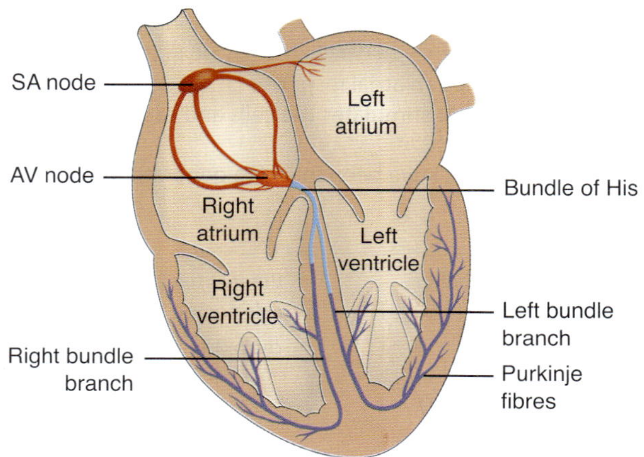

FIGURE 45.1 The conducting system of the heart. Impulses originating in the sinoatrial (SA) node are transmitted through the atrial bundles to the atrioventricular (AV) node and down the bundle of His and the bundle branches by way of the Purkinje fibres through the ventricles.

Automaticity

All cardiac cells possess some degree of automaticity (see Chapter 42) in which the cells undergo a spontaneous depolarisation during diastole or rest because they decrease the flow of potassium ions out of the cell and probably leak sodium into the cell, causing an action potential.

The action potential of the cardiac muscle cell consists of five phases:

- *Phase 0* occurs when the cell reaches a point of stimulation. The sodium gates open along the cell membrane and sodium rushes into the cell; this positive flow of electrons into the cell results in an electrical potential. This is called depolarisation.
- *Phase 1* is a very short period during which the sodium ion concentration equalises inside and outside the cell.
- *Phase 2*, or the plateau stage, occurs as the cell membrane becomes less permeable to sodium, calcium slowly enters the cell and potassium begins to leave the cell. The cell membrane is trying to return to its resting state, a process called repolarisation.
- *Phase 3* is a time of rapid repolarisation as the sodium gates are closed and potassium flows out of the cell.
- *Phase 4* occurs when the cell comes to rest; the sodium–potassium pump returns the membrane to its resting membrane potential and spontaneous depolarisation begins again.

Each area of the heart has a slightly different-appearing action potential that reflects the complexity of the cells in that area. Because of these differences in the action potential, each area of the heart has a slightly different rate of rhythmicity. The SA node generates an impulse about 60–100 times per minute, the atrioventricular (AV) node about 40–50 times per minute and the complex ventricular muscle cells about 10–20 times per minute.

Haemodynamics

The study of the forces that move blood throughout the cardiovascular system is called **haemodynamics**. The ability of the heart to effectively pump blood depends on the coordinated contraction of the atrial and ventricular muscles, which are stimulated to contract via the conduction system. The conduction system is designed so that atrial stimulation is followed by total atrial contraction and ventricular stimulation is followed by total ventricular contraction.

To pump effectively, these muscles need to contract together. If this orderly initiation and conduction of impulses is altered, the result can be a poorly coordinated contraction of the ventricles that is unable to deliver an adequate supply of oxygenated blood to the brain and other organs, including the heart muscle. If these haemodynamic alterations are severe, serious complications can occur. For example, lack of sufficient blood flow to the brain can cause syncope or precipitate stroke; lack of sufficient blood flow to the myocardium can exacerbate atherosclerosis and cause angina or myocardial infarction (MI).

Types of arrhythmias

Various factors can change the cardiac rate and rhythm, resulting in an arrhythmia. Arrhythmias can be caused by changes in rate (**tachycardia**, which is a faster-than-normal heart rate, or **bradycardia**, which is a slower-than-normal heart rate); by stimulation from

BOX 45.1 Understanding atrial fibrillation

Atrial fibrillation (AF) is a relatively common arrhythmia of the atria. It has been associated with coronary artery disease (CAD), myocardial inflammation, valvular disease, cardiomegaly and rheumatic heart disease. The cells of the atria are connected side to side and top to bottom, and are relatively simple cells. In contrast, the cells of the ventricles are connected only from top to bottom, with one cell connected only to one or two other cells. It is much easier, therefore, for an ectopic focus in the atria to spread that impulse throughout the entire atria, setting up a cycle of chaotic depolarisation and repolarisation. It is more difficult to stimulate fibrillation in the ventricles, because one ectopic site cannot rapidly spread impulses to many other cells, only to the cells connected in its two- or three-cell set.

Fibrillation results in lack of any coordinated pumping action, because the muscles are not stimulated to contract and pump out blood. In the ventricles, this is a life-threatening situation. If the ventricles do not pump blood, no blood is delivered to the brain, the tissues of the body, or the heart muscle itself. However, loss of pumping action in the atria per se does not usually cause much of a problem. The atrial contraction is like an extra kick of blood into the ventricles; it provides a nice backup to the system, but the blood will still flow normally without that kick.

DANGER OF BLOOD CLOTS

One of the problems with AF occurs when it exists for longer than 1 week. The auricles (those appendages hanging on the atria to collect blood; see Chapter 42) fill with blood that is not effectively pumped into the ventricles. Over time, this somewhat stagnant blood tends to clot. Because the auricles are sacks of striated muscle fibres, blood clots form around these fibres. In this situation, if the atria were to contract in a coordinated manner, there is a substantial risk that those clots or emboli would be pumped into the ventricles and then into the lungs (from the right auricle), which could lead to pulmonary emboli, or to the brain or periphery (from the left auricle), which could cause a stroke or occlusion of peripheral vessels.

TREATMENT CHOICES

Treatment of AF can be complicated if the length of time the person has been in AF is not known. If a person goes into AF acutely, drug therapy is available for rapid conversion. In some situations, digoxin has been effective in converting AF. Electrocardioversion, a DC current shock to the chest, may break the cycle of fibrillation and convert a person to sinus rhythm, after which the rhythm will need to be stabilised with drug therapy.

If the onset of AF is not known and it is suspected that the atria may have been fibrillating for longer than 1 week, the person is better off staying in AF without drug therapy or electrocardioversion. Prophylactic oral anticoagulants are given to decrease the risk of clot formation and emboli being pumped into the system. Conversion in this case could result in potentially life-threatening embolisation of the lungs, brain or other tissues.

SVT: ANOTHER DANGER

The other danger of AF is rapid ventricular response to the atrial stimuli, a condition called supraventricular tachycardia (SVT). With the atria firing impulses, possibly 200–300 a minute, the number of stimuli conducted into the ventricles is erratic and irregular. If the ventricle is responding too rapidly – more than 120 times a minute – the filling time of the ventricles is greatly reduced, causing cardiac output to fall dramatically. In these situations, and when AF is anticipated (such as with atrial flutter or paroxysmal atrial tachycardia), drugs may be given to slow conduction and protect the ventricles from rapid rates. Flecainide and propranolol are often used to convert rapid SVT. Esmolol and adenosine are used intravenously to convert SVT with rapid ventricular response, which could progress to AF.

IMPLICATIONS FOR HEALTH PROFESSIONALS

Careful assessment is essential before beginning treatment for AF. If the person's history cannot be established from information and medical records are not available, it is usually recommended that AF be left untreated and anticoagulant therapy started. This can pose a challenge for the nurse or midwife in trying to teach people about why their rapid and irregular heart rate will not be treated and explaining all of the factors involved in the long-term use of oral anticoagulants.

an ectopic focus, such as **premature atrial contractions** (**PACs**) or **premature ventricular contractions** (**PVCs**), atrial flutter, atrial fibrillation (Box 45.1) or ventricular fibrillation; or by alterations in conduction through the muscle, such as **heart blocks** and bundle-branch blocks. Figure 45.2 displays an electrocardiogram (ECG) strip showing normal sinus rhythm; Figures 45.3–45.5 depict various arrhythmias.

KEY POINTS

- Arrhythmias (also called dysrhythmias) are disruptions in the normal rate or rhythm of the heart.
- The cardiac conduction system determines the heart's rate and rhythm. The property by which the cardiac cells generate an action potential internally to stimulate the cardiac muscle without other stimulation is known as automaticity.
- Electrolyte disturbances, decreases in the oxygen delivered to the cells, structural damage in the conduction pathway, drug effects, acidosis or the accumulation of waste products can trigger arrhythmias.
- Changes in the heart rate, uncoordinated heart muscle contractions or blocks that alter the movement of impulses through the system can disrupt heart rhythm.
- Arrhythmias change the mechanics of blood circulation (haemodynamics), which can interrupt delivery of blood to the brain, other tissues and the heart.

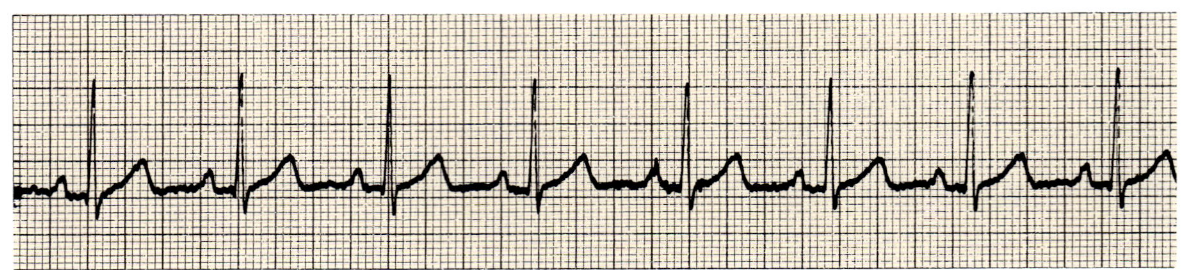

FIGURE 45.2 Normal sinus rhythm. Rhythm: regular. Rate: 60–100 beats/minute. P–R interval: 0.12–0.20 seconds. QRS: 0.06–0.10 seconds.

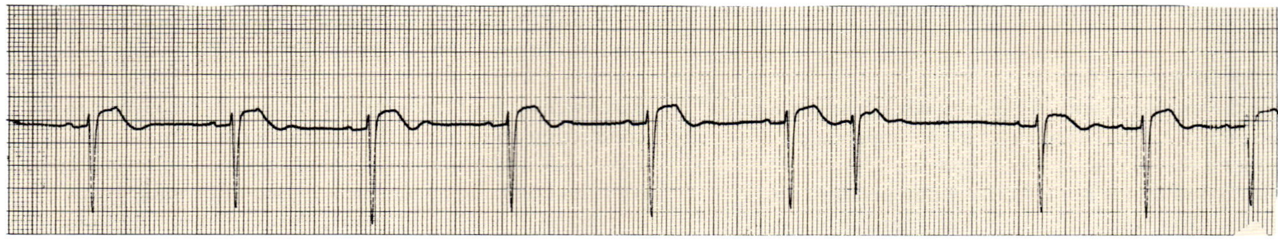

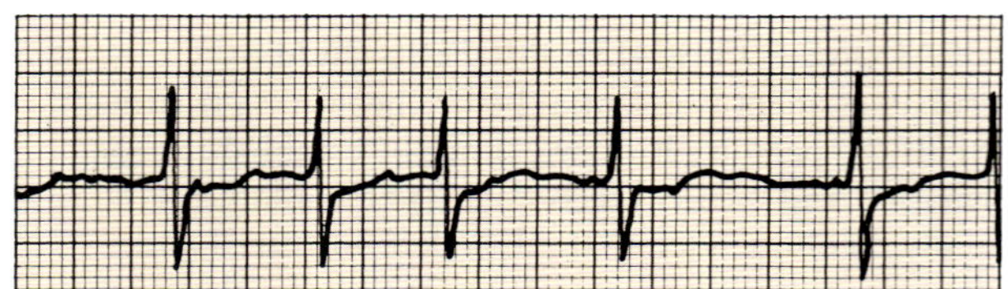

FIGURE 45.3 Atrial arrhythmias: premature atrial contractions (PACs). Rhythm: irregular due to the origination of a beat outside the normal conduction system (ectopic). Rate: normal sinus rate, except for PACs. P–R interval: P wave is abnormal, and interval may be slightly shortened in ectopic beat. QRS: normal. Atrial fibrillation. Rhythm: irregularly irregular. Rate: variable; usually rapid on initiation of rhythm; decreases when controlled by medication. P–R interval: no P waves are seen, replaced by an irregular wavy baseline. The atria are fibrillating because impulses are arising at a rate greater than 350 per minute. The ventricles respond when the atrioventricular (AV) node is stimulated to threshold and can receive the impulse. QRS: normal.

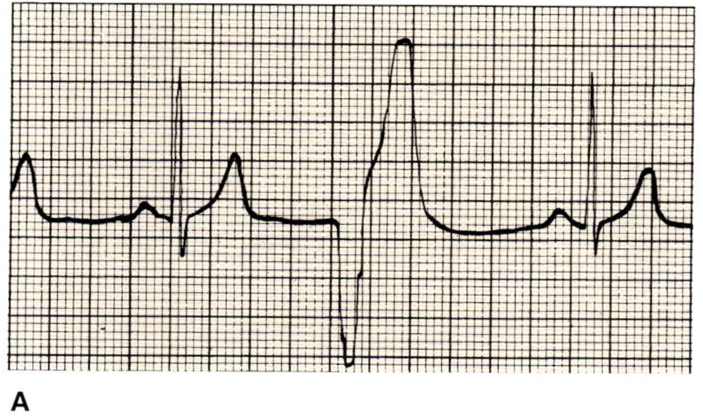

A

Premature ventricular contraction (PVC).

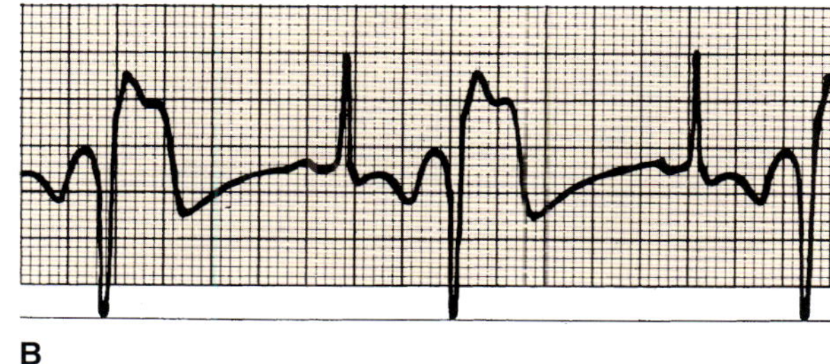

B

Ventricular bigeminy. (Every other beat is a PVC.)

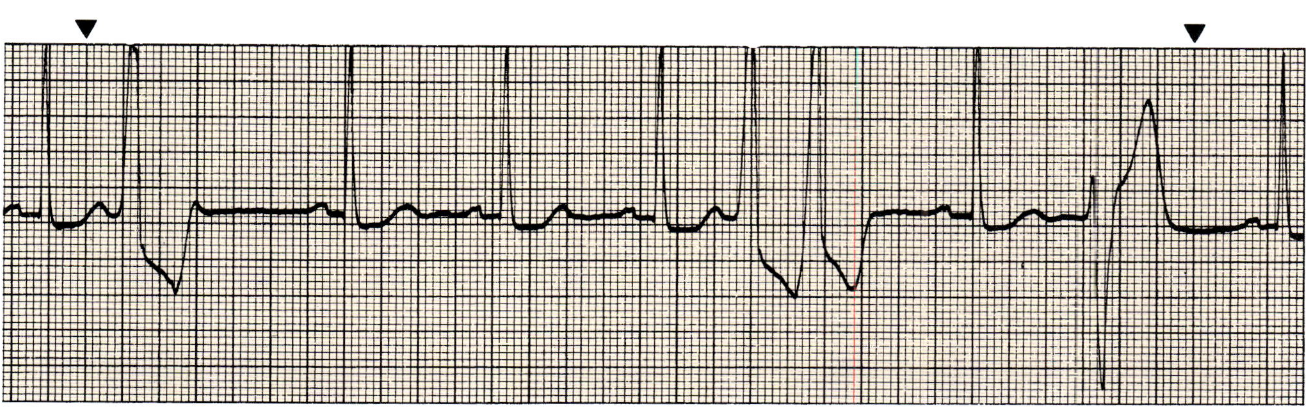

C

Multiformed PVCs.

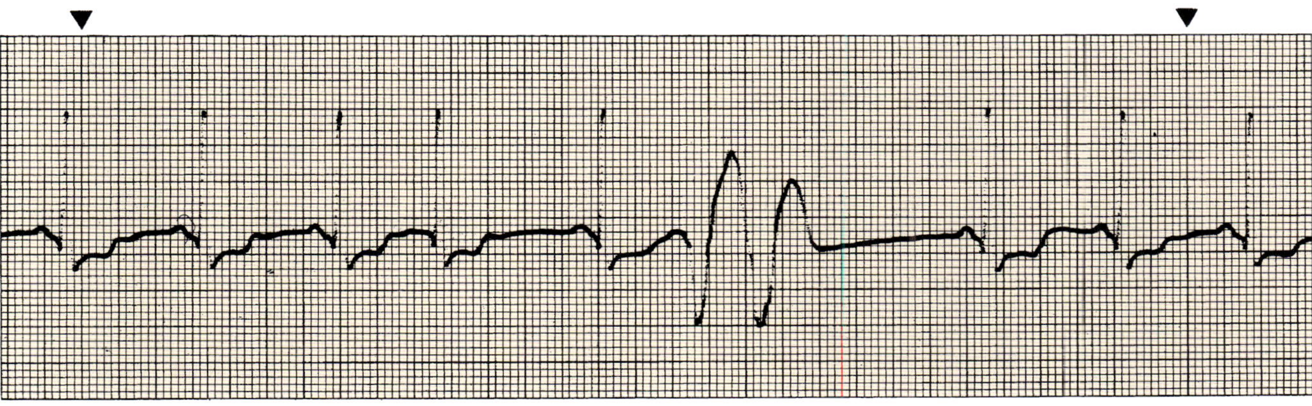

D

Heart block with PVCs.

FIGURE 45.4 Premature ventricular contractions (PVCs) or ventricular premature beats (VPBs). Rhythm: irregular. Rate: variable; only interrupts the cycle of the ectopic, ventricular contraction. P–R interval: normal in sinus beats, not measurable in PVCs. QRS: wide, bizarre, greater than 0.12 seconds.

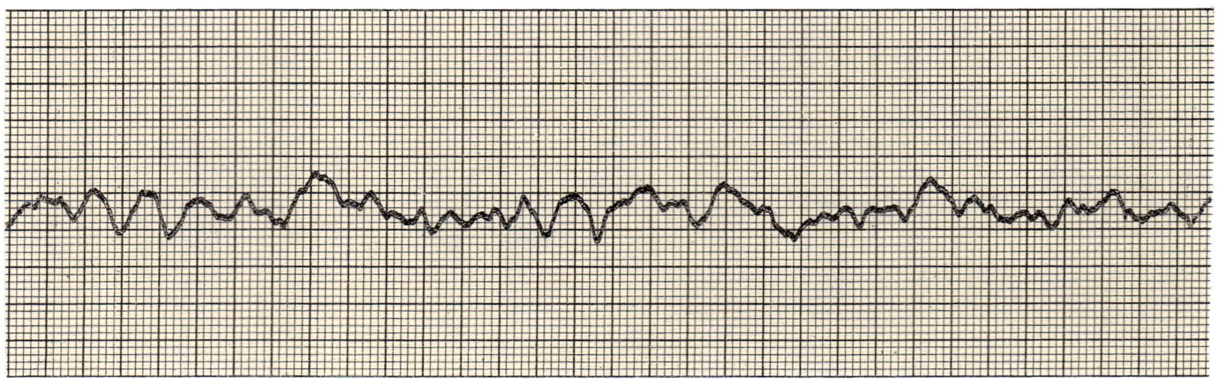

FIGURE 45.5 Ventricular fibrillation. Rhythm: irregular. Rate: not measurable. P–R interval: not measurable. QRS: not measurable, replaced by an irregular wavy baseline. No coordinated electrical or mechanical activity in the ventricle, no cardiac output.

ANTIARRHYTHMIC AGENTS

Antiarrhythmics affect the action potential of the cardiac cells by altering their automaticity, conductivity or both. Because of this effect, antiarrhythmic drugs can also produce new arrhythmias – that is, they are **proarrhythmic**. Antiarrhythmics are used in emergency situations when the haemodynamics arising from the person's arrhythmia are severe and could potentially be fatal. Box 45.2 contains information regarding use of antiarrhythmic agents across the lifespan.

Antiarrhythmics were widely used on a long-term basis to suppress any abnormal arrhythmia, until the publication of the **Cardiac Arrhythmia Suppression Trial** (**CAST**) in the early 1990s. This multicentre, randomised, long-term study conducted by the US National

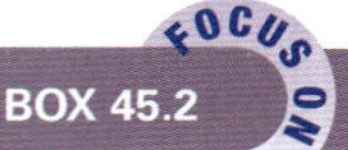

BOX 45.2 **Drug therapy across the lifespan**

Antiarrhythmic agents

CHILDREN

Antiarrhythmic agents are not used as often in children as they are in adults. Children who do require these drugs, after cardiac surgery or because of congenital heart problems, need to be monitored very closely to deal with the related adverse effects that can occur with these drugs.

Digoxin is approved for use in children to treat arrhythmias and has an established recommended dose. If other antiarrhythmics are used, the dose should be carefully calculated using weight and age and should be independently checked by another health care professional before administration.

Adenosine, propranolol and digoxin have been successfully used to treat supraventricular arrhythmias, with propranolol and digoxin being the drugs of choice for long-term management. Verapamil should be avoided in children.

Many arrhythmias in children are now treated by ablation techniques to destroy the arrhythmia-producing cells. This has been very successful in treating Wolff–Parkinson–White and related syndromes in children. If lidocaine (lignocaine) is used for ventricular arrhythmias related to cardiac surgery or digoxin toxicity, serum levels should be monitored regularly to determine the appropriate dose and to avoid the potential for serious proarrhythmias and other adverse effects. The child should receive continuous cardiac monitoring.

ADULTS

Adults receive these drugs most often as emergency measures. Monitoring and careful evaluation of the total drug regimen should be a routine procedure to ensure the most effective treatment with the least chance of adverse effects. Frequent monitoring and medical follow-up is very important for these people.

PREGNANCY AND BREASTFEEDING

The safety for the use of these drugs during pregnancy has not been established. They should not be used in pregnancy unless the benefit to the mother clearly outweighs the potential risk to the fetus. The drugs enter breast milk, and some have been associated with adverse effects on the neonate. Class I, III and IV agents should not be used during breastfeeding; if they are needed, another method of feeding the baby should be used.

OLDER ADULTS

Older adults frequently are prescribed one of these drugs. Older adults are more likely to develop adverse effects associated with the use of these drugs, including arrhythmias, hypotension and congestive heart failure. They are also more likely to have renal and/or hepatic impairment related to underlying medical conditions, which could interfere with the metabolism and excretion of these drugs.

The dose for older adults should be started at a lower level than that recommended for other adults. The person should be monitored very closely and the dose adjusted based on response. If other drugs are added to or removed from the drug regimen, appropriate dose adjustments may need to be made.

Heart, Lung and Blood Institute looked at the mortality rate of people with asymptomatic, non-life-threatening arrhythmias being treated with antiarrhythmics. The results showed that long-term use of some antiarrhythmics was associated with an increased risk of death. In fact, the risk of death for some people was two to three times greater than that for untreated individuals. These results prompted more clinical trials to look at the effectiveness of long-term use of antiarrhythmics.

It was found that antiarrhythmics may block some reflex arrhythmias that help to keep the cardiovascular system in balance, or they may precipitate new, deadly arrhythmias. Therefore, it is important to document the arrhythmia being treated and the rationale for treatment and to monitor a person regularly when using these drugs.

Class I antiarrhythmics

Class I antiarrhythmics (Table 45.1) are drugs that block the sodium channels in the cell membrane during an action potential. These drugs are further broken down into three subclasses, reflecting the manner in which their blockage of sodium channels affects the action potential. These subclasses include the following:

- Class Ia antiarrhythmics: disopyramide (*Rythmodan*)
- Class Ib antiarrhythmics: lidocaine (lignocaine) (*Xylocard* and others)
- Class Ic antiarrhythmics: flecainide (*Flecatab*, *Tambocor*) and propafenone (*Rytmonorm* [not available in Australia])

Therapeutic actions and indications

The class I antiarrhythmics stabilise the cell membrane by binding to sodium channels, depressing phase 0 of the action potential and changing the duration of the action potential (Figure 45.6). *Class Ia drugs* depress phase 0 of the action potential and prolong the duration of the action potential. *Class Ib drugs* depress phase 0 somewhat and actually shorten the duration of the action potential. *Class Ic drugs* markedly depress phase 0, with a resultant extreme slowing of conduction, but have little effect on the duration of the action potential.

These drugs are local anaesthetics or membrane-stabilising agents. They bind more quickly to sodium channels that are open or inactive – ones that have been stimulated and are not yet repolarised. This characteristic makes these drugs preferable in conditions such as tachycardia, in which the sodium gates are open frequently. These drugs are indicated for the treatment of potentially life-threatening ventricular arrhythmias and should not be used to treat other arrhythmias because of the risk of a proarrhythmic effect. See Table 45.1 for usual indications for each class I antiarrhythmic agent.

Pharmacokinetics

These drugs are widely distributed after injection or after rapid absorption through the gastrointestinal (GI) tract. They undergo extensive hepatic metabolism and are excreted in urine. These drugs cross the placenta and are found in breast milk (see Contraindications and cautions).

Disopyramide is available in oral form. Lidocaine (lignocaine) is administered by the IM or IV route, and can also be given as a bolus injection in emergencies when monitoring is not available to document the exact arrhythmia. Flecainide is available in oral form.

Contraindications and cautions

Class I antiarrhythmics are contraindicated in the presence of allergy to any of these drugs; with bradycardia or heart block unless an artificial pacemaker is in place, *because changes in conduction could lead to complete heart block*; with heart failure (HF), hypotension or shock, *which could be exacerbated by effects on the action potential*; and with electrolyte disturbances, *which could alter the effectiveness of these drugs*. Caution should be used in people with renal or hepatic dysfunction, *which could interfere with the biotransformation and excretion of these drugs*.

These drugs cross the placenta, and although no specific adverse effects have been associated with their use, it is suggested that they be used in pregnancy only if the benefits to the mother clearly outweigh the potential risks to the fetus. Class I antiarrhythmics enter breast milk, and *because of the potential for adverse effects on the neonate*, they should not be used during breast-feeding. Another method of feeding the baby should be chosen.

TABLE 45.1 *DRUGS IN FOCUS* Antiarrhythmic agents

Drug name	Dosage/route	Usual indications
Class I antiarrhythmics		
Class Ia		
disopyramide (*Rythmodan*)	Adult: 300–800 mg/day PO in 3 divided doses	Treatment of life-threatening ventricular arrhythmias

Continued on following page

TABLE 45.1 DRUGS IN FOCUS Antiarrhythmic agents *(continued)*

Drug name	Dosage/route	Usual indications
Class I antiarrhythmics *(continued)*		
Class Ib		
(P) lidocaine (lignocaine) (*Xylocard*)	Adult: preinfusion, 1 mg/kg to a maximum of 100 mg slowly IV over 1–2 min; after 15 minutes either repeated or followed by IV infusion, 20–50 micrograms/kg/min to a total of 50–100 mg under ECG monitoring. Repeat after 5 minutes to a maximum of 200–300 mg within 1 hour	Treatment of life-threatening ventricular arrhythmias during myocardial infarction or cardiac surgery; also used as bolus injection in emergencies when monitoring is not available to document exact arrhythmia
Class Ic		
flecainide (*Flecatab, Tambocor*)	50–100 mg PO q 12 hours. Maximum dose: supraventricular arrhythmias, 300 mg/day; ventricular arrhythmias, 400 mg/day Reduce dose as needed with older people or people with renal impairment to a maximum of 100 mg/day	Treatment of life-threatening ventricular arrhythmias in adults; prevention of paroxysmal atrial tachycardia (PAT) in symptomatic people with no structural heart defect
propafenone (*Rytmonorm*)	Adult: 150 mg tid or 300 mg bd PO based on the individual's response; start with lower dose and increase slowly with older people. Maximum 900 mg/day	Treatment of life-threatening ventricular arrhythmias in adults; prevention of PAT in symptomatic people with no structural heart defect
Class II antiarrhythmics		
esmolol (*Brevibloc*)	Adult: 50–200 micrograms/kg/min IV infusion as per protocol	Short-term management of supraventricular tachycardia in adults and tachycardia that is not responding to other measures
(P) propranolol (*Inderal, Deralin*)	Arrhythmia: 10–40 mg tid–qid	Treatment of supraventricular tachycardias caused by digoxin or catecholamines in adults; also used as an antihypertensive, antianginal and antimigraine headache drug
Class III antiarrhythmics		
(P) amiodarone (*Aratac, Cordarone X, Cardinorm*)	Oral, initiation: 200 mg tds for 1 week, then 200 mg twice daily. Oral, maintenance: usually 200 mg daily IV infusion: 5 mg/kg in 20 min to 2 hours; may repeat to a maximum of 1200 mg/24 hours (15 mg/kg/day)	Treatment of adults with life-threatening ventricular arrhythmias not responding to any other drug; preferred antiarrhythmic in Advanced Cardiac Life Support protocol
sotalol (*Cardol, Sotacor*)	80 mg/day PO in 2 divided doses; may be titrated to 160–320 mg/day PO; maximum 640 mg/day. Reduce dose in people with renal impairment	Treatment of adults with life-threatening ventricular arrhythmias not responding to any other drug
Class IV antiarrhythmics		
(P) diltiazem (*Cardizem CD, Dilzem*)	Adult, oral, immediate release: 60 mg tid; maximum 360 mg daily in 3–4 divided doses Adult, oral, modified release: 120–180 mg daily, maximum 360 mg daily. Swallow whole, do not crush or chew	IV to treat paroxysmal supraventricular tachycardia in adults
verapamil (*Anpec, Cordilox SR, Isoptin, Isoptin SR*)	Adult, oral, immediate release: 80 mg bd–tid, up to 160 mg bd–tid Adult, oral, sustained release: 180–240 mg in the morning to a maximum of 480 mg/day in 2 divided doses. Paediatric: 0.1–0.3 mg/kg (maximum 5 mg) IV over 2–3 minutes with ECG and blood pressure monitoring; may repeat in 30 minutes if needed	IV to treat paroxysmal supraventricular tachycardia; temporarily controls the ventricular response to rapid atrial rates

TABLE 45.1 DRUGS IN FOCUS Antiarrhythmic agents (continued)

Drug name	Dosage/route	Usual indications
Other antiarrhythmics		
adenosine (*Adenocor*)	Adults: initially 3 mg of 6 mg/2 mL solution; if necessary administer 6 mg after 1–2 minutes; if necessary administer 12 mg after a further 1–2 minutes *Note*: adenosine (*Adenoscan*) 30 mg/10 mL is for coronary vasodilation	Treatment of supraventricular tachycardias, including those caused by the use of alternative conduction pathways in adults
digoxin (*Lanoxin*)	Adult, oral loading: 0.75–1.5 mg over 24 hours in divided doses; maintenance (according to renal function, clinical response and therapeutic drug monitoring), 62.5–250 micrograms once daily Paediatric: complex dosing, refer to prescriber information	Treatment of atrial flutter, atrial fibrillation, paroxysmal atrial tachycardia

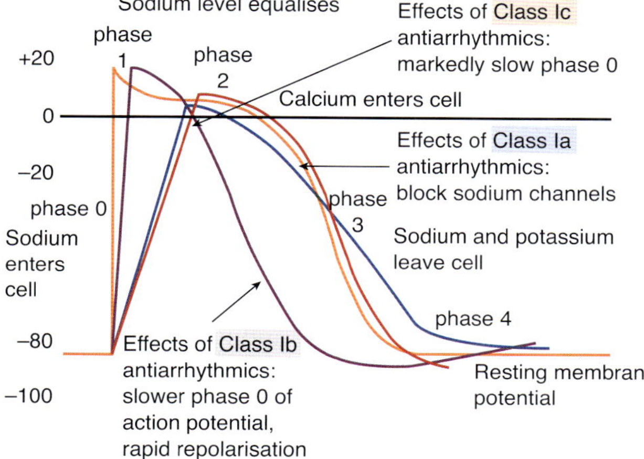

FIGURE 45.6 The cardiac action potentials, showing the effects of class Ia, Ib and Ic antiarrhythmics.

Adverse effects

The adverse effects of the class I antiarrhythmics are associated with their membrane-stabilising effects and effects on action potentials. Central nervous system (CNS) effects can include dizziness, drowsiness, fatigue, twitching, mouth numbness, slurred speech, vision changes and tremors that can progress to convulsions. GI symptoms include changes in taste, nausea and vomiting. Cardiovascular effects include the proarrhythmic effects that lead to the development of arrhythmias (including heart blocks), hypotension, vasodilation and the potential for cardiac arrest. Respiratory depression progressing to respiratory arrest can also occur. Other adverse effects include rash, hypersensitivity reactions, loss of hair and potential bone marrow depression.

Flecainide is a class Ic drug that was found to increase the risk of death in the CAST study.

Clinically important drug–drug interactions

Several drug–drug interactions have been reported with these agents, so the possibility of an interaction should always be considered before any drug is added to a regimen containing an antiarrhythmic. Amiodarone has a high potential for drug–drug interactions. The half-life of amiodarone is long and with chronic oral dosing can be 14–110 days but is usually in the range 14–59 days. Amiodarone may interact with a wide range of other medicines for a couple of months after therapy is complete, including medications that prolong the QT interval, antiarrhythmics, agents that cause hypokalaemia, beta blockers, calcium channel blockers, cardiac glycosides, HMG-CoA reductase inhibitors (statins), phenytoin, theophylline, thyroid hormones and warfarin.

The risk of bleeding effects of these drugs increases if they are combined with oral anticoagulants; people receiving this combination should be monitored closely and have their anticoagulant dose reduced as needed. Check individual drug monographs for specific interactions associated with each drug.

Prototype summary: lidocaine (lignocaine)

Indications: management of acute ventricular arrhythmias during cardiac surgery or MI.

Actions: decreases depolarisation, decreasing automaticity of the ventricular cells; increases ventricular fibrillation threshold.

Pharmacokinetics:

Route	Onset	Peak	Duration
IM	5–10 min	5–15 min	2 hours
IV	Immediate	Immediate	10–20 min

$T_{1/2}$: 10 minutes, then 1.5–3 hours; metabolised in the liver and excreted in urine.

Adverse effects: dizziness, light-headedness, fatigue, arrhythmias, cardiac arrest, nausea, vomiting, anaphylactoid reactions, hypotension, vasodilation.

KEY POINTS

- Antiarrhythmics are drugs that alter the action potential of the heart cells and interrupt arrhythmias. The CAST study found that the long-term treatment of arrhythmias may actually cause cardiac death, so these drugs are now indicated only for the short-term treatment of potentially life-threatening ventricular arrhythmias.
- Class I antiarrhythmics block sodium channels, depress phase 0 of the action potential and generally prolong the action potential, leading to a slowing of conduction and automaticity.
- Class I antiarrhythmics are membrane stabilisers; the adverse effects seen are related to the stabilisation of cell membranes, including those in the CNS and the GI tract.

Class II antiarrhythmics

The class II antiarrhythmics are beta-adrenergic blockers that block beta receptors, causing a depression of phase 4 of the action potential (Figure 45.7). Several beta-adrenergic blockers, such as esmolol (*Brevibloc*) and propranolol (*Deralin*, *Inderal*), are used as antiarrhythmics.

Therapeutic actions and indications

The class II antiarrhythmics competitively block beta-receptor sites in the heart and kidneys. The result is a decrease in heart rate, cardiac excitability and cardiac output, a slowing of conduction through the AV node and a decrease in the release of renin. These effects stabilise excitable cardiac tissue and decrease blood pressure, which decreases the heart's workload and may further stabilise hypoxic cardiac tissue. These drugs are indicated for the treatment of supraventricular tachycardias and PVCs. See Table 45.1 for usual indications for each drug.

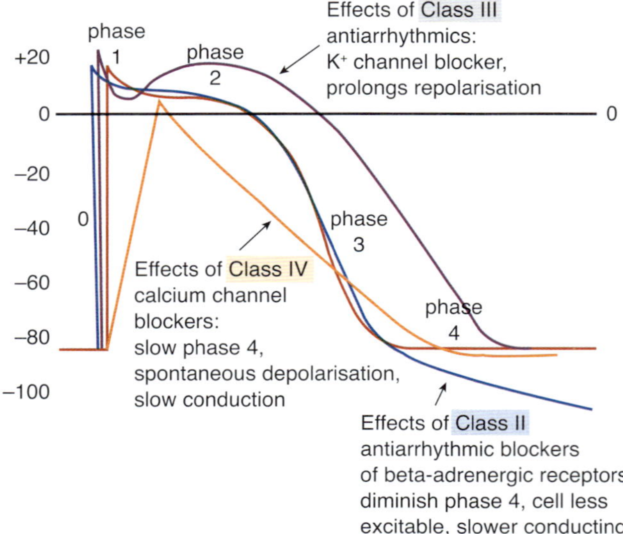

FIGURE 45.7 The cardiac action potentials, showing the effects of class II, III and IV antiarrhythmics.

Pharmacokinetics

Esmolol is administered intravenously (IV). Propranolol may be administered orally or IV. These drugs are absorbed from the GI tract or have an immediate effect when given IV and undergo hepatic metabolism. They are excreted in the urine. Food has been found to increase the bioavailability of propranolol, although this effect has not been found with other beta-adrenergic-blocking agents.

Contraindications and cautions

The use of these drugs is contraindicated in the presence of sinus bradycardia (rate less than 45 beats/minute) and AV block, *which could be exacerbated by the effects of these drugs*; with cardiogenic shock, HF, asthma or respiratory depression, *which could worsen due to blockage of beta receptors*; and with pregnancy and breastfeeding *because of the potential for adverse effects on the fetus or neonate.*

Caution should be used in people with diabetes and thyroid dysfunction, *which could be altered by the blockade of the beta receptors*, and in people with renal and hepatic dysfunction, *which could alter the metabolism and excretion of these drugs.*

Adverse effects

The adverse effects associated with class II antiarrhythmics are related to the effects of blocking beta receptors in the sympathetic nervous system. CNS effects include dizziness, insomnia, nightmares and fatigue. Cardiovascular symptoms can include hypotension, bradycardia, AV block, arrhythmias and alterations in peripheral perfusion. Respiratory effects can include bronchospasm and dyspnoea. GI problems frequently include nausea, vomiting, anorexia, constipation and diarrhoea. Other effects to anticipate include a loss of libido, decreased exercise tolerance and alterations in blood glucose levels.

Clinically important drug–drug interactions

The risk of adverse effects increases if these drugs are taken with verapamil; if this combination is used, dose adjustment will be needed.

There is a possibility of increased hypoglycaemia if these drugs are combined with insulin; individuals should be monitored closely.

Other specific drug interactions may occur with each drug; check a drug reference before combining these drugs with any others.

 **Prototype summary: propranolol**

Indications: treatment of cardiac arrhythmias, especially supraventricular tachycardia; treatment of ventricular tachycardia induced by digitalis or catecholamines.

Actions: competitively blocks beta-adrenergic receptors in the heart and kidney, has a membrane-stabilising effect, and decreases the influence of the sympathetic nervous system.

Pharmacokinetics:

Route	Onset	Peak	Duration
Oral	20–30 min	60–90 min	6–12 hours
IV	Immediate	1 min	4–6 hours

$T_{1/2}$: 3–5 hours; metabolised in the liver and excreted in urine.

Adverse effects: bradycardia, HF, cardiac arrhythmias, heart blocks, cerebrovascular accident (CVA), pulmonary oedema, gastric pain, flatulence, nausea, vomiting, diarrhoea, impotence, decreased exercise tolerance, antinuclear antibody (ANA) development.

KEY POINTS

- Class II antiarrhythmics are beta-adrenergic-receptor blockers that prevent sympathetic stimulation.
- Adverse effects related to class II antiarrhythmics are associated with blocking of the sympathetic response.

Class III antiarrhythmics

The class III antiarrhythmics include amiodarone (*Aratac*, *Cordarone X*) and sotalol (*Cardol*, *Sotacor*).

Therapeutic actions and indications

The class III antiarrhythmics block potassium channels and slow the outward movement of potassium during phase 3 of the action potential, prolonging it (Figure 45.7). All of these drugs are proarrhythmic and have the potential of inducing arrhythmias. Although amiodarone has been associated with such serious and even fatal toxic reactions, in 2005 the American Heart Association issued new guidelines for Advanced Cardiac Life Support (ACLS) that named amiodarone the drug of choice for treating ventricular fibrillation or pulseless ventricular tachycardia in cardiac arrest situations. See Table 45.1 for usual indications for each drug.

Pharmacokinetics

Amiodarone is available in an oral or IV form. Sotalol is administered only in oral form. These drugs are well absorbed after oral administration. Absorption of sotalol is decreased by the presence of food. This drug is metabolised in the liver and excreted in urine.

Contraindications and cautions

When these drugs are used to treat life-threatening arrhythmias for which no other drug has been effective, there are no contraindications. *Because sotalol is known to be proarrhythmic*, individuals should be monitored very closely at the initiation of therapy and periodically during therapy. Caution should be used with all of these drugs in the presence of shock, hypotension or respiratory depression; with a prolonged QTc interval, *which could worsen due to the depressive effects on action potentials*; and with renal or hepatic disease, *which could alter the biotransformation and excretion of these drugs*.

Adverse effects

The adverse effects associated with these drugs are related to the changes they cause in action potentials. Nausea, vomiting and GI distress; weakness and dizziness; and hypotension, HF and arrhythmia are common. Amiodarone has been associated with a potentially fatal liver toxicity, ocular abnormalities and the development of very serious cardiac arrhythmias.

Clinically important drug–drug interactions

These drugs can cause serious toxic effects if they are combined with digoxin. There is an increased risk of proarrhythmias if they are combined with antihistamines, phenothiazines or tricyclic antidepressants.

 **Prototype summary: amiodarone**

Indications: treatment of life-threatening ventricular arrhythmias.

Actions: acts directly on heart muscle cells to prolong repolarisation and the refractory period, increasing the threshold for ventricular fibrillation; also acts on peripheral smooth muscle to decrease peripheral resistance.

Pharmacokinetics:

Route	Onset	Peak	Duration
Oral	2–3 days	3–7 hours	6–8 hours
IV	Immediate	20 min	Infusion

$T_{1/2}$: 10 days; metabolised in the liver and excreted in urine.

Adverse effects: malaise, fatigue, dizziness, HF, cardiac arrhythmias, cardiac arrest, constipation, nausea, vomiting, hepatotoxicity, pulmonary toxicity, corneal microdeposits and vision changes.

Sotalol may have a loss of effectiveness if it is combined with non-steroidal anti-inflammatory drugs, aspirin or antacids. Other specific drug–drug interactions have been reported with individual drugs; a drug reference should always be consulted when adding a new drug to a regimen containing any of these agents.

KEY POINTS

- Class III antiarrhythmics block potassium channels and prolong phase 3 of the action potential.
- Amiodarone is the drug recommended for use during life support measures. It is associated with serious to potentially fatal hepatotoxicity.

Class IV antiarrhythmics

Class IV antiarrhythmics include two calcium channel blockers: diltiazem (*Cardizem*) and verapamil (*Anpec, Cordilox SR, Isoptin*).

Therapeutic actions and indications

The class IV antiarrhythmics block the movement of calcium ions across the cell membrane, depressing the generation of action potentials and delaying phases 1 and 2 of repolarisation, which slows automaticity and conduction (see Figure 45.7). Both diltiazem and verapamil are used as antihypertensives (see Chapter 43) and to treat angina (see Chapter 46). Table 45.1 describes usual indications for each drug.

Pharmacokinetics

Diltiazem is administered IV. When used as an antiarrhythmic, verapamil is used IV. These drugs are well absorbed after IV administration. They are highly protein bound, metabolised in the liver and excreted in the urine. They cross the placenta and enter breast milk.

Contraindications and cautions

These drugs are contraindicated with known allergy to any calcium channel blocker *to avoid hypersensitivity reactions*; with sick sinus syndrome or heart block (unless an artificial pacemaker is in place) *because the block could be exacerbated by these drugs*; with pregnancy or breastfeeding *because of the potential for adverse effects on the fetus or neonate*; and with HF or hypotension *because of the hypotensive effects of these drugs*. Caution should be used in cases of idiopathic hypertrophic subaortic stenosis (IHSS), *which could be exacerbated*, or impaired renal or liver function, *which could affect the metabolism or excretion of these drugs*.

Adverse effects

The adverse effects associated with these drugs are related to their vasodilation of blood vessels throughout the body. CNS effects include dizziness, weakness, fatigue, depression and headache. GI upset, nausea and vomiting can occur. Hypotension, HF, shock, arrhythmias and oedema have also been reported.

Prototype summary: diltiazem

Indications: treatment of paroxysmal supraventricular tachycardia, atrial fibrillation and atrial flutter.

Actions: blocks the movement of calcium ions across the cell membrane, depressing the generation of action potentials, delaying phases 1 and 2 of repolarisation, and slowing conduction through the AV node.

Pharmacokinetics:

Route	Onset	Peak	Duration
Oral	30–60 min	2–3 hours	6–8 hours
IV	Immediate	2–3 min	unknown

$T_{1/2}$: 3.5–6 hours; metabolised in the liver and excreted in urine.

Adverse effects: dizziness, light-headedness, headache, asthenia, peripheral oedema, bradycardia, AV block, flushing, nausea, hepatic injury.

Clinically important drug–drug interactions

Verapamil has been associated with many drug–drug interactions, including increased risk of cardiac depression with beta blockers; additive AV slowing with digoxin; increased serum levels and toxicity of digoxin, carbamazepine and prazosin; increased respiratory depression with atracurium, pancuronium and vecuronium; and decreased effects if combined with calcium products or rifampicin.

There is a risk of severe cardiac effects if these drugs are given IV within 48 hours of IV beta-adrenergic drugs. The combination should be avoided.

Diltiazem can increase the serum levels and toxicity of ciclosporin if the drugs are taken concurrently.

KEY POINTS

- Class IV antiarrhythmics are calcium channel blockers that shorten the action potential, disrupting ineffective rhythms and rates.
- Whichever type of antiarrhythmic is used, the person receiving an antiarrhythmic drug needs

TABLE 45.2 Types of arrhythmias and drugs of choice for treatment

Arrhythmia	Antiarrhythmic drugs
Atrial	
Flutter or fibrillation	Class Ic: flecainide Class III: amiodarone, sotalol Class IV: diltiazem Other: adenosine Other: digoxin
Paroxysmal atrial tachycardia (PAT)	Other: digoxin
Supraventricular tachycardia (SVT)	Class Ic: flecainide, propafenone* Class II: esmolol* (short-term), propranolol Class IV: diltiazem, verapamil (IV) Other: adenosine* (SVT, including those caused by using alternative conduction pathways)
Ventricular	
Premature ventricular contractions (PVCs)	Class Ib: lidocaine (lignocaine)*
Tachycardia or fibrillation	Class Ib: lidocaine (lignocaine)
Life-threatening ventricular arrhythmias	Class Ia: disopyramide Class Ic: flecainide (X), propafenone Class III: amiodarone*, sotalol (X)

*Drug of choice; (X) not drug of choice; proarrhythmic.

to be constantly monitored while being stabilised and throughout the course of therapy to detect the development of arrhythmias or other adverse effects associated with alteration of the action potentials of other muscles or nerves.

OTHER ANTIARRHYTHMICS

Drugs other than those classified as class I, II, III or IV may be used to treat arrhythmias. Table 45.2 provides a summary of types of arrhythmias and the specific drugs used to treat each type. Additional antiarrhythmics include adenosine (*Adenocor*, *Adenoscan*) and digoxin (*Lanoxin*). For dosages and usual indications see also Table 45.1.

Adenosine is another antiarrhythmic agent that is used to convert supraventricular tachycardia to sinus rhythm if vagal manoeuvres have been ineffective. It is often the drug of choice for terminating supraventricular tachycardias, including those associated with the use of alternative conduction pathways around the AV node (eg, Wolff–Parkinson–White syndrome), for two reasons: (1) it has a very short duration of action (about 15 seconds), after which it is picked up by circulating red blood cells and cleared through the liver; and (2) it is associated with very few adverse effects (headache, flushing and dyspnoea of short duration). This drug slows conduction through the AV node, prolongs the refractory period and decreases automaticity in the AV node. It is given IV with continuous monitoring of the person.

Digoxin (see Chapter 44) is also used at times to treat arrhythmias. This drug slows calcium from leaving the cell, prolonging the action potential and slowing conduction and heart rate. Digoxin is effective in the treatment of atrial arrhythmias. The drug exerts a positive inotropic effect, leading to increased cardiac output, which increases perfusion of the coronary arteries and may eliminate the cause of some arrhythmias as hypoxia is resolved and waste products are removed more effectively.

Care considerations for people receiving antiarrhythmic agents

Assessment: history and examination

- Assess for contraindications or cautions: any known allergies to these drugs *to avoid hypersensitivity reactions*; impaired liver or kidney function, *which could alter the metabolism and excretion of the drug*; any condition that could be exacerbated by the depressive effects of the drugs (eg, heart block, HF, hypotension, shock, respiratory dysfunction, electrolyte disturbances) *to avoid exacerbation of these conditions*; and current status of pregnancy and breastfeeding *to prevent potential adverse effects on the fetus or baby.*
- Perform a physical assessment *to establish a baseline before beginning therapy and during therapy to determine the effectiveness of therapy and evaluate for any potential adverse effects.*
- Assess the person's neurological status, including level of alertness, speech and vision and reflexes, *to identify possible CNS effects.*
- Assess cardiac status closely, including pulse, blood pressure, heart rate and rhythm, *to identify changes requiring a change in the dosage of the drug or the presence of adverse effects*; auscultate heart sounds, noting any evidence of abnormal sounds, *for early detection of heart failure*; and

anticipate cardiac monitoring *to evaluate heart rate and rhythm and aid in identifying arrhythmia.*

- Monitor respiratory rate and depth, and auscultate lungs, for evidence of adventitious sounds *to identify respiratory depression and detect changes associated with heart failure.*
- Inspect abdomen *for evidence of distension*; auscultate bowel sounds *to evaluate GI motility.*
- Evaluate skin for colour, lesions and temperature *to detect adverse reactions and to assess cardiac output.*
- Obtain a baseline ECG *to evaluate heart rate and rhythm*; monitor the results of laboratory tests, including full blood count, *to identify possible bone marrow suppression*, and renal and liver function tests, *to determine the need for possible changes in dose and identify toxic effects.*

Implementation with rationale

- Titrate the dose to the smallest amount needed to achieve control of the arrhythmia *to decrease the risk of severe adverse effects.*
- Continually monitor cardiac rhythm when initiating or changing dose *to detect potentially serious adverse effects and to evaluate drug effectiveness.*
- Ensure that emergency life support equipment is readily available *to treat severe adverse reactions that might occur.*
- Administer parenteral forms as ordered only if the oral form is not feasible; expect to switch to the oral form as soon as possible *to decrease the potential for severe adverse effects.*
- Consult with the prescriber to reduce the dose in people with renal or hepatic dysfunction; reduced dose may be needed *to ensure therapeutic effects without increased risk of toxic effects.*
- Establish safety precautions, including side rails, lighting and noise control, if CNS effects occur *to ensure the person's safety.*
- Arrange for periodic monitoring of cardiac rhythm when the person is receiving long-term therapy *to evaluate effects on cardiac status.*
- Provide comfort measures *to help the person tolerate drug effects.* These include small, frequent meals to minimise nausea and vomiting; access to bathroom facilities; bowel program as needed *to deal with nausea, vomiting and constipation*; administration of food with drug if GI upset is severe *to alleviate the discomfort*; environmental controls, such as temperature regulation, light control and decreased noise, *to alleviate overstimulation if CNS effects occur*; and reorientation as needed.
- Offer support and encouragement *to help the person to deal with the diagnosis and the drug regimen.*
- Provide thorough teaching, including the name of the drug, dosage prescribed, measures to avoid adverse effects, warning signs of problems and the need for periodic monitoring and evaluation, *to enhance knowledge about drug therapy and to promote compliance.*

Evaluation

- Monitor response to the drug (stabilisation of cardiac rhythm and output).
- Monitor for adverse effects (sedation, hypotension, cardiac arrhythmias, respiratory depression, CNS effects).
- Evaluate the effectiveness of the teaching plan (person can name drug, dosage, adverse effects to watch for, specific measures to avoid them and the importance of continued follow-up).
- Monitor the effectiveness of comfort measures and compliance with the regimen.

See the Critical thinking scenario for information on managing the person on chronic antiarrhythmic therapy.

CRITICAL THINKING SCENARIO

Managing people on chronic antiarrhythmic therapy

THE SITUATION

R.A., a 63-year-old man, developed atrial fibrillation 2 years ago, with a rapid drop in blood pressure and a rapid pulse of 160 beats/minute, irregularly irregular. He was cardioverted within a few hours of onset to normal sinus rhythm with a heart rate of 74 beats/minute. He was started on digoxin (*Lanoxin*) and remained stable for more than a year. It was decided to stop the drug and monitor R.A. He did well, but on a long-awaited trip to Italy, he again developed atrial fibrillation, with rapid pulse and drop in blood pressure. He was treated at an Italian clinic with cardioversion and seen by his cardiologist on his return to Australia. He was again placed on digoxin to maintain his conversion to sinus rhythm. He called the clinic with complaints of palpitations and a severe headache and was told to immediately come in to be evaluated. He was found to be in sinus rhythm with PVCs. He stated that he felt that the headache was related to gastroenteritis and a urinary tract infection (UTI) he had been fighting. He has been taking levofloxacin that was prescribed for his wife, as she had some left-over tablets from her previous course.

CRITICAL THINKING

Based on your knowledge of the drug digoxin and the symptoms reported by R.A, what do you think happened?
What actions should be taken at this time to make sure that R.A.'s heart rhythm remains stable?
What teaching points will be essential to convey to R.A. before he goes home?
What other screening should be done at this time to prevent problems in the future?

DISCUSSION

R.A. has the signs and symptoms of increased digoxin levels – headache and ventricular arrhythmias. Initially, R.A. should be placed on a cardiac monitor and supported to ensure that the ventricular arrhythmias do not progress. His digoxin should be stopped until the situation is stabilised. Emergency life support equipment should be readily available in case the situation deteriorates.

R.A. stabilised rapidly and was given IV fluids to dilute the drug effects and encourage excretion. His PVCs became less and less frequent, and he remained in normal sinus rhythm. R.A. should be questioned about how and when he takes his drug and any other drugs he might be taking. Levofloxacin is a quinolone antibiotic. Potential adverse effects include prolongation of the QT interval, ventricular arrhythmia and *torsades des pointes*. R.A. should be reminded about checking with the doctor or a pharmacist about taking any medication, including over-the-counter medications, not sharing medications with others and properly disposing of unused medications. It is a good idea to keep a complete list of drugs being taken – including over-the-counter drugs and herbal remedies – so the health care provider can check and make sure that there is no potential reaction to be concerned about. He should also be reminded about the importance of regular medical follow-up, which will include an electrocardiogram and blood tests, to evaluate the effects of the drug on his body.

While R.A. is within the health care system, it would be a good idea to do a full electrocardiogram and to get blood tests to measure his creatinine levels, as well as serum electrolytes, which have an effect on cardiac conduction.

CARE GUIDE FOR R.A.: DIGOXIN (ANTIARRHYTHMIC AGENTS)

Assessment: history and examination

Assess the person's health history for allergies to digoxin; for any heart block or prolonged QT intervals; history of atrial fibrillation, including onset of last episode; and drug history for use of drugs that could prolong the QT interval, other antiarrhythmics or tricyclic antidepressants.
Focus the physical examination on the following areas:
Cardiovascular: blood pressure, pulse, heart rhythm, perfusion
Neurological (CNS): orientation, affect, reflexes
Respiratory system: respiratory rate and character, adventitious sounds
Laboratory tests: renal function tests, serum electrolytes, electrocardiogram (hypokalaemia, hypomagnesaemia and hypercalcaemia increase the risk of digoxin toxicity.)

Implementation

Continually monitor cardiac rhythm when initiating or changing dose.
Ensure that emergency life support equipment is readily available.
Establish safety precautions, including side rails, lighting and noise control, if CNS effects occur
Arrange for periodic monitoring of cardiac rhythm when the person is receiving long-term therapy.
Provide comfort measures, including small, frequent meals to minimise nausea and vomiting; access to bathroom facilities; and environmental controls, such as temperature regulation, light control and decreased noise.
Offer support and encouragement to help the person deal with the diagnosis and the drug regimen.
Provide teaching regarding drug name, dosage, schedule of administration, measures to reduce adverse effects, other drugs to avoid, what to report, and the need for regular, periodic monitoring.

Evaluation

Monitor response to the drug (stabilisation of cardiac rhythm and output).
Monitor for adverse effects (sedation, hypotension, cardiac arrhythmias, respiratory depression, CNS effects).
Monitor for drug–drug interactions.
Evaluate the effectiveness of the teaching plan (person can name drug, dosage, adverse effects to watch for, specific measures to avoid them, and the importance of continued follow-up).
Monitor the effectiveness of comfort measures and compliance with the regimen.

TEACHING FOR R.A.

- An antiarrhythmic drug, such as digoxin, acts to stop the irregular rhythm in your heart, helping it to beat more regularly and therefore more efficiently.
- When taking digoxin, you should remember to take it once a day. If you miss a dose, do not make up the dose, just return to your regular schedule. Never take more than one dose a day.
- Do not take any other medications without checking with your doctor or a pharmacist, as some medications can increase the adverse effects, which can be quite serious. There are other drugs that should be avoided; make sure you give your health care provider a complete list of the drugs that you are taking, including over-the-counter drugs and herbal remedies, so thesafety of any combinations can be checked.
- Some adverse effects that might occur include the following:

- *Headache*: medication may be available to help if this is a problem.
- *Dizziness, light-headedness*: avoid driving a car or operating dangerous machinery until you know how this drug will affect you.
- *Nausea, diarrhoea, flatulence*: small, frequent meals may help to alleviate these problems.
- Report any of the following to your health care provider: *chest pain, difficulty breathing, palpitations, numbness or tingling*.
- Tell any doctor, nurse or other health provider involved in your care that you are taking this drug.
- Keep this drug, and all medications, out of the reach of children.
- Schedule regular medical appointments while you are on this drug to evaluate your heart rhythm and your response to the drug and to monitor your blood levels of important electrolytes that affect heart function.
- Do not stop taking this medication. If you have to stop the medication, contact your health care provider immediately.

CHAPTER SUMMARY

- Disruptions in the normal rate or rhythm of the heart are called arrhythmias (also known as dysrhythmias).
- Electrolyte disturbances, decreases in the oxygen delivered to the cells leading to hypoxia or anoxia, structural damage that changes the conduction pathway, acidosis or the accumulation of waste products or drug effects can lead to disruptions in the automaticity of the cells or in the conduction of the impulse that result in arrhythmias. The result can be changes in heart rate (tachycardias or bradycardias); stimulation from ectopic foci in the atria or ventricles that cause an uncoordinated muscle contraction; or blocks in the conduction system (eg, AV heart block, bundle-branch blocks) that alter the normal movement of the impulse through the system.
- Arrhythmias cause problems because they alter the haemodynamics of the cardiovascular system. They can cause a decrease in cardiac output related to the uncoordinated pumping action of the irregular rhythm, leading to lack of filling time for the ventricles. Any of these effects can interfere with the delivery of blood to the brain, to other tissues or to the heart muscle.
- Antiarrhythmics are drugs that alter the action potential of the heart cells and interrupt arrhythmias. The CAST study found that the long-term treatment of arrhythmias may actually cause cardiac death, so these drugs are now indicated only for the short-term treatment of potentially life-threatening ventricular arrhythmias.
- Class I antiarrhythmics block sodium channels, depress phase 0 of the action potential and generally prolong the action potential, leading to a slowing of conduction and automaticity.
- Class II antiarrhythmics are beta-adrenergic-receptor blockers that prevent sympathetic stimulation.
- Class III antiarrhythmics block potassium channels and prolong phase 3 of the action potential.
- Class IV antiarrhythmics are calcium channel blockers that shorten the action potential, disrupting ineffective rhythms and rates.
- A person receiving an antiarrhythmic drug needs to be constantly monitored while being stabilised and throughout the course of therapy to detect the development of arrhythmias or other adverse effects associated with alteration of the action potentials of other muscles or nerves.

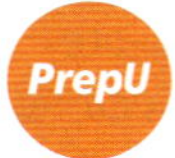

Knowing your strengths and weaknesses helps you to study more effectively. Take a PrepU Practice Quiz to find out how you measure up!

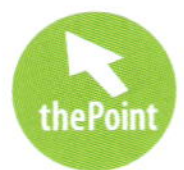

ONLINE RESOURCES

An extensive range of additional resources to enhance teaching and learning and to facilitate understanding of this chapter may be found online at the text's accompanying website, located on thePoint at http://thepoint.lww.com. These include Watch and Learn videos, Concepts in Action animations, journal articles, review questions, case studies, discussion topics and quizzes.

BIBLIOGRAPHY

Braunwald, E. & Bonow, R. O., MD Consult LLC (2012). *Braunwald's Heart Disease: A Textbook of Cardiovascular Medicine* (9th edn). Philadelphia: Elsevier Saunders.

Epstein, A. E., Hallstrom, A. P., Rogers, W. J., Liebson, P. R., Seals, A. A., Anderson, J. L., et al. (1993). Mortality following ventricular arrhythmia suppression by encainide, flecainide, and moricizine after myocardial infarction. The original design concept of the Cardiac Arrhythmia Suppression Trial (CAST). *JAMA, 270*, 2451–2455.

Farrell, M. & Dempsey, J. (2014). *Smeltzer & Bare's Textbook of Medical-Surgical Nursing* (3rd edn). Sydney: Lippincott Williams & Wilkins.

Goodman, L. S., Brunton, L. L., Chabner, B. & Knollmann, B. C. (2011). *Goodman and Gilman's Pharmacological Basis of Therapeutics* (12th edn). New York: McGraw-Hill.

Greener, M. (2010). The nurse's role in the management of atrial fibrillation. *Nurse Prescribing, 8(11)*, 532, 534–537.

Hurst, J. W., Fuster, V., Walsh, R. A. & Harrington, R. A. (Eds.). (2011). *Hurst's the Heart* (13th edn). New York: McGraw-Hill.

McKenna, L. & Mirkov, S. (2019). *McKenna's Drug Handbook for Nursing and Midwifery* (8th edn). Sydney: Wolters Kluwer Health Australia.

Mosher, M. C. (2011). Amiodarone-induced hypothyroidism and other adverse effects. *Dimensions of Critical Care Nursing, 30(2)*, 87–93.
Naganathan, V. (2013). Cardiovascular drugs in older people. *Australian Prescriber, 36(6)*, 190–194.
O'Donovan, K. (2012). Amiodarone and its role in arrhythmia. *Nurse Prescribing, 10(5)*, 241–246.
Porth, C. M. (2011). *Essentials of Pathophysiology: Concepts of Altered Health States* (3rd edn). Philadelphia: Lippincott Williams & Wilkins.
Porth, C. M. (2009). *Pathophysiology: Concepts of Altered Health States* (8th edn). Philadelphia: Lippincott Williams & Wilkins.
Samardhi, H., Santos, M., Denman, R., Walters, D. L. & Bett, N. (2011). Current management of atrial fibrillation. *Australian Prescriber, 34(4)*, 100–104.
Swift, J. (2013). Assessment and treatment of patients with acute tachyarrhythmia. *Nursing Standard, 28(5)*, 50–59.

CHECK YOUR UNDERSTANDING

Answers to the questions in this chapter can be found in Appendix A at the back of this book.

MULTIPLE CHOICE

Select the best response to the following.

1. Cardiac contraction and relaxation are controlled by:
   a. a specific area in the brain.
   b. the sympathetic nervous system.
   c. the autonomic nervous system.
   d. spontaneous impulses arising within the heart.
2. Antiarrhythmic drugs alter the action potential of the cardiac cells. Because they alter the action potential, antiarrhythmic drugs often:
   a. cause heart failure.
   b. alter blood flow to the kidney.
   c. cause new arrhythmias.
   d. cause electrolyte disturbances.
3. Because of the results of the CAST study:
   a. antiarrhythmics are now more widely used.
   b. antiarrhythmics are used as prophylactic measures in situations that might lead to an arrhythmia.
   c. antiarrhythmics are no longer used in Australia.
   d. antiarrhythmics are reserved for use in cases of life-threatening arrhythmias.
4. The drug of choice for the treatment of a supraventricular tachycardia associated with Wolff–Parkinson–White syndrome is:
   a. digoxin.
   b. verapamil.
   c. lidocaine (lignocaine).
   d. adenosine.
5. A person who is receiving an antiarrhythmic drug needs:
   a. constant cardiac monitoring until stabilised.
   b. frequent blood tests, including drug levels.
   c. an antidepressant to deal with the psychological depression.
   d. dietary changes to prevent irritation of the heart muscle.
6. A person is brought into the emergency department with a potentially life-threatening ventricular arrhythmia. Immediate treatment might include:
   a. a loading dose of digoxin.
   b. injection of labetalol.
   c. bolus and titrated doses of lidocaine (lignocaine).
   d. a loading dose of esmolol.

MULTIPLE RESPONSE

Select all that apply.

1. The conduction system of the heart includes which of the following?
   a. sinoatrial node
   b. sinuses of Valsalva
   c. atrial bundles
   d. Purkinje fibres
   e. coronary sinus
   f. bundle of His
2. Arrhythmias (or dysrhythmias) can be caused by which of the following?
   a. lack of oxygen to the heart muscle cells
   b. acidosis near a cell
   c. structural damage in the conduction pathway through the heart
   d. vasodilation in the myocardial vascular bed
   e. thyroid hormone imbalance
   f. electrolyte imbalances

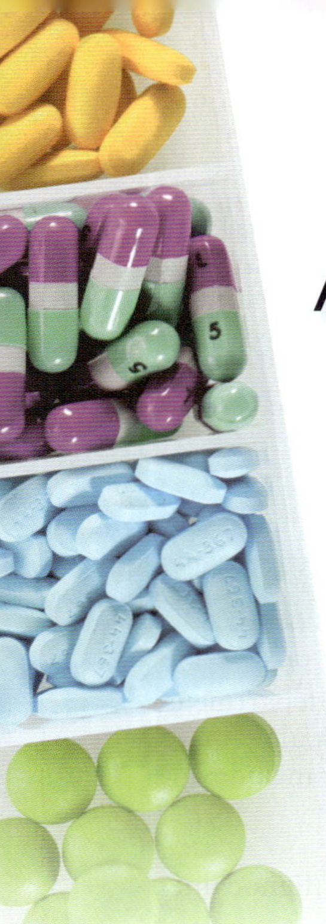

46 Antianginal agents

Learning objectives

On completing this chapter you should be able to:

1. Describe coronary artery disease, including identified risk factors and clinical presentation.
2. Describe the therapeutic actions, indications, pharmacokinetics, contraindications and cautions, most common adverse reactions and important drug–drug interactions associated with the nitrates, beta blockers and calcium channel blockers used to treat angina.
3. Discuss the use of antianginal agents across the lifespan.
4. Compare and contrast the prototype drugs glyceryl trinitrate, metoprolol and diltiazem with other agents used to treat angina.
5. Outline the care considerations, including important teaching points, for people receiving drugs used to treat angina.

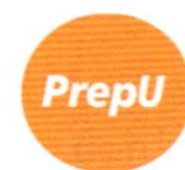

Test your current knowledge of antianginal agents with a PrepU Practice Quiz!

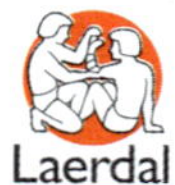

Simulation-based learning
On completion of the chapter, consider the scenario of Carl Shapiro (Part 2) who arrives in the emergency department. Consider the medication management of Carl's condition, as it relates to your learning in this chapter.

Glossary of key terms

angina pectoris: 'suffocation of the chest'; pain caused by the imbalance between oxygen being supplied to the heart muscle and demand for oxygen by the heart muscle

atheroma: plaque in the endothelial lining of arteries; contains fats, blood cells, lipids, inflammatory agents and platelets; leads to narrowing of the lumen of the artery, stiffening of the artery and loss of distensibility and responsiveness

atherosclerosis: narrowing of the arteries caused by build-up of atheromas, swelling and accumulation of platelets; leads to a loss of elasticity and responsiveness to normal stimuli

coronary artery disease (CAD): characterised by progressive narrowing of coronary arteries, leading to a decreased delivery of oxygen to cardiac muscle cells; leading killer of adults in the Western world

myocardial infarction: end result of vessel blockage in the heart; leads to ischaemia and then necrosis of the area cut off from the blood supply; it can heal, with the dead cells replaced by scar tissue

nitrates: drugs used to cause direct relaxation of smooth muscle, leading to vasodilation and decreased venous return to the heart with decreased resistance to blood flow; this rapidly decreases oxygen demand in the heart and can restore the balance between blood delivered and blood needed in the heart muscle of people with angina

pulse pressure: the systolic blood pressure minus the diastolic blood pressure; reflects the filling pressure of the coronary arteries

stable angina: predictable pain due to the imbalance of myocardial oxygen supply and demand that is relieved by rest or stoppage of activity

unstable angina: unpredictable episode of myocardial ischaemia with pain due to the imbalance of myocardial oxygen supply and demand when the person is at rest

variant (Prinzmetal or vasospastic) angina: drop in blood flow through the coronary arteries caused by a vasospasm in the artery, not by atherosclerosis

ANTIANGINAL AGENTS	Beta blockers	Calcium channel blockers	Potassium channel opener
Nitrates	atenolol	amlodipine	nicorandil
(P) glyceryl trinitrate	(P) metoprolol	(P) diltiazem	
isosorbide dinitrate	oxprenolol	nifedipine	
isosorbide mononitrate	pindolol	perhexiline	
	propranolol	verapamil	

Antianginal agents are used to help restore the appropriate supply-and-demand ratio in oxygen delivery to the myocardium. An imbalance in this ratio, manifested by pain, is most commonly due to **coronary artery disease (CAD)**. CAD has, for many years, been a leading cause of death in Australia and New Zealand and most Western nations. Despite great strides in understanding the contributing causes of this disease and ways to prevent it, CAD claims more lives than any other disease. The drugs discussed in this chapter are used to prevent myocardial cell death when the coronary vessels are already seriously damaged and are having trouble maintaining the blood flow to the heart muscle. Chapters 47 and 48 discuss drugs that are used to prevent the blocking of the coronary arteries before they become narrowed and damaged or to restore blood flow through narrowed vessels.

CORONARY ARTERY DISEASE

The myocardium must receive a constant supply of blood to have the oxygen and nutrients needed to maintain a constant pumping action. The myocardium receives all of its blood from two coronary arteries that exit the sinuses of Valsalva at the base of the aorta. These vessels divide and subdivide to form the capillaries that deliver oxygen to heart muscle fibres.

Unlike other tissues in the body, the heart muscle receives its blood supply during diastole, while it is at rest. This is important because when the heart muscle contracts, it becomes tight and clamps the blood vessels closed, rendering them unable to receive blood during systole, which is when all other tissues receive fresh blood. The openings in the sinuses of Valsalva, which are the beginnings of the coronary arteries, are positioned so that they can be filled when the blood flows back against the aortic valve when the heart is at rest. The pressure that fills these vessels is the **pulse pressure** (the systolic pressure minus the diastolic pressure) – the pressure of the column of blood falling back onto the closed aortic valve. The heart has just finished contracting and using energy and oxygen. The acid and carbon dioxide built up in the muscle cause a local vasodilation, and the blood flows freely through the coronary arteries and into the muscle cells.

In CAD, the lumen of the blood vessels becomes narrowed so that blood is no longer able to flow freely to the muscle cells. The narrowing of the vessels is caused by the development of **atheromas**, or fatty tumours in the intima of the vessels, in a process called **atherosclerosis** (Figure 46.1A). These deposits cause damage to

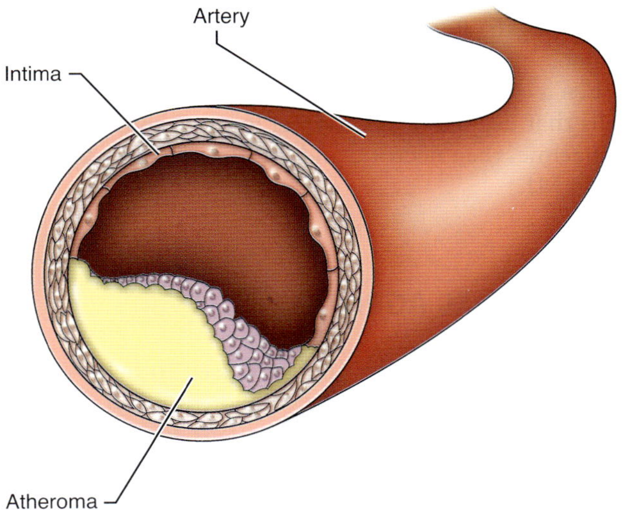

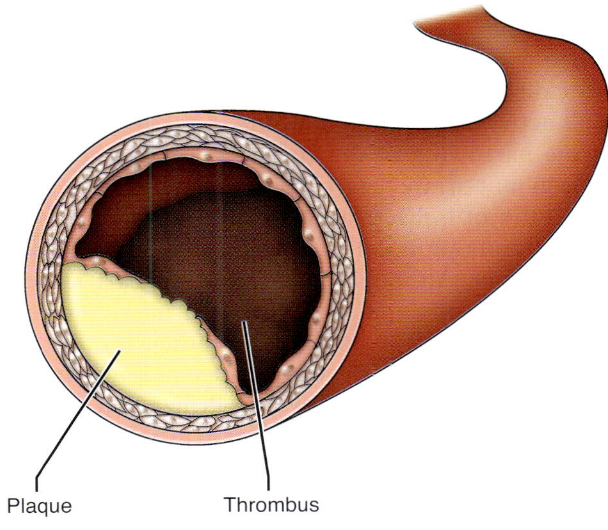

FIGURE 46.1 **A.** Schematic illustration of atheromatous plaque. **B.** Thrombosis of atherosclerotic plaque. It may partially or completely occlude the lumen of the vessel.

the intimal lining of the vessels, attracting platelets and immune factors and causing swelling and the development of a larger deposit. Over time, these deposits severely decrease the size of the vessel. While the vessel is being narrowed by the deposits in the intima, it is also losing its natural elasticity and becoming unable to respond to the normal stimuli to dilate or constrict to meet the needs of the tissues.

The person with atherosclerosis has a classic supply-and-demand problem. The heart may function without a problem until increases in activity or other stresses place a demand on it to beat faster or harder. Normally, the heart would stimulate the vessels to deliver more blood when this occurs, but the narrowed vessels are not able to respond and cannot supply the blood needed by the working heart (Figure 46.1B). The heart muscle then becomes hypoxic. This imbalance between oxygen supply and demand is manifested as pain, or **angina pectoris**, which literally means 'suffocation of the chest'.

Angina

The pain of angina is thus body's response to a lack of oxygen in the heart muscle. Although the heart muscle does not have any pain fibres, a chemical mediator called factor P is released from ischaemic myocardial cells, and pain is felt wherever factor P reacts with a pain receptor. For many people this is the chest, for some it is the left arm, while others have pain in the jaw and teeth. The basic response to this type of pain is to stop whatever one is doing and to wait for the pain to go away. In cases of minor limitations to the blood flow through vessels, stopping activity may bring the supply and demand for blood back into balance. This predictable condition is called **stable angina**. There is no damage to heart muscle and the basic reflexes surrounding the pain restore blood flow to the heart muscle. This process can go on for a long time with no resultant myocardial infarction. This is also called chronic angina, and can severely limit a person's activities and quality of life.

If the narrowing of the coronary arteries becomes more pronounced, the heart may experience unpredictable episodes of ischaemia even when the person is at rest. This condition is called **unstable angina** or pre-infarction angina. Although no damage to heart muscle occurs, the person is at increased risk of a complete blockage of blood supply to the heart muscle if the heart needs to work harder or the oxygen demand increases.

Variant angina (also known as **Prinzmetal** angina or **vasospastic** angina) is an unusual form of angina because it seems to be caused by spasm of the coronary blood vessels and not just by vessel narrowing. The person with this type of angina has angina at rest, often at the same time each day and usually with an associated electrocardiogram (ECG) pattern change.

Acute myocardial infarction

If a coronary vessel becomes completely occluded and is unable to deliver blood to the cardiac muscle, the area of muscle that depends on that vessel for oxygen becomes ischaemic and then necrotic. This is called a **myocardial infarction (MI)**. The pain associated with this event can be excruciating. Nausea and a severe sympathetic stress reaction may also be present. A serious danger of an MI is that arrhythmias can develop in nearby tissue that is ischaemic and very irritable. Most of the deaths caused by MI occur as a result of fatal arrhythmias. If the heart muscle has a chance to heal, within 6–10 weeks, scar tissue will form in the necrotic area and the muscle will compensate for the injury. If the area of the muscle that is damaged is very large, however, the muscle may not be able to compensate for the loss, and heart failure and even cardiogenic shock may occur. These conditions can be fatal or can leave a person severely limited by the weakened heart muscle.

KEY POINTS

- CAD involves changes in the coronary vessels that promote atheromas (tumours), which narrow the coronary arteries and decrease their elasticity and responsiveness to normal stimuli.
- Angina pectoris occurs when the narrowed vessels cannot accommodate the myocardial demand for oxygen.
- Stable angina occurs when the heart muscle is perfused adequately except during exertion or increased demand.
- Unstable or pre-infarction angina occurs when the vessels are so narrow that the myocardial cells are deprived of sufficient oxygen even at rest.
- Variant angina is a spasm of a coronary vessel that decreases the flow of blood through the narrowed lumen.
- When a coronary vessel is completely occluded, the cells that depend on that vessel for oxygen become ischaemic, then necrotic and die. The result is known as an MI.

ANTIANGINAL AGENTS

Antianginal drugs (Table 46.1) are used to help restore the appropriate supply-and-demand ratio in oxygen delivery to the myocardium when rest is not enough. These drugs can work to improve blood delivery to the heart muscle in one of two ways: (1) by dilating blood vessels (i.e. increasing the supply of oxygen) or (2) by decreasing the work of the heart (i.e. decreasing the demand for oxygen). Nitrates, beta-adrenergic blockers

TABLE 46.1 DRUGS IN FOCUS Antianginal agents

Drug name	Dosage/route	Usual indications
Nitrates		
(P) glyceryl trinitrate (*Anginine, Nitroderm TTS, Nitro-Dur, Nitrolingual*)	Sublingual tablets: 600–900 micrograms SL or buccal; maximum 1200 micrograms/dose Sublingual spray: 400–800 micrograms (1–2 sprays) repeat if no relief within 5 minutes; IV Infusion: initially 5 micrograms/min, increase by 5 micrograms/min q 3–5 minutes until response; if no response at 20 micrograms/min, increase by 10–20 micrograms/min Transdermal patch: one patch daily (5–15 mg/24 hours); a patch-off period of 8–12 hours, usually at night, every 24 hours is recommended to overcome tolerance	Nitrate of choice for treatment of acute angina attack; prevention of anginal attacks
isosorbide dinitrate (*Isordil, Sorbidin*)	Sublingual tablets: 5–10 mg sublingually q 2–3 hours or as necessary Oral tablets: 5–30 mg qid; usually 10 mg qid	Taken before chest pain begins in situations in which exertion or stress can be anticipated for prevention of angina in adults; taken daily for management of chronic angina
isosorbide mononitrate (*Duride, Imdur, ISMO 20, ISMO 40 Retard*)	Adult, oral, immediate release: 10 mg bd for 2 days, then 20 mg bd; maximum 20 mg tid Adult, oral, modified release: 40–60 mg once daily; maximum 120 mg/day	Prevention and treatment of angina pectoris
Beta blockers		
atenolol (*Noten, Tenormin*)	100 mg daily in 1 or 2 divided doses	Treatment of angina pectoris in adults
(P) metoprolol succinate (*Betaloc CR, Minax*)	Adult 95–190 mg once daily in the morning	Treatment of angina in adults; prevention of reinfarction within 3–10 days after MI
metoprolol tartarate (*Betaloc, Lopressor, Slow Lopressor, Minax*)	Oral, immediate release: 50–100 mg bd–tid; oral, modified release: 100–200 mg once daily in the morning; if necessary, dose may be repeated in the evening	Treatment of angina pectoris in adults
oxprenolol (*Corbeton*)	20–40 mg tid up to 320 mg daily	Treatment of angina pectoris in adults
pindolol (*Barbloc*)	7.5–20 mg daily in 3 divided doses	Treatment of angina pectoris in adults
propranolol (*Inderal*)	40 mg bd–tid; maximum 120–320 mg/day	Long-term management of angina and prevention of reinfarction in people 1–4 weeks after MI
Calcium channel blockers		
amlodipine (*Norvasc*)	2.5–5 mg/day PO; maximum 10 mg/day; reduce dose with hepatic impairment or in elderly people	Treatment of chronic, stable angina and of variant angina in adults
(P) diltiazem (*Cardizem CD, Dilzem*)	Adult, oral, immediate release: 30 mg tid–qid, usually 18–240 mg in 4 divided doses; maximum 360 mg/day in 4 divided doses Adult, oral, modified release: 120–180 mg/day; maximum 360 mg/day. Swallow whole, do not crush or chew	Treatment of angina in adults
nifedipine Sustained-release twice-daily preparation (*Adalat Modified Release, Nyefax, Retard*) Sustained-release once-daily preparation (*Adalat OROS, Adefin XL*)	Sustained-release twice-daily preparation: 10–20 mg bd; maximum 30 mg bd Sustained-release once-daily preparation: 30 mg once daily, increased if necessary to 60 mg once daily; angina, maximum 90 mg/day	Treatment of angina in adults
perhexiline (*Pexsig*)	Initially, 100 mg PO daily, up to 400 mg/day PO	Treatment of moderate to severe angina in adults who have not responded to other treatment

Continued on following page

TABLE 46.1 DRUGS IN FOCUS Antianginal agents *(continued)*

Drug name	Dosage/route	Usual indications
Calcium channel blockers *(continued)*		
verapamil (*Cordilox SR, Isoptin, Isoptin SR, Verapamil, Verapamil SR*)	Immediate release: 80–160 mg bd; maximum 160 mg tid Sustained release: 180–240 mg in the morning; maximum 480 mg in 2 divided doses	Treatment of angina in adults; treatment of tachyarrhythmias
Potassium channel opener		
nicorandil (*Ikorel*)	10-20 mg PO bd	Treatment of chronic stable angina pectoris

and calcium channel blockers are used to treat angina (Figure 46.2).

All antianginal agents are effective and may be used in combination to achieve good pain control. The type of drug that is best for a person is determined by tolerance of adverse effects and response to the drug. The use of antianginal agents with different age groups is discussed in Box 46.1.

Nitrates

Nitrates are drugs that act directly on smooth muscle to cause relaxation and to depress muscle tone. Because the action is direct, these drugs do not influence any nerve or other activity and the response is usually quite fast.

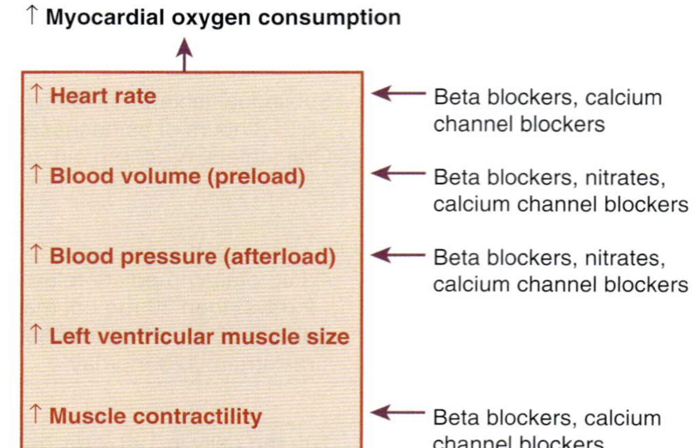

FIGURE 46.2 Interaction of antianginal agents with factors affecting myocardial oxygen demand.

BOX 46.1 FOCUS ON Drug therapy across the lifespan

Antianginal agents

CHILDREN

The antianginals are not indicated for any condition commonly found in children. In some situations, particularly congenital heart defects or cardiac surgery, glyceryl trinitrate may be used. The dose of the drug should be determined by considering age and weight. The child should be very carefully monitored for adverse reactions, including potentially dangerous changes in blood pressure.

ADULTS

Adults who receive these drugs should be instructed in their proper administration, particularly if varying forms of glyceryl trinitrate are used. Individuals should also be encouraged to determine what activities or situations tend to precipitate an anginal attack so that they can take measures to avoid those circumstances or take an antianginal agent before the event occurs.

With glyceryl trinitrate use, it is important that the person knows how to use the drug, how to store the drug, how to determine whether it is still effective and how much to take before seeking emergency medical care.

People should know that regular medical follow-up is important and should be instructed in non-pharmacological measures – weight loss, smoking cessation, activity changes, diet changes – that could decrease their risk of coronary artery disease and improve the effectiveness of the antianginal therapy.

PREGNANCY AND BREASTFEEDING

The safety for the use of these drugs during pregnancy has not been established. There is a significant potential for adverse effects on the fetus related to blood flow changes and direct drug effects when the drugs cross the placenta. The drugs do enter breast milk, and it is advised that another method of feeding the baby be used if one of these drugs is prescribed during breastfeeding.

OLDER ADULTS

Older adults frequently are prescribed one of these drugs. Older adults are more likely to develop adverse effects associated with the use of these drugs – arrhythmias, hypotension and heart disease. Safety measures may be needed if these effects occur and interfere with the person's mobility and balance.

Older adults are also more likely to have renal and/or hepatic impairment related to underlying medical conditions, which could interfere with the metabolism and excretion of these drugs. The dose for older adults should be started at a lower level than that recommended for younger adults. The person should be monitored very closely and dose adjusted based on response.

If other drugs are added to, or removed from, the drug regimen, appropriate dose adjustments may need to be made. If the person is using a different form of glyceryl trinitrate, special care should be taken to make sure that the proper administration, storage and timing of use are understood.

Nitrates include isosorbide dinitrate (*Isordil*, *Sorbidin*), isosorbide mononitrate (*Duride*, *Imdur* and others) and glyceryl trinitrate (*Anginine*, *Nitro-Dur*, *Nitrolingual* and others).

Therapeutic actions and indications

The nitrates relax and dilate veins, arteries and capillaries, allowing increased blood flow through the vessels and lowering systemic blood pressure because of a drop in resistance. Because CAD causes a stiffening and lack of responsiveness in the coronary arteries, the nitrates probably have very little effect on increasing blood flow through these arteries. However, they do increase blood flow through healthy coronary arteries. Therefore, the blood supply through any healthy vessels in the heart increases, possibly helping the heart to compensate somewhat.

The main effect of nitrates, however, seems to be related to the drop in blood pressure that occurs. The vasodilation causes blood to pool in veins and capillaries, decreasing preload, while the relaxation of the vessels decreases afterload. The combination of these effects greatly reduces the cardiac workload and the demand for oxygen, thus bringing the supply-and-demand ratio back into balance. Nitrates are indicated for the prevention and treatment of attacks of angina pectoris. See Table 46.1 for usual indications for each of these drugs.

Pharmacokinetics

Glyceryl trinitrate is available as a sublingual tablet, a translingual spray, an intravenous solution (for bolus injection or infusion), a transdermal patch or a transmucosal agent. It can be carried with the person, who then can use it when the need arises. Slow-release forms also are available for use in preventing anginal attacks.

Isosorbide dinitrate and isosorbide mononitrate are available in oral form.

Nitrates are very rapidly absorbed, metabolised in the liver and excreted in urine. They cross the placenta and enter breast milk. Glyceryl trinitrate is available in many forms; absorption, onset of action and duration vary with the form used (see Prototype summary). Isosorbide dinitrate and isosorbide mononitrate, when given orally, have an onset of action in 14–45 minutes, or up to 4 hours if the sustained-release (SR) form is used. The drug may have a duration of action of 4–6 hours, or 6–8 hours if the SR form is used.

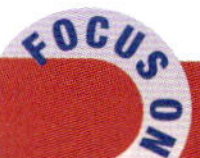

Safe medication administration

Sublingual, transbuccal and transdermal administration of glyceryl trinitrate

Sublingual administration: *individuals often prefer this route of administration, opting to administer the drug themselves even in the institutional setting. Make sure that the drug is given correctly:*

- *Check under the tongue to make sure there are no lesions or abrasions that could interfere with the absorption of the drug. Have the person take a sip of water to moisten the mucous membranes so the tablet will dissolve quickly. Then instruct the person to place the tablet under the tongue, close the mouth and wait until it has dissolved.*
- *Caution the person not to swallow the tablet; its effectiveness would be lost if the tablet entered the stomach. If the person uses sublingual and transbuccal drugs often, encourage them to alternate sides of the tongue – placing it under the left side for one dose, and under the right side for the next dose.*
- *Here's a tip to help in administering sublingual medications to people who cannot do it themselves or who cannot open their mouths: use a tongue depressor to move the tongue aside and place the tablet, or slide the tablet down through a straw to the underside of the tongue.*

Transbuccal administration: *make sure that the tablet the person is going to use is designed for buccal administration:*

- *Check the inside of the cheeks to be sure there are no ulcerations or abrasions that could interfere with the absorption of the drug. Have the person place the tablet between their gums and cheek pocket and then hold it in place until the tablet dissolves.*
- *Again, caution the person not to swallow the tablet. Swallowing the tablet will cause systemic absorption. Instruct the person to rotate the site of placement from side to side with each dose.*

Transdermal administration: *errors have been reported with inappropriate use of glyceryl trinitrate patches. The patch should be removed before defibrillation, cardioversion, diathermy, or MRI (Nitroderm TTS only). Make sure to discuss safe administration with the person:*

- *It is very important to teach people to remove the old transdermal system after 16 hours and to wash the area before placing a new system to prevent adverse effects such as severe hypotension.*
- *Wait for at least 8 hours before applying a new patch. The patch should be applied to a clean, hairless area of skin at the same time each day and to a different area of skin, to prevent skin irritation. Do not cut the patch. Dispose of the patch by folding it in half with the sticky sides together. Keep out of reach of children.*

Contraindications and cautions

Nitrates are contraindicated in the presence of any allergy to nitrates. These drugs are also contraindicated in the following conditions: severe anaemia *because the decrease in cardiac output could be detrimental in a person who already has a decreased ability to deliver oxygen because of a low red blood cell count*; head trauma or cerebral haemorrhage *because the relaxation of cerebral vessels could cause intracranial bleeding*;

and pregnancy or breastfeeding *because of potential adverse effects on the neonate and ineffective blood flow to the fetus*.

Caution should be used in people with hepatic or renal disease, *which could alter the metabolism and excretion of these drugs*. Caution is also required for people with hypotension, hypovolaemia and conditions that limit cardiac output (eg, tamponade, low ventricular filling pressure, low pulmonary capillary wedge pressure) *because these conditions could be exacerbated, resulting in serious adverse effects*.

Adverse effects

The adverse effects associated with these drugs are related to vasodilation and the decrease in blood flow that occurs. Central nervous system (CNS) effects include headache, dizziness and weakness. Gastrointestinal (GI) symptoms can include nausea, vomiting and incontinence. Cardiovascular problems include: hypotension, which can be severe and must be monitored; reflex tachycardia that occurs when blood pressure falls; syncope; and angina, which could be exacerbated by the hypotension and changes in cardiac output. Skin-related effects include flushing, pallor and increased perspiration. With the transdermal preparation, there is a risk of contact dermatitis and local hypersensitivity reactions.

Clinically important drug–drug interactions

There is a risk of hypertension and decreased anti-anginal effects if these drugs are given with ergot derivatives. There is also a risk of decreased therapeutic effects of heparin if these drugs are given together with heparin; if this combination is used, the person should be monitored and appropriate dose adjustments made. Individuals should be warned not to combine nitrates with avanafil, sildenafil, tadalafil or vardenafil (drugs used to treat erectile dysfunction) because serious hypotension and cardiovascular events could occur.

Prototype summary: glyceryl trinitrate

Indications: treatment of acute angina, prophylaxis of angina, intravenous treatment of angina unresponsive to beta blockers or organic nitrates, perioperative hypertension, and heart failure (HF) associated with acute MI; to produce controlled hypotension during surgery.

Actions: relaxes vascular smooth muscle with a resultant decrease in venous return and decrease in arterial blood pressure, reducing the left ventricular workload and decreasing myocardial oxygen consumption.

Pharmacokinetics:

Route	Onset	Duration
IV	1–2 min	3–5 min
Sublingual tablet	1–3 min	30–60 min
Translingual spray	2 min	30–60 min
Transmucosal tablet	1–2 min	3–5 min
Oral, SR tablet	20–45 min	8–12 hours
Transdermal	30–60 min	24 hours

$T_{1/2}$: 1–4 minutes; metabolised in the liver and excreted in urine.

Adverse effects: hypotension, headache, dizziness, tachycardia, rash, flushing, nausea, vomiting, sweating, chest pain.

Care considerations for people receiving nitrates

Assessment: history and examination

- Assess for contraindications or cautions: any known allergies to nitrates *to avoid hypersensitivity reactions*; impaired liver or kidney function, *which could alter the metabolism and excretion of the drug; any condition that could be exacerbated by the hypotension and change in blood flow caused by these drugs*, such as early MI, head trauma, cerebral haemorrhage, hypotension, hypovolaemia, anaemia or low cardiac-output states; and current status of pregnancy or breastfeeding *because of the potential for adverse effects on the fetus or breastfeeding baby*.
- Perform a physical assessment *to establish baseline status before beginning therapy* and *during therapy to determine effectiveness and to evaluate for any potential adverse effects*.
- Inspect the skin for colour, intactness and any signs of redness, irritation or breakdown, especially if the person is using the transdermal or topical form of the drug, *to prevent possible skin reaction and ensure adequate surface for application and absorption of transdermal or topical drug*. Also check the person's oral or buccal mucosa (including the area under the tongue) if sublingual or buccal forms are ordered *to reduce the risk of irritation and ensure adequate surface for absorption*.
- Assess the person's complaint of pain, including onset, duration, intensity, location and measures used to relieve it. Investigate activity level before and after the onset of pain *to aid in identifying possible contributing factors to the pain and its progression*.

- Assess neurological status, including level of alertness, affect and reflexes, *to evaluate for CNS effects.*
- Monitor respirations and auscultate lungs *to evaluate changes in cardiac output.*
- Assess cardiopulmonary status closely, including pulse rate, blood pressure, heart rate and rhythm, *to determine the effects of therapy and identify any adverse effects.*
- Obtain an ECG as ordered *to evaluate heart rate and rhythm, which could indicate changes in cardiac perfusion.*
- Monitor laboratory test results, including liver and renal function tests, full blood count and haemoglobin level, *to determine the need for possible dose adjustment.*

Implementation with rationale

- Give sublingual preparations under the tongue or in the buccal pouch, and encourage the person not to swallow, *to ensure that therapeutic effectiveness is achieved* (see Pharmacokinetics for discussion of safe medication administration).
- Ask the person if the tablet 'fizzles' or burns, which indicates potency. Always check the expiration date on the bottle and protect the medication from heat and light *because these drugs are volatile and lose their potency.*
- Instruct the person that a sublingual dose may be repeated in 5 minutes if relief is not felt, for a total of three doses, if pain persists. They should go to an emergency department *to ensure proper medical support if an MI should occur.*
- Give sustained-release forms with water, and caution the person not to chew or crush tablets or capsules *because these preparations need to reach the GI tract intact.*
- Rotate the sites of topical forms *to decrease the risk of skin abrasion and breakdown*; monitor for signs of skin breakdown *to arrange for appropriate skin care as needed.*
- Make sure that sublingual spray is used under the tongue and not inhaled *to ensure that the therapeutic effects can be achieved.*
- Break an amyl nitrate capsule and wave it under the nose of the person with angina *to provide rapid relief using the inhalation form of the drug*; this may be repeated with another capsule in 3–5 minutes if needed.
- Keep a record of the number of sprays used if a sublingual spray form is used, *to prevent running out of medication and episodes of untreated angina.*
- Have emergency life support equipment readily available *in case of severe reaction to the drug or MI.*
- Taper the dose gradually (over 4–6 weeks) after long-term therapy *because abrupt withdrawal could cause a severe reaction, including MI.*
- Provide comfort measures *to help the person tolerate drug effects.* These include small, frequent meals *to alleviate GI upset*; access to bathroom facilities if GI upset is severe or the person experiences incontinence; environmental controls such as temperature, controlled lighting and noise reduction *to decrease stresses that could aggravate cardiac workload*; safety precautions such as lying or sitting down after taking the drug and assistance with ambulation *to reduce the risk of injury*; reorientation; and appropriate skin care as needed.
- Offer support and encouragement *to help the person deal with the diagnosis and the drug regimen.*
- Provide thorough teaching, including the name of the drug; dosage prescribed; proper technique for administration (oral, sublingual, sublingual spray, transbuccal, transdermal, or topical); need for removal of transdermal or topical drug before application of the next dose; the importance of having an adequate supply of drug (eg, teaching the individual to count the number of sprays used for a translingual spray so as not to run short); measures to prevent anginal attacks and actions to take when an attack occurs; use of medication during an attack (such as the number of tablets and time span that the person can take sublingual tablets); measures to avoid adverse effects, warning signs of problems and signs and symptoms to report immediately; and the need for periodic monitoring and evaluation *to enhance knowledge about drug therapy and to promote compliance.*

Evaluation

- Monitor response to the drug (alleviation of signs and symptoms of angina, prevention of angina).
- Monitor for adverse effects (hypotension, cardiac arrhythmias, GI upset, skin reactions, headache).
- Evaluate the effectiveness of the teaching plan (person can name drug, dosage, proper administration, adverse effects to watch for, specific measures to avoid them and the importance of continued follow-up).
- Monitor the effectiveness of comfort measures and compliance with the regimen.

See the Critical thinking scenario for measures for handling an angina attack.

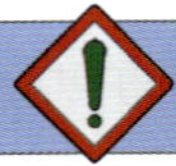

CRITICAL THINKING SCENARIO

Handling an angina attack

THE SITUATION

S.W. is a 48-year-old Caucasian woman with a 2-year history of angina pectoris. She was given sublingual glyceryl trinitrate to use when she had chest pain. For the past 6 months, she has been stable, experiencing little chest pain. This morning after her exercise class, S.W. had an argument with her daughter and experienced severe chest pain that was unrelieved by four glyceryl trinitrate tablets taken over a 20-minute period. S.W.'s daughter rushed her to the hospital, where she was given oxygen through nasal cannula and placed on a cardiac monitor, which showed a sinus tachycardia of 110 beats/min. A 12-lead electrocardiogram (ECG) showed no changes from her previous ECG of 7 months ago.

S.W. did not have elevated troponin levels. The chest pain subsided within 3 minutes after she received another sublingual glyceryl trinitrate. It was decided that S.W. should stay in the emergency department (ED) for a few hours for observation. The diagnosis of an acute angina attack was made.

CRITICAL THINKING

What care interventions are appropriate for S.W. while she is still in the ED? *Consider the progression of coronary artery disease (CAD) and the ways in which that progression can be delayed and chest pain avoided.* What teaching points should be stressed with this person?

What type of feeling may the daughter experience after the disagreement with S.W.? *What interventions would be useful in dealing with mother and daughter during this crisis?*

Should any further tests or treatments be addressed with S.W. when discussing her heart disease?

DISCUSSION

S.W.'s vital signs should be monitored closely while she is in the ED. If her attack subsides, she will be discharged, and teaching points about CAD will be reviewed with her. It would be a good time to discuss angina with S.W. and her daughter, explaining the pathophysiology of the disease and ways to avoid disrupting the supply-and-demand ratio in the heart muscle.

Because S.W. took four glyceryl trinitrate tablets with no effect before coming to the ED, it would be important to find out the age and potency of her drug. Review the storage requirements for the drug, ways to tell whether it is potent, and the importance of replacing the pills at least every 6 months.

S.W. and her daughter should be encouraged to air their feelings about this episode; for example, guilt or anger may be precipitated by this scare. They should have the opportunity to explore other ways of handling their problems, try to pace activities to avoid excessive demand for oxygen and plan what to do if this happens again. They should both receive support and encouragement to cope with the angina and its implications.

Written information, including drug information, should be given to S.W. Once her condition is stabilised, further studies may be indicated to monitor the progress of her disease. The use of dietary interventions, avoidance of smoking as appropriate, blood pressure control and monitoring of activity should be considered.

CARE GUIDE FOR S.W.: ANTIANGINAL NITRATES

Assessment: history and examination

Assess S.W. for allergies to any nitrates, renal or hepatic dysfunction, pregnancy and breastfeeding (if appropriate), early MI, head trauma, hypotension and hypovolaemia.

Focus the physical examination on the following areas:

Cardiovascular: blood pressure, pulse, perfusion, ECG

Neurological (CNS): orientation, affect, reflexes, vision

Skin: colour, lesions, texture

Respiratory system: respiratory rate and character, adventitious sounds

GI: abdominal examination, bowel sounds

Laboratory tests: liver and renal function tests, full blood count, haemoglobin

Implementation

Ensure proper administration of drug, and protect the drug from heat and light.

Provide comfort and safety measures:

- Offer environmental control for headaches.
- Give drug with food if GI upset occurs.
- Provide skin care as needed.
- Taper dose after long-term use.

Provide support and reassurance to deal with drug effects.

Provide teaching regarding drug, dosage, adverse effects, what to report and safety precautions.

Evaluation

Evaluate drug effects: relief of signs and symptoms of angina, prevention of angina.

Monitor for adverse effects: headache, dizziness; arrhythmias; GI upset; skin reactions; hypotension; and cardiovascular effects.

Monitor for drug–drug interactions as indicated for each drug.

Evaluate the effectiveness of the teaching program and comfort and safety measures.

TEACHING FOR S.W.

- A nitrate is given to people with chest pain that occurs because the heart muscle is not receiving enough oxygen. The nitrates act by decreasing the heart's workload and thus its need for oxygen, which it uses for energy. This relieves the pain of angina.
- Besides taking the drug as prescribed, you can also help your heart by decreasing the work that it must do. For example, you can do the following:
  - Reduce weight, if necessary.
  - Decrease or avoid the use of coffee, cigarettes or alcoholic beverages.
  - Avoid going outside in very cold weather; if this cannot be avoided, dress warmly and avoid exertion while outside.
  - Avoid stressful activities, especially in combination. For example, if you eat a big meal, do not drink coffee or alcoholic beverages with that meal. If you have just eaten a big meal, do not climb stairs; rest for a while.
  - Determine which social interactions are stressful or anxiety producing; then find ways to limit or avoid these situations.
  - Learn to slow down, rest periodically, and schedule your activities to allow your heart to pace its use of energy throughout the day and to help you to maintain your activities without pain.
- Glyceryl trinitrate tablets are taken sublingually. Place one tablet under your tongue. Do not swallow until the tablet has dissolved. The tablet should burn slightly or 'fizzle' under your tongue; if this does not occur, the tablet is not effective and you should get a fresh supply of tablets.
- Ideally, take the glyceryl trinitrate before your chest pain begins. If you know that a certain activity usually causes pain (eg, eating a big meal, attending a business meeting, engaging in sexual intercourse), take the tablet before undertaking that activity.
- Sublingual glyceryl trinitrate is a very unstable compound. Do not buy large quantities at a time because it does not store well. Keep the drug in a dark, dry place and in a dark-coloured glass container, not a plastic bottle, with a tight lid. Leave it in its own bottle. Do not combine it with other drugs.
- Some of the following adverse effects may occur:
  - *Dizziness, light-headedness*: this often passes as you adjust to the drug. Use great care if you are taking sublingual or transmucosal forms of the drug. Sit or lie down to avoid dizziness or falls. Change position slowly to help decrease the dizziness.
  - *Headache*: this is a common problem. Over-the-counter headache remedies often provide no relief for the pain. Lying down in a cool environment and resting may help alleviate some of the discomfort.
  - *Flushing of the face and neck*: this is usually a very minor problem that passes as the drug's effects pass.
  - (Report any of the following to your health care provider): *blurred vision, persistent or severe headache, skin rash, more frequent or more severe angina attacks, or fainting.*
- Sublingual glyceryl trinitrate usually relieves chest pain within 3–5 minutes. One glyceryl trinitrate tablet should be placed (or one spray of Nitrolingual sprayed) under the tongue. If pain is not relieved within 5 minutes, take another tablet or spray. If pain continues, take another tablet or spray in 5 minutes. If there is no pain relief, call an ambulance – 000 in Australia or 111 in New Zealand.
- Tell any doctor, nurse or other health care provider involved in your care that you are taking this drug.
- Keep this drug, and all medications, out of the reach of children.
- Avoid taking over-the-counter medications while you are taking this drug. If you feel that you need one of these, consult with your health care provider for the best choice. Many over-the-counter drugs can change the effects of this drug and cause problems.
- Avoid alcohol while you are taking this drug because the combination can cause serious problems.
- If you are taking this drug for a prolonged period of time, do not stop taking it suddenly. Your body will need time to adjust to the loss of the drug. The dose must be gradually reduced to prevent serious problems.

KEY POINTS

- Nitrates cause blood vessels to relax and dilate. This results in a drop in peripheral resistance and blood pressure and a decrease in venous return to the heart. These actions will decrease myocardial workload and can restore the appropriate balance in the supply–demand ratio in the heart.
- Nitrates are available in many forms that vary in time of onset and duration of action. Fast-acting nitrates are used to treat acute anginal attacks. Slower-acting nitrates are used to prevent anginal attacks from occurring.

BETA-ADRENERGIC BLOCKERS

As discussed in Chapter 31, beta-adrenergic blockers are used to block the stimulatory effects of the sympathetic nervous system. The beta blockers recommended for use in angina include atenolol (*Noten*, *Tenormin*), metoprolol (*Betaloc, Minax*), oxprenolol (*Corbeton*), pindolol (*Barbloc*) and propranolol (*Inderal*).

Therapeutic actions and indications

The beta blockers competitively block beta-adrenergic receptors in the heart and juxtaglomerular apparatus, decreasing the influence of the sympathetic nervous system on these tissues. The result is a decrease in the excitability of the heart, a decrease in cardiac output, a decrease in cardiac oxygen consumption and a lowering of blood pressure. They are indicated for the long-term management of angina pectoris caused by atherosclerosis. These drugs are sometimes used in combination with nitrates to increase exercise tolerance. See Table 46.1 for usual indications for each of these drugs.

Beta blockers are not indicated for the treatment of variant angina because they could cause vasospasm due to blocking of beta-receptor sites. Propranolol and metoprolol can also be used to prevent reinfarction in stable individuals 1–4 weeks after an MI. This effect is thought to be caused by the suppression of myocardial oxygen demand for a prolonged period.

Pharmacokinetics

These drugs are absorbed from the GI tract after oral administration and undergo hepatic metabolism. They reach peak levels in 60–90 minutes and have varying duration of effects, ranging from 6 to 19 hours. Food has been found to increase the bioavailability of propranolol, but this effect has not been found with other beta-adrenergic-blocking agents.

Contraindications and cautions

The beta blockers are contraindicated in individuals with bradycardia, heart block and cardiogenic shock *because blocking of the sympathetic response could exacerbate these diseases*. They are also contraindicated with pregnancy and breastfeeding *because of the potential for adverse effects on the fetus or neonate*.

Caution should be used in individuals with diabetes, peripheral vascular disease, asthma, chronic obstructive pulmonary disease (COPD) or thyrotoxicosis *because the blockade of the sympathetic response blocks normal reflexes that are necessary for maintaining homeostasis in people with these diseases*. Many people with these complicating disorders receive beta blockers, and these individuals need to be monitored carefully to avoid serious adverse effects.

Adverse effects

Beta blockers have many adverse effects associated with the blockade of the sympathetic nervous system. However, the dose used to prevent angina is lower than doses used to treat hypertension. Therefore, there is a decreased incidence of adverse effects associated with this specific use of beta blockers.

Adverse effects do occur. CNS effects include dizziness, fatigue, emotional depression and sleep disturbances. GI problems include gastric pain, nausea, vomiting, colitis and diarrhoea. Cardiovascular effects can include heart failure, reduced cardiac output and arrhythmias. Respiratory effects can include bronchospasm, dyspnoea and cough. Decreased exercise tolerance and malaise are also common complaints.

Clinically important drug–drug interactions

A paradoxical hypertension occurs when clonidine is given with beta blockers, and an increased rebound hypertension with clonidine withdrawal may also occur; it is best to avoid this combination.

A decreased antihypertensive effect occurs when beta blockers are given with non-steroidal anti-inflammatory drugs; if this combination is used, the person should be monitored closely and a dose adjustment made.

An initial hypertensive episode followed by bradycardia occurs if these drugs are given with noradrenaline, and a possibility of peripheral ischaemia exists if beta blockers are taken in combination with ergot alkaloids.

There also is a potential for a change in blood glucose levels if these drugs are given with insulin or antidiabetic agents, and the individual will not have the

---

Prototype summary: metoprolol

Indications: treatment of stable angina pectoris; also used for treatment of hypertension, prevention of reinfarction in people with MI, and treatment of stable, symptomatic HF.

Actions: competitively blocks beta-adrenergic receptors in the heart and kidneys, decreasing the influence of the sympathetic nervous system on these tissues and the excitability of the heart; decreases cardiac output, which results in a lowered blood pressure and decreased cardiac workload.

Pharmacokinetics:

Route	Onset	Peak	Duration
Oral	15 min	90 min	15–19 hours
IV	Immediate	60–90 min	15–19 hours

$T_{1/2}$: 3–4 hours; metabolised in the liver and excreted in urine.

Adverse effects: dizziness, vertigo, HF, arrhythmias, gastric pain, flatulence, diarrhoea, vomiting, impotence, decreased exercise tolerance.

---

usual signs and symptoms of hypoglycaemia or hyperglycaemia to alert them to potential problems. If this combination is used, the person should monitor blood glucose frequently throughout the day and be alert to new warnings about glucose imbalance.

Care considerations for people receiving beta blockers

See Chapter 31 for the care considerations associated with beta blockers.

KEY POINTS

- Beta blockers are used in the treatment of angina to help restore the balance between supply of oxygen and demand for oxygen.
- Beta blockers prevent the activation of sympathetic receptors, which normally would increase heart rate, increase blood pressure and increase cardiac contraction. All of these actions would increase the demand for oxygen; blocking these actions decreases the demand for oxygen.

Calcium channel blockers

Calcium channel blockers include amlodipine (*Norvasc*), diltiazem (*Cardizem*), nifedipine (*Adalat, Nyefax*), perhexiline (*Pexsig*), and verapamil (*Cordilox SR*, *Isoptin*).

Therapeutic actions and indications

Calcium channel blockers inhibit the movement of calcium ions across the membranes of myocardial and arterial muscle cells, altering the action potential and blocking muscle cell contraction. A loss of smooth muscle tone, vasodilation and decreased peripheral resistance occur. Subsequently, preload and afterload are decreased, which in turn decreases cardiac workload and oxygen consumption.

Calcium channel blockers are indicated for the treatment of variant angina, chronic angina, effort-associated angina and hypertension. In variant angina, these agents relieve coronary artery vasospasm, increasing blood flow to the muscle cells. Research also indicates that these drugs block the proliferation of cells in the endothelial layer of the blood vessel, slowing the progress of the atherosclerosis. Verapamil is also used to treat cardiac tachyarrhythmias because it slows conduction more than the other calcium channel blockers do. The drug of choice depends on the person's diagnosis and ability to tolerate adverse drug effects. See Table 46.1 for usual indications for each of these drugs.

Pharmacokinetics

These drugs are generally well absorbed after oral administration, metabolised in the liver and excreted in urine. They have an onset of action of 20 minutes and duration of action of 2–4 hours. These drugs cross the placenta and enter breast milk.

Contraindications and cautions

Calcium channel blockers are contraindicated in the presence of allergy to any of these drugs *to avoid hypersensitivity reactions* and with pregnancy or breast-feeding *because of the potential for adverse effects on the fetus or neonate.*

Caution should be used with heart block or sick sinus syndrome, *which could be exacerbated by the conduction-slowing effects of these drugs*; with renal or hepatic dysfunction, *which could alter the metabolism and excretion of these drugs*; and with heart failure, *which could be exacerbated by the decrease in cardiac output that could occur.* People with diabetes should be careful when taking perhexiline, as this drug can cause hypoglycaemia, and dose adjustment may be necessary in the first few days.

Adverse effects

The adverse effects associated with these drugs are related to their effects on cardiac output and on smooth muscle. CNS effects include dizziness, light-headedness, headache and fatigue. GI effects can include nausea and hepatic injury related to direct toxic effects on hepatic cells. Cardiovascular effects include hypotension, bradycardia, peripheral oedema and heart block. Skin effects include flushing and rash.

Clinically important drug–drug interactions

Drug–drug interactions vary with each of the calcium channel blockers. Potentially serious effects to keep in mind include increased serum levels and toxicity of ciclosporin if this is taken with diltiazem and increased risk of heart block and digoxin toxicity if this is combined with verapamil (because verapamil increases digoxin serum levels). Both verapamil and digoxin depress myocardial conduction. If any combinations of these drugs must be used, the individual should be monitored very closely and appropriate dose adjustments made. Verapamil has also been associated with serious respiratory depression when given with general anaesthetics or as an adjunct to anaesthesia.

 **Prototype summary: diltiazem**

Indications: treatment of variant angina, effort-associated angina and chronic stable angina; also used to treat essential hypertension and paroxysmal supraventricular tachycardia.

Actions: inhibits the movement of calcium ions across the membranes of myocardial and arterial muscle cells, altering the action potential and blocking muscle cell contraction, which depresses myocardial contractility; slows cardiac impulse formation in the conductive tissues, and relaxes and dilates arteries, causing a fall in blood pressure and a decrease in venous return; decreases the workload of the heart and myocardial oxygen consumption; relieves the vasospasm of the coronary artery, increasing blood flow to the muscle cells (variant angina).

Pharmacokinetics:

Route	Onset	Peak
Oral	30–60 min	2–3 hours
SR, extended release (ER)	30–60 min	6–11 hours
IV	Immediate	2–3 min

$T_{1/2}$: 3.5–6 hours (SR), 5–7 hours (ER); metabolised in the liver and excreted in urine.

Adverse effects: dizziness, light-headedness, headache, asthenia, peripheral oedema, bradycardia, atrioventricular block, flushing, rash, nausea.

Potassium channel opener

There is one other drug group used in the treatment of angina pectoris, namely potassium channel openers of which one, nicorandil (*Ikorel*), is currently available.

Therapeutic actions and indications

Potassium channel openers promote opening of ATP-dependent potassium channels located in vascular smooth muscle, where they cause hyperpolarisation. This effect leads to dilation of arteries and reduction in afterload. The effect also leads to vascular smooth muscle relaxation, enhancing pooling of blood and reducing preload.

Pharmacokinetics

Nicorandil is rapidly absorbed after oral administration, mainly through the GI system. Peak levels are achieved in 30–60 minutes. The drug and its metabolites are excreted in urine. Effects during pregnancy and breastfeeding are unknown so the drug is not recommended during these periods.

Contraindications and cautions

Nicorandil is contraindicated in the presence of allergy to the drug, nicotinamide or nicotinic acid *to avoid hypersensitivity reactions* and with pregnancy or breastfeeding *because of the potential for adverse effects on the fetus or neonate.*

The drug should not be used in individuals with cardiogenic shock, hypotension or acute MI, *which could be exacerbated by the conduction-slowing effects of the drug.*

Adverse effects

The adverse effects associated with nicorandil are related to their effects on cardiac output and smooth muscle. CNS effects include dizziness, light-headedness, headache and fatigue. GI effects can include nausea, dyspepsia and abdominal pain. Cardiovascular effects include hypotension, tachycardia, palpitations and vasodilation. Skin effects include flushing and rash.

Clinically important drug–drug interactions

Nicorandil has been found to have few drug–drug interactions. However, caution should be taken when using the drug concurrently with other drugs that *lower blood pressure, as this effect may be enhanced.* Use of corticosteroids with nicorandil has been found to *increase risk of GI perforation.*

Care considerations for people receiving calcium channel blockers and potassium channel openers

Assessment: history and examination

- Assess for contraindications or cautions: known allergies to any of these drugs *to avoid hypersensitivity reactions*; impaired liver or kidney function, *which could alter the metabolism and excretion of the drug*; heart block, *which could be exacerbated by the conduction depression of these drugs*; and current status of pregnancy or breastfeeding *because of the risk of adverse effects to the fetus or breastfeeding baby.*
- Perform a physical assessment to establish baseline status before beginning therapy and during therapy *to determine the effectiveness and evaluate for any potential adverse effects.*
- Inspect skin for colour and integrity *to identify possible adverse skin reactions.*

- Assess the person's complaint of pain, including onset, duration, intensity and location, and measures used to relieve the pain. Investigate activity level before and after the onset of pain *to aid in identifying possible contributing factors to the pain and its progression.*
- Assess cardiopulmonary status closely, including pulse rate, blood pressure, heart rate and rhythm, *to determine the effects of therapy and identify any adverse effects.*
- Obtain an ECG as ordered *to evaluate heart rate and rhythm.*
- Monitor respirations and auscultate lungs *to evaluate changes in cardiac output.*
- Monitor laboratory test results, including liver and renal function tests, *to determine the need for possible dose adjustment.*

Implementation with rationale

- Monitor the person's blood pressure, cardiac rhythm, and cardiac output closely while the drug is being titrated or dose is being changed *to ensure early detection of potentially serious adverse effects.*
- Monitor blood pressure very carefully if the person is also taking nitrates *because there is an increased risk of hypotensive episodes.*
- If a person is on long-term therapy, periodically monitor blood pressure and cardiac rhythm while using these drugs *because of the potential for adverse cardiovascular effects.*
- Provide comfort measures *to help the person tolerate drug effects.* These include small, frequent meals *to alleviate GI upset*; environmental controls, such as limiting light, maintaining temperature and avoiding excessive noise and interruptions, *which could aggravate stress and increase myocardial demand*; and taking safety precautions, such as providing periodic rests and assisting with ambulation if dizziness occurs, *to prevent injury.*
- Offer support and encouragement *to help the person deal with the diagnosis and the drug regimen.*
- Provide thorough teaching, including the name of the drug and dosage prescribed; measures to avoid adverse effects and prevent anginal attacks; actions to take when an attack occurs; warning signs of problems, and signs and symptoms to report immediately; and the need for periodic monitoring and evaluation *to enhance knowledge about drug therapy and to promote compliance.*

Evaluation

- Monitor response to the drug (alleviation of signs and symptoms of angina, prevention of angina).
- Monitor for adverse effects (hypotension, cardiac arrhythmias, GI upset, skin reactions, headache).
- Monitor the effectiveness of comfort measures and compliance with the regimen.
- Evaluate the effectiveness of the teaching plan (person can name drug, dosage, proper administration, adverse effects to watch for, specific measures to avoid them and the importance of continued follow-up).

KEY POINTS

- Calcium channel blockers block muscle contraction in smooth muscle and decrease the heart's workload, relax vasospasm in variant angina and possibly block the proliferation of the damaged endothelium in coronary vessels.
- Individuals taking calcium channel blockers need to be monitored for signs of decreased cardiac output and response, including slow heart rate, hypotension, dizziness and headache.
- The potassium channel opener, nicorandil, promotes arterial dilation and vascular smooth muscle relaxation, reducing both preload and afterload.

CHAPTER SUMMARY

- CAD, a leading cause of death in Australia and New Zealand and most Western nations, develops when changes in the intima of coronary vessels lead to the development of atheromas or fatty tumours, accumulation of platelets and debris, and a thickening of arterial muscles, resulting in a loss of elasticity and responsiveness to normal stimuli.
- Narrowing of the coronary arteries secondary to the atheroma buildup is called atherosclerosis.
- Narrowed coronary arteries eventually become unable to deliver all the blood that is needed by the myocardial cells, causing a problem of supply and demand.
- Angina pectoris, or 'suffocation of the chest', occurs when the myocardial demand for oxygen cannot be met by the narrowed vessels. Pain, anxiety and fatigue develop when the supply-and-demand ratio is upset. Types of angina include stable, unstable and variant angina.

- MI occurs when a coronary vessel is completely occluded and the cells that depend on that vessel for oxygen become ischaemic, then necrotic and die.
- Angina can be treated by drugs that either increase the supply of oxygen or decrease the heart's workload, which decreases the demand for oxygen.
- Nitrates and beta blockers are used to cause vasodilation and to decrease venous return and arterial resistance – effects that decrease cardiac workload and oxygen consumption.
- Glyceryl trinitrate is the drug of choice for treating an acute anginal attack. It is available in various forms.
- Beta blockers prevent the activation of sympathetic receptors, which would normally increase heart rate, increase blood pressure and increase cardiac contraction. All of these actions would increase the demand for oxygen; blocking these actions decreases the demand for oxygen.
- Calcium channel blockers block muscle contraction in smooth muscle and decrease the heart's workload, relax vasospasm in variant angina and possibly block the proliferation of the damaged endothelium in coronary vessels.
- The potassium channel opener, nicorandil, promotes arterial dilation and vascular smooth muscle relaxation, reducing both preload and afterload.

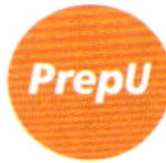

Knowing your strengths and weaknesses helps you to study more effectively. Take a PrepU Practice Quiz to find out how you measure up!

ONLINE RESOURCES

An extensive range of additional resources to enhance teaching and learning and to facilitate understanding of this chapter may be found online at the text's accompanying website, located on thePoint at http://thepoint.lww.com. These include Watch and Learn videos, Concepts in Action animations, journal articles, review questions, case studies, discussion topics and quizzes.

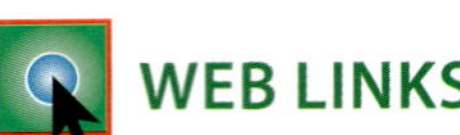

WEB LINKS

Health care providers and students may want to explore information from the following web resources:

www.heartfoundation.org.au
Heart Foundation in Australia, information on angina, drug therapy and current research.

www.heartfoundation.org.nz
Heart Foundation in New Zealand, information on angina, drug therapy and current research.

www.healthnavigator.org.nz/health-a-z/a/angina/#Medicines
Health Navigator New Zealand patient teaching resources about angina

BIBLIOGRAPHY

Cruden, N. & Fox, K. (2011). Current approaches to the management of stable angina. *Prescriber, 22(3)*, 22, 25, 28–31.

Farrell, M. & Dempsey, J. (2014). *Smeltzer & Bare's Textbook of Medical-Surgical Nursing* (3rd edn). Sydney: Lippincott Williams & Wilkins.

Fox, K. (2011). The medical management of stable angina. *British Journal of Cardiology, 18*(supp 3), s1–s12.

Goodman, L. S., Brunton, L. L., Chabner, B. & Knollmann, B. C. (2011). *Goodman and Gilman's Pharmacological Basis of Therapeutics* (12th edn). New York: McGraw-Hill.

Hawley, C. L. (2013). Guidance on optimal management of stable angina in general practice. *Primary Care Cardiovascular Journal, 6(3)*, 112–116.

Hurst, J. W., Fuster, V., Walsh, R. A. & Harrington, R. A. (Eds.). (2011). *Hurst's the Heart* (13th edn). New York: McGraw-Hill.

McKenna, L. & Mirkov, S. (2019). *McKenna's Drug Handbook for Nursing and Midwifery* (8th edn). Sydney: Wolters Kluwer Health Australia.

Porth, C. M. (2011). *Essentials of Pathophysiology: Concepts of Altered Health States* (3rd edn). Philadelphia: Lippincott Williams & Wilkins.

Porth, C. M. (2009). *Pathophysiology: Concepts of Altered Health States* (8th edn). Philadelphia: Lippincott Williams & Wilkins.

Sargent, A. (2011). Prescribing calcium channel blockers. *Nurse Prescribing, 9(3)*, 137–142.

Shah, A. & Fox, K. (2013). Stable angina: Current guidelines and advances in management. *Prescriber, 24(17)*, 35–44.

CHECK YOUR UNDERSTANDING

Answers to the questions in this chapter can be found in Appendix A at the back of this book.

MULTIPLE CHOICE

Select the best answer to the following.

1. Coronary artery disease results in:
   a. an imbalance in cardiac muscle oxygen supply and demand.
   b. delivery of blood to the heart muscle during systole.
   c. increased pulse pressure.
   d. a decreased workload on the heart.
2. Angina:
   a. causes death of heart muscle cells.
   b. is pain due to lack of oxygen to myocardial cells.
   c. cannot occur at rest.
   d. is not treatable.
3. Nitrates are commonly used antianginal drugs that act to:
   a. increase the preload on the heart.
   b. increase the afterload on the heart.
   c. dilate coronary vessels to increase the delivery of oxygen through those vessels.
   d. decrease venous return to the heart, decreasing the myocardial workload.
4. Calcium channel blockers are effective in treating angina because they:
   a. prevent any cardiovascular exercise, preventing strain on the heart.
   b. block strong muscle contractions, causing vasodilation.
   c. alter the electrolyte balance of the heart, preventing arrhythmias.
   d. increase the heart rate, making it more efficient.
5. A nurse or midwife would question an order for which of the following if the person was also receiving verapamil?
   a. oral contraceptives
   b. ciclosporin
   c. digoxin
   d. barbiturate anaesthetics
6. Variant angina occurs as a result of:
   a. electrolyte imbalance.
   b. a spasm of a coronary vessel.
   c. decreased venous return to the heart.
   d. a ventricular arrhythmia.

MULTIPLE RESPONSE

Select all that apply.

1. Treating angina involves modifying factors that could decrease myocardial oxygen consumption. It could be expected that this might include:
   a. weight loss.
   b. use of nitrates.
   c. use of angiotensin-converting-enzyme (ACE) inhibitors.
   d. activity modification.
   e. use of aspirin every day.
   f. use of a calcium channel blocker.
2. An acute myocardial infarction is usually associated with which of the following?
   a. permanent injury to the heart muscle
   b. potentially serious arrhythmias
   c. pain
   d. development of hypertension
   e. loss of consciousness
   f. a feeling of anxiety
3. When describing the action of antianginal drugs to a person, which of the following would the nurse or midwife include?
   a. decrease the workload on the heart
   b. increase the supply of oxygen to the heart
   c. change the metabolic pathway in the heart muscle to remove the need for oxygen
   d. restore the supply-and-demand balance of oxygen in the heart
   e. decrease venous return to the heart
   f. alter the coronary artery filling pathway
4. A person who has glyceryl trinitrate to avert an acute anginal attack would need to be taught:
   a. to take five or six tablets and then seek medical help if no relief occurs.
   b. to buy the tablets in bulk to decrease the cost.
   c. to protect tablets from light and humidity.
   d. to store the tablets in a clearly marked, clear container in open view.
   e. to use the glyceryl trinitrate before an event or activity that will most likely precipitate an anginal attack.
   f. to discard them if they do not fizzle when placed under the tongue.

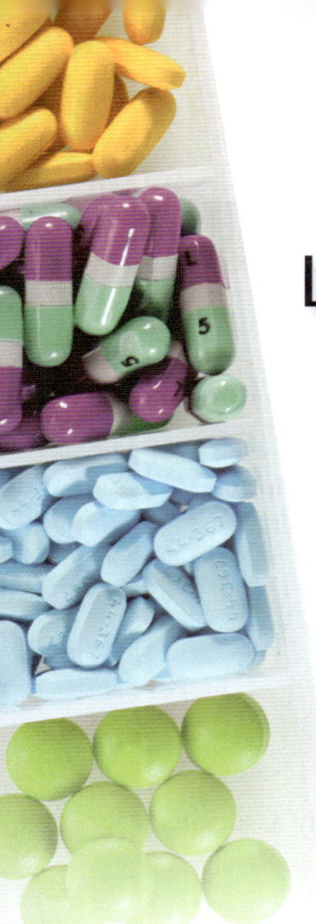

47 Lipid–lowering agents

Learning objectives

On completing this chapter you should be able to:

1. Outline the mechanisms of fat metabolism in the body and discuss the role of hyperlipidaemia as a risk factor for coronary artery disease.
2. Describe the therapeutic actions, indications, pharmacokinetics, contraindications and cautions, most common adverse reactions and important drug–drug interactions associated with the bile acid sequestrants, HMG-CoA reductase inhibitors, cholesterol absorption inhibitors and other agents used to lower lipid levels.
3. Discuss the use of drugs that lower lipid levels across the lifespan.
4. Compare and contrast the prototype drugs colestyramine, atorvastatin and ezetimibe with various other agents used to lower lipid levels.
5. Outline the care considerations, including important teaching points, for people receiving drugs used to lower lipid levels.

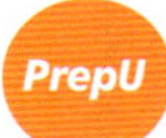

Test your current knowledge of lipid-lowering agents with a PrepU Practice Quiz!

Glossary of key terms

antihyperlipidaemic agents: general term used for drugs used to lower lipid levels in the blood

bile acids: cholesterol-containing acids found in the bile that act like detergents to break up fats in the small intestine

cholesterol: necessary component of human cells that is produced and processed in the liver, then stored in the bile until stimulus causes the gallbladder to contract and send the bile into the duodenum via the common bile duct; a fat that is essential for the formation of steroid hormones and cell membranes; it is produced in cells and taken in by dietary sources

chylomicron: carrier for lipids in the bloodstream, consisting of proteins, lipids, cholesterol, and other molecules

endocannabinoids: endogenous substances that activate nervous system receptors that are important in the regulation of appetite, food intake and metabolism

high-density lipoprotein (HDL): loosely packed chylomicron containing fats, able to absorb fats and fat remnants in the periphery; thought to have a protective effect, decreasing the development of coronary artery disease

hydroxymethylglutaryl-coenzyme A (HMG-CoA) reductase: enzyme that regulates the last step in cellular cholesterol synthesis

hyperlipidaemia: increased levels of lipids in the serum, associated with increased risk of coronary artery disease development

low-density lipoprotein (LDL): tightly packed fats that are thought to contribute to the development of coronary artery disease when remnants left over from the LDL are processed in the arterial lining

metabolic syndrome: a collection of factors, including insulin resistance, abdominal obesity, low high-density lipoprotein and high triglyceride levels, hypertension and proinflammatory and prothrombotic states that increase the incidence of coronary artery disease

risk factors: factors that have been identified as increasing the risk of the development of a disease; for coronary artery disease, risk factors include genetic predisposition, gender, age, high-fat diet, sedentary lifestyle, gout, hypertension, diabetes and oestrogen deficiency

LIPID-LOWERING AGENTS

Bile acid sequestrants

(P) colestyramine
colestipol

HMG-CoA reductase inhibitors

(P) atorvastatin
fluvastatin
pravastatin
rosuvastatin
simvastatin

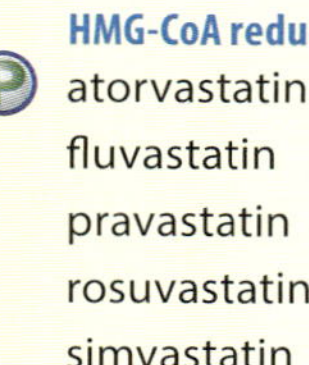

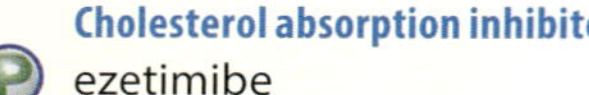

Cholesterol absorption inhibitor

(P) ezetimibe

OTHER LIPID-LOWERING AGENTS

Fibrates

fenofibrate
gemfibrozil

Vitamin B

nicotinic acid

The drugs discussed in this chapter lower serum levels of cholesterol and various lipids. These drugs are sometimes called **antihyperlipidaemic agents** used to treat **hyperlipidaemia** – an increase in the level of lipids in the blood. There is mounting evidence that the incidence of coronary artery disease (CAD), the leading killer of adults in the Western world, is higher among people with high serum lipid levels. The cause of CAD is poorly understood, but some evidence indicates that cholesterol and fat may play a major role in disease development. Lipid and triglyceride levels play a role in **metabolic syndrome**, a collection of factors, including insulin resistance, abdominal obesity, low high-density lipoprotein and high triglyceride levels, hypertension and proinflammatory and prothrombotic states, that has been shown to increase the incidence of CAD. See Table 47.1.

TABLE 47.1 Clinical aspects of the metabolic syndrome

Parameter	Significant values
Insulin resistance	Fasting blood glucose > 7.0 mmol/L
Abdominal obesity	Waist measurement > 94 cm in men; > 80 cm in women; > 90 cm in men from Middle Eastern, South Asian, Chinese, Asian-Indian, South and Central American backgrounds
Lipid abnormalities	High density lipoproteins (HDLs) > 1.0 mmol/L; any triglycerides (TG) > 2.0 mmol/L
Hypertension	Blood pressure > 130/85 mmHg
Proinflammatory state	Increased macrophage levels, increased levels of interleukin-6 and tumour necrosis factor (TNF)
Prothrombotic state	Increased plasminogen activator levels

CORONARY ARTERY DISEASE

As explained in Chapter 46, CAD is characterised by the progressive growth of atheromatous plaques, or atheromas, in the coronary arteries. These plaques, which begin as fatty streaks in the endothelium, eventually injure the endothelial lining of the artery, causing an inflammatory reaction. This inflammatory process triggers the development of characteristic foam cells containing fats and white blood cells that further injure the endothelial lining. Over time, platelets, fibrin, other fats and remnants collect on the injured vessel lining and cause the atheroma to grow, further narrowing the interior of the blood vessel and limiting blood flow.

The injury to the vessel also causes scarring and a thickening of the vessel wall. As the vessel thickens, it becomes less distensible and less reactive to many neurological and chemical stimuli that would ordinarily dilate or constrict it. As a result, the coronary vessels are no longer able to balance the myocardial demand for oxygen with increased blood supply. More recent evidence indicates that the makeup of the core of the atheroma may be a primary determinant of which atheromas might rupture and cause acute blockage of a vessel. The softer, more lipid-filled atheromas appear to be more likely to rupture than the stable, harder cores.

BOX 47.1 Risk factors for coronary artery disease

Unmodifiable risk factors

- *Genetic predispositions*: CAD is more likely to occur in people who have a family history of the disease, particularly if the disease occurs in relatives younger than the age of 55 years.
- *Age*: the incidence of CAD increases with age.
- *Gender*: men are more likely than premenopausal women to have CAD; however, the incidence is almost equal in men and postmenopausal women, possibly because of a protective effect of oestrogens (see Box 47.3).

Modifiable risk factors

- *Gout*: increased uric acid levels seem to injure vessel walls.
- *Cigarette smoking*: nicotine causes vasoconstriction and may have an effect on the endothelium of blood vessels; over time, smoking can lower oxygen levels in the blood.
- *Sedentary lifestyle*: exercise increases the levels of chemicals that seem to protect the coronary arteries.
- *High stress levels*: constant sympathetic reactions increase the myocardial oxygen demand while causing vasoconstriction and may contribute to a remodelling of the blood vessel endothelium, leading to an increased susceptibility to atheroma development.
- *Hypertension*: high pressure in the arteries causes endothelial injury and increases afterload and myocardial oxygen demand.
- *Obesity*: this may reflect altered fat metabolism and will increase the heart's workload.
- *Diabetes*: people with diabetes have a capillary membrane thickening, which accelerates the effects of atherosclerosis and abnormal fat metabolism, which increases lipid levels.
- *Other factors* that, if untreated, may contribute to CAD include bacterial infections (*Chlamydia* infections have been correlated with onset of CAD, and treatment with tetracycline and fluororoentgenography has been associated with decreased incidence of CAD, indicating a possible bacterial link) and autoimmune processes (some plaques contain antibodies and other products of immune reactions, making autoimmune reactions a possibility).

Risk factors

Strong evidence exists that atheroma development occurs more quickly in individuals with elevated cholesterol and lipid levels. People who consume high-fat diets are more likely to develop high lipid levels. However, individuals without increased lipid levels can also develop atheromas leading to CAD, so other factors evidently contribute to this process. Although the exact mechanism of atherogenesis (atheroma development) is not understood, certain **risk factors** increase the likelihood that a person will develop CAD. Metabolic syndrome occurs when a person has several risk factors: increased insulin resistance, high blood pressure, altered lipid levels and a proinflammatory and prothrombotic state, which seem to increase the risk of CAD development dramatically. Unmodifiable and modifiable risk factors are presented in Box 47.1. Different ethnic groups also have different risk factors, as discussed in Box 47.2, as do different genders, as discussed in Box 47.3.

Treatment

Because an exact cause of CAD is not known, successful treatment involves manipulating a number of these risk factors (see Table 47.2). Overall treatment and prevention of CAD should include the following measures: decreasing dietary fats (decreasing total fat intake and limiting saturated fats seems to have the most impact on serum lipid levels); losing weight, which helps to decrease insulin resistance and the development of type 2 diabetes; eliminating smoking; increasing exercise levels; decreasing stress; and treating hypertension, diabetes and gout.

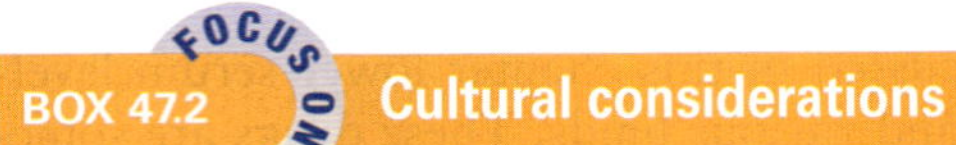

BOX 47.2 Cultural considerations

Variations in lipoprotein levels

Australia and New Zealand both have high incidences of coronary artery disease. Certain risk factors are known to place particular cultural groups at higher risk than national averages. Among the ethnic groups in New Zealand, death rates of Pacific people are higher than in Māori in hypertensive disease, cerebrovascular disease and cardiomyopathy (males). The CHD death rate in Māori men has fallen since 1996, but risen in women, while rates in Pacific people have increased in both men and women. (Source: www.heartfoundation.org.nz. Technical Report 82: Cardiovascular Disease in New Zealand, 2004: A Summary of Recent Statistical Information.)

In Australia, Indigenous Australians have been reported to have three times the rate of death from major coronary events than other Australians. (AIHW 2010. Australia's health 2010. Cat. no. AUS 122. Canberra: AIHW.)

There are identified cultural variations in lipid levels as well. Cultural variations in key lipid parameters have been identified in the specific ethnic groups below; however, currently no data exist for Pacific Islander, Māori people or Indigenous Australians in relation to lipid profiles.

Cultural variations in key lipid parameters include:

- serum cholesterol levels: whites > African Americans, Native Americans
- high-density lipoprotein (HDL) levels: African Americans, Asians > whites
- low-density lipoprotein (LDL) levels: African Americans < whites
- HDL: cholesterol ratio: African Americans < whites

KEY POINTS

- CAD is the leading cause of death in the Western world. It is associated with the development of atheromas or plaques in arterial linings that lead to narrowing of the lumen of the artery and hardening of the artery wall, with loss of distensibility and responsiveness to stimuli for contraction or dilation.
- The cause of CAD is not known, but many contributing risk factors have been identified, including increasing age, male gender, genetic predisposition, high-fat diet, sedentary lifestyle, smoking, obesity, high stress levels, bacterial infections, diabetes, hypertension, gout and menopause. The presence of many of these factors constitutes metabolic syndrome.
- Treatment and prevention of CAD are aimed at manipulating the known risk factors to decrease CAD development and progression.

FAT AND BIOTRANSFORMATION (METABOLISM)

Fats are taken into the body as dietary fats, then broken down in the stomach to fatty acids, lipids and cholesterol (Figure 47.1). The presence of these products in the duodenum stimulates contraction of the gallbladder and the release of bile. **Bile acids**, which contain high levels of **cholesterol** (a fat), act like a detergent in the small intestine and break up the fats into small units, called micelles, which can be absorbed into the wall of the small intestine. (Imagine ads for dishwashing detergents that break up the grease and fats in the dishwashing water; bile acids do much the same thing.) The bile acids are then reabsorbed and recycled to the gallbladder, where they remain until the gallbladder is again stimulated to release them to facilitate fat absorption.

Fats and water do not mix and cannot be absorbed directly into the plasma. To allow absorption, micelles are carried on a **chylomicron**, a package of fats and proteins.

BOX 47.3 FOCUS ON **Gender considerations**

Women and heart disease

Until the late 1990s, heart disease was considered to be a condition that primarily affected men. Because of that belief, women were seldom screened for heart disease, and when they did experience acute cardiac events, they were not treated promptly or adequately. However, recent research has shown that heart disease is the leading cause of death among women, surpassing such diseases as breast and colon cancers. This finding has led to further research, still ongoing, about women and heart disease.

Women enjoy a protective hormone effect against the development of coronary artery disease (CAD) until menopause, when oestrogen loss seems to rapidly increase the production of atheromas and the development of CAD. In several studies, women who received hormone replacement therapy (HRT) at menopause had a significantly reduced risk of CAD and myocardial infarction (MI) in the first few years after the onset of menopause. Research showed, however, that after 5 years of HRT the incidence of MI and stroke rose sharply, leading to an early closure of the study. Studies have found that women experience different symptoms of heart disease – jaw and neck pain, fatigue and insomnia – and sometimes these are overlooked.

HRT is not recommended as a means of reducing the risk of heart disease or stroke, although it is still recommended for the treatment of severe menopausal symptoms in the first few years after menopause. Women should be advised to reduce other cardiac risk factors by eating a diet low in saturated fats, exercising regularly, not smoking, controlling weight, managing stress, and seeking treatment for gout, hypertension and diabetes.

Clearly, heart disease is not just a disease of men. Research will continue to offer health care professionals new information on preventing and treating heart disease in women.

TABLE 47.2 Risk factors for coronary artery disease

Unmodifiable risks	Modifiable risks	Suggested modifications
Family history	Sedentary lifestyle	Exercise
Age	High-fat diet	Low-fat diet (polyunsaturated and monounsaturated fats)
Gender	Smoking	Smoking cessation
	Obesity	Weight loss
	High stress levels	Stress management
	Bacterial infections	Antibiotic treatment
	Diabetes	Control of blood glucose levels
	Hypertension	Control of blood pressure
	Gout	Control of uric acid levels
	Menopause	Hormone replacement therapy (first few years of menopause only)

This packaging is done by brush enzymes in all of the small intestine. The chylomicrons pass through the wall of the small intestine, are picked up by the surrounding intestinal lymphatic system, travel through the system to the heart, and are then sent out into circulation. The proteins that are exposed on the chylomicron, called apoproteins, determine the fate of the lipids or fats being carried. For example, some of these packages are broken down in the tissues to be used for energy, some are stored in fat deposits for future use as energy and some continue to the liver, where they are further processed into lipoproteins.

Lipoproteins

The lipoproteins produced in the liver that have well-known clinical implications are the **low-density lipoproteins (LDLs)** and the **high-density lipoproteins (HDLs)**. LDLs enter the circulation as tightly packed cholesterol, triglycerides and lipids – all of which are carried by proteins that enter the circulation to be broken down for energy or stored for future use as energy. When an LDL package is broken down, many remnants or leftovers need to be returned to the liver for recycling. If a person has many of these remnants in the blood vessels, it is thought that the inflammatory process is initiated to help remove this debris. Some experts believe that this is the underlying process involved in atherogenesis.

HDLs enter the circulation as loosely packed lipids that are used for energy and to pick up remnants of fats and cholesterol that are left in the periphery by LDL breakdown. HDLs serve a protective role in cleaning up remnants in blood vessels. It is known that HDL levels increase during exercise, which could explain why people who exercise regularly lower their risk of CAD. HDL levels also increase in response to oestrogen, which could explain some of the protective effect of oestrogen before menopause.

Cholesterol

The body needs fats, particularly cholesterol, to maintain normal function. Cholesterol is the base unit for the formation of the steroid hormones (the sex hormones, as well as the adrenal cortical hormones). It is also a basic

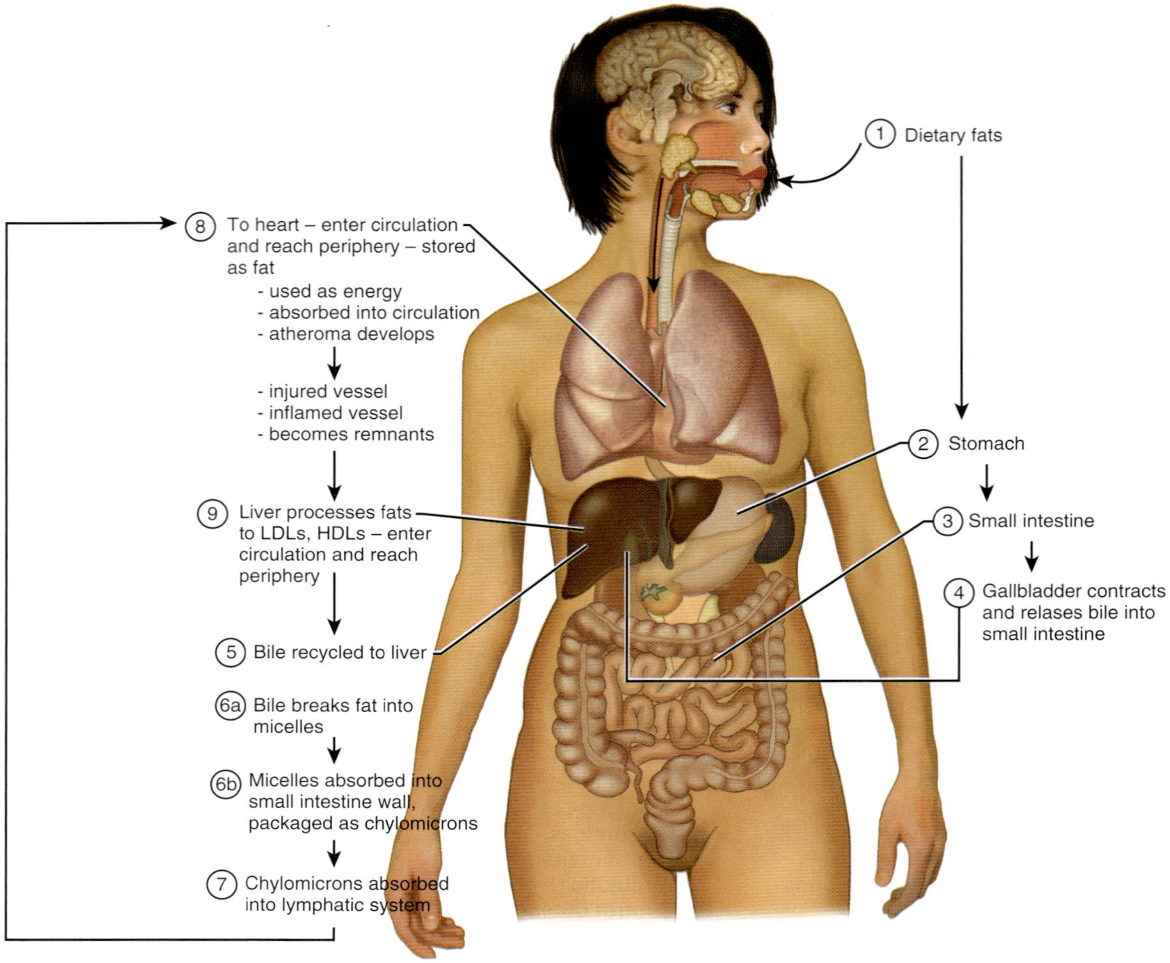

FIGURE 47.1 Metabolism of fats in the body.

unit in the formation and maintenance of cell membranes. Cholesterol is usually provided through the diet and the fat metabolism process just described. If dietary cholesterol falls off, the body is prepared to produce cholesterol to ensure that the cell membranes and the endocrine system are intact.

Every cell in the body has the metabolic capability of producing cholesterol. The enzyme **hydroxymethylglutaryl-coenzyme A (HMG-CoA) reductase** regulates the early, rate-limiting step in the cellular synthesis of cholesterol. If dietary cholesterol is severely limited, the cellular synthesis of cholesterol will increase.

Hyperlipidaemias

When the levels of lipids in the blood increase, hyperlipidaemia occurs. This can result from excessive dietary intake of fats or from genetic alterations in fat metabolism leading to a variety of elevated fats in the blood (eg, hypercholesterolaemia, hypertriglyceridaemia, alterations in LDL and HDL concentrations). Cultural variations related to lipid levels have also been identified (see Box 47.4).

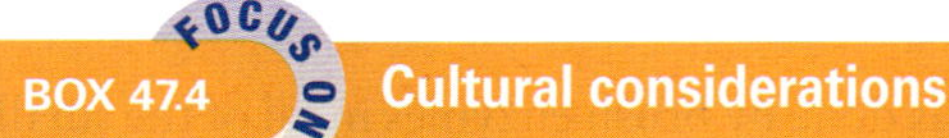

BOX 47.4 Cultural considerations

Rosuvastatin and Asian people

Rosuvastatin reaches higher serum levels in Asian people than in other populations. Higher serum levels are associated with an increased risk for rhabdomyolysis. It is recommended that this drug be reserved for use in non-Asian people.

Dietary modifications are often successful in treating hyperlipidaemia that is caused by excessive dietary intake of fats. Drug therapy is needed if the cause is genetically linked alterations in lipid levels or if dietary limits do not decrease the serum lipid levels to an acceptable range. The NHF (2012) recommends the following standard goals for lipid levels: LDL–cholesterol (LDL-c) < 1.8; HDL-c > 1.0; TG < 2.0; and non-HDL-c < 2.5. Antihyperlipidaemic agents such as bile acid sequestrants, HMG-CoA reductase inhibitors, fibrates, niacin, cholesterol absorption inhibitors and, in some cases, hormones (in women) may be used. These drugs are often used in combination and should be part of an overall health care regimen that includes exercise, dietary restrictions and lifestyle changes.

See the Critical thinking scenario for additional information on treating hyperlipidaemia.

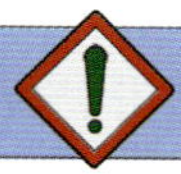

CRITICAL THINKING SCENARIO

Treating hyperlipidaemia

THE SITUATION

M.M., a 55-year-old Caucasian businessman, was seen for a routine insurance physical examination. He was found to be obese and borderline hypertensive, with a non-fasting LDL level of above 4.0 mmol/L (very high). M.M. reported smoking two packs of cigarettes a day and noted in his family history that both of his parents died of heart attacks before the age of 50. He described himself as a 'workaholic' with no time to exercise and a tendency to eat most of his meals in restaurants. The primary medical regimen suggested for M.M. included stopping or decreasing smoking, weight loss, dietary changes to eliminate saturated fats and decreased stress. On a return visit after 4 weeks, M.M. had lost 3.5 kg and reported a decrease in smoking, but his LDL levels were unchanged. The use of an antihyperlipidaemic drug was discussed. He was started on atorvastatin and advised to continue the diet and exercise program and to return in 3 months for follow-up.

CRITICAL THINKING

What care interventions are appropriate at this point? *Consider all of the known risk factors for CAD; then rank M.M's risk based on those factors.*

What lifestyle changes can help M.M. to reduce his risk of heart disease?

What support services should be consulted to help M.M.?

Should other tests be done before considering any drug therapy for M.M.? *Think about the kind of teaching that would help M.M. to cope with the overwhelming lifestyle changes that have been suggested, yet remain compliant with his medical regimen.*

DISCUSSION

M.M.'s description of himself as a workaholic should alert the health care provider to the possibility that he will have trouble adapting to any prescribed lifestyle changes. (Workaholics tend to be very organised, goal-driven and somewhat controlling individuals.) M.M. should first receive extensive teaching about CAD, his risk factors and his options. The benefits of decreasing or eliminating risk factors should be discussed. Drug therapy is intended as an adjunct to diet and exercise, and the effectiveness of drug therapy improves remarkably when diet and exercise changes are made. M.M. may be more compliant if he exercises some control over his situation, so he should be invited to suggest possible lifestyle changes or adaptations. M.M. also should be encouraged to set short-range goals that are achievable, to help him feel successful. He needs to understand that beginning drug therapy does not mean that exercise and diet are no longer important.

M.M. also needs to understand that antihyperlipidaemic drugs can cause dizziness, headaches, gastrointestinal (GI) upset and constipation. Because of his busy lifestyle, M.M. may have trouble coping with these adverse effects. M.M.'s health care provider may need to try a variety of different drugs or combinations of drugs to find ones that are effective but do not cause unacceptable adverse effects.

The Australian National Heart Foundation has numerous booklets, diets, support groups and counsellors who can help M.M. as he tries to adapt to his medical regimen. He can contact the Foundation online at www.heartfoundation.org.au for a quick reference and referrals to other sources. M.M. will benefit from having a consistent health care provider who can offer him encouragement, answer any questions and allow him to vent his feelings. Often, lifestyle changes are the most difficult part of this medical regimen, so M.M. will need constant support.

CARE GUIDE FOR M.M.: HMG-CoA REDUCTASE INHIBITORS

Assessment: history and examination

Assess M.M.'s health history for allergies to any HMG-CoA reductase inhibitor or fungal byproducts; hepatic dysfunction; or endocrine disorders.

Focus the physical examination on the following areas:

Cardiovascular: blood pressure, pulse, perfusion

Neurological (CNS): orientation, affect, reflexes, vision

Skin: colour, lesions, texture

Respiratory system: rate, adventitious sounds

GI: abdominal examination, bowel sounds

Laboratory tests: liver and renal function tests, serum lipids

Implementation

Administer the drug at bedtime.

Monitor serum lipids before therapy and periodically during therapy.

Provide comfort and safety measures: give small meals.

Arrange for periodic ophthalmic examinations to screen for cataracts.

Give the drug with food if GI upset occurs.

Institute bowel program as needed.

Provide safety measures if needed.

Monitor liver function, and arrange to stop the drug if liver impairment occurs.

Provide support and reassurance to deal with drug effects and the need to make lifestyle, diet and exercise changes.

Provide teaching regarding drug, dosage, adverse effects, what to report and safety precautions.

Evaluation

Evaluate drug effects: lowering of serum cholesterol and lipid levels, prevention of first MI, slowed progression of CAD.

Monitor for adverse effects: sedation, dizziness, headache, cataracts, GI upset; hepatic or renal dysfunction; rhabdomyolysis.

Monitor for drug–drug interactions as indicated for each drug.

Evaluate the effectiveness of the teaching program.

Evaluate the effectiveness of comfort and safety measures.

TEACHING FOR M.M.

- An HMG-CoA reductase inhibitor, or 'statin', is an antihyperlipidaemic agent, which means that it works to decrease the levels of certain lipids, or fats, in your blood. An increase in serum lipid levels has been associated with the development of many blood vessel disorders, including coronary artery disease, which can lead to a heart attack. This drug must be used in conjunction with a low-calorie, low-saturated-fat diet and an exercise program.
- Some of the following adverse effects may occur:
  - *Headache, blurred vision, nervousness, insomnia*: avoid driving or performing hazardous or delicate tasks that require concentration; these effects may pass with time.
  - *Nausea, vomiting, flatulence, constipation*: small, frequent meals may help. If constipation becomes a problem, consult with your health care provider for appropriate interventions.
  - Report any of the following to your health care provider: *severe GI upset, vision changes, unusual bleeding, dark urine or light-coloured stools, or sudden muscle pain accompanied by fever.*
- You will need to have regular medical examinations to monitor the effectiveness of this drug on your lipid levels and to detect any adverse effects. These examinations will include blood tests and eye examinations.
- Avoid grapefruit juice while you are taking this drug.
- Tell any doctor, nurse or other health care provider that you are taking this drug.
- Keep this drug, and all medications, out of the reach of children.
- To help to decrease your risk of heart disease, follow these guidelines; adhere to a diet that is low in calories and saturated fat, exercise regularly, stop smoking and reduce stress.

KEY POINTS

- CAD is associated with arterial atheromas or plaques, narrowed arterial lumens and hardening of the artery wall, all of which lead to impaired contraction and vascular dilatation.
- Risk factors for CAD include increasing age, male gender, genetic predisposition, high-fat diet, sedentary lifestyle, smoking, obesity, high stress levels, bacterial infections, diabetes, hypertension, gout and menopause.
- CAD prevention and treatment aim at decreasing risk factors to delay disease or decrease its progress.
- Hyperlipidaemia refers to an increase in the level of lipids (cholesterol and triglycerides) in the blood.
- Hyperlipidaemia increases a person's risk for the development of CAD.
- Fats are taken into the body as dietary fats, then broken down in the stomach to fatty acids, lipids and cholesterol.
- Bile acids act like detergents to break down or metabolise fats into small molecules called micelles, which are absorbed into the intestinal wall and combined with proteins to become chylomicrons, to allow transport throughout the circulatory system.
- Cholesterol is a fat that is used to make bile acids; all cells can produce cholesterol, which is the base for steroid hormones and cell membrane structure.
- The enzyme HMG-CoA reductase controls the final step that produces cellular cholesterol; HMG-CoA is active in every cell.

LIPID-LOWERING AGENTS

Lipid-lowering agents lower serum levels of cholesterol and various lipids. These include bile acid sequestrants, HMG-CoA reductase inhibitors and a cholesterol absorption inhibitor. Other drugs that are used to affect lipid levels do not fall into any of these classes but are approved for use in combination with changes in diet and exercise (see section on Other lipid-lowering agents). Box 47.5 summarises the use of lipid-lowering agents in different age groups.

Bile acid sequestrants

Bile acid sequestrants are used to decrease plasma cholesterol levels. Two bile acid sequestrants currently (but rarely) in use are colestyramine (*Questran*) and colestipol (*Colestid*).

Therapeutic actions and indications

Bile acid sequestrants bind with bile acids in the intestine to form an insoluble complex that is then excreted in the faeces (Figure 47.2). Bile acids contain high levels

BOX 47.5 FOCUS ON

Drug therapy across the lifespan

Lipid-lowering agents

CHILDREN

Familial hypercholesterolaemia may be seen in children. Because of the importance of lipids in the developing nervous system, treatment is usually restricted to tight dietary restrictions to limit fats and calories.

The HMG-CoA reductase inhibitors simvastatin and atorvastatin can be used in postmenarchal girls and boys 10–17 years of age for treating familial hypercholesterolaemia. Pravastatin has been approved for use in children older than 8 years of age, but these children should be monitored very closely.

ADULTS

Lifestyle changes, including dietary restrictions, exercise, smoking cessation and stress reduction, should be tried before any antihyperlipidaemic drug is used.

HMG-CoA reductase inhibitors are the first drug of choice in the treatment of hypercholesterolaemia in people who are at risk for, or who have already developed, CAD. The drugs are well tolerated and less expensive than some of the other antihyperlipidaemic drugs. Combination therapy with a bile acid sequestrant, a fibrate, or nicotinic acid may be necessary if lipid levels still cannot be reduced.

PREGNANCY AND BREASTFEEDING

Women of childbearing age should not take HMG-CoA reductase inhibitors (Pregnancy Category X). Bile acid sequestrants are the drug of choice for these women if a lipid-lowering agent is needed.

OLDER ADULTS

Lifestyle changes, including dietary restrictions, exercise, smoking cessation and stress reduction, should be tried before any antihyperlipidaemic drug is used.

Lower doses of HMG-CoA reductase inhibitors should be used in elderly people and in any person with renal dysfunction. Care must be taken with those drugs that cannot be cut, crushed or chewed. People should be alerted about these restrictions.

Lipid-lowering agents have little value for a frail elder with limited life expectancy and living in long-term care, and therefore should be discontinued.

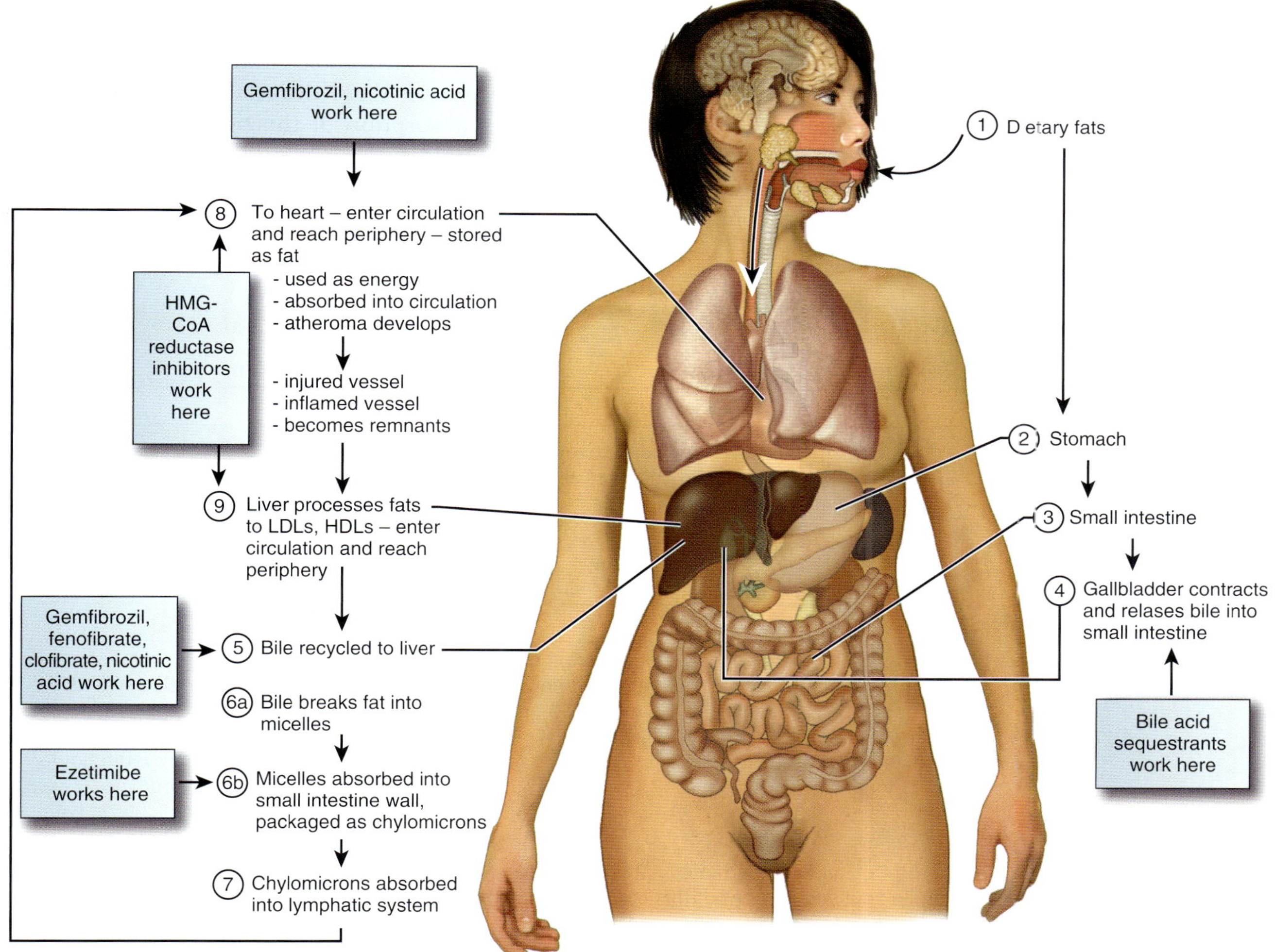

FIGURE 47.2 Sites of action of lipid-lowering agents.

of cholesterol. As a result, the liver must use cholesterol to make more bile acids. The hepatic intracellular cholesterol level falls, leading to an increased absorption of cholesterol-containing LDL segments from the circulation to replenish the cell's cholesterol. The serum levels of cholesterol and LDL decrease as the circulating cholesterol is used to provide the cholesterol that the liver needs to make bile acids. These drugs are used to reduce serum cholesterol in individuals with primary hypercholesterolaemia (manifested by high cholesterol and high LDL levels) as an adjunct to diet and exercise. Colestyramine is also used to treat pruritus associated with partial biliary obstruction. See Table 47.3 for usual indications for each of these drugs.

Pharmacokinetics

Bile acid sequestrants are not absorbed systemically. They act while in the intestine and are excreted directly in the faeces. Their action is limited to their effects while they are present in the intestine. Colestyramine is a powder that must be mixed with liquids and taken up to six times a day. Colestipol is available in both powder and tablet form and is taken only four times a day.

Contraindications and cautions

Bile acid sequestrants are contraindicated in the presence of allergy to any bile acid sequestrant *to prevent hypersensitivity reactions*. These drugs also are contraindicated in the following conditions: complete biliary obstruction, *which would prevent bile from being secreted into the intestine*; abnormal intestinal function, *which could be aggravated by the presence of these drugs*; and pregnancy or breastfeeding *because the potential decrease in the absorption of fat and fat-soluble vitamins could have a detrimental effect on the fetus or neonate*. If a lipid-lowering drug is needed, however, a bile acid sequestrant is the drug of choice.

Adverse effects

Adverse effects associated with the use of these drugs include headache, anxiety, fatigue and drowsiness, which could be related to changes in serum cholesterol levels. Direct GI irritation, including nausea, constipation that may progress to faecal impaction, and aggravation of haemorrhoids may occur. Other effects include increased bleeding times related to a decreased absorption of vitamin K and consequent decreased production of clotting factors; vitamin A and D deficiencies related to decreased absorption of fat-soluble vitamins; rash; and muscle aches and pains.

Clinically important drug–drug interactions

Malabsorption of fat-soluble vitamins occurs when they are combined with these drugs. These drugs decrease or delay the absorption of thiazide diuretics, digoxin, warfarin, thyroid hormones and corticosteroids. Consequently, any of these drugs should be taken 1 hour before or 4–6 hours after the bile acid sequestrant.

TABLE 47.3 *DRUGS IN FOCUS* Lipid-lowering drugs

Drug name	Dosage/route	Usual indications
Bile acid sequestrants		
(P) colestyramine (*Questran*)	4 g PO 1–2 times a day, maximum dose 24 g/day; must be mixed with water or other non-carbonated fluids	Adjunctive treatment of primary hypercholesterolaemia; treatment of pruritus associated with partial biliary obstruction
colestipol (*Colestid*)	15–30 g/day PO in 2–4 divided doses Must be mixed with 100–150 mL of fluid	Adjunctive treatment of primary hypercholesterolaemia
HMG-CoA reductase inhibitors		
(P) atorvastatin (*Lipitor, Lorstat, Zarator*)	10 mg/day PO with a possible dose range of 10–80 mg/day; may be taken at any time of day Children (10–18 years): 10 mg/day PO, maximum dose 20 mg/day	Adjunctive therapy for reduction of increased cholesterol and low-density lipoprotein (LDL) levels, triglycerides; prevention of CAD in adults with multiple risk factors; approved to lower cholesterol levels in children 10–17 years of age who meet specific criteria with genetic hyperlipidaemias
fluvastatin (*Lescol*)	80 mg PO, taken at bedtime; > 2 hours after a bile acid sequestrant, if this combination is being used	Adjunctive therapy for reduction of increased cholesterol and LDL levels; to slow the progression of CAD in people with known CAD; reduction of the risk of undergoing revascularisation procedures

TABLE 47.3 DRUGS IN FOCUS Lipid-lowering drugs *(continued)*

Drug name	Dosage/route	Usual indications
HMG-CoA reductase inhibitors *(continued)*		
pravastatin (*Cholstat, Cholvastin, Pravachol*)	10–40 mg/day PO taken at bedtime; start with 10 mg/day in elderly people and people with hepatic or renal impairment Children (8–13 years): 10 mg daily at night, up to 20 mg/day PO; children (14–18 years): 10 mg daily at night, up to 40 mg/day PO	Only statin with outcome data to show effectiveness in decreasing CAD and incidence of MI; prevents first MI even in people who do not have a documented increased cholesterol concentration (an effect possibly related to blocking of the formation of foam cells in injured arteries); adjunctive therapy for reduction of increased cholesterol and LDL levels; approved for use with children > 8 years of age with genetically linked hyperlipidaemia, as an adjunct to diet and exercise
rosuvastatin (*Crestor*)	5–10 mg/day PO initial dose range; maximum 40 mg/day	Adjunctive therapy for reduction of increased cholesterol, LDL levels and triglycerides; with diet to slow the progression of atherosclerosis; raises HDL level slightly better than the other statins and at a lower price
simvastatin (*Lipex, Simvar, Zocor*)	10–80 mg/day PO taken once a day in the evening; start with 10 mg/day in elderly people and in people with hepatic or renal impairment Children (10–17 years): 10 mg/day PO, up to 40 mg/day based on response	Prevention of first MI in people with known hypercholesterolaemia and CAD; adjunctive therapy for reduction of increased cholesterol and LDL levels; approved to lower cholesterol levels in children 10–17 years of age who meet specific criteria with genetic hyperlipidaemias
Cholesterol absorption inhibitor		
(P) ezetimibe (*Ezetrol*)	10 mg/day PO	Adjunct to diet and exercise to reduce cholesterol as monotherapy or combined with an HMG-CoA reductase inhibitor or a bile acid sequestrant; adjunct to diet to reduce elevated sitoterol and campesterol levels in homozygous sitosterolaemia (to reduce elevated sitosterol and campesterol levels, the enzymes that are elevated when people have this rare disorder); used in combination with atorvastatin or simvastatin as treatment for homozygous familial hypercholesterolaemia
Other lipid-lowering agents		
Fibrates		
fenofibrate (*Lipidil*)	145 mg/day PO given with a meal. Patients with renal impairment: initially 48 mg/day up to 96 mg/day; monitor people with impaired renal function and the elderly very carefully; contraindicated for creatinine clearance < 30 mL/min	Treatment of very high triglyceride levels in adults who are at risk for pancreatitis if not responsive to dietary measures
gemfibrozil (*Lipazil*)	600 mg bd, on an empty stomach; maximum 1.5 g/day	Treatment of very high triglyceride levels with abdominal pain and potential pancreatitis in adults
Vitamin B		
nicotinic acid (generic)	Initially 100 mg tid, increased to usual dose of 1 g tid; maximum 3 g tid	Treatment of hyperlipidaemia not responding to diet and weight loss; to slow progression of coronary artery disease when combined with a bile acid sequestrant

Prototype summary: colestyramine

Indications: reduction of elevated serum cholesterol in people with primary hypercholesterolaemia; pruritus associated with partial biliary obstruction.

Actions: binds with bile acids in the intestine, allowing excretion in faeces instead of reabsorption, causing cholesterol to be oxidised in the liver and serum cholesterol levels to fall.

Pharmacokinetics: not absorbed systemically.

$T_{1/2}$: not absorbed systemically, excreted in faeces.

Adverse effects: rash, headache, anxiety, vertigo, dizziness, constipation due to faecal impaction, exacerbation of haemorrhoids, cramps, flatulence, nausea, increased bleeding tendencies, vitamin A and D deficiencies, muscle and joint pain.

Care considerations for people receiving bile acid sequestrants

Assessment: history and examination

- Assess for contraindications or cautions: known allergies to these drugs *to avoid hypersensitivity reactions*; impaired intestinal function, *which could be exacerbated by these drugs*; biliary obstruction, *which could block the effectiveness of these drugs*; and current status related to pregnancy and breastfeeding *because of the potential for adverse effects on the fetus or breastfeeding baby.*
- Perform a physical assessment *to establish a baseline before beginning therapy and during therapy to determine the effectiveness of therapy and evaluate for any potential adverse effects.*
- Weigh the person *to establish a baseline and evaluate for changes reflecting lifestyle changes that accompany drug therapy.*
- Inspect the person's skin for colour, bruising and rash *to evaluate for possible adverse effects.*
- Assess neurological status, including level of orientation and alertness, *to determine any central nervous system effects.*
- Monitor pulse and blood pressure *for changes related to changes in CAD risk factors.*
- Inspect the abdomen for distension and auscultate bowel sounds *for changes in GI motility.*
- Assess bowel elimination patterns, including frequency of stool passage and stool characteristics, *to identify possible constipation and faecal impaction.*
- Monitor the results of laboratory tests, including serum cholesterol and lipid levels, *to evaluate the effectiveness of drug therapy.*

Implementation with rationale

- Do not administer powdered agents in dry form; *these drugs must be mixed in fluids to be effective.* Mix with fruit juices, soups, liquids, cereals or pulpy fruits. Mix colestipol, but not colestyramine, with carbonated beverages. Stir, and encourage the person to swallow all of the dose.
- If the person is taking tablets, ensure that tablets are not cut, chewed or crushed *because they are designed to be broken down in the GI tract; if they are crushed, the active ingredients will not be effective.* Urge the person to swallow tablets whole with plenty of fluid.
- Give the drug before meals *to ensure that the drug is in the GI tract with food.*
- Administer other oral medications 1 hour before or 4–6 hours after the bile sequestrant *to avoid drug–drug interactions.*
- Arrange for a bowel program as appropriate *to effectively deal with constipation if it occurs.*
- Provide comfort measures *to help the person tolerate the drug effects.* These include small, frequent meals to reduce the risk of nausea; ready access to bathroom facilities to prevent constipation; safety precautions to prevent injury if dizziness, central nervous system (CNS) changes or bleeding is a problem; replacement of fat-soluble vitamins; skin care as needed; and analgesics for headache.
- Offer support and encouragement *to help the person deal with the diagnosis and the drug regimen and lifestyle changes that may be necessary;* refer to services that might help with the high cost of these drugs.
- Provide thorough teaching, including the name of the drug, dosage prescribed and schedule for administration; method to administer the drug, such as mixing the powder form in fluids or taking tablets whole (without crushing, chewing or cutting); appropriate fluids for mixing the drug; measures to avoid adverse effects, warning signs of problems, and the need for follow-up laboratory testing *to monitor cholesterol and lipid levels; dietary and lifestyle changes for risk reduction*; and monitoring and evaluation *to enhance knowledge about drug therapy and to promote compliance.*

Evaluation

- Monitor response to the drug as appropriate (reduction in serum cholesterol levels).
- Monitor for adverse effects (headache, vitamin deficiency, increased bleeding times, constipation, nausea, rash).
- Evaluate the effectiveness of the teaching plan (person can name drug, dosage, adverse effects to watch for and specific measures to avoid them; person understands the importance of continued follow-up).
- Monitor the effectiveness of comfort measures and compliance with the regimen.

KEY POINTS

- Bile acid sequestrants prevent the reabsorption of bile salts, which are very high in cholesterol. Consequently, the liver will pull cholesterol from the blood to make new bile acids, lowering the serum cholesterol level.
- People receiving bile acid sequestrants need to learn how to mix the powders or, if taking the tablet form, the importance of swallowing the tablet whole and not cutting, crushing or chewing it. Doses should not be taken with other drugs to avoid problems with absorption.
- GI problems are often reported when using bile acid sequestrants, including nausea, bloating and constipation.

HMG-CoA REDUCTASE INHIBITORS

The HMG-CoA reductase inhibitors include atorvastatin (*Lipitor*), fluvastatin (*Lescol*), pravastatin (*Cholstat*, *Pravachol*), rosuvastatin (*Crestor*) and simvastatin (*Simvar*, *Zocor*).

Therapeutic actions and indication

The early rate-limiting step in the synthesis of cellular cholesterol involves the enzyme HMG-CoA reductase. If this enzyme is blocked, serum cholesterol and LDL levels decrease because more LDLs are absorbed by the cells for processing into cholesterol. In contrast, HDL levels increase slightly with this alteration in fat metabolism. HMG-CoA reductase inhibitors block HMG-CoA reductase from completing the synthesis of cholesterol (see Figure 47.2). Most of these drugs are chemical modifications of compounds produced by fungi. As a group, they are frequently referred to as 'statins'. Because these drugs undergo a marked first-pass effect in the liver, most of their effects are seen in the liver (see Adverse effects). These drugs may also have some effects on the process that generates atheromas in vessel walls. That exact mechanism of action is not understood. These drugs are indicated as adjuncts with diet and exercise for the treatment of increased cholesterol and LDL levels that are unresponsive to dietary restrictions alone.

Pravastatin and simvastatin are indicated for individuals with documented CAD to slow progression of the disease. These two agents and atorvastatin are used to prevent a first MI in people who have multiple risk factors for developing CAD. Table 47.3 discusses usual indications for each of the HMG-CoA reductase inhibitors. Several of the statin drugs have been formulated as combination therapy. Examples of combination therapy are highlighted in Box 47.6.

BOX 47.6 Combination therapy for lowering cholesterol levels

In recent years, combination therapy for reducing the risk of atherosclerosis in people with multiple risk factors has been introduced in Australia. It has been thought that the convenience of taking one tablet each day would improve compliance with the lipid-lowering therapy and other complementary medicines.

Newer combination drugs for treating CAD

- *Azotet*, *Caduet* and *Rosuzet* are combinations of 5 or 10 mg amlodipine and 10, 20, 40 or 80 mg atorvastatin. The person should first be stabilised on the individual drugs before the correct combination is selected. The combination provides the blood pressure–lowering and antianginal effect of the amlodipine with the lipid-lowering effects of the atorvastatin. The usual adult dose is 5–10 mg amlodipine with 10–80 mg atorvastatin, based on the individual's response. The recommended dose in children 10–17 years of age is 2.5–5 mg amlodipine with 10–20 mg atorvastatin.
- *Vytorin* and *Zimybe** are combinations of ezetimibe and simvastatin, and was approved to help lower lipid levels in people who did not have good results with single-drug therapy. Ezetimibe decreases the absorption of cholesterol, and simvastatin decreases the body's production of cholesterol. The drug is available in tablets that contain 10 mg ezetimibe and 10, 20, 40 or 80 mg simvastatin. Dose should be determined based on lipid levels.

**Only Zimybe is available in New Zealand at time of publication.*

Pharmacokinetics

The statins are all absorbed from the GI tract and undergo first-pass metabolism in the liver. They are excreted through faeces and urine. The peak effect of these drugs is usually seen within 2–4 weeks. These drugs are most effective when taken at night when the liver is processing the most lipids. These drugs cross the placenta, and most have been found in breast milk.

Contraindications and cautions

These drugs are contraindicated in the presence of allergy to any of the statins or to fungal byproducts or compounds *to avoid hypersensitivity reactions.* Statins are also contraindicated in people with active liver disease or a history of alcoholic liver disease, *which could be exacerbated, leading to severe liver failure,* and with pregnancy or breastfeeding, *because of the potential for adverse effects on the fetus or neonate.* These drugs are labelled as pregnancy category D.

Atorvastatin levels are not affected by renal disease, but individuals with renal impairment who are taking other statins require close monitoring. Caution should be used in individuals with impaired endocrine function *because of the potential alteration in the formation of steroid hormones.*

Adverse effects

The most common adverse effects associated with these drugs reflect their effects on the GI system: flatulence, abdominal pain, cramps, nausea, vomiting and constipation. CNS effects can include headache, dizziness, blurred vision, insomnia, fatigue and cataract development, and may reflect changes in the cell membrane and synthesis of cholesterol. Increased concentrations of liver enzymes commonly occur, and acute liver failure has been reported with the use of atorvastatin and fluvastatin. Pravastatin and simvastatin are not associated with some of the severe liver toxicity that is seen with the other agents. Rhabdomyolysis, a breakdown of muscles whose waste products can injure the glomerulus and cause acute renal failure, is a rare adverse effect but has been known to occur with the use of all of these drugs. MEDSAFE New Zealand has also warned that high dose (80 mg) of simvastatin increases the risk of myopathies.

Clinically important drug–drug interactions

The risk of rhabdomyolysis increases if any of these drugs is combined with erythromycin, ciclosporin, gemfibrozil, niacin or antifungal drugs; such combinations should be avoided.

Increased serum levels and resultant toxicity can occur if these drugs are combined with digoxin or warfarin; if this combination is used, serum digoxin levels and/or clotting times should be monitored carefully and the prescriber consulted for appropriate dose changes.

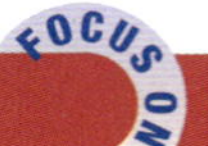

Safe medication administration

Individuals who are taking HMG-CoA reductase inhibitors need to be cautioned to avoid using grapefruit juice while taking these drugs. Grapefruit juice alters the metabolism of the drugs, leading to an increased serum level of the drug and increased risk for adverse effects, such as the potentially fatal rhabdomyolysis with renal failure. The effects of the juice may last for several days, so just drinking the juice at a different time of day does not protect the person from risk.

Increased oestrogen levels can occur if these drugs are taken with oral contraceptives; the person should be monitored carefully if this combination is used.

Serum levels of the drug and the risk of toxicity increase if the drug is combined with grapefruit juice.

Prototype summary: atorvastatin

Indications: adjunct to diet in the treatment of elevated levels of cholesterol, triglycerides and LDL; to increase HDL–cholesterol level in people with primary hypercholesterolaemia; treatment of boys and postmenarchal girls age 10–17 years of age with familial hypercholesterolaemia and two or more risk factors for CAD; prevention of CAD in adults without clinically evident heart disease but with multiple risk factors to reduce the risk of cardiovascular events.

Actions: inhibits HMG-CoA reductase, causing a decrease in serum cholesterol levels, LDLs and triglycerides and an increase in HDL levels.

Pharmacokinetics:

Route	Onset	Peak	Duration
Oral	Slow	1–2 hours	20–30 hours

$T_{1/2}$: 14 hours; metabolised in the liver and cells and excreted in bile.

Adverse effects: headache, flatulence, abdominal pain, cramps, constipation, rhabdomyolysis with acute renal failure.

Care considerations for people receiving HMG-CoA reductase inhibitors

Assessment: history and examination

- Assess for contraindications and cautions: any known allergies to these drugs or to fungal byproducts to avoid hypersensitivity reactions; active liver disease or history of alcoholic liver disease, *which could be exacerbated by the effects of these drugs*; current status of pregnancy or breastfeeding *because of potential adverse effects on the fetus or neonate*; and impaired endocrine function, *which could be exacerbated by effects on steroid hormones*.

- Perform a physical assessment *to establish a baseline before beginning therapy and during therapy to determine the drug's effectiveness and evaluate for any potential adverse effects*.
- Weigh the person *to establish a baseline and evaluate for changes reflecting lifestyle changes that accompany drug therapy*.
- Assess the person's neurological status, including level of orientation, affect and reflexes, which show early changes related to CNS function, *to evaluate for possible CNS effects of the drug*.
- Obtain vital signs, including pulse and blood pressure, *to identify changes*.
- Inspect the abdomen for distension and auscultate bowel sounds *for changes in GI motility*.
- Assess bowel elimination patterns, including frequency of stool passage and stool characteristics, *to identify possible constipation*.
- Monitor the results of laboratory tests, including renal and liver function tests, *to identify possible toxicity and serum lipid levels to evaluate the drug's effectiveness*.

Implementation with rationale

- Administer the drug at bedtime *because the highest rates of cholesterol synthesis occur between midnight and 5 a.m., and the drug should be taken when it will be most effective*; give atorvastatin at any time during the day.
- Monitor serum cholesterol and LDL levels before and periodically during therapy *to evaluate the effectiveness of this drug*.
- Arrange for periodic ophthalmic examinations *to monitor for cataract development*.
- Monitor liver function tests before and periodically during therapy *to monitor for liver damage*; consult with the prescriber to discontinue the drug if the aspartate aminotransferase (AST) or alanine aminotransferase (ALT) level increases to three times normal.
- Ensure that the person has attempted a cholesterol-lowering diet and exercise program for at least 3–6 months before beginning therapy *to ensure the need for drug therapy*.
- Encourage the person to make the lifestyle changes necessary *to decrease the risk of CAD and to increase the effectiveness of drug therapy*.
- Withhold atorvastatin or fluvastatin in any acute, serious medical condition (eg, infection, hypotension, major surgery or trauma, metabolic endocrine disorders, seizures) *that might suggest myopathy or serve as a risk factor for the development of renal failure*.
- Suggest the use of barrier contraceptives for women of childbearing age *because there is a risk of severe fetal abnormalities if these drugs are taken during pregnancy*.
- Provide comfort measures *to help the person tolerate drug effects*. These include small, frequent meals *to minimise nausea and vomiting*; access to bathroom facilities *to ensure adequate bowel evacuation*; bowel program as needed *to address constipation*; use of food with the drug if GI upset is severe *to decrease direct irritating effects*; environmental controls, such as temperature and lighting controls, *to help deal with headaches*; and safety precautions, such as lighting control and activity restrictions, *to protect the person if vision changes and muscle effects occur*.
- Offer support and encouragement *to help the person deal with the diagnosis, needed lifestyle changes and the drug regimen*.
- Provide thorough teaching, including the name of the drug, dosage prescribed and administration at bedtime for best effectiveness; measures to avoid adverse effects, warning signs of problems and the need for follow-up laboratory testing to monitor cholesterol and lipid levels; importance of follow-up renal and liver function testing; dietary and lifestyle changes for risk reduction; and monitoring and evaluation, *to enhance knowledge about drug therapy and to promote compliance*.

See the Critical thinking scenario for discussion of a person receiving an HMG-CoA reductase inhibitor.

Evaluation

- Monitor response to the drug (lowering of serum cholesterol and LDL levels, prevention of first MI, slowing of progression of CAD).
- Monitor for adverse effects (headache, dizziness, blurred vision, cataracts, GI upset, liver failure, rhabdomyolysis).
- Monitor the effectiveness of comfort measures and compliance with the regimen.
- Evaluate the effectiveness of the teaching plan (person can name drug, dosage, adverse effects to watch for and specific measures to avoid them; individual understands the importance of continued follow-up).

KEY POINTS

- HMG-CoA reductase inhibitors, or statins, block the enzyme HMG-CoA reductase, resulting in lower serum cholesterol levels, a resultant breakdown of LDLs and a slight increase in HDL levels.
- Individuals receiving HMG-CoA reductase inhibitors should avoid pregnancy because of serious fetal adverse effects; take the drug in the evening to mimic the normal patterns of lipid formation; have liver function monitored regularly; and be instructed to report any sudden muscle pain, especially if accompanied by fever.

Cholesterol absorption inhibitors

The first drug in this class of drugs to lower cholesterol levels was approved in 2003 – ezetimibe (*Ezetrol*). Addition of ezetimibe to statin combination therapy is an effective treatment option that leads to additional LDL–cholesterol (LDL-c) lowering, recommended when LDL-c targets cannot be achieved with maximal or maximally tolerated statin monotherapy treatment. It leads to additional risk reduction, without raising significant safety concerns. Benefits associated with this therapy are discussed in Box 47.7.

Therapeutic actions and indications

Ezetimibe works in the brush border of the small intestine to decrease the absorption of dietary cholesterol from the small intestine. As a result, less dietary cholesterol is delivered to the liver, and the liver increases the clearance of cholesterol from the serum to make up for the drop in dietary cholesterol, causing the total serum cholesterol level to drop. See Table 47.3 for usual indications.

Pharmacokinetics

Ezetimibe is absorbed well after oral administration, reaching peak levels in 4–6 hours. It is metabolised in the liver and the small intestine, with a half-life of 22 hours. Excretion is through faeces and urine. It is not known whether the drug crosses the placenta or enters breast milk.

Contraindications and cautions

Ezetimibe is contraindicated in people with an allergy to any component of the drug *to avoid hypersensitivity reactions*. If it is used in combination with a statin, it should not be used during pregnancy or breastfeeding or with severe liver disease *because of the known effects of statins, including possible liver problems and renal failure*.

The drug should be used with caution as monotherapy during pregnancy or breastfeeding *because the effects on the fetus or neonate are not known* and with elderly people or individuals with liver disease *because of the potential for adverse reactions*.

Adverse effects

The most common adverse effects associated with ezetimibe are mild abdominal pain and diarrhoea. It is not associated with the bloating and flatulence that occurs with the bile acid sequestrants and another class of lipid-lowering drugs called fibrates. Other adverse effects that have been reported include headache, dizziness, fatigue, upper respiratory tract infection (URTI), back pain and muscle aches and pains.

Clinically important drug–drug interactions

The risk of elevated serum levels of ezetimibe increases if it is given with colestyramine, fenofibrate, gemfibrozil

BOX 47.7 FOCUS ON The evidence

SHARP and IMPROVE-IT

The two landmark studies were the SHARP and IMPROVE-IT randomised controlled trials. The Study of Heart and Renal Protection (SHARP) (simvastatin plus ezetimibe compared with placebo) was a randomised double-blind trial conducted among high-risk patients with diabetes and chronic kidney disease. The combination therapy demonstrated superiority over statin monotherapy in reducing LDL-c levels, translating to reduced incidence of the primary endpoint of the first major atherosclerotic cardiovascular disease event – non-fatal myocardial infarction or cardiovascular death, non-haemorrhagic stroke, or any arterial revascularisation procedure. Reducing LDL-c with simvastatin–ezetimibe safely reduced the incidence of major atherosclerotic events in patients with advanced chronic kidney disease.

The IMPROVE-IT (simvastatin plus ezetimibe compared with simvastatin monotherapy) was the first randomised double-blind controlled trial to show a significant reduction in cardiovascular events when ezetimibe is added to statin therapy, demonstrating a significant add-on effect of ezetimibe to statins in terms of both reduced LDL-c levels and reduced incidence of cardiovascular events.

or antacids. If these drugs are used in combination, ezetimibe should be taken at least 2 hours before or 4 hours after the other drugs.

The risk of toxicity also increases if ezetimibe is combined with ciclosporin. If this combination cannot be avoided, the person should be monitored very closely.

If ezetimibe is combined with any fibrate, the risk of cholethiasis increases. The person should be monitored closely. Warfarin levels increase in a person who is also taking ezetimibe; if this combination is used, the person should be monitored very closely.

Prototype summary: ezetimibe

Indications: adjunct to diet and exercise to lower serum cholesterol levels; in combination with atorvastatin or simvastatin for the treatment of homozygous familial hypercholesterolaemia; with diet for the treatment of homozygous sitosterolaemia to lower sitosterol and campesterol levels.

Actions: works in the brush border of the small intestine to inhibit the absorption of cholesterol.

Pharmacokinetics:

Route	Onset	Peak
Oral	Moderate	4–12 hours

$T_{1/2}$: 22 hours; metabolised in the liver and small intestine and excreted in faeces and urine.

Adverse effects: headache, dizziness, abdominal pain, diarrhoea, URTI, back pain, myalgia, arthralgia.

Care for people receiving cholesterol absorption inhibitors

Assessment: history and examination

- Assess for contraindications or cautions: any known allergies to any component of the drug *to avoid hypersensitivity reactions*; liver dysfunction or advanced age *because the processing of the drug may differ from the norm*; current status of pregnancy or breastfeeding *because the possible effects on the fetus or neonate are not known.*
- Perform a physical assessment to establish a baseline before beginning therapy and during therapy *to determine its effectiveness and evaluate for any potential adverse effects.*
- Monitor orientation and reflexes *to detect changes in CNS function, such as dizziness, that could require safety measures.*
- Monitor respirations and auscultate lungs for *evidence of adventitious sounds to monitor changes in cardiac output.*
- Inspect the abdomen for distension and auscultate bowel sounds *for changes in GI motility.*
- Assess bowel elimination patterns, including frequency of stool passage and stool characteristics, *to identify possible changes that could require intervention.*
- Monitor the results of laboratory tests, including serum cholesterol and lipid levels, *to evaluate the effectiveness of drug therapy*, and liver function studies *to monitor for toxic effects.*

Implementation with rationale

- Monitor serum cholesterol, triglyceride and LDL levels before and periodically during therapy *to evaluate the effectiveness of this drug.*
- Monitor liver function tests before and periodically during therapy *to detect possible liver damage.*
- Ensure that the person has attempted a cholesterol-lowering diet and exercise program for at least several months before beginning therapy *to ensure the need for drug therapy.*
- Encourage the person to make the lifestyle changes necessary *to decrease the risk of CAD and to increase the effectiveness of drug therapy.*
- Suggest the use of barrier contraceptives for women of childbearing age if the drug is being used in combination with a statin *because there is a risk of severe fetal abnormalities if these drugs are taken during pregnancy.*
- Provide comfort measures *to help the person tolerate drug effects.* These include readily available access to bathroom facilities *to help with episodes of diarrhoea*; safety precautions *to protect the individual if dizziness is an issue*; and analgesics for headache and muscle aches if appropriate.
- Offer support and encouragement *to help the person deal with the diagnosis, needed lifestyle changes and the drug regimen.*
- Provide thorough teaching, including the name of the drug, dosage prescribed and schedule for administration; measures to avoid adverse effects, warning signs of problems, and the need for follow-up laboratory testing to monitor cholesterol and lipid levels; dietary and lifestyle changes for reducing the risk of CAD and increasing the effectiveness of drug therapy; and monitoring and evaluation *to enhance knowledge about drug therapy and to promote compliance.*

Evaluation

- Monitor response to the drug (lowering of serum cholesterol and LDL levels, lowering of sitosterol and campesterol levels).
- Monitor for adverse effects (headache, dizziness, GI pain, muscle aches and pains, URTI).
- Monitor the effectiveness of comfort measures and compliance with the regimen.
- Evaluate the effectiveness of the teaching plan (person can name drug, dosage, adverse effects to watch for and specific measures to avoid them; individual understands the importance of continued follow-up).

KEY POINTS

- The cholesterol absorption inhibitor ezetimibe works in the brush border of the small intestine to prevent the absorption of dietary cholesterol, which leads to increased clearance of cholesterol by the liver and a resultant fall in serum cholesterol.
- Change in diet and increased exercise are very important parts of the overall treatment of a person receiving a cholesterol absorption inhibitor.

OTHER LIPID-LOWERING AGENTS

Other drugs that are used to affect lipid levels do not fall into any of the classes discussed previously. They are approved for use in combination with changes in diet and exercise. They include the fibrates (derivatives of fibric acid), the vitamin niacin and the peroxisome-proliferator-receptor-alpha activator, fenofibric acid.

Fibrates

The fibrates stimulate the breakdown of lipoproteins from the tissues and their removal from the plasma. They lead to a decrease in lipoprotein and triglyceride synthesis and secretion. The fibrates are absorbed from the GI tract and are metabolised in the liver and excreted in urine. Fibrates in use today include the following agents:

- Fenofibrate (*Lipidil*): inhibits triglyceride synthesis in the liver, resulting in reduction of LDL levels; increases uric acid secretion; and may stimulate triglyceride breakdown. It is used for adults with very high triglyceride levels who are not responsive to strict dietary measures and who are at risk for pancreatitis. Peak effects are usually seen within 4 weeks, and the person's serum lipid levels should be re-evaluated at that time.
- Gemfibrozil (*Lipazil*): inhibits peripheral breakdown of lipids, reduces production of triglycerides and LDLs and increases HDL concentrations. It is associated with GI and muscle discomfort. This drug should not be combined with statins. There is an increased risk of rhabdomyolysis from 3 weeks to several months after therapy if this combination is used. If this combination cannot be avoided, the individual should be monitored very closely.

Vitamin B

Vitamin B_3, known as nicotinic acid (generic), inhibits the release of free fatty acids from adipose tissue, increases the rate of triglyceride removal from plasma, and generally reduces LDL and triglyceride levels and increases HDL levels. It may also decrease the levels of apoproteins needed to form chylomicrons. The initial effect on lipid levels is usually seen within 5–7 days, with the maximum effect occurring in 3–5 weeks. Nicotinic acid is associated with intense cutaneous flushing, nausea and abdominal pain, making its use somewhat limited. It also increases serum levels of uric acid and may predispose people to the development of gout. Nicotinic acid is often combined with bile acid sequestrants for increased effect. It is given at bedtime to make maximum use of night time cholesterol synthesis, and it must be given 4–6 hours after the bile sequestrant to ensure absorption.

Peroxisome-proliferator-receptor-alpha activator

In 2009, the U.S. Food and Drug Administration (FDA) approved the first drug in a new class of drugs called peroxisome-proliferator-receptor-alpha activators. Fenofibric acid (*Trilipix*) is the first drug in this class. This drug is not available in New Zealand or Australia. It works to activate a specific hepatic receptor that results in increased breakdown of lipids, elimination of triglyceride-rich particles from the plasma, and reduction in the production of an enzyme that naturally inhibits lipid breakdown. The result is seen as a decrease in triglyceride levels, changes in LDL production that makes them more easily broken down in the body, and an increase in HDL levels. Fenofibric acid is used in combination with a statin to reduce triglyceride levels and increase HDL levels in people with mixed lipid disorders; as monotherapy to decrease triglyceride levels in people with severe hypertriglyceridaemia; and as monotherapy to reduce LDL, total cholesterol and triglycerides and to increase HDL levels in individuals with primary hyperlipidaemia or mixed lipid disorders. Fenofibric acid is slowly absorbed from the GI tract, with peak levels occurring in 4–5 hours; metabolised in the liver, it has a half-life of 20 hours and is excreted in the urine. Caution should be used in people with renal impairment, and the drug should be avoided in individuals with severe renal impairment. The most common adverse effects that have been reported are headache, back pain, nausea, diarrhoea, muscle pain, runny nose and respiratory infections. Gallstones have also been reported with this drug. Individuals complaining of gallstone-type pain should be screened carefully. There is an increased risk of muscle breakdown and rhabdomyolysis if taken with a statin, and people using this combination need to be monitored closely. Caution must be used with warfarin anticoagulants; increased bleeding can occur. The person should be monitored closely and the dose of the anticoagulant regulated to achieve therapeutic anticoagulation.

COMBINATION THERAPY

Frequently, if the person shows no response to strict dietary modification, exercise, and lifestyle changes and the use of one lipid-lowering agent, combination therapy may be initiated to achieve desirable serum LDL and cholesterol levels. For example, a bile acid sequestrant might be combined with niacin; the combination would decrease the synthesis of LDLs while lowering the serum levels of LDLs. This combination is thought to help slow the progression of CAD. Numerous fixed-dose combination therapies are available (see Box 47.6). However, care must be taken not to combine agents that increase the risk of rhabdomyolysis. For example, HMG-CoA reductase inhibitors are not usually combined with nicotinic acid or gemfibrozil.

FUTURE THERAPIES

Despite advances in treatment, CAD remains the number one killer of adults in Australia. New drugs are being investigated that would address multiple risk factors simultaneously with hopes of cutting risk successfully. The **endocannabinoids** are substances present in the body that activate various neurological receptors that seem to be very important in the body's regulation of appetite, satiety and lipid metabolism. With blocking of the endocannabinoid system, a series of changes occur that would seem to have a very profound effect on many components of the metabolic syndrome. Blocking the endocannabinoid system results in feelings of satiety and decreased appetite, leading to weight loss; decreased release of growth hormone, increased oxygen and glucose use in the muscle, decreased fat synthesis in the liver, decreased levels of triglycerides and LDLs and increased levels of HDLs, improving the lipid profile; increased sensitivity of insulin receptor sites, leading to decreased blood glucose levels; decreased fat production and storage; increased levels of adiponectin; and decreased activity of tumour necrosis factor, a proinflammatory agent, and decreased activity of C-reactive protein, which is associated with proinflammatory and prothrombotic states.

Rimonabant is an endocannabinoid blocker that has been used in Europe as a weight loss agent. In early studies in the US, it was shown to significantly reduce weight and abdominal adiposity and improve lipid profiles while increasing insulin sensitivity and reducing the proinflammatory and prothrombotic markers. US approval of the drug was denied at one point because of some significant CNS changes that occur, leading to questions of safety. It has since been removed from the market.

KEY POINTS

- Other agents used to lower cholesterol include fibrates, peroxisome-proliferator-receptor-alpha activator and niacin. Often lipid-lowering agents are used in combination to lower the cholesterol at different sites.
- Research is being done on the effects of blocking the endocannabinoid system, resulting in weight loss, improved lipid profiles and decreased proinflammatory and prothrombotic states. Questions have not been answered about the safety or effectiveness of drugs that block this system.

CHAPTER SUMMARY

- CAD is the leading cause of death in the Western world. It is associated with the development of atheromas or plaques in arterial linings that lead to narrowing of the lumen of the artery and hardening of the artery wall, with loss of distensibility and responsiveness to stimuli for contraction or dilation.
- The cause of CAD is not known, but many contributing risk factors have been identified, including increasing age, male gender, genetic predisposition, high-fat diet, sedentary lifestyle, smoking, obesity, high stress levels, bacterial infections, diabetes, hypertension, gout and menopause. The presence of many of these factors constitutes the metabolic syndrome.
- Treatment and prevention of CAD is aimed at manipulating the known risk factors to decrease CAD development and progression.
- Fats are metabolised with the aid of bile acids, which act as a detergent to break fats into small molecules called micelles. Micelles are absorbed into the intestinal wall and combined with proteins to become chylomicrons, which can be transported throughout the circulatory system.
- Some fats are used immediately for energy or are stored in adipose tissue; others are processed in the liver to LDLs, which are associated with the development of CAD. LDLs are broken down in the periphery and leave many remnants (eg, fats) that must be removed from blood vessels. This process

involves the inflammatory reaction and may initiate or contribute to atheroma production.

- Some fats are processed into HDLs, which are able to absorb fats and remnants from the periphery and offer a protective effect against the development of CAD.
- Cholesterol is an important fat that is used to make bile acids. It is the base for steroid hormones and provides the necessary structure for cell membranes. All cells can produce cholesterol.
- HMG-CoA reductase is an enzyme that controls the production of cellular cholesterol.
- People taking lipid-lowering drugs need to include diet, exercise and lifestyle changes to reduce the risk of CAD.
- Bile acid sequestrants bind with bile acids in the intestine and lead to their excretion in faeces. This results in lower bile acid levels as the liver uses cholesterol to produce more bile acids. The end result is a decrease in serum cholesterol and LDL levels as the liver changes its metabolism of these fats to meet the need for more bile acids.
- HMG-CoA reductase inhibitors, or statins, block the enzyme HMG-CoA reductase, resulting in lower serum cholesterol levels, a resultant breakdown of LDLs and a slight increase in HDL levels.
- The cholesterol absorption inhibitor ezetimibe works in the brush border of the small intestine to prevent the absorption of dietary cholesterol, which leads to increased clearance of cholesterol by the liver and a resultant fall in serum cholesterol.
- Other agents used to lower cholesterol include fibrates and nicotinic acid. Often lipid-lowering agents are used in combination to lower the cholesterol at different sites.
- Research is being done on the effects of blocking the endocannabinoid system, resulting in weight loss, improved lipid profiles and decreased proinflammatory and prothrombotic states. Questions have not been answered about the safety or effectiveness of drugs that block this system.

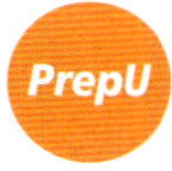

Knowing your strengths and weaknesses helps you to study more effectively. Take a PrepU Practice Quiz to find out how you measure up!

ONLINE RESOURCES

An extensive range of additional resources to enhance teaching and learning and to facilitate understanding of this chapter may be found online at the text's accompanying website, located on thePoint at http://thepoint.lww.com. These include Watch and Learn videos, Concepts in Action animations, journal articles, review questions, case studies, discussion topics and quizzes.

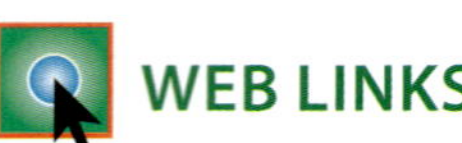

WEB LINKS

Health care providers and students may want to consult the following web resources:

www.heartfoundation.org.au
Information on research, alternative methods of therapy and pharmacology.

www.heartfoundation.org.nz
Information on research, alternative methods of therapy and pharmacology.

www.medsafe.govt.nz/profs/puarticles/simvastinsept2011.htm
New Zealand Medicines and Medical Devices Authority. *High-dose simvastatin increases myopathy risk.*

BIBLIOGRAPHY

Australian Institute of Health and Welfare (AIHW). (2010). *Cardiovascular disease mortality: Trends at Different Ages.* Cat. no. CVD 47. Canberra: AIHW.

Ayer, J. G. & Sholler, G. F. (2012). Cardiovascular risk factors in Australian children: Hypertension and lipid abnormalities. *Australian Prescriber, 35(2)*, 51–55.

Colquhoun, D. (2008). How to treat hypercholesterolaemia. *Australian Prescriber, 31*, 119–122.

Farrell, M. & Dempsey, J. (2014). *Smeltzer & Bare's Textbook of Medical-Surgical Nursing* (3rd edn). Sydney: Lippincott Williams & Wilkins.

Goodman, L. S., Brunton, L. L., Chabner, B. & Knollmann, B. C. (2011). *Goodman and Gilman's Pharmacological Basis of Therapeutics* (12th edn). New York: McGraw-Hill.

Hamilton-Craig, I., Kostner, K. M., Woodhouse, S. & Colquhoun, D. (2012). Use of fibrates in clinical practice: Queensland Lipid Group consensus recommendations. *International Journal of Evidence-Based Healthcare, 10(3)*, 181–190.

Hossain, P., Kawar, B. & El Nahas, M. (2007). Obesity and diabetes in the developing world—A growing challenge. *New England Journal of Medicine, 356*, 213–215.

Kastelen, J. P., Akdim, F., Stroes, E. & Zwinderman, A. H. (2008). Simvastatin with or without ezetimibe in familial hypercholesterolemia. *New England Journal of Medicine,* 358, 1431–1443.

McKenna, L. & Mirkov, S. (2019). *McKenna's Drug Handbook for Nursing and Midwifery* (8th edn). Sydney: Wolters Kluwer Health Australia.

National Heart Foundation (NHF). (2012). Reducing risk in heart disease: An expert guide to clinical practice for secondary prevention of coronary heart disease. www.heartfoundation.org.au/SiteCollectionDocuments/Reducing-risk-in-heart-disease.pdf.

Nissen, S. E., Nicholls, S. J., Wolski, K., Rodes-Cabau, J., Cannon, C. P., Deanfield, J. E., et al. (2008). Effect of rimonabant on progression of atherosclerosis in patients with abdominal obesity and coronary artery disease. *JAMA, 229*, 1547–1560.

Porth, C. M. (2011). *Essentials of Pathophysiology: Concepts of Altered Health States* (3rd edn). Philadelphia: Lippincott Williams & Wilkins.

Porth, C. M. (2009). *Pathophysiology: Concepts of Altered Health States* (8th edn). Philadelphia: Lippincott Williams & Wilkins.

Schwartz, G., Ander, G. O., Ezekowitz, M. E., Ganz, P., Oliver, M. F., Waters, D., et al. (2001). Effects of atorvastatin in early recurrent ischemic events in acute coronary syndrome. The MIRACL study: A randomized controlled trial. *JAMA, 285*, 1711–1718.

Smith, J. (2011). Appropriate primary prevention of cardiovascular disease: Does this mean more or less statin use? *Australian Prescriber, 34(6)*, 169–172.

Spinler, S. A. (2006). Challenges associated with metabolic syndrome. *Pharmacotherapy*, 26, 209S–217S.

Zhu, Y. Y., Hayward, P. A., Hare, D. L., Stewart, A. G. & Buxton, B. F. (2012). Lipid management in high risk coronary patients: How effective are we at secondary prevention? *Heart, Lung & Circulation, 21(2)*, 82–87.

CHECK YOUR UNDERSTANDING

Answers to the questions in this chapter can be found in Appendix A the back of this book.

MULTIPLE CHOICE

Select the best answer to the following.

1. After describing to a community group the ways in which the body uses cholesterol, which of the following, if stated by the group as a way, indicates successful teaching?
   a. the production of water-soluble vitamins
   b. the formation of steroid hormones
   c. the mineralisation of bones
   d. the development of dental plaques

2. The formation of atheromas in blood vessels precedes the signs and symptoms of:
   a. hepatitis.
   b. coronary artery disease.
   c. diabetes mellitus.
   d. chronic obstructive pulmonary disease (COPD).

3. Hyperlipidaemia is considered to be:
   a. a normal finding in adult males.
   b. related to stress levels.
   c. a treatable CAD risk factor.
   d. a side effect of cigarette smoking.

4. The bile acid sequestrants:
   a. are absorbed into the liver.
   b. take several weeks to show an effect.
   c. have no associated adverse effects.
   d. prevent bile salts from being reabsorbed.

5. HMG-CoA reductase inhibitors work in the:
   a. process of bile secretion.
   b. process of cholesterol formation in the cell.
   c. intestinal wall to block fat absorption.
   d. kidney to block fat excretion.

6. Which of the following would the health care provider include when teaching a person about HMG-CoA reductase inhibitors?
   a. The person will not have a heart attack.
   b. The person will not develop CAD.
   c. The person might develop cataracts as a result.
   d. The person might stop absorbing fat-soluble vitamins.

7. Which of the following would the nurse expect the health care provider to prescribe for a person who has high lipid levels and cannot take fibrates or HMG-CoA reductase inhibitors?
   a. nicotine
   b. vitamin C
   c. nicotinic acid
   d. nitrates

8. Which of the following would alert the health care provider to suspect that a person receiving HMG-CoA reductase inhibitors is developing rhabdomyolysis?
   a. flatulence and abdominal bloating
   b. increased bleeding and bruising
   c. the development of cataracts and blurred vision
   d. muscle pain and weakness

MULTIPLE RESPONSE

Select all that apply.

1. A bile acid sequestrant is a drug of choice for a person who has which of the following?
   a. a high LDL concentration
   b. a high triglyceride concentration
   c. biliary obstruction
   d. vitamin K deficiency
   e. a high HDL concentration
   f. intolerance to statins

2. Teaching a person who is prescribed an HMG-CoA reductase inhibitor to treat high cholesterol and high lipid levels should include which of the following?
   a. the importance of exercise
   b. the need for dietary changes to alter cholesterol levels
   c. that taking a statin will allow a full, unrestricted diet
   d. that drug therapy is always needed when these levels are elevated
   e. the importance of controlling blood pressure and blood glucose levels
   f. that stopping smoking may also help to lower lipid levels

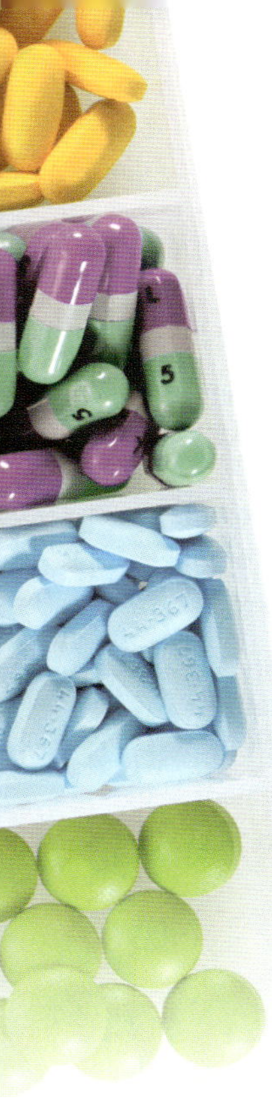

Drugs affecting blood coagulation

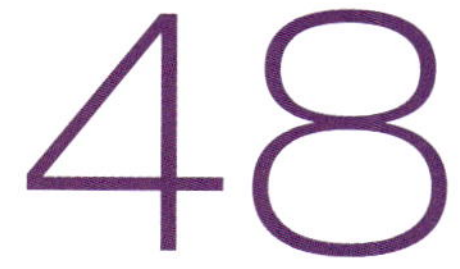

Learning objectives

On completing this chapter you should be able to:

1. Outline the mechanisms by which blood clots dissolve in the body, correlating this information with the actions of drugs used to affect blood clotting.
2. Describe the therapeutic actions, indications, pharmacokinetics, contraindications, most common adverse reactions and important drug–drug interactions associated with drugs affecting blood coagulation.
3. Discuss the use of drugs that affect blood coagulation across the lifespan.
4. Compare and contrast the prototype drugs aspirin, heparin and antihaemophilic factor with other agents used to affect blood coagulation.
5. Outline the care considerations, including important teaching points, for people receiving drugs used to affect blood coagulation.

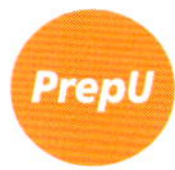

Test your current knowledge of drugs affecting blood coagulation with a PrepU Practice Quiz!

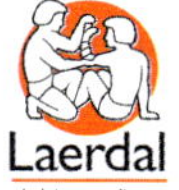

Simulation-based learning

On completion of the chapter, consider the scenario of Carl Shapiro (Part 1) who arrives in the emergency department. Consider the medication management of Carl's condition, as it relates to your learning in this chapter.

Then, work through the second scenario of Vernon Watkins (Part 2) who underwent a hemicolectomy 5 days ago and now has abdominal and leg pain. Consider how the concepts learnt in this chapter relating to medication management apply to his case.

Glossary of key terms

anticoagulants: drugs that block or inhibit any step of the coagulation process, preventing or slowing clot formation

antiplatelet agents: drugs that interfere with the aggregation or clumping of platelets to form the platelet plug

clotting factors: substances formed in the liver – many requiring vitamin K – that react in a cascading sequence to cause the formation of thrombin from prothrombin; thrombin then breaks down fibrin threads from fibrinogen to form a clot

coagulation: the process of blood changing from a fluid state to a solid state to plug injuries to the vascular system

extrinsic pathway: cascade of clotting factors in blood that has escaped the vascular system to form a clot on the outside of the injured vessel

haemorrhagic disorders: disorders characterised by a lack of clot-forming substances, leading to states of excessive bleeding

haemostatic agents: drugs that stop blood loss, usually by blocking the plasminogen mechanism and preventing clot dissolution

Hageman factor: first factor activated when a blood vessel or cell is injured; starts the cascading reaction of the clotting factors, activates the conversion of plasminogen to plasmin to dissolve clots and activates the kinin system responsible for the activation of the inflammatory response

intrinsic pathway: cascade of clotting factors leading to the formation of a clot within an injured vessel

plasminogen: natural clot-dissolving system; converted to plasmin (also called fibrinolysin) by many substances to dissolve clots that have formed and to maintain the patency of injured vessels

platelet aggregation: property of platelets to adhere to an injured surface and then attract other platelets, which clump together or aggregate at the area, plugging up an injury to the vascular system

thromboembolic disorders: disorders characterised by the formation of clots or thrombi on injured blood vessels with potential breaking of the clot to form emboli that can travel to smaller vessels, where they become lodged and occlude the vessel

thrombolytic agents: drugs that lyse, or break down, a clot that has formed; these drugs activate the plasminogen mechanism to dissolve fibrin threads

DRUGS AFFECTING CLOT FORMATION AND RESOLUTION

Antiplatelet agents
- abciximab
- anagrelide
- (P) aspirin
- cilostazol
- clopidogrel
- dipyridamole
- eptifibatide
- prasugrel
- ticagrelor
- tirofiban

Anticoagulants
- antithrombin III
- apixaban
- bivalirudin
- dabigatran
- fondaparinux
- (P) heparin
- rivaroxaban
- warfarin

Thrombolytic agents
- alteplase
- reteplase
- tenecteplase

Other drugs affecting clot formation

Low-molecular-weight heparins
- dalteparin
- enoxaparin

Heparinoid
- danaparoid

Haemorheological agent
- pentoxifylline (oxpentifylline)

DRUGS USED TO CONTROL BLEEDING

Anticoagulant reversal agents
- idarucizumab
- protamine sulfate
- vitamin K (phytomenadione)

Antihaemophilic agents
- (P) antihaemophilic factor, recombinant
- coagulation factor VIIa
- coagulation factor VIII
- factor IX complex

Haemostatic agents
- absorbable gelatine
- aprotinin
- human fibrin sealant
- tranexamic acid

The cardiovascular system is a closed system, and blood remains in a fluid state while in it. Because the blood is trapped in a closed space, it maintains the difference in pressure required to keep the system moving along. Everything in the cardiovascular system moves from higher pressure to lower pressure. If the vascular system is injured – from a cut, a puncture or capillary destruction – the fluid blood could leak out, causing the system in that area to lose pressure and changing the flow in the system, potentially shutting it down entirely. To deal with the problem of blood leaking and potentially shutting down the system, blood that is exposed to an injury in a vessel almost immediately forms into a solid state, or clot, which plugs the hole in the system and keeps the required pressure differences intact.

BLOOD COAGULATION

People injure blood vessels all the time (eg, by coughing too hard, by knocking into the corner of the desk when sitting down). Consequently, the vascular system must maintain an intricate balance between the tendency to clot or form a solid state, called **coagulation**, and the need to 'unclot', or reverse coagulation, to keep the vessels open and the blood flowing. If a great deal of vascular damage occurs, such as with a major cut or incision, the balance in the area shifts to a procoagulation mode and a large clot is formed. At the same time, the enzymes in the plasma work to dissolve this clot before blood flow to tissues is lost, which otherwise would lead to hypoxia and potential cell death.

Drugs that affect blood coagulation work at various steps in the blood clotting and clot-dissolving processes to restore the balance that is needed to maintain the cardiovascular system. Box 48.1 discusses the uses of these drugs in various age groups.

Clotting process

Blood coagulation is a complex process that involves vasoconstriction, platelet clumping or aggregation and a cascade of **clotting factors** produced in the liver that eventually react to break down fibrinogen (a protein also produced in the liver) into insoluble fibrin threads. When a clot is formed, plasmin (another blood protein) acts to break it down. Blood coagulation can be affected at any step in this complicated process to alter the way that blood clotting occurs.

Vasoconstriction

The first reaction to a blood vessel injury is local vasoconstriction (Figure 48.1). If the injury to the blood vessel is very small, this vasoconstriction can seal off any break and allow the area to heal.

Platelet aggregation

Injury to a blood vessel exposes blood to the collagen and other substances under the endothelial lining of the vessel. This exposure causes platelets in the circulating blood to stick or adhere to the site of the injury. Once they stick, the platelets release adenosine diphosphate (ADP) and other chemicals that attract other platelets, causing them to gather or aggregate and to stick as well. ADP is also a precursor of the prostaglandins, from which thromboxane A_2 is formed. Thromboxane A_2 causes local vasoconstriction and further **platelet aggregation** and adhesion. This series of events forms a platelet plug at the site of the vessel injury. In many injuries, the combination of vasoconstriction and platelet aggregation is enough to seal off the injury and keep the cardiovascular system intact (Figure 48.2).

Intrinsic pathway

As blood comes in contact with the exposed collagen of the injured blood vessel, one of the clotting factors,

BOX 48.1 FOCUS ON **Drug therapy across the lifespan**

Drugs affecting blood coagulation

CHILDREN

Little research is available on the use of anticoagulants in children. If they are used, the child needs to be monitored very carefully to avoid excessive bleeding related to drug interactions or alterations in gastrointestinal or liver function. People who interact with the child need to understand the importance of preventing injuries and providing safety precautions. They should be aware of what to do if the child is injured and begins to bleed.

If heparin is used, the dose should be carefully calculated based on weight and age and checked by another person before being administered.

Warfarin is used with children who are to undergo cardiac surgery. Again, the dose must be determined based on weight and age, and the child should be monitored closely.

The safety of low-molecular-weight heparins has not been established in children.

At this time, there are no indications for the use of antiplatelet or thrombolytic drugs with children.

ADULTS

Adults receiving these drugs need to be instructed in ways to prevent injury – such as using an electric razor instead of a straight razor, using a soft-bristled toothbrush to protect the gums, and avoiding contact sports – and instructed in what to do if bleeding does occur (apply constant, firm pressure and contact a health care provider). They should receive a written list of signs of bleeding to watch for and to report to their health care provider.

Because so many drugs and alternative therapies are known to interact with these agents, it is very important that these people be urged to report the use of this drug to any other health care provider and to consult with one before using any over-the-counter drugs or alternative therapies.

It is prudent to advise any person using one of these drugs in the home setting to carry or wear a MedicAlert notification in case of emergency.

The person also needs to understand the importance of regular, periodic blood tests to evaluate the effects of the drug.

PREGNANCY AND BREASTFEEDING

Because of the many risks associated with increased bleeding or increased blood clotting during pregnancy, these drugs should not be used during pregnancy unless the benefit to the mother clearly outweighs the potential risk to the fetus and to the mother at delivery. Risks of altered blood clotting in the neonate make these drugs generally inadvisable for use during breastfeeding.

OLDER ADULTS

Older adults may have many underlying medical conditions that require the need for drugs that alter blood clotting (eg, coronary artery disease, cerebrovascular accident, peripheral vascular disease, transient ischaemic attacks). Statistically, older adults also take more medications, making them more likely to encounter drug–drug interactions associated with these drugs. The older adult is also more likely to have impaired liver and kidney function, conditions that can alter the metabolism and excretion of these drugs.

The older adult should be carefully evaluated for liver and kidney function, use of other medications, and ability to follow through with regular blood testing and medical evaluation before therapy begins. Therapy should be started at the lowest possible level and adjusted accordingly after the person's response has been noted.

Careful attention needs to be given to the person's total drug regimen. Starting, stopping or changing the dose of another drug may alter the body's metabolism of the drug that is being used to affect coagulation, leading to increased risk of bleeding or ineffective anticoagulation.

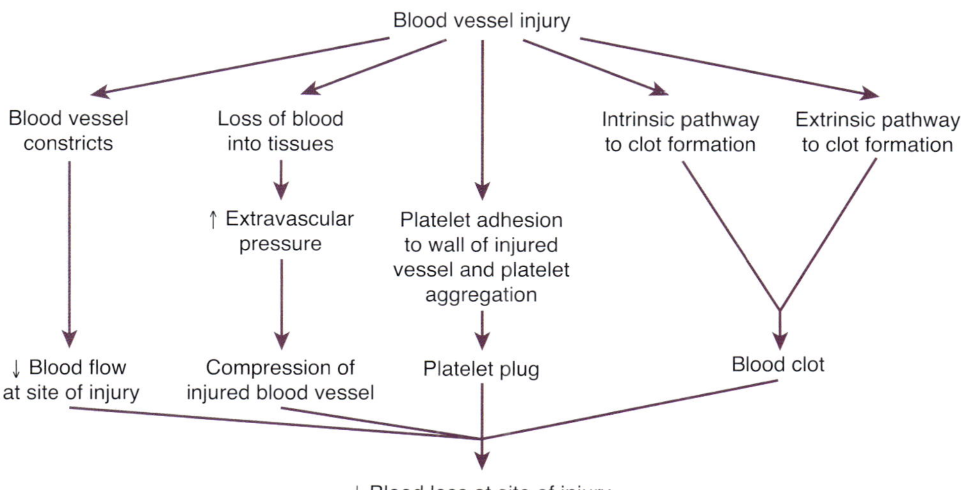

FIGURE 48.1 Process of blood coagulation.

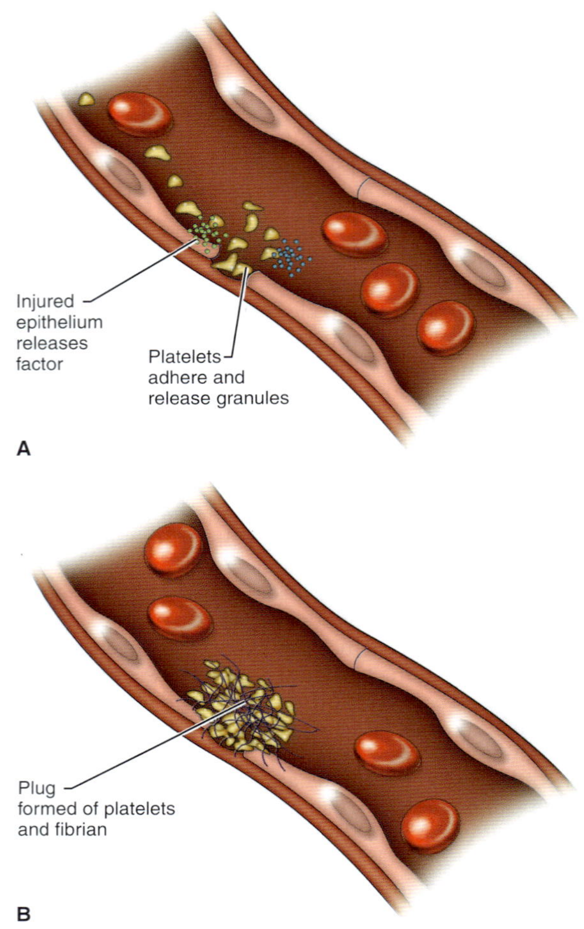

FIGURE 48.2 **A.** Damaged vessel endothelium is a stimulus to circulating platelets, causing platelet adhesion. **B.** Platelets release mediators, and platelet aggregation results.

Hageman factor (also called factor XII), a chemical substance that is found circulating in the blood, is activated. (Clotting factors are often known by a name and by a Roman numeral. When one of these factors becomes activated, the lowercase letter 'a' is added; eg, activated Hageman factor is also called factor XIIa.) The activation of Hageman factor starts a number of reactions in the area: the clot formation process is activated, the clot-dissolving process is activated and the inflammatory response is started (see Chapter 15). The activation of Hageman factor first activates clotting factor XI (plasma thromboplastin antecedent [PTA]) and then activates a cascading series of coagulant substances called the **intrinsic pathway** (Figure 48.3) that ends with the conversion of prothrombin to thrombin. Activated thrombin breaks down fibrinogen to form insoluble fibrin threads, which form a clot inside the blood vessel. The clot, called a thrombus, acts to plug the injury and seal the system.

Extrinsic pathway

While the coagulation process is going on inside the blood vessel via the intrinsic pathway, the blood that has leaked out of the vascular system and into the surrounding tissues is caused to clot by the **extrinsic pathway.** Injured cells release a substance called tissue thromboplastin, which activates clotting factors in the blood and starts the clotting cascade to form a clot on the outside of the blood vessel. The injured vessel is now vasoconstricted and has a platelet plug, as well as a clot on both the inside and the outside of the blood vessel in

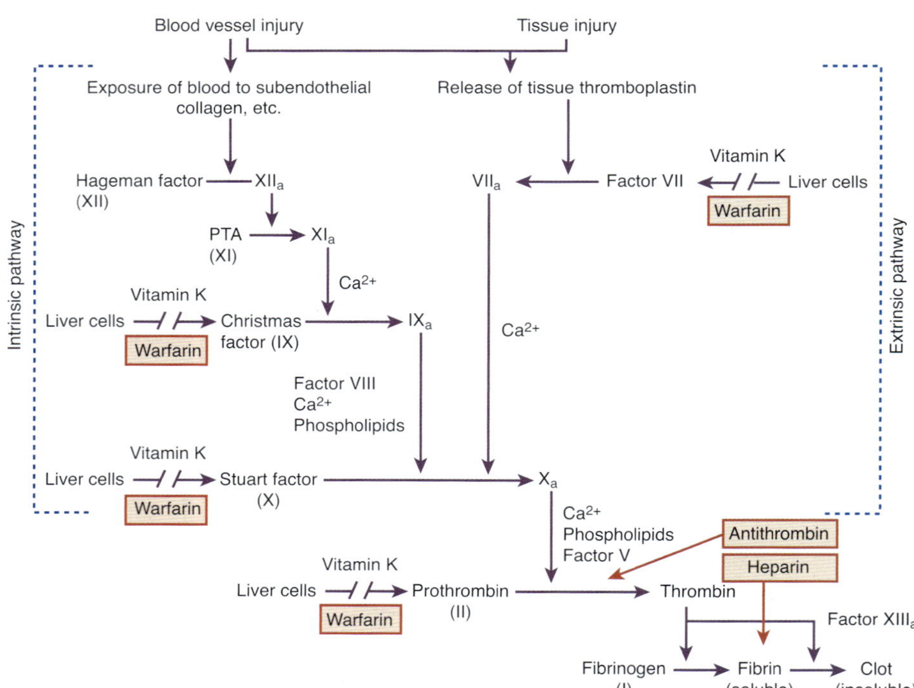

FIGURE 48.3 Details of the intrinsic and extrinsic clotting pathways. The sites of action of some of the drugs that can influence these processes are shown in red.

the area of the injury. These actions maintain the closed nature of the cardiovascular system (see Figure 48.3).

Clot resolution and anticlotting process

Blood plasma also contains anticlotting substances that inhibit clotting reactions that might otherwise lead to an obstruction of blood vessels by blood clots. For example, antithrombin III prevents the formation of thrombin, thus stopping the breakdown of the fibrin threads.

Another substance in the plasma, called plasmin or fibrinolysin, dissolves clots to ensure free movement of blood through the system. Plasmin is a protein-dissolving substance that breaks down the fibrin framework of blood clots and opens up vessels. Its precursor, called **plasminogen**, is made in the liver and is found in the plasma. The conversion of plasminogen to plasmin begins with the activation of Hageman factor and is facilitated by a number of other factors, including antidiuretic hormone (ADH), adrenaline, pyrogens, emotional stress, physical activity and urokinase. Plasmin helps to keep blood vessels open and functional. Very high levels of plasmin are found in the lungs (which contain millions of tiny, easily injured capillaries) and in the uterus (which in pregnancy must maintain a constant blood flow for the developing fetus). The action of plasmin is evident in the female menstrual flow, in that clots do not form rapidly when the lining of the uterus is shed; the blood oozes slowly over a period of days (Figure 48.4).

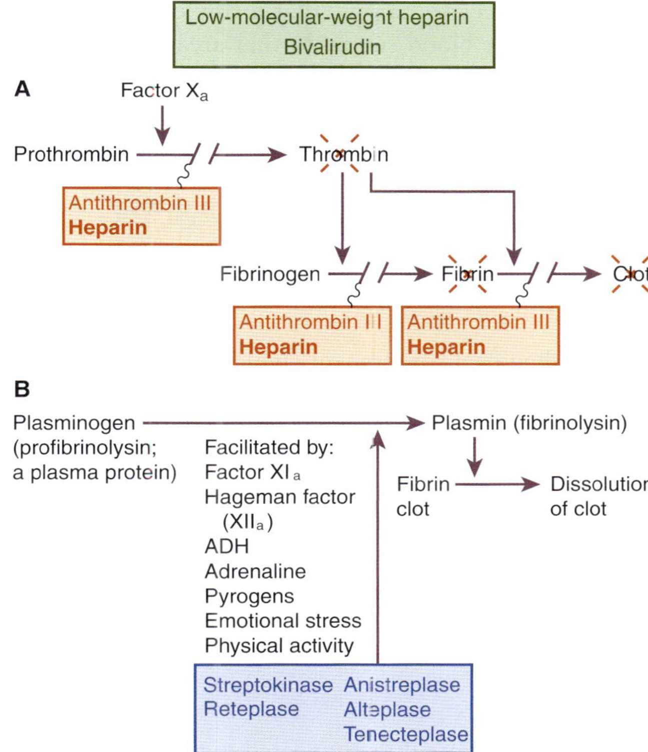

FIGURE 48.4 **A.** Anticlotting process. Antithrombin III (in plasma) inhibits the activity of Stuart factor (factor Xa) and thrombin; the drug heparin enhances the activity of antithrombin III. Steps in clot formation that are inhibited by heparin are shown in red. **B.** Fibrinolytic process: clots are dissolved. The step that is facilitated by the clot-dissolving drugs and by other agents is shown in blue.

KEY POINTS

- The transformation of fluid blood into a solid state to seal breaks in the vascular system is known as coagulation.
- The coagulation process involves vasoconstriction, platelet aggregation to form a plug and intrinsic and extrinsic clot formation initiated by Hageman factor to plug any breaks in the system.
- The conversion of prothrombin to thrombin, which results in insoluble fibrin threads, is the final step of clot formation.
- To prevent the occlusion of blood vessels and the blocking of blood flow to the tissues, a formed clot must be dissolved.
- The base of the clot-dissolving system is the conversion of plasminogen to plasmin (fibrinolysin) by several factors, including Hageman factor. Plasmin dissolves fibrin threads and resolves the clot.

DISORDERS AFFECTING BLOOD COAGULATION

Disorders that directly affect the coagulation process are referred to as haemorrhagic disorders. These disorders fall into two main categories: (1) conditions that involve overproduction of clots, or thromboembolic disorders; and (2) conditions in which the clotting process is not working effectively, resulting in risk for excess bleeding.

Thromboembolic disorders

Medical conditions that involve the formation of thrombi result in decreased blood flow through, or total occlusion of, a blood vessel. These conditions are marked by the signs and symptoms of hypoxia, anoxia or even necrosis in areas affected by the decreased blood flow. In some of these disorders, pieces of the thrombus, called emboli, can break off and travel through the cardiovascular system until they become lodged in a tiny vessel, plugging it up.

Conditions that predispose a person to the formation of clots and emboli are called **thromboembolic disorders**. Coronary artery disease (CAD) involves a narrowing of the coronary arteries caused by damage to the endothelial lining of these vessels. Thrombi tend to form along the damaged endothelial lining. As the damage builds up, the lumens of the vessels become narrower and narrower. Over time, the coronary arteries are unable to deliver enough blood to meet the needs of the heart muscle and hypoxia develops. If a vessel becomes so narrow that a tiny clot occludes it completely, the blood supply to that area is cut off and anoxia occurs, followed by infarction and necrosis. With age, many of the vessels in the body can be damaged and develop similar problems with narrowing and blood delivery. These disorders are treated with drugs that interfere with the normal coagulation process to prevent the formation of clots in the system.

Haemorrhagic disorders

Haemorrhagic disorders, in which excess bleeding occurs, are less common than thromboembolic disorders. These disorders include haemophilia, in which there is a genetic lack of clotting factors; liver disease, in which clotting factors and proteins needed for clotting are not produced; and bone marrow disorders, in which platelets are not formed in sufficient quantity to be effective. These disorders are treated with clotting factors and drugs that promote the coagulation process.

KEY POINT

- Disorders that are directly related to the clotting process include thromboembolic disorders, in which too much clotting can lead to emboli and occlusion of blood vessels, and haemorrhagic disorders, including haemophilia, in which lack of efficient clotting can lead to excessive blood loss.

DRUGS AFFECTING CLOT FORMATION AND RESOLUTION

Drugs that affect clot formation include **antiplatelet** drugs, which alter platelet aggregation and the formation of the platelet plug; anticoagulants, which interfere with the clotting cascade and thrombin formation; and thrombolytic agents, which break down the thrombus or clot that has been formed by stimulating the plasmin system (see Table 48.1). Box 48.2 discusses the interaction of herbal remedies with these agents.

ANTIPLATELET AGENTS

Antiplatelet agents decrease the formation of the platelet plug by decreasing the responsiveness of the platelets to stimuli that would cause them to stick and aggregate on a vessel wall. Antiplatelet agents available for use include abciximab (*ReoPro*), anagrelide (*Agrylin*), aspirin, cilostazol (*Pletal* [not available in New Zealand]), clopidogrel (*Plavix*), dipyridamole (*Persantin*), eptifibatide (*Integrilin*), prasugrel (*Effient*), ticagrelor (*Brilinta*), ticlopidine (*Tilodene*), and tirofiban (*Aggrastat*).

Therapeutic actions and indications

Most antiplatelet agents inhibit platelet adhesion and aggregation by blocking receptor sites on the platelet membrane, preventing platelet–platelet interaction or

TABLE 48.1 DRUGS IN FOCUS Drugs affecting clot formation and resolution

Drug name	Dosage/route	Usual indications
Antiplatelet agents		
abciximab (*ReoPro*)	0.25 mg/kg IV bolus 10–60 minutes before procedure, then continuous infusion of 10 micrograms per minute for 12 hours Angina: 0.25 mg/kg by IV bolus, then 10 micrograms per minute IV for 18–24 hours	Prevention of acute cardiac events during transluminal coronary angioplasty when used in conjunction with heparin and aspirin; early treatment of unstable angina and non-Q-wave myocardial infarction (MI)
anagrelide (*Agrylin*)	Initially 0.5 mg bd, increasing by 0.5 mg weekly; usual dose 1.5–3 mg daily; maximum 2.5 mg/dose or 10 mg/day	Treatment of essential thrombocythaemia to reduce elevated platelet count and decrease the risk of thrombosis
(P) aspirin (*Astrix, Cardiprin, Cartia*)	75–150 mg/day PO to reduce platelet aggregation	Reduction of the incidence of TIAs and strokes in men; reduction of the risk of death or non-fatal MI in people with a past history of MI or with angina
cilostazol (*Pletal*)	100 mg PO bd half an hour before or 2 hours after meals	Reduction of symptoms of intermittent claudication, allowing increased walking distance in adults
clopidogrel (*Plavix*)	Prevention: 75 mg/day PO Treatment: 300 mg loading dose then 75 mg/day	Treatment of people who are at risk for ischaemic events; people with a history of MI, peripheral artery disease, or ischaemic stroke; and people with acute coronary syndrome

TABLE 48.1 DRUGS IN FOCUS Drugs affecting clot formation and resolution *(continued)*

Drug name	Dosage/route	Usual indications
Antiplatelet agents *(continued)*		
dipyridamole (*Persantin, Persantin SR, Pytazen SR*)	Angina: 50 mg PO tid; 75–100 mg PO qid for people with heart valve problems Sustained release: 200 mg bd or 150 mg bd Immediate release: 300–450 mg daily in 3–4 divided doses, maximum 600 mg daily Injection, perfusion imaging: 0.142 mg/kg/min (0.56 mg/kg total) IV over 4 minutes for diagnosis; maximum 60 mg Injection, stress echo: 0.56 mg/kg over 4 minutes, followed by 4 minutes of no dose, then if echo monitoring shows no changes, 0.28 mg/kg over 2 minutes, yielding a cumulative dosage of 0.84 mg/kg over 10 minutes	Prevention of thromboembolism in people with artificial heart valves when used in combination with warfarin; aids diagnosis of coronary artery disease (CAD) in people who cannot exercise; may be used in treatment of angina (found to be only 'possibly effective' by the US FDA)
eptifibatide (*Integrilin*)	180 micrograms/kg bolus IV over 1–2 minutes, then 2 micrograms/kg/min IV for up to 72 hours for acute coronary syndrome; second bolus 180 micrograms/kg 10 minutes after first bolus	Treatment of acute coronary syndrome; prevention of ischaemic episodes in people undergoing percutaneous coronary interventions
prasugrel (*Effient*)	Single 60 mg PO loading dose, then 10 mg/day PO	Prevention of atherothrombotic events in individuals with acute coronary syndromes, in conjunction with aspirin
ticagrelor (*Brilinta*)	180 mg PO loading dose, then 90 mg PO bd	Prevention of atherothrombotic events in individuals with acute coronary syndromes, in conjunction with aspirin
tirofiban (*Aggrastat*)	0.4 microgram/kg per minute IV over 30 minutes, then continuous infusion of 0.1 microgram/kg per minute	Treatment of acute coronary syndrome and prevention of cardiac ischaemic events during percutaneous coronary intervention; used in combination with heparin
Anticoagulants		
antithrombin III (*Thrombotrol-VF*)	Dose must be calculated using body weight and baseline levels. Exact loading dose and maintenance intervals individualised for each patient, based on individual's clinical condition, response to therapy and actual plasma ATIII levels achieved	Replacement in hereditary antithrombin III deficiency; treatment of people with this deficiency who are to undergo surgery or obstetric procedures that might put them at risk for thromboembolism
apixaban (*Eliquis*)	Prophylaxis: 2.5 mg bd Treatment of DVT and PE: 10 mg bd for 7 days, followed by 5 mg bd	Prevention of thromboembolic events in individuals who have undergone elective total hip or total knee replacement; prevention of stroke and embolism in individuals with atrial fibrillation and one or more risk factors
bivalirudin (*Angiomax*)	0.1–0.75 mg/kg bolus, depending on condition, followed by 0.25–1.75 mg/kg/hour infusion, depending on condition	Prevention of ischaemic events in people undergoing transluminal coronary angioplasty when used in combination with aspirin
dabigatran (*Pradaxa*)	Prophylaxis of stroke, embolism or DVT: 110–150 mg bd depending on condition and age of patient	Prevention of thromboembolic events in individuals who have undergone elective total hip or total knee replacement; prevention of stroke and embolism in individuals with atrial fibrillation and one or more risk factors
fondaparinux (*Arixtra*)	Prevention: 2.5 mg/day by SC injection starting 6 hours after surgical closure and continuing for 7–9 days Treatment: 5–10 mg/day by SC injections for 5 days depending on patient's body weight	Prevention and treatment of venous thromboembolic events following surgery for hip fracture, hip replacement or knee replacement; used with warfarin when appropriate

Continued on following page

TABLE 48.1 DRUGS IN FOCUS Drugs affecting clot formation and resolution *(continued)*

Drug name	Dosage/route	Usual indications
Anticoagulants *(continued)*		
(P) heparin (generic)	Adults, prophylaxis: 5000 units SC 2 hours before surgery and every 8–12 hours for 7 days Adults, intermittent IV treatment: 5000 units or 75 units/kg as bolus, followed by continuous IV infusion of 18 units/kg/hour (monitor APTT and adjust dose accordingly) Adults, SC treatment: following 5000 units IV bolus, 15,000 units SC every 12 hours (monitor APTT and adjust dose accordingly) Paediatric: 50 units/kg IV bolus, then 100 units/kg IV q 4 hours	Prevention and treatment of venous thrombosis, pulmonary embolus, atrial fibrillation with embolisation; prevention of clotting in blood samples, dialysis and venous tubing; diagnosis and treatment of disseminated intravascular coagulation (DIC) (Box 48.3); also used as an adjunct in the treatment of MI and stroke
rivaroxaban (*Xarelto*)	Prevention: 10–20 mg once daily, depending on condition Treatment of DVT and PE and prevention of recurrent DVT and PE: 15 mg bd for the first 3 weeks followed by 20 mg once daily	Prevention of thromboembolic events in individuals who have undergone elective total hip or total knee replacement; prevention of stroke and embolism in individuals with atrial fibrillation and one or more risk factors; prevention of deep vein thrombosis (DVT) and pulmonary embolism
warfarin (*Coumadin*, *Marevan*)	Adult, day 1: 5–10 mg once daily (5 mg for elderly people or those with high bleeding risk); day 2: 5 mg once daily, then adjusted according to INR; usual maintenance dose 1–10 mg/day PO, based on INR, then 2–10 mg/day PO, based on PT ratio or INR; use lower doses with elderly people Adult, low dose initiation: 3 mg once daily for 2 days, then adjusted according to INR	Treatment of people with atrial fibrillation, artificial heart valves or valvular damage that makes them susceptible to thrombus and embolus formation; prevention and treatment of venous thrombosis, pulmonary embolus, embolus with atrial fibrillation, systemic emboli after MI
Thrombolytic agents		
alteplase (*Actilyse*)	Adult: 10 mg IV bolus then 50 mg IV over 1 hour, then 40 mg IV over another 2 hours	Treatment of MI, acute pulmonary embolism and acute ischaemic stroke; restoration of function in occluded central venous access devices
reteplase (*Rapilysin*)	10 International Units bolus IV over 2 minutes then, after 30 minutes, 10 International Units double-bolus IV each over 2 minutes, 30 minutes apart	Treatment of coronary artery thrombosis associated with an acute MI
tenecteplase (*Metalyse*)	Adult: 30–50 according to body weight (maximum 50 mg) IV over 5–10 seconds, started as soon as possible and within 12 hours of symptom onset	Reduction of mortality associated with acute MI
Other drugs affecting clot formation		
Low-molecular-weight heparins		
dalteparin (*Fragmin*)	DVT: 2500–5000 International Units/day SC starting 1–2 hours before surgery and then for 5–7 days Orthopaedic surgery (eg, hip replacement): 5000 International Units SC daily for 5 weeks Angina: 120 International Units/kg SC q 12 hours with aspirin therapy for 5–8 days	Prevention of DVT that may lead to PE after abdominal surgery or hip replacement; treatment of unstable angina and non-Q-wave MI
enoxaparin (*Clexane*)	Hip surgery: 40 mg SC 12 hours before surgery then 40 mg SC daily for 30 days Abdominal surgery: 40 mg/day SC for 7–10 days DVT or PE: 1 mg/kg SC q 12 hours Angina: 1 mg/kg SC q 12 hours Prevention of DVT in high-risk people: 40 mg/day SC for 7–10 days Reduce dose in people with renal impairment	Prevention of DVT that may lead to PE after hip replacement or abdominal surgery; with warfarin to treat acute DVT or PE; prevention of ischaemic complications of unstable angina or non-Q-wave MI; prevention of DVT in people with severely restricted mobility due to illness

TABLE 48.1 DRUGS IN FOCUS Drugs affecting clot formation and resolution *(continued)*

Drug name	Dosage/route	Usual indications
Heparinoids		
Danaparoid (*Orgaran*)	Adult: 750 anti-Factor Xa units bd for 7–10 days	Prevention of postoperative VTE in patients undergoing general or orthopaedic surgery
vitamin K (*Konakion Adult, Konakion MM*)	Konakion Adult, adult: 2.5–10 mg PO or IV Konakion MM, neonatal prophylaxis: 2 mg PO at birth, repeated at 3–5 days and 4 weeks, or 1 mg IM at birth	Treatment of anticoagulant-induced prothrombin deficiency
Haemorheological agent		
oxypentifylline (*Trental*)	400 mg PO tds with meals	Treatment of intermittent claudication to improve function and reduce symptoms; improve blood flow in vascular diseases

BOX 48.2 FOCUS ON Herbal and alternative therapies

Many herbal therapies can cause problems when used with drugs that affect blood coagulation. People taking these drugs should be cautioned to avoid angelica, cat's claw, chamomile, chondroitin, feverfew, garlic, ginkgo, goldenseal, grape seed extract, green leaf tea, horse chestnut seed, psyllium and turmeric. If a person who is taking an anticoagulant presents with increased bleeding and no other interaction or cause is found, question the person about the possibility of use of herbal therapies.

the interaction of platelets with other clotting chemicals. One drug, anagrelide, blocks the production of platelets in the bone marrow. These agents are used effectively to treat cardiovascular diseases that are prone to produce occluded vessels; for the maintenance of venous and arterial grafts; to prevent cerebrovascular occlusion; and as adjuncts to thrombolytic therapy in the treatment of myocardial infarction (MI) and the prevention of reinfarction after MI. The prescriber's choice of drug depends on the intended use and the person's tolerance of the associated adverse effects. See Table 48.1 for usual indications for each of these agents.

Pharmacokinetics

Abciximab, eptifibatide and tirofiban are administered intravenously (IV). Antiplatelet agents that are administered orally include anagrelide, aspirin, cilostazol, clopidogrel, prasugrel and ticagrelor. Dipyridamole is used orally or as an IV agent.

These drugs are generally well absorbed and highly bound to plasma proteins. They are metabolised in the liver and excreted in urine, and they tend to enter breast milk (see Contraindications and cautions).

Contraindications and cautions

Antiplatelet agents are contraindicated in the presence of allergy to the specific drug *to avoid hypersensitivity reactions*. Caution should be used in the following conditions: the presence of any known bleeding disorder *because of the risk of excessive blood loss*; recent surgery *because of the risk of increased bleeding in unhealed vessels*; and closed head injuries *because of the risk of bleeding from the injured vessels in the brain*.

Although there are no adequate studies of these drugs in pregnancy, they are contraindicated *because of the potential for increased bleeding* (see Adverse effects); they should be used during pregnancy only if the benefits to the mother clearly outweigh the potential risks to the fetus. These drugs are also contraindicated during breastfeeding *because of the potential adverse effects on the fetus or neonate*; if they are needed by a breastfeeding woman, she should find another method of feeding the baby.

Anagrelide should be used with caution with any history of thrombocytopenia *because it decreases the production of platelets in the bone marrow*. Platelet levels should be checked regularly to monitor for thrombocytopenia if a person is on this drug.

Adverse effects

The most common adverse effect seen with these drugs is bleeding, which often occurs as increased bruising and bleeding while brushing the teeth. Other common problems include headache, dizziness and weakness; the cause of these reactions is not understood. Nausea and gastrointestinal (GI) distress may occur because of direct irritating effects of the oral drug on the GI tract. Skin rash, another common effect, may be related to direct drug effects on the dermis.

Clinically important drug–drug interactions

The risk of excessive bleeding increases if any of these drugs is combined with another drug that affects blood clotting.

Prototype summary: aspirin

Indications: reduction of risk of recurrent transient ischaemic attacks (TIAs) or strokes in men with a history of TIA due to fibrin or platelet emboli; reduction of death or non-fatal MI in people with a history of infarction or unstable angina; MI prophylaxis; also used for its anti-inflammatory, analgesic and antipyretic effects.

Actions: inhibits platelet aggregation by inhibiting platelet synthesis of thromboxane A_2.

Pharmacokinetics:

Route	Onset	Peak	Duration
Oral	5–30 min	0.25–2 hours	3–6 hours

$T_{1/2}$: 15 minutes to 12 hours; metabolised in the liver and excreted in urine.

Adverse effects: acute aspirin toxicity with hyperpnoea, possibly leading to fever, coma and cardiovascular collapse; nausea, dyspepsia, heartburn, epigastric discomfort, GI bleeding, occult blood loss, dizziness, tinnitus, difficulty hearing, anaphylactoid reaction.

Care considerations for people receiving antiplatelet agents

Assessment: history and examination

- Assess for the following conditions, *which could be cautions or contraindications to use of the drug*: any known allergies to these drugs; pregnancy or breastfeeding *because of the potential adverse effects on the fetus or neonate*; and bleeding disorders, recent surgery or closed head injury *because of the potential for excessive bleeding.*
- Assess baseline status before beginning therapy *to determine any potential adverse effects.* This includes body temperature; skin colour, lesions and temperature; affect, orientation and reflexes; pulse, blood pressure and perfusion; respirations and adventitious sounds; full blood count (FBC); and clotting studies (see Table 48.2).

Implementation with rationale

- Provide small, frequent meals *to relieve GI discomfort* if GI upset is a problem.
- Provide comfort measures and analgesia for headache *to relieve pain and improve compliance with the drug regimen.*
- Suggest safety measures, including the use of an electric razor and avoidance of contact sports, *to decrease the risk of bleeding.*
- Monitor platelet count if the person is using anagrelide *to detect thrombocytopenia and increased risk of bleeding.*
- Provide increased precautions against bleeding during invasive procedures; use pressure dressings and ice *to decrease excessive blood loss caused by anticoagulation.*
- Mark the chart of any person receiving this drug *to alert medical staff that there is a potential for increased bleeding.*
- Provide thorough teaching, including the name of the drug, dosage prescribed, measures to avoid adverse effects, warning signs of problems, the need for periodic monitoring and evaluation, and the need to wear or carry a MedicAlert notification, *to enhance knowledge about drug therapy and to promote compliance.*
- Offer support and encouragement *to help the person deal with the diagnosis and the drug regimen.*

Evaluation

- Monitor response to the drug (increased bleeding time, prevention of occlusive events).
- Monitor for adverse effects (bleeding, GI upset, dizziness, headache).
- Evaluate the effectiveness of the teaching plan (person can name drug, dosage, adverse effects to watch for and specific measures to avoid them; individual understands the importance of continued follow-up).
- Monitor the effectiveness of comfort measures and compliance with the regimen.

Anticoagulants

Anticoagulants are drugs that interfere with the normal coagulation process by interfering with the clotting cascade and thrombin formation. Drugs in this class include antithrombin III (*Thrombotrol-VF*), apixaban (*Eliquis*), bivalirudin (*Angiomax*), dabigatran etexilate (*Pradaxa*), fondaparinux (*Arixtra* [not available in New Zealand]), heparin (generic), rivaroxaban (*Xarelto*) and warfarin (*Coumadin*, *Marevan*).

Therapeutic actions and indications

As noted previously, the anticoagulants interfere with the normal cascade of events involved in the clotting process. Warfarin causes a decrease in the production of vitamin K–dependent clotting factors in the liver. The eventual effect is a depletion of these clotting factors and a prolongation of clotting times. It is used to maintain a state of anticoagulation in situations in which the person is susceptible to potentially dangerous clot formation (see Table 48.1 for usual indications for warfarin). *See the Critical thinking scenario for additional care for people taking warfarin.*

Heparin, bivalirudin, apixaban, dabigatran and rivaroxaban block the formation of thrombin from prothrombin. The usual indications for heparin include acute treatment and prevention of venous thrombosis and pulmonary embolism; treatment of atrial fibrillation with embolisation; prevention of clotting in blood samples, and in dialysis and venous tubing; and diagnosis and treatment of disseminated intravascular coagulation (DIC) (Box 48.3). Because heparin must be injected, it is often not the drug of choice for outpatients, who would be responsible for injecting the drug several times during the day. Individuals may be started on heparin in the acute situation and then switched to the oral drug warfarin. Apixaban, dabigatran and rivaroxaban are commonly used to prevent thrombosis following total hip or knee replacement and in individuals with atrial fibrillation.

Antithrombin interferes with the formation of thrombin from prothrombin; it is a naturally occurring anticoagulant, as mentioned earlier, and a natural safety feature in the clotting system. Fondaparinux is a selective inhibitor of activated factor Xa, approved in 2002. It inhibits factor Xa and blocks the clotting cascade to prevent clot formation. It is supplied in prefilled syringes, making it convenient for people who self-administer the drug at home.

Pharmacokinetics

Heparin is injected IV or subcutaneously (SC) and has an almost immediate onset of action. It is excreted in urine. Warfarin, apixaban, dabigatran and rivaroxaban are used orally. All other drugs in this class (heparin, antithrombin, fondaparinux and bivalirudin) are given parenterally. Warfarin is readily absorbed through the GI tract, metabolised in the liver and excreted in urine and faeces. Warfarin's onset of action is about 3 days;

BOX 48.3 Understanding disseminated intravascular coagulation

Disseminated intravascular coagulation (DIC) is a syndrome in which bleeding and thrombosis are found together. It can occur as a complication of many problems, including severe infection with septic shock, traumatic childbirth or missed abortion, and massive injuries. In these disorders, local tissue damage causes the release of coagulation-stimulating substances into the circulation. These substances then stimulate the coagulation process, causing fibrin clot formation in small vessels in the lungs, kidneys, brain and other organs. This continuing reaction consumes excessive amounts of fibrinogen, other clotting factors and platelets. The end result is increased bleeding. In essence, the person clots too much, resulting in the possibility of bleeding to death.

The first step in treating this disorder is to control the problem that initially precipitated it. For example, treating the infection, performing dilation and curettage to clear the uterus, or stabilising injuries can help stop this continuing process. Whole-blood infusions or the infusion of fibrinogen may be used to buy some time until the person is stable and can form clotting factors again. There are associated problems with giving whole blood (eg, development of hepatitis or AIDS), and there is a risk that fibrinogen may set off further intravascular clotting. Paradoxically, the treatment of choice for DIC is the anticoagulant heparin. Heparin prevents the clotting phase from being completed, thus inhibiting the breakdown of fibrinogen. It may also help avoid haemorrhage by preventing the body from depleting its entire store of coagulation factors.

Because heparin is usually administered to prevent blood clotting, and the adverse effects that are monitored with heparin therapy include signs of bleeding, it can be a real challenge for the health care providers to feel comfortable administering heparin to a person who is bleeding to death. Understanding of the disease process can help alleviate any doubts about the treatment.

CRITICAL THINKING SCENARIO

Oral anticoagulant therapy

THE SITUATION

G.R. is a 68-year-old woman with a history of severe mitral valve disease. For the last several years, she has been able to manage her condition with digoxin, a diuretic and a potassium supplement. However, on a recent visit to her doctor she disclosed that she had been experiencing periods of breathlessness, palpitations and dizziness. Tests showed that she was having frequent periods of atrial fibrillation (AF), with a heart rate of up to 140 beats/minute. Because of the danger of emboli as a result of her valve disease and the bouts of AF, warfarin therapy was begun.

CRITICAL THINKING

What care interventions should be done at this point?

Why do people with mitral valve disease frequently develop AF? *Think about why emboli form when the atria fibrillate.*

Stabilising G.R. on warfarin may take several weeks of blood tests and dose adjustments. How can this process be made easier?

What teaching points should be covered with G.R. to ensure that she is protected from emboli and does not experience excessive bleeding?

DISCUSSION

G.R.'s situation is complex. She has a progressive degenerative valve disease that usually leads to heart failure (HF) and frequently to other complications, such as AF and emboli formation. Her digoxin and potassium levels should be checked to determine whether her HF has stabilised or the digoxin is causing the AF because of excessive doses or potassium imbalance. If these tests are within normal limits, G.R. may be experiencing AF because of irritation to the atrial cells caused by the damaged mitral valve and associated swelling and scarring. If this is the case, an anticoagulant will help protect G.R. against emboli, which form in the auricles when blood pools there while the atria are fibrillating. There is less chance of emboli formation if clotting is slowed.

G.R. will need extensive teaching about warfarin, including the need for frequent blood tests, the list of potential drug–drug interactions, the importance of being alert to the many factors that can affect dose needs (including illness and diet) and how to monitor for subtle blood loss. This can also be a good opportunity to review teaching about valvular disease and HF and to answer any questions that she might have about how all of these things interrelate. If possible, it would be useful to teach G.R. or a responsible carer how to take a pulse so that G.R. can be alerted to potential arrhythmias and avert problems before they begin. It also would be a good idea to check on support services for G.R. to ensure that her blood tests can be done and that her response to the drug is monitored carefully.

CARE GUIDE FOR G.R.: WARFARIN

Assessment: history and examination

Assess G.R.'s health history for allergies to warfarin, subacute bacterial endocarditis (SBE), haemorrhagic disorders, tuberculosis, renal or hepatic dysfunction, gastric ulcers, thyroid disease, uncontrolled hypertension, severe trauma or a long-term indwelling catheter (which increases the risk of bleeding). Also assess concurrent use of numerous drugs and herbal therapies.

Focus the physical examination on the following areas:

Cardiovascular: blood pressure, pulse, perfusion, baseline electrocardiogram (ECG)

Neurological (CNS): orientation, affect, reflexes, vision

Skin: colour, lesions, texture

Respiratory system: respiratory rate and character, adventitious sounds

GI: abdominal examination, guaiac stool test results (for occult blood)

Laboratory tests: liver and renal function tests, prothrombin time (PT), International Normalised Ratio (INR)

Implementation

Ensure proper administration of the drug.

Provide comfort and safety measures, such as small meals, protection from injury during invasive and other procedures, bowel program as needed, standby antidotes (eg, vitamin K) and careful skin care.

Provide support and reassurance to deal with drug effects.

Provide teaching regarding drug, dosage, adverse effects, what to report and safety precautions.

Evaluation

Evaluate drug effects: increased bleeding times, PT 1.5–2.5 times control or PT/INR ratio of 2:3.

Monitor for adverse effects: bleeding, alopecia, rash, GI upset, excessive bleeding.

Monitor for drug–drug interactions (numerous).

Evaluate the effectiveness of the teaching program and comfort and safety measures.

TEACHING FOR G.R.

- An anticoagulant slows the body's normal blood clotting processes to prevent harmful blood clots from forming. This type of drug is often called a 'blood thinner'; however, it cannot dissolve any clots that have already formed.
- *Never* change any medication that you are taking – such as adding or stopping another drug, taking a new over-the-counter medication, or stopping one that you have been taking regularly – without consulting with your health care provider. Many other drugs affect the way that your anticoagulant works; starting or stopping another drug can cause excessive bleeding or interfere with the desired effects of the drug.
- Some of the following adverse effects may occur:
  - *Stomach bloating, cramps:* these problems often pass with time; consult your health care provider if they persist or become too uncomfortable.
  - *Loss of hair, skin rash:* these problems can be very frustrating; you may wish to discuss these with your health care provider.
  - *Orange-yellow discolouration of the urine:* this can be frightening, but it may just be an effect of the drug. If you are concerned that this might be blood, simply add vinegar to your urine; the colour should disappear. If the colour does not disappear, it may be caused by blood, and you should contact your health care provider.
  - Report any of the following to your health care provider: *unusual bleeding (when brushing your teeth, excessive bleeding from an injury, excessive bruising); black or tarry*

stools; cloudy or dark urine; sore throat, fever or chills; severe headache or dizziness.
- Tell any doctor, nurse or other health care provider involved in your care that you are taking this drug. You should carry or wear medical identification stating that you are taking this drug to alert emergency medical personnel that you are at increased risk for bleeding.
- Avoid situations in which you could be easily injured – for example, engaging in contact sports or games with children or using a straight razor.
- Keep this drug, and all medications, out of the reach of children.
- Avoid the use of over-the-counter medications while you are taking this drug. If you feel that you need one of these, consult with your health care provider for the best choice. Many of these drugs can interfere with your anticoagulant.
- Schedule regular, periodic blood tests while you are taking this drug to monitor the effects of the drug on your body and adjust your dose as needed.

its effects last for 4–5 days. Because of the time delay, warfarin is not the drug of choice in an acute situation, but it is convenient and useful for prolonged effects.

Because antithrombin is an exogenous form of a naturally occurring anticoagulant, the body handles it in the same way that it handles naturally occurring antithrombin. Fondaparinux is absorbed quickly from SC sites and metabolised and excreted by the kidneys. Bivalirudin is given IV and is excreted through the kidneys.

Contraindications and cautions

The anticoagulants are contraindicated in the presence of known allergy to the drugs *to avoid hypersensitivity reactions*. They also should not be used with any conditions *that could be compromised by increased bleeding tendencies*, including haemorrhagic disorders, recent trauma, spinal puncture, GI ulcers, recent surgery, intrauterine device placement, tuberculosis, presence of indwelling catheters and threatened abortion. Warfarin is contraindicated in pregnancy *because fetal injury and death have occurred*; in breastfeeding, *because of the potential risk to the baby*; and in renal or hepatic disease, *which could interfere with the metabolism and effectiveness of these drugs*. Although some adverse fetal effects have been reported with its use during pregnancy, heparin does not enter breast milk, and so it is the anticoagulant of choice if one is needed during breastfeeding. Dabigatran is renally cleared and accumulates in people with poor renal function. Therefore, dabigatran must not be given to people with a creatinine clearance (CrCl) of less than 30 mL/minute.

Caution should be used in people with heart failure (HF), thyrotoxicosis, senility or psychosis *because of the potential for unexpected effects* and in individuals with diarrhoea or fever, *which could alter the normal clotting process by, respectively, loss of vitamin K from the intestine or activation of plasminogen*. Caution should be used in pregnancy with anticoagulants other than warfarin *because of the potential for adverse effects*; benefit should outweigh potential risks.

Adverse effects

The most commonly encountered adverse effect of the anticoagulants is bleeding, ranging from bleeding gums with tooth brushing to severe internal haemorrhage. Individuals will need teaching about administration, disposal of the syringes and signs of bleeding to watch for. Periodic blood tests will be needed to assess the effects of the drug on the body. Clotting times should be monitored closely to avoid these problems. Table 48.2 reviews clotting studies that should be monitored. The person should also be monitored for warfarin overdose.

Serious adverse effects may occur when adding or taking away a drug from the regimen of a person receiving warfarin without careful monitoring and adjustment of the warfarin dose (see Clinically important drug–drug interactions). Warfarin has been associated with alopecia and dermatitis, as well as bone marrow depression and, less frequently, prolonged and painful erections. The Focus on safe medication administration discusses treatment of heparin overdose. Nausea, GI upset, diarrhoea and hepatic dysfunction also may occur secondary to direct drug toxicity.

Clinically important drug–drug interactions

Increased bleeding can occur if heparin is combined with oral anticoagulants, salicylates, penicillins or cefalosporins. Decreased anticoagulation can occur if heparin is combined with glyceryl trinitrate.

Warfarin has documented drug–drug interactions with a vast number of other drugs (Table 48.3). It is a wise practice never to add or take away a drug from the regimen of the person receiving warfarin without careful monitoring and adjustment of the warfarin dose to prevent serious adverse effects. Because of the many factors that can affect the therapeutic levels of warfarin, it is often very difficult to reach a stable level and maintain that level.

TABLE 48.2 Review of clotting studies

Test	Measure	Therapeutic range	Uses
Activated partial thromboplastin time (aPTT) Partial thromboplastin time (PTT)	Activity of intrinsic pathway of coagulation	1.5–2.5 times baseline	Dose adjustment for heparin, low-molecular-weight heparins, bivalirudin
International Normalised Ratio (INR)	Standardised measure of prothrombin levels	2–3.5	Warfarin dose adjustment, fondaparinux dose adjustment
Prothrombin time (PT)	Time required for clotting to occur; extrinsic pathway activity	1.3–1.5	Warfarin dose adjustment

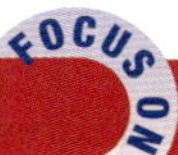

Safe medication administration

Injectable vitamin K (phytomenadione) is used to reverse the effects of warfarin. Vitamin K promotes the liver synthesis of several clotting factors. When these pathways have been inhibited by warfarin, clotting time is increased. If an increased level of vitamin K is provided, more of these factors are produced, and the clotting time can be brought back within a normal range. Because of the way in which vitamin K exerts its effects on clotting, there is a delay of at least 24 hours from the time the drug is given until some change can be seen. This occurs because there is no direct effect on the warfarin, but rather an increased stimulation of the liver, which must then produce the clotting factors. The usual dose for the treatment of anticoagulant-induced prothrombin deficiency is 0.5–10 mg by IV injection over 30 seconds. Oral doses can be used if injection is not feasible. A prothrombin time (PT) response within 6–8 hours after parenteral doses or 12–48 hours after oral doses will determine the need for a repeat dose. If a response is not seen and the person is bleeding excessively, fresh-frozen plasma or an infusion of whole blood may be needed.

 **Prototype summary: heparin**

Indications: prevention and treatment of venous thrombosis and pulmonary emboli; treatment of atrial fibrillation with embolisation; diagnosis and treatment of DIC; prevention of clotting in blood samples and heparin locksets.

Actions: inhibits thrombus and clot production by blocking the conversion of prothrombin to thrombin and fibrinogen to fibrin.

Pharmacokinetics:

Route	Onset	Peak	Duration
IV	Immediate	Minutes	2–6 hours
SC	20–60 min	2–4 hours	8–12 hours

$T_{1/2}$: 30–180 minutes; metabolised in the cells and excreted in urine.

Adverse effects: loss of hair, bruising, chills, fever, osteoporosis, suppression of renal function (with long-term use).

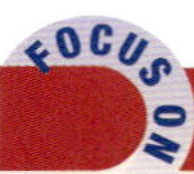

Safe medication administration

In cases of a heparin overdose, the antidote is protamine sulfate (generic). This basic protein drug forms stable salts with heparin as soon as the two drugs come in contact, immediately reversing heparin's anticoagulant effects. Paradoxically, if protamine is given to a person who has not received heparin, it has anticoagulant effects. The dose is determined by the amount of heparin that was given and the time that elapsed since then. A dose of 1 mg IV protamine neutralises 80–100 units of heparin and approximately 100 units of low-molecular-weight heparin. The drug must be administered very slowly – not to exceed 50 mg IV in any 10-minute period. Care must be taken to calculate the amount of heparin that has been given to the person. Potentially fatal anaphylactic reactions have been reported with the use of protamine sulfate and so life support equipment should be readily available when it is used.

Care considerations for people receiving anticoagulants

Assessment: history and examination

- Assess for any known allergies to these drugs. Also screen for conditions *that could be exacerbated by increased bleeding tendencies*, including haemorrhagic disorders, recent trauma, spinal puncture, GI ulcers, recent surgery, intrauterine device placement, tuberculosis, presence of indwelling catheters and threatened abortion. Also screen for pregnancy *to ensure that benefits outweigh any potential risks (contraindicated with warfarin)*; breastfeeding, *because of the potential for risks to the baby* (use of heparin is suggested if an anticoagulant is needed during breastfeeding); renal or hepatic disease, *which could interfere with the metabolism and effectiveness of these drugs*; HF; thyrotoxicosis; senility or psychosis *because of the potential for unexpected effects*; and diarrhoea or fever, *which could alter the normal clotting process*.

- Assess baseline status before beginning therapy *to determine any potential adverse effects.* This includes body temperature; skin colour, lesions and temperature; affect, orientation and reflexes; pulse, blood pressure and perfusion; respirations and adventitious sounds; clotting studies, renal and liver function tests, FBC and stool guaiac; and electrocardiogram (ECG), if appropriate.

Implementation with rationale

- Evaluate for therapeutic effects of warfarin – prothrombin time (PT) 1.5–2.5 times the control value or ratio of PT to INR (international normalised ratio) of 2–3 – *to evaluate the effectiveness of the drug dose.*
- Evaluate for therapeutic effects of heparin – whole blood clotting time (WBCT) 2.5–3 times control or activated partial thromboplastin time (APTT) 1.5–3 times the control value – *to evaluate the effectiveness of the drug dose.*
- Evaluate the person regularly for any sign of blood loss (petechiae, bleeding gums, bruises, dark-coloured stools, dark-coloured urine) *to evaluate the effectiveness of the drug dose and to determine the need to consult with the prescriber if bleeding becomes apparent.*
- Establish safety precautions *to protect the person from injury.*
- Provide safety measures, such as use of an electric razor and avoidance of contact sports, *to decrease the risk of bleeding.*
- Provide increased precautions against bleeding during invasive procedures; use pressure dressings; avoid IM injections; and do not rub SC injection sites *because the state of anticoagulation increases the risk of blood loss.*
- Mark the chart of any individual receiving this drug *to alert the medical staff that there is a potential for increased bleeding.*
- Maintain antidotes on standby (protamine sulfate for heparin, vitamin K for warfarin) *in case of overdose.*
- Monitor the person carefully when any drug is added to or withdrawn from the drug regimen of a person taking warfarin *because of the risk of drug–drug interactions that would change the effectiveness of the anticoagulant.*
- Make sure that the person receives regular follow-up and monitoring, including measurement of clotting times, *to ensure maximum therapeutic effects.*
- Provide thorough teaching, including the name of the drug, dosage prescribed, measures to avoid adverse effects, warning signs of problems, the need for periodic monitoring and evaluation, and the need to wear or carry a MedicAlert notification, *to enhance knowledge about drug therapy and to promote compliance with the drug regimen.*
- Offer support and encouragement *to help the person deal with the diagnosis and the drug regimen.*

Evaluation

- Monitor response to the drug: increased bleeding time (warfarin, PT 1.5–2.5 times the control value or PT/INR ratio of 2–3; heparin, WBCT of 2.5–3 times the control value or APTT of 1.5–3 times the control value).
- Monitor for adverse effects (bleeding, bone marrow depression, alopecia, GI upset, rash).
- Evaluate the effectiveness of the teaching plan (person can name drug, dosage, adverse effects to watch for and specific measures to avoid them; the individual understands the importance of continued follow-up).
- Monitor the effectiveness of comfort measures and compliance with the regimen.

TABLE 48.3 Clinically important drug–drug reactions with warfarin

↑Bleeding effects	↓Anticoagulation	↑Activity and effects of other drug
salicylates	barbiturates	phenytoin
chloral hydrate	griseofulvin	
disulfiram	rifampicin	
chloramphenicol	phenytoin	
metronidazole	carbamazepine	
cimetidine	vitamin K	
ranitidine	vitamin E	
trimethoprim with sulfamethoxazole	colestyramine	
quinine		
thyroid drugs		
glucagon		
danazol		
erythromycin		
androgens		
amiodarone		
cefazolin		
cefoxitin		
ceftriaxone		
mefenamic acid		
famotidine		
nizatidine		

THROMBOLYTIC AGENTS

Thrombolytic agents break down formed thrombi by stimulating the plasmin system. This process is called clot resolution. Thrombolytic agents include alteplase (*Actilyse*), reteplase (*Rapilysin*) and tenecteplase (*Metalyse*).

Therapeutic actions and indications

If a thrombus has already formed in a vessel (eg, during an acute MI), it may be necessary to dissolve that clot to open the vessel and restore blood flow to the dependent tissue. All of the drugs that are available for this purpose work to activate the natural anticlotting system – conversion of plasminogen to plasmin. The activation of this system breaks down fibrin threads and dissolves any formed clot. The thrombolytics are effective only if the person has plasminogen in the plasma. See Table 48.1 for usual indications for each of these agents.

Pharmacokinetics

These drugs are given IV and are cleared from the body after liver metabolism. They cross the placenta, but it is not known whether they enter breast milk (see Contraindications and cautions).

Contraindications and cautions

The use of thrombolytic agents is contraindicated in the presence of allergy to any of these drugs *to prevent hypersensitivity reactions.* They should also not be used with any condition *that could be worsened by the dissolution of clots*, including recent surgery, active internal bleeding, cerebrovascular accident (CVA) within the last 2 months, aneurysm, vaginal or caesarean birth, organ biopsy, recent serious GI bleeding, rupture of a non-compressible blood vessel, recent major trauma (including cardiopulmonary resuscitation), known blood clotting defects, cerebrovascular disease, uncontrolled hypertension and liver disease (*which could affect normal clotting factors and the production of plasminogen*).

These drugs are also contraindicated in pregnancy *because of the possible adverse effects on the fetus or neonate.* These drugs should not be used during pregnancy unless the benefits to the mother clearly outweigh the potential risks to the fetus. Caution should be used during breastfeeding *because of the potential risk of bleeding effects in the breastfeeding baby.*

Adverse effects

The most common adverse effect associated with the use of thrombolytic agents is bleeding. People should be monitored closely for the occurrence of cardiac arrhythmias (with coronary reperfusion) and hypotension. Hypersensitivity reactions are not uncommon; they range from rash and flushing to bronchospasm and anaphylactic reaction.

Clinically important drug–drug interactions

The risk of haemorrhage increases if thrombolytic agents are used with any anticoagulant or antiplatelet drug.

Care considerations for people receiving thrombolytic agents

Assessment: history and examination

- Assess for any known allergies to these drugs *to prevent hypersensitivity reactions.* Also screen for any conditions *that could be worsened by the dissolution of clots*, including recent surgery, active internal bleeding, CVA within the last 2 months, aneurysm, obstetric delivery, organ biopsy, recent serious GI bleeding, rupture of a non-compressible blood vessel, recent major trauma (including cardiopulmonary resuscitation), known blood clotting defects, cerebrovascular disease, uncontrolled hypertension, liver disease (*which could affect normal clotting factors and the production of plasminogen*) and pregnancy or breastfeeding (*because of the possible adverse effects on the neonate*).
- Assess baseline status before beginning therapy *to determine any potential adverse effects.* Assess the following: body temperature; skin colour, lesions and temperature; affect, orientation and reflexes; pulse, blood pressure and perfusion; respirations and adventitious sounds; and clotting studies, renal and liver function tests, FBC, guaiac test for occult blood in stool and ECG.

Implementation with rationale

- Arrange to administer tenecteplase to reduce mortality associated with acute MI as soon as possible after the onset of symptoms *because the timing for the administration of tenecteplase is critical to resolve the clot before permanent damage occurs to the myocardial cells.*
- Discontinue heparin if it is being given before administration of a thrombolytic agent, unless specifically ordered for coronary artery infusion, *to prevent excessive loss of blood.*
- Evaluate the person regularly for any sign of blood loss (petechiae, bleeding gums, bruises, dark-coloured stools, dark-coloured urine) *to evaluate drug effectiveness and for the need to consult with the prescriber if blood loss becomes apparent.*
- Monitor coagulation studies regularly; consult with the prescriber *to adjust the drug dose appropriately.*

- Institute treatment within 6 hours after the onset of symptoms of acute MI *to achieve optimal therapeutic effectiveness.*
- Arrange to type and cross-match blood *in case of serious blood loss that requires whole-blood transfusion.*
- Monitor cardiac rhythm continuously if the drug is being given for acute MI *because of the risk of alteration in cardiac function;* have life support equipment on standby as needed.
- Provide increased precautions against bleeding during invasive procedures, use pressure dressings and ice, avoid IM injections and do not rub SC injection sites *because of the risk of increased blood loss in the anticoagulated state.*
- Mark the chart of any person receiving this drug *to alert medical staff that there is a potential for increased bleeding.*
- Provide thorough teaching, including the name of the drug, dosage prescribed, measures to avoid adverse effects, warning signs of problems and the need for periodic monitoring and evaluation, *to enhance knowledge about drug therapy and to promote compliance with the drug regimen.*
- Offer support and encouragement *to help the person deal with the diagnosis and the drug regimen.*

Evaluation

- Monitor response to the drug (dissolution of the clot and return of blood flow to the area).
- Monitor for adverse effects (bleeding, arrhythmias, hypotension, hypersensitivity reaction).
- Evaluate the effectiveness of the teaching plan (person can name drug, adverse effects to watch for and specific measures to avoid them).
- Monitor the effectiveness of comfort measures and compliance with the regimen.

OTHER DRUGS AFFECTING CLOT FORMATION

Other drugs that affect clot formation are also effective in preventing thromboembolic episodes. These drugs include the low-molecular-weight heparins, adjunctive agents used to help alleviate adverse reactions to these drugs and a haemorrheologic agent.

Low-molecular-weight heparins

In the late 1990s, a series of low-molecular-weight heparins were developed. These drugs inhibit thrombus and clot formation by blocking factors Xa and IIa. Because of the size and nature of the molecules, these drugs do not greatly affect thrombin, clotting or the PT; therefore, they cause fewer systemic adverse effects. They have also been found to block angiogenesis, the process that allows cancer cells to develop new blood vessels. They are being studied as possible adjuncts to cancer chemotherapy. These drugs are indicated for very specific uses in the prevention of clots and emboli formation after certain surgeries or prolonged bed rest. The care of a person receiving one of these drugs is similar to that of a person receiving heparin. The drug is given just before (or just after) the surgery and then is continued for 7–14 days during the postoperative recovery process. Caution must be used to avoid combining these drugs with standard heparin therapy; serious bleeding episodes and deaths have been reported when this combination was inadvertently used. Low-molecular-weight heparins include dalteparin (*Fragmin*) and enoxaparin (*Clexane*). See Table 48.1 for additional information about these agents.

Haemorrheological agent

Pentoxifylline (oxpentifylline) (*Trental*) is known as a haemorrheologic agent, or a drug that can induce haemorrhage. It is a xanthine that, like caffeine and theophylline, decreases platelet aggregation and fibrinogen concentration in the blood. These effects can decrease blood clot formation and increase blood flow through narrowed or damaged vessels. The mechanism of action by which pentoxifylline does these things is not known. It is one of the very few drugs found to be effective in treating intermittent claudication, a painful vascular problem of the legs.

Because pentoxifylline is a xanthine, it is associated with many cardiovascular stimulatory effects; people with underlying cardiovascular problems need to be monitored carefully when taking this drug. Pentoxifylline can also cause headache, dizziness, nausea and upset stomach. It is taken orally three times a day for at least 8 weeks to evaluate its effectiveness. See Table 48.1 for additional information about this drug.

KEY POINTS

- To keep blood from coagulating, anticoagulants block blood aggregates or interfere with the mechanisms that cause blood to clot.
- Thrombolytic drugs activate the plasminogen system to dissolve clots naturally.

DRUGS USED TO CONTROL BLEEDING

Drugs used to control bleeding include anticoagulant reversal agents, antihaemophilic and haemostatic agents. Anticoagulant reversal agents include idarucizumab (*Praxbind*), used for rapid reversal of anticoagulation with dabigatran (*Pradaxa*); protamine sulfate (generic), an antidote to heparin; and vitamin K (*phytomenadione*), an antidote for warfarin.

On the other end of the spectrum of coagulation problems are various bleeding disorders. These include:

- haemophilia, in which there is a genetic lack of clotting factors that leaves the person vulnerable to excessive bleeding with any injury.
- liver disease, in which clotting factors and proteins needed for clotting are not produced.
- bone marrow disorders, in which platelets are not formed in sufficient quantity to be effective.

Bleeding disorders are treated with clotting factors and drugs that promote the coagulation process. These include antihaemophilic agents and haemostatic agents (systemic and topical). (See Table 48.4.)

ANTIHAEMOPHILIC AGENTS

The drugs used to treat haemophilia are replacement factors for the specific clotting factors that are genetically missing in that particular type of haemophilia. These drugs include antihaemophilic factor, recombinant (*Recombinate* [not available in New Zealand]), coagulation factor VIII (*Biostate*) and factor IX complex (*MonoFIX-VF*).

Therapeutic actions and indications

The antihaemophilic drugs replace clotting factors that are either genetically missing or low in a particular type of haemophilia. The drug of choice depends on the particular haemophilia that is being treated.

TABLE 48.4 *DRUGS IN FOCUS* Drugs used to control bleeding

Drug name	Dosage/route	Usual indications
Anticoagulant reversal agents		
Idarucizumab (*Praxbind*)	Adult: 5 g IV followed by another 5 g IV if required; administer either as 2 consecutive 2.5 g IV infusions, each given over 5–10 minutes, or as an IV bolus injection, as 2 consecutive 2.5 g IV injections	Rapid reversal of dabigatran anticoagulation
protamine sulfate (generic)	Adult Overdose with IV unfractionated heparin: 25–50 mg IV after heparin infusion stopped (rate not exceeding 5 mg/min) Overdose with SC unfractionated heparin or LMWH: 1 mg neutralises 100 units heparin or LMWH; 25–50 mg IV (max 5 mg/min), then IV over 8–16 hours; maximum total dose 50 mg	Treatment of heparin or low-molecular-weight heparin (LMWH) overdose
vitamin K (phytomenadione) (*Konakion MM*)	Adult, asymptomatic individuals with high INR: 1–5 mg PO (give the injection orally) or 0.5–1mg IV Neonatal prophylaxis: 1 mg IM at birth Severe or life-threatening haemorrhage during anticoagulant therapy: withdraw coumadin anticoagulant then give 5–10 mg IV over 30 seconds with fresh frozen plasma (FFP) or prothrombin complex concentrate (PCC); repeated as needed	Treatment of anticoagulant-induced prothrombin deficiency
Antihaemophilic agents		
(P) Antihaemophilic factor, recombinant (*Recombinate*)	IV dose based on serum factor VIII levels and body weight	Prevention and control of bleeding episodes in haemophilia A; perioperative management of bleeding in people with haemophilia A
coagulation factor VIIa (*NovoSeven RT*)	90 micrograms/kg IV q 3 hours for 2–3 doses or 270 micrograms/kg single dose	Treatment of bleeding episodes in people with haemophilia A or B
factor IX complex (*MonoFIX-VF*)	IV dose based on factor levels, weight and desired response	Treatment or prevention of haemophilia B (Christmas disease, a deficiency of factor IX); treatment of bleeding episodes in people with factor VII and factor VIII deficiencies; controls bleeding episodes in people with haemophilia A

TABLE 48.4 **DRUGS IN FOCUS** **Drugs used to control bleeding *(continued)***

Drug name	Dosage/route	Usual indications
Haemostatic agents		
Topical		
absorbable gelatine (*Gelfoam*)	Smear or press onto surface; do not remove, will be absorbed	Controls bleeding from surface cuts or injury
human fibrin sealant (aprotinin, factor XIII, fibrinogen, thrombin) (*Artiss, Tisseel*)	Apply thin layer on to site	Adheres autologous skin grafts to surgically prepared wound beds resulting from burns in adults and children
tranexamic acid (*Cyklokapron*)	Adult: local fibrinolysis: PO: 1–1.5 g (or 15–25 mg/kg) PO bd–tid; IV: 0.5–1 g IV bd–tid Menorrhagia: 1 g PO tid starting when menstruation begins, for up to 4 days; maximum 4 g daily	Local fibrinolysis, reduction of bleeding in surgery, dental extraction in patients with coagulopathies, epistaxis, menorrhagia, hereditary angioedema

Antihaemophilic factor is factor VIII, the clotting factor that is missing in classic haemophilia (haemophilia A). This recombinant (genetically engineered product that does not use human blood) antihaemophilic factor is used to correct or prevent bleeding episodes or to allow necessary surgery.

Coagulation factor VIIa (*NovoSeven*) and factor IX complex are used for people with haemophilia A or B (see Table 48.4 for usual indications for each of these agents). Coagulation factor VIIa is a preparation made from mouse, hamster and bovine proteins that contains variable amounts of preformed clotting factors (see Contraindications and cautions). Factor IX complex contains plasma fractions of many of the clotting factors and increases blood levels of factors II, VII, IX and X. The drug of choice for any given person is determined by his or her particular coagulation abnormalities.

Pharmacokinetics

These agents replace normal clotting factors and are processed as such by the body. They must be given intravenously and are processed by the body in the same way that naturally occurring clotting factors are processed in the plasma, usually with a half-life of 24–36 hours.

Contraindications and cautions

Antihaemophilic factor is contraindicated in the presence of known allergy to mouse proteins *to prevent hypersensitivity reactions*. Factor IX is contraindicated in the presence of liver disease with signs of intravascular coagulation or fibrinolysis *to prevent serious aggravation of these disorders*. Coagulation factor VIIa is contraindicated with known allergies to mouse, hamster or bovine products *to prevent hypersensitivity reactions*. These drugs are not recommended for use during breastfeeding, and caution should be used during pregnancy *because of the potential for adverse effects on the baby or fetus*. They should be used during pregnancy only if the benefit to the mother clearly outweighs the potential risk to the fetus. It is recommended that another method of feeding the baby be used if these drugs are needed during breastfeeding. Because these drugs are used to prevent serious bleeding problems or to treat bleeding episodes, there are few contraindications to their use.

Adverse effects

The most common adverse effects associated with antihaemophilic agents involve risks associated with the use of blood products (eg, hepatitis, AIDS). Headache, flushing, chills, fever and lethargy may occur as a reaction to the injection of a foreign protein. Nausea and vomiting may also occur, as may stinging, itching and burning at the site of the injection.

Prototype summary: antihaemophilic factor

Indications: treatment of classic haemophilia to provide temporary replacement of clotting factors to correct or prevent bleeding episodes or to allow necessary surgery.

Actions: normal plasma protein that is needed for the transformation of prothrombin to thrombin, the final step in the clotting pathway.

Pharmacokinetics:

Route	Onset	Peak	Duration
IV	Immediate	Unknown	Unknown

$T_{1/2}$: 12 hours; cleared from the body by normal protein metabolism.

Adverse effects: allergic reaction, stinging at injection site, headache, rash, chills, nausea, hepatitis, AIDS (risks associated with the use of blood products).

Care considerations for people receiving antihaemophilic agents

Assessment: history and examination

- Assess for the following conditions, *which could be cautions or contraindications to use of the drug*: any known allergies to these drugs or to mouse proteins with antihaemophilic factor; liver disease.
- Assess for baseline status before beginning therapy *to determine any potential adverse effects*.
- Assess the following: body temperature; skin colour, lesions and temperature; affect, orientation and reflexes; pulse, blood pressure and perfusion; respirations and adventitious sounds; clotting studies; and liver function tests.

Implementation with rationale

- Administer by the IV route only *to ensure therapeutic effectiveness*.
- Monitor clinical response and clotting factor levels regularly *to arrange to adjust dose as needed*.
- Monitor the person for any sign of thrombosis *to arrange to use comfort and support measures as needed (eg, support hose, positioning, ambulation, exercise)*.
- Decrease the rate of infusion if headache, chills, fever or tingling occurs *to prevent severe drug reaction;* in some individuals the drug will need to be discontinued.
- Arrange to type and crossmatch blood *in case of serious blood loss that will require whole-blood transfusion*.
- Mark the chart of any person receiving this drug *to alert medical staff that there is a potential for increased bleeding*.
- Provide thorough teaching, including the name of the drug, dosage prescribed, measures to avoid adverse effects, warning signs of problems and the need for periodic monitoring and evaluation, *to enhance knowledge about drug therapy and to promote compliance with the drug regimen*.
- Offer support and encouragement *to help the person deal with the diagnosis and the drug regimen*.

Evaluation

- Monitor response to the drug (control of bleeding episodes, prevention of bleeding episodes).
- Monitor for adverse effects (thrombosis, CNS effects, nausea, hypersensitivity reaction, hepatitis, AIDS).
- Evaluate the effectiveness of the teaching plan (person can name drug, dosage of drug, adverse effects to watch for, specific measures to avoid them and warning signs to report).
- Monitor the effectiveness of comfort measures and compliance with the regimen.

HAEMOSTATIC AGENTS

Some situations result in a fibrinolytic state with excessive plasminogen activity and risk of bleeding from clot dissolution. For example, people undergoing repeat coronary artery bypass graft (CABG) surgery are especially prone to excessive bleeding and may require blood transfusion. **Haemostatic agents** are used to stop bleeding. Haemostatic drugs may be either systemic or topical.

The haemostatic drug that is used systemically is aminocaproic acid which is not yet available in New Zealand and Australia. Topical haemostatic agents include absorbable gelatine (*Gelfoam*), human fibrin sealant (*Artiss*, *Tisseel* [not available in New Zealand]).

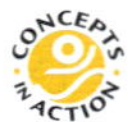

Haematology: Haemostasis

Therapeutic actions and indications

Systemic haemostatic agents

The systemic haemostatic agents are used to prevent body-wide or systemic clot breakdown, thus preventing blood loss in situations in which serious systemic bleeding could occur, or hyperfibrinolysis. There is only one systemic haemostatic agent available for use in the US. This drug is currently not available in New Zealand and Australia.

Aminocaproic acid inhibits plasminogen-activating substances and has some antiplasmin activity. When taking the oral form of aminocaproic acid, the person may need to take 10 tablets in the first hour and then continue taking the drug around the clock. Aprotinin (*Tisseel VH*), another systemic haemostatic agent used to reduce blood loss and need for transfusions associated with coronary artery bypass graft surgery, was withdrawn from the market in 2008 after reports of increased risk of cardiovascular events in people who had been treated with this drug. It is still available for topical use during surgical procedures.

Topical haemostatic agents

Some surface injuries involve so much damage to the small vessels in the area that clotting does not occur and blood is slowly and continually lost. For these situations, topical or local haemostatic agents are often used. The use of these drugs is also incorporated into the care of wounds or decubitus ulcers as adjunctive therapy. The drug of choice depends on the nature of the injury and the prescriber's preference. The newest topical haemostatic agent is human fibrin sealant. Thrombin recombinant is the first topical haemostatic agent approved to be made using recombinant DNA technology (this will decrease many of the potential allergic reactions associated with bovine thrombin; see Contraindications and cautions). See Table 48.4 for additional information about these agents.

Pharmacokinetics

Systemic haemostatic agents

Aminocaproic acid is available in oral and IV forms. It is rapidly absorbed and widely distributed throughout the body. It is excreted largely unchanged in urine, with a half-life of 2 hours.

Topical haemostatic agents

Absorbable gelatine and microfibrillar collagen are available in sponge form and are applied directly to the injured area until the bleeding stops. These formulations are not yet available in the Australian and New Zealand market.

Other forms of human fibrin sealant are spray form, applied in a thin layer onto the graft bed or sprayed directly onto any active bleeding site. These are not yet available in Australia and New Zealand.

Thrombin, which is derived from bovine sources, is a solution that is applied topically and mixed in with the blood. Thrombin recombinant is also a solution and is applied directly to the bleeding site surface in conjunction with absorbable gelatine sponge; the amount needed varies with the area of tissue to be treated.

Contraindications and cautions

Systemic haemostatic agents

Aminocaproic acid is contraindicated in the presence of allergy to the drug *to prevent hypersensitivity reactions* and with acute DIC *because of the risk of tissue necrosis*. Caution should be used in cardiac disease *because of the risk of arrhythmias* and in renal and hepatic dysfunction, *which could alter the excretion of this drug and the normal clotting processes*. Although the safety for use of this drug during pregnancy has not been established, it should be used only if the benefits to the mother clearly outweigh the potential risks to the neonate *because of the potential for adverse effects on the fetus*. It is recommended that nursing mothers use a different method for feeding the baby if this drug is used *because of the potential for adverse effects on the baby*.

Topical haemostatic agents

Use thrombin with caution for those people with an allergy to bovine products. *Because thrombin comes from animal sources, it may precipitate an allergic response; the person needs to be carefully monitored for such a reaction*. Many of the potential allergic reactions associated with bovine thrombin will be decreased as a result of approval for thrombin recombinant to be made using recombinant DNA technology. Safety for use of thrombin recombinant in children has not been established.

Adverse effects

Systemic haemostatic agents

The most common adverse effect associated with systemic haemostatic agents is excessive clotting. In 2007, there were many reports of increased cardiovascular events, including fatalities in people who received aprotinin. Some of the events occurred months after the drug was used. The drug was removed from the market in 2008. CNS effects of aminocaproic acid can include hallucinations, drowsiness, dizziness, headache and psychotic states, all of which could be related to changes in cerebral blood flow associated with changes in clot dissolution. GI effects, including nausea, cramps and diarrhoea, may be related to excessive clotting in the GI tract, causing reflex GI stimulation. Weakness, fatigue, malaise and muscle pain can occur as small clots build up in muscles. Intrarenal obstruction and renal dysfunction have also been reported.

Topical haemostatic agents

Use of absorbable gelatine and microfibrillar collagen can pose a risk of infection *because bacteria can become trapped in the vascular area when the sponge is applied*. Immediate removal of the sponge and cleaning of the area can help to decrease this risk.

Clinically important drug–drug interactions

Systemic haemostatic agents

Aminocaproic acid is associated with the development of hypercoagulation states if it is combined with oral contraceptives or oestrogens. The risk of bleeding increases if it is given with heparin.

Topical haemostatic agents

There are no reported drug–drug interactions with the topically applied haemostatic agents.

Care considerations for people receiving systemic haemostatic

Care considerations for a person receiving topical haemostatic agents are similar to those with the use of any topical drug (see Appendix C).

Assessment: history and examination

- Assess for the following conditions, *which could be cautions or contraindications to the use of systemic haemostatic agents*: any known allergies to any component of the drug *to prevent hypersensitivity reactions*; acute DIC *because of the risk of tissue necrosis*; renal and hepatic dysfunction, *which could alter the excretion of these drugs and the normal clotting processes*; and breastfeeding *because of the potential for adverse effects on the neonate*.
- Assess baseline status before beginning therapy *to determine any potential adverse effects*. Assess the following: body temperature; skin colour, lesions and temperature; affect, orientation and reflexes; pulse, blood pressure and perfusion; respirations and adventitious sounds; bowel sounds and normal output; urinalysis and clotting studies; and renal and liver function tests.

Implementation with rationale

- Monitor clinical response and clotting factor levels regularly *to arrange to adjust dose as needed*.
- Monitor the person for any sign of thrombosis *to arrange to use comfort and support measures as needed (eg, support hose, positioning, ambulation, exercise)*.
- Orient the person and offer support and safety measures if hallucinations or psychoses occur *to prevent injury*.
- Offer comfort measures *to help the person deal with the effects of the drug*. These include small, frequent meals; mouth care; environmental controls; and safety measures.
- Provide thorough teaching, including the name of the drug, dosage prescribed, measures to avoid adverse effects, warning signs of problems and the need for periodic monitoring and evaluation, *to enhance knowledge about drug therapy and to promote compliance with the drug regimen*.
- Offer support and encouragement *to help the person deal with the diagnosis and the drug regimen*.

Evaluation

- Monitor response to the drug (control of bleeding episodes).
- Monitor for adverse effects (thrombosis, CNS effects, nausea, hypersensitivity reaction).
- Evaluate the effectiveness of the teaching plan (person can name drug, dosage of drug, adverse effects to watch for, specific measures to avoid them and warning signs to report).
- Monitor the effectiveness of comfort measures and compliance with the regimen.

KEY POINTS

- Haemostatic agents are used to stop bleeding from occurring. They are used in situations that result in a fibrinolytic state with excessive plasminogen activity and the risk of bleeding from clot dissolution. For example, people undergoing repeat coronary artery bypass graft surgery are especially prone to excessive bleeding and may require blood transfusion.
- Aminocaproic acid is a systemic haemostatic agent used to treat conditions resulting from systemic hyperfibrinolysis. Several topical agents are also available for local use on active bleeding sites, often during surgery or with severe injury.

CHAPTER SUMMARY

- Coagulation is the transformation of fluid blood into a solid state to plug up breaks in the vascular system.
- Coagulation involves several processes, including vasoconstriction, platelet aggregation to form a plug, and intrinsic and extrinsic clot formation initiated by Hageman factor to plug any breaks in the system.
- The final step of clot formation is the conversion of prothrombin to thrombin, which breaks down fibrinogen to form insoluble fibrin threads.
- Once a clot is formed, it must be dissolved to prevent the occlusion of blood vessels and loss of blood supply to tissues.
- Plasminogen is the basis of the clot-dissolving system. It is converted to plasmin (fibrinolysin) by several factors, including Hageman factor. Plasmin dissolves fibrin threads and resolves the clot.
- Anticoagulants block blood coagulation by interfering with one or more of the steps involved, such as blocking platelet aggregation or inhibiting the intrinsic or extrinsic pathways to clot formation.
- Thrombolytic drugs dissolve clots or thrombi that have formed. They activate the plasminogen system to stimulate natural clot dissolution.
- Haemostatic drugs are used to stop bleeding. They may replace missing clotting factors or prevent the plasminogen system from dissolving formed clots.
- Haemophilia, a genetic lack of essential clotting factors, results in excessive bleeding. It is treated by replacing missing clotting factors.

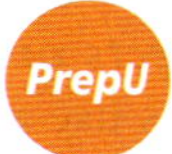

Knowing your strengths and weaknesses helps you to study more effectively. Take a PrepU Practice Quiz to find out how you measure up!

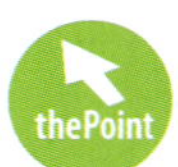

ONLINE RESOURCES

An extensive range of additional resources to enhance teaching and learning and to facilitate understanding of this chapter may be found online at the text's accompanying website, located on thePoint at http://thepoint.lww.com. These include Watch and Learn videos, Concepts in Action animations, journal articles, review questions, case studies, discussion topics and quizzes.

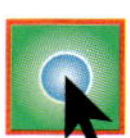

WEB LINKS

Health care providers and students may want to explore the following web resources:

www.haemophilia.org.au
The Haemophilia Foundation Australia.

ww2.health.wa.gov.au/~/media/Files/Corporate/general%20documents/Quality/PDF/Living-with-Warfarin.pdf
Department of Health Western Australia publication 'Living with Warfarin'.

www.pharmac.govt.nz/2011/06/10/Dabigatran%20bleeding%20management.pdf
Guidelines for management of bleeding with dabigatran – for possible inclusion into local management protocols. PHARMAC New Zealand.

www.saferx.co.nz/full/dabigatran.pdf
Safer Use of High Risk Medicines – Waitemata District Health Board New Zealand.

BIBLIOGRAPHY

Chapman, N. H., Brighton, T., Harris, M., Caplan, G. A., Braithwaite, J. (2009). Venous thromboembolism: management in general practice. *Australian Family Physician, 38(1–2)*, 36–40.

Farrell, M. & Dempsey, J. (2014). *Smeltzer & Bare's Textbook of Medical-Surgical Nursing* (3rd edn). Sydney: Lippincott Williams & Wilkins.

Goodman, L. S., Brunton, L. L., Chabner, B. & Knollmann, B. C. (2011). *Goodman and Gilman's Pharmacological Basis of Therapeutics* (12th edn). New York: McGraw-Hill.

Hassan, S. S., Feng, S. R., Ahmadi, K., Ahmad, K. M., Chong, D. W. K., Anwar, M. & Badarudin, N. Z. (2010). Factors influencing concomitant use of complementary and alternative medicines with warfarin. *Journal of Pharmacy Practice & Research, 40(4)*, 294–299.

Hicks, R. W., Wanzer, L. J. & Goeckner, B. (2011). Perioperative pharmacology: Blood coagulation modifiers. *AORN Journal, 93(6)*, 726–736.

Ho, W. K. (2010). Deep vein thrombosis: Risks and diagnosis. *Australian Family Physician, 39(7)*, 468–474.

Lankshear, A., Harden, J. & Simms, J. (2010). Safe practice for patients receiving anticoagulant therapy. *Nursing Standard, 24(20)*, 47–56.

Leung, E. S., Hamilton-Bruce, M. A. & Koblar, S. A. (2010). Warfarin: indications, risks and drug interactions. *Australian Family Physician, 39(11)*, 820–824.

Lowinger, J. S. & Maxwell, D. J. (2009). Heparins for venous thromboembolism prophylaxis—safety issues. *Australian Prescriber, 32(4)*, 108–112.

McKenna, L. & Mirkov, S. (2019). *McKenna's Drug Handbook for Nursing and Midwifery* (8th edn). Sydney: Wolters Kluwer Health Australia.

McRae, S. (2010). Pulmonary embolism. *Australian Family Physician, 39(7)*, 462–466.

Merriman, E. (2011). Antiplatelet drugs, anticoagulants and elective surgery. *Australian Prescriber, 34(5)*, 139–143.

Myers, S. P. (2002). Interactions between complementary medicines and warfarin. *Australian Prescriber, 25*, 54–56.

Nguyen, T., Yacoub, M., Chan, T-I. & Quach, K. (2012). Atrial fibrillation: Focus on anticoagulant pharmacotherapy. *Journal for Nurse Practitioners, 8(7)*, 560–565.

Nutescu, E. A. (2013). Oral anticoagulant therapies: Balancing the risks. *American Journal of Health-System Pharmacy, 70(10)*, S3–S11.

Pickering, A. & Thomas, D. P. (2007). An audit of INR control in the Australian indigenous setting. *Australian Family Physician, 36(11)*, 959–969.

Porth, C. M. (2011). *Essentials of Pathophysiology: Concepts of Altered Health States* (3rd edn). Philadelphia: Lippincott Williams & Wilkins.

Porth, C. M. (2009). *Pathophysiology: Concepts of Altered Health States* (8th edn). Philadelphia: Lippincott Williams & Wilkins.

Samardhi, H. (2011). Current management of atrial fibrillation. *Australian Prescriber, 34(4)*, 100–104.

Tadros, R. & Shakib, S. (2010). Clot prevention: Common questions about medications. *Australian Family Physician, 39(7)*, 480–483.

Tadros, R. & Shakib, S. (2010). Warfarin: indications, risks and drug interactions. *Australian Family Physician, 39(7)*, 476–479.

CHECK YOUR UNDERSTANDING

Answers to the questions in this chapter can be found in Appendix A at the back of this book.

MULTIPLE CHOICE

Select the best answer to the following.

1. Blood coagulation is a complex reaction that involves:
   a. vasoconstriction, platelet aggregation and plasminogen action.
   b. vasodilation, platelet aggregation and activation of the clotting cascade.
   c. vasoconstriction, platelet aggregation and conversion of prothrombin to thrombin.
   d. vasodilation, platelet inhibition, and action of the intrinsic and extrinsic clotting cascades.
2. Warfarin, an oral anticoagulant, acts:
   a. to directly prevent the conversion of prothrombin to thrombin.
   b. to decrease the production of vitamin K clotting factors in the liver.
   c. as a catalyst in the conversion of plasminogen to plasmin.
   d. immediately, so it is the drug of choice in emergency situations.
3. Heparin reacts to prevent the conversion of prothrombin to thrombin. Heparin:
   a. is available in oral and parenteral forms.
   b. takes about 72 hours to have a therapeutic effect.
   c. has its effects reversed with the administration of protamine sulfate.
   d. has its effects reversed with the injection of vitamin K.
4. The low-molecular-weight heparin of choice for preventing deep venous thrombosis after hip replacement therapy is:
   a. protamine sulfate.
   b. dalteparin.
   c. heparin.
   d. enoxaparin.
5. A thrombolytic agent could be safely used in:
   a. CVA within the last 2 months.
   b. acute MI within the last 3 hours.
   c. recent, serious GI bleeding.
   d. caesarean birth.
6. Antihaemophilic agents are used to replace missing clotting factors to prevent severe blood loss. The most common side effect or side effects associated with the use of these drugs are:
   a. bleeding.
   b. dark stools and urine.
   c. hepatitis and AIDS.
   d. constipation.

MULTIPLE RESPONSE

Select all that apply.

1. Hageman factor is known to activate which of the following?
   a. the clotting cascade
   b. the anticlotting process
   c. the inflammatory response
   d. platelet aggregation
   e. thromboxane A_2
   f. troponin coupling
2. Plasminogen is converted to plasmin, a clot-dissolving substance, by which of the following?
   a. nicotine
   b. Hageman factor
   c. tenecteplase
   d. pyrogens
   e. thrombin
   f. Christmas factor
3. Antiplatelet drugs block the aggregation of platelets and keep vessels open. These drugs would be useful in which of the following?
   a. maintaining the patency of grafts
   b. decreasing the risk of fatal MI
   c. preventing reinfarction after MI
   d. dissolving a pulmonary embolus and improving oxygenation
   e. decreasing damage in a subarachnoid bleed
   f. preventing thromboembolic strokes
4. Evaluating a person who is taking an anticoagulant for blood loss would usually include assessing for which of the following?
   a. the presence of petechiae
   b. bleeding gums while brushing the teeth
   c. dark-coloured urine
   d. yellow colour to the sclera or skin
   e. the presence of ecchymotic areas
   f. loss of hair

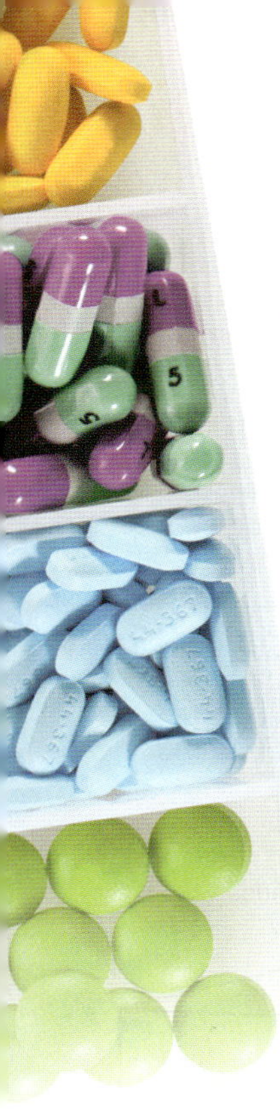

Drugs used to treat anaemias

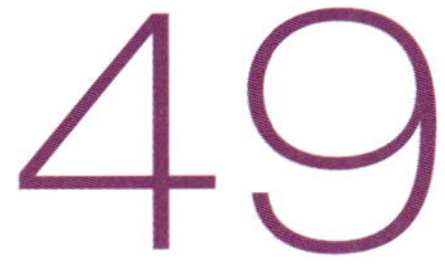

Learning objectives

On completing this chapter you should be able to:

1. Explain the process of erythropoiesis and its correlation with the development of three types of anaemias.
2. Describe the therapeutic actions, indications, pharmacokinetics, contraindications and cautions, most common adverse reactions and important drug–drug interactions associated with drugs used to treat anaemias.
3. Discuss the use of drugs used to treat anaemias across the lifespan.
4. Compare and contrast the prototype drugs epoetin alfa, ferrous sulfate, folic acid, hydroxocobalamin and hydroxycarbamide (hydroxyurea) with other agents in their class.
5. Outline the considerations, including important teaching points, for people receiving drugs used to treat anaemias.

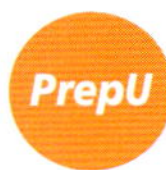

Test your current knowledge of drugs used to treat anaemias with a PrepU Practice Quiz!

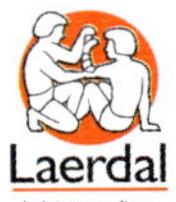

Simulation-based learning

On completion of the chapter, consider the scenario of Lloyd Bennett (Part 1) who has been ordered a blood transfusion for low haemoglobin postoperatively. Consider whether medication management, and if so, which products may also assist in raising his haemoglobin levels.

Glossary of key terms

anaemia: disorder involving too few red blood cells (RBCs) or ineffective RBCs that can alter the blood's ability to carry oxygen

erythrocytes: RBCs, responsible for carrying oxygen to the tissues and removing carbon dioxide; they have no nucleus and live approximately 120 days

erythropoiesis: process of RBC production and life cycle; formed by megaloblastic cells in the bone marrow, using iron, folic acid, carbohydrates, vitamin B12 and amino acids; they circulate in the vascular system for about 120 days and then are lysed and recycled

erythropoietin: glycoprotein produced by the kidneys, released in response to decreased blood flow or oxygen tension in the kidney; controls the rate of RBC production in the bone marrow

iron deficiency anaemia: low RBC count with low iron available because of high demand, poor diet or poor absorption; treated with iron replacement

megaloblastic anaemia: anaemia caused by lack of vitamin B12 and/or folic acid, in which RBCs are fewer in number and have a weak stroma and a short lifespan; treated by replacement of folic acid and vitamin B12

pernicious anaemia: type of megaloblastic anaemia characterised by lack of vitamin B12 secondary to low production of intrinsic factor by gastric cells; vitamin B12 must be replaced by intramuscular injection or nasal spray because it cannot be absorbed through the gastrointestinal tract

plasma: the liquid part of the blood; consists mostly of water and plasma proteins, glucose and electrolytes

reticulocyte: RBC that has only recently lost its nucleus and entered circulation; not yet fully matured

ERYTHROPOIESIS-STIMULATING AGENTS	AGENTS USED FOR IRON DEFICIENCY ANAEMIA	AGENTS USED FOR OTHER ANAEMIAS	
darbepoetin alfa	ferric carboxymaltose	**Agents for megaloblastic anaemias**	**Vitamin B12**
(P) epoetin alfa	ferrous fumarate	**Folic acid derivatives**	mecobalamin (co-methylcobalamin)
epoetin beta	(P) ferrous sulfate	calcium folinate	cyanocobalamin
epoetin lambda	iron polymaltose	(P) folic acid	(P) hydroxocobalamin
methoxy polyethylene glycol-epoetin beta	iron sucrose		**Agent for sickle cell anaemia**
			(P) hydroxycarbamide (hydroxyurea)

Blood is essential for cell survival because it carries oxygen and nutrients and removes waste products that could be toxic to the tissues. It also contains clotting factors that help to maintain the vascular system and keep it sealed. In addition, blood contains the important components of the immune and inflammatory systems that protect the body from infection.

Blood is composed of liquid and formed elements. The liquid part of blood is called **plasma**. Plasma is mostly water, but it also contains proteins that are essential for the immune response and for blood clotting. The formed elements of the blood include leucocytes (white blood cells), which are an important part of the immune system (see Chapter 15); **erythrocytes** (red blood cells [RBCs]), which carry oxygen to the tissues and remove carbon dioxide for delivery to the lungs; and platelets, which play an important role in coagulation (see Chapter 48). This chapter discusses drugs that are used to treat **anaemias**, which are disorders that involve too few RBCs or ineffective RBCs that can alter the blood's ability to carry oxygen.

ANAEMIA

Anaemia results from an alteration in **erythropoiesis**, the process of RBC production, which occurs in the myeloid tissue of the bone marrow. The rate of RBC production is controlled by the glycoprotein **erythropoietin**, which is released from the kidneys in response to decreased blood flow or decreased oxygen tension in the kidneys. Under the influence of erythropoietin, an undifferentiated cell in the bone marrow becomes a haemocytoblast. This cell uses certain amino acids, lipids, carbohydrates, vitamin B12, folic acid and iron to become an immature RBC. In the last phase of RBC production, the cell loses its nucleus and enters circulation. This cell, called a **reticulocyte**, finishes its maturing process in circulation (see Figure 49.1).

Although the mature RBC has no nucleus, it does have a vast surface area to improve its ability to transport oxygen and carbon dioxide. Because it lacks a nucleus, the RBC cannot reproduce or maintain itself, and so it will eventually wear out. The average lifespan of an RBC is about 120 days. At that time, the elderly

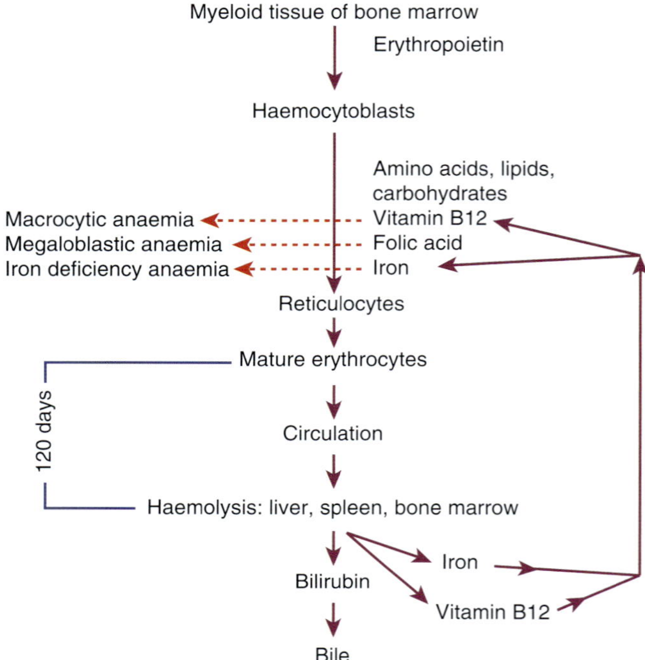

FIGURE 49.1 Erythropoiesis. Red blood cells are produced in the myeloid tissue of the bone marrow in response to the hormone erythropoietin. The haemocytoblasts require various essential factors to produce mature erythrocytes. A lack of any one of these can result in an anaemia of the type indicated opposite each factor. Mature erythrocytes survive for about 120 days and are then lysed in the liver, spleen or bone marrow.

RBC is lysed in the liver, spleen or bone marrow. The building blocks of the RBC (eg, iron, vitamin B12) are then recycled and returned to the bone marrow for the production of new RBCs. The only part of the RBC that cannot be recycled is the toxic pigment bilirubin, which is conjugated in the liver, passed into the bile and excreted from the body in the faeces or the urine. Bilirubin is what gives colour to both of these excretions. Erythropoiesis is a constant process by which about 1% of the body's RBCs are destroyed and replaced each day.

Aetiology of anaemia

Anaemia can occur if erythropoietin levels are low. This is seen in renal failure, when the kidneys are no longer able to produce erythropoietin. It can also occur if the body does not have enough of the building blocks necessary to form RBCs or if a person has a genetic predisposition to forming abnormal RBCs, as in sickle cell anaemia. To produce healthy RBCs, the bone marrow must have:

- adequate amounts of iron, which are used in forming haemoglobin rings to carry the oxygen
- minute amounts of vitamin B12 and folic acid, to form a strong supporting structure that can survive being battered through blood vessels for 120 days
- essential amino acids and carbohydrates to complete the haemoglobin rings, cell membrane and basic structure.

Normally, an individual's diet supplies adequate amounts of all of these substances, which are absorbed from the gastrointestinal (GI) tract and transported to the bone marrow. However, when the diet cannot supply enough of a nutrient, or enough of the nutrient cannot be absorbed, the person can develop a deficiency anaemia. Fewer RBCs are produced, and the ones that are produced are immature and inefficient iron carriers. This type of anaemia is called a deficiency anaemia.

Another type of anaemia is megaloblastic anaemia, which involves decreased production of RBCs and ineffectiveness of those RBCs that are produced (they do not usually survive for the 120 days that is normal for the life of an RBC). People with megaloblastic anaemia usually have a lack of vitamin B12 or folic acid.

A third type of anaemia is haemolytic anaemia, which involves a lysing of RBCs because of genetic factors or from exposure to toxins. Sickle cell anaemia is a type of haemolytic anaemia.

Iron deficiency anaemia

All cells in the body require some amount of iron, but iron can be very toxic to cells, especially neurons. To maintain the needed iron levels and avoid toxic levels, the body has developed a system for controlling the amount of iron that can enter the body through intestinal absorption. Only enough iron is absorbed to replace the amount of iron that is lost each day. Once iron is absorbed, it is carried by a plasma protein called transferrin, a beta-globulin. This protein carries iron to various tissues to be stored and transports iron from RBC lysis back to the bone marrow for recycling.

Only about 1 mg of iron is actually lost each day in sweat, in sloughed skin, and from GI and urinary tract linings. Because of the body's efficient iron recycling, very little iron is usually needed in the diet, and most diets adequately replace the iron that is lost. However, in situations in which blood is being lost, a negative iron balance might occur, and the person could develop **iron deficiency anaemia**. This can occur in certain rare GI diseases in which the person is unable to absorb iron from the GI tract, but iron deficiency anaemia is also a relatively common problem in certain groups, including:

- menstruating women, who lose RBCs monthly
- pregnant and breastfeeding women, who have increased demands for iron
- rapidly growing adolescents, especially those who do not have a nutritious diet
- people with GI bleeding, including individuals with slow bleeding associated with use of non-steroidal anti-inflammatory drugs (NSAIDs)

The person with this type of anaemia may complain of being tired because there is insufficient oxygen delivery to the tissues. These conditions are usually treated with iron replacement therapy (see section on iron preparations).

Megaloblastic anaemias

Megaloblastic anaemias result from insufficient amounts of folic acid or vitamin B12 to adequately create the stromal structure needed in a healthy RBC, causing a slowing of nuclear DNA synthesis. This effect occurs in rapidly dividing cells such as the bone marrow. The bone marrow contains a large number of megaloblasts, or large, immature RBCs, and because these RBCs are so large, they become crowded in the bone marrow and fewer RBCs are produced, increasing the amount of immature cells in circulation. Cells in the GI tract are additional examples of cells that are often affected. When the GI tract is involved, this can result in the appearance of a characteristic red and glossy tongue, and diarrhoea.

Folic acid deficiency

Folic acid is essential for cell division in all types of tissue. Deficiencies in folic acid are noticed first in rapidly growing cells, such as those in cancerous tissues, in the GI tract and in the bone marrow. Folic acid is very important for the developing fetus, a site of very rapidly growing cells. Pregnant women are urged to take folic acid supplements to help prevent fetal abnormalities, particularly neural tube defects. Most people can get all the folic acid they need from their diet. For example, folic acid is found in green leafy vegetables, milk, eggs and liver. Deficiency in folic acid may occur in certain malabsorption states, such as sprue and coeliac diseases. Malnutrition that accompanies alcoholism is also a common cause of folic acid deficiency. Repeated pregnancies and extended treatment with certain anti-epileptic medications can also contribute to folic acid deficiency. Folic acid deficiency is treated by the administration of folic acid or folate.

Vitamin B12 deficiency

Vitamin B12 is used in minute amounts by the body and is stored for use if dietary intake falls. It is necessary not only for the health of the RBCs, but also for the formation and maintenance of the myelin sheath in the central nervous system (CNS). It is found in the diet in meats, seafood, eggs and cheese. Strict vegetarians who eat nothing but vegetables may develop a vitamin B12 deficiency. Such individuals with a dietary insufficiency of vitamin B12 typically respond to vitamin B12 replacement therapy to reverse their anaemia.

The most common cause of this deficiency, however, is inability of the GI tract to absorb the needed amounts of the vitamin. Gastric mucosal cells produce a substance called intrinsic factor, which is necessary for the absorption of vitamin B12 by the upper intestine.

Pernicious anaemia occurs when the gastric mucosa cannot produce intrinsic factor and vitamin B12 cannot be absorbed. The person with pernicious anaemia will complain of fatigue and lethargy, and will also have CNS effects because of damage to the myelin sheath. Individuals will also complain of numbness, tingling, and eventually lack of coordination and motor activity. Pernicious anaemia was once a fatal disease, but it is now treated with parenteral or nasal vitamin B12 to replace the amount that can no longer be absorbed.

Sickle cell anaemia

Sickle cell anaemia is a chronic haemolytic anaemia that occurs almost exclusively in black people ('haemolytic' means that the anaemia involves a lysing or destruction of RBCs). It is characterised by a genetically inherited haemoglobin S, which gives the RBCs a sickle-shaped appearance. The person with sickle cell anaemia produces fewer than normal RBCs, and the RBCs that are produced are unable to carry oxygen efficiently. The sickle-shaped RBCs can become lodged in tiny blood vessels, where they stack up on one another and occlude the vessel. This occlusion leads to anoxia and infarction of the tissue in that area, which is characterised by severe pain and an acute inflammatory reaction, the person may even have ulcers on the extremities as a result of such occlusions. Severe, acute episodes of sickling with vessel occlusion may be associated with acute infections as well as the body's reactions to the immune and inflammatory responses. In the past, sickle cell anaemia was treated only with pain medication and support for the person. Now hydroxycarbamide (hydroxyurea) has been found to be effective in treating this disease in adults.

KEY POINTS

- RBCs are produced in the bone marrow in a process called erythropoiesis, which is controlled by the glycoprotein erythropoietin, produced in the kidneys. The bone marrow uses iron, amino acids, carbohydrates, folic acid and vitamin B12 to produce healthy, efficient RBCs.
- Anaemia is a state of too few RBCs or ineffective RBCs. Anaemia can be caused by a lack of erythropoietin or a lack of the components needed to produce RBCs.
- Anaemia can be categorised as deficiency (iron deficiency anaemia), megaloblastic (folic acid or vitamin B12 deficiency) or haemolytic (sickle cell).

ERYTHROPOIESIS-STIMULATING AGENTS

Individuals who are no longer able to produce enough erythropoietin in the kidneys may benefit from treatment with exogenous erythropoietin (EPO), which is available as the drugs epoetin alfa (*Eprex*), epoetin beta (*NeoRecormon*), epoetin lambda (*Novicrit* [not available in New Zealand]), darbepoetin alfa (*Aranesp*) and methoxy polyethylene glycol-epoetin beta (*Mircera*). When agents are used to stimulate the bone marrow to make more RBCs, it is important to ensure that the person has adequate levels of the components required to make RBCs, including adequate iron. See Table 49.1 for additional information about each of these agents. Box 49.1 highlights important considerations for different age groups when this group of drugs and other drugs used to treat anaemia are administered.

Therapeutic actions and indications

Epoetin alfa acts like the natural glycoprotein erythropoietin to stimulate the production of RBCs in the bone marrow (see Figure 49.2). This drug is indicated in the treatment of anaemia associated with renal failure and for people on dialysis; for anaemia associated with AIDS therapy; and for anaemia associated with cancer chemotherapy when the bone marrow is depressed and the kidneys may be affected by the toxic drugs. It is not approved to treat other anaemias and is not a replacement for whole blood in the emergency treatment of anaemia. See Table 49.1 for additional indications.

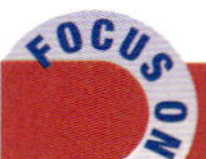

Safe medication administration

With any of these drugs, there is a risk of decreasing the normal levels of erythropoietin if this drug is given to people who have normal renal functioning and adequate levels of erythropoietin (see Adverse effects for important safety information related to medication administration). Negative feedback occurs with the renal cells and less endogenous erythropoietin is produced if exogenous erythropoietin is given. Administration of this drug to a person with anaemia and normal renal function can actually cause a more severe anaemia if the endogenous levels fall and no longer stimulate RBC production.

TABLE 49.1 **DRUGS IN FOCUS** **Erythropoiesis-stimulating agents**

Drug name	Dosage/route	Usual indications
darbepoetin alfa (*Aranesp*)	0.45 microgram/kg SC once weekly, or 0.75 microgram/kg SC once q 2 weeks, or 1.5 micrograms/kg SC once monthly, then titrate according to response	Treatment of anaemia associated with chronic renal failure, including people on dialysis; treatment of chemotherapy-induced anaemia
(P) epoetin alfa (*Eprex*)	Initially: 50 IU/kg SC or slow IVI 3 times/week; may increase by 25 IU/kg at monthly intervals to a maximum of 200 IU/kg 3 times/week Maintenance: 75–300 IU/kg/week	Treatment of anaemia associated with renal failure, and people on dialysis; reduction in need for people undergoing surgical procedures; treatment of anaemia associated with AIDS therapy; treatment of anaemia associated with cancer chemotherapy
epoetin beta (*NeoRecormon*)	SC: initially 60 IU/kg/week; may increase by 60 IU/kg/week every 4 weeks IV: initially 120 IU/kg/week in 3 divided doses; may increase after 4 weeks to 240 IU/kg/week	Treatment of anaemia associated with chronic renal failure, individuals with non-myeloid malignancy, or to augment autologous blood transfusion
epoetin lambda (*Novicrit*)	Elective surgery: 600 IU/kg SC weekly for 3 weeks. Autologous predonation program: 300–600 IU/kg IV twice weekly for 3 weeks Chronic renal failure: 75–300 IU/kg IV or SC weekly	Treatment of anaemia associated with chronic renal failure, individuals with non-myeloid malignancy, or to augment autologous blood transfusion
methoxy polyethylene glycol-epoetin beta (*Mircera*)	Initially SC: 0.6 microgram/kg q 2 weeks or 1.2 micrograms/kg q 1 month. Double the fortnightly dose can be given monthly after target haemoglobin level is reached	Treatment of anaemia associated with chronic renal failure, including people undergoing dialysis treatment

Darbepoetin alfa is an erythropoietin-like protein produced in Chinese hamster ovary cells with the use of recombinant DNA technology. This drug gained negative publicity after it was used by athletes to increase their RBC count in the hope that it would give them more endurance and strength. Many athletic governing bodies now screen for the presence of darbepoetin among other banned drugs. This drug has the advantage of once-weekly administration, compared with two to three times a week administration for epoetin. Methoxy polyethylene glycol-epoetin beta, the newest drug in this class, has the advantage of dosing once every 2 weeks or once a month. Both darbepoetin alfa and methoxy polyethylene glycol-epoetin beta are approved to treat anaemias associated with chronic renal failure, including people receiving dialysis. Darbepoetin alfa is also used for treatment of anaemia induced by cancer chemotherapy. (See also Table 49.1.)

Pharmacokinetics

All of these drugs can be given IV or by subcutaneous (SC) injection. Epoetin alfa, which is like endogenous erythropoietin, is metabolised in the serum through the normal process that the body uses to clear erythropoietin. It has a slow onset and peaks in 5–24 hours, and its duration of effect is usually 24 hours. It has a half-life of 4–13 hours and is excreted in the urine. Darbepoetin alfa has a half-life of 21 hours after intravenous (IV) administration or 49 hours after SC administration. It reaches peak effects in 14 hours (if given IV) or 34 hours (SC). Duration of effects is 24–72 hours and excretion is through the urine. Methoxy polyethylene glycol-epoetin beta has a half-life of 67 hours. It has a slow onset and reaches peak effects in 48–72 hours. It is also cleared in the serum and excreted in the urine. It is not known whether epoetin alfa or methoxy polyethylene glycol-epoetin enters breast milk; however, darbepoetin alfa does cross into breast milk.

Contraindications and cautions

All three of these drugs are contraindicated in the presence of uncontrolled hypertension *because of the risk of even further hypertension when RBC numbers increase and the pressure within the vascular system also increases*; with known hypersensitivity to any component of the drug *to avoid hypersensitivity reactions*; and with breastfeeding *because of the potential for allergic-type reactions with the neonate*. There are no adequate studies in pregnancy, and so use should be limited to situations in which the benefit to the mother clearly outweighs the potential risk to the fetus.

Use caution when administering any of these drugs to people with normal renal functioning and adequate levels of erythropoietin *because of the rebound decrease in erythropoietin that will occur* and when administering them to a person with anaemia and normal renal function *because this can cause more severe anaemia* (see Figure 49.3).

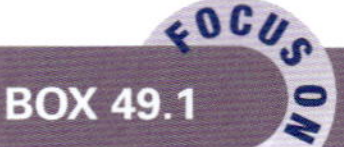

BOX 49.1 Drug therapy across the lifespan

Drugs used to treat anaemias

CHILDREN

Proper nutrition should be established for children to provide the essential elements needed for the formation of RBCs. The cause of the anaemia should be determined to avoid prolonged problems.

The safety and efficacy of epoetin alfa use have not been established for children. If the drug is used, careful dose calculation should be done based on weight and age, and the child should be monitored very closely for response, iron levels and nutrition.

Iron doses for replacement therapy are determined by age. If a liquid solution is being used, the child should drink it through a straw to avoid staining of the teeth. Periodic blood counts should be performed; it may take 4–6 months of oral therapy to reverse an iron deficiency. Remember that iron can be toxic to children. Iron supplements should be kept out of their reach and administration monitored.

Maintenance doses for folic acid have been established for children, based on age. Nutritional means should be used to establish folic acid levels whenever possible.

Children with pernicious anaemia require a monthly injection of vitamin B12; the nasal form has not been approved for use with children.

ADULTS

The underlying cause of the anaemia should be established and appropriate steps taken to reverse the cause if possible. Adults receiving epoetin alfa or darbepoetin alfa should be monitored closely for response, for the need for iron or other RBC building blocks, and for the possibility of development of pure red-cell aplasia.

Advertised heavily in the mass media, epoetin is often requested by adults to help restore energy. Careful teaching about the drug and how and why it is administered may be needed.

Adults receiving iron replacement may experience GI upset and frequently experience constipation. Appropriate measures to maintain bowel function may be needed.

Adults also need to know that periodic blood tests will be needed to evaluate response.

Adults being treated for pernicious anaemia may opt for the nasal vitamin B12. These people need to receive careful instructions about the proper administration of the drug and should have nasal mucous membranes evaluated periodically.

PREGNANCY AND BREASTFEEDING

Proper nutrition during pregnancy and breastfeeding is often still not an adequate way to meet the increased demands of those states. Prenatal vitamins contain iron and folic acid and are usually prescribed for pregnant women. Folic acid is known to be very important for the development of the neural tube, and often women who are considering becoming pregnant are encouraged to take folic acid to build up levels for the planned pregnancy. Use of epoetin alfa or darbepoetin alfa is not recommended during pregnancy or breastfeeding because of the potential for adverse effects on the fetus or baby. Iron replacement is frequently needed postpartum to provide the iron lost during delivery. The new mother should be reminded to keep the drug out of the reach of children and not to combine prescribed iron with an over-the-counter preparation containing high levels of iron.

Women maintained on vitamin B12 before pregnancy should continue the treatment during pregnancy. Increased doses may be needed due to changes associated with the pregnancy.

OLDER ADULTS

Older adults may have nutritional problems related to age and may lose more iron through cellular sloughing. Older adults should be assessed for anaemia and possible causes should be evaluated.

Replacement therapy in the older adult can cause the same adverse effects as are seen in the younger person. Bowel training programs may be needed to prevent severe constipation.

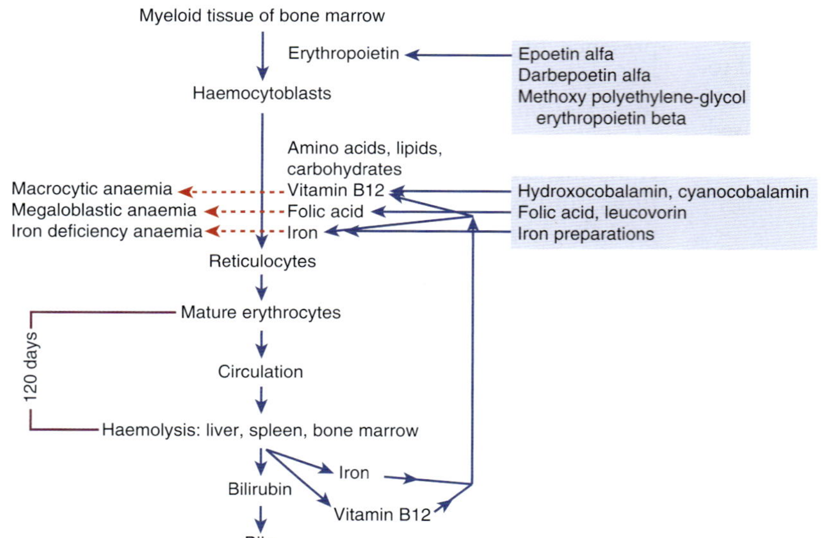

FIGURE 49.2 Sites of action of drugs used to treat anaemia.

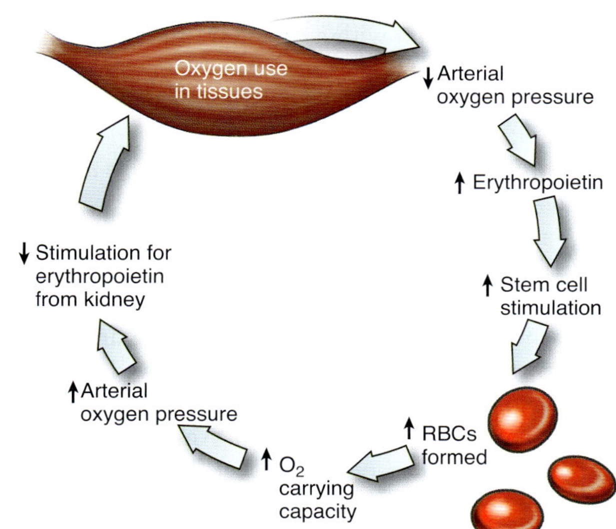

FIGURE 49.3 Erythropoiesis controls the rate of blood cell production.

Adverse effects

The adverse effects most commonly associated with these drugs include the CNS effects of headache, fatigue, asthenia and dizziness and the potential for serious seizures. These effects may be the result of a cellular response to the glycoprotein. Nausea, vomiting and diarrhoea are also common effects. Cardiovascular symptoms can include hypertension, oedema and possible chest pain, all of which may be related to the increase in RBC numbers changing the balance within the cardiovascular system. People receiving IV administration must also be monitored for possible clotting of the access line related to direct cellular effects of the drug. In 2005, postmarketing studies showed that pure red-cell aplasia associated with erythropoietin-neutralising antibodies could occur with all of these products. In 2008, after analyses of several postmarketing studies, these drugs were required to add *black-box warnings* to their prescribing information.

Clinically important drug–drug interactions

These drugs should never be mixed in solution with any other drugs because of a risk of interactions in the solution.

Prototype summary: epoetin alfa

Indications: treatment of anaemia associated with chronic renal failure, related to treatment of HIV infection or to chemotherapy in people with cancer; to reduce the need for allogenic blood transfusion in people undergoing surgical procedures.

Actions: natural glycoprotein that stimulates RBC production in the bone marrow.

Pharmacokinetics:

Route	Onset	Peak	Duration
SC	7–14 days	5–24 hours	24 hours

$T_{1/2}$: 4–13 hours; metabolised in serum and excreted in urine.

Adverse effects: headache, arthralgias, fatigue, asthenia, dizziness, hypertension, oedema, chest pain, nausea, vomiting, diarrhoea.

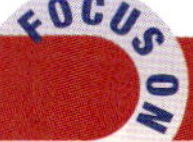

Safe medication administration

*In late 2005, the makers of epoetin and darbepoetin sent out warning letters to health care professionals to bring attention to serious adverse effects that had been noted in postmarketing studies. Cases of pure red-cell aplasia (defective or insufficient production) and severe anaemias, with or without cytopenias (decreased levels of other blood cells), had been reported. These cases were associated with the development of neutralising antibodies to erythropoietin. Use of any therapeutic protein brings with it the risk of antibody production. All of the erythropoietic proteins (*Aranesp, Eprex*) now carry a warning about the potential for this problem. If a person is being treated with one of these drugs and develops a sudden loss of response accompanied by severe anaemia and low reticulocyte count, they should be assessed for the possible causes. Assays for binding and neutralising antibodies should be done. If an antibody-mediated anaemia is confirmed, the drug should be permanently stopped and the person should not be switched to another erythropoietic protein because cross-reaction could occur. Most of the people in the reported cases had chronic renal failure and were being treated with SC injections. It is now recommended that people on haemodialysis receive the drug IV rather than SC. If the drug is started and there is no response, or if a person fails to maintain a response, the dose should not be increased, and red blood cell aplasia should be suspected. The person should be evaluated with the appropriate tests and supported.*

A target haemoglobin of no more than 12 g/dL is sought when using these drugs. Higher levels have been associated with cardiovascular events, including death, and increased rates of tumour progression death in people with cancer in whom the drug was being used to treat anaemia associated with toxic drug therapy. Monitoring the haemoglobin levels is critical for safe and therapeutic use of the erythropoiesis-stimulating agents. An increase in tumour growth was also found in people with cancer treated with these drugs when haemoglobin levels were not kept within the guidelines of no more than 12 g/dL. This has been added to the warnings for these drugs to alert carers to carefully monitor haemoglobin levels to assure safety.

Care considerations for people receiving erythropoiesis-stimulating agents

Assessment: history and examination

- Assess for contraindications or cautions: any known allergies to any component of the drug *to avoid hypersensitivity reactions*; severe hypertension, *which could be exacerbated*; and breastfeeding *because of potential adverse effects on the neonate*. These drugs should be used with caution in people with anaemia and normal renal function *to prevent rebound decrease in normal erythropoietin production* and in people with cancer receiving the drugs to increase haematocrit after antineoplastic chemotherapy *because of the risk of rapid tumour progression if haemoglobin levels exceed guidelines*.
- Perform a physical assessment to establish a *baseline before beginning therapy and during therapy to determine drug effectiveness and evaluate any potential adverse effects*.
- Assess neurological status, including affect, orientation and muscle strength, *to identify possible adverse CNS effects*.
- Monitor vital signs, including pulse and blood pressure, *for changes*, and assess cardiovascular status, *to identify possible cardiovascular effects*; and inspect lower extremities *for evidence of oedema, which could indicate a change in cardiovascular function*.
- Assess respirations and auscultate lungs for adventitious breath sounds *for early detection of changes in cardiovascular function*.
- Monitor the results of laboratory tests, including renal function tests, full blood count (FBC), haematocrit, iron concentration, transferrin and electrolyte levels, *to evaluate the effectiveness of therapy*. Be aware of variations in haematological test results due to race (see Box 49.2).

Implementation with rationale

- Confirm the chronic, renal nature of the person's anaemia before administering the drug to treat renal failure anaemia *to ensure proper use of the drug*.
- Give epoetin alfa three times per week, either IV or SC, *to achieve appropriate therapeutic drug levels*. Administer darbepoetin alfa once per week, SC or IV. Administer methoxy polyethylene glycol-epoetin beta once every 2 weeks, and then once a month when the person is stabilised, by SC injection *to achieve appropriate therapeutic drug levels*.
- Provide the person with a calendar of marked days *to aid in remembering dates for injection and promote increased compliance with the drug regimen*.
- Do not mix with any other drug solution *to avoid potential incompatibilities*
- Monitor access lines for clotting and *arrange to clear line as needed*.
- Ensure that prescribed laboratory testing, such as haematocrit levels, is completed before drug administration *to determine correct dose*. If the person does not respond within 8 weeks, re-evaluate the cause of anaemia. Anticipate a target haemoglobin range between 10 and 12 g/dL.
- Evaluate iron stores before and periodically during therapy *because supplemental iron may be needed as the person makes more RBCs*.
- Maintain seizure precautions on standby *in case seizures occur as a reaction to the drug*.
- Provide comfort measures *to help the person tolerate the drug effects*. These include small, frequent meals to help minimise nausea and vomiting; readily available access to bathroom facilities if diarrhoea occurs; and analgesia for headache or arthralgia.
- Offer support and encouragement *to help the person deal with the diagnosis and the drug regimen*.
- Provide thorough teaching, including the name of the drug, dosage prescribed, administration technique and frequency of administration, measures to avoid adverse effects, warning signs of problems and need to notify health care provider, and the need for follow-up laboratory testing, *to enhance knowledge about drug therapy and to promote compliance*.

Evaluation

- Monitor response to the drug (alleviation of anaemia, target haemoglobin level a maximum of 12 g/dL).
- Monitor for adverse effects (headache, hypertension, nausea, vomiting, seizures, dizziness).
- Monitor the effectiveness of comfort measures and compliance with the regimen.
- Evaluate the effectiveness of the teaching plan (person can name drug, dosage, adverse effects to watch for and specific measures to avoid them; person understands the importance of continued follow-up).

BOX 49.2 FOCUS ON Cultural considerations

Haematological laboratory test variations

There are racial variations in haematological laboratory test results:

Haemoglobin/haematocrit – levels in African Americans are generally 1 g lower than in other groups.

Serum transferrin levels (children aged 1–3.5 years) – the mean value for African American children is 22 mg/100 mL higher than that for Caucasian children. (This may be because African Americans have lower haematocrit and haemoglobin; transferrin levels increase normally in the presence of anaemia.)

Because of these variations, the diagnosis and treatment of anaemia in African Americans should be based on a different norm to that of other ethnic groups.

KEY POINTS

- Erythropoiesis-stimulating drugs are used to act like erythropoietin and stimulate the bone marrow to produce more RBCs.
- These drugs must be given IV or by SC injection. Individuals must have an adequate supply of the other components of RBCs, including iron, for these drugs to be effective.
- Erythropoiesis-stimulating drugs should be used with a target haemoglobin level of no more than 12 g/dL. Higher levels are associated with an increased risk of cardiovascular events and increased tumour growth in people with cancer.

AGENTS USED FOR IRON DEFICIENCY ANAEMIA

Although most people get all of the iron they need through diet, in some situations diet alone may not be adequate. The iron preparations that are available include ferrous fumarate (*Ferro-tab*), ferrous sulfate (*Fefol, Ferro-Gradumet*), iron polymaltose (*Ferrosig, Ferrum H*) and iron sucrose (*Venofer*). See also Table 49.2

Therapeutic actions and indications

Iron preparations elevate the serum iron concentration (see Figure 49.2). They are then either converted

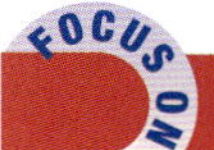

Safe medication administration

Z-track injections

The Z-track method is used when injecting iron to reduce the risk of SC staining and irritation. It is a good idea to review the method of giving Z-track injections before giving one. The area to be injected is prepped for the injection. Place your gloved finger on the skin surface and pull the skin and the SC layers out of alignment with the muscle lying beneath. Try to move the skin about 1 cm. Insert the needle at a 90-degree angle at the point where you originally placed your finger. Inject the drug and then withdraw the needle. Remove your finger from the skin, which will allow the layers to slide back into their normal position. The track that the needle made when inserting into the muscle is now broken by the layers, and the drug is trapped in the muscle (see Figure 49.4).

TABLE 49.2 DRUGS IN FOCUS Agents used for iron deficiency anaemia

Drug name	Dosage/route	Usual indications
ferric carboxymaltose (*Ferinject*)	Undiluted solution IV up to a maximum single dose of 1000 mg iron (20 mg iron/kg body weight) over 15 minutes. Maximum 1000 mg iron per week Body weight: 35–70 kg: Hb < 100 g/L: 1500 mg IV; Hb > 100 g/L: 1000 mg IV Body weight > 70 kg: Hb < 100 g/L: 2000 mg IV; Hb > 100 g/L: 1500 mg IV	Treatment of iron deficiency anaemia
ferrous fumarate (*Ferro-tab*)	1 tablet PO tid before food; each tablet contains 65 mg elemental iron	Treatment of iron deficiency anaemia
(P) ferrous sulfate (*Ferro-Gradumet*)	325 mg/day PO; each tablet contains 105 mg elemental iron	Treatment of iron deficiency anaemia
iron polymaltose complex (*Ferrosig, Ferrum H*)	2 mL IM alternate days, using Z-track technique (contains 100 mg/2 mL)	Treatment of iron deficiency anaemia (parenteral)
iron sucrose (*Venofer*)	Venofer is 100 mg elemental iron per 5 mL. 100 mg IV infusion in 100 mL normal saline over 15 minutes, or IV injection into venous line of dialysis machine over 5 minutes (maximum 200 mg over 10 minutes) 500 mg IV infusion in 500 mL normal saline is given over 3.5 hours	Treatment of iron deficiency in people undergoing chronic haemodialysis or non-dialysis people with renal failure who are also receiving supplemental erythropoietin therapy

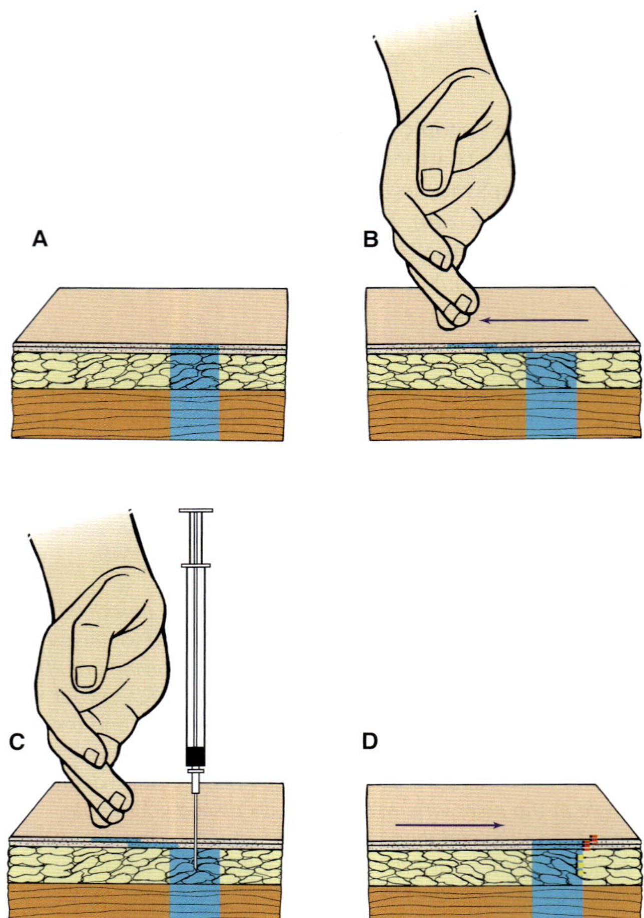

FIGURE 49.4 Use of the Z-track, or zigzag, technique for injections. **A.** Normal skin and tissues. **B.** Move the skin to one side. **C.** Insert the needle at a 90-degree angle and aspirate for blood. **D.** Withdraw the needle, and allow the displaced tissue to return to normal position, thereby keeping the solution from leaving the muscle tissue.

to haemoglobin or trapped in reticuloendothelial cells for storage and eventual release and conversion into a usable form of iron for RBC production. Oral iron preparations are often used to help these people regain a positive iron balance; these preparations need to be supplemented with adequate dietary intake of iron. They are indicated for the treatment of iron deficiency anaemias and may also be used as adjunctive therapy in people receiving an erythropoiesis-stimulating drug. The drug of choice depends on the prescriber's personal preference and experience, and often on what kinds of samples are available to give the person. See Table 49.2 for usual indications.

Pharmacokinetics

Ferrous fumarate and ferrous sulfate are available for oral administration. Iron polymaltose is a parenteral form of iron given by the Z-track method.

Individuals should be switched to the oral form if at all possible because of the pain associated with IM administration of iron. Iron polymaltose is given IV specifically for people who are undergoing chronic haemodialysis or who are in renal failure and not on dialysis but are receiving supplemental erythropoietin therapy.

Iron is primarily absorbed from the small intestine by an active transport system. It is transported in the blood, bound to transferrin. Small amounts are lost daily in the sweat, urine, sloughing of skin and mucosal cells, and sloughing of intestinal cells, as well as in the menstrual flow of women. Most of the oral drug that is taken is lost in the faeces, but slowly some of the metal is absorbed into the intestine and transported to the bone marrow. It can take 2–3 weeks to see improvement and up to 6–10 months for a return to a stable iron level once a deficiency exists. It is used during pregnancy and breastfeeding to help the mother meet the increased demands for iron that occur at those times.

Contraindications and cautions

These drugs are contraindicated for people with known allergy to any of these preparations *because severe hypersensitivity reactions have been associated with the parenteral form of iron.* They also are contraindicated in the following conditions: haemochromatosis (excessive iron); haemolytic anaemias, *which may increase serum iron levels and cause toxicity*; normal iron balance *because the drug will not be absorbed and will just pass through the body*; and peptic ulcer, colitis or regional enteritis *because the drug can be directly irritating to these tissues and can cause exacerbation of the diseases.*

Adverse effects

The most common adverse effects associated with oral iron are related to direct GI irritation; these include GI upset, anorexia, nausea, vomiting, diarrhoea, dark stools and constipation. With increasing serum levels, iron can be directly toxic to the CNS, causing coma and even death. Box 49.3 discusses iron toxicity and drugs that are used to counteract this effect. Parenteral iron is associated with severe anaphylactic reactions, local irritation, staining of the tissues and phlebitis. *See the Critical thinking scenario for additional information about iron preparations and toxicity.*

Clinically important drug–drug interactions

Iron absorption decreases if iron preparations are taken with antacids, tetracyclines or cimetidine; if these drugs must be used, they should be spaced at least 2 hours apart.

Anti-infective response to ciprofloxacin, norfloxacin or ofloxacin can decrease if these drugs are taken with iron because of a decrease in absorption; they should also be administered at least 2 hours apart. Increased iron levels occur if iron preparations are taken with

BOX 49.3 Chelating agents

Heavy metals, including iron, lead, arsenic, mercury, copper and gold, can cause toxicity in the body by their ability to tie up chemicals in living tissues that need to be free in order for the cell to function normally. When these vital substances (thiols, sulfurs, carboxyls and phosphoryls) are bound to the metal, certain cellular enzyme systems become deactivated, resulting in failure of cellular function and eventual cell death. Drugs that have been developed to counteract metal toxicity are called chelating agents (from the Greek word for 'claw').

Chelating agents grasp and hold a toxic metal so that it can be carried out of the body before it has time to harm the tissues. The chelating agent binds the molecules of the metal, preventing it from damaging the cells within the body. The complex that is formed by the chelating agent and the metal is non-toxic and is excreted by the kidneys.

Chelating agent	Toxic metal	Notes
desferrioxamine mesylate (*Desferal*)	iron	Given IM, SC or IV; rash and vision changes are common
penicillamine (*D-Penamine*)	copper, gold, mercury, lead, zinc	Administered orally on an empty stomach, and at least 2 hours before a meal or 1 hour after other drugs, food or milk
sodium calcium edetate (*Calcium Disodium Edetate*)	lead	Given by IV infusion over 3–4 hours; monitor renal and hepatic function, because serious and even fatal toxicity can occur

chloramphenicol; people receiving this combination should be monitored closely for any sign of iron toxicity. The effects of levodopa may decrease if it is taken with iron preparations; people receiving both of these drugs should take them at least 2 hours apart.

Clinically important drug–food interactions

Iron is not absorbed if taken with antacids, eggs, milk, coffee or tea. These substances should not be administered concurrently. Acidic liquids may enhance the absorption of iron and should not be given concurrently.

CRITICAL THINKING SCENARIO

Iron preparations and toxicity

THE SITUATION

L.L., a 28-year-old woman, experienced a miscarriage 6 weeks ago. She lost a great deal of blood during the miscarriage and underwent a dilation and curettage to control the bleeding. On her 6-week routine follow-up visit, she was found to have recovered physically from the event but was still depressed over her loss. Her haematocrit was 31%, and she admitted feeling tired and weak. She was offered emotional support and given a supply of ferrous sulfate tablets, with instructions to take one tablet three times a day.

At home, L.L. transferred the pills to a decorative bottle that had once held vitamins and left it on her table as a reminder to take the tablets. The next day, she discovered her 2-year-old daughter eating the tablets and punished her for getting into them. About 1 hour later, the toddler complained of a really bad 'tummy ache' and started vomiting. She then became lethargic, and L.L. called the paediatrician, who told them to go immediately to the emergency department and bring the remaining tablets with them. The toddler was found to have a weak, rapid pulse (156 beats/minute), rapid, shallow respirations (32 per minute), and a low blood pressure (60/42 mmHg). When a diagnosis of acute iron toxicity was made, L.L. became distraught. She said she had no idea that iron could be dangerous because it can be bought over-the-counter (OTC) in so many preparations. She had not read the written information given to her because it was 'just iron'.

CRITICAL THINKING

What interventions should be done at this point?

What sort of crisis intervention would be most appropriate for L.L.? *Think about the combined depression from the miscarriage, fear and anxiety related to this crisis, and L.L.'s iron-depleted state.*

What kind of reserve does she have for dealing with this crisis? Which measures would be appropriate for helping the mother cope with this crisis and for treating the toddler?

DISCUSSION

The first priority is to support and detoxify the child who has iron toxicity. In cases of acute iron poisoning, eggs and milk are given to bind the iron and prevent absorption. Gastric lavage, using a 1% sodium bicarbonate solution, can be done in a medical facility. This procedure is safe for about the first hour after ingestion. After that time, there is an increased risk of gastric erosion caused by the corrosive iron, making the lavage very dangerous. Because this toddler is well beyond the first hour, other measures will be needed. Supportive measures to deal with shock, dehydration and GI damage will be necessary. In addition, an iron-chelating agent such as desferrioxamine mesylate may be tried.

During this crisis, L.L. will need a great deal of support, including a responsible relative or friend or other person who can stay with her. She also will need reassurance and a place to rest. After the situation is stabilised, L.L. will need teaching and additional support. For example, she should be reassured that most people do not take OTC drugs seriously and many do not even read the labels. However, the health care professional can use this opportunity to stress the importance of reading all of the labels and following the directions that come with OTC drugs. L.L. also should be commended for calling the paediatrician and getting medical care for the toddler quickly. Finally, she should receive a review of the iron teaching information and be encouraged to ask questions.

This case is a good example for a staff in-service program, stressing not only the dangers of iron toxicity, but also the vital importance of providing good education before sending the person home with a new drug. Simply giving the person written information is often not enough. The care guide and teaching guidelines for L.L. when she was given the iron supplement should have included the following.

CARE GUIDE FOR L.L.: IRON PREPARATIONS

Assessment: history and examination

Assess L.L.'s health history for allergies to any iron preparation, colitis, enteritis, hepatic dysfunction or peptic ulcer.

Then focus the physical examination on the following areas:

Cardiovascular: blood pressure, pulse, perfusion

Neurological (CNS): orientation, affect, reflexes, vision

Skin: colour, lesions, gums, teeth

Respiratory system: respiratory rate and character, adventitious sounds

GI: abdominal examination, bowel sounds

Laboratory tests: full blood count, haemoglobin, haematocrit, serum ferritin assays

Implementation

Confirm iron deficiency anaemia before administering the drug.

Provide comfort and safety measures; for example, give small meals; ensure access to bathroom facilities; give the drug with food if GI upset occurs; and institute a bowel program as needed.

Arrange for the treatment of the underlying cause of anaemia.

Provide support and reassurance to deal with drug effects.

Provide teaching regarding drug, dosage, adverse effects, what to report and safety precautions.

Evaluation

Evaluate drug effects (relief of signs and symptoms of anaemia, haematocrit within normal limits).

Monitor for adverse effects: GI upset, CNS toxicity, coma.

Monitor haematocrit and haemoglobin periodically.

Monitor for drug–drug interactions as indicated for each drug.

Evaluate the effectiveness of the teaching program and comfort and safety measures.

TEACHING FOR L.L.

- Iron is a naturally occurring mineral found in many foods. It is used by the body to make red blood cells, which carry oxygen to all parts of the body. Supplemental iron needs to be taken when the body does not have enough iron available to make healthy red blood cells, a condition called anaemia.
- Iron is a toxic substance if too much is taken. You must avoid self-medicating with over-the-counter preparations containing iron while you are taking this drug.
- You will need to return for regular medical checkups while taking this drug to determine its effectiveness.
- Take your medication as follows, depending on the specific iron preparation that has been prescribed:
  - Dissolve *ferrous salts* in orange juice to improve the taste.
  - Take *liquid iron preparations* with a straw to prevent the iron from staining teeth.
  - Place iron drops on the back of the tongue to prevent staining of the teeth.
- Some of the following adverse effects may occur:
  - *Dark, tarry or green stools*: the iron preparations stain the stools; the colour remains as long as you are taking the drug and should not cause concern.
  - *Constipation*: this is a common problem; if it becomes too uncomfortable, consult with your health care provider for an appropriate remedy.
  - *Nausea, indigestion, vomiting*: these problems can often be solved by taking the drug with food, making sure to avoid eggs, milk, coffee and tea.
  - Report any of the following to your health care provider: *severe diarrhoea, severe abdominal pain or cramping, unusual tiredness or weakness, or bluish tint to the lips or fingernail beds.*
- Tell any doctor, nurse or other health care provider that you are taking this drug.
- Keep this drug, and all medications, out of the reach of children. Because iron can be very toxic, seek emergency medical help immediately if you suspect that a child has taken this preparation unsupervised.
- Because iron can interfere with the absorption of some drugs, do not take iron at the same time as *tetracycline* or *antacids*. These drugs must be taken during intervals when iron is not in the stomach.

Prototype summary: ferrous sulfate

Indications: prevention and treatment of iron deficiency anaemia; dietary supplement for iron.

Actions: elevates the serum iron concentration and is then converted into haemoglobin or stored for eventual conversion to a usable form of iron.

Pharmacokinetics:

Route	Onset	Peak	Duration
Oral	4 days	7–10 days	2–4 months

$T_{1/2}$: not known; recycled for use, not excreted.

Adverse effects: GI upset, anorexia, nausea, vomiting, constipation, diarrhoea, CNS toxicity progressing to coma and death with overdose.

Care considerations for people receiving iron preparations

Assessment: history and examination

- Assess for contraindications or cautions: any known allergies to this drug *to avoid hypersensitivity reactions*; hyperchromatosis *to avoid increasing already increased iron levels*; colitis, enteritis or peptic ulcer, *which could lead to increased GI irritation from the drug and exacerbation of the disorder*; and haemolytic anaemias, *which could increase serum iron levels and lead to toxicity.*
- Perform a physical assessment *to establish a baseline before beginning therapy and during therapy to determine drug effectiveness and to evaluate for any potential adverse effects.*
- Inspect the colour and integrity of the skin and mucous membranes *to identify potential signs and symptoms associated with anaemia and evaluate for possible adverse effects of the parenteral form.*
- Assess the person's neurological status, including level of orientation, affect and reflexes, *to identify possible CNS effects and early signs of possible toxicity.*
- Monitor pulse, blood pressure and perfusion, and respirations and adventitious sounds, *to check cardiovascular function and detect early signs of toxicity.*
- Inspect abdomen for distension and auscultate bowel sounds *to evaluate GI motility.*
- Inspect the skin integrity of the intended parenteral administration site *to ensure intactness and evaluate for possible staining.*
- Monitor the results of laboratory tests, including FBC haematocrit, haemoglobin and serum ferritin assays, *to determine drug effectiveness and identify toxic levels.*

Implementation with rationale

- Ensure that iron deficiency anaemia is confirmed before administering drugs *to ensure proper use of the drug.*
- Consult with the doctor to arrange for the treatment of the underlying cause of anaemia if possible *because iron replacement will not correct the cause of the iron loss.*
- Administer the oral form with meals that do not include eggs, milk, coffee and tea *to relieve GI irritation and nausea if GI upset is severe and to prevent drug–food interactions*; have the person drink oral solutions through a straw *to prevent staining of teeth.*
- Caution the person that stool may be dark or green *to prevent undue alarm if this occurs.*
- Take measures to help alleviate constipation *to prevent discomfort and the adverse effects of severe constipation.*
- Administer intramuscularly only by Z-track technique *to ensure proper administration and to avoid staining of the tissues brown.* Warn the person that the injection can be painful.
- Arrange for haematocrit and haemoglobin measurements before administration and periodically during therapy *to monitor drug effectiveness.*
- Provide comfort measures *to help the person tolerate drug effects.* These include small, frequent meals to minimise nausea and readily available access to bathroom facilities should constipation occur, and increased fibre and fluid intake and increased exercise *to help alleviate constipation.*
- Offer support and encouragement *to help the person deal with the diagnosis and the drug regimen.*
- Provide thorough teaching, including the drug name, dosage and route of administration; administration technique, such as parenteral Z-track injection or oral solution through a straw, and frequency of administration; foods and fluids to avoid and to include to ensure proper absorption; need for increased fluids and fibre in diet, and exercise to prevent constipation; notification of change in stool colour and consistency; potential for pain at site and staining of skin with parenteral administration; measures to avoid adverse effects; warning signs of problems and need to notify health care provider; and the need for follow-up laboratory testing, *to enhance knowledge about drug therapy and to promote compliance.*

Evaluation

- Monitor response to the drug (alleviation of anaemia).
- Monitor for adverse effects (GI upset and reaction, CNS toxicity, coma).

- Monitor the effectiveness of comfort measures and compliance with the regimen.
- Evaluate the effectiveness of the teaching plan (person can name drug, dosage, adverse effects to watch for and specific measures to avoid them; person understands the importance of continued follow-up).

KEY POINTS

- Iron products are used to replace iron in cases of iron deficiency anaemia, which can occur because of deficient iron intake or because of blood loss leading to lower iron levels.
- Iron products commonly cause constipation, nausea, green stools and GI upset.
- Iron toxicity can cause severe CNS toxicity, coma and even death because high iron levels are very toxic to nerve cell membranes.

AGENTS USED FOR OTHER ANAEMIAS

This section discusses treatment for megaloblastic anaemias and sickle cell anaemia. Table 49.3 gives a complete list of agents.

AGENTS FOR MEGALOBLASTIC ANAEMIAS

Megaloblastic anaemia is treated with folic acid and vitamin B12. Folate deficiencies usually occur secondary to increased demand (as in pregnancy or growth spurts); as a result of absorption problems in the small intestine; because of drugs that cause folate deficiencies; or secondary to the malnutrition of alcoholism. Vitamin B12 deficiencies can result from poor diet or increased demand, but the usual cause is lack of intrinsic factor in the stomach, which is necessary for absorption. The drugs are usually given together to ensure that the problem is addressed and the blood cells can be formed properly (see Table 49.3). Folic acid derivatives include folic acid (*Fefol*) and calcium folinate (*Leucovorin*). B12 includes hydroxocobalamin (*Hydroxo-B12, Neo-B12*), mecobalamin (co-methylcobalamin) (*Methylcobalamin*) and cyanocobalamin (generic).

Therapeutic actions and indications

Folic acid and vitamin B12 are essential for cell growth and division and for the production of a strong stroma in RBCs (see Figure 49.3). Vitamin B12 is also necessary for maintenance of the myelin sheath in nerve tissue. Both are given as replacement therapy

TABLE 49.3 DRUGS IN FOCUS Agents used for other anaemias

Drug name	Dosage/route	Usual indications
Agents for megaloblastic anaemias		
Folic acid derivatives		
calcium folinate (*Leucovorin*)	Megaloblastic anaemia: 1 mg IM or IV/day or 5–15 mg/day PO Methotrexate rescue: 10 mg/m^2 IM, IV, or PO every 6 hours for 10 doses starting 24 hours after the beginning of the methotrexate infusion	Replacement therapy and treatment of megaloblastic anaemia; used as 'leucovorin rescue' after chemotherapy, allowing non-cancerous cells to survive the chemotherapy; used with fluorouracil for palliative treatment of colorectal cancer (see Chapter 14)
(P) folic acid (*Ferro-F-tab, FGF*)	1 tablet daily	Replacement therapy and treatment of megaloblastic anaemia
Vitamin B12		
mecobalamin (co-methylcobalamin) (*Methylcobalamin*)	10 mg/2 mL slow IM; inform people with pernicious anaemia that they will require monthly injections of vitamin B12 for the rest of their lives	Replacement therapy: treatment of pernicious anaemia
cyanocobalamin (generic)	Adult: 5 mg/day deep IM for short periods Neonatal: 1 mg/day IM	Replacement therapy; treatment of megaloblastic anaemia, pernicious anaemia
(P) hydroxocobalamin (*Hydroxo-B12, Neo-B12*)	250–1000 micrograms IM on alternate days for 1–2 weeks, then 250 micrograms/week IM; maintenance: 1000 micrograms q 2–3 months	Replacement therapy; treatment of megaloblastic anaemia, pernicious anaemia
Agent for sickle cell anaemia		
(P) hydroxycarbamide (hydroxyurea) (*Hydrea*)	Initially 15 mg/kg/day PO as a single dose; increase by 5 mg/kg/day every 12 weeks to a maximum dose of 35 mg/kg/day PO	Off-label use to reduce of frequency of painful crises and decrease the need for blood transfusions in adults with sickle cell anaemia

for dietary deficiencies, as replacement in high-demand states such as pregnancy and breastfeeding, and to treat megaloblastic anaemia. Folic acid is used as a rescue drug for cells exposed to some toxic chemotherapeutic agents. Calcium folinate is used as a rescue drug following methotrexate therapy to decrease the toxicity of methotrexate caused by decreased elimination or overdose of folic acid antagonists such as trimethoprim and for the treatment of various megaloblastic anaemias.

Pharmacokinetics

Folic acid can be given in oral, intramuscular, IV and SC forms. The parenteral drugs are preferred for people with potential absorption problems; others should be given the oral form if at all possible. Calcium folinate is a reduced form of folic acid that is available for oral, intramuscular and IV use.

Hydroxocobalamin must be given intramuscularly every day for 5–10 days to build up levels, then once a month for life. It cannot be taken orally because the problem with pernicious anaemia is the inability to absorb vitamin B12 secondary to low levels of intrinsic factor. It can be used in states of increased demand (eg, pregnancy, growth spurts) or dietary deficiency, but oral vitamins are preferred in most of those cases. Cyanocobalamin is not as tightly bound to proteins and does not last in the body as long as hydroxocobalamin does. This drug is primarily stored in the liver and slowly released as needed for metabolic functions.

Folic acid and vitamin B12 are well absorbed after injection, metabolised mainly in the liver and excreted in urine. These vitamins are considered essential during pregnancy and breastfeeding because of the increased demands of the mother's metabolism.

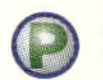 **Prototype summary: folic acid**

Indications: treatment of megaloblastic anaemia due to sprue, nutritional deficiency.

Actions: reduced form of folic acid, required for nucleoprotein synthesis and maintenance of normal erythropoiesis.

Pharmacokinetics:

Route	Onset	Peak
Oral, IM, SC, IV	Varies	30–60 min

$T_{1/2}$: unknown; metabolised in the liver and excreted in urine.

Adverse effects: allergic reactions, pain and discomfort at injection site.

 **Prototype summary: hydroxocobalamin**

Indications: treatment of vitamin B12 deficiency; to meet increased vitamin B12 requirements related to disease, pregnancy or blood loss.

Actions: essential for nucleic acid and protein synthesis; used for growth, cell reproduction, haematopoiesis, and nucleoprotein and myelin synthesis.

Pharmacokinetics:

Route	Onset	Peak
IM	Intermediate	60 min

$T_{1/2}$: 24–36 hours; metabolised in the liver and excreted in urine.

Adverse effects: itching, transitory exanthema, mild diarrhoea, anaphylactic reaction, heart failure, pulmonary oedema, hypokalaemia, pain at injection site.

Contraindications and cautions

These drugs are contraindicated in the presence of known allergies to these drugs or to their components *to avoid hypersensitivity reactions*. They should be used cautiously in people who are pregnant or breastfeeding or who have other anaemias *to ensure that the correct doses of the drug are used to provide the best therapeutic effect and decrease the risk of toxic effects.*

Adverse effects

These drugs have relatively few adverse effects because they are used as replacement for required chemicals. Hydroxocobalamin has been associated with itching, rash and signs of excessive vitamin B levels, which can also include peripheral oedema and heart failure. Mild diarrhoea has been reported with these drugs. Pain and discomfort can occur at injection sites. Nasal irritation can occur with the use of intranasal spray.

Care considerations for people receiving folic acid derivatives or vitamin B12

Assessment: history and examination

- Assess *for contraindications or cautions*: any known allergies to these drugs or drug components, other anaemias, pregnancy, breastfeeding and nasal erosion.
- Assess baseline status before beginning therapy *to determine any potential adverse effects.* This includes affect, orientation and reflexes; pulse, blood pressure and perfusion; respirations and adventitious

sounds; and FBC, haematocrit and iron levels, *to determine the effectiveness of drug therapy.*

Implementation with rationale

- Confirm the nature of the megaloblastic anaemia *to ensure that the proper drug regimen is being used.*
- Give both types of drugs in cases of pernicious anaemia *to ensure therapeutic effectiveness.*
- Parenteral vitamin B12 must be given intramuscularly each day for 5–10 days and then once a month for life *if used to treat pernicious anaemia.*
- Arrange for nutritional consultation *to ensure a well-balanced diet.*
- Monitor for the possibility of hypersensitivity reactions; *have life support equipment on standby in case reactions occur.*
- Arrange for haematocrit readings before and periodically during therapy *to monitor drug effectiveness.*
- Provide comfort measures *to help the person tolerate drug effects.* These include small, frequent meals, access to bathroom facilities and analgesia for muscle or nasal pain.
- Provide thorough teaching, including the name of the drug, dosage prescribed, measures to avoid adverse effects, warning signs of problems, and the need for periodic monitoring and evaluation, *to enhance knowledge about drug therapy and to promote compliance with the drug regimen.*
- Offer support and encouragement *to help the person deal with the diagnosis and the drug regimen.*

Evaluation

- Monitor response to the drug (alleviation of anaemia).
- Monitor for adverse effects (nasal irritation, pain at injection site, nausea).
- Evaluate the effectiveness of the teaching plan (person can name drug, dosage, adverse effects to watch for and specific measures to avoid them; individual understands the importance of continued follow-up).
- Monitor the effectiveness of comfort measures and compliance with the regimen.

Agent for sickle cell anaemia

People with sickle cell anaemia are treated with antibiotics to help fight the infections that can occur when blood flow is decreased to any area; with pain-relieving activities to help alleviate the pain associated with the anoxia to tissues, which can range from heat applied to the area to OTC pain medications to prescription opioids; and now, for adults, with hydroxycarbamide (hydroxyurea) (*Hydrea*). Hydroxycarbamide is a cytotoxic antineoplastic drug that is also used to treat leukaemia, ovarian cancer and melanoma.

Therapeutic actions and indications

Hydroxycarbamide, taken for several months, increases the amount of fetal haemoglobin produced in the bone marrow and dilutes the formation of the abnormal haemoglobin S in adults who have sickle cell anaemia. This results in less clogging of small vessels and the painful, anoxic effects associated with the RBC sickling or stacking. See Table 49.3 for usual indications.

Pharmacokinetics

Given orally, hydroxycarbamide is absorbed well from the GI tract, reaching peak levels in 1–4 hours. It is metabolised in the liver and excreted in the urine with a half-life of 3–4 hours. It is known to cross the placenta and to enter breast milk.

Contraindications and cautions

Hydroxycarbamide is contraindicated with known allergy to any component of the drug *to prevent hypersensitivity reactions* and with severe anaemia or leucopenia *because it can cause further bone marrow suppression.* It should be used with caution in the presence of impaired liver or renal function, *which could interfere with metabolism and excretion of the drug,* and it should only be used in pregnancy and breastfeeding if the benefit to the mother clearly outweighs the potential risk to the fetus or baby *because this drug crosses the placenta and enters breast milk and could cause serious effects in the fetus or baby.*

Prototype summary: hydroxycarbamide (hydroxyurea)

Indications: reduction of frequency of painful crisis and need for blood transfusions in adult people with sickle cell anaemia.

Actions: increases fetal haemoglobin production in the bone marrow and dilutes the formation of abnormal haemoglobin S.

Pharmacokinetics:

Route	Onset	Peak	Duration
Oral	Varied	1–4 hours	18–20 hours

$T_{1/2}$: 3–4 hours; metabolised in the liver and excreted in urine.

Adverse effects: dizziness, headache, rash, erythema, anorexia, nausea, vomiting, stomatitis, bone marrow depression, cancer.

Adverse effects

Hydroxycarbamide is cytotoxic and is associated with adverse effects associated with the death of cells, especially in cells that are rapidly turning over. GI effects include anorexia, nausea, vomiting, stomatitis, diarrhoea or constipation; dermatological effects include rash or erythema; and bone marrow suppression usually occurs. Headache, dizziness, disorientation, fever, chills and malaise have been reported, possibly related to the effects of cell death in the body. As with other cytotoxic drugs, there is an increased risk of cancer development.

Clinically important drug–drug interactions

There is an increased risk of uric acid levels if this drug is combined with any uricosuric agents; if this combination must be used, dose adjustments will be needed for the uricosuric agent.

Care considerations for people receiving hydroxycarbamide (hydroxyurea)

See Chapter 14, Antineoplastic agents, for considerations for a person receiving hydroxycarbamide.

KEY POINTS

- Megaloblastic anaemia is treated with folic acid and vitamin B12.
- Calcium folinate is used as rescue drugs for methotrexate therapy when folate inhibition is high.
- People receiving these drugs require periodic blood tests to ensure therapeutic effects and avoid toxicity associated with high serum levels.
- Sickle cell anaemia is a genetic disorder in haemoglobin formation that can lead to clogging of blood vessels, with resulting anoxia and severe pain.
- Hydroxycarbamide (hydroxyurea), an antineoplastic drug, is useful in reducing the painful crises and need for blood transfusions in adults with sickle cell anaemia. It is associated with many adverse effects because it is a cytotoxic drug.

CHAPTER SUMMARY

- Blood is composed of liquid plasma and formed elements (white blood cells, RBCs and platelets) and contains oxygen and nutrients that are essential for cell survival; it delivers these to the cells and removes waste products from the tissues.
- RBCs are produced in the bone marrow in a process called erythropoiesis, which is controlled by the glycoprotein erythropoietin, produced by the kidneys.
- RBCs do not have a nucleus, and their lifespan is about 120 days, at which time they are lysed and their building blocks are recycled to make new RBCs.
- The bone marrow uses iron, amino acids, carbohydrates, folic acid and vitamin B12 to produce healthy, efficient RBCs.
- An insufficient number or immaturity of RBCs results in low oxygen levels in the tissues, with tiredness, fatigue and loss of energy reserves.
- Anaemia is a state of too few RBCs or ineffective RBCs. Anaemia can be caused by a lack of erythropoietin or by a lack of the components needed to produce RBCs.
- Iron deficiency anaemia occurs when there is inadequate iron intake in the diet or an inability to absorb iron from the GI tract. Iron is needed to produce haemoglobin, which carries oxygen. Iron deficiency anaemia is treated with iron replacement.
- Iron is a very toxic mineral at high levels. The body controls the absorption of iron and carefully regulates its storage and movement in the body.
- Folic acid and vitamin B12 are needed to produce a strong supporting structure in the RBC so that it can survive 120 days of being propelled through the vascular system. Deficiencies are usually caused by inadequate amounts in the diet. Deficiencies are treated with folic acid and vitamin B12 replacement.
- A dietary lack of or inability to absorb folic acid, vitamin B12 or both will produce a megaloblastic anaemia, in which the RBCs are large and immature, and have a short lifespan.
- Pernicious anaemia is a lack of vitamin B12, which is also used by the body to maintain the myelin sheath on nerve axons. If vitamin B12 is lacking, these neurons will degenerate and cause many CNS effects.
- Pernicious anaemia is caused by the deficient production of intrinsic factor by gastric cells.
- Intrinsic factor is needed to allow the body to absorb vitamin B12. If intrinsic factor is lacking, vitamin B12 must be given parenterally for life to ensure absorption.
- Sickle cell anaemia is a genetic disorder characterised by the production of S haemoglobin. The RBCs have a sickle shape and can stack up in blood vessels and cause anoxia, pain and even cell death.
- Sickle cell anaemia is treated with antibiotics, pain-relieving measures and the cytotoxic drug hydroxycarbamide (hydroxyurea), which causes increased fetal haemoglobin production in the bone marrow and dilution of the S haemoglobin with a resultant reduction in RBC stacking and clogging of blood vessels.

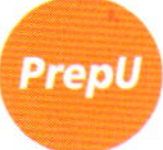

Knowing your strengths and weaknesses helps you to study more effectively. Take a PrepU Practice Quiz to find out how you measure up!

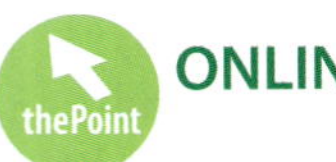

ONLINE RESOURCES

An extensive range of additional resources to enhance teaching and learning and to facilitate understanding of this chapter may be found online at the text's accompanying website, located on thePoint at http://thepoint.lww.com. These include Watch and Learn videos, Concepts in Action animations, journal articles, review questions, case studies, discussion topics and quizzes.

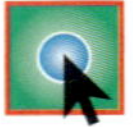

WEB LINKS

Health care providers and students may want to explore the following web resources:

www.aamds.org/aplastic
Information on various forms of anaemias – causes, characteristics, diagnosis and treatment.

www.anaemia.com
Information designed for patients and families regarding anaemias.

www.medsafe.govt.nz
New Zealand Medicines and Medical Devices Safety Authority.

www.nlm.nih.gov/medlineplus/druginfo/medmaster/a692034.html
Information on erythropoietin – action, uses and warnings.

http://nzformulary.org
New Zealand Formulary.

www.rch.org.au/clinicalguide/cpg.cfm?doc_id=5245
Royal Children's Hospital Melbourne Clinical Practice Guidelines for Sickle Cell Disease.

www.transfusion.com.au/transfusion_practice/anaemia_management/iron_deficiency_anaemia
Australian Red Cross Blood Bank information for health professionals on iron deficiency anaemia.

BIBLIOGRAPHY

Bar-Zeev, S. J., Kruske, S. G., Barclay, L. M., BarZeev, N. & Kildea, S. V. (2013). Adherence to management guidelines for growth faltering and anaemia in remote dwelling Australian Aboriginal infants and barriers to health service delivery. *BMC Health Services Research, 13*, 250.

Bennett, C. L., Silver, S. M., Djulbegovic, B., Sammas, A. T., Blau, C. A., Gleason, K. J., et al. (2008). Venous thromboembolism and mortality associated with recombinant erythropoietin and darbepoetin administration for the treatment of cancer-associated anemia. *JAMA, 299*, 914–924.

Benson, J., Maldari, T. & Turnbull, T. (2010). Vitamin B12 deficiency: Why refugee patients are at high risk. *Australian Family Physician, 39(4)*, 215–217.

Farrell, M. & Dempsey, J. (2014). *Smeltzer & Bare's Textbook of Medical-Surgical Nursing* (3rd edn). Sydney: Lippincott Williams & Wilkins.

Goodman, L. S., Brunton, L .L., Chabner, B. & Knollmann, B. C. (2011). *Goodman and Gilman's Pharmacological Basis of Therapeutics* (12th edn). New York: McGraw-Hill.

McKenna, L. & Mirkov, S. (2019). *McKenna's Drug Handbook for Nursing and Midwifery* (8th edn). Sydney: Wolters Kluwer Health Australia.

Metcalfe, S. A., Barlow-Stewart, K., Campbell, J. & Emery, J. (2007). Genetics and blood: Haemoglobinopathies and clotting disorders. *Australian Family Physician, 36(10)*, 812–819.

Minck, S., Robinson, K., Saxon, B., Spigiel, T. & Thomson, A. (2013). Patient blood management: The GP's guide. *Australian Family Physician, 42(5)*, 291–297.

Naim, M. & Hunter, J. (2010). Intravenous iron replacement: Management in general practice. *Australian Family Physician, 39(11)*, 839–841.

Porth, C. M. (2011). *Essentials of Pathophysiology: Concepts of Altered Health States* (3rd edn). Philadelphia: Lippincott Williams & Wilkins.

Porth, C. M. (2009). *Pathophysiology: Concepts of Altered Health States* (8th edn). Philadelphia: Lippincott Williams & Wilkins.

Roger, S. D. (2009). Managing the anaemia of chronic kidney disease. *Australian Prescriber, 32*, 129–131.

Stevens, P. E. (2012). Anaemia, diabetes and chronic kidney disease: where are we now? *Journal of Renal Care, 38*(supp 1), 67–77.

CHECK YOUR UNDERSTANDING

Answers to the questions in this chapter can be found in Appendix A at the back of this book.

MULTIPLE CHOICE

Select the best answer to the following.

1. After teaching a group of students about red blood cell production, the instructor determines that the teaching was effective when the group states that the rate of red blood cell production is controlled by:
   a. iron.
   b. folic acid.
   c. erythropoietin.
   d. vitamin B12.
2. Red blood cells must be continually produced by the body because:
   a. the iron within the RBC wears out and must be replaced.
   b. RBCs cannot maintain themselves and wear out.
   c. RBCs are continuously entering and being lost from the gastrointestinal (GI) tract.
   d. RBCs are processed into bile salts and must be replaced.
3. Which of the following would the nurse include in the teaching plan when describing anaemia to a person?
   a. a decreased number of or abnormal red blood cells
   b. a lack of iron in the body
   c. a lack of vitamin B12 in the body
   d. an excessive number of platelets
4. Megaloblastic anaemia is a result of insufficient folic acid or vitamin B12, affecting which of the following?
   a. white blood cell production
   b. vegetarians
   c. rapidly turning over cells
   d. slow-growing cells
5. The nurse/midwife would expect the doctor to prescribe epoetin alfa (*Eprex*) as the drug of choice:
   a. for acute blood loss during surgery.
   b. to replace blood loss from traumatic injury.
   c. for treatment of anaemia during breastfeeding.
   d. for treatment of anaemia associated with renal failure.
6. A person with anaemia who is given iron salts could expect to show a therapeutic increase in haematocrit:
   a. within 72 hours.
   b. within 2–3 weeks.
   c. within 6–10 months.
   d. within 1–2 weeks.
7. To ensure maximum absorption, a nurse instructs a person receiving oral iron therapy to avoid taking the iron with:
   a. protein.
   b. antibiotics.
   c. dairy products.
   d. any other drugs.
8. After teaching a person with pernicious anaemia about vitamin B12, therapy. which person's statement would indicate that the teaching was successful?
   a. I can take this pill with breakfast.
   b. I should take this pill at bedtime.
   c. I need to inject this drug SC every day.
   d. I need to inject this drug intramuscularly every 5–10 days.

MULTIPLE RESPONSE

Select all that apply.

1. People are often given iron pills by their clinic. Instructions in giving these pills should include:
   a. taking the drug with milk to avoid GI problems.
   b. the potential for constipation.
   c. keeping these potentially toxic pills away from children.
   d. taking the drug with antacids to alleviate the GI upset.
   e. having periodic blood tests to evaluate the drug effect.
   f. being aware that stools may be coloured green.
2. In a healthy person, very little iron is needed on a daily basis. Loss of iron is associated with which of the following?
   a. heavy menstrual flow
   b. bile duct obstruction
   c. internal bleeding
   d. penetrating traumatic injury
   e. bone marrow suppression
   f. alcoholic cirrhosis

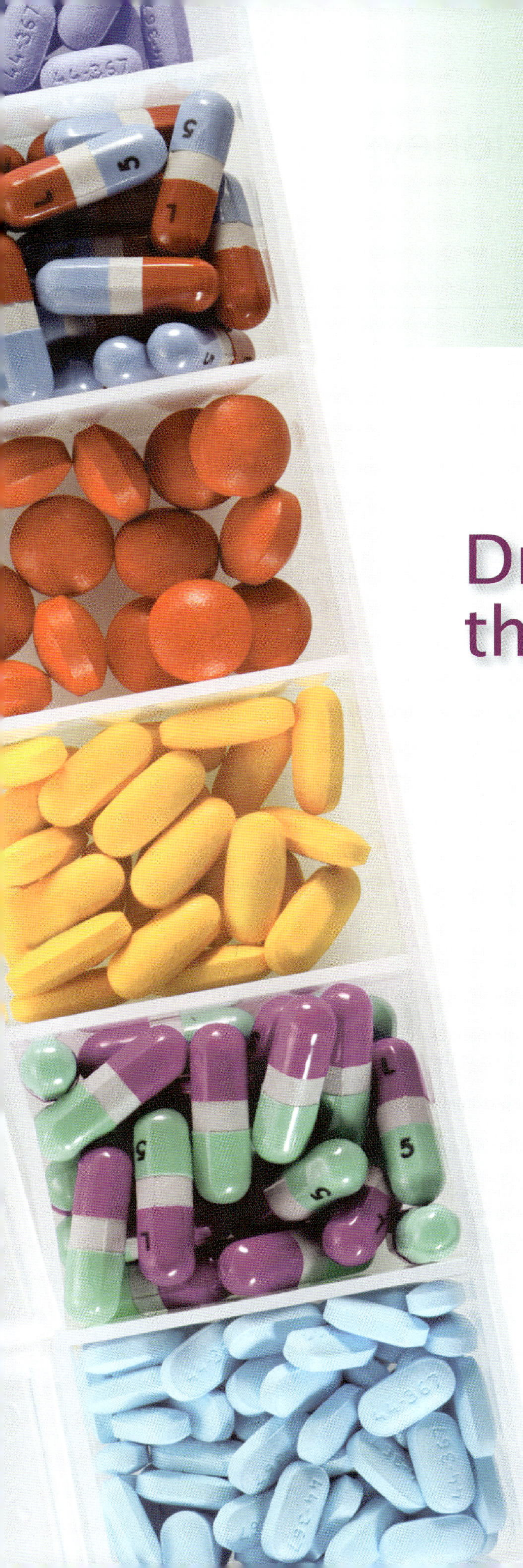

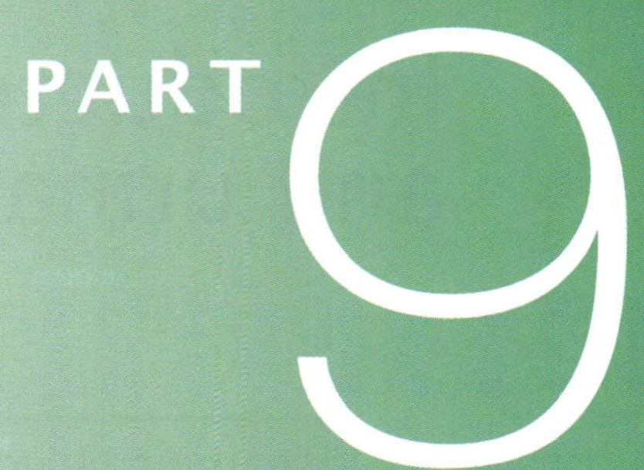

PART 9

Drugs acting on the renal system

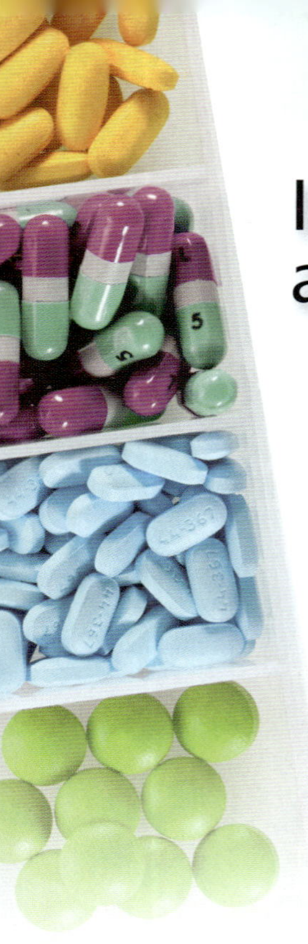

Introduction to the kidneys and urinary tract

Learning objectives

On completing this chapter you should be able to:

1. Review the anatomy of the kidney, including the structure of the nephron.
2. Explain the basic processes of the kidney and where these processes occur.
3. Explain the control of calcium, sodium, potassium and chloride in the nephron.
4. Discuss the countercurrent mechanism and the control of urine concentration and dilution, applying these effects to various clinical scenarios.
5. Describe the renin–angiotensin–aldosterone system, including controls and clinical situations where this system is active.
6. Discuss the roles of the kidney in acid–base balance, calcium regulation and red blood cell production, integrating this information to explain the clinical manifestations of renal failure.

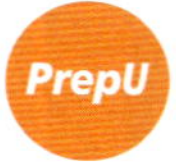

Test your current knowledge of the kidneys and urinary tract with a PrepU Practice Quiz!

Glossary of key terms

aldosterone: hormone produced by the adrenal gland that causes the distal tubule to retain sodium, and therefore water, while losing potassium into the urine

antidiuretic hormone (ADH): hormone produced by the hypothalamus and stored in the posterior pituitary gland; important in maintaining fluid balance; causes the distal tubules and collecting ducts of the kidney to become permeable to water, leading to an antidiuretic effect and fluid retention

carbonic anhydrase: a catalyst that speeds up the chemical reaction combining water and carbon dioxide, which react to form carbonic acid and immediately dissociate to form sodium bicarbonate

countercurrent mechanism: process used by medullary nephrons to concentrate or dilute the urine in response to body stimuli to maintain fluid and electrolyte balance

filtration: passage of fluid and small components of the blood through the glomerulus into the nephron tubule

glomerulus: the tuft of blood vessel between the afferent and efferent arterioles in the nephron; the fenestrated membrane of the glomerulus allows filtration of fluid from the blood into the nephron tubule

nephron: functional unit of the kidney, composed of Bowman's capsule, the proximal and distal convoluted tubules and the collecting duct

prostate gland: gland located around the male urethra; responsible for producing an acidic fluid that maintains sperm and lubricates the urinary tract

reabsorption: the movement of substances from the renal tubule back into the vascular system

renin–angiotensin–aldosterone system: compensatory process that leads to increased blood pressure and blood volume to ensure perfusion of the kidneys; important in the continual regulation of blood pressure

secretion: the active movement of substances from the blood into the renal tubule

The renal system is composed of the kidneys and the structures of the urinary tract: the ureters, the urinary bladder and the urethra. This system has four major functions in the body:

- maintaining the volume and composition of body fluids within normal ranges, including the following functions:
  - clearing nitrogenous wastes from protein metabolism
  - maintaining acid–base balance and electrolyte levels
  - excreting various drugs and drug metabolites
- regulating vitamin D activation, which helps to maintain and regulate calcium levels
- regulating blood pressure through the renin–angiotensin–aldosterone system
- regulating red blood cell production through the production and secretion of erythropoietin.

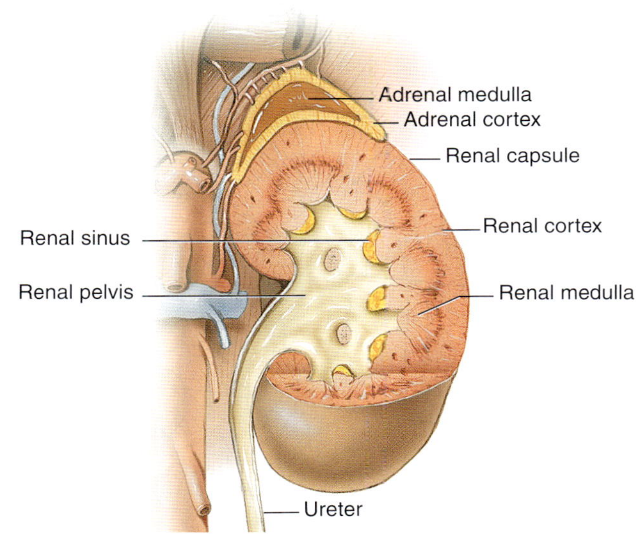

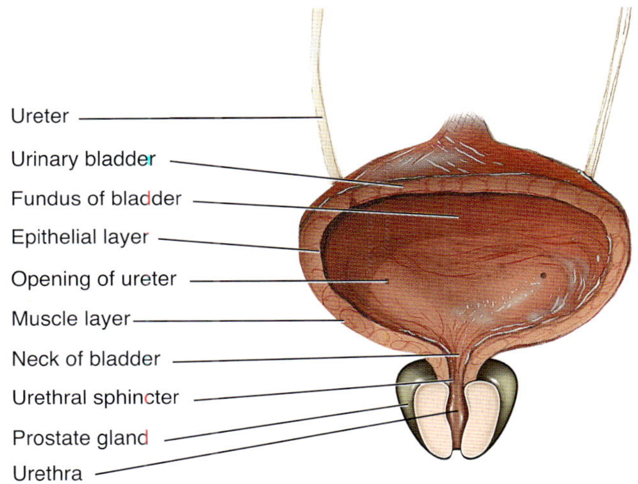

FIGURE 50.1 The kidney and organs of the urinary tract.

THE KIDNEYS

The kidneys are two small organs that make up about 0.5% of total body weight but receive about 25% of the cardiac output. Approximately 1600 L of blood flows through these two small organs each day for cleansing. Most of the fluid that is filtered out by the kidneys is returned to the body, and the waste products that remain are excreted in a relatively small amount of water as urine.

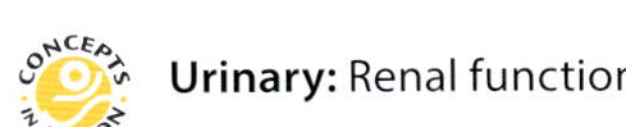
Urinary: Renal function

Structure

The kidneys are located under the ribs, for protection from injury. They have three protective layers that make up the renal capsule: a fibre layer, a perirenal, or brown fat, layer and the renal parietal layer. The capsule contains pain fibres, which are stimulated if the capsule is stretched secondary to an inflammatory process.

The kidneys have three identifiable regions: the outer cortex, the inner medulla and the renal pelvises. The renal pelvises drain the urine into the ureters. The ureters are muscular tubes that lead into the urinary bladder, where urine is stored until it is excreted (Figure 50.1).

Nephron

The functional unit of the kidneys is called the **nephron.** There are approximately 2.4 million nephrons in an adult. All of the nephrons filter fluid and make urine, but only the medullary nephrons can concentrate or dilute urine. It is estimated that only about 25% of the total number of nephrons are necessary to maintain healthy renal function. That means that the renal system is well protected from failure with a large backup system. However, it also means that by the time a person manifests signs and symptoms, suggesting failure of the kidneys, extensive kidney damage has already occurred.

The nephron is basically a tube that begins at Bowman's capsule and becomes the proximal and then distal convoluted tubule (Figure 50.2). Bowman's capsule has a fenestrated or 'window-like' epithelium that works like a sieve or a strainer to allow fluid to flow through but keep large components (eg, proteins) from entering. The tube exits the capsule curling around in a section called the proximal convoluted tubule. From there, it narrows to form the descending and ascending loop of Henle. It widens as the distal convoluted tubule and then flows into the collecting ducts, which meet at the renal pelvises. Each section of the tubule functions in a slightly different manner to maintain fluid and electrolyte balance in the body.

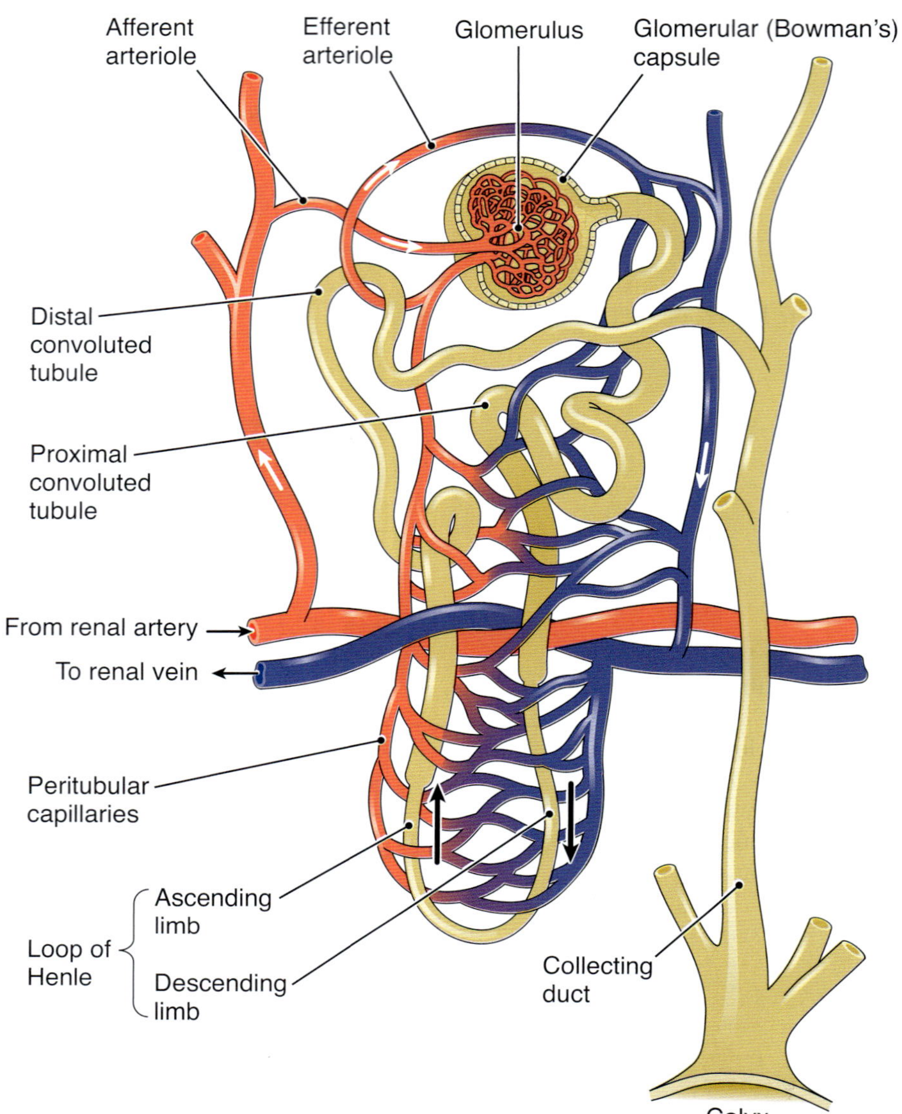

FIGURE 50.2 The nephron – the functional unit of the kidneys. Secretion and reabsorption of water, electrolytes and other solutes in the various segments of the renal tubule, the loop of Henle, and the collecting duct can be influenced by diuretics, other drugs and endogenous substances, including certain hormones. In the kidneys, the distal convoluted tubule wraps around and is actually next to the afferent arteriole.

Blood supply

The blood flow to the nephron is unique. The renal arteries come directly off the aorta and enter each kidney. As a renal artery enters each of the kidneys, it divides to form interlobar arteries, which become smaller arcuate (bowed) arteries and then afferent arterioles. The afferent arterioles branch to form the **glomerulus** inside Bowman's capsule. The glomerulus is like a tuft of blood vessels with a capillary-like endothelium that allows easy passage of fluid and waste products. The efferent arteriole exits from the glomerulus and branches into the peritubular capillary system, which returns fluid and electrolytes that have been reabsorbed from the tubules to the bloodstream. These capillaries flow into the vasa recta, which flows into intralobar veins, which in turn drain into the inferior vena cava. The two arterioles around the glomerulus work together to closely regulate the flow of fluid into the glomerulus, increasing or decreasing pressure on either side of the glomerulus as needed.

Other structures

A small group of cells, called the juxtaglomerular apparatus, connects the afferent arteriole to the distal convoluted tubule. This is where erythropoietin and renin are produced. Because of their proximity to the afferent arteriole, these cells are especially sensitive to the volume and quality of blood flow into the glomerulus. Surrounding the nephrons is an area called the macula densa, which consists of immune system cells and chemicals that can respond quickly to any cellular damage or injury.

Nephron function

The nephrons function by using three basic processes: glomerular **filtration** (passage of fluid and small components of the blood through the glomerulus into the nephron tubule), tubular **secretion** (active movement of substances from the blood into the renal tubule) and tubular **reabsorption** (movement of substances from the renal tubule back into the vascular system).

Glomerular filtration

The glomerulus acts as an ultrafine filter for all of the blood that flows into it. The semipermeable membrane keeps blood cells, proteins and lipids inside the vessel, whereas the hydrostatic pressure from the blood pushes water and smaller components of the plasma into the tubule. The resulting fluid is called the filtrate. Scarring, or swelling of, or damage to the semipermeable membrane leads to the escape of larger plasma components, such as blood cells or protein, into the filtrate. The large size of these components prevents them from being reabsorbed by the tubule, and they are lost in the urine. Thus a clinical sign of renal damage is the presence of blood cells or protein in the urine.

Approximately 125 mL of fluid is filtered out each minute, or 180 L/day. About 99% of the filtered fluid is returned to the bloodstream as the filtrate continues its movement through the renal tubule. Approximately 1% of the filtrate – less than 2 L of fluid – is excreted each day in the form of urine.

Tubular secretion

The epithelial cells that line the renal tubule can secrete substances from the blood into the tubular fluid. This is an energy-using process that allows active transport systems to remove electrolytes, some drugs and drug metabolites, and uric acid from the surrounding capillaries and secrete them into the filtrate. For example, the epithelial cells can use tubular secretion to help maintain acid–base levels by secreting hydrogen ions as needed.

Tubular reabsorption

The cells lining the renal tubule reabsorb water and various essential substances from the filtrate back into the vascular system. About 99% of the water filtered at the glomerulus is reabsorbed. Other filtrate components that are reabsorbed regularly include vitamins, glucose, electrolytes, sodium bicarbonate and sodium chloride. The reabsorption process uses a series of transport systems that exchange needed ions for unwanted ones (see Chapter 7 for a review of cellular transport systems). Drugs that affect renal function frequently overwhelm one of these transport systems or interfere with its normal activity, leading to an imbalance in acid–base or electrolyte levels. The precision of the reabsorption process allows the body to maintain the correct extracellular fluid volume and composition.

Maintenance of volume and composition of body fluids

The kidneys regulate the composition of body fluids by balancing the levels of the key electrolytes, secreting or absorbing these electrolytes to maintain the desired levels. The volume of body fluids is controlled by diluting or concentrating the urine.

Sodium regulation

Sodium is one of the body's major cations (positively charged ions). It filters through the glomerulus and enters the renal tubule; then it is actively reabsorbed in the proximal convoluted tubule to the peritubular capillaries. As sodium is actively moved out of the filtrate, it takes chloride ions and water with it. This occurs by passive diffusion as the body maintains the osmotic and electrical balances on both sides of the tubule.

Sodium ions are also reabsorbed via a transport system that functions under the influence of the catalyst **carbonic anhydrase**. This enzyme speeds the combining of carbon dioxide and water to form carbonic acid. The carbonic acid immediately dissociates to form sodium bicarbonate, using a sodium ion from the renal tubule and a free hydrogen ion (an acid). The hydrogen ion remains in the filtrate, causing the urine to be slightly acidic. The bicarbonate is stored in the renal tubule as the body's alkaline reserve for use when the body becomes too acidic and a buffer is needed.

The distal convoluted tubule acts to further adjust the sodium levels in the filtrate under the influence of **aldosterone** (a hormone produced by the adrenal gland) and natriuretic hormone (probably produced by the hypothalamus). Aldosterone is released into the circulation in response to high potassium levels, sympathetic stimulation or angiotensin III. Aldosterone stimulates a sodium–potassium exchange pump in the cells of the distal tubule, causing reabsorption of sodium in exchange for potassium (see Chapter 7 for a review of the sodium–potassium pump). As a result of aldosterone stimulation, sodium is reabsorbed into the system and potassium is lost in the filtrate.

Natriuretic hormone causes a decrease in sodium reabsorption from the distal tubules with a resultant diluted urine or increased volume. Natriuretic hormone is released in response to fluid overload or haemodilution.

Countercurrent mechanism

Sodium is further regulated in the medullary nephrons in what is known as the **countercurrent mechanism** in the loop of Henle. In the descending loop of Henle, the cells are freely permeable to water and sodium. Sodium is actively reabsorbed into the surrounding peritubular tissue, and water flows out of the tubule into this sodium-rich tissue to maintain osmotic balance. The filtrate at the end of the descending loop of Henle is concentrated in comparison to the rest of the filtrate.

In contrast, the ascending loop of Henle is impermeable to water, and so water that remains in the tubule is trapped there. Chloride is actively transported out of the tubule using energy in a process that is referred to as the chloride pump; sodium leaves with the chloride to maintain electrical neutrality. As a result, the fluid in the ascending loop of Henle becomes hypotonic in comparison to the hypertonic situation in the peritubular tissue.

Antidiuretic hormone (ADH), which is produced by the hypothalamus and stored in the posterior pituitary gland, is important in maintaining fluid balance. ADH is released in response to falling blood volume, sympathetic stimulation, or rising sodium levels (a concentration that is sensed by the osmotic cells of the hypothalamus).

If ADH is present at the distal convoluted tubule and the collecting duct, the permeability of the membrane to water is increased. Consequently, the water remaining in the tubule rapidly flows into the hypertonic tissue surrounding the loop of Henle, where it either is absorbed by the peritubular capillaries or re-enters the descending loop of Henle in a countercurrent style. The resulting urine is hypertonic and of small volume. If ADH is not present, the tubule remains impermeable to water. The water that has been trapped in the ascending loop of Henle passes into the collection duct, resulting in hypotonic urine of greater volume. This countercurrent mechanism allows the body to finely regulate fluid volume by regulating the control of sodium and water (Figure 50.3).

Chloride regulation

Chloride is an important negatively charged ion that helps to maintain electrical neutrality with the movement of cations across the cell membrane. Chloride is primarily reabsorbed in the loop of Henle, where it promotes the movement of sodium out of the cell.

Potassium regulation

Potassium is another cation that is vital to proper functioning of the nervous system, muscles and cell membranes. About 65% of the potassium that is filtered at the glomerulus is reabsorbed at Bowman's capsule and the proximal convoluted tubule. Another 25%–30% is reabsorbed in the ascending loop of Henle. The fine-tuning of potassium levels occurs in the distal convoluted tubule, where aldosterone activates the sodium–potassium exchange, leading to a loss of potassium. If potassium levels are very high, the retention of sodium in exchange for potassium also leads to a retention of water and a dilution of blood volume, which further decreases the potassium concentration (see Figure 50.3).

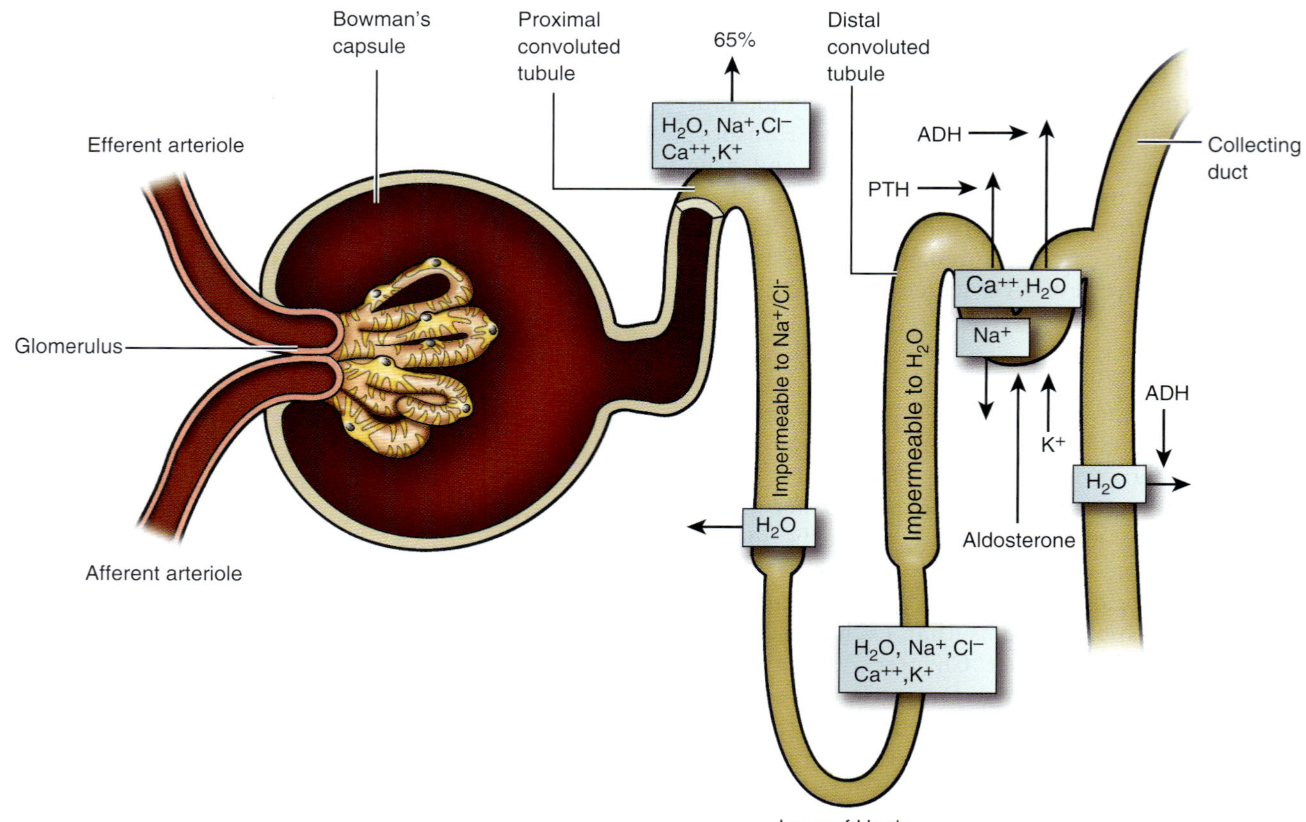

FIGURE 50.3 Nephron and points of regulation of sodium, chloride, potassium, calcium and water. ADH, antidiuretic hormone; PTH, parathyroid hormone.

Calcium regulation

Calcium is important in muscle function, blood clotting, bone formation, contraction of cell membranes and muscle movement, and is another important cation that is regulated by the kidneys. The absorption of calcium from the gastrointestinal (GI) tract is regulated by vitamin D ingested as part of the diet. The vitamin then must be activated in the kidneys to a form that will promote calcium absorption. Once absorbed from the GI tract, calcium levels are maintained within a very tight range by the activity of parathyroid hormone (PTH) and calcitonin.

Calcium is filtered at the glomerulus and mostly reabsorbed in the proximal convoluted tubule and ascending loop of Henle. Fine-tuning of calcium reabsorption occurs in the distal convoluted tubule, where the presence of PTH stimulates reabsorption of calcium to increase serum calcium levels when they are low (see Figure 50.3 and Chapter 37).

Blood pressure control

The fragile nephrons require a constant supply of blood and are equipped with a system to ensure that they are perfused. This mechanism, called the **renin–angiotensin–aldosterone system**, involves a total body reaction to decreased blood flow to the nephrons.

Whenever blood flow or oxygenation to the nephron is decreased (due to haemorrhage, shock, heart failure or hypotension), renin is released from the juxtaglomerular cells. (These cells, which are positioned next to the glomerulus, are stimulated by decreased stretch and decreased oxygen levels.) The released renin is immediately absorbed into the capillary system and enters circulation.

The released renin activates angiotensinogen, a substrate produced in the liver, which becomes angiotensin I. Angiotensin I is then converted into angiotensin II by angiotensin-converting enzyme (ACE), found in the lungs and some blood vessels. Angiotensin II is a very powerful vasoconstrictor, reacting with angiotensin II–receptor sites in blood vessels to cause vasoconstriction. This powerful vasoconstriction raises blood pressure and should increase blood flow to the kidneys.

Angiotensin II is converted in the adrenal gland to angiotensin III, which stimulates the release of aldosterone from the adrenal gland. Aldosterone acts on the renal tubules to retain sodium and therefore water. This increases blood volume and further increases blood pressure, which should increase blood flow to the kidneys. The osmotic centre in the brain senses the increased sodium levels and releases ADH, leading to a further retention of water and a further increase in blood volume and pressure, which should again increase blood flow to the kidneys.

The renin–angiotensin–aldosterone system constantly works to maintain blood flow to the kidneys. For example, an individual rising from a lying position experiences a drop in blood flow to the kidneys as blood pools in the legs because of gravity. This causes a massive release of renin and activation of this system to ensure that blood pressure is maintained and the kidneys are perfused. Blood loss from injury or during surgery also activates this system to increase blood flow through the kidneys.

Drugs that interfere with any aspect of this system will cause a reflex response. For example, taking a drug such as a diuretic to decrease fluid volume can lead to decreased blood flow to the kidneys as blood volume drops. This in turn leads to rebound retention of fluid as part of the effects of the renin–angiotensin–aldosterone system (Figure 50.4).

Regulation of red blood cell production

Whenever blood flow or oxygenation to the nephron is decreased (due to haemorrhage, shock, heart failure or hypotension), the hormone erythropoietin is also released from the juxtaglomerular cells. This hormone stimulates the bone marrow to increase the production of red blood cells, which bring oxygen to the kidneys. Erythropoietin is the only known factor that can regulate the rate of red blood cell production. When

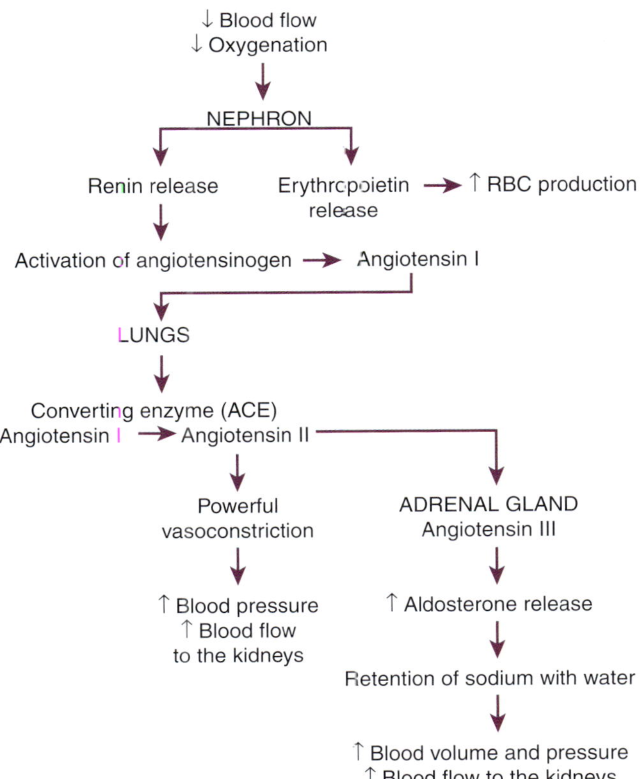

FIGURE 50.4 The renin–angiotensin–aldosterone system for reflex maintenance of blood pressure control.

a person develops renal failure and the production of erythropoietin drops, the production of red blood cells falls and the person becomes anaemic.

KEY POINTS

- The kidneys are two small, bean-shaped organs that receive about 25% of the cardiac output.
- The nephron is the functional unit of the kidneys and is involved in three processes: glomerular filtration, tubular secretion and tubular reabsorption.
- The kidney plays a key role in regulating body fluid volume and maintaining blood pressure, red blood cell production, acid–base balance and electrolyte stability.
- The renin–angiotensin–aldosterone system is activated when blood flow to the nephron is decreased and renin is released. The end result is increased vasoconstriction and increased blood pressure and sodium and water retention, which increase blood volume and pressure.
- Red blood cell production is controlled by erythropoietin released from the juxtaglomerular apparatus when oxygen delivery to the nephron is decreased. Erythropoietin stimulates the bone marrow to produce red blood cells to increase oxygen delivery to the nephrons.

THE URINARY TRACT

As noted previously, the urinary tract is composed of the ureters, urinary bladder and urethra (see Figure 50.1).

Ureters

One ureter exits each kidney, draining the filtrate from the collecting ducts. The ureters have a smooth endothelial lining and circular muscular layers. Urine entering the ureter stimulates a peristaltic wave that pushes the urine down towards the urinary bladder.

Urinary bladder

The urinary bladder is a muscular pouch that stretches and holds the urine until it is excreted from the body. Urine is usually a slightly acidic fluid; this acidity helps to maintain the normal transport systems and to destroy bacteria that may enter the bladder. Control of bladder emptying is learned control over the urethral sphincter; once it is established, a functioning nervous system is necessary to maintain control.

Urethra

In the female, the urethra is a very short tube that leads from the bladder to an area populated by normal flora, including *Escherichia coli*, which can cause frequent bladder infections or cystitis. In the male, the urethra is much longer and passes through the **prostate gland,** a small gland that produces an alkaline fluid that is important in maintaining sperm and lubricating the tract. Enlargement and infection in the prostate gland are often problems in older men.

KEY POINTS

- The ureters, urinary bladder and urethra make up the rest of the urinary tract.
- The shorter female urethra leads from the urinary bladder to the outer body into an area rich in gram-negative bacteria. Cystitis, or infection of the urinary bladder, is a common problem for women.
- The longer male urethra passes through the prostate gland, which may enlarge or become infected, a problem often associated with advancing age.

CHAPTER SUMMARY

- The functional unit of the kidneys is called the nephron; it is composed of Bowman's capsule, the proximal convoluted tubule, the loop of Henle, the distal convoluted tubule and the collecting duct.
- The blood flow to the nephron is unique, allowing autoregulation of blood flow through the glomerulus.
- Sodium levels are regulated throughout the tubule by active and passive movement and are fine tuned by the presence of aldosterone in the distal tubule.
- The countercurrent mechanism in the medullary nephrons allows for the concentration or dilution of urine under the influence of ADH secreted by the hypothalamus.
- Potassium concentration is regulated throughout the tubule, with aldosterone being the strongest influence for potassium loss.
- The kidneys play a key role in the regulation of calcium by activating vitamin D to allow GI calcium reabsorption and by reabsorbing or excreting calcium from the tubule under the influence of parathyroid hormone.
- The kidneys influence blood pressure control, releasing renin to activate the renin–angiotensin system, which leads to increased blood pressure and volume and a resultant increased blood flow to the kidney. The balance of this reflex system can lead to water retention or excretion and has an impact on drug therapy that promotes water or sodium loss.
- The ureters, urinary bladder and urethra make up the rest of the urinary tract. The longer male urethra passes through the prostate gland, which may enlarge or become infected, a problem often associated with advancing age.

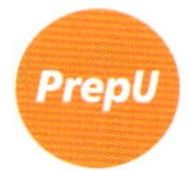

Knowing your strengths and weaknesses helps you to study more effectively. Take a PrepU Practice Quiz to find out how you measure up!

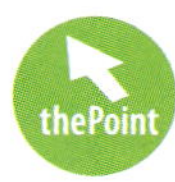

ONLINE RESOURCES

An extensive range of additional resources to enhance teaching and learning and to facilitate understanding of this chapter may be found online at the text's accompanying website, located on thePoint at http://thepoint.lww.com. These include Watch and Learn videos, Concepts in Action animations, journal articles, review questions, case studies, discussion topics and quizzes.

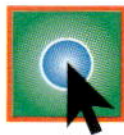

WEB LINK

For a virtual tour of the kidneys and urinary tract, visit the following web resources:

www.InnerBody.com

BIBLIOGRAPHY

Barrett, K. E. & Ganong, W. F. (2010). *Ganong's Review of Medical Physiology* (23rd edn). New York: McGraw-Hill.

Danziger, J., Zeidel, M. D., Parker, M. J. & Schwartzstein, R. M. (2012). *Renal Physiology: A Clinical Approach*. Philadelphia: Lippincott Williams & Wilkins.

Eaton, D. C., Pooler, J. P. & Vander, A. J. (2013). *Vander's Renal Physiology* (8th edn). New York: McGraw-Hill.

Goodman, L. S., Brunton, L. L., Chabner, B. & Knollmann, B. C. (2011). *Goodman and Gilman's Pharmacological Basis of Therapeutics* (12th edn). New York: McGraw-Hill.

Guyton, A. & Hall, J. (2011). *Textbook of Medical Physiology* (12th edn). Philadelphia: Saunders Elsevier.

Porth, C. M. (2011). *Essentials of Pathophysiology: Concepts of Altered Health States* (3rd edn). Philadelphia: Lippincott Williams & Wilkins.

Porth, C. M. (2009). *Pathophysiology: Concepts of Altered Health States* (8th edn). Philadelphia: Lippincott Williams & Wilkins.

Rennke, H. G. & Denker, B. M. (2013). *Renal Pathophysiology: The Essentials* (4th edn). Philadelphia: Lippincott Williams & Wilkins.

CHECK YOUR UNDERSTANDING

Answers to the questions in this chapter can be found in Appendix A at the back of this book.

MULTIPLE CHOICE

Select the best answer to the following.

1. During severe exertion, a man may lose up to 4 L of hypotonic sweat per hour. This loss would result in:
   a. decreased plasma volume.
   b. decreased plasma osmolarity.
   c. decreased circulating levels of ADH.
   d. return of body fluid balance to normal after ingestion of 100 mL of water.
2. Urine passes through the ureter by:
   a. osmosis.
   b. air pressure.
   c. filtration.
   d. peristalsis
3. When describing renal reabsorption to a group of students, the instructor would identify it as the movement of which of the following?
   a. substances from the renal tubule into the blood
   b. substances from the blood into the renal tubule
   c. water that is increased in the absence of ADH
   d. sodium occurring only in the proximal tubule
4. Considering the functions of the kidney, if a person lost kidney function, a nurse or midwife would expect to see:
   a. increased red blood cell count.
   b. decreased fluid volume.
   c. electrolyte disturbances.
   d. decreased blood pressure.
5. Blood flow to the nephron differs from blood flow to other tissues in that:
   a. the venous system is not involved in blood flow around the nephron.
   b. there are no capillaries in the nephron allowing direct flow from artery to vein.
   c. efferent and afferent arterioles allow for autoregulation of blood flow.
   d. the capillary bed has a fenestrated membrane to allow passage of fluid and small particles.
6. Concentration and dilution of urine is controlled by:
   a. afferent arterioles.
   b. the renin–angiotensin system.
   c. aldosterone release.
   d. the countercurrent mechanism.

7. Women tend to have more problems with bladder infections than men because:
   a. women have *E. coli* in the urinary tract.
   b. women have a short urethra, making access to the bladder easier for bacteria.
   c. the prostate gland secretes a substance that protects men from bladder infections.
   d. women's urine is more acidotic, encouraging the growth of bladder bacteria.

MULTIPLE RESPONSE

Select all that apply.

1. Considering the metabolic functions of the kidneys, renal failure would be expected to cause which of the following?
   a. anaemia
   b. loss of calcium regulation
   c. urea buildup on the skin
   d. respiratory alkalosis
   e. metabolic acidosis
   f. changes in the function of blood cells

2. During severe diarrhoea, there is a loss of water, bicarbonate and sodium from the gastrointestinal tract. Physiological compensation for this would probably include which of the following?
   a. increased alveolar ventilation
   b. decreased hydrogen ion secretion by the renal tubules
   c. decreased urinary excretion of sodium and water
   d. increased renin secretion
   e. increased hydrogen ion secretion by the renal tubules
   f. increased ADH levels

3. Maintenance of blood pressure is important in maintaining the fragile nephrons. Reflex systems that work to ensure blood flow to the kidneys include:
   a. the renin–angiotensin system causing vasoconstriction.
   b. baroreceptor monitoring of the renal artery.
   c. aldosterone release secondary to angiotensin stimulation.
   d. ADH release in response to decreased blood volume with increased osmolarity.
   e. release of erythropoietin.
   f. local response of the afferent arterioles.

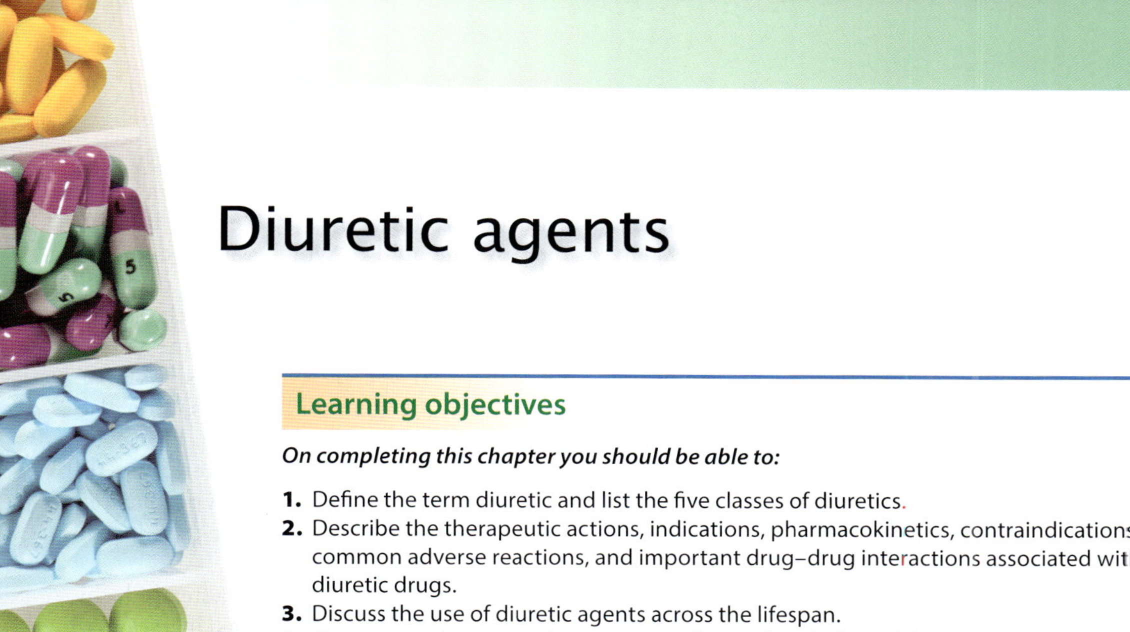

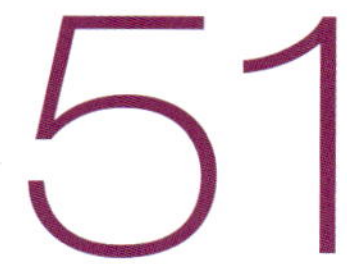

51

Diuretic agents

Learning objectives

On completing this chapter you should be able to:

1. Define the term diuretic and list the five classes of diuretics.
2. Describe the therapeutic actions, indications, pharmacokinetics, contraindications and cautions, most common adverse reactions, and important drug–drug interactions associated with the various classes of diuretic drugs.
3. Discuss the use of diuretic agents across the lifespan.
4. Compare and contrast the prototype drugs of each class of diuretic drugs, hydrochlorothiazide, furosemide (frusemide), mannitol and spironolactone with other agents in their class.
5. Outline the care considerations, including important teaching points, for people receiving diuretic agents.

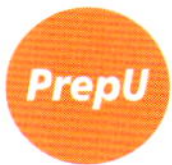

Test your current knowledge of diuretic agents with a PrepU Practice Quiz!

Glossary of key terms

alkalosis: state of not having enough acid to maintain normal homeostatic processes; seen with loop diuretics, which cause loss of bicarbonate in the urine

fluid rebound: reflex reaction of the body to the loss of fluid or sodium; the hypothalamus causes the release of antidiuretic hormone, which promotes water retention, and stress related to fluid loss combines with decreased blood flow to the kidneys to activate the renin–angiotensin–aldosterone system, leading to further water and sodium retention

high-ceiling diuretics: powerful diuretics that work in the loop of Henle to inhibit the reabsorption of sodium and chloride, leading to a sodium-rich diuresis

hyperaldosteronism: excessive output of aldosterone from the adrenal gland, leading to increased sodium and water retention and loss of potassium

hypokalaemia: low potassium in the blood, which often occurs after diuretic use; characterised by weakness, muscle cramps, trembling, nausea, vomiting, diarrhoea and cardiac arrhythmias

oedema: movement of fluid into the interstitial spaces; occurs when the balance between osmotic pull (from plasma proteins) and hydrostatic push (from blood pressure) is disturbed

osmotic pull: drawing force of large molecules on water, pulling it into a tubule or capillary; essential for maintaining normal fluid balance within the body; used to draw out excess fluid into the vascular system or the renal tubule

saluretic effect: relating to or causing excretion of salt

DIURETICS

Thiazide diuretics and thiazide-like diuretics

Thiazide diuretics

bendroflumethiazide (bendrofluazide)

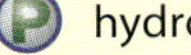 hydrochlorothiazide

Thiazide-like diuretics

chlortalidone

indapamide

Loop diuretics

bumetanide

etacrynic acid

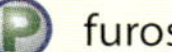 furosemide (frusemide)

Carbonic anhydrase inhibitors

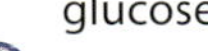 acetazolamide

brinzolamide

Potassium-sparing diuretics

amiloride

eplerenone

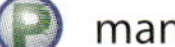 spironolactone

triamterene

Osmotic diuretics

glucose

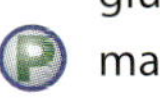 mannitol

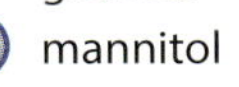

Diuretic agents are commonly thought of simply as drugs that increase the amount of urine produced by the kidneys. Most diuretics do increase the volume of urine produced to some extent, but the greater clinical significance of diuretics is their ability to increase sodium excretion.

Most diuretics prevent the cells lining the renal tubules from reabsorbing an excessive proportion of the sodium ions (Na^+) in the glomerular filtrate. As a result, sodium and other ions (and the water in which they are dissolved) are lost in the urine instead of being returned to the blood, where they would cause increased intravascular volume and therefore increased hydrostatic pressure.

Diuretics are indicated for the treatment of **oedema** associated with heart failure (HF), acute pulmonary oedema, liver disease (including cirrhosis) and renal disease, and for the treatment of hypertension. They are also used to decrease fluid pressure in the eye (intraocular pressure), which is useful in treating glaucoma. Diuretics that decrease potassium levels may also be indicated in the treatment of conditions that cause hyperkalaemia.

HF can cause oedema as a result of several factors. The failing heart muscle does not supply sufficient blood to the kidneys, causing activation of the renin–angiotensin system and resulting in increases in blood volume and sodium retention. Because the failing heart muscle cannot respond to the usual reflex stimulation, the increased volume is slowly pushed out into the capillary level as venous pressure increases because the blood is not being pumped effectively (see Chapter 44).

Pulmonary oedema, or left-sided HF, develops when the increased volume of fluids is pushed out into the capillaries in the lungs and interferes with gas exchange. If this condition develops rapidly, it can be life-threatening.

People with liver failure and cirrhosis often present with oedema and ascites. This is caused by (1) reduced plasma protein production, which results in less oncotic pull in the vascular system and fluid loss at the capillary level, and (2) obstructed blood flow through the portal system, which is caused by increased pressure from congested hepatic vessels.

In renal disease where there is damage to glomerular basement membrane, oedema occurs because of the loss of plasma proteins into the urine. Other types of renal disease produce oedema because of activation of the renin–angiotensin system as a result of decreasing volume (associated with the loss of fluid into the urine), which causes a drop in blood pressure, or because of failure of the renal tubules to regulate electrolytes effectively.

Hypertension is predominantly an idiopathic disorder; in other words, the underlying pathology is not known. Treatment of hypertension is aimed at reducing the higher-than-normal blood pressure, which can damage end organs and lead to serious cardiovascular disorders. Diuretics were once the key element in antihypertensive therapy, the goal of which was to decrease volume and sodium, which would then decrease pressure in the system. Now several other classes of drugs, including angiotensin-converting enzyme (ACE) inhibitors, angiotensin II–receptor blockers (ARBs), beta blockers and calcium channel blockers, are also used for the initial treatment of hypertension. However, some studies have found that the use of diuretics is still the most effective way of treating initial hypertension. Diuretics are also often used as an adjunct to improve the effectiveness of these other drugs.

Glaucoma is an eye disease characterised by increased pressure in the eye – known as intraocular pressure (IOP) – which can cause optic nerve atrophy and blindness. Diuretics are used to provide osmotic pull to remove some of the fluid from the eye, which decreases the IOP, or as adjunctive therapy to reduce fluid volume and pressure in the cardiovascular system, which also somewhat decreases pressure in the eye.

DIURETICS

There are five classes of diuretics, each working at a slightly different site in the nephron or using a different mechanism. Diuretic classes include the thiazide and thiazide-like diuretics, loop diuretics, carbonic anhydrase inhibitors, potassium-sparing diuretics and osmotic diuretics (Table 51.1). For the most part, the overall nursing care of a person receiving any diuretic is similar, although there are specific differences. Adverse effects associated with diuretics are also specific to the particular class used. For details, see the section on adverse effects for each class of diuretics discussed in this chapter, and refer to Table 51.1. The most common adverse effects seen with diuretics include gastrointestinal (GI) upset, fluid and electrolyte imbalances, hypotension and electrolyte disturbances.

This chapter presents each class in the order of frequency of use, beginning with the most frequent. Box 51.1 highlights important considerations related to diuretic use based on the person's age.

KEY POINTS

- Diuretics increase sodium excretion, and therefore water excretion, from the kidneys.
- Diuretics help to relieve oedema associated with HF and pulmonary oedema, liver failure and cirrhosis, and various types of renal disease. They are also used in treating hypertension.

TABLE 51.1 **DRUGS IN FOCUS** Diuretics

Drug name	Dosage/route	Usual indications
Thiazide diuretics		
Thiazide diuretics		
bendroflumethiazide (bendrofluazide) (*Neo-Naclex*)	2.5–10 mg/day PO for oedema; 2.5–15 mg/day PO for hypertension alone or in combination with other antihypertensive agents	Treatment of oedema caused by heart failure (HF), liver disease or renal disease; monotherapy or as adjunctive treatment of hypertension
(P) hydrochlorothiazide (*Dithiazide*)	Adult: 25–50 mg/day PO as a single dose or 2 divided doses; maximum 100 mg/day Paediatric (< 6 months): up to 3.5 mg/kg/day PO in 2 divided doses Paediatric (6 months–2 years): 12.5–37.5 mg/day PO in 2 divided doses Paediatric (2–12 years): 37.6–100 mg/day PO in 2 divided doses	Treatment of oedema caused by HF, liver disease or renal disease; monotherapy or as adjunctive treatment of hypertension
Thiazide-like diuretics		
chlortalidone (*Hygroton*)	Adults: 12.5–50 mg/day PO	Treatment of oedema caused by HF or by liver or renal disease; adjunctive treatment of hypertension
indapamide (*Insig, Natrilix, Natrilix SR, Odaplix SR*)	Immediate-release tablet: 2.5 mg PO in the morning Sustained-release tablet: 1.5 mg PO in the morning	Treatment of oedema caused by HF or by liver or renal disease; adjunctive treatment of hypertension
Loop diuretics		
bumetanide (*Burinex*)	1 mg/day PO up to maximum daily dose of 10 mg	Treatment of acute HF; acute pulmonary oedema; hypertension; and oedema of HF, renal disease or liver disease
etacrynic acid (*Edecrin*)	Adult: 50 mg/day PO in the morning, up to maximum 400 mg/day PO Children > 2 years: 25 mg/day after breakfast, may increase to 50 mg/day	Treatment of acute HF; acute pulmonary oedema; hypertension; and oedema of HF, renal disease or liver disease
(P) furosemide (frusemide) (*Lasix, Urex*)	20–80 mg/day PO, up to 400 mg/day; 20–50 mg IM or IV given slowly; doses > 50 mg by IV infusion only 50–250 mg IV infusion over 60 minutes, for doses > 80 mg, maximum rate 4 mg/min, maximum 1.5 g Elderly or renally impaired: 250 mg q 4 hours; maximum 1 g/day PO Children: 1–2 mg/kg/day PO once or twice daily for hypertension, not to exceed 6 mg/kg/dose; 1 mg/kg IV or IM for oedema, increased by 1 mg/kg as needed; not to exceed 6 mg/kg	Treatment of acute HF; acute pulmonary oedema; hypertension; and oedema of HF, renal disease or liver disease
Carbonic anhydrase inhibitors		
(P) acetazolamide (*Diamox*)	Glaucoma, adult: Open-angle: 0.25–1 g PO daily in divided doses Secondary glaucoma, perioperatively in angle-closure glaucoma: 250 mg PO q 4 hours; acute therapy: 500 mg PO then 125–250 mg q 4 hours IV, glaucoma: 500 mg IV repeated in 2–4 hours, then 250 mg–1 g/day in divided doses q 6–8 hours Epilepsy, adult: 0.25–1 g daily in divided doses; children: 8–30 mg/kg/day in divided doses, maximum 750 mg/day Diuresis: 250–375 mg PO once daily or on alternate days	Treatment of glaucoma; adjunctive treatment of epilepsy, mountain sickness

Continued on following page

TABLE 51.1 DRUGS IN FOCUS Diuretics *(continued)*

Drug name	Dosage/route	Usual indications
Carbonic anhydrase inhibitors *(continued)*		
brinzolamide (*Azopt*)	1 drop in affected eye bd	Treatment of ocular hypertension, open-angle glaucoma
Potassium-sparing diuretics		
amiloride (*Kaluril*)	5–10 mg/day PO to maximum 20 mg/day	Adjunctive treatment of oedema caused by HF, liver disease or renal disease; hypertension; hyperkalaemia; and hyperaldosteronism **Special consideration:** not for use in children
eplerenone (*Inspra*)	25 mg/day PO titrated to 50 mg/day PO within 4 weeks	Risk reduction in people with heart failure and left ventricular impairment after acute myocardial infarction
(P) spironolactone (*Aldactone*)	Adjunctive therapy of resistant hypertension: 25 mg once daily Adjunctive therapy of heart failure: 25 mg once daily, maximum 50 mg daily Oedema: 100–200 mg/day PO Hyperaldosteronism: 100–400 mg/day PO Female hirsutism: 50–100 mg/day PO Paediatric: 1–3 mg/kg/day PO in divided doses	Adjunctive treatment of oedema caused by HF, liver disease or renal disease; hypertension; hyperkalaemia; and hyperaldosteronism **Special consideration:** can be used in children with careful monitoring of electrolytes
Osmotic diuretics		
glucose (generic)	IV; depends on individual	Treatment of oedematous states, including cerebral oedema
(P) mannitol (*Osmitrol*)	Oliguria: 20–100 g/day IV; maximum dose 50 g Reducing intracranial pressure: 0.25–2 g/kg IV over 30–60 minutes; repeated if required 1–2 times after 4–8 hours; dose not established for children < 12 years	Treatment of elevated intracranial pressure, acute renal failure, acute glaucoma; also used to decrease intracranial pressure, prevent oliguric phase of renal failure, and to promote movement of toxic substances through the kidneys

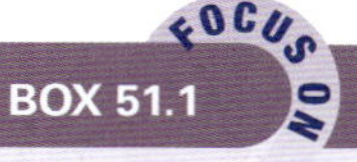

Drug therapy across the lifespan

Diuretic agents

CHILDREN

Diuretics are often used in children to treat oedema associated with heart defects, to control hypertension, and to treat oedema associated with renal and pulmonary disorders.

Hydrochlorothiazide has established paediatric dosing guidelines. Furosemide (frusemide) is often used when a stronger diuretic is needed; care should be taken not to exceed 6 mg/kg/day when using this drug. Etacrynic acid may be used orally in some situations but should not be used in infants. Bumetanide, although not recommended for use in children, may be used for children who are taking other ototoxic drugs, including antibiotics, and may cause less hypokalaemia, making it preferable to furosemide for children also taking digoxin. Spironolactone is the only potassium-sparing diuretic that is recommended for use in children, but, as with adults, it should not be used in the presence of severe renal impairment.

Because of the size and rapid metabolism of children, the effects of diuretics may be rapid and adverse effects may occur suddenly. The child receiving a diuretic should be monitored for serum electrolyte changes; for evidence of fluid volume changes; for rapid weight gain or loss, which could reflect fluid volume; and for signs of ototoxicity.

ADULTS

Adults may be taking diuretics for prolonged periods and need to be aware of the signs and symptoms of fluid imbalance to report to their health care provider. Adults receiving chronic diuretic therapy should weigh themselves on the same scale, in the same clothes, and at the same time each day to monitor for fluid retention or sudden fluid loss. They should be alerted to situations that could aggravate fluid loss, such as diarrhoea, vomiting, or excessive heat and sweating, which could change their need for the diuretic. They should also be urged to maintain their fluid intake to help balance their body's compensatory mechanisms and to prevent fluid rebound.

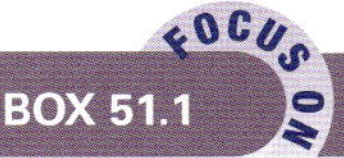

BOX 51.1 Drug therapy across the lifespan *(continued)*

People taking potassium-losing diuretics should be encouraged to eat foods that are high in potassium and to have their serum potassium levels checked periodically. People taking potassium-sparing diuretics should be cautioned to avoid those same foods.

PREGNANCY AND BREASTFEEDING

The use of diuretics to change the fluid shifts associated with pregnancy is not appropriate. Women maintained on these drugs for underlying medical reasons should not stop taking them, but they need to be aware of the potential for adverse effects on the fetus. Breastfeeding women who need a diuretic should find another method of feeding the baby because of the potential for adverse effects on the baby as well as the breastfeeding mother.

OLDER ADULTS

Older adults often have conditions that are treated with diuretics. They are also more likely to have renal or hepatic impairment, which requires cautious use of these drugs.

Older adults should be started on the lowest possible dose of the drug and the dose should be titrated slowly based on individual response. Frequent serum electrolyte measurements should be done to monitor for adverse reactions.

The intake and activity level of the person can alter the effectiveness and need for the diuretic. High-salt diets and inactivity can aggravate conditions that lead to oedema, and people should be encouraged to follow activity and dietary guidelines if possible.

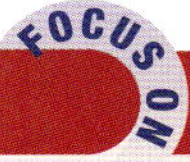

Safe medication administration

Explaining fluid rebound

Care must be taken when using diuretics to avoid **fluid rebound***, which is associated with fluid loss. If a person stops taking in water and takes the diuretic, the result will be concentrated plasma of smaller volume. The decreased volume is sensed by the nephrons, which activate the renin–angiotensin system. When the concentrated blood is sensed by the osmotic centre in the brain, antidiuretic hormone (ADH) is released to hold water and dilute the blood. The result can be a 'rebound' oedema as fluid is retained.*

Many people who are taking a diuretic markedly decrease their fluid intake so as to decrease the number of trips to the bathroom. The result is a rebound of water retention after the diuretic effect. This effect can also be seen in many diets that promise 'immediate results'; they frequently contain a key provision to increase fluid intake to 8–10 full glasses of water daily. The reflex result of diluting the system with so much water is a drop in ADH release and fluid loss.

Some people can lose 2–3 kg in a few days by doing this. However, the body's reflexes are quickly activated, causing rebound retention of fluid to re-establish fluid and electrolyte balance. People can become frustrated at this point and give up the fad diet. It is important to be able to explain this effect. Teaching people about balancing the desired diuretic effect with the actions of the normal reflexes is a clinical skill.

THIAZIDE AND THIAZIDE-LIKE DIURETICS

The thiazide diuretics belong to a chemical class of drugs called the sulfonamides. Thiazide-like diuretics have a slightly different chemical structure but work in the same way as thiazide diuretics.

Thiazide diuretics include hydrochlorothiazide (*Dithiazide*) and bendroflumethiazide (bendrofluazide) (*Neo-Naclex*). Thiazide-like diuretics include chlortalidone (*Hygroton*) and indapamide (*Dapa-Tabs, Natrilix*). Thiazide and thiazide-like diuretics are among the most frequently used diuretics.

Therapeutic actions and indications

Thiazide and thiazide-like diuretics act to block the chloride pump. Chloride is actively pumped out of the tubule by cells lining the ascending limb of the loop of Henle and the distal tubule. Sodium passively moves with the chloride to maintain electrical neutrality. (Chloride is a negative ion, and sodium is a positive ion.) Blocking of the chloride pump keeps the chloride and the sodium in the tubule to be excreted in the urine, thus preventing the reabsorption of both chloride and sodium in the vascular system (see Figure 51.1). Because

Prototype summary: hydrochlorothiazide

Indications: adjunctive therapy for oedema associated with HF, cirrhosis, corticosteroid or oestrogen therapy, and renal dysfunction; treatment of hypertension as monotherapy or in combination with other antihypertensives.

Actions: inhibits reabsorption of sodium and chloride in distal renal tubules, increasing the excretion of sodium, chloride and water by the kidneys.

Pharmacokinetics:

Route	Onset	Peak	Duration
Oral	2 hours	4–6 hours	6–12 hours

$T_{1/2}$: 5.6–14 hours; metabolised in the liver and excreted in urine.

Adverse effects: dizziness, vertigo, orthostatic hypotension, nausea, anorexia, vomiting, dry mouth, diarrhoea, polyuria, nocturia, muscle cramps or spasms.

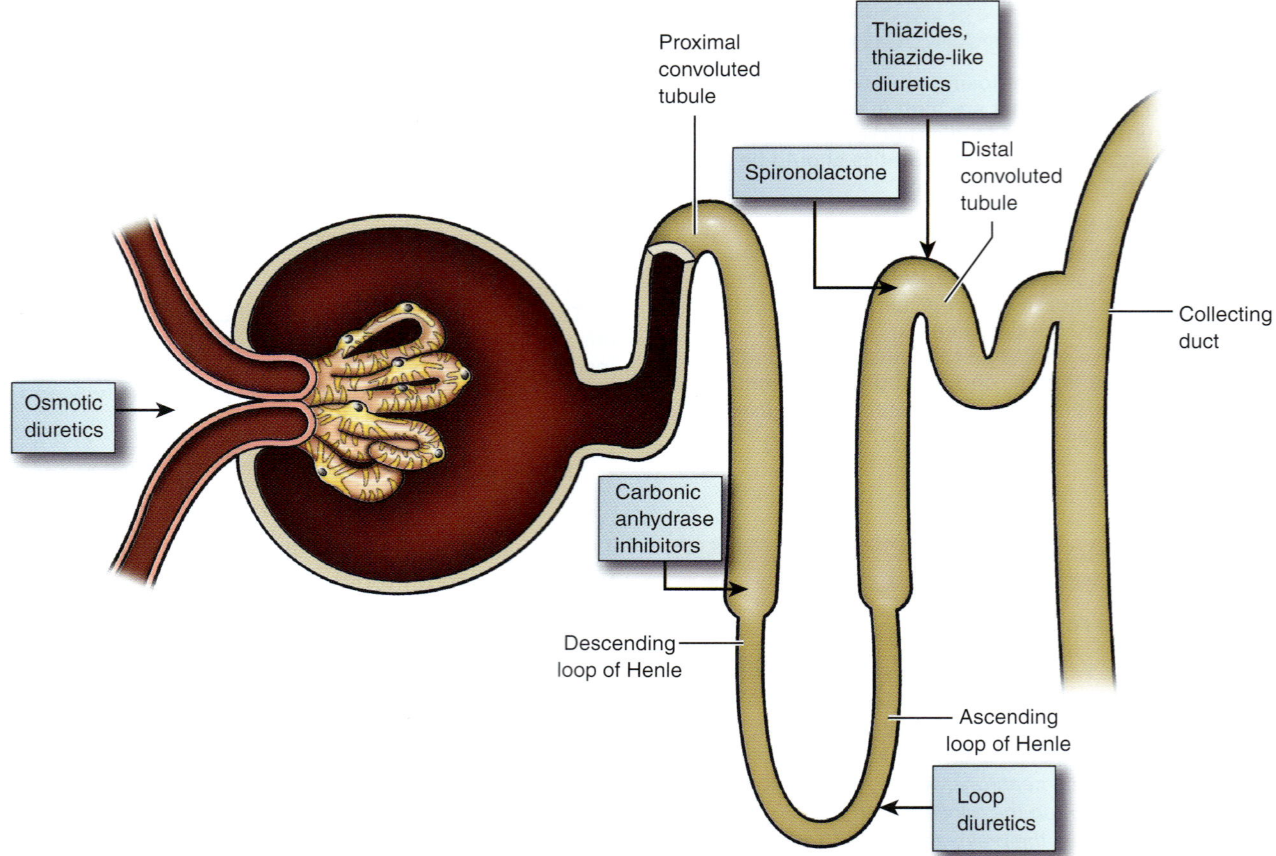

FIGURE 51.1 Sites of action of diuretics in the nephron.

these segments of the tubule are impermeable to water, there is little increase in the volume of urine produced, but it will be sodium rich, a **saluretic effect**. Thiazides are considered to be mild diuretics compared with the more potent loop diuretics. These drugs are the first-line drugs used to manage essential hypertension when drug therapy is needed. See Table 51.2 for usual indications for these agents.

Pharmacokinetics

These drugs are well absorbed from the GI tract after oral administration, with onset of action ranging from 1 to 3 hours. They have peak effects within 4–6 hours and duration of effects of 6–12 hours. They are metabolised in the liver and excreted in the urine. These diuretics cross the placenta and enter breast milk. Hydrochlorothiazide is the most frequently used of the thiazide diuretics and the prototype of this class.

Contraindications and cautions

Thiazide and thiazide-like diuretics are contraindicated with allergy to thiazides or sulfonamides *to prevent hypersensitivity reactions*; fluid and electrolyte imbalances, *which can be potentiated by the fluid and electrolyte changes caused by these diuretics*; and severe renal disease, *which may prevent the diuretic from working or precipitate a crisis stage due to the blood flow changes brought about by the diuretic.*

Caution should be used with the following conditions: systemic lupus erythematosus (SLE), *which frequently causes glomerular changes and renal dysfunction that could precipitate renal failure in some cases*; glucose tolerance abnormalities or diabetes mellitus, *which is worsened by the glucose elevating effects of many diuretics*; gout, *which reflects an abnormality in normal tubule reabsorption and secretion*; liver disease, *which could interfere with the normal metabolism of the drugs, leading to an accumulation of the drug or toxicity*; hyperparathyroidism, *which could be exacerbated by the renal effects of these drugs*; and bipolar disorder, *which could be exacerbated by the changes in calcium levels that occur with these drugs*. Routine use during pregnancy is not appropriate; these drugs should be reserved for situations in which the mother has pathological reasons for use, not pregnancy manifestations or complications, and only if

TABLE 51.2 Comparison of diuretics

Diuretic class	Major site of action	Usual indications	Major adverse effects
Thiazide, thiazide-like	Distal convoluted tubule	Oedema of HF, liver and renal disease Adjunct for hypertension	GI upset, CNS complications, hypovolaemia
Loop	Loop of Henle	Acute HF Acute pulmonary oedema Hypertension Oedema of HF, renal and liver disease	Hypokalaemia, volume depletion, hypotension, CNS effects, GI upset, hyperglycaemia
Carbonic anhydrase inhibitors	Proximal tubule	Glaucoma Diuresis in HF Mountain sickness Epilepsy	GI upset, urinary frequency
Potassium-sparing	Distal tubule and collecting duct	Adjunct for oedema of HF, liver and renal disease Treatment of hypokalaemia Adjunct for hypertension Hyperaldosteronism	Hyperkalaemia, CNS effects, diarrhoea
Osmotic	Glomerulus, tubule	Reduction of intracranial pressure Prevention of oliguric phase of renal failure Reduction of intraocular pressure Renal clearance of toxic substances	Hypotension, GI upset, fluid and electrolyte imbalances

the benefit to the mother clearly outweighs the risk to the fetus. If one of these drugs is needed during breastfeeding, another method of feeding the baby should be used *because of the potential for adverse effects on fluid and electrolyte changes in the baby.*

Adverse effects

The most common adverse effects associated with diuretic agents include GI upset, fluid and electrolyte imbalances, hypotension and electrolyte disturbances. Adverse effects associated with the use of thiazide and thiazide-like diuretics are related to interference with the normal regulatory mechanisms of the nephron. Potassium is lost at the distal tubule because of the actions on the pumping mechanism, and **hypokalaemia** (low blood levels of potassium) may result. Signs and symptoms of hypokalaemia include weakness, muscle cramps and arrhythmias. Another adverse effect is decreased calcium excretion, which leads to increased calcium levels in the blood. Uric acid excretion is also decreased because the thiazides interfere with its secretory mechanism. High levels of uric acid can result in gout.

If these drugs are used over a prolonged period, blood glucose levels may increase. This may result from the change in potassium levels (which keeps glucose out of the cells), or it may relate to some other mechanism of glucose control.

Urine is slightly alkalinised when the thiazides or thiazide-like diuretics are used because they block the reabsorption of bicarbonate. This effect can cause problems for individuals who are susceptible to bladder infections.

Clinically important drug–drug interactions

Decreased absorption of these drugs may occur if they are combined with colestyramine or colestipol. If this combination is used, the drugs should be taken separated by at least 2 hours.

The risk of digoxin toxicity increases due to potential changes in potassium levels; serum potassium should be monitored if this combination is used.

Decreased effectiveness of agents to control elevated blood glucose levels may occur related to the changes in glucose metabolism; dose adjustment of those agents may be needed.

The risk of lithium toxicity may increase if these drugs are combined. Serum lithium levels should be monitored and appropriate dose adjustment made as needed.

LOOP DIURETICS

Loop diuretics are so named because they work in the loop of Henle. Loop diuretics are also referred to as **high-ceiling diuretics** because they cause a greater degree of diuresis than other diuretics do. Three loop diuretics are available: etacrynic acid (*Edecrin* [not available in New Zealand]) the first loop diuretic introduced; bumetanide (*Burinex*); and furosemide (frusemide) (*Lasix*), the most commonly used loop diuretic.

Therapeutic actions and indications

Loop diuretics block the chloride pump in the ascending loop of Henle, where normally 30% of all filtered sodium is reabsorbed. This action decreases the reabsorption of sodium and chloride. The loop diuretics have a similar effect in the descending loop of Henle and in the distal convoluted tubule, resulting in the production of a copious amount of sodium-rich urine. These drugs work even in the presence of acid–base disturbances, renal failure, electrolyte imbalances or nitrogen retention.

Because they can produce a loss of fluid of up to 10 L/day, loop diuretics are the drugs of choice when a rapid and extensive diuresis is needed. In cases of severe oedema or acute pulmonary oedema, it is important to remember that these drugs can have an effect only on the blood that reaches the nephrons. A rapid diuresis occurs, producing a more hypertonic intravascular fluid. In pulmonary oedema, this fluid then circulates back to the lungs, pulls fluid out of the interstitial spaces by its oncotic pull, and delivers this fluid to the kidneys, where the water is filtered out, completing the cycle. In the treatment of pulmonary oedema, it can sometimes take hours to move all of the fluid out of the lungs because the fluid must be removed from the interstitial spaces in the lungs before it can be circulated to the kidneys for removal. Remembering how the drugs work and the way in which fluid moves in the vascular system will make it easier to understand the effects to anticipate.

Loop diuretics are commonly indicated for the treatment of acute HF, acute pulmonary oedema, oedema associated with HF or with renal or liver disease and hypertension. See Table 51.1 for usual indications for each of these agents. Furosemide (frusemide) is less powerful than bumetanide and therefore has a larger margin of safety for home use. *See the Critical thinking scenario for additional information about using furosemide in HF.*

Etacrynic acid is used less frequently in the clinical setting because of the improved potency and reliability of the other drugs.

Pharmacokinetics

Loop diuretics are available for oral or IV use. Furosemide may also be given IM. They reach peak levels in 60–120 minutes (orally) or 30 minutes (parenterally) and are metabolised with a half-life of 30–60 minutes and excreted primarily through urine.

Contraindications and cautions

Among the contraindications to these drugs are allergy to a loop diuretic *to prevent hypersensitivity reactions*; electrolyte depletion, *which could be aggravated by the electrolyte effects of these drugs*; anuria – severe renal failure, *which may prevent the diuretic from working or precipitate a crisis stage due to the blood flow changes brought about by the diuretic*; and hepatic coma, *which could be exacerbated by the fluid shifts associated with drug use*. Routine use during pregnancy is not appropriate; these drugs should be reserved for situations in which the mother has pathological reasons for use, not pregnancy manifestations or complications, and only if the benefit to the mother clearly outweighs the risk to the fetus.

Caution should be used with the following conditions: SLE, *which frequently causes glomerular changes and renal dysfunction that could precipitate renal failure in some cases*; glucose tolerance abnormalities or diabetes mellitus, *which are worsened by the glucose-elevating effects of many diuretics*; and gout, *which reflects an abnormality in normal tubule reabsorption and secretion*.

Safety for use in children younger than 18 years of age has not been established. If one of these drugs is used for a child, careful monitoring of the child's fluid and electrolyte balance is needed, and emergency support measures should be on standby.

Adverse effects

Adverse effects are related to the imbalance in electrolytes and fluid that these drugs cause. Hypokalaemia is a very common adverse effect because potassium is lost when the transport systems in the tubule try to save some of the sodium being lost. **Alkalosis**, a rise in serum pH to an alkaline state, may occur as bicarbonate is lost in the urine. Calcium is also lost in the tubules along with the bicarbonate, which may result in hypocalcaemia and tetany. The rapid loss of fluid can result in hypotension and dizziness if it causes a rapid imbalance in fluid levels. Long-term use of these drugs may also result in hyperglycaemia because of the diuretic effect on blood glucose levels, so susceptible individuals need to be monitored for this effect. Ototoxicity and even deafness have been reported with these drugs, but the loss of hearing is usually reversible after the drug is stopped. This may

Prototype summary: furosemide (frusemide)

Indications: treatment of oedema associated with HF, acute pulmonary oedema, hypertension.

Actions: inhibits the reabsorption of sodium and chloride from the distal renal tubules and the loop of Henle, leading to a sodium-rich diuresis.

Pharmacokinetics:

Route	Onset	Peak	Duration
Oral	60 min	60–120 min	6–8 hours
IV, IM	5 min	30 min	2 hours

$T_{1/2}$: 120 minutes; metabolised in the liver and excreted in urine.

Adverse effects: dizziness, vertigo, paraesthesias, orthostatic hypotension, rash, urticaria, nausea, anorexia, vomiting, glycosuria, urinary bladder spasm.

be an effect of electrolyte changes on the conduction of fragile nerves in the central nervous system.

Clinically important drug–drug interactions

The risk of ototoxicity increases if loop diuretics are combined with aminoglycosides or cisplatin. Anticoagulation effects may increase if these drugs are given with anticoagulants. There may also be a decreased loss of sodium and decreased antihypertensive effects if these drugs are combined with indometacin, ibuprofen, salicylates or other non-steroidal anti-inflammatory agents; a person receiving this combination should be monitored closely, and appropriate dose adjustments should be made.

CARBONIC ANHYDRASE INHIBITORS

The carbonic anhydrase inhibitors are relatively mild diuretics. Available agents include acetazolamide (*Diamox*) and brinzolamide (*Azopt*) used as eye drops to treat glaucoma.

Therapeutic actions and indications

The enzyme carbonic anhydrase is a catalyst for the formation of sodium bicarbonate, which is stored as the alkaline reserve in the renal tubule, and for the excretion of hydrogen, which results in a slightly acidic urine. Carbonic anhydrase inhibitors block the effects of carbonic anhydrase, slowing down the movement of hydrogen ions; as a result, more sodium and bicarbonate are lost in the urine. These drugs are used as adjuncts to other diuretics when a more intense diuresis is needed. Most often, carbonic anhydrase inhibitors are used to treat glaucoma because the inhibition of carbonic anhydrase results in decreased secretion of aqueous humour of the eye. See Table 51.2 for usual indications for each of these agents.

Pharmacokinetics

Acetazolamide is rapidly absorbed and widely distributed. It is available orally and for IV use. Peak serum concentration occurs 2–4 hours (15 minutes if given IV) and have a 6–12-hour duration. It is excreted in urine and dose adjustment is required in people with impaired renal function. Acetazolamide has been shown to be teratogenic in animals. As there are no adequate well-controlled studies in pregnant women, it should not be used in pregnancy, especially during the first trimester. Acetazolamide has been detected in low levels in the milk of lactating women. Because of the potential for adverse effects on the baby, another method of feeding should be used if one of these drugs is needed during breastfeeding.

Contraindications and cautions

Carbonic anhydrase inhibitors are contraindicated in individuals with allergy to the drug, to antibacterial sulfonamides or thiazides *to prevent hypersensitivity reactions*, or in individuals with chronic non-congestive angle-closure glaucoma, *which would not be effectively treated by these drugs*. Routine use during pregnancy is not appropriate; these drugs should be reserved for situations in which the mother has pathological reasons for use, not pregnancy manifestations or complications, and only if the benefit to the mother clearly outweighs the risk to the fetus.

Cautious use is recommended in people who have fluid or electrolyte imbalances, renal or hepatic disease, adrenocortical insufficiency, respiratory acidosis or chronic obstructive pulmonary disease, *which could be exacerbated by the fluid and electrolyte changes caused by acetazolamide.*

Adverse effects

Adverse effects of acetazolamide are related to the disturbances in acid–base and electrolyte balances. Metabolic acidosis is a relatively common and potentially dangerous effect that occurs when bicarbonate is lost. Hypokalaemia is also common because potassium excretion is increased as the tubule loses potassium in an attempt to retain some of the sodium that is being excreted. People also complain of paraesthesias (tingling) of the extremities, confusion and drowsiness, all of which are probably related to the neural effect of the electrolyte changes.

Clinically important drug–drug interactions

There may be an increased excretion of salicylates and lithium if they are combined with acetazolamide.

 **Prototype summary: acetazolamide**

Indications: adjunctive treatment of open-angle glaucoma, secondary glaucoma; preoperative use in acute angle-closure glaucoma when delay of surgery is indicated; oedema caused by HF; drug-induced oedema.

Actions: inhibits carbonic anhydrase, which decreases aqueous humour formation in the eye, intraocular pressure and hydrogen secretion by the renal tubules.

Pharmacokinetics:

Route	Onset	Peak	Duration
Oral	1 hour	2–4 hours	6–12 hours
Sustained-release oral	2 hours	8–12 hours	18–24 hours
IV	1–2 min	15–18 min	4–5 hours

$T_{1/2}$: 5–6 hours; excreted unchanged in urine.

Adverse effects: weakness, fatigue, rash, anorexia, nausea, urinary frequency, renal calculi, bone marrow suppression, weight loss.

CRITICAL THINKING SCENARIO

Using furosemide (frusemide) (*Lasix*) in heart failure

THE SITUATION

M.R. is a 68-year-old woman with rheumatic mitral valve heart disease. She has refused any surgical intervention and has developed progressively worsening heart failure (HF). Recently furosemide (frusemide) (*Lasix*), 40 mg/day PO, was prescribed for her along with digoxin. After 10 days with the new prescription, M.R. calls to tell you that she is allergic to the new medicine and cannot take it anymore. She reports extensive ankle swelling and difficulty breathing. You refer her to a cardiologist for immediate review.

CRITICAL THINKING

Think about the physiology of mitral valve disease and the progression of HF in this person. How does furosemide work in the body?

What additional activities will be important to help maintain some balance in this person's cardiac status?

What is the nature of M.R.'s reported allergy and what other options could be tried?

DISCUSSION

Over time, an incompetent mitral valve leads to an enlarged and overworked left ventricle as the backup of blood 'waiting to be pumped' continues to progress. Drug therapy for a person with this disorder is usually aimed at decreasing the workload of the heart as much as possible to maintain cardiac output. Digoxin increases the contractility of the heart muscle, which should lead to better perfusion of the kidneys. Furosemide – a loop diuretic – acts on the loop of Henle to block the reabsorption of sodium and water, and lead to a diuresis, which decreases the volume of blood the heart needs to pump and concentrates the blood that is pumped. This blood then has an oncotic pull to move fluid from the tissue into circulation, where it can be acted on by the kidney, leading to further diuresis.

M.R. should be encouraged to maintain fluid intake and to engage in activity as much as possible but to take frequent rest periods. Her potassium level should be monitored regularly (this is especially important because she is also taking digoxin, which is very sensitive to potassium levels), her oedematous limbs should be elevated periodically during the day, and she should monitor her sodium intake.

When M.R. was questioned about her reported allergy, it was discovered that her 'allergic reaction' was actually increased urination (a therapeutic effect). M.R. needs to learn about the actions of the drug. She also needs information about the timing of administration so that the resultant diuresis will not interfere with rest or with her daily activities. HF is a progressive, incurable disease, so education is a very important part of the overall management regimen.

CARE GUIDE FOR M.R.: DIURETIC AGENTS

Assessment: history and examination

Assess M.R.'s health history, including allergies to diuretics, fluid or electrolyte disturbances, gout, glucose tolerance abnormalities, liver disease, systemic lupus erythematosus, pregnancy and breastfeeding.

Focus the physical examination on the following areas:

Neurological: orientation, reflexes, strength

Skin: colour, texture, oedema

Cardiovascular: blood pressure, pulse, cardiac auscultation

Gastrointestinal: liver evaluation

Genitourinary: urinary output

Laboratory tests: haematology; serum electrolytes, glucose, uric acid; liver function tests

Implementation

Obtain daily weight and monitor urine output.

Provide comfort and safety measures: sugarless lozenges, mouth care, safety precautions, skin care, nutrition.

Administer the drug with food early in the day.

Provide support and reassurance to deal with drug effects and lifestyle changes.

Provide teaching regarding drug name, dosage, side effects, precautions, warnings to report, daily weighing and recording dietary changes as needed.

Evaluation

Evaluate drug effects: urinary output, weight changes, status of oedema, blood pressure changes.

Monitor for adverse effects: hypotension, hypokalaemia, hyperkalaemia, hypocalcaemia, hypercalcaemia, hyperglycaemia, increased uric acid levels.

Monitor for drug–drug interactions as indicated.

Evaluate the effectiveness of the teaching program and comfort and safety measures.

TEACHING FOR M.R.

- A diuretic, or 'water pill', such as furosemide (*Lasix*) will help to reduce the amount of fluid that is in your body by causing the kidneys to pass larger amounts of water and salt into your urine. By removing this fluid, the diuretic helps to decrease the work of the heart, lower blood pressure, and get rid of oedema or swelling in your tissues.
- This drug can be taken with food, which may eliminate possible stomach upset. When taking a diuretic, you

should maintain your usual fluid intake and try to avoid excessive intake of salt.
- Furosemide is a diuretic that causes potassium loss, so you should eat foods that are high in potassium (eg, orange juice, raisins, bananas).
- Weigh yourself each day, at the same time of day and in the same clothing. Record these weights on a calendar. Report any loss or gain of 2 kg or more in 1 day.
- Common effects of this drug include the following:
  - *Increased volume and frequency of urination*: have ready access to bathroom facilities. Once you are used to the drug, you will know how long the effects last for you.
  - *Dizziness, feeling faint on rising, drowsiness*: loss of fluid can lower blood pressure and cause these feelings. Change positions slowly; if you feel drowsy, avoid driving or other dangerous activities. These feelings are often increased if alcohol is consumed; avoid this combination or take special precautions if you combine them.
  - *Increased thirst*: as fluid is lost, you may experience a feeling of thirst. Sucking on sugarless lozenges and frequent mouth care might help to alleviate this feeling. Do not drink an excessive amount of fluid while taking a diuretic. Try to maintain your usual fluid intake.
  - Report any of the following to your health care provider: *muscle cramps or pain, loss or gain of more than 2 kg in 1 day, swelling in your fingers or ankles, nausea or vomiting, unusual bleeding or bruising, trembling or weakness.*
- Avoid the use of any over-the-counter (OTC) medication without first checking with your health care provider. Several OTC medications can interfere with the effectiveness of this drug.
- Tell any doctor, nurse or other health care provider involved in your care that you are taking this drug.
- Keep this drug, and all medications, out of the reach of children.

Caution should be used to monitor serum levels of individuals taking lithium.

Potassium-sparing diuretics

The potassium-sparing diuretics are not as powerful as the loop diuretics, but they retain potassium instead of wasting it. Drugs include amiloride (*Kaluril*), spironolactone (*Aldactone*), eplerenone (*Inspra*) and triamterene with hydrochlorothiazide (*Hydrene* [not available in New Zealand]). These diuretics are used for individuals who are at high risk for hypokalaemia associated with diuretic use (eg, individuals receiving digoxin or individuals with cardiac arrhythmias).

Therapeutic actions and indications

Potassium-sparing diuretics cause a loss of sodium while promoting the retention of potassium. Spironolactone acts as an aldosterone antagonist, blocking the actions of aldosterone in the distal tubule. Amiloride and triamterene block potassium secretion through the tubule. The diuretic effect of these drugs comes from the balance achieved in losing sodium to offset the potassium retained.

Potassium-sparing diuretics are often used as adjuncts with thiazide or loop diuretics or in people who are especially at risk if hypokalaemia develops, such as individuals taking certain antiarrhythmics or digoxin and those who have particular neurological conditions. Spironolactone, the most frequently prescribed of these drugs, is the drug of choice for treating **hyperaldosteronism**, a condition seen in cirrhosis of the liver and nephrotic syndrome (see Table 51.2).

Pharmacokinetics

These drugs are well absorbed after oral administration, are protein bound and widely distributed. They are metabolised in the liver and primarily excreted in urine. These diuretics cross the placenta and enter breast milk. Spironolactone has a slow onset of action, 24–48 hours, reaches peak effects in 48–72 hours and has a duration of effect of 72 hours. Amiloride and triamterene reach peak effects in 6–10 hours and have a duration effect of 16–24 hours.

Contraindications and cautions

These drugs are contraindicated for use in individuals with allergy to the drug *to prevent hypersensitivity reactions*, and hyperkalaemia, renal disease or anuria, *which could be exacerbated by the effects of these drugs.* Routine use during pregnancy is not appropriate; these drugs should be reserved for situations in which the mother has pathological reasons for use, not pregnancy manifestations or complications, and only if the benefit to the mother clearly outweighs the risk to the fetus.

Adverse effects

The most common adverse effect of potassium-sparing diuretics is hyperkalaemia, which can cause lethargy, confusion, ataxia, muscle cramps and cardiac arrhythmias. People taking these drugs need to be evaluated regularly for signs of increased potassium levels and informed about the signs and symptoms to watch for. They also should be advised to avoid foods that are high in potassium (Box 51.2). Because these drugs work much like aldosterone, they are associated with various androgen (another similar hormone) effects such as

BOX 51.2 Potassium-rich foods

avocados	lima beans	prunes
bananas	navy beans	rhubarb
broccoli	nuts	spinach
cantaloupe	oranges	sunflower seeds
dried fruits	peaches	tomatoes
grapefruit	potatoes	watermelon

hirsutism, gynaecomastia, deepening of the voice and irregular menses.

Clinically important drug–drug interactions

The diuretic effect decreases if potassium-sparing diuretics are combined with salicylates. Dose adjustment may be necessary to achieve therapeutic effects.

Prototype summary: spironolactone

Indications: primary hyperaldosteronism, adjunctive therapy in the treatment of oedema associated with HF, nephrotic syndrome, hepatic cirrhosis; treatment of hypokalaemia or prevention of hypokalaemia in people at high risk if hypokalaemia occurs; essential hypertension.

Actions: competitively blocks the effects of aldosterone in the renal tubule, causing loss of sodium and water and retention of potassium.

Pharmacokinetics:

Route	Onset	Peak	Duration
Oral	24–48 hours	48–72 hours	48–72 hours

$T_{1/2}$: 20 hours; metabolised in the liver and excreted in urine.

Adverse effects: dizziness, headache, drowsiness, rash, cramping, diarrhoea, hyperkalaemia, hirsutism, gynaecomastia, deepening of the voice, irregular menses.

OSMOTIC DIURETICS

Osmotic diuretics pull water into the renal tubule without sodium loss. The osmotic diuretics include glucose and mannitol (*Osmitrol*).

Therapeutic actions and indications

Some non-electrolytes are used intravenously to increase the volume of fluid produced by the kidneys. Mannitol, for example, is a sugar that is not well reabsorbed by the tubules; it acts to pull large amounts of fluid into the urine due to the **osmotic pull** exerted by the large sugar molecule. Because the tubule is not able to reabsorb all of the sugar pulled into it, large amounts of fluid are lost in the urine. The effects of these osmotic drugs are not limited to the kidneys because the injected substance pulls fluid into the vascular system from extravascular spaces, including the aqueous humour. Therefore, these drugs are often used in acute situations when it is necessary to decrease intraocular pressure before eye surgery or during acute attacks of glaucoma. They also are the diuretics of choice in cases of increased cranial pressure or acute renal failure due to shock, drug overdose or trauma. See Table 51.2 for usual indications for each of these agents.

Pharmacokinetics

Mannitol is only available for intravenous use. This drug is freely filtered at the renal glomerulus, poorly reabsorbed by the renal tubule, not secreted by the tubule and resistant to metabolism. Its action depends on the concentration of the osmotic activity in the solution. It is not known whether it can cause fetal harm. In addition, the effects of mannitol during breastfeeding are not well understood.

Contraindications and cautions

These drugs are contraindicated in individuals with renal disease and anuria from severe renal disease, pulmonary congestion, intracranial bleeding, dehydration

Prototype summary: mannitol

Indications: prevention and treatment of the oliguric phase of renal failure; reduction of intracranial pressure and treatment of cerebral oedema; reduction of elevated intraocular pressure; promotion of urinary excretion of toxic substances; diagnostic use for measurement of glomerular filtration rate; also available as an irrigant in transurethral prostatic resection and other transurethral procedures.

Actions: elevates the osmolarity of the glomerular filtrate, leading to a loss of water, sodium and chloride; creates an osmotic gradient in the eye, reducing intraocular pressure; creates an osmotic effect that decreases swelling after transurethral surgery.

Pharmacokinetics:

Route	Onset	Peak	Duration
IV	30–60 min	1 hour	6–8 hours
Irrigation	Rapid	Rapid	Short

$T_{1/2}$: 15–100 minutes; excreted unchanged in urine.

Adverse effects: dizziness, headache, hypotension, rash, nausea, anorexia, dry mouth, thirst, diuresis, fluid and electrolyte imbalances.

and HF, *which could be exacerbated by the large shifts in fluid related to use of these drugs.* Routine use during pregnancy is not appropriate; these drugs should be reserved for situations in which the mother has pathological reasons for use, not pregnancy manifestations or complications, and only if the benefit to the mother clearly outweighs the risk to the fetus.

Adverse effects

The most common and potentially dangerous adverse effect related to osmotic diuretics is the sudden drop in fluid levels. Nausea, vomiting, hypotension, lightheadedness, confusion and headache can be accompanied by cardiac decompensation and even shock. People receiving these drugs should be closely monitored for fluid and electrolyte imbalance.

Care considerations for people receiving diuretics

Assessment: history and examination

- Assess for contraindication or cautions: any known allergies to thiazides or sulfonamides *to prevent hypersensitivity reactions*; fluid or electrolyte disturbances, *which could be exacerbated by the diuretic or render the diuretic ineffective*; gout, *which reflects an abnormal tubule function and could be worsened by the diuretic or reflect a condition that would render the diuretic ineffective*; glucose tolerance abnormalities, *which may be exacerbated by the glucose-elevating effects*; liver disease, *which could alter the metabolism of the drug, leading to toxic levels*; systemic lupus erythematosus, *which frequently affects the glomerulus and could be exacerbated by the use of a thiazide or thiazide-like diuretic*; hyperparathyroidism and bipolar disorder, *which could be exacerbated due to increased serum concentrations of calcium*; and current status of pregnancy or breastfeeding *because of the potential for adverse effects on the fetus or baby.*
- Perform a physical assessment *to establish baseline data before beginning therapy, to determine the effectiveness of therapy and to evaluate for occurrence of any adverse effects associated with drug therapy.*
- Inspect the skin carefully for signs and symptoms of oedema; note the extent and degree of oedema, including evidence of pitting, *to provide a baseline as a reference for drug effectiveness*; check skin turgor *to determine hydration status.*
- Assess cardiopulmonary status, including blood pressure and pulse, and auscultate heart and lung sounds for abnormalities *to evaluate fluid movement and state of hydration and monitor the effects on the heart and lungs.*
- Obtain an accurate body weight *to provide a baseline to monitor fluid balance.*
- Monitor intake and output and assess voiding patterns *to evaluate fluid balance and renal function.*
- Evaluate liver status *to determine potential problems in drug metabolism.*
- Monitor the results of laboratory tests, including serum electrolyte levels, especially potassium and calcium, uric acid and glucose levels, *to determine the drug's effect*, and renal and liver function tests *to identify the need for possible dose adjustment and toxic effects.*

Implementation with rationale

- Administer oral drug with food or milk *to buffer the drug effect on the stomach lining if GI upset is a problem.*
- Administer intravenous diuretics slowly *to prevent severe changes in fluid and electrolytes.*
- Continuously monitor urinary output, cardiac response and heart rhythm of individuals receiving intravenous diuretics *to monitor for rapid fluid switch and potential electrolyte disturbances leading to cardiac arrhythmia.* Switch to the oral form, *which is less potent and easier to monitor,* as soon as possible, as appropriate.
- Administer the oral form early in the day *so that increased urination will not interfere with sleep.*
- Monitor the dose carefully and reduce the dose of one or both drugs if given with antihypertensive agents; *loss of fluid volume can precipitate hypotension.*
- Monitor the response to the drug (eg, blood pressure, urinary output, weight, serum electrolytes, hydration, periodic blood glucose monitoring) *to evaluate the effectiveness of the drug and monitor for adverse effects.*
- Assess weight daily *to evaluate fluid balance.*
- Check skin turgor *to evaluate for possible fluid volume deficit*, and assess oedematous areas for changes, including a decrease in amount or degree of pitting.
- Provide comfort measures, including skin care and nutrition consultation, *to increase compliance with drug therapy and decrease the severity of adverse effects;* provide safety measures if dizziness and weakness are a problem *to prevent injury.*
- Provide potassium-rich or low-potassium diet as appropriate *to maintain electrolyte balance and replace lost potassium or prevent hyperkalaemia.*

- Provide thorough teaching, including the name of the drug and dosage prescribed, *to enhance knowledge about drug therapy and to promote compliance.* Additional teaching includes the:
  - importance of taking the diuretic early in the day to avoid interference with sleep
  - administration of the drug with food or meals if GI upset occurs
  - need to weigh oneself daily and report any increase in weight of 2 kg or more in 1 day
  - importance of maintaining an adequate fluid intake to prevent fluid rebound (see Focus on safe medication administration in this chapter's introduction to diuretic agents)
  - need to have readily available access to bathroom facilities after taking the prescribed dose
  - signs and symptoms of adverse effects, including hypo- and hyperkalaemia and hypocalcaemia, and the need to notify the health care provider should any occur
  - danger signs and symptoms to be reported immediately
  - safety measures, such as moving slowly if dizziness is an issue and avoiding very hot environments and other situations potentially leading to extra loss of fluid
  - dietary sources of foods high in potassium, with an emphasis on the need for intake of these foods or the need to avoid these foods
  - need for compliance with therapy to achieve intended results
  - importance of continued follow-up and monitoring, including laboratory testing to determine the effectiveness of therapy.

Evaluation

- Monitor response to the drug (weight, urinary output, oedema changes, blood pressure).
- Monitor for adverse effects (electrolyte imbalance, orthostatic hypotension, rebound oedema, hyperglycaemia, increased uric acid levels, acid–base disturbances, dizziness).
- Monitor the effectiveness of comfort measures and compliance with the regimen.
- Evaluate the effectiveness of the teaching plan (person can name drug, dosage, adverse effects to watch for and specific measures to avoid them).

CHAPTER SUMMARY

- Diuretics – drugs that increase the excretion of sodium, and therefore water, from the kidneys – are used in the treatment of oedema associated with HF and pulmonary oedema, liver failure, cirrhosis and various types of renal disease, and as adjuncts in the treatment of hypertension.
- Classes of diuretics differ in their site of action and intensity of effects. Thiazide diuretics work to block the chloride pump in the distal convoluted tubule. This effect leads to a loss of sodium and potassium and a minor loss of water. Thiazides are frequently used alone or in combination with other drugs to treat hypertension. They are considered to be mild diuretics.
- Loop diuretics work in the loop of Henle and have a powerful diuretic effect, leading to the loss of water, sodium and potassium. These drugs are the most potent diuretics and are used in acute situations, as well as in chronic conditions not responsive to milder diuretics.
- Carbonic anhydrase inhibitors work to block the formation of carbonic acid and bicarbonate in the renal tubule. These drugs can cause an alkaline urine and loss of the bicarbonate buffer. Carbonic anhydrase inhibitors are used in combination with other diuretics when a stronger diuresis is needed, and they are frequently used to treat glaucoma, either orally or as eye drops, because they decrease the amount of aqueous humour produced in the eye.
- Potassium-sparing diuretics are mild diuretics that act to spare potassium in exchange for the loss of sodium and water in the urine. These diuretics are preferable if potassium loss could be detrimental to a person's cardiac or neuromuscular condition. People must be careful not to become hyperkalaemic while taking these drugs.
- Osmotic diuretics use hypertonic pull to remove fluid from the intravascular spaces and to deliver large amounts of water into the renal tubule. There is a danger of sudden change of fluid volume and massive fluid loss with some of these drugs. These drugs are used to decrease intracranial pressure, to treat glaucoma and to help push toxic substances through the kidney.

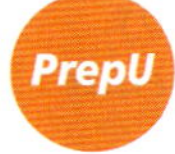

Knowing your strengths and weaknesses helps you to study more effectively. Take a PrepU Practice Quiz to find out how you measure up!

ONLINE RESOURCES

An extensive range of additional resources to enhance teaching and learning and to facilitate understanding of this chapter may be found online at the text's accompanying website, located on thePoint at http://thepoint.lww.com. These include Watch and Learn videos, Concepts in Action animations, journal articles, review questions, case studies, discussion topics and quizzes.

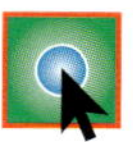

WEB LINKS

Health care providers and students may want to consult the following web resources:

www.heartfoundation.org.au
Information on HF, pathophysiology, treatment and research.

www.heartfoundation.org.nz
Information on HF, pathophysiology, treatment and research.

www.medsafe.govt.nz
New Zealand Medicines and Medical Devices Safety Authority.

http://nzformulary.org
New Zealand Formulary.

BIBLIOGRAPHY

Bennett, S. (2008). Diuretics: Use, actions and prescribing rationale. *Nurse Prescribing, 6(2)*, 72–77.

Berry, S. D., Mittleman, M. A., Zhang, Y., Solomon, D. H., Lipsitz, L. A., Mostofsky, E., Goldense, D. & Kiel, D. P. (2012). New loop diuretic prescriptions may be an acute risk factor for falls in the nursing home. *Pharmacoepidemiology & Drug Safety, 21(5)*, 560–563.

Farrell, M. & Dempsey, J. (2014). *Smeltzer & Bare's Textbook of Medical-Surgical Nursing* (3rd edn). Sydney: Lippincott Williams & Wilkins.

Goodman, L. S., Brunton, L. L., Chabner, B. & Knollmann, B. C. (2011). *Goodman and Gilman's Pharmacological Basis of Therapeutics* (12th edn). New York: McGraw-Hill.

Harvey, S. & Jordan, S. (2010). Diuretic therapy: Implications for nursing practice. *Nursing Standard, 24(43)*, 40–49.

Hurst, J. W., Fuster, V., Walsh, R. A. & Harrington, R. A. (Eds.). (2011). *Hurst's the Heart* (13th edn). New York: McGraw-Hill.

Khatib, R. (2011). Prescribing diuretics in the management of heart failure. *Nurse Prescribing, 9(9)*, 435, 437–441.

McKenna, L. & Mirkov, S. (2019). *McKenna's Drug Handbook for Nursing and Midwifery* (8th edn). Sydney: Wolters Kluwer Health Australia.

Porth, C. M. (2011). *Essentials of Pathophysiology: Concepts of Altered Health States* (3rd edn). Philadelphia: Lippincott Williams & Wilkins.

Porth, C. M. (2009). *Pathophysiology: Concepts of Altered Health States* (8th edn). Philadelphia: Lippincott Williams & Wilkins.

Roberts, M. E. & Epstein, B. J. (2009). Optimizing management of hypertension with combination therapy: Considerations for the nurse practitioner. *Journal of Cardiovascular Nursing, 24(5)*, 380–389.

Shannon, G. (2011). Severe hyponatraemia—recognition and management. *Australian Prescriber, 34(2)*, 42–45.

Sumnall, R. (2007). Fluid management and diuretic therapy in acute renal failure. *Nursing in Critical Care, 12(1)*, 27–33.

Watson, C. & Annus, C. (2013). Intravenous diuretic delivery in the home. *Nursing Times, 109(14)*, 20–21.

CHECK YOUR UNDERSTANDING

Answers to the questions in this chapter can be found in Appendix A at the back of this book.

MULTIPLE CHOICE

Select the best answer to the following.

1. Most diuretics act in the body to cause:
   a. loss of calcium.
   b. loss of sodium.
   c. retention of potassium.
   d. retention of chloride.
2. Diuretics cause a loss of fluid volume in the body. The drop in volume activates compensatory mechanisms to restore the volume, including:
   a. suppression of ADH release and stimulation of the countercurrent mechanism.
   b. suppression of aldosterone release and increased ADH release.
   c. activation of the renin–angiotensin–aldosterone system with increased ADH and aldosterone.
   d. stimulation of the countercurrent mechanism with reflex drop in renin release.
3. Thiazide diuretics are considered mild diuretics because:
   a. they block the sodium pump in the loop of Henle.
   b. they cause loss of sodium and chloride but little water.
   c. they do not cause a fluid rebound when they work in the kidneys.
   d. they have little or no effect on electrolyte levels.
4. The nurse or midwife would anticipate an order for a loop diuretic as the drug of choice for a person with:
   a. hypertension.
   b. shock.
   c. pulmonary oedema.
   d. fluid retention of pregnancy.
5. When providing care to a person who is receiving a loop diuretic, the nurse would determine the need to regularly monitor which of the following?
   a. sodium levels
   b. bone marrow function
   c. calcium levels
   d. potassium levels

6. When developing the plan of care for a person with hyperaldosteronism, the nurse or midwife would expect the doctor to prescribe which agent?
   a. spironolactone
   b. furosemide (frusemide)
   c. hydrochlorothiazide
   d. acetazolamide

7. A person with severe glaucoma who is about to undergo eye surgery would benefit from a decrease in intraocular fluid. This is often best accomplished by giving the person:
   a. a loop diuretic.
   b. a thiazide diuretic.
   c. a carbonic anhydrase inhibitor.
   d. an osmotic diuretic.

8. The nurse or midwife would instruct a person receiving a loop diuretic to report:
   a. yellow vision.
   b. weight loss of 1 kg in 2 days.
   c. muscle cramping.
   d. increased urination.

MULTIPLE RESPONSE

Select all that apply.

1. Diuretics are currently recommended for the treatment of which of the following?
   a. hypertension
   b. renal disease
   c. obesity
   d. severe liver disease
   e. fluid retention of pregnancy
   f. heart failure

2. Routine care of a person receiving a diuretic would include which of the following?
   a. daily weighing
   b. tight fluid restrictions
   c. periodic electrolyte evaluations
   d. monitoring of urinary output
   e. regular intraocular pressure testing
   f. teaching the person to report muscle cramping

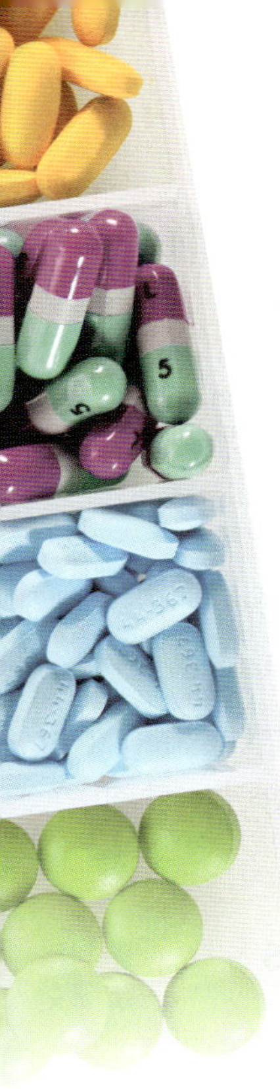

Drugs affecting the urinary tract and bladder

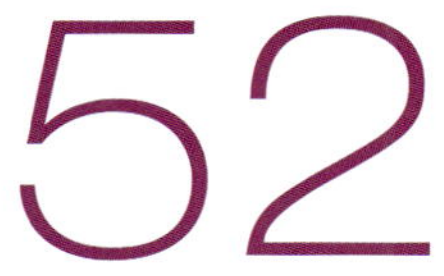

Learning objectives

On completing this chapter you should be able to:

1. Describe four common problems associated with the urinary tract, including the clinical manifestations of these problems.
2. Describe the therapeutic actions, indications, pharmacokinetics, contraindications and cautions, most common adverse reactions and important drug–drug interactions associated with urinary tract anti-infectives, antispasmodics and analgesics, bladder protectants and drugs used to treat benign prostatic hyperplasia (BPH).
3. Discuss the use of drugs affecting the urinary tract and bladder across the lifespan.
4. Compare and contrast the prototype drugs norfloxacin, oxybutynin and pentosan polysulfate sodium with other agents in their class.
5. Outline the care considerations, including important teaching points, for people receiving drugs affecting the urinary tract and bladder.

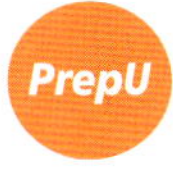

Test your current knowledge of drugs affecting the urinary tract and bladder with a PrepU Practice Quiz!

Glossary of key terms

acidification: the process of increasing the acid level; used to treat bladder infections, making the bladder an undesirable place for bacteria
antispasmodics: agents that block muscle spasm associated with irritation or neurological stimulation
benign prostatic hyperplasia (BPH): enlargement of the prostate gland, associated with age and inflammation; also called benign prostatic hypertrophy
cystitis: inflammation of the bladder, caused by infection or irritation
dysuria: painful urination
interstitial cystitis: chronic inflammation of the interstitial connective tissue of the bladder; may extend into deeper tissue
nocturia: getting up to void at night, reflecting increased renal perfusion with fluid shifts in the supine position when a person has gravity-dependent oedema related to heart failure; other medical conditions, including urinary tract infection, increase the need to get up and void
pyelonephritis: inflammation of the pelvises of the kidney, frequently caused by backward flow problems or by bacteria ascending the ureter
urgency: the feeling that one needs to void immediately; associated with infection and inflammation in the urinary tract
urinary frequency: the need to void often; usually seen in response to irritation of the bladder, age and inflammation

URINARY TRACT ANTI-INFECTIVES
cefalexin
methenamine (hexamine) hippurate
nitrofurantoin
(P) norfloxacin
trimethoprim

URINARY TRACT ANTISPASMODICS
darifenacin
(P) oxybutynin
solifenacin
tolterodine

OTHER DRUGS USED THAT AFFECT THE URINARY TRACT AND BLADDER
Bladder protectant
(P) pentosan polysulfate sodium

DRUGS FOR TREATING BENIGN PROSTATIC HYPERPLASIA
Alpha-adrenergic blockers
alfuzosin
tamsulosin
terazosin

Drugs that block testosterone production
dutasteride
finasteride

Conditions affecting the urinary tract and bladder are common problems. These conditions include acute urinary tract infections (UTIs), bladder spasms, bladder pain and benign prostatic hyperplasia (BPH).

Females, with shorter urethras, are particularly vulnerable to repeated urinary tract, bladder and even kidney infections. Children also may have frequent urinary tract problems. People with indwelling catheters or intermittent catheterisations often develop bladder infections or **cystitis**, which can result from bacteria introduced into the bladder by these devices. Blockage anywhere in the urinary tract can lead to backflow problems and the spread of bladder infections into the kidney (**pyelonephritis**). The signs and symptoms of a UTI are uncomfortable and include **urinary frequency**, **urgency**, burning on urination (associated with cystitis), and chills, fever, flank pain and tenderness (associated with acute pyelonephritis). To treat these infections, clinicians use specific urinary tract anti-infectives, which include antibiotics, as well as specific agents that reach antibacterial levels only in the kidney and bladder and are thought to sterilise the urinary tract.

Drugs also are available to block spasms of the urinary tract muscles, decrease urinary tract pain, protect the cells of the bladder from irritation, and treat enlargement of the prostate gland in men. Table 52.1 summarises urinary tract problems and the drugs of choice to treat them. Box 52.1 highlights important considerations related to urinary tract drugs based on the person's age.

TABLE 52.1

Urinary tract problem	Drugs of choice
Infection	Urinary tract anti-infectives: methenamine (hexamine) hippurate, nitrofurantoin, norfloxacin, trimethoprim
Spasm	Antispasmodics: oxybutynin, tolterodine
Pain	Bladder protectant for interstitial cystitis: pentosan
Benign prostatic hyperplasia	Alpha-adrenergic blockers: alfuzosin, tamsulosin, terazosin
	Testosterone inhibitors: finasteride, dutasteride

URINARY TRACT ANTI-INFECTIVES

Urinary tract anti-infectives (Table 52.2) are of two types. One type comprises the antibiotics, which are particularly effective against the Gram-negative bacteria that cause most UTIs. The antibiotics used specifically to treat UTIs include norfloxacin (*Roxin*) and nitrofurantoin (*Macrodantin*). Ciprofloxacin (*Cifran, Ciproxin*) and trimethoprim (*Alprim, Triprim*) are also used frequently to treat UTIs but are not specific to urinary tract

BOX 52.1 FOCUS ON **Drug therapy across the lifespan**

Urinary tract agents

CHILDREN

Children may develop urinary tract infections (UTIs), including cystitis, and need to be treated with a urinary tract anti-infective. Some children, because of congenital problems or indwelling catheters, require other urinary tract agents such as urinary tract analgesics or antispasmodics. The older anti-infectives – such as nitrofurantoin and methenamine (hexamine) hippurate – have established paediatric guidelines. A child with repeated urinary tract infections should be evaluated for potential sexual abuse.

Children need to be instructed in proper hygiene and should not be given bubble baths if urinary tract infections occur. They should be encouraged to avoid the alkaline ash juices such as orange or grapefruit juice and urged to drink lots of water.

If an antispasmodic is needed, oxybutynin is indicated for children older than 5 years of age.

ADULTS

Adults need to be cautioned about the various measures that can be used to decrease the likelihood of urinary tract infections. They should be encouraged to drink plenty of fluids to maintain bladder health.

If they are taking an anticholinergic to block spasm, adults need to be advised of other precautions to take when the parasympathetic system is blocked.

Adult men being treated for benign prostatic hyperplasia need to be aware of the possibility of decreased sexual function, as well as fatigue, lethargy and the potential for dizziness, which could interfere with working or activities of daily living.

PREGNANCY AND BREASTFEEDING

The use of urinary tract agents during pregnancy should be approached with caution. Women who are breastfeeding should use these agents with caution because of the potential for adverse effects on the baby, or they should find another method of feeding the baby.

OLDER ADULTS

Older adults often have conditions that are treated with the urinary tract agents. They are also more likely to have renal or hepatic impairment, which requires caution in the use of these drugs. Older adults should be started on the lowest possible dose of the drug, and it should be titrated slowly based on response. Special precautions to monitor cardiac function, intraocular pressure, blood pressure and bladder emptying need to be taken when using alpha-adrenergic blockers with these people. Older people may have a difficult time maintaining fluid intake and might benefit from extra encouragement to drink fluids, including cranberry juice, and to avoid alkaline ash drinks.

TABLE 52.2 DRUGS IN FOCUS Urinary tract anti-infectives

Drug name	Dosage/route	Usual indications
methenamine (hexamine) hippurate (*Hiprex*)	1 g bd PO Paediatric (6–12 years): 0.5–1 g PO bd	Suppression or elimination of bacteriuria associated with UTIs and anatomical abnormalities
nitrofurantoin (*Macrodantin*)	50–100 mg PO qid for 10–14 days; 50–100 mg PO at bedtime for chronic suppressive therapy Paediatric: 5–7 mg/kg/day in four divided doses	Treatment of UTIs caused by susceptible bacteria
(P) norfloxacin (*Roxin*)	400 mg q 12 hours PO, length of therapy dependent on site and intensity of infection	Treatment of UTIs caused by susceptible bacteria (broad-spectrum agent); treatment of uncomplicated urethral and cervical gonorrhoea and prostatitis
trimethoprim (*Alprim, Triprim*)	Treatment of acute uncomplicated UTI, women: 300 mg PO daily at night for 3 days; pregnant women (avoid in first trimester): 300 mg PO daily at night for 7 days; men: 300 mg PO daily at night for 7 days UTI prophylaxis: 150 mg PO at night	Prophylaxis and treatment of UTI

infections and are also used for treating other infections (see Chapter 9).

The other type of urinary tract anti-infective works to acidify the urine, killing bacteria that might be in the bladder. This group includes methenamine (hexamine) hippurate (*Hiprex*).

Therapeutic actions and indications

Urinary tract anti-infectives act specifically within the urinary tract to destroy bacteria, either through a direct antibiotic effect or through **acidification** of the urine. They do not generally have an antibiotic effect systemically, being activated or effective only in the urinary tract (Figure 52.1). Those drugs with an antibiotic effect interfere with reproduction of the Gram-negative bacteria and cause bacterial cell death. Those that cause acidification of the urine produce an environment that is not conducive to bacterial survival, leading to bacterial cell death. They are used to treat chronic UTIs, as adjunctive therapy in acute cystitis and pyelonephritis, and as prophylaxis with urinary tract anatomical abnormalities and residual urine disorders. *See the Critical thinking scenario for additional information regarding teaching the person about treatment with methenamine hippurate for cystitis.*

Table 52.2 discusses usual indications for each of the urinary tract anti-infectives.

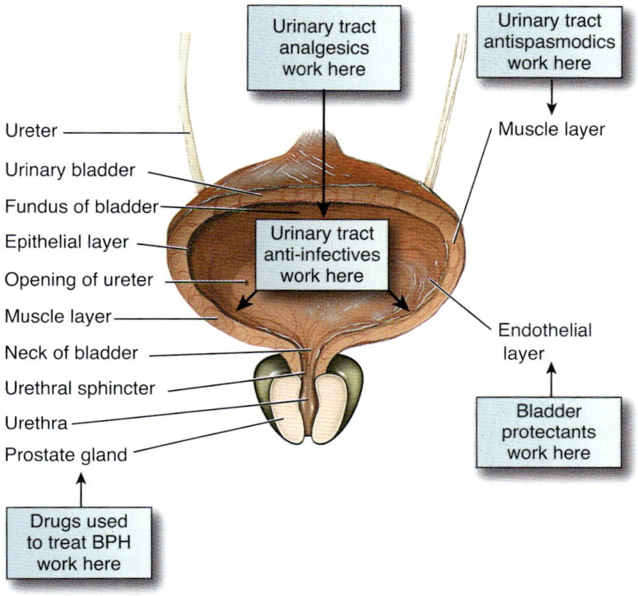

FIGURE 52.1 Sites of action of drugs acting on the urinary tract.

Pharmacokinetics

Norfloxacin, a newer and broader-spectrum drug, is effective against even more Gram-negative strains. This drug is rapidly absorbed when taken orally and undergoes hepatic metabolism and renal excretion. The dose of norfloxacin must also be reduced in the presence of renal impairment.

Nitrofurantoin is another older drug with a very short half-life (20–60 minutes). It is not effective against as many Gram-negative bacteria as the newer drugs are, but it has been successfully used for suppression therapy in adults and children with chronic UTIs. It is well absorbed when taken orally, metabolised in the liver and excreted in urine. No dose adjustment is needed with renal impairment.

Methenamine hippurate, taken orally, is well absorbed, undergoes metabolism in the liver and is excreted in urine.

Norfloxacin, nitrofurantoin and methenamine hippurate cross the placenta and enter breast milk.

Contraindications and cautions

These drugs are contraindicated in the presence of any known allergy to any of these drugs *to prevent hypersensitivity reactions.* They should be used with caution in the presence of renal dysfunction, *which could interfere with the excretion and action of these drugs,* and with pregnancy and breastfeeding *because of the potential for adverse effects on the fetus or neonate.*

Adverse effects

Adverse effects associated with these drugs include nausea, vomiting, diarrhoea, anorexia, bladder irritation and dysuria. Infrequent symptoms include pruritus, urticaria, headache, dizziness, nervousness and confusion. These effects may result from gastrointestinal (GI) irritation caused by the agent, which may be somewhat alleviated if the drug is taken with food, or from a systemic reaction to the urinary tract irritation.

Clinically important drug–drug interactions

Because these drugs are from several different chemical classes, the drug–drug interactions that can occur are very specific to the drug being used. Consult a drug guide for specific interactions.

Prototype summary: norfloxacin

Indications: treatment of adults with UTIs caused by susceptible strains of bacteria; uncomplicated urethral and cervical gonorrhoea; prostatitis caused by *Escherichia coli.*

Actions: interferes with DNA replication in susceptible Gram-negative bacteria, leading to cell death.

Pharmacokinetics:

Route	Onset	Peak	Duration
Oral	Varies	2–3 hours	12 hours

$T_{1/2}$: 3–4.5 hours; metabolised in the liver and excreted in urine.

Adverse effects: headache, dizziness, nausea, vomiting, dry mouth, fever, rash, photosensitivity.

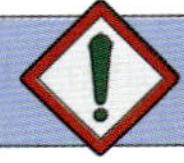

CRITICAL THINKING SCENARIO

Teaching about cystitis treatment

THE SITUATION

J.K. is a 6-year-old girl with a history of repeated urinary tract infections (UTIs). She was screened for potential sexual abuse, which may present as repeated urinary tract infections, and no evidence of abuse was found. She is seen today with complaints of dysuria, frequency, urgency and a low-grade fever. A urine sample is sent for culture and sensitivity testing. The doctor prescribes methenamine (hexamine) hippurate (*Hiprex*), 1 g bid, and refers J.K. and her mother to the nurse for teaching.

CRITICAL THINKING

What is the best approach for J.K.?

What key teaching points (at least five) should be emphasised to assist the pharmacological therapy in treating this infection? *Think about the following points: what the drug is doing, how it works and how it works best.*

DISCUSSION

Cystitis is very difficult to treat in young girls and can become a chronic problem. Person and parent education is very important for blocking the growth of bacteria and curing the infection. Teaching points should emphasise activities that will decrease the number of bacteria introduced into the bladder, acidify the urine to make the bladder an inhospitable environment for bacterial growth, and flush the bladder to prevent stagnant urine from encouraging bacterial growth.

To decrease the number of bacteria introduced into the bladder, education should cover the following hygiene measures: always wipe from front to back and never from back to front to avoid the introduction of intestinal bacteria into the urethra; avoid baths, particularly bubble baths, which facilitate the entry of bacteria into the urethra on the bubbles; and wear dry, cotton underwear to discourage bacterial growth.

Education also should stress the importance of avoiding alkaline ash foods (eg, citrus fruits, certain vegetables) and antacids and encouraging foods that acidify the urine. Cranberry juice is often recommended as a choice for fruit juice because it helps to prevent the bacteria from adhering to the bladder wall, which in turn aids infection prevention. Fluid intake, especially water, should be encouraged as much as possible to keep the bladder flushed. Finally, the person should be encouraged to complete the full course of medication prescribed and not to stop taking the drug when symptoms disappear.

CARE GUIDE FOR J.K.: URINARY TRACT ANTI-INFECTIVE METHENAMINE HIPPURATE

Assessment: history and examination

Assess J.K.'s health history, particularly any allergies to antibacterial medications, and liver or renal dysfunction. (If J.K. were of childbearing age, you would assess pregnancy and breastfeeding status.)

Focus the physical examination on the following areas:

Neurological: orientation, reflexes, strength

Skin: colour, texture, oedema

Gastrointestinal: liver evaluation

Genitourinary: urinary output

Laboratory tests: liver function tests, urinalysis, urine culture, and sensitivity testing

Implementation

Obtain urine sample for culture and sensitivity test.

Provide comfort and safety measures: safety precautions, skin care, nutrition.

Encourage eating acidifying foods and drinking lots of fluids.

Teach hygiene measures.

Administer medication with food if GI upset is a problem.

Provide support and reassurance to deal with drug effects and lifestyle changes.

Provide teaching to J.K. and her parents or carers regarding drug name, dosage, adverse effects, precautions, warnings to report, hygiene measures and dietary changes as needed.

Evaluation

Evaluate drug effects: relief of symptoms, resolution of infection.

Monitor for adverse effects: GI upset, headache, dizziness, confusion, dysuria, pruritus, urticaria.

Monitor for drug–drug interactions as indicated, especially use of antacids.

Evaluate the effectiveness of teaching program and comfort and safety measures.

TEACHING FOR J.K.

- A urinary tract anti-infective such as methenamine hippurate treats UTIs by destroying bacteria and by helping to produce an environment that is not conducive to bacterial growth.
- If this drug causes stomach upset, it can be taken with food. It is important to avoid foods that alkalinise the urine, such as citrus fruits and milk. because they decrease the effectiveness of the drug. Cranberry juice is one juice that can be used. As much fluid as possible (8–10 glasses of water a day) should be taken to help flush out the bacteria and treat the infection.
- Avoid using any over-the-counter (OTC) medication that might contain sodium bicarbonate (eg, antacids, baking soda) because these drugs alkalinise the urine and interfere with the ability of methenamine hippurate to treat the infection. Check with your health care provider before using any OTC drug.
- Take the full course of your prescription. Do not use this drug to self-treat any other infection.
- Common adverse effects of this drug may include the following:
  - *Stomach upset, nausea*: taking the drug with food or eating small, frequent meals may help.
  - *Painful urination*: if this occurs, report it to your health care provider. A dose adjustment may be needed.
- Report any of the following to your health care provider: *skin rash or itching, severe GI upset, GI upset that prevents adequate fluid intake, very painful urination and pregnancy in older women.*
- The following can help to decrease UTIs:
  - Avoid bubble baths.
  - Void whenever you feel the urge; try not to wait.
  - Always wipe from front to back, never from back to front.
- Tell any doctor, nurse or other health care provider involved in your care that you are taking this drug.

Care considerations for people receiving urinary tract anti-infectives

Assessment: history and examination

- Assess for *contraindications or cautions*: any history of allergy to antibiotics or anti-infectives *to avoid hypersensitivity reactions*; liver or renal dysfunction *that might interfere with the drug's metabolism and excretion*; and current status of pregnancy and breastfeeding, *which require cautious use of the drug.*
- Perform a physical assessment before therapy *to establish baseline data* and during therapy *to determine the effectiveness of the drug and the occurrence of any adverse effects associated with drug therapy.*
- Inspect the skin *to evaluate for the development of rash or hypersensitivity reactions.*
- Assess level of consciousness and monitor orientation and reflexes *to evaluate any central nervous system (CNS) effects of the drug.*
- Assess urinary elimination patterns, including amount and episode frequency, and for complaints of frequency, urgency, pain or difficulty voiding *to determine the effectiveness of therapy.*
- Monitor laboratory test results, including urinalysis and urine culture and sensitivity, *to evaluate effectiveness* and renal and liver function tests *to determine the need for possible dose adjustment and to identify possible toxicity.*

Implementation with rationale

- Ensure that culture and sensitivity tests are performed before therapy begins and are repeated if the response is not as expected *to ensure appropriate treatment of the infection.*
- Administer the drugs with food *to decrease GI adverse effects if they occur.*
- Institute safety precautions if the person experiences CNS effects *to prevent injury.*
- Advise people to continue the full course of the drug ordered and not to stop taking it as soon as the uncomfortable signs and symptoms pass *to ensure eradication of the infection and prevent the emergence of resistant strains of bacteria.*
- Encourage the person to drink lots of fluids (unless contraindicated by other conditions) *to promote flushing of the bladder and prevent urinary stasis*, and to avoid citrus juices and antacids, *which promote an alkaline urine and provide opportunity for bacteria growth.*
- Provide or assist with perineal hygiene as indicated *to reduce the risk of re-infection or prevent transmission of infection.*
- Explain to people with chronic UTIs about additional activities that can facilitate an acidic urine *to increase the effectiveness of urinary tract anti-infectives.*
- Provide thorough teaching, including drug name, dosage, intended effect and schedule for administration; measures to prevent or alleviate adverse effects; the need to avoid foods that cause alkaline ash and produce an alkaline urine (eg, citrus juices, antacids); the need to take the drug with food or meals to reduce GI effects; the importance of increasing fluid intake, including the use of cranberry juice; measures to prevent the recurrence of UTIs; and the need for periodic monitoring and laboratory testing such as urinalysis, urine culture and sensitivity *to enhance knowledge about drug therapy and to promote compliance.*

Evaluation

- Monitor the person's response to the drug (resolution of UTI and relief of signs and symptoms); repeat culture and sensitivity tests as recommended for evaluation of the effectiveness of all of these drugs.
- Monitor for adverse effects (skin evaluation, orientation and reflexes, GI effects).
- Evaluate the effectiveness of the teaching plan (person can name drug, dosage, adverse effects to watch for, specific measures to avoid them and measures to take to increase the effectiveness of the drug).
- Monitor the effectiveness of comfort and safety measures and compliance with the therapeutic regimen.

KEY POINTS

- Urinary tract anti-infectives destroy bacteria in the urinary tract that could be causing infections.
- Urinary tract–specific antibiotics prevent bacterial reproduction and cause bacterial cell death.
- Some urinary tract anti-infectives kill urinary tract bacteria by acidifying the urine, making the tract a poor host for bacterial growth, or by killing the bacteria outright.
- Hygiene measures, proper diet and extra hydration are activities that help to decrease harmful bacteria in the urinary tract, which promotes the effect of urinary tract anti-infective agents.

URINARY TRACT ANTISPASMODICS

Urinary tract **antispasmodics** (Table 52.3) block the spasms of urinary tract muscles caused by various conditions. The antispasmodics that are available include darifenacin (*Enablex*), oxybutynin (*Ditropan*), tolterodine (*Detrusitol*) and solifenacin (*Vesicare*).

Therapeutic actions and indications

Inflammation in the urinary tract, such as cystitis, prostatitis, urethritis and urethrocystitis/urethrotrigonitis, causes smooth muscle spasms along the urinary tract. Irritation of the urinary tract leading to muscle spasm also occurs in individuals with neurogenic bladder. These spasms lead to the uncomfortable effects of **dysuria** (pain or discomfort with urination), urgency, incontinence, **nocturia** (recurrent night time urination) and suprapubic pain. The urinary tract antispasmodics relieve these spasms by blocking parasympathetic activity, thus suppressing overactivity, which leads to relaxation of the detrusor and other urinary tract muscles (see Figure 52.1). Because the parasympathetic system uses acetylcholine to cause its effects, these drugs are called anticholinergic drugs. See Table 52.3 for usual indications of urinary tract antispasmodics.

Pharmacokinetics

All of these agents are administered orally only, with the exception of oxybutynin, which is not only given orally but is also available as a dermal patch. These drugs are rapidly absorbed, have a slow onset of action and have a duration of action of 6–12 hours. Oxybutynin, when given by the transdermal system, has a duration of action of 96 hours. The system has to be replaced every 4 days. These drugs are metabolised in the liver and excreted in urine. They cross the placenta and are found in breast milk.

TABLE 52.3 DRUGS IN FOCUS Urinary tract antispasmodics

Drug name	Dosage/route	Usual indications
darifenacin (*Enablex*)	7.5 mg/day PO; may be increased to 15 mg/day	Treatment of overactive bladder in people with urinary urgency, incontinence or frequency
(P) oxybutynin (*Ditropan, Oxytrol*)	Adult: 5 mg PO tid–qid; transdermal patch: apply 1 patch twice weekly (every 3–4 days) to dry, intact skin Paediatric > 5 years: 5 mg PO bd, up to a maximum of 5 mg PO tid	Symptomatic relief of urinary bladder spasm; treatment of overactive bladder
solifenacin (*Vesicare*)	5–10 mg/day PO	Treatment of overactive bladder in people with urinary urgency, incontinence or frequency
tolterodine (*Detrusitol*)	1–2 mg PO bd; reduce dose in people with hepatic impairment to 1 mg PO bd	Treatment of overactive bladder in people with urinary urgency, frequency or incontinence

Contraindications and cautions

These drugs are contraindicated in the presence of known allergy to the drugs *to avoid hypersensitivity reactions*; with pyloric or duodenal obstruction or recent surgery *because the anticholinergic effects can cause serious complications*; with obstructive urinary tract problems, *which could be further aggravated by the blocking of muscle activity*; and with glaucoma, myasthenia gravis or acute haemorrhage, *which could all be exacerbated by the anticholinergic effects of these drugs*. Caution should be used in people with renal or hepatic dysfunction, *which could alter the metabolism and excretion of the drugs*, and in pregnant and breast-feeding women *because of potential adverse effects on the fetus or neonate secondary to the anticholinergic effects of the drugs*.

Adverse effects

Adverse effects of urinary tract antispasmodics are related to the blocking of the parasympathetic system and include nausea, vomiting, dry mouth, nervousness, tachycardia and vision changes.

Oxybutynin has numerous anticholinergic effects, making it undesirable in certain conditions or situations that might be aggravated by decreased sweating, urinary retention, tachycardia and changes in GI activity.

Clinically important drug–drug interactions

Decreased effectiveness of phenothiazines and haloperidol has been associated with the combination of these drugs with oxybutynin. If any such combinations must be used, the person should be monitored closely and appropriate dose adjustments made. There is a risk of increased QT interval and serious cardiac arrhythmias if solifenacin is combined with other drugs that prolong the QT interval (antihistamines, antipsychotics); the person must be monitored closely if this combination is used. There is also a risk of increased serum levels and toxic effects if solifenacin is combined with cytochrome P450 (CYP) 3A4 inhibitors; the dose of solifenacin must be reduced and the person monitored closely. Tolterodine levels and toxicity can increase if it is taken with CYP 2D6 inhibitors (fluoxetine); the dose of tolterodine must be reduced if this combination is used.

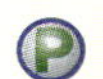
Prototype summary: oxybutynin

Indications: relief of symptoms of bladder instability associated with uninhibited neurogenic and reflex neurogenic bladder; treatment of signs and symptoms of overactive bladder.

Actions: acts directly to relax smooth muscle in the bladder; inhibits the effects of acetylcholine at muscarinic receptors.

Pharmacokinetics:

Route	Onset	Peak	Duration
Oral	30–60 min	3–6 hours	6–10 hours
Transdermal system	Varies	6–8 hours	96 hours

$T_{1/2}$: unknown; metabolised in the liver and excreted in urine.

Adverse effects: drowsiness, dizziness, blurred vision, tachycardia, dry mouth, nausea, urinary hesitancy, decreased sweating.

Care considerations for people receiving urinary tract antispasmodics

Assessment: history and examination

- Assess for *contraindications or cautions*: any history of allergy to these drugs *to prevent hypersensitivity reactions*; pyloric or duodenal obstruction or other GI lesions or obstructions or obstructions of the lower urinary tract, *which could be dangerously exacerbated by these drugs*; glaucoma, *which could increase intraocular pressure due to blockage of the parasympathetic nervous system*; and current status of pregnancy or breastfeeding, *which would require cautious use.*
- Perform a physical assessment before therapy *to establish baseline data* and during therapy *to determine the effectiveness of the drug and the occurrence of any adverse effects associated with drug therapy.*
- Inspect the skin *to evaluate for the development of rash or hypersensitivity reactions.*
- Assess level of consciousness, orientation and reflexes *to evaluate for any CNS effects of the drug.*
- Assess urinary elimination pattern, including amount and frequency of episodes, and for any complaints of frequency, urgency, pain or difficulty voiding *to monitor for excessive parasympathetic blockade or development of underlying UTI.*
- Arrange for ophthalmological examination, including intraocular pressure, *to assess for any developing glaucoma.*
- Assess vital signs, including pulse, *to establish a baseline for evaluating the extent of parasympathetic blockade.*
- Monitor the results of laboratory tests such as urinalysis and urine culture and sensitivity *to evaluate the effectiveness if UTI is the problem* and renal and liver function tests *to determine the need for possible dose adjustment and to evaluate for possible toxicity.*

Implementation with rationale

- Arrange for the appropriate treatment of any underlying UTI, *which may be causing the spasm.*
- Arrange for an ophthalmological examination at the beginning of therapy and periodically during long-term treatment *to evaluate drug effects on intraocular pressure so that the drug can be stopped if intraocular pressure increases.*
- Administer the drug with food if GI upset occurs *to alleviate GI discomfort.*
- Encourage fluid intake *to maintain urinary flow, flush the bladder and prevent urinary stasis.*
- Offer frequent sips of water or use of sugarless hard lollies *to alleviate dry mouth.*
- Monitor urinary output *to ensure adequate renal function and bladder emptying.*
- Institute safety precautions if the person experiences CNS effects *to prevent injury.*
- Encourage the person to continue treatment for the underlying cause of the spasm *to treat the cause and prevent the return of the signs and symptoms.*
- Offer support and encouragement *to help the person deal with the discomfort of the drug therapy.*
- Provide thorough teaching, including drug name, dosage, rationale for use and schedule for administration; signs and symptoms of adverse effects; measures to alleviate or prevent adverse effects; use of fluids and sugarless hard lollies *to combat dry mouth*; danger signs and symptoms to report immediately; appropriate perineal hygiene measures *to reduce the risk of infection if that is the underlying cause*; and the importance of periodic monitoring, including laboratory testing and evaluation, *to enhance knowledge about drug therapy and to promote compliance.*

Evaluation

- Monitor the person's response to the drug (resolution of urinary tract spasms and relief of signs and symptoms); repeat culture and sensitivity tests as recommended for evaluation of the effectiveness of all of these drugs.
- Monitor for adverse effects (skin evaluation, orientation and reflexes, intraocular pressure).
- Monitor the effectiveness of comfort and safety measures and compliance with the regimen.
- Evaluate the effectiveness of the teaching plan (person can name drug, dosage, adverse effects to watch for and specific measures to avoid them).

KEY POINTS

- Smooth muscle spasms affecting the urinary tract may be caused by inflammation and irritation; effects of the spasms include dysuria, urinary urgency, incontinence, nocturia and suprapubic pain.
- Antispasmodics block parasympathetic activity, thereby relaxing detrusor and other urinary tract muscles.

BLADDER PROTECTANT AGENT

Another type of drug frequently used to alleviate problems in the urinary tract and bladder is the bladder protectant pentosan, used to prevent irritation to the

TABLE 52.4 DRUGS IN FOCUS Other drugs affecting the urinary tract and bladder

Drug name	Dosage/route	Usual indications
Bladder protectant		
(P) pentosan polysulfate sodium (*Elmiron*)	100 mg PO tds	Relief of bladder pain or discomfort associated with interstitial cystitis

bladder wall. Pentosan polysulfate sodium (*Elmiron*) is used to coat or adhere to the bladder mucosal wall and protect it from irritation related to solutes in urine. It is not available in New Zealand.

Therapeutic actions and indications

Pentosan polysulfate sodium, available for oral administration, is a heparin-like compound that has anticoagulant and fibrinolytic effects. This drug adheres to the bladder wall mucosal membrane and acts as a buffer to control cell permeability, preventing irritating solutes in the urine from reaching the bladder wall cells (see Figure 52.1). It is used specifically to decrease the pain and discomfort associated with **interstitial cystitis**, a chronic inflammation of the interstitial connective tissue of the bladder that may extend into deeper tissue. See Table 52.4.

Pharmacokinetics

After oral administration, very little of this drug is absorbed (3%). It is distributed to the GI tract, liver, spleen, skin, bone marrow and periosteum. It undergoes metabolism in the liver and spleen and is excreted in urine. It has a half-life of 4.8 hours. It is not known whether the drug crosses the placenta or enters breast milk because of the lack of adequate studies of the effects of the drug during pregnancy or breastfeeding; caution should be used if the drug is needed during pregnancy or breastfeeding.

Contraindications and cautions

Pentosan should not be used with any condition that involves an increased risk of bleeding (surgery, pregnancy, anticoagulation, haemophilia) *because of its heparin-like effects*. It is also contraindicated in the presence of a history of heparin-induced thrombocytopenia, *which could recur with use of this drug*.

Caution should be used in people with bleeding disorders, those taking anticoagulants, elderly people or individuals with hepatic dysfunction (eg, people with alcohol dependence), *which could be affected by the heparin-like actions of the drug*, and in pregnant or breastfeeding women *because of the potential for adverse effects on the fetus or neonate*.

Adverse effects

Adverse effects associated with pentosan use include bleeding that may progress to haemorrhage (related to the drug's heparin-like effects), headache, alopecia (seen with heparin-type drugs) and GI disturbances related to local irritation of the GI tract with administration.

Clinically important drug–drug interactions

There is a potential for increased bleeding risks if this drug is combined with anticoagulants, aspirin or non-steroidal anti-inflammatory drugs (NSAIDs). If such a combination is used, the person should be monitored very closely for any signs of bleeding, and appropriate dose adjustments should be made to the anticoagulants, aspirin or NSAID.

(P) Prototype summary: pentosan polysulfate sodium

Indications: relief of bladder pain associated with interstitial cystitis.

Actions: adheres to the bladder wall mucosal membrane and acts as a buffer to control cell permeability, preventing irritating solutes in the urine from reaching the bladder wall cells.

Pharmacokinetics:

Route	Onset
Oral	Varies

$T_{1/2}$: 4.8 hours; metabolised in the liver and spleen and excreted in urine.

Adverse effects: bleeding, headache, alopecia, GI disturbances.

Care considerations for people receiving a bladder protectant

Assessment: history and examination

- Assess for *contraindications or cautions*: history of allergy to these drugs *to prevent hypersensitivity reactions* or renal insufficiency, *which could interfere with excretion of the drug*; history of bleeding abnormalities, splenic disorders or hepatic dysfunction, *which could be exacerbated by the heparin-like effects*; and current status of pregnancy and breastfeeding, *which require cautious use of this drug.*

- Perform a physical assessment before therapy *to establish baseline data* and during therapy *to determine the effectiveness of the drug and the occurrence of any adverse effects associated with drug therapy.*
- Inspect the skin for colour and note any evidence of petechiae or bruising *that may suggest coagulation problems and possible hypersensitivity reactions.*
- Assess vital signs for changes *to provide early evidence of bleeding.*
- Assess the urinary elimination pattern *to evaluate the effects of the underlying condition and the effectiveness of therapy.*
- Monitor laboratory test results, including liver function tests and coagulation studies, *to establish a baseline for monitoring safe use of the drug and the occurrence of adverse effects.*

Implementation with rationale

- Assist with establishing the presence of interstitial cystitis by biopsy or cystoscopy before beginning therapy *to ensure that appropriate therapy is being used.*
- Administer the drug on an empty stomach, 1 hour before or 2 hours after meals, *to relieve GI discomfort and improve absorption.*
- Obtain specimens for coagulation studies as ordered *to assess for excessive heparin-like effect.*
- Monitor urinary elimination for amount and characteristics and person's complaints of pain or difficulty voiding *to evaluate the effectiveness of therapy.*
- Arrange for a wig or appropriate head covering *if alopecia develops as a result of drug therapy.*
- Inspect the skin frequently for evidence of petechiae, bruising or oozing from insertion sites *to identify increased risk for bleeding.*
- Institute safety precautions such as minimising invasive procedures and protection from injury *to minimise the person's risk for injury.*
- Provide thorough teaching, including drug name, dosage, rationale for use and schedule for administration; signs and symptoms of adverse effects; measures to alleviate or prevent adverse effects; danger signs and symptoms to report immediately; comfort measures, such as taking the drug on an empty stomach, use of a wig if alopecia occurs, and analgesics for headache; measures to prevent or reduce the risk of recurrent interstitial cystitis; and the importance of periodic monitoring, including laboratory testing and evaluation, *to enhance knowledge about drug therapy and to promote compliance.*

Evaluation

- Monitor response to the drug (relief of bladder pain and discomfort).
- Monitor for adverse effects (skin evaluation, GI upset and complaints, headache, coagulation studies).
- Evaluate the effectiveness of the teaching plan (person can name drug, dosage, adverse effects to watch for and specific measures to avoid them).
- Monitor the effectiveness of comfort measures and compliance with the regimen.

KEY POINTS

- Pentosan is a bladder protectant. It is a heparin-like drug that protects the inner lining of the bladder from irritation by solutes in the urine. Because it is a heparin-like drug, the risk of bleeding must be considered.

DRUGS FOR TREATING BENIGN PROSTATIC HYPERPLASIA

Benign prostatic hyperplasia (BPH), also called benign prostatic hypertrophy or enlarged prostate, is a common problem in men, and it increases in incidence with age. The prostate completely encircles the urethra. The enlargement of the gland surrounding the urethra leads to discomfort, difficulty in initiating a stream of urine, feelings of bloating and an increased incidence of cystitis.

Two types of drugs are used to relieve the symptoms of BPH. These drugs include the alpha-adrenergic blockers alfuzosin (*Xatral SR*), tamsulosin (*Flomaxtra*) and terazosin (*Hytrin*) and drugs that block testosterone production – dutasteride (*Avodart*) and finasteride (*Proscar*). Box 52.2 discusses an alternative therapy used to treat BPH.

BOX 52.2 FOCUS ON **Herbal and alternative therapies**

Saw palmetto is a herbal therapy that has been used very successfully for the relief of symptoms associated with benign prostatic hyperplasia (BPH). People with BPH should be cautioned not to combine saw palmetto with finasteride because serious toxicity can occur. People should also be cautioned that random studies of various saw palmetto products have shown a huge variation in contents and activity of the tablets. If people choose to use this alternative therapy, they should be cautioned to check products carefully and to avoid switching products once they have success with one.

Therapeutic actions and indications

Before any of these drugs are used, it is important to make sure that the prostate enlargement is benign and not caused by cancer, infection, stricture or hypotonic bladder, which would require a different treatment. Individuals receiving long-term therapy need to be reassessed periodically to make sure that they have not developed a serious underlying problem like prostate cancer. Alpha-adrenergic blockers block postsynaptic alpha-1-adrenergic receptors, which results in a dilation of arterioles and veins and a relaxation of sympathetic effects on the bladder and urinary tract. In addition to treating BPH, most of these drugs are also indicated for treating hypertension (see Chapter 43).

Drugs that block testosterone production – dutasteride and finasteride – inhibit the intracellular enzyme that converts testosterone to the potent androgen dihydrotestosterone (DHT), which the prostate gland depends on for its development and maintenance (see Figure 52.1).

See Table 52.5 for usual indications for alpha-adrenergic blockers and drugs that block testosterone production.

Pharmacokinetics

The alpha-1-selective adrenergic-blocking agents are well absorbed after oral administration, reaching peak levels in 2–8 hours, and undergo extensive hepatic metabolism. They are excreted in urine. Finasteride and dutasteride are rapidly absorbed from the GI tract after oral administration, undergo hepatic metabolism, and are excreted in faeces and urine.

Contraindications and cautions

Both groups of drugs are contraindicated in individuals who are allergic to the drugs *to prevent hypersensitivity reactions*. Caution should be used in individuals with hepatic or renal dysfunction, *which could alter the metabolism and excretion of the drugs*. The adrenergic blockers should be used with caution in individuals with heart failure or known coronary disease, *which could be aggravated by the drop in blood pressure or tachycardia*. Finasteride and dutasteride have no indications for women and are rated pregnancy category X *because of androgen effects*. Women must be cautioned not to touch finasteride or dutasteride tablets *because of the risk of absorption through the skin*.

Adverse effects

Adverse effects of alpha-adrenergic blockers include headache, fatigue, dizziness, postural dizziness, lethargy, tachycardia, hypotension, GI upset and sexual dysfunction, all of which are effects seen with blockade of the alpha-receptors. Tamsulosin is not associated with as many adverse adrenergic-blocking effects as the other agents. Finasteride and dutasteride are associated with decreased libido, impotence and sexual dysfunction, all of which are related to decreased levels of DHT. People using either finasteride or dutasteride cannot donate blood for 6 months after the last dose to protect potential blood recipients from exposure to the testosterone-blocking effects.

Clinically important drug–drug interactions

There is a possibility of increased antihypertensive effects if the alpha-adrenergic blockers are combined

TABLE 52.5 *DRUGS IN FOCUS* Drugs for treating benign prostatic hyperplasia (BPH)

Drug name	Dosage/route	Usual indications
Alpha-adrenergic blockers		
alfuzosin (*Xatral SR*)	10 mg/day PO, take after the same meal each day	Relief of symptoms of BPH
tamsulosin (*Flomaxtra*)	400 micrograms/day PO, 30 minutes after the same meal each day	Treatment of BPH
terazosin (*Hytrin*)	1–20 mg/day PO based on the person's response	Relief of symptoms of BPH; hypertension
Drugs that block testosterone production		
dutasteride (*Avodart*)	500 micrograms/day PO	Long-term treatment of symptomatic BPH to shrink the prostate and relieve symptoms of hyperplasia
finasteride (*Proscar, Propecia*)	5 mg/day PO for BPH, 1 mg/day PO for male-pattern baldness (*Propecia*)	Long-term treatment of symptomatic BPH to shrink the prostate and relieve symptoms of hyperplasia; prevention of male-pattern baldness in people with strong family history

with any other antihypertensives. The person should be monitored and appropriate dose adjustments made to the antihypertensive agent if this combination is used.

Care considerations for people receiving drugs to treat benign prostatic hypertrophy

Assessment: history and examination

- Assess for *contraindications or cautions*: history of allergy to the drug *to prevent hypersensitivity reaction*; renal or hepatic failure, *which could alter the metabolism and excretion of the drug*; or history of heart failure or coronary heart disease (with alpha-adrenergic blockers), which could *be exacerbated by the effects of the alpha-adrenergic blockers.*
- Perform a physical assessment before therapy *to establish baseline data* and during therapy *to determine the effectiveness of the drug and the occurrence of any adverse effects associated with drug therapy.*
- Inspect the skin *to evaluate for the development of rash or hypersensitivity reactions.*
- Assess cardiopulmonary status, including vital signs especially blood pressure and pulse rate, and auscultate heart sounds and assess tissue perfusion, *to determine possible cardiovascular effects of alpha-adrenergic blockade.*
- Assess urinary elimination pattern and renal function *to assure adequate kidney function and evaluate for potential changes in drug excretion.*
- Assist with prostate examination and palpation *to establish hyperplasia and rule out other potential medical problems.*
- Monitor laboratory test results, including urinalysis, *to evaluate for possible changes*; renal and liver function tests *to determine the need for dose adjustment*; and prostate-specific antigen (PSA) levels *to eliminate the diagnosis of prostate cancer.*

Implementation with rationale

- Determine the presence of BPH and periodically evaluate through prostate examination and measurement of PSA levels *to reconfirm that no other problem is occurring.*
- Administer the drug without regard to meals, but give with meals *if GI upset is a problem.*
- Arrange for analgesics, *if needed, for headache.*
- Encourage the person to change positions slowly and to sit at the edge of the bed or chair for a few minutes before rising *if low blood pressure becomes a problem.*
- Offer support and encouragement and refer for counselling if appropriate *to help the person cope with potential decreases in sexual functioning.*
- Provide thorough teaching, including drug name, dosage, rationale for use and schedule for administration; signs and symptoms of adverse effects; measures to alleviate or prevent adverse effects, such as changing positions slowly and taking drug with food if GI upset occurs; and the importance of periodic monitoring, including laboratory testing and evaluation, *to enhance knowledge about drug therapy and to promote compliance.*

Evaluation

- Monitor response to the drug (relief of signs and symptoms of BPH, improved urine flow, decrease in discomfort).
- Monitor for adverse effects (skin evaluation, GI upset and complaints, headache, cardiovascular effects).
- Monitor the effectiveness of comfort measures and compliance with the regimen.
- Evaluate the effectiveness of the teaching plan (person can name drug, dosage, adverse effects to watch for and specific measures to avoid them).

KEY POINTS

- Benign prostatic hyperplasia (BPH) is a common enlargement of the prostate gland in older men.
- Drugs frequently used to relieve the signs and symptoms of prostate enlargement include alpha-adrenergic blockers, which relax the sympathetic effects on the bladder and sphincters, and finasteride and dutasteride, which block the body's production of a powerful androgen. The prostate is dependent on testosterone for its maintenance and development; blocking the androgen leads to shrinkage of the gland and relief of symptoms.

CHAPTER SUMMARY

- Urinary tract anti-infectives include two groups of drugs: antibiotics that are particularly effective against Gram-negative bacteria, and drugs that work to acidify the urine, ultimately killing the bacteria that might be in the bladder.
- Many activities are necessary to help decrease the bacteria in the urinary tract (eg, hygiene measures, proper diet, forcing fluids) to facilitate the treatment of UTIs and help the urinary tract anti-infectives to be more effective.

- Inflammation and irritation of the urinary tract can cause smooth muscle spasms along the urinary tract. These spasms lead to the uncomfortable effects of dysuria, urgency, incontinence, nocturia and suprapubic pain.
- The urinary tract antispasmodics act to relieve spasms of the urinary tract muscles by blocking parasympathetic activity and relaxing the detrusor and other urinary tract muscles.
- Pentosan polysulfate sodium is a heparin-like compound that has anticoagulant and fibrinolytic effects and adheres to the bladder wall mucosal membrane to act as a buffer to control cell permeability. This action prevents irritating solutes in the urine from reaching the cells of the bladder wall. It is used specifically to decrease the pain and discomfort associated with interstitial cystitis.
- Benign prostatic hyperplasia (BPH) is a common enlargement of the prostate gland in older men.
- Drugs frequently used to relieve the signs and symptoms of prostate enlargement include alpha-adrenergic blockers, which relax the sympathetic effects on the bladder and sphincters, and finasteride and dutasteride, which block the body's production of a powerful androgen. The prostate is dependent on testosterone for its maintenance and development; blocking the androgen leads to shrinkage of the gland and relief of symptoms.

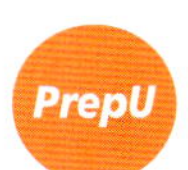

Knowing your strengths and weaknesses helps you to study more effectively. Take a PrepU Practice Quiz to find out how you measure up!

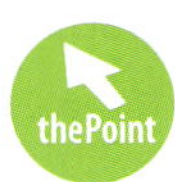

ONLINE RESOURCES

An extensive range of additional resources to enhance teaching and learning and to facilitate understanding of this chapter may be found online at the text's accompanying website, located on thePoint at http://thepoint.lww.com. These include Watch and Learn videos, Concepts in Action animations, journal articles, review questions, case studies, discussion topics and quizzes.

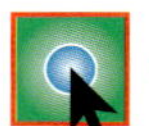

WEB LINKS

Health care providers and students may want to consult the following web resources:

www.healthymale.org.au
Healthy Male. Andrology Australia information on benign prostatic hyperplasia (BPH), support groups, research and treatment for patients.

www.usanz.org.au
The Urological Society of Australia and New Zealand.

BIBLIOGRAPHY

Farrell, M. & Dempsey, J. (2014). *Smeltzer & Bare's Textbook of Medical-Surgical Nursing* (3rd edn). Sydney: Lippincott Williams & Wilkins.

Gilchrist, K. (2004). Benign prostatic hyperplasia: Is it a precursor to prostate cancer? *Nurse Practitioner, 29(6)*, 30–37.

Goodman, L. S., Brunton, L. L., Chabner, B. & Knollmann, B. C. (2011). *Goodman and Gilman's Pharmacological Basis of Therapeutics* (12th edn). New York: McGraw-Hill.

Kirby, R. S. (2004). Selecting long-term medical therapy for BPH. *Contemporary Urology, 16(1)*, 12, 15–16, 18.

Kuteesa, W. (2006). Anticholinergic drugs for overactive bladder. *Australian Prescriber, 29*, 22–24.

McKenna, L. & Mirkov, S. (2019). *McKenna's Drug Handbook for Nursing and Midwifery* (8th edn). Sydney: Wolters Kluwer Health Australia.

McMurdo, M. E., Bissett, L. Y., Price, R. J., Phillips, G. & Crombie, I. K. (2005). Does ingestion of cranberry juice reduce symptomatic urinary tract infections in older people in the hospital? A double-blind, placebo-controlled trial. *Age and Ageing, 34(3)*, 256–261.

Mehnert-Kay, S. A. (2005). Diagnosis and management of uncomplicated urinary tract infections. *American Family Physician, 72*, 451–456.

Porth, C. M. (2011). *Essentials of Pathophysiology: Concepts of Altered Health States* (3rd edn). Philadelphia: Lippincott Williams & Wilkins.

Porth, C. M. (2009). *Pathophysiology: Concepts of Altered Health States* (8th edn). Philadelphia: Lippincott Williams & Wilkins.

Wu, C. & Kapoor, A. (2013). Dutasteride for the treatment of benign prostatic hyperplasia. *Expert Opinion on Pharmacotherapy, 14(10)*, 1399–1408.

CHECK YOUR UNDERSTANDING

Answers to the questions in this chapter can be found in Appendix A at the back of this book.

MULTIPLE CHOICE

Select the best answer to the following.

1. The antibiotic of choice for a person with cystitis who has great difficulty following medical regimens is:
   a. finasteride.
   b. oxybutynin.
   c. nitrofurantoin.
   d. norfloxacin.
2. Urinary tract antispasmodics block the pain and discomfort associated with spasm in the smooth muscle of the urinary tract. The numerous adverse effects associated with these drugs are related to:
   a. their blockade of sympathetic beta-receptors.
   b. their stimulation of cholinergic receptors.
   c. their stimulation of sympathetic receptors.
   d. their blockade of cholinergic receptors.
3. When planning the care for an older male diagnosed with BPH, which two types of drugs would the nurse most likely expect the doctor to prescribe?
   a. alpha-adrenergic blockers and anticholinergic drugs
   b. alpha-adrenergic blockers and testosterone production blockers
   c. anticholinergic drugs and alpha-adrenergic stimulators
   d. testosterone production stimulators and adrenal androgens
4. The drug of choice for treatment of BPH in a man with known hypertension might be:
   a. finasteride.
   b. terazosin.
   c. tamsulosin.
   d. propranolol.
5. Before administering a drug for the treatment of BPH, the nurse or midwife should ensure that:
   a. the person has had a prostate examination, including measurement of the PSA level.
   b. the person has not had a vasectomy.
   c. the person is still sexually active.
   d. the person is hypertensive.
6. A male who is very concerned about his hair loss and who is being treated for BPH might prefer treatment with:
   a. alfusozin.
   b. finasteride.
   c. tamsulosin.
   d. terazosin.

MULTIPLE RESPONSE

Select all that apply.

1. In evaluating a person for the presence of a bladder infection, one would expect to find reports of which of the following?
   a. frequency of urination
   b. painful urination
   c. oedema of the fingers and hands
   d. urgency of urination
   e. feelings of abdominal bloating
   f. itching, scaly skin
2. Important educational points for people with cystitis include which of the following?
   a. avoidance of bubble baths
   b. voiding immediately after sexual intercourse
   c. always wiping from back to front
   d. avoidance of foods high in alkaline ash
   e. tight fluid restriction
   f. always wiping from front to back

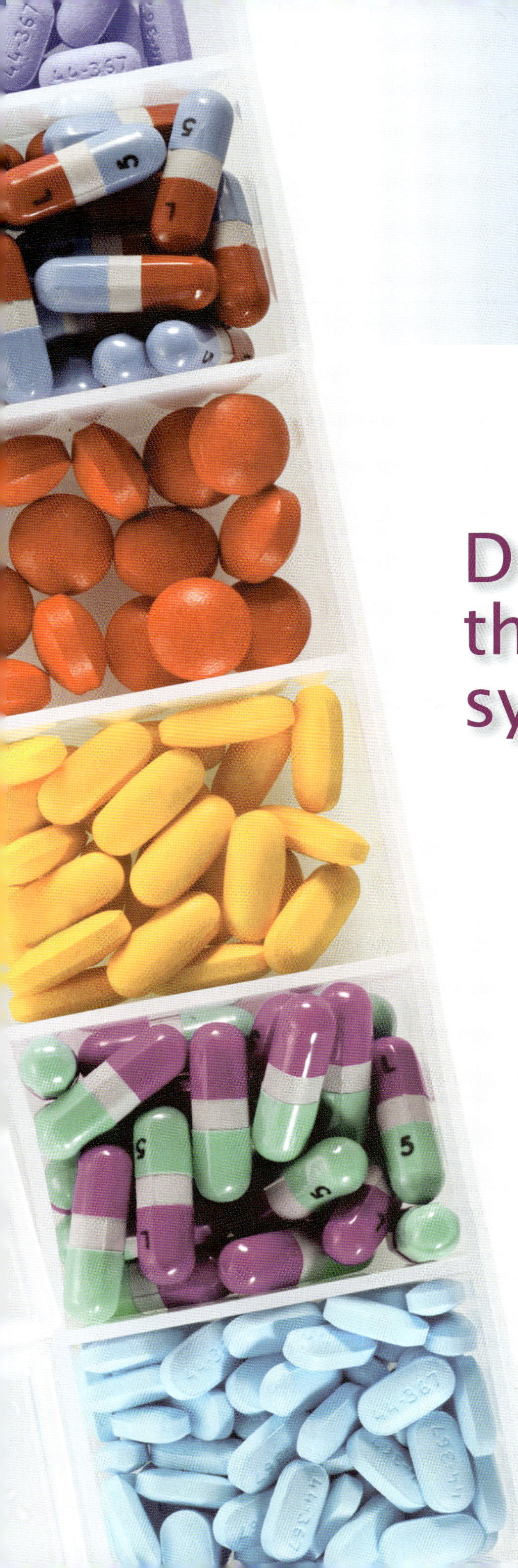

PART 10

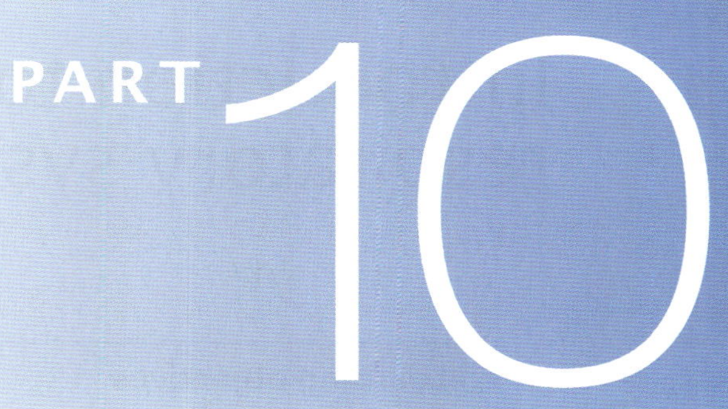

Drugs acting on the respiratory system

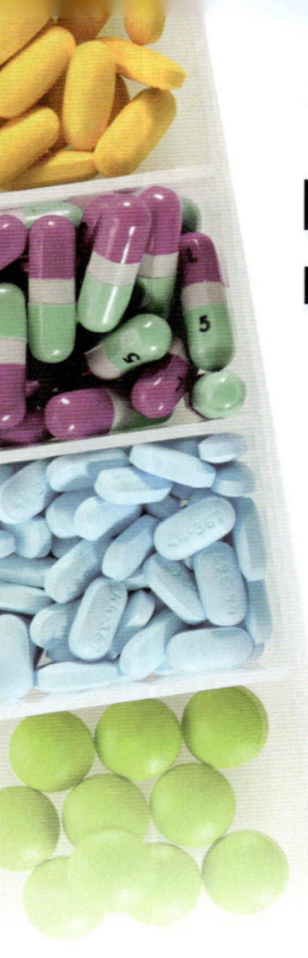

Introduction to the respiratory system

Learning objectives

On completing this chapter you should be able to:

1. Describe the major structures of the respiratory system, including the role of each in respiration.
2. Describe the process of respiration, with clinical examples of problems that can arise with alterations in the respiratory membrane.
3. Differentiate between the common conditions that affect the upper respiratory system.
4. Identify three conditions involving the lower respiratory tract, including the clinical presentations of these conditions.
5. Discuss the process involved in obstructive respiratory diseases, correlating this to the signs and symptoms of these diseases.

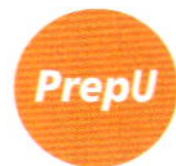

Test your current knowledge of the respiratory system with a PrepU Practice Quiz!

Glossary of key terms

alveoli: the respiratory sac, the smallest unit of the lungs, where gas exchange occurs

asthma: disorder characterised by recurrent episodes of bronchospasm (i.e. bronchial muscle spasm leading to narrowed or obstructed airways)

atelectasis: collapse of once-expanded alveoli

bronchial tree: the conducting airways leading into the alveoli; the branches become smaller and smaller, appearing much like a tree

chronic obstructive pulmonary disease (COPD): chronic condition that occurs over time; often the result of chronic bronchitis or repeated and severe asthma attacks; leads to destruction of the respiratory defence mechanisms and physical structure

cilia: microscopic, hair-like projections of the epithelial cell membrane lining the upper respiratory tract, which are constantly moving and directing the mucus and any trapped substance towards the throat

common cold: viral infection of the upper respiratory tract that initiates the release of histamine and prostaglandins and causes an inflammatory response

cough: reflex response to irritation in the respiratory membrane, results in expelling of forced air through the mouth

cystic fibrosis: a hereditary disease that results in the accumulation of copious amounts of very thick secretions in the lungs, which leads to obstruction of the airways and destruction of lung tissue

larynx: the vocal cords and the epiglottis, which close during swallowing to protect the lower respiratory tract from any foreign particles

lower respiratory tract: the bronchi and the alveoli that make up the lungs; the area where gas exchange takes place

pneumonia: inflammation of the lungs that can be caused by bacterial or viral invasion of the tissue or by aspiration of foreign substances

pneumothorax: air in the pleural space exerting high pressure against the alveoli

respiration: the act of breathing to allow the exchange of gases, a basic process for living things

respiratory distress syndrome (RDS): disorder found in premature neonates whose lungs have not had time to mature and who are lacking sufficient surfactant to maintain open airways to allow for respiration

respiratory membrane: area through which gas exchange must be made; made up of the capillary endothelium, the capillary basement membrane, the interstitial space, the alveolar basement membrane, the alveolar endothelium and the surfactant layer

seasonal rhinitis: inflammation of the nasal cavity, commonly called hay fever; caused by reaction to a specific antigen

sinuses: air-filled passages through the skull that open into the nasal passage

sinusitis: inflammation of the epithelial lining of the sinus cavities

sneeze: reflex response to irritation to receptors in the nares, results in expulsion of forced air through the nose

surfactant: lipoprotein that reduces surface tension in the alveoli, allowing them to stay open to allow gas exchange
trachea: the main conducting airway leading into the lungs
upper respiratory tract: the nose, mouth, pharynx, larynx and trachea – the conducting airways where no gas exchange occurs
ventilation: the movement of gases in and out of the lungs

The respiratory system is essential for survival. It brings oxygen into the body, allows for the exchange of gases and leads to the expulsion of carbon dioxide and other waste products. The normal functioning of the respiratory system depends on an intricate balance of the nervous, cardiovascular and musculoskeletal systems. Numerous conditions can affect the respiratory tract and interfere with the body's ability to ensure adequate oxygenation and gas exchange.

STRUCTURE AND FUNCTION OF THE RESPIRATORY SYSTEM

The respiratory system consists of two major components: the **upper respiratory tract** and the **lower respiratory tract**. The upper portion, or conducting airways, is composed of the nose, mouth, pharynx, larynx and trachea. The lower portion is made up of the **bronchial tree** (Figure 53.1). The smallest bronchi and the **alveoli** (respiratory sacs), which make up the lungs, where gas exchange takes place, are called the respiratory airways.

The upper respiratory tract

The upper respiratory tract is primarily involved in the movement of air in and out of the body, called **ventilation**. Air usually moves into the body through the nose and into the nasal cavity. The nasal hairs catch and filter foreign substances that may be present in the inhaled air. The air is warmed and humidified as it passes by blood vessels close to the surface of the epithelial lining in the nasal cavity. The epithelial lining contains goblet cells that produce mucus. This mucus traps dust, microorganisms, pollen and any other foreign substances. The epithelial cells of the lining also contain **cilia** – microscopic, hair-like projections of the cell membrane – which are constantly moving and directing the mucus and any trapped substances down towards the throat

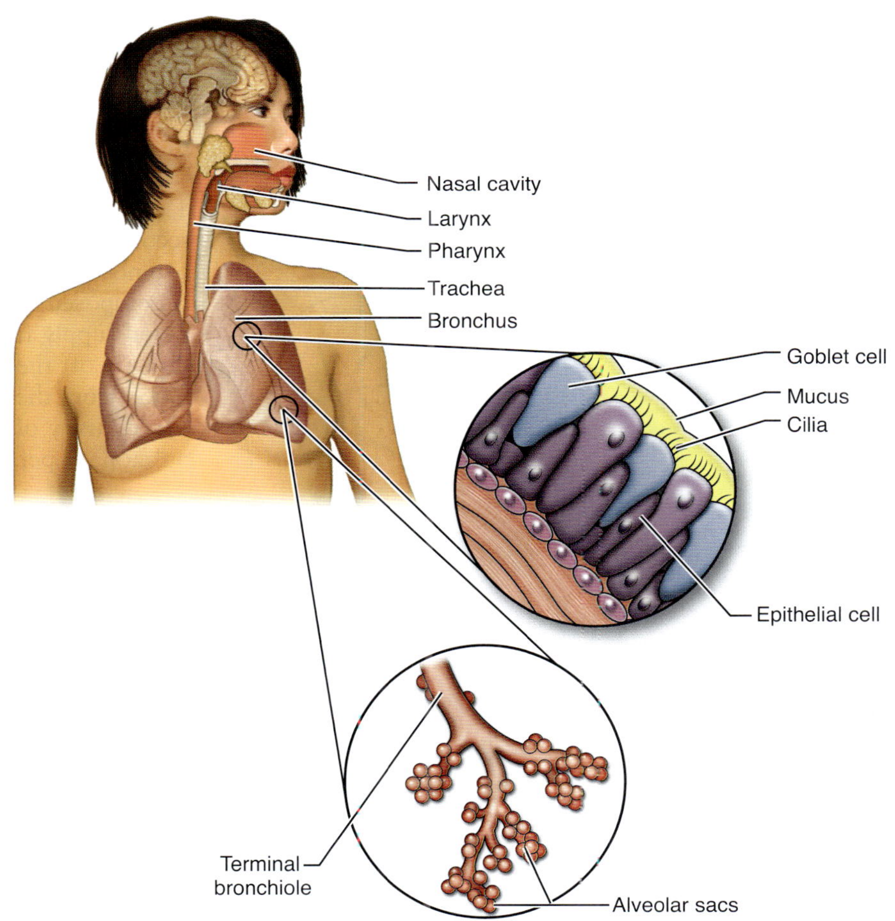

FIGURE 53.1 The respiratory tract.

(Figure 53.2). The action of the goblet cells and cilia is commonly called the mucociliary escalator.

Pairs of **sinuses** (air-filled passages through the skull) open into the nasal cavity. Because the epithelial lining of the nasal passage is continuous with the lining of the sinuses, the mucus produced in the sinuses drains into the nasal cavity. From there, the mucus drains into the throat and is swallowed into the gastrointestinal tract, where stomach acid destroys foreign materials.

Air moves from the nasal cavity into the pharynx and **larynx**. The larynx contains the vocal cords and the epiglottis, which closes during swallowing to protect the lower respiratory tract from any foreign particles. From the larynx, air proceeds to the **trachea**, the main conducting airway into the lungs. The trachea bifurcates, or divides, into two main bronchi, which further divide into smaller and smaller branches. All of these tubes contain mucus-producing goblet cells and cilia to entrap any particles that may have escaped the upper protective mechanisms. The cilia in these tubes move the mucus up the trachea and into the throat, where again it is swallowed.

The walls of the trachea and conducting bronchi are highly sensitive to irritation. When receptors in the walls are stimulated, a central nervous system reflex is initiated and a **cough** results. The cough causes air to be pushed through the bronchial tree under tremendous pressure, cleaning out any foreign irritant. This reflex, along with the similar **sneeze** reflex (which is initiated by receptors in the nasal cavity), forces foreign materials directly out of the system, opening it for more efficient flow of gas.

Throughout the airways, many macrophage scavengers freely move about the epithelium and destroy invaders. Mast cells are present in abundance and release histamine, serotonin, adenosine triphosphate (ATP) and other chemicals to ensure a rapid and intense inflammatory reaction to any cell injury. The end result of these various defence mechanisms is that the lower respiratory tract is virtually sterile – an important protection against respiratory infection that could interfere with essential gas exchange.

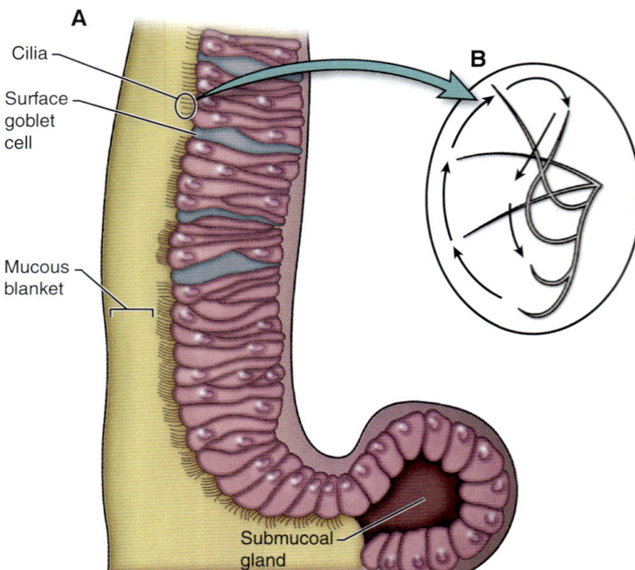

FIGURE 53.2 **A.** The mucociliary escalator. **B.** Conceptual scheme of ciliary movement, which allows forward motion to move the viscous gel layer and backward motion to occur entirely within the less viscous layer of the mucous blanket.

The lower respiratory tract

The lower respiratory tract (i.e. the respiratory airways) is composed of the bronchial tree, the smallest bronchioles and the alveoli (see Figure 53.1). The bronchial tubes are composed of three layers: cartilage, muscle and epithelial cells. The cartilage keeps the tube open, but it becomes progressively less abundant as the bronchi divide and get smaller. The muscles keep the bronchi open; the muscles in the bronchi become smaller and less abundant, with only a few muscle fibres remaining in the terminal bronchi and alveoli. The epithelial cells are very similar in structure and function to the epithelial cells in the nasal passage. The alveoli at the end of the bronchioles form the respiratory membrane. These structures are the functional units of the lungs where gas exchange occurs.

The lungs are two spongy organs that fill the chest cavity. They are separated by the mediastinum, which contains the heart, oesophagus, thymus gland and various blood vessels and nerves. The lungs are made up of the bronchial tree, the alveoli, the blood supply to the lungs and the blood coming from the right ventricle to the alveoli for gas exchange and elastic tissue. This tissue is important in allowing the expansion and recoil of the lungs to allow ventilation. The left lung is composed of two lobes or sections, and the right lung is composed of three lobes. The lung tissue receives its blood supply from the bronchial artery, which branches directly off the aorta. The alveoli receive unoxygenated blood from the right ventricle via the pulmonary artery. The delivery of this blood to the alveoli is referred to as pulmonary perfusion.

Gas exchange

Gas exchange occurs in the alveoli. In this process, carbon dioxide is lost from the blood and oxygen is transferred to the blood. The exchange of gases at the alveolar level is called **respiration**. The alveolar sac holds the gas, allowing needed oxygen to diffuse across the **respiratory membrane** into the capillary while carbon dioxide, which is more abundant in the capillary blood, diffuses across the membrane and enters the alveolar sac to be expired.

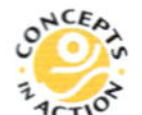

Respiratory: Asthma Respiratory: Gas exchange

The respiratory membrane is made up of the capillary endothelium, the capillary basement membrane, the interstitial space, the alveolar basement membrane, the alveolar epithelium and the surfactant layer (Figure 53.3). The sac is able to stay open because the surface tension of the cells is decreased by the lipoprotein **surfactant**. Absence of surfactant leads to alveolar collapse. Surfactant is produced by the type II cells in the alveoli. These cells have other metabolic functions, including the conversion of angiotensin I to angiotensin II, the degradation of serotonin and possibly the metabolism of various hormones.

The oxygenated blood is returned to the left atrium via the pulmonary veins; from there it is pumped throughout the body to deliver oxygen to the cells and to pick up waste products.

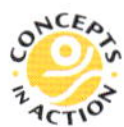

Respiratory: Oxygen transport

Respiration

Respiration, or the act of breathing to allow gas exchange, is controlled by the central nervous system. The inspiratory muscles – diaphragm, external intercostals and abdominal muscles – are stimulated to contract by the respiratory centre in the medulla. The medulla receives input from chemoreceptors (neuroreceptors sensitive to carbon dioxide and acid levels) to increase the rate and/or depth of respiration to maintain homeostasis in the body.

The vagus nerve, a predominantly parasympathetic nerve, plays a key role in stimulating diaphragm contraction and inspiration. Vagal stimulation also leads to a bronchoconstriction or tightening. The sympathetic system also innervates the respiratory system. Stimulation of the sympathetic system leads to increased rate and depth of respiration, and dilation of the bronchi to allow freer flow of air through the system.

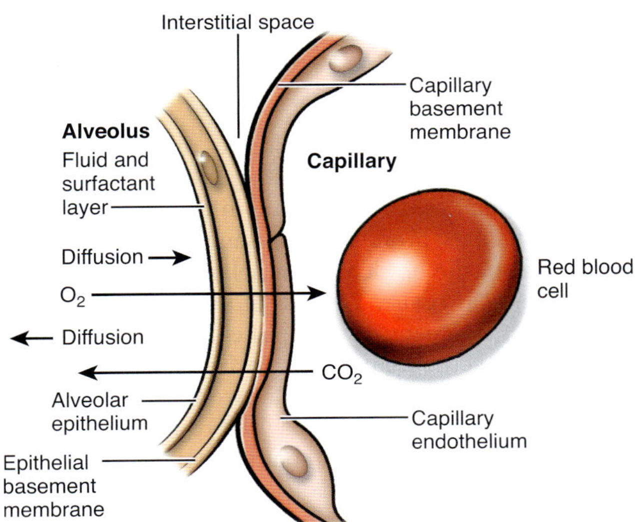

FIGURE 53.3 The respiratory membrane.

KEY POINTS

- The respiratory system has two parts: the upper respiratory tract, which includes the nose, pharynx, larynx and trachea, and the lower respiratory tract, which includes the bronchial tree and alveoli. Gas exchanges occur in the alveoli.
- Nasal hairs, mucus-producing goblet cells, cilia, the superficial blood supply of the upper respiratory tract and the cough and sneeze reflexes all work to keep foreign substances from entering the lower respiratory tract.
- Gas exchange occurs across the respiratory membrane in the alveolar sac. The alveoli produce surfactant, which reduces surface tension, among other functions.
- The medulla controls respiration, which depends on a functioning muscular system and a balance between the sympathetic and parasympathetic systems.

RESPIRATORY PATHOPHYSIOLOGY

Several conditions or disorders of the upper and lower respiratory tracts can interfere with the functioning of the respiratory system. These problems can range from generalised discomfort to life-threatening changes in gas exchange. Having a basic understanding of the processes at work will facilitate the understanding of the drugs that are used to treat these disorders.

Upper respiratory tract conditions

The most common conditions that affect the upper respiratory tract involve the inflammatory response and its effects on the mucosal layer of the conducting airways.

The common cold

A number of viruses cause the **common cold**. These viruses invade the tissues of the upper respiratory tract, initiating the release of histamine and prostaglandins, and causing an inflammatory response. As a result of the inflammatory response, the mucous membranes become engorged with blood, the tissues swell and the goblet cells increase the production of mucus. These effects cause the person with a common cold to complain of sinus pain, nasal congestion, runny nose, sneezing, watery eyes, scratchy throat and headache. In susceptible people, this swelling can block the outlet of the eustachian tube, which drains the inner ear and equalises pressure across the tympanic membrane. If this outlet becomes blocked, feelings of ear stuffiness and pain can occur, and the individual is more likely to develop an ear infection (otitis media).

Seasonal rhinitis

A similar condition that afflicts many people is allergic or **seasonal rhinitis** (an inflammation of the nasal cavity), commonly called hay fever. This condition occurs when the upper airways respond to a specific antigen (eg, pollen, mould, dust) with a vigorous inflammatory response, resulting again in nasal congestion, sneezing, stuffiness and watery eyes.

Sinusitis

Other areas of the upper respiratory tract can become irritated or infected, with a resultant inflammation of that particular area. **Sinusitis** occurs when the epithelial lining of the sinus cavities becomes inflamed. The resultant swelling often causes severe pain due to pressure against the bone, which cannot stretch, leading to blockage of the sinus passage. The danger of a sinus infection is that, if it is left untreated, microorganisms can travel up the sinus passages and into brain tissue.

Pharyngitis and laryngitis

Pharyngitis and laryngitis are infections of the pharynx and larynx, respectively. These infections are frequently caused by common bacteria or viruses. Pharyngitis and laryngitis are frequently seen with influenza, which is caused by a variety of different viruses and produces uncomfortable respiratory symptoms or other inflammations along with fever, muscle aches and pains, and malaise.

Lower respiratory tract conditions

A number of disorders affect the lower respiratory tract, including atelectasis, pneumonia (bacterial, viral or aspiration), bronchitis or inflammation of the bronchi (acute and chronic), bronchiectasis and the obstructive disorders – asthma, chronic obstructive pulmonary disease (COPD), cystic fibrosis and respiratory distress syndrome (RDS). Tuberculosis, discussed in Chapter 9, is a bacterial infection. Once known as consumption, this disease has been responsible for many respiratory deaths throughout the centuries. All of these disorders involve, to some degree, an alteration in the ability to move gases into and out of the lungs.

Atelectasis

Atelectasis, the collapse of once-expanded alveoli, can occur as a result of outside pressure against the alveoli – for example, from a pulmonary tumour, a **pneumothorax** (air in the pleural space exerting high pressure against the alveoli) or a pleural effusion. Atelectasis most commonly occurs as a result of airway blockage, which prevents air from entering the alveoli, keeping the lung expanded. This occurs when a mucus plug, oedema of the bronchioles, or a collection of pus or secretions occludes the airway and prevents the movement of air. People may experience atelectasis after surgery, when the effects of anaesthesia, pain and decreased coughing reflexes can lead to a decreased tidal volume and accumulation of secretions in the lower airways. People may present with crackles, dyspnoea, fever, cough, hypoxia and changes in chest wall movement. Treatment may involve clearing the airways, delivering oxygen and assisting ventilation. In the case of a pneumothorax, treatment also involves the insertion of a chest tube to restore the negative pressure to the space between the pleura.

Pneumonia

Pneumonia is an inflammation of the lungs caused either by bacterial or viral invasion of the tissue or by aspiration of foreign substances into the lower respiratory tract. The rapid inflammatory response to any foreign presence in the lower respiratory tract leads to localised swelling, engorgement and exudation of protective sera. The respiratory membrane is affected, resulting in decreased gas exchange. People complain of difficulty breathing and fatigue, and they present with fever, noisy breath sounds and poor oxygenation.

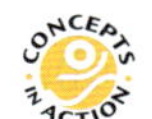

Respiratory: Change in breathing sounds

Bronchitis

Acute bronchitis occurs when bacteria, viruses or foreign materials infect the inner layer of the bronchi. There is an immediate inflammatory reaction at the site of the infection, resulting in swelling, increased blood flow in that area and changes in capillary permeability, leading to leakage of proteins into the area. The person with bronchitis may have a narrowed airway during the inflammation; this condition can be very serious in a person with obstructed or narrowed airflow. Chronic bronchitis is an inflammation of the bronchi that does not clear.

Bronchiectasis

Bronchiectasis is a chronic disease that involves the bronchi and bronchioles. It is characterised by dilation of the bronchial tree and chronic infection and inflammation of the bronchial passages. With chronic inflammation, the bronchial epithelial cells are replaced by a fibrous scar tissue. The loss of the protective mucus and ciliary movement of the epithelial cell membranes, combined with the dilation of the bronchial tree, leads to chronic infections in the now-unprotected lower areas of the lung tissue. People with bronchiectasis often have an underlying medical condition that makes them more susceptible to infections (eg, immune suppression, acquired immune deficiency syndrome, chronic inflammatory conditions). These people present with the signs and symptoms of acute infection, including fever, malaise, myalgia, arthralgia and a purulent, productive cough.

Obstructive pulmonary diseases

As noted previously, the obstructive pulmonary diseases include asthma, cystic fibrosis, COPD and RDS.

Asthma

Asthma is characterised by reversible bronchospasm, inflammation and hyperactive airways (Figure 53.4). The hyperactivity is triggered by allergens or non-allergic inhaled irritants or by factors such as exercise and emotions. The trigger causes an immediate release of histamine, which results in bronchospasm in about 10 minutes. The later response (3–5 hours) is cytokine-mediated inflammation, with mucus production and oedema contributing to obstruction. Appropriate treatment depends on understanding the early and late responses. The extreme case of asthma is called status asthmaticus; this is a life-threatening bronchospasm that does not respond to usual treatment and occludes airflow into the lungs.

Chronic obstructive pulmonary disease

Chronic obstructive pulmonary disease (COPD) is a permanent, chronic obstruction of airways, often related to cigarette smoking. It is caused by two related disorders – emphysema and chronic bronchitis – both of which result in airflow obstruction on expiration, as well as over-inflation of the lungs and poor gas exchange. Emphysema is characterised by loss of the elastic tissue of the lungs, destruction of alveolar walls and a resultant alveolar hyperinflation with a tendency to collapse with expiration. Chronic bronchitis is a permanent inflammation of the airways, with mucus secretion, oedema and poor inflammatory defences. Characteristics of both disorders are often present in a person with COPD (Figure 53.5).

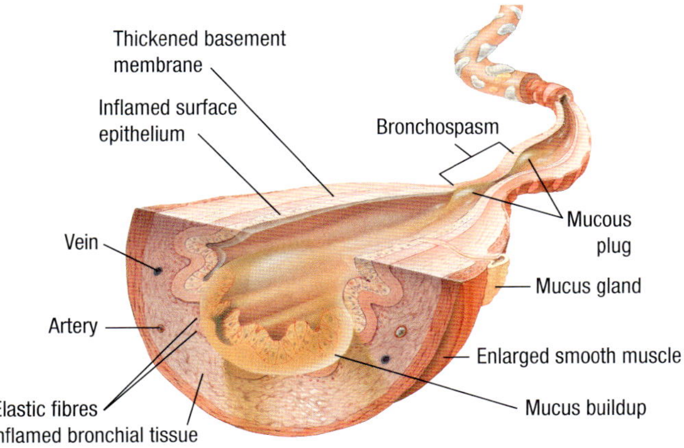

FIGURE 53.4 Asthma. The bronchiole is obstructed on expiration, particularly by muscle spasm, oedema of the mucosa, and thick secretions.

Cystic fibrosis

Cystic fibrosis (CF) is a hereditary disease involving the exocrine glands of the respiratory, gastrointestinal and reproductive tracts. CF results in the accumulation of copious amounts of very thick secretions in the lungs. Eventually, the secretions obstruct the airways, leading to destruction of the lung tissue. Treatment is aimed at keeping the secretions fluid and moving, and maintaining airway patency as much as possible.

Respiratory distress syndrome

Respiratory distress syndrome (RDS) causes obstruction at the alveolar level. It is frequently seen in premature infants who are born before their lungs have fully developed and while surfactant levels are still very low. Surfactant is necessary for lowering the surface tension in the alveoli so that they can stay open to allow the flow of gases. If surfactant levels are low, the alveoli do not expand and cannot receive air, leading to decreased gas exchange, low oxygen levels and generalised distress throughout the body as cells do not receive the oxygen that they need to survive. Treatment is aimed at instilling surfactant to prevent atelectasis and to allow the lungs to expand.

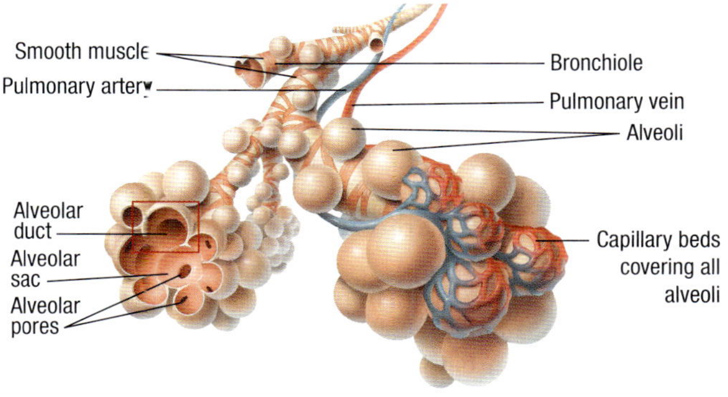

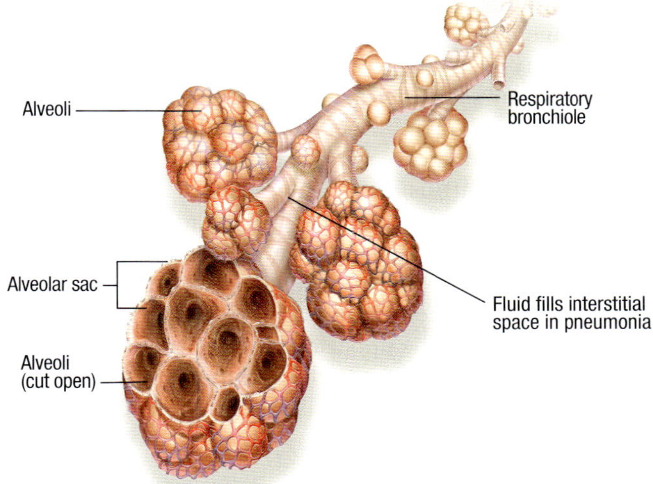

FIGURE 53.5 Distended and destroyed alveoli versus normal alveoli.

Acute respiratory distress syndrome (ARDS) is characterised by progressive loss of lung compliance and increasing hypoxia. This syndrome typically results from a severe insult to the body, such as cardiovascular collapse, major burns, severe trauma or rapid depressurisation. Treatment of ARDS involves reversal of the underlying cause of the problem combined with ventilatory support.

KEY POINTS

- Inflammation of the lower respiratory tract can result in serious disorders that interfere with gas exchange, including bronchitis and pneumonia.
- Obstructive disorders interfere with the ability to deliver gases to the alveoli because of obstructions in the conducting airways and eventually in the respiratory airways. These disorders include asthma, chronic obstructive pulmonary disease (COPD), cystic fibrosis and respiratory distress syndrome (RDS).

CHAPTER SUMMARY

- The respiratory system is composed of the upper respiratory tract, which includes the nose, pharynx, larynx and trachea, and the lower respiratory tract, which includes the bronchial tree and the alveoli.
- The respiratory system is essential for survival; it brings oxygen into the body, allows for the exchange of gases and expels carbon dioxide and other waste products.
- The upper airways have many features to protect the fragile alveoli: hairs filter the air; goblet cells produce mucus to trap foreign material; cilia move the trapped material towards the throat for swallowing; the blood supply close to the surface warms the air and adds humidity to improve gas movement and gas exchange; and the cough and sneeze reflexes clear the airways.
- The alveolar sac is where gas exchange occurs across the respiratory membrane. The alveoli produce surfactant to decrease surface tension within the sac and facilitate diffusion.
- Respiration is controlled through the medulla in the central nervous system and depends on a balance between the sympathetic and parasympathetic systems and a functioning muscular system.
- Inflammation of the upper respiratory tract is seen in many disorders, including the common cold, seasonal rhinitis, sinusitis, pharyngitis and laryngitis.
- Inflammation of the lower respiratory tract can result in serious disorders that interfere with gas exchange, including bronchitis and pneumonia.
- Obstructive disorders interfere with the ability to deliver gases to the alveoli because of obstructions in the conducting airways and eventually in the respiratory airways. These disorders include asthma, chronic obstructive pulmonary disease (COPD), cystic fibrosis and respiratory distress syndrome (RDS).

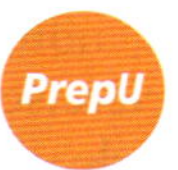

Knowing your strengths and weaknesses helps you to study more effectively. Take a PrepU Practice Quiz to find out how you measure up!

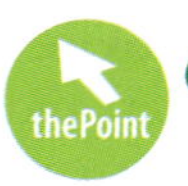

ONLINE RESOURCES

An extensive range of additional resources to enhance teaching and learning and to facilitate understanding of this chapter may be found online at the text's accompanying website, located on thePoint at http://thepoint.lww.com. These include Watch and Learn videos, Concepts in Action animations, journal articles, review questions, case studies, discussion topics and quizzes.

BIBLIOGRAPHY

Barrett, K. E. & Ganong, W. F. (2010). *Ganong's Review of Medical Physiology* (23rd edn). New York: McGraw-Hill.

George, R. B., Light, R. W., Matthay, M. A. & Matthay, R. A. (Eds.). (2006). *Chest Medicine: Essentials of Pulmonary and Critical Care Medicine*. Philadelphia: Lippincott Williams & Wilkins.

Goodman, L. S., Brunton, L. L., Chabner, B. & Knollmann, B. C. (2011). *Goodman and Gilman's Pharmacological Basis of Therapeutics* (12th edn). New York: McGraw-Hill.

Guyton, A. & Hall, J. (2011). *Textbook of Medical Physiology* (12th edn). Philadelphia: Saunders Elsevier.

Levitzky, M. G. (2007). *Pulmonary Physiology*. New York: McGraw-Hill.

Porth, C. M. (2011). *Essentials of Pathophysiology: Concepts of Altered Health States* (3rd edn). Philadelphia: Lippincott Williams & Wilkins.

Porth, C. M. (2009). *Pathophysiology: Concepts of Altered Health States* (8th edn). Philadelphia: Lippincott Williams & Wilkins.

Simon, S. (2007). *Lungs: Your Respiratory System*. New York: Collins.

Weinberger, S. E., Cockrill, B. A. & Mandel, J. (2014). *Principles of Pulmonary Medicine*. Philadelphia: Elsevier Saunders.

West, J. B. (2013). *Pulmonary Physiology: The Essentials* (8th edn). Philadelphia: Lippincott Williams & Wilkins.

Zevitz, M. & Leonhardt, R. (2005). *Pulmonary Medicine Review*. New York: McGraw-Hill.

CHECK YOUR UNDERSTANDING

Answers to the questions in this chapter can be found in Appendix A at the back of this book.

MULTIPLE CHOICE

Select the best answer to the following.

1. The health professional emphasises the need to take sinusitis very seriously because:
   a. it can cause a loss of sleep and exhaustion.
   b. it can lead to a painful otitis media.
   c. if it is left untreated, microorganisms can travel to brain tissue.
   d. drainage from infected sinus membranes often leads to pneumonia.
2. Diffusion of CO_2 from the tissues into the capillary blood:
   a. occurs if the tissue concentration of CO_2 is greater than that in the blood.
   b. decreases as blood acidity increases.
   c. increases in the absence of carbonic anhydrase.
   d. is accompanied by a decrease in plasma bicarbonate.
3. The type II cells of the walls of the alveoli function to:
   a. replace mucus in the alveoli.
   b. produce serotonin.
   c. secrete surfactant.
   d. protect the lungs from bacterial invasion.
4. A person who coughs is experiencing a reflex caused by:
   a. inflammation irritating the sinuses in the skull.
   b. irritants affecting receptor sites in the nasal cavity.
   c. pressure against the eustachian tube.
   d. irritation to receptors in the trachea and conducting airways.
5. Which of the following is most critical for respiration to occur?
   a. low levels of oxygen
   b. low levels of CO_2
   c. functioning inspiratory muscles
   d. an actively functioning autonomic system
6. After teaching a community group about the common cold, the instructor determines that the teaching was successful when the group states which of the following as the cause?
   a. bacteria that grow best in the cold
   b. allergens in the environment
   c. irritation of the delicate mucous membrane
   d. a number of different viruses
7. A person with chronic obstructive pulmonary disease would be expected to have:
   a. an acute viral infection of the respiratory tract.
   b. loss of protective respiratory mechanisms due to prolonged irritation or damage.
   c. localised swelling and inflammation within the lungs.
   d. inflammation or swelling of the sinus membranes over a prolonged period.

MULTIPLE RESPONSE

Select all that apply.

1. Which of the following would a nurse expect to assess if a person has inflammation of the upper respiratory tract?
   a. a runny nose
   b. laryngitis
   c. sneezing
   d. hypoxia
   e. rales
   f. wheezing
2. For gas exchange to occur in the lungs, oxygen must pass through which of the following?
   a. the conducting airways
   b. the alveolar epithelium
   c. the pleural fluid
   d. the interstitial alveolar wall
   e. the capillary basement membrane
   f. the interstitial space
3. The nose performs which of the following functions in the respiratory system?
   a. serves as a passageway for air movement
   b. warms and humidifies the air
   c. cleanses the air using hair fibres
   d. stimulates surfactant release from the alveoli
   e. initiates the cough reflex
   f. initiates the sneeze reflex

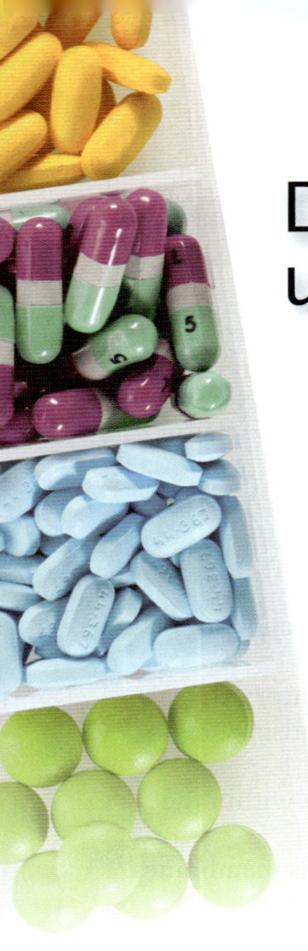

Drugs acting on the upper respiratory tract

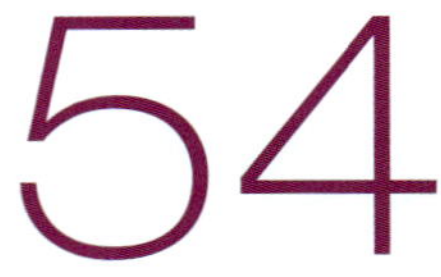

Learning objectives

On completing this chapter you should be able to:

1. Outline the underlying physiological events that occur with upper respiratory disorders.
2. Describe the therapeutic actions, indications, pharmacokinetics, contraindications, most common adverse reactions and important drug–drug interactions associated with drugs acting on the upper respiratory tract.
3. Discuss the use of drugs that act on the upper respiratory tract across the lifespan.
4. Compare and contrast the prototype drugs with other agents in their class and with other classes of drugs that act on the upper respiratory tract.
5. Outline the care considerations, including important teaching points, for people receiving drugs acting on the upper respiratory tract.

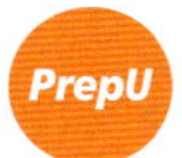

Test your current knowledge of drugs acting on the upper respiratory tract with a PrepU Practice Quiz!

Glossary of key terms

antihistamines: drugs that block the release or action of histamine, a chemical released during inflammation that increases secretions and narrows airways

antitussives: drugs that block the cough reflex

decongestants: drugs that decrease the blood flow to the upper respiratory tract and decrease the overproduction of secretions

drug vehicle: substance added to a drug to produce the final delivery form such as tablet; also known as excipient

expectorants: drugs that increase productive cough to clear the airways

mucolytics: drugs that increase or liquefy respiratory secretions to aid the clearing of the airways

rebound congestion: a process that occurs when the nasal passages become congested as the effect of a decongestant drug wears off; people tend to use more drug to decrease the congestion, and a vicious circle of congestion, drug and congestion develops, leading to abuse of the decongestant; also called rhinitis medicamentosa

rhinitis medicamentosa: reflex reaction to vasoconstriction caused by decongestants; a rebound vasodilation that often leads to prolonged overuse of decongestants; also called rebound congestion

ANTITUSSIVES
codeine
(P) dextromethorphan
pentoxyverine
pholcodine

DECONGESTANTS
Topical nasal decongestants
(P) ephedrine
oxymetazoline
phenylephrine
xylometazoline

Oral decongestants
phenylephrine
(P) pseudoephedrine

Topical nasal steroid decongestants
beclomethasone
budesonide
fluticasone
triamcinolone

ANTIHISTAMINES
First-generation
brompheniramine
chlorphenamine (chlorpheniramine)
cyproheptadine
dexchlorpheniramine
(P) diphenhydramine
pheniramine
promethazine

Second-generation (non-sedating)
azelastine
cetirizine
desloratadine
fexofenadine
loratadine

EXPECTORANT
(P) guaifenesin

MUCOLYTICS
(P) acetylcysteine
bromhexine
dornase alfa

Drugs that affect the respiratory system work to keep the airways open and gases moving efficiently. The classes discussed in this chapter mainly act on the upper respiratory tract. Figure 54.1 shows structures of the upper respiratory tract. Figure 54.2 displays the sites of action of these drugs.

ANTITUSSIVES

Antitussives are drugs that suppress the cough reflex (Table 54.1). Many disorders of the respiratory tract, including the common cold, sinusitis, pharyngitis and pneumonia, are accompanied by an uncomfortable, unproductive

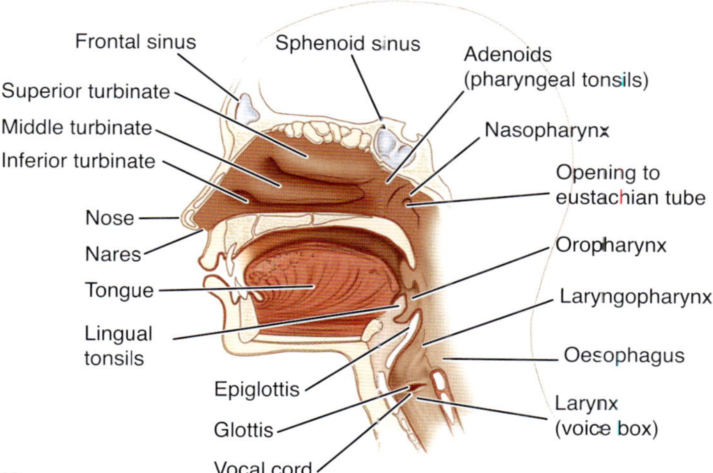

FIGURE 54.1 Structures of the upper respiratory tract.

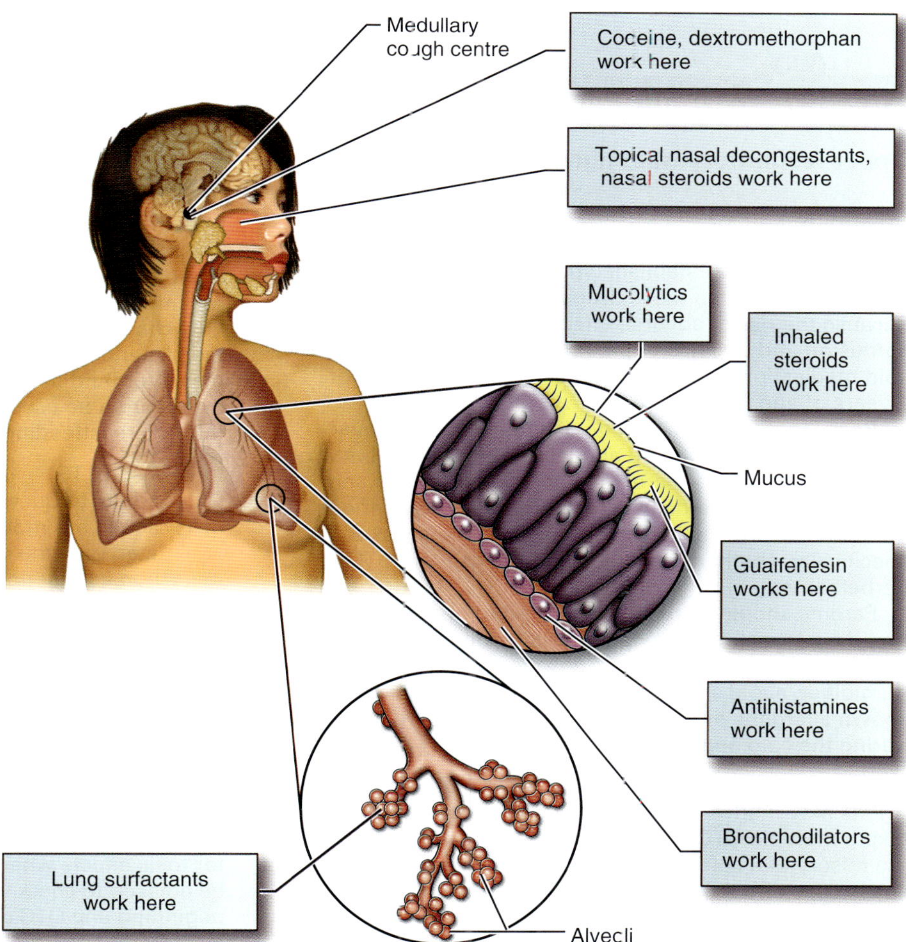

FIGURE 54.2 Sites of action of drugs acting on the upper respiratory tract.

TABLE 54.1 DRUGS IN FOCUS Antitussives

Drug name	Dosage/route	Usual indications
codeine (*Actacode*)	Linctus 5 mg/mL: adults 5 mL (25 mg) q 4–6 hours; contraindicated in children < 12 years Oral tablets: adults 15–30 mg q 6–8 hours; not indicated for children < 12 years	Treatment of non-productive cough
P dextromethorphan (*Bisolvon Dry, Robitussin Dry*)	Adult: 10–30 mg; maximum 4 doses a day Paediatric: 6–11 years: 5–15 mg; maximum 4 doses a day; use in children aged 6–11 years only on the advice of a doctor, pharmacist or nurse practitioner; do not use in children < 6 years	Treatment of non-productive cough
pentoxyverine (*Nyal Dry Cough Medicine*)	Adults: 10 mL tds or qid Paediatric (6–12 years): 5 mL on medical advice only	Treatment of non-productive cough
pholcodine (*Duro-Tuss*)	Adult: 5–15 mg; maximum 4 doses /day Paediatric, 6–12 years: 6–9 mg; maximum 4 doses/day (only on medical advice); do not use in children < 6 years	Treatment of non-productive cough

cough. Persistent coughing can be exhausting and can cause muscle strain and further irritation of the respiratory tract. A cough that occurs without the presence of any active disease process or persists after treatment may be a symptom of another disease process and should be investigated before any medication is given to alleviate it. Box 54.1 discusses the use of antitussives and other drugs acting on the upper respiratory tract in various age groups.

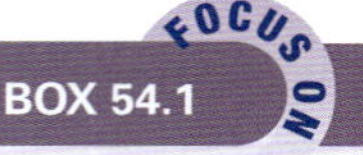

BOX 54.1 Drug therapy across the lifespan

Upper respiratory tract agents

CHILDREN

These drugs are used frequently with children. Most of these agents have established paediatric guidelines. Care must be taken when these drugs are used with children because the risk of adverse effects – including sedation, confusion and dizziness – are more common. Cough and cold medications should not be used in children under 2 years of age.

Because many of these agents are available in over-the-counter (OTC) cold, flu and allergy remedies, it is very important to educate parents about reading labels and following dosing guidelines to avoid potentially serious accidental overdose. Parents should always be asked specifically whether they are giving the child an OTC or herbal remedy.

Parents should also be encouraged to implement non-drug measures to help the child cope with the upper respiratory problem – drink plenty of fluids, use a humidifier, avoid smoke-filled areas, avoid contact with known allergens or irritants, and wash hands frequently during the cold and flu season.

ADULTS

Adults may inadvertently overdose on these agents when taking multiple OTC preparations to help them get through the misery of a cold or flu. They need to be questioned specifically about the use of OTC or herbal remedies before any of these drugs are advised or administered. Adults can also be encouraged to use non-drug measures to help them cope with the signs and symptoms.

PREGNANCY AND BREASTFEEDING

The safety for the use of these drugs during pregnancy and breastfeeding has not been established. There is a potential for adverse effects on the fetus related to blood flow changes and direct drug effects when the drugs cross the placenta. The drugs may enter breast milk and also may alter fluid balance and milk production. It is advised that caution be used if one of these drugs is prescribed during breastfeeding.

OLDER ADULTS

Older adults frequently are prescribed one of these drugs. Older adults are more likely to develop adverse effects associated with the use of these drugs, including sedation, confusion and dizziness. Safety measures may be needed if these effects occur and interfere with the person's mobility and balance.

Older adults are also more likely to have renal and/or hepatic impairment related to underlying medical conditions, which could interfere with the metabolism and excretion of these drugs. The dose for older adults should be started at a lower level than recommended for younger adults. The person should be monitored very closely, and dose adjustment should be based on the person's response.

These people also need to be alerted to the potential for toxic effects when using OTC preparations and should be advised to check with their health care provider before beginning any OTC drug regimen.

Therapeutic actions and indications

The traditional antitussives include codeine (*Actacode*), dextromethorphan (*Bisolvon Dry*, *Robitussin Dry* and many others) and pholcodine (*Duro-Tuss*), which act directly on the medullary cough centre of the brain to depress the cough reflex. Because they are centrally acting, they are not the drugs of choice for anyone who has a head injury or who could be impaired by central nervous system (CNS) depression.

Other antitussives have a direct effect on the respiratory tract. All of these drugs are indicated for the treatment of non-productive cough.

Pharmacokinetics

Codeine and dextromethorphan are rapidly absorbed, metabolised in the liver and excreted in urine. They cross the placenta and enter breast milk. These drugs should not be used in pregnancy and breastfeeding (see Contraindications and cautions).

Contraindications and cautions

Antitussives are contraindicated in people who need to cough to maintain the airways (eg, postoperative persons and those who have undergone abdominal or thoracic surgery) *to avoid respiratory distress*. Careful use is recommended for people with asthma and emphysema *because cough suppression in these people could lead to an accumulation of secretions and a loss of respiratory reserve*. Caution should also be used in people who are hypersensitive to, or have a history of, addiction to narcotics (codeine). *Codeine is a narcotic and has addiction potential*. People who need to drive or to be alert should use codeine and dextromethorphan with extreme caution *because these drugs can cause sedation and drowsiness*. This drug should not be used during pregnancy and breastfeeding *because of the potential for adverse effects on the fetus or baby, including sedation and CNS depression*.

Adverse effects

Traditional antitussives have a drying effect on the mucous membranes and can increase the viscosity of respiratory tract secretions. Because they affect centres in the brain, these antitussives are associated with CNS adverse effects, including drowsiness and sedation. Their drying effect can lead to nausea, constipation and complaints of dry mouth. The locally acting antitussives are associated with gastrointestinal (GI) upset, headache, feelings of congestion and sometimes dizziness.

Drug–drug interactions

Dextromethorphan should not be used with monoamine oxidase (MAO) inhibitors; hypotension, fever, nausea, myoclonic jerks and coma could occur.

Prototype summary: dextromethorphan

Indications: control of non-productive cough.

Actions: depresses the cough centre in the medulla to control cough spasms.

Pharmacokinetics:

Route	Onset	Peak	Duration
Oral	25–30 min	2 hours	3–6 hours

$T_{1/2}$: 2–4 hours; metabolised in the liver and excreted in urine.

Adverse effects: dizziness, respiratory depression, dry mouth.

Pholcodine increases the risk of intraoperative anaphylaxis due to neuromuscular-blocking agents (NMBAs) (eg, suxamethonium). Anaphylactic reactions to NMBAs have been observed in patients without previous exposure to NMBAs. The quaternary ammonium ion in NMBAs was found to be the allergenic portion (epitope) that allows binding of immunoglobulin E (IgE), causing IgE-mediated anaphylaxis. Pholcodine contains a tertiary ammonium ion that can cause production of IgE against the quaternary ammonium ions in NMBAs. Consumption of pholcodine therefore has a potential sensitising effect to NMBAs.

Care considerations for people receiving antitussives

Assessment: history and examination

- Assess for *possible contraindications or cautions*: any history of allergy to any component of the drug or **drug vehicle** *to avoid allergic reactions*; cough that persists longer than 1 week or is accompanied by other signs and symptoms, *which could indicate a serious underlying medical condition that should be addressed before suppressing symptoms*; and pregnancy or breastfeeding *because of the potential for adverse effects on the fetus or baby*.
- Perform a physical examination *to establish baseline data for assessing the effectiveness of the drug and the occurrence of any adverse effects associated with drug therapy*.
- Monitor temperature *to evaluate for possible underlying infection*.
- Assess respirations and adventitious sounds *to assess drug effectiveness and to monitor for accumulation of secretions*.
- Evaluate orientation and affect *to monitor for CNS effects of the drug*.

Implementation with rationale

- Ensure that the drug is not taken any longer than recommended *to prevent serious adverse effects and increased respiratory tract problems.*
- Arrange for further medical evaluation for coughs that persist or are accompanied by high fever, rash or excessive secretions *to detect the underlying cause and to arrange for appropriate treatment of the underlying problem.*
- Provide other measures *to help relieve cough* (eg, humidity, cool temperatures, fluids, use of topical lozenges) as appropriate.
- Provide thorough teaching, including the drug name and prescribed dosage, measures to help avoid adverse effects, warning signs that may indicate problems and the need for periodic monitoring and evaluation, *to enhance knowledge about drug therapy and to promote compliance.*
- Offer support and encouragement *to help the person cope with the disease and the drug regimen.*

Evaluation

- Monitor response to the drug (control of non-productive cough).
- Monitor for adverse effects (respiratory depression, dizziness, sedation).
- Evaluate the effectiveness of the teaching plan (person can name drug, dosage, adverse effects to watch for, specific measures to avoid them and measures to take to increase the effectiveness of the drug).
- Monitor the effectiveness of other measures to relieve cough.

KEY POINTS

- Antitussive drugs suppress the cough reflex by acting centrally to suppress the medullary cough centre to increase secretion and buffer irritation.
- Antitussive drugs can cause CNS depression, including drowsiness and sedation.
- Antitussive drugs should be used with caution in any situation in which coughing could be important for clearing the airways.

DECONGESTANTS

Decongestants decrease the overproduction of secretions by causing local vasoconstriction to the upper respiratory tract (Table 54.2). This vasoconstriction leads to a shrinking of swollen mucous membranes and tends to open clogged nasal passages, providing relief from the discomfort of a blocked nose and promoting drainage of secretions and improved airflow. An adverse effect that accompanies frequent or prolonged use of these drugs is a **rebound congestion**, technically called **rhinitis medicamentosa**. The reflex reaction to vasoconstriction is a rebound vasodilation, which often leads to prolonged overuse of decongestants.

Decongestants are usually adrenergics or sympathomimetics (see Chapter 30). Topical steroids are also used as decongestants, although they take several weeks to be really effective and are more often used in cases of chronic rhinitis.

TOPICAL NASAL DECONGESTANTS

The topical nasal decongestants include ephedrine (*generic*), oxymetazoline (*Dimetapp*, *Drixine* and others), phenylephrine (*Nyal*) and xylometazoline (*FLO Xylo-POS*). Many of these are available as over-the-counter (OTC) preparations. The choice of a topical nasal decongestant varies with the individual. Some people may have no response to one and respond very well to another.

Therapeutic actions and indications

Topical decongestants are sympathomimetics, meaning that they imitate the effects of the sympathetic nervous system to cause vasoconstriction, leading to decreased oedema and inflammation of the nasal membranes. They are available as nasal sprays that are used to relieve the discomfort of nasal congestion that accompanies the common cold, sinusitis and allergic rhinitis. These drugs can also be used when dilation of the nares is desired to facilitate medical examination or to relieve the pain and congestion of otitis media. Opening the nasal passage allows better drainage of the eustachian tube, relieving pressure in the middle ear. See Table 54.2 for usual indications for each of these agents.

Pharmacokinetics

Because these drugs are applied topically, the onset of action is almost immediate and there is less chance of systemic effects. Although they are not generally absorbed systemically, any portion of these topical decongestants that is absorbed is metabolised in the liver and excreted in urine. See Box 54.2 for tips on how to teach a person to use these medications.

Contraindications and cautions

Caution should be used when there is any lesion or erosion in the mucous membranes *that could lead to systemic absorption*. Caution should also be used in

TABLE 54.2 DRUGS IN FOCUS Decongestants

Drug name	Dosage/route	Usual indications
Topical nasal decongestants		
(P) ephedrine (extemporaneous preparation)	Instil solution in each nostril q 4 hours, do not use for children < 6 years unless advised by doctor	Relieves discomfort of nasal congestion associated with the common cold, sinusitis, allergic rhinitis; relieves pressure of otitis media
oxymetazoline (*Dimetapp, Drixine*)	Adults and paediatric > 6 years: nasal spray and pump spray, 1–3 sprays in each nostril bd; maximum 2 doses/24 hours for a maximum of 3 days	Relieves discomfort of nasal congestion associated with the common cold, sinusitis, allergic rhinitis
phenylephrine (*Nyal*)	Adults and paediatric > 12 years: nasal spray, 1 spray, each nostril q 3–4 hours	Relieves discomfort of nasal congestion associated with the common cold, sinusitis, allergic rhinitis
xylometazoline (*FLO Xylo-POS*)	Adult, spray: 1 spray bid–tid Adult, drops: 2–3 drops bid–tid Paediatric, 6–11 years: junior spray, 2 sprays bid–tid; or junior drops, 2–3 drops bid–tid All forms: no more than q 8–10 hours	Relieves discomfort of nasal congestion associated with the common cold, sinusitis, allergic rhinitis; relieves pressure of otitis media
Oral decongestant		
(P) pseudoephedrine (*Sudafed*)	Adult and paediatric > 12 years: oral tablets (60 mg): 1 tablet tid–qid; maximum 4 tablets per 24 hours for a maximum of 7 days; prolonged-release tablets (120 mg): 1 tablet q 12 hours; maintenance: 1 tablet q 24 hours for for a maximum of 7 days	Decreases nasal congestion associated with the common cold, allergic rhinitis; relief of pain and congestion of otitis media
Topical steroid nasal decongestants		
beclomethasone (*Alanase, Becloclear, Beconase, Beconase Hayfever*)	Adult: 1–2 inhalations in each nostril bd Paediatric (6–11 years): one inhalation in each nostril bd	Treatment of seasonal allergic rhinitis in people who are not obtaining a response with other decongestants or preparations; relieves inflammation following removal of nasal polyps
budesonide (*Butacort, Butamax, Eltair Forte, Rhinocort*)	Adults and paediatric > 6 years: nasal spray, 32 micrograms/dose, 2 sprays in each nostril morning and evening or 4 sprays in each nostril in the morning; nasal spray, 64 micrograms/dose, 1 spray in each nostril morning and evening or 2 sprays in each nostril in the morning	Treatment of seasonal allergic rhinitis in people who are not obtaining a response with other decongestants or preparations; relieves inflammation following removal of nasal polyps
fluticasone (*Avamys, Flixonase*)	Adults and paediatric > 12 years: initially 2 sprays in each nostril once daily Paediatric 2–11 years: 1 spray in each nostril per day (*Avamys* only)	Treatment of seasonal allergic rhinitis in people who are not obtaining a response with other decongestants or preparations; relieves inflammation following removal of nasal polyps
triamcinolone (*Telnase*)	Adult: two sprays in each nostril every day	Treatment of seasonal allergic rhinitis in people who are not obtaining a response with other decongestants or preparations; relieves inflammation following removal of nasal polyps

people with any condition that might be exacerbated by sympathetic activity, such as glaucoma, hypertension, diabetes, thyroid disease, coronary disease or prostate problems, *because these agents have adrenergic properties. Because there are no studies regarding the effects of these topical drugs in pregnancy or breastfeeding,* if used during pregnancy or breastfeeding, caution is advised.

Adverse effects

Adverse effects associated with topical decongestants include local stinging and burning, which may occur the first few times the drug is used. If the sensation does not pass, the drug should be discontinued because this may indicate lesions or erosion of the mucous membranes. Use for longer than 3–5 days can lead to rebound

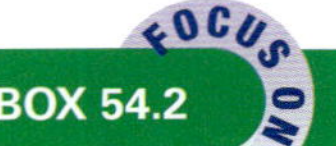

BOX 54.2 Individual and family teaching

Administering nasal medications

Proper administration technique is very important for assuring that drugs given nasally have the desired therapeutic effect. It is important to periodically check the nares for any signs of erosion or lesions, which could allow systemic absorption of the drug. Most people prefer to self-administer nasal drugs, so teaching is very important. Explain the technique, and then observe the person using the technique.

NASAL SPRAY

Teach the person to sit upright and press a finger over one naris to close it. Hold the spray bottle upright and place the tip of the bottle about 10–15 mm into the open naris. Firmly squeeze the bottle to deliver the drug. Caution the person not to squeeze too forcefully, which could send the drug up into the sinuses, causing more problems. Repeat with the other naris.

NASAL AEROSOL

Teach the person to place the medication cartridge into the plastic nasal adapter and shake it well. Remove the plastic cap from the applicator and place the tip inside the nostril. Have the person sit upright and tilt the head back. The person should firmly press on the canister once to deliver the drug, inhale, hold their breath for a few seconds, and then exhale. The person should be encouraged to keep the head tilted back for a few minutes and reminded not to blow their nose for at least 2 minutes.

congestion. (Rebound congestion occurs when the nasal passages become congested as the drug effect wears off. As a result, people tend to use more drug to decrease the congestion, thus initiating a vicious cycle of congestion–drug–congestion, which leads to abuse of the decongestant.) Sympathomimetic effects (eg, increased pulse and blood pressure; urinary retention) should be monitored because some systemic absorption may occur, although these effects are less likely with topical administration than with other routes.

Clinically important drug–drug interactions

The use of topical nasal decongestants is contraindicated with concurrent use of cyclopropane or halothane anaesthesia because serious cardiovascular effects could occur. Combined use with any other sympathomimetic drug or sympathetic-blocking drug could result in toxic or non-effective responses. Monitor the use of these combinations carefully.

Ⓟ Prototype summary: ephedrine

Indications: symptomatic relief of nasal and nasopharyngeal mucosal congestion due to the common cold, hay fever or other respiratory allergies; adjunctive therapy of middle-ear infections to decrease congestion around the eustachian ostia.

Actions: sympathomimetic effects, partly due to release of noradrenaline from nerve terminals; vasoconstriction leads to decreased oedema and inflammation of the nasal membranes.

Pharmacokinetics:

Route	Onset	Duration
Topical (nasal drops)	Immediate	4–6 hours

$T_{1/2}$: 0.4–0.7 hours; metabolised in the liver and excreted in urine; little is usually absorbed for systemic metabolism.

Adverse effects: disorientation, confusion, light-headedness, nausea, vomiting, fever, dyspnoea, rebound congestion.

Care considerations for people receiving topical nasal decongestants

Assessment: history and examination

- Assess for *possible contraindications or cautions*: any history of allergy to the drug or a component of the drug vehicle; glaucoma, hypertension, diabetes, thyroid disease, coronary disease and prostate problems, *all of which could be exacerbated by the sympathomimetic effects*; and pregnancy or breastfeeding, *which require cautious use of the drug.*
- Perform a physical examination *to establish baseline data for assessing the effectiveness of the drug and the occurrence of any adverse effects associated with drug therapy.*
- Assess skin colour and temperature *to assess sympathetic response.*
- Evaluate orientation and reflexes *to evaluate CNS effects of the drug.*
- Monitor pulse, blood pressure and cardiac auscultation *to assess cardiovascular and sympathomimetic effects.*
- Evaluate respirations and adventitious breath sounds *to assess the effectiveness of the drug and potential excess effect.*
- Perform bladder percussion *to monitor for urinary retention related to sympathomimetic effects.*
- Evaluate nasal mucous membranes *to monitor for lesions that could lead to systemic absorption and to evaluate decongestant effect.*

Implementation with rationale

- Teach person the proper administration of the drug *to ensure therapeutic effect* (see Box 54.2). The person should be instructed to clear the nasal passages before use, to tilt the head back when applying the drops or spray and to keep it tilted back for a few seconds after administration. This technique *helps to ensure contact with the affected mucous membranes and decreases the chances of letting the drops trickle down the back of the throat, which may lead to more systemic effects.*
- Caution the person not to use the drug for longer than 5 days and to seek medical care if signs and symptoms persist after that time *to facilitate detection of underlying medical conditions that may require treatment.*
- Caution the person that these drugs are found in many OTC preparations and that care should be taken not to inadvertently combine drugs with the same ingredients, *which could lead to overdose.*
- Provide safety measures if dizziness or sedation occurs as a result of drug therapy *to prevent injury.*
- Institute other measures *to help relieve the discomfort of congestion* (eg, humidity, increased fluid intake, cool environment, avoidance of smoke-filled areas) as appropriate.
- Provide thorough teaching, including the drug name and prescribed dosage, measures to help avoid adverse effects, warning signs that may indicate problems, and the need for periodic monitoring and evaluation, *to enhance knowledge about drug therapy and to promote compliance.*
- Offer support and encouragement *to help the person cope with the disease and the drug regimen.*

Evaluation

- Monitor response to the drug (relief of nasal congestion).
- Monitor for adverse effects (local burning and stinging; adrenergic effects such as increased pulse, blood pressure, urinary retention, cool and clammy skin).
- Evaluate the effectiveness of the teaching plan (person can name drug, dosage, adverse effects to watch for, specific measures to avoid them, measures to take to increase the effectiveness of the drug, proper administration technique).
- Monitor the effectiveness of comfort and safety measures and compliance with the regimen.

ORAL DECONGESTANTS

Oral decongestants currently available for use are phenylephrine (*Nyal*) and pseudoephedrine (*Sudafed* [and other forms with multiple active ingredients, eg, *Codral*, *Demazin* and *Logicin*]) (Table 54.2).

Therapeutic actions and indications

Oral decongestants are drugs that are taken orally to decrease nasal congestion related to the common cold, sinusitis and allergic rhinitis. They are also used to relieve the pain and congestion of otitis media. Opening of the nasal passage allows better drainage of the eustachian tube, relieving pressure in the middle ear.

Oral decongestants shrink the nasal mucous membrane by stimulating the alpha-adrenergic receptors in the nasal mucous membranes. This shrinkage results in a decrease in membrane size, promoting drainage of the sinuses and improving airflow.

Pharmacokinetics

Pseudoephedrine is generally well absorbed and reaches peak levels quickly – in 20–45 minutes. It is widely distributed in the body, metabolised in the liver and primarily excreted in urine.

Contraindications and cautions

Because pseudoephedrine has adrenergic properties, caution should be used in people with any condition *that might be exacerbated by sympathetic activity*, such as glaucoma, hypertension diabetes, thyroid disease, coronary disease and prostate problems. *Because there are no adequate studies about its use during pregnancy and breastfeeding*, such use should be reserved for situations in which the benefit to the mother outweighs any potential risk to the fetus or neonate.

Adverse effects

Adverse effects associated with pseudoephedrine include rebound congestion. Because this drug is taken systemically, adverse effects related to the sympathomimetic effects are more likely to occur, including feelings of anxiety, tenseness, restlessness, tremors, hypertension, arrhythmias, sweating and pallor. This drug is found in many OTC cold and flu preparations, and care must be taken to avoid inadvertent overdose when more than one such drug is used.

Clinically important drug–drug interactions

Many OTC products, including cold remedies, allergy medications and flu remedies, may contain pseudoephedrine. Taking many of these products concurrently can cause serious adverse effects. Educate people to read the OTC labels to avoid inadvertent overdose.

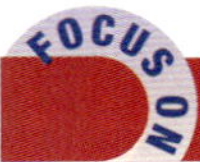

Safe medication administration

In 2001, preparations containing the oral decongestant phenylpropanolamine (PPA) were removed from the Australian market. This drug, which had been the centre of controversy for many years, was found to be associated with an increased number of strokes in young women in the US and many reports of severe high blood pressure in Australia. Some products reappeared on the market with the drug pseudoephedrine taking the place of PPA. This drug, a sympathomimetic, is also known to cause sympathetic effects, including increased blood pressure and increased heart rate. Close follow-up of the effects of this drug will be done to monitor for any increased risk associated with its use.

Prototype summary: pseudoephedrine

Indications: temporary relief of nasal congestion caused by the common cold, hay fever, sinusitis; promotion of nasal and sinus drainage; relief of eustachian tube congestion.

Actions: sympathomimetic effects, causes vasoconstriction in mucous membranes of nasal passages resulting in their shrinkage, which promotes drainage and improvement in ventilation.

Pharmacokinetics:

Route	Onset	Duration
Oral	30 min	4–6 hours

$T_{1/2}$: 7 hours; metabolised in the liver and excreted in urine.

Adverse effects: anxiety, restlessness, headache, dizziness, drowsiness, vision changes, seizures, hypertension, arrhythmias, pallor, nausea, vomiting, urinary retention, respiratory difficulty.

Care considerations for people receiving an oral decongestant

Assessment: history and examination

- Assess for *possible contraindications or cautions*: any history of allergy to the drug and pregnancy or breastfeeding, *which are contraindications to drug use*; hypertension or coronary artery disease, *which require cautious use*; and hyperthyroidism, diabetes mellitus or prostate enlargement, *all of which could be exacerbated by these drugs.*

BOX 54.3 Use of cough and cold medicines in children – Medsafe advice

The Cough and Cold Review Group have recommended to Medsafe that oral cough and cold medicines containing the following substances should not be used in children under six years of age:

- guaifenesin
- phenylephrine
- doxylamine
- ipecacuanha
- brompheniramine
- promethazine
- dextromethorphan
- chlorphenamine (chlorpheniramine)
- triprolidine
- pholcodine
- diphenhydramine
- pseudoephedrine

The Cough and Cold Review Group considered that the use of cough and cold medicines containing only bromhexine, or intranasal decongestants (such as oxymetazoline and xylometazoline) should be restricted to adults and children two years of age and over.

Source: New Zealand Formulary, http://nzformulary.org

- Perform a physical examination *to establish baseline data for assessing the effectiveness of the drug and the occurrence of any adverse effects associated with drug therapy.*
- Assess skin colour and lesions *to monitor for adverse reactions.*
- Evaluate orientation, reflexes and affect *to monitor CNS effects of the drug.*
- Monitor blood pressure, pulse and auscultation *to assess cardiovascular stimulations.*
- Evaluate respiration and adventitious sounds *to monitor drug effectiveness.*
- Monitor urinary output *to evaluate for urinary retention.*

Implementation with rationale

- Note that this drug is found in many OTC products, especially combination cold and allergy preparations; *care should be taken to prevent inadvertent overdose or excessive adverse effects.*
- Provide safety measures as needed if CNS effects occur *to prevent injury.*
- Monitor pulse, blood pressure and cardiac response to the drug, especially in people who are at risk for cardiac stimulation, *to detect adverse effects early and arrange to reduce dose or discontinue the drug.*

- Encourage the person not to use this drug for longer than 1 week, and to seek medical evaluation if symptoms persist after that time, *to encourage the detection of underlying medical conditions that could be causing these symptoms and to arrange for appropriate treatment.*
- Provide thorough teaching, including the drug name and prescribed dosage, measures to help avoid adverse effects, warning signs that may indicate problems and the need for periodic monitoring and evaluation, *to enhance knowledge about drug therapy and to promote compliance.*
- Offer support and encouragement *to help the person cope with the disease and the drug regimen.*

Evaluation

- Monitor response to the drug (improvement in nasal congestion).
- Monitor for adverse effects (sympathomimetic reactions, including increased pulse, blood pressure, pallor, sweating, arrhythmias, feelings of anxiety, tension, dry skin).
- Evaluate the effectiveness of the teaching plan (person can name drug, dosage, adverse effects to watch for, specific measures to avoid them and measures to take to increase the effectiveness of the drug).
- Monitor the effectiveness of comfort and safety measures and compliance with the regimen.

Topical nasal steroid decongestants

The topical nasal steroid decongestants (Table 54.2) include beclomethasone (*Beconase* and others), budesonide (*Butacort, Butamax, Eltair Forte, Rhinocort*), fluticasone (*Avamys, Flixonase*) and triamcinolone (*Telnase*).

Therapeutic actions and indications

Topical nasal steroid decongestants are very popular for the treatment of allergic rhinitis and to relieve inflammation after the removal of nasal polyps. They have been found to be effective in people who are no longer getting a response with other decongestants. The exact mechanism of action of topical steroids is not known. Their anti-inflammatory action results from their ability to produce a direct local effect that blocks many of the complex reactions responsible for the inflammatory response.

Pharmacokinetics

The onset of action is not immediate, and these drugs may actually require up to 1 week to cause any changes. If no effects are seen after 3 weeks, the drug should be discontinued. Because these drugs are not generally absorbed systemically, their pharmacokinetics are not reported. If they were to be absorbed systemically, they would have the same pharmacokinetics as other steroids (see Chapter 36).

Contraindications and cautions

Because nasal steroids block the inflammatory response, their use is contraindicated in the presence of acute infections. Increased incidence of *Candida albicans* infection has been reported with their use, related to the anti-inflammatory and anti-immune activities associated with steroids. Caution should be used in any person who has an active infection, including tuberculosis, *because systemic absorption would interfere with the inflammatory and immune responses.* People using nasal steroids should avoid exposure to any airborne infection, such as chickenpox or measles. As with all drugs, caution should always be used when taking these drugs during pregnancy or breastfeeding. Because the systemic absorption of these drugs is minimal, they are often used during pregnancy and breastfeeding.

Adverse effects

Because they are applied topically, there is less chance of systemic absorption and associated adverse effects. The most common adverse effects are local burning, irritation, stinging, dryness of the mucosa and headache. Because healing is suppressed by steroids, people who have recently experienced nasal surgery or trauma should be monitored closely until healing has occurred.

Care considerations for people receiving topical steroid nasal decongestants

Assessment: history and examination

- Assess for *possible contraindications or cautions*: any history of allergy to steroid drugs or any components of the drug vehicle, *which would be a contraindication*, and acute infection, *which would require cautious use.*
- Perform a physical examination *to establish baseline data for assessing the effectiveness of the drug and the occurrence of any adverse effects associated with drug therapy.*
- Perform an intranasal examination *to determine the presence of any lesions that would increase the risk of systemic absorption of the drug.*
- Assess respiration and adventitious sounds *to evaluate drug effectiveness.*
- Monitor temperature *to monitor for the possibility of acute infection.*

Implementation with rationale

- Teach the person how to administer these drugs properly, *which is very important to ensure effectiveness and prevent systemic effects.* A variety of preparations are available (eg, sprays, aerosols, powder discs). Advise the person about the proper administration technique for whichever preparation is recommended.
- Have the person clear the nasal passages before using the drug *to improve its effectiveness.*
- Encourage the person to continue using the drug regularly, even if results are not seen immediately, *because benefits may take 2–3 weeks to appear.*
- Monitor the person for the development of acute infection which would require medical intervention. Encourage the person to avoid areas where airborne infections could be a problem *because steroid use decreases the effectiveness of the immune and inflammatory responses.*
- Provide thorough teaching, including the drug name and prescribed dosage, measures to help avoid adverse effects, warning signs that may indicate problems and the need for periodic monitoring and evaluation, *to enhance knowledge about drug therapy and to promote compliance.*
- Offer support and encouragement *to help the person cope with the disease and the drug regimen.*

Evaluation

- Monitor response to the drug (relief of nasal congestion).
- Monitor for adverse effects (local burning and stinging).
- Evaluate the effectiveness of the teaching plan (person can name drug, dosage, adverse effects to watch for, specific measures to avoid them and measures to take to increase the effectiveness of the drug).
- Monitor the effectiveness of comfort and safety measures and compliance with the regimen.

KEY POINTS

- Decongestants cause local vasoconstriction, thereby reducing blood flow to the mucous membranes of the nasal passages and sinus cavities.
- Rebound vasodilation (rhinitis medicamentosa) is an adverse effect of excessive or long-term decongestant use.
- Topical nasal decongestants are preferred for people who need to avoid systemic adrenergic effects associated with oral decongestants.
- Topical nasal steroid decongestants block the inflammatory response and are preferred for people with allergic rhinitis for whom systemic steroid therapy is undesirable.

ANTIHISTAMINES

Antihistamines (Table 54.3) block the release or action of histamine, a chemical released during inflammation that increases secretions and narrows airways. Antihistamines are found in multiple OTC preparations that are designed to relieve respiratory symptoms and to treat allergies. When choosing an antihistamine, the individual person's reaction to the drug is usually the governing factor. Because first-generation antihistamines have greater anticholinergic effects, with resultant drowsiness, a person who needs to be alert should be given one of the second-generation, less-sedating antihistamines. Because of their OTC availability, these drugs are often misused to treat colds and influenza (see Box 54.4).

First-generation antihistamines include brompheniramine (*Dimetapp*), chlorphenamine (chlorpheniramine) (*Codral*, *Demazin* and others), cyproheptadine (*Periactin*), dexchlorpheniramine (*Polaramine*), diphenhydramine (*Benadryl* and others), pheniramine (*Avil)* and promethazine (*Avomine*, *Phenergan*).

Second-generation antihistamines include azelastine (*Azep*), cetirizine (*Razene*, *Zyrtec*), desloratadine (*Aerius*), fexofenadine (*Telfast*) and loratadine (*Claratyne*, *Lora-Tabs*).

Therapeutic actions and indications

The antihistamines selectively block the effects of histamine at the histamine-1-receptor sites, decreasing the allergic response. They also have anticholinergic (atropine-like) and antipruritic effects. Antihistamines are used for the relief of symptoms associated with seasonal and perennial allergic rhinitis, allergic conjunctivitis, uncomplicated urticaria and angioedema. They are also used for the reducing allergic reactions to blood or blood products, for relief of discomfort associated with dermographism and as adjunctive therapy in anaphylactic reactions. See Table 54.3 for usual indications for each of these agents. Other uses that are being explored include relief of exercise- and hyperventilation-induced asthma and histamine-induced bronchoconstriction in people with asthma. They are most effective if used before the onset of symptoms.

Pharmacokinetics

The antihistamines are well absorbed orally, with an onset of action ranging from 1 to 3 hours. They are generally metabolised in the liver, with excretion in faeces

TABLE 54.3 DRUGS IN FOCUS Antihistamines

Drug name	Dosage/route	Usual indications
First-generation		
brompheniramine (*Dimetapp*)	Adult and paediatric (> 12 years): multiple actives, no common dose: see manufacturer's instructions	Relief of symptoms of seasonal and perennial allergic rhinitis
chlorphenamine (chlorpheniramine) (*Codral*, *Demazin*)	Adult and paediatric (> 12 years): multiple actives, no common dose: see manufacturer's instructions	Relief of symptoms of seasonal and perennial allergic rhinitis, allergic conjunctivitis, uncomplicated urticaria and angioedema; reducing allergic reactions; relief of discomfort associated with dermographism; used as adjunctive therapy in anaphylactic reactions
cyproheptadine (*Periactin*)	Adult: 4–20 mg/day PO in divided doses Paediatric: 7–14 years: 4 mg PO tds; maximum 16 mg/day 2–6 years: 2 mg PO bd–tds	Relief of symptoms of seasonal and perennial allergic rhinitis, allergic conjunctivitis, uncomplicated urticaria and angioedema; reducing allergic reactions; relief of discomfort associated with dermographism; used as adjunctive therapy in anaphylactic reactions
dexchlorpheniramine (*Polaramine*)	Tablets, 2 mg, adults and paediatric > 12 years: 2 mg every 6 hours Syrup 2 mg/5 mL: adults and paediatric > 12 years: 5 mL q 6 hours; paediatric 2–4 years: 1.25–1.75 mL q 6–8 hours; paediatric 4–6 years: 1.75–2 mL q 6–8 hours; paediatric 6–12 years: 2–4 mL q 6–8 hours	Relief of symptoms of seasonal and perennial allergic rhinitis, allergic conjunctivitis, uncomplicated urticaria and angioedema; reducing allergic reactions; relief of discomfort associated with dermographism; used as adjunctive therapy in anaphylactic reactions
(P) diphenhydramine (*Benadryl*, others)	Adults, paediatric > 12 years: 25 mg of 12.5 mg/5 mL mixture Children 6–12 years: 12.5 mg of 12.5 mg/5 mL mixture Use caution with elderly people	Relief of symptoms of seasonal and perennial allergic rhinitis, allergic conjunctivitis, uncomplicated urticaria, and angioedema; reducing allergic reactions; relief of discomfort associated with dermographism; also used as adjunctive therapy in anaphylactic reactions, as a sleeping aid, and for parkinsonism
pheniramine (*Avil*)	Adult: half of 45.3 mg tablet PO up to tds increased to one tablet tds if necessary Paediatric (5–10 years): half of 45.3 mg tablet PO up to tds	Relief of symptoms of seasonal and perennial allergic rhinitis and conditions of the respiratory tract when increased secretions are present.
promethazine (*Phenergan*, *Avomine*)	Adult: 25–50 mg PO, IM or IV Paediatric: 6–12 years: 10–25 mg PO at night or 10 mg PO bid–tid	Relief of symptoms of seasonal and perennial allergic rhinitis, allergic conjunctivitis, uncomplicated urticaria, and angioedema; reducing allergic reactions; relief of discomfort associated with dermographism; used as adjunctive therapy in anaphylactic reactions; also used for sedation
Second-generation (non-sedating)		
azelastine (*Azep*)	One spray per nostril bd	Relief of symptoms of seasonal and perennial allergic rhinitis
cetirizine (*Zyrtec*, *Alzene*)	Adults, paediatric > 12 years: 10 mg once daily; may increase to a maximum of 20 mg once daily Paediatric 6–12 years: 5–10 mg daily Paediatric 2–6 years: 5 mg daily	Relief of symptoms of seasonal and perennial allergic rhinitis; management of chronic urticaria

Continued on following page

TABLE 54.3 DRUGS IN FOCUS Antihistamines *(continued)*

Drug name	Dosage/route	Usual indications
Second-generation *(continued)*		
desloratadine (*Aerius*)	Adults, paediatric > 12 years: 5 mg once daily; hepatic or renal impairment: 5 mg PO every other day Children 6–11 years: 2.5 mg once daily Children 1–5 years: 1.25 mg once daily Children 6 months–1 year: 1 mg once daily	Relief of symptoms of seasonal allergic rhinitis, chronic idiopathic urticaria
fexofenadine (*Telfast*)	Oral tablet 60 mg, 80 mg, 120 mg Suspension 6 mg/mL Adults, paediatric > 12 years: allergic rhinitis, 60 mg bd; seasonal allergic rhinitis, 120–180 mg once daily; urticaria, 180 mg once daily Children 6–11 years: 30 mg bd	Relief of symptoms of seasonal and perennial allergic rhinitis
loratadine (*Claratyne Lora-Tabs*)	Adult and paediatric (> 6 years): 10 mg/day PO Elderly or liver-impaired person: 5 mg PO daily or 10 mg every 2nd day Paediatric 2–12 years, > 30 kg: 10 mg/day; ≤ 30 kg: 5 mg/day Paediatric 1–2 years: 2.5 mg/day	Relief of symptoms of seasonal and perennial allergic rhinitis, allergic conjunctivitis, uncomplicated urticaria and angioedema; reducing allergic reactions; relief of discomfort associated with dermographism; and as an adjunctive therapy in anaphylactic reactions

and urine. These drugs cross the placenta and enter breast milk (see Contraindications and cautions).

Contraindications and cautions

Antihistamines are contraindicated during pregnancy or breastfeeding *unless the benefit to the mother clearly outweighs the potential risk to the fetus or baby*. They should be used with caution in renal or hepatic impairment, *which could alter the metabolism and excretion of the drug*. Antihistamines are excreted in human milk and so are not recommended in breastfeeding women. Box 54.4 presents topics for parent education in the use of these OTC products.

Adverse effects

The adverse effects most often seen with antihistamine use are drowsiness and sedation (*see Critical thinking scenario for additional information*), although second-generation antihistamines are less sedating in many people. The anticholinergic effects that can be anticipated include drying of the respiratory and GI mucous membranes, GI upset and nausea, arrhythmias, dysuria, urinary hesitancy, and skin eruption and itching

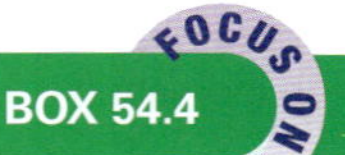

BOX 54.4 Individual and family teaching

Following reports of serious and even fatal adverse effects when OTC cough and cold medicines were used in children under the age of 2 years, the U.S. Food and Drug Administration (FDA) held meetings to evaluate the safety and efficacy of the use of these products in young children. In early 2008, it completed its review and came out with recommendations that these products should not be used in children 2 years of age and younger. While continued research looks at the efficacy and safety of these products for children 2–11 years of age, the FDA suggests that parents be instructed in the safe use of OTC cough and cold products. Parents should be taught the following:

- Do not give OTC cough and cold products to children younger than 2 years of age unless specifically instructed to do so by a health care provider.
- Do not give your child OTC cough and cold medicines made for adults; look for the children's, infant's or paediatric use on the label.
- Always check the 'active ingredients' on the drug label.
- Be very careful if you are giving your child more than one cough and cold medicine; they may contain the same active ingredients and overdose can occur.
- Carefully follow the directions in the 'drug facts' section of the label and follow the directions for how often you can give the drug.
- Use the measuring spoons or cups that come with the medicine; do not use household spoons, which can vary widely in the amount of medicine they hold.
- Use OTC cough and cold medicines with childproof caps and keep them out of the reach of children to avoid possible overdose.
- Consult with your health care provider; these drugs only treat signs and symptoms and do not cure any disease; contact your health care provider if the symptoms get worse.
- Do not use these products to make your child sleepy.
- Tell any health care provider taking care of your child the names of any OTC products that you are giving your child.

associated with dryness. Children and the elderly are more susceptible to adverse effects; paradoxical stimulation may occur, although rarely.

Drug–drug interactions

Drug–drug interactions vary among the antihistamines; for example, anticholinergic effects may be prolonged if diphenhydramine is taken with an MAO inhibitor, and the interaction of fexofenadine with erythromycin may raise fexofenadine concentrations to toxic levels. For more information, consult a nursing drug handbook or package insert for individual details.

Prototype summary: diphenhydramine

Indications: symptomatic relief of perennial and seasonal rhinitis, vasomotor rhinitis, allergic conjunctivitis, urticaria, and angioedema; also used for treating motion sickness and parkinsonism and as a night-time sleep aid and to suppress coughs.

Actions: competitively blocks the effects of histamine at H_1-receptor sites; has atropine-like antipruritic and sedative effects.

Pharmacokinetics:

Route	Onset	Peak	Duration
Oral	15–30 min	1–4 hours	4–7 hours
IM	20–30 min	1–4 hours	4–8 hours
IV	Rapid	30–60 min	4–8 hours

$T_{1/2}$: 2.5–7 hours; metabolised in the liver and excreted in urine.

Adverse effects: drowsiness, sedation, dizziness, epigastric distress, thickening of bronchial secretions, urinary frequency, rash, bradycardia.

Care considerations for people receiving antihistamines

Assessment: history and examination

- Assess for *possible contraindications or cautions*: any history of allergy to antihistamines; pregnancy or breastfeeding, *which are contraindications to the use of the drug*; and renal or hepatic impairment, *which requires cautious use of the drug.*
- Perform a physical examination *to establish baseline data for assessing the effectiveness of the drug and the occurrence of any adverse effects associated with drug therapy.*
- Assess the skin colour, texture and lesions *to monitor for anticholinergic effects or allergy.*
- Evaluate orientation, affect and reflexes *to monitor for changes due to CNS effects.*
- Assess respirations and adventitious sounds *to monitor drug effects.*
- Evaluate liver and renal function tests *to monitor for factors that could affect the metabolism or excretion of the drug.*

Implementation with rationale

- Administer drug on an empty stomach, 1 hour before or 2 hours after meals, *to increase the absorption of the drug*; the drug may be given with meals if GI upset is a problem.
- Note that person may have poor response to one of these agents but a very effective response to another; the prescriber may need to try several different agents *to find the one that is most effective.*
- Because of the drying nature of antihistamines, people often experience dry mouth, which may lead to nausea and anorexia; suggest sugarless lollies or lozenges *to relieve some of this discomfort.*
- Provide safety measures as appropriate if CNS effects occur *to prevent injury.*
- Increase humidity and push fluids *to decrease the problem of thickened secretions and dry nasal mucosa.*
- Have person void before each dose *to decrease urinary retention if this is a problem.*
- Provide skin care as needed if skin dryness and lesions become a problem *to prevent skin breakdown.*
- Caution the person to avoid excessive doses and to check OTC drugs for the presence of antihistamines, *which are found in many OTC preparations and could cause toxicity.*
- Caution the person to avoid alcohol while taking these drugs *because serious sedation can occur.*
- Provide thorough teaching, including the drug name and prescribed dosage, measures to help avoid adverse effects, warning signs that may indicate problems and the need for periodic monitoring and evaluation, *to enhance knowledge about drug therapy and to promote compliance.*
- Offer support and encouragement *to help the person cope with the disease and the drug regimen.*

Evaluation

- Monitor response to the drug (relief of the symptoms of allergic rhinitis).
- Monitor for adverse effects (skin dryness, GI upset, sedation and drowsiness, urinary retention, thickened secretions, glaucoma).

- Evaluate the effectiveness of the teaching plan (person can name drug, dosage, adverse effects to watch for, specific measures to avoid them and measures to take to increase the effectiveness of the drug).
- Monitor the effectiveness of comfort and safety measures and compliance with the regimen.

KEY POINTS

- The antihistamines selectively block the effects of histamine at the histamine-1-receptor sites, decreasing the allergic response. Antihistamines are used for the relief of symptoms associated with seasonal and perennial allergic rhinitis, allergic conjunctivitis, uncomplicated urticaria and angioedema.
- People taking antihistamines may react to dryness of the skin and mucous membranes. The carer should encourage them to drink plenty of fluids, use a humidifier if possible, avoid smoke-filled rooms, and use good skin care and moisturisers.
- Antihistamines should be avoided with any person who has a prolonged QT interval because serious cardiac complications and even death have occurred.

EXPECTORANTS

Expectorants (Table 54.4) increase productive cough to clear the airways. They liquefy lower respiratory tract secretions, reducing the viscosity of these secretions and making it easier for the person to cough them up. Expectorants are available in many OTC preparations, making them widely available without advice from a health care provider. The only available expectorant is guaifenesin (*Robitussin* and others), although a number of plant-derived preparations, such as liquorice and senega, are also used for this purpose.

Therapeutic actions and indications

Guaifenesin enhances the output of respiratory tract fluids by reducing the adhesiveness and surface tension of these fluids, allowing easier movement of the less viscous

CRITICAL THINKING SCENARIO

Dangers of self-medicating for seasonal rhinitis

THE SITUATION

K.E. is a 46-year-old businessman who has been self-treating for seasonal rhinitis and a cold. His wife calls the doctor's office; she is concerned that her husband is dizzy, has lost his balance several times and is very drowsy. He is unable to drive to work or to stay awake. She wants to take him to the emergency department of the local hospital.

CRITICAL THINKING

What is the best approach for this person?

What crucial personal history questions should you ask before proceeding any further?

If you do not know this person, given his presenting story, what medical conditions would need to be ruled out before proceeding further?

If K.E. is self-medicating for the signs and symptoms of seasonal rhinitis, what could be causing his drowsiness and dizziness?

What teaching points should be emphasised with this person and his wife?

DISCUSSION

The first impression of K.E.'s condition is that it is a neurological disorder. K.E. should be evaluated by a health care provider to rule out significant neurological problems. However, after a careful history and physical examination, K.E.'s condition seemed to be related to high levels of OTC medications.

There are a multitude of OTC cold and allergy remedies, most of which contain the same ingredients in varying proportions. A person may be taking one to stop nasal drip, another to help a cough, another to relieve congestion, and so on. By combining OTC medications like this, a person is at great risk for inadvertently overdosing or at least allowing the medication to reach toxic levels.

In this situation, the first thing to determine is exactly what medication is being taken and how often. K.E. seems to have received toxic levels of antihistamines, decongestants or other upper respiratory tract agents. The nurse should encourage K.E. – and everyone seen – to check the labels of any OTC medications being taken and to check with the health care provider if there are any questions. K.E. and his wife should receive written information about the drugs that K.E. is taking. They also should be shown how to read OTC bottles or boxes for information on the contents of various preparations. In addition, they should be encouraged to use alternative methods to relieve the discomfort of seasonal rhinitis (eg, using a humidifier, drinking lots of liquids, avoiding smoky areas) to allay the belief that many OTC drugs are needed. Finally, K.E. and his wife should be advised to check with their health care provider if they have any questions about OTC or prescription drugs or if they have continued problems coping with seasonal allergic reactions. Other prescription medication may prove more effective.

CARE GUIDE FOR K.E.: ANTIHISTAMINES

Assessment: history and examination

Assess K.E.'s health history for allergies and GI stenosis or obstruction, bladder obstruction, narrow-angle glaucoma, benign prostatic hypertrophy, and concurrent use of MAO inhibitors and OTC allergy or cold products.

Focus the physical examination on the following areas:

Neurological: orientation, reflexes, affect, coordination

Skin: lesions

Cardiovascular: blood pressure, pulse, peripheral perfusion

Gastrointestinal: bowel sounds, abdominal examination

Haematological: full blood count

Respiratory: respiratory rate and character, nares, adventitious sounds

Genitourinary: urinary output

Implementation

Provide comfort and safety measures, for example, give drug with meals; teach about mouth care; increase humidity; institute safety measures if dizziness occurs.

Provide support and reassurance to deal with drug effects and allergy.

Provide teaching regarding drug name, dosage, adverse effects, precautions and warning signs to report.

Evaluation

Evaluate drug effects, that is, relief of respiratory symptoms.

Monitor for adverse effects: CNS effects, thickening of secretions, urinary retention, glaucoma.

Monitor for drug–drug interactions as indicated.

Evaluate the effectiveness of support and encouragement strategies, teaching program, and comfort and safety measures.

TEACHING FOR K.E.

- Antihistamines are commonly used to treat the signs and symptoms of various allergic reactions. Because these drugs work throughout the body, the first generation of antihistamines were associated with many systemic effects (eg, dry mouth, dizziness, drowsiness).
- Take this drug only as prescribed. Do not increase the dose if symptoms are not relieved. Instead, consult your health care provider.
- Common effects of this drug include:
  - *Drowsiness, dizziness:* do not drive or operate dangerous machinery if this occurs. Use caution to prevent injury.
  - *Gastrointestinal upset, nausea, vomiting, heartburn:* taking the drug with food may help this problem.
  - *Dry mouth:* frequent mouth care and sucking sugarless lozenges may help.
  - *Thickening of the mucus, difficulty coughing, tightening of the chest:* use a humidifier or, if you do not have one, place pans of water throughout the house to increase the humidity of the room air; avoid smoke-filled areas; drink plenty of fluids.
- Report any of the following to your health care provider: *difficulty breathing, rash, hives, difficulty in voiding, abdominal pain, visual changes, disorientation or confusion.*
- Avoid the use of alcoholic beverages while you are taking this drug. Serious drowsiness or sedation can occur if these are combined.
- Avoid the use of any OTC medication without first checking with your health care provider. Several of these medications contain drugs that can interfere with the effectiveness of this drug or they can contain very similar drugs and you could experience toxic effects.
- Tell any doctor, nurse or other health care provider involved in your care that you are taking this drug.
- Take this drug only as prescribed. Do not give this drug to anyone else, and do not take similar preparations that have been prescribed for someone else. Keep this drug, and all medications, out of the reach of children.

secretions. The result of this thinning of secretions is a more productive cough and thus decreased frequency of coughing. See Table 54.4 for usual indications.

Pharmacokinetics

Guaifenesin is rapidly absorbed, with an onset of 30 minutes and duration of 4–6 hours. Sites of metabolism and excretion have not been reported.

Contraindications

This drug should not be used in people with a known allergy to the drug *to prevent hypersensitivity reactions*, and it should be used with caution in pregnancy and breastfeeding *because of the potential for adverse effects on the fetus or baby* and with persistent coughs, *which could be indicative of underlying medical problems.*

Adverse effects

The most common adverse effects associated with expectorants are GI symptoms (eg, nausea, vomiting, anorexia). Some people experience headache or dizziness, or both; occasionally, a mild rash develops. The most important consideration in the use of these drugs is discovering the cause of the underlying cough. Prolonged

TABLE 54.4 **DRUGS IN FOCUS** Expectorant

Drug name	Dosage/route	Usual indications
Ⓟ guaifenesin (*Robitussin, Vicks*)	Adults, paediatric > 12 years: 200–400 mg q 4 hours; maximum 1200 mg/day Children 6–11 years: 166 mg (Vicks), or 200 mg (Robitussin) q 4 hours; maximum 6 doses in 24 hours	Symptomatic relief of respiratory conditions characterised by a dry, non-productive cough, including the common cold, acute bronchitis and influenza

use of the OTC preparations could result in the masking of important symptoms of a serious underlying disorder. These drugs should not be used for more than 1 week; if the cough persists, encourage the person to seek health care.

Ⓟ Prototype summary: guaifenesin

Indications: symptomatic relief of respiratory conditions characterised by dry, non-productive cough and in the presence of mucus in the respiratory tract.

Actions: enhances the output of respiratory tract fluid by reducing the adhesiveness and surface tension of the fluid, facilitating the removal of viscous mucus.

Pharmacokinetics:

Route	Onset	Peak	Duration
Oral	30 min	Unknown	4–6 hours

$T_{1/2}$: unknown; metabolism and excretion are also unknown.

Adverse effects: nausea, vomiting, headache, dizziness, rash.

Care considerations for people receiving expectorants

Assessment: history and examination

- Assess for *possible contraindications or cautions*: any history of allergy to the drug; persistent cough due to smoking, asthma or emphysema, *which would be cautions to the use of the drug*; and very productive cough, *which would indicate an underlying problem that should be evaluated.*
- Perform a physical examination *to establish baseline data for assessing the effectiveness of the drug and the occurrence of any adverse effects associated with drug therapy.*
- Assess the skin *for the presence of lesions and colour to monitor for any adverse reactions.*
- Monitor temperature *to assess for an underlying infection.*
- Assess respirations and adventitious sounds *to evaluate the respiratory response to the drug effects.*
- Monitor orientation and affect *to monitor CNS effects of the drug.*

Implementation with rationale

- Caution the person not to use these drugs for longer than 1 week and to seek medical attention if the cough persists after that time *to evaluate for any underlying medical condition and to arrange for appropriate treatment.*
- Advise the person to take small, frequent meals *to alleviate some of the GI discomfort associated with these drugs.*
- Advise the person to avoid driving or performing dangerous tasks if dizziness and drowsiness occur *to prevent injury.*
- Alert the person that these drugs may be found in OTC preparations and that care should be taken *to avoid excessive doses.*
- Provide thorough teaching, including the drug name and prescribed dosage, measures to help avoid adverse effects, warning signs that may indicate problems and the need for periodic monitoring and evaluation, *to enhance knowledge about drug therapy and to promote compliance.*
- Offer support and encouragement *to help the person cope with the disease and the drug regimen.*

Evaluation

- Monitor response to the drug (improved effectiveness of cough).
- Monitor for adverse effects (skin rash, GI upset, CNS effects).
- Evaluate the effectiveness of the teaching plan (person can name drug, dosage, adverse effects to watch for, specific measures to avoid them and measures to take to increase the effectiveness of the drug).
- Monitor the effectiveness of comfort and safety measures and compliance with the regimen.

KEY POINTS

- Expectorants are drugs that liquefy the lower respiratory tract secretions. They are used for the symptomatic relief of respiratory conditions characterised by a dry, non-productive cough.
- Guaifenesin is the only expectorant currently available. Care should be taken to avoid inadvertent overdose when using OTC products that might contain this drug.

MUCOLYTICS

Mucolytics (Table 54.5) increase or liquefy respiratory secretions to aid the clearing of the airways in high-risk respiratory people who are coughing up thick, tenacious secretions. People may be suffering from conditions such as chronic obstructive pulmonary disease (COPD), cystic fibrosis, pneumonia or tuberculosis. Mucolytics include acetylcysteine (*Mucomyst* and others), bromhexine (*Bisolvon*) and dornase alfa (*Pulmozyme*).

Therapeutic actions and indications

Acetylcysteine is used orally to protect liver cells from being damaged during episodes of paracetamol toxicity because it normalises hepatic glutathione levels and binds with a reactive hepatotoxic metabolite of acetaminophen. Acetylcysteine affects the mucoproteins in the respiratory secretions by splitting apart disulfide bonds that are responsible for holding the mucus material together. The result is a decrease in the tenacity and viscosity of the secretions. See Table 54.5 for usual indications.

Bromhexine reduces viscosity of secretions and activates ciliated epithelium, facilitating expectoration.

Dornase alfa is a mucolytic prepared by recombinant DNA techniques that selectively breaks down respiratory tract mucus by separating extracellular DNA from proteins. It is used in cystic fibrosis, which is characterised by thick, tenacious mucus production. See Table 54.5 for usual indications.

Pharmacokinetics

The medication may be administered by nebulisation or by direct instillation into the trachea via an endotracheal tube or tracheostomy.

Acetylcysteine is metabolised in the liver and excreted somewhat in urine. It is not known whether it crosses the placenta or enters breast milk. Bromhexine is completely absorbed in the GI tract. It crosses the blood brain barrier and a small amount crosses the placenta. Dornase alfa has a long duration of action, and its fate in the body is not known.

Contraindications and cautions

Caution should be used in cases of acute bronchospasm, peptic ulcer and oesophageal varices *because the increased secretions could aggravate the problem*. There are no data on the effects of the drugs in pregnancy or breastfeeding. Use cautiously in people with gastric ulceration and those with renal or hepatic impairment.

Adverse effects

Adverse effects most commonly associated with mucolytic drugs include GI upset, stomatitis, rhinorrhoea, bronchospasm and occasionally a rash.

Prototype summary: acetylcysteine

Indications: mucolytic adjunctive therapy for abnormal, viscid or inspissated mucus secretions in acute and chronic bronchopulmonary disorders; to lessen hepatic injury in cases of paracetamol toxicity.

Actions: splits sulfur bonds in mucoproteins contained in respiratory mucus secretions, decreasing the viscosity of the secretions; protects liver cells from effects of paracetamol toxicity.

Pharmacokinetics:

Route	Onset	Peak	Duration
Instillation/ inhalation	1 min	5–10 min	2–3 hours
Oral	30–60 min	1–2 hours	Unknown

$T_{1/2}$: 6.25 hours; metabolised in the liver and excreted in urine.

Adverse effects: nausea, stomatitis, urticaria, bronchospasm, rhinorrhoea.

Care considerations for people receiving mucolytics

Assessment: history and examination

- Assess for *possible contraindications or cautions*: any history of allergy to the drugs and the presence of acute bronchospasm, *which are contraindications to the use of these drugs*; and peptic ulcer and oesophageal varices, *which would require careful monitoring and cautious use*.
- Perform a physical examination *to establish baseline data for assessing the effectiveness of the drug and the occurrence of any adverse effects associated with drug therapy*.
- Assess skin colour and lesions *to monitor for adverse reactions*.

TABLE 54.5 DRUGS IN FOCUS Mucolytics

Drug name	Dosage/route	Usual indications
bromhexine (*Bisolvon*)	Adults: 8 mg PO tds increased to 16 mg PO tds if required Paediatric (6–11 years): 8 mg PO tds	Liquefaction of secretions in respiratory conditions where excess mucus is produced
dornase alfa (*Pulmozyme*)	2.5 mg inhaled once daily through nebuliser may increase to 2.5 mg bd in people over 21 years	To relieve the buildup of secretions in people with high-risk respiratory conditions who have difficulty moving secretions, including postoperatively (eg, people with tracheostomies to facilitate airway clearance and suctioning); clearing of secretions for diagnostic tests (eg, diagnostic bronchoscopy); treatment of atelectasis from thick mucus secretions as in cystic fibrosis

- Monitor blood pressure and pulse *to evaluate cardiac response to drug treatment.*
- Evaluate respirations and adventitious sounds *to monitor drug effectiveness.*

Implementation with rationale

- Avoid combining with other drugs in the nebuliser *to avoid the formation of precipitates and potential loss of effectiveness of either drug.*
- Dilute concentrate with sterile water for injection *if buildup becomes a problem that could impede drug delivery.*
- Note that people receiving acetylcysteine by face mask should have the residue wiped off the facemask and off their face with plain water *to prevent skin breakdown.*
- Review use of the nebuliser with people receiving dornase alfa at home *to ensure the most effective use of the drug.* People should be cautioned to store the drug in the refrigerator, protected from light.
- Caution people with cystic fibrosis who are receiving dornase alfa about the need to continue all therapies for their cystic fibrosis *because dornase alfa is only a palliative therapy that improves respiratory symptoms, and other therapies are still needed.*
- Provide thorough teaching, including the drug name and prescribed dosage, measures to help avoid adverse effects, warning signs that may indicate problems and the need for periodic monitoring and evaluation, *to enhance knowledge about drug therapy and to promote compliance.*
- Offer support and encouragement *to help the person cope with the disease and the drug regimen.*

Evaluation

- Monitor response to the drug (improvement of respiratory symptoms, loosening of secretions).
- Monitor for adverse effects (CNS effects, skin rash, bronchospasm, GI upset).
- Evaluate the effectiveness of the teaching plan (person can name drug, dosage, adverse effects to watch for, specific measures to avoid them and measures to take to increase the effectiveness of the drug).
- Monitor the effectiveness of comfort and safety measures and compliance with the regimen.

KEY POINTS

- Mucolytics work to break down mucus to aid people with high-risk respiratory conditions in coughing up thick, tenacious secretions.
- Dornase alfa is specific for the treatment of people with cystic fibrosis, which is characterised by copious, thick, tenacious mucus production that can block airways.

CHAPTER SUMMARY

- The classes of drugs that affect the upper respiratory system work to keep the airways open and gases moving efficiently.
- Antitussives are drugs that suppress the cough reflex. They can act centrally to suppress the medullary cough centre or locally to increase secretion and buffer irritation. These drugs should not be used for longer than 1 week; people with persistent cough after that time should seek medical evaluation.
- Decongestants are drugs that cause local vasoconstriction and therefore decrease the blood flow to the irritated and dilated capillaries of the mucous membranes lining the nasal passages and sinus cavities.

- An adverse effect that accompanies frequent or prolonged use of decongestants is rebound vasodilation, called rhinitis medicamentosa. The reflex reaction to vasoconstriction is a rebound vasodilation, which often leads to prolonged overuse of decongestants.
- Topical nasal decongestants are preferable in people who need to avoid systemic adrenergic effects. Oral decongestants are associated with systemic adrenergic effects and require caution in people with cardiovascular disease, hyperthyroidism or diabetes mellitus.
- Topical nasal steroid decongestants block the inflammatory response from occurring. These drugs, which take several days to weeks to reach complete effectiveness, are preferred for people with allergic rhinitis who need to avoid the complications of systemic steroid therapy.
- Antihistamines selectively block the effects of histamine at the histamine-1-receptor sites, decreasing the allergic response. Antihistamines are used for the relief of symptoms associated with seasonal and perennial allergic rhinitis, allergic conjunctivitis, uncomplicated urticaria or angioedema.
- People taking antihistamines may react to dryness of the skin and mucous membranes. The carer should encourage them to drink plenty of fluids, use a humidifier if possible, avoid smoke-filled rooms, and use good skin care and moisturisers.
- The antihistamines terfenadine and astemizole are no longer marketed in Australia and New Zealand because of their effect of prolonging the QT interval. Cetirizine and loratadine have minimal risk for QT prolongation.
- Expectorants are drugs that liquefy the lower respiratory tract secretions. They are used for the symptomatic relief of respiratory conditions characterised by a dry, non-productive cough.
- Mucolytics work to break down mucus to aid people with high-risk respiratory conditions in coughing up thick, tenacious secretions.
- Many of the drugs that act on the upper respiratory tract are found in various OTC cough and allergy preparations. People need to be advised to always read the labels carefully to avoid inadvertent overdose and toxicity.

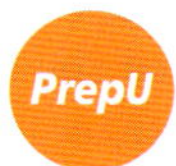

Knowing your strengths and weaknesses helps you to study more effectively. Take a PrepU Practice Quiz to find out how you measure up!

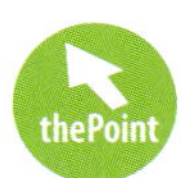

ONLINE RESOURCES

An extensive range of additional resources to enhance teaching and learning and to facilitate understanding of this chapter may be found online at the text's accompanying website, located on thePoint at http://thepoint.lww.com. These include Watch and Learn videos, Concepts in Action animations, journal articles, review questions, case studies, discussion topics and quizzes.

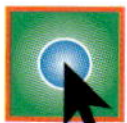

WEB LINKS

Health care providers and students may want to consult the following web resources:

www.allergy.org.au
The Australasian Society of Clinical Immunology and Allergy. Provides information on allergic diseases.

www.aihw.gov.au/reports/chronic-respiratory-conditions/allergic-rhinitis-hay-fever/contents/allergic-rhinitis-by-the-numbers
Australian Institute of Health and Welfare information on allergic rhinitis.

www.cysticfibrosis.org.au
Cystic Fibrosis National Website. Provides information and resources.

http://nzformulary.org
New Zealand Formulary.

BIBLIOGRAPHY

Bostock-Cox, B. (2012). Recognising and managing allergic disease in the community. *British Journal of Community Nursing, 17(7)*, 302–308.

Brusch, A.M., Clarke, R.C., Platt, P.R. & Phillips, E.J. (2014). Exploring the link between pholcodine exposure and neuromuscular blocking agent anaphylaxis. *British Journal of Clinical Pharmacology, 78(1)*, 14–23.

Burns, D. (2012). Management of patients with asthma and allergic rhinitis. *Nursing Standard, 26(32)*, 41–46.

Crilly, H. & Rose, M. (2014). Anaphylaxis and anaesthesia – can treating a cough kill? *Australian Prescriber, 37*, 74–76.

Farrell, M. & Dempsey, J. (2014). *Smeltzer & Bare's Textbook of Medical-Surgical Nursing* (3rd edn). Sydney: Lippincott Williams & Wilkins.

Goodman, L. S., Brunton, L. L., Chabner, B. & Knollmann, B. C. (2011). *Goodman and Gilman's Pharmacological Basis of Therapeutics* (12th edn). New York: McGraw-Hill.

Graudins, L. V. (2009). Preventing motion sickness in children. *Australian Prescriber, 32*, 61–63.

Irwin, R. S., Baumann, M. H., Bolser, D. C., Boulet, L. P., Braman, S. S., Brightling, C. E., et al. (2006). Diagnosis and management of cough executive summary: ACCP evidence-based clinical practice guidelines. *Chest, 129* (1 Supplement), 1S–23S.

Masel, P. (2012). Management of cystic fibrosis in adults. *Australian Prescriber, 35*, 118–121.

McKenna, L. & Mirkov, S. (2019). *McKenna's Drug Handbook for Nursing and Midwifery* (8th edn). Sydney: Wolters Kluwer Health Australia.

Plaut, M. & Valentine, M. D. (2005). Allergic rhinitis. *New England Journal of Medicine, 353(18)*, 1934–1944.

Porth, C. M. (2011). *Essentials of Pathophysiology: Concepts of Altered Health States* (3rd edn). Philadelphia: Lippincott Williams & Wilkins.

Porth, C. M. (2009). *Pathophysiology: Concepts of Altered Health States* (8th edn). Philadelphia: Lippincott Williams & Wilkins.

Salisbury-Afshar, E. (2012). Oral antihistamine/decongestant/analgesic combinations for the common cold. *American Family Physician, 86(9)*, 812–813.

Sung, V. (2009). Cough and cold remedies for children. *Australian Prescriber, 32*, 122–124.

CHECK YOUR UNDERSTANDING

Answers to the questions in this chapter can be found in Appendix A at the back of this book.

MULTIPLE CHOICE

Select the best answer to the following.

1. A person with sinus pressure and pain related to a seasonal rhinitis would benefit from taking:
   a. an antitussive.
   b. an expectorant.
   c. a mucolytic.
   d. a decongestant.
2. Antitussives are useful in blocking the cough reflex and preserving the energy associated with prolonged, non-productive coughing. Antitussives are best used:
   a. postoperatively.
   b. in people with asthma.
   c. in people with a dry, irritating cough.
   d. in people with COPD who tire easily.
3. People with seasonal rhinitis experience irritation and inflammation of the nasal passages and passages of the upper airways. Treatment for these people might include:
   a. systemic corticosteroids.
   b. mucolytic agents.
   c. an expectorant.
   d. topical nasal steroids.
4. A person taking an OTC cold medication and an OTC allergy medicine is found to be taking double doses of pseudoephedrine. As a result, the person might exhibit:
   a. ear pain and eye redness.
   b. restlessness and palpitations.
   c. sinus pressure and ear pain.
   d. an irritating cough and nasal drainage.
5. Antihistamines should be used very cautiously in people with:
   a. a history of arrhythmias or prolonged QT intervals.
   b. COPD or bronchitis.
   c. asthma or seasonal rhinitis.
   d. angioedema or low blood pressure.
6. A person is not getting a response to the antihistamine that was prescribed. Appropriate action might include:
   a. switching to a decongestant.
   b. stopping the drug and increasing fluids.
   c. trying a different antihistamine.
   d. switching to a corticosteroid.
7. Dornase alfa (*Pulmozyme*), because of its mechanism of action, is reserved for use in:
   a. clearing secretions before diagnostic tests.
   b. facilitating the removal of secretions postoperatively.
   c. protecting the liver from paracetamol toxicity.
   d. relieving the buildup of secretions in cystic fibrosis.

MULTIPLE RESPONSE

Select all that apply.

1. Common adverse effects associated with the use of topical nasal steroids would include which of the following?
   a. local burning and stinging
   b. dryness of the mucosa
   c. headache
   d. constipation and urinary retention
   e. fungal infections
   f. osteonecrosis
2. An antihistamine would be the drug of choice for treating which of the following?
   a. itchy eyes
   b. irritating cough
   c. nasal congestion
   d. runny nose
   e. idiopathic urticaria
   f. thick, tenacious secretions
3. Additional care interventions for people receiving antihistamines probably would include which of the following?
   a. using a humidifier
   b. advising person to suck sugarless lozenges to help to relieve dry mouth
   c. limiting fluid intake to decrease swelling
   d. providing safety measures to prevent falls or injury
   e. encouraging pushing fluids, if allowed
   f. leaving bowls of water around the house to increase humidity

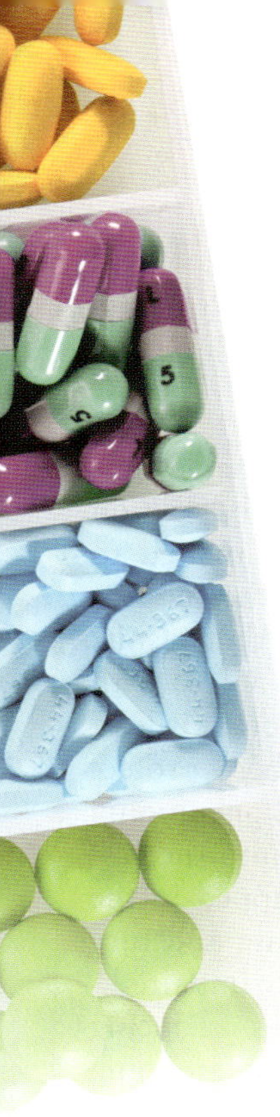

Drugs acting on the lower respiratory tract

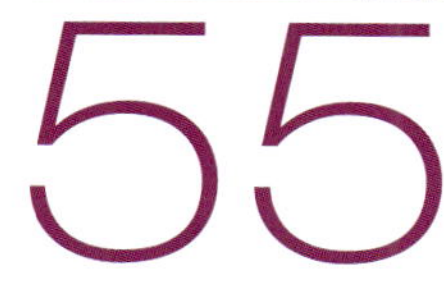

Learning objectives

On completing this chapter you should be able to:

1. Describe the underlying pathophysiology involved in obstructive pulmonary disease and correlate this information with the presenting signs and symptoms.
2. Describe the therapeutic actions, indications, pharmacokinetics, contraindications, most common adverse reactions and important drug–drug interactions associated with drugs used to treat lower respiratory tract disorders.
3. Discuss the use of drugs used to treat obstructive pulmonary disorders across the lifespan.
4. Compare and contrast the prototype drugs used to treat obstructive pulmonary disorders with other agents in their class and with other classes of drugs used to treat obstructive pulmonary disorders.
5. Outline the care considerations, including important teaching points, for people receiving drugs used to treat obstructive pulmonary disorders.

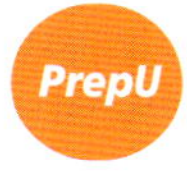

Test your current knowledge of drugs acting on the lower respiratory tract with a PrepU Practice Quiz!

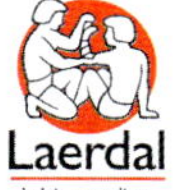

Simulation-based learning

On completion of the chapter, consider the scenario of Jennifer Hoffman (Part 1) who arrives in the emergency room with respiratory distress. Continue to Part 2. Consider the medication management of Jennifer's condition throughout her episode of care, as it relates to your learning in this chapter.

Then, work through the scenarios of Vincent Brody (Parts 1 and 2) and consider how the concepts learnt in this chapter relating to airway medication management apply to his case. What learning can be applied?

Glossary of key terms

bronchodilator: medication used to facilitate respirations by dilating the airways; helpful in symptomatic relief or prevention of bronchial asthma and bronchospasm associated with chronic obstructive pulmonary disease

Cheyne–Stokes respiration: abnormal pattern of breathing characterised by apnoeic periods followed by periods of tachypnoea; may reflect delayed blood flow through the brain

leukotriene-receptor antagonists: drugs that selectively and competitively block or antagonise receptors for the production of leukotrienes D_4 and E_4, components of slow-reacting substance of anaphylaxis (SRSA)

mast cell stabiliser: drug that works at the cellular level to inhibit the release of histamine (released from mast cells in response to inflammation or irritation) and inflammatory mediators

sympathomimetics: drugs that mimic the effects of the sympathetic nervous system

xanthines: naturally occurring substances, including caffeine and theophylline, that have a direct effect on the smooth muscle of the respiratory tract, both in the bronchi and in the blood vessels

BRONCHODILATORS/ ANTIASTHMATICS

Xanthines
- (P) aminophylline
- caffeine
- theophylline

Sympathomimetics
- (P) adrenaline (epinephrine)
- formoterol (eformoterol)
- ephedrine
- olodaterol
- indacaterol
- salbutamol
- salmeterol
- terbutaline
- vilanterol

Anticholinergics
- aclidinium
- (P) ipratropium
- tiotropium

DRUGS AFFECTING INFLAMMATION

Inhaled steroids
- beclometasone
- (P) budesonide
- ciclesonide
- fluticasone

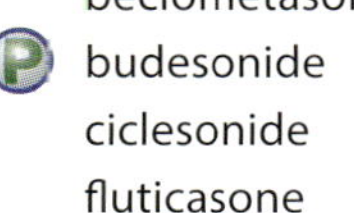

Leukotriene-receptor antagonist
(P) montelukast

Mast cell stabilisers
nedocromil sodium
(P) sodium cromoglycate

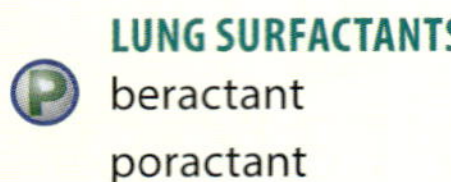

LUNG SURFACTANTS
(P) beractant
poractant

The lower respiratory tract includes the bronchial tree and the alveoli, where gas exchange occurs (see Figure 55.1). Disorders of the lower respiratory tract can have a direct impact on gas exchange and oxygenation and can include infections such as bronchiectasis, bronchitis and pneumonia and obstructive disorders that directly interfere with airflow to the alveoli.

Pulmonary obstructive diseases include asthma and chronic obstructive pulmonary disease (COPD), which includes emphysema. (See Chapter 53 for detailed pathophysiology.) These diseases cause obstruction of the major airways and may lead to complications such as infections, pneumonia and movement of inhaled substances deep into the respiratory system. The obstruction of asthma, emphysema and COPD can be related to inflammation that results in narrowing of the interior of the airway and to muscular constriction that results in narrowing of the conducting tube (Figure 55.2). With chronic inflammation, muscular and cilial action is lost, and complications related to the loss of these protective processes can occur, such as infections, pneumonia and movement of inhaled substances deep into the respiratory system. In severe COPD, air is trapped in the lower respiratory tract, the alveoli degenerate and fuse together, and the exchange of gases is greatly impaired.

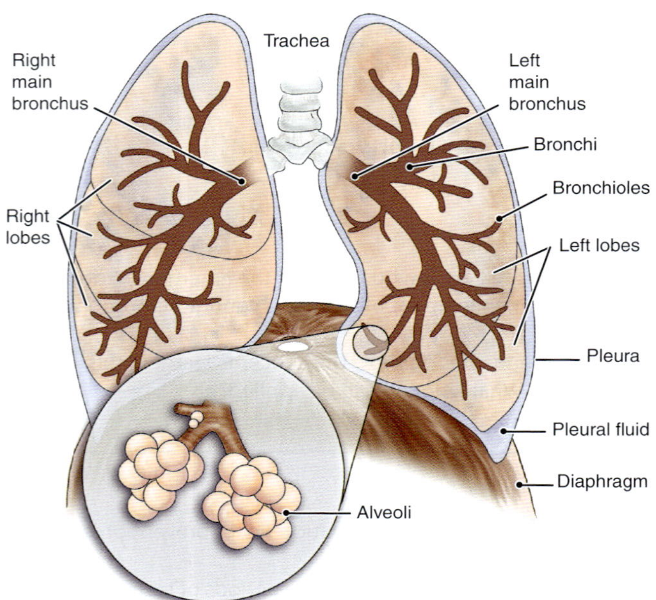

FIGURE 55.1 The lower respiratory tract.

The first step for treatment includes reducing environmental exposure to irritants such as stopping smoking, filtering allergens from the air, and avoiding exposure to known irritants and allergens. If these efforts are not sufficient to prevent problems, treatment is aimed at either opening the conducting airways through muscular bronchodilation or decreasing the effects of inflammation on the lining of the airway.

Additional obstructive pulmonary diseases are respiratory distress syndrome (RDS), which causes obstruction at the alveolar level, and adult respiratory distress syndrome (ARDS), which is characterised by progressive loss of lung compliance and increasing hypoxia. This syndrome occurs as a result of a severe insult to the body, such as cardiovascular collapse, major burns, severe trauma and rapid depressurisation. The obstruction of RDS in the neonate is related to a lack of the lipoprotein surfactant, which leads to an inability to maintain an open alveolus. Surfactant is essential in decreasing the surface tension in the tiny alveolus, allowing it to expand and remain open. If surfactant is

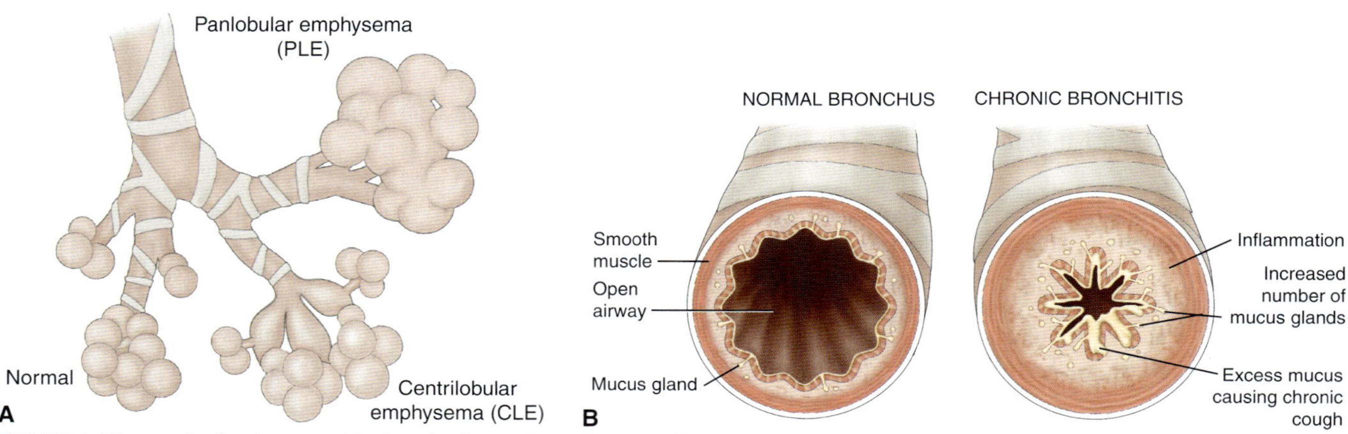

FIGURE 55.2 Changes in the airways with chronic obstructive pulmonary disease.

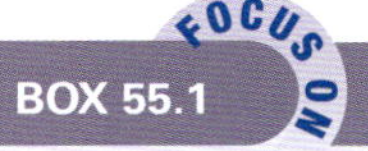

BOX 55.1 **Drug therapy across the lifespan**

Lower respiratory tract agents

CHILDREN

Antiasthmatics are frequently used in children. The incidence of asthma in children has rapidly increased in the 21st century. The leukotriene-receptor antagonists have been found to be especially effective for long-term prophylaxis in children. Acute episodes are best treated with a β-agonist and then a long-acting inhaled steroid or a mast cell stabiliser.

Parents need to be encouraged to take measures to prevent acute attacks, including avoidance of known allergens, smoke-filled rooms, and crowded or dusty areas. Parents should be cautioned about the proper way to measure liquid preparations to avoid inadvertent toxic doses or lack of therapeutic effects.

Theophylline has been used in children, but because of its many adverse effects and the better control afforded by newer agents, its use is reserved for cases that do not respond to other therapies.

As the child grows and matures, the disease will need to be re-evaluated and dose adjustments made to meet the needs of the growing child. Teenagers need to learn the proper administration and use of inhaled steroids for prevention of exercise-induced asthma.

As with other classes of medications, children may be more susceptible to the adverse effects associated with these drugs and need to be carefully monitored and evaluated. Over-the-counter (OTC) drugs and herbal remedies should be avoided if possible; if they are used, they should be reported to the health care provider so that appropriate dose adjustments can be made when needed.

The parents of premature babies undergoing surfactant therapy will require consistent support and education to help them to cope with the stress of this event.

ADULTS

Adults may be able to manage their asthma quite well with the use of inhalers and avoidance of aggravating situations. Periodic review of the proper use of the various inhalers should be part of routine evaluation of these people. Periodic spirometry readings should be done to evaluate the effectiveness of the therapy.

PREGNANCY AND BREASTFEEDING

The safety of these drugs during pregnancy and breastfeeding has not been established. There is a potential for adverse effects on the fetus related to blood flow changes and direct drug effects when the drugs cross the placenta. Use should be reserved for those situations in which the benefit to the mother outweighs the potential risk to the fetus. The drugs may enter breast milk and also may alter fluid balance and milk production. It is advised that caution be used if one of these drugs is prescribed during breastfeeding.

OLDER ADULTS

Older adults frequently are prescribed one or more of these drugs. Older adults are more likely to develop adverse effects associated with the use of these drugs, such as sedation, confusion, dizziness, urinary retention and cardiovascular effects. Safety measures may be needed if these effects occur and interfere with the person's mobility and balance.

Older adults are also more likely to have renal and/or hepatic impairment related to underlying medical conditions, which could interfere with the metabolism and excretion of these drugs. The dose for older adults should be started at a lower level than that recommended for young adults. People should be monitored very closely and dose adjustment made based on the person's response.

These people also need to be alerted to the potential for toxic effects when using OTC preparations and should be advised to check with their health care provider before beginning any OTC drug regimen. Older adults with progressive chronic obstructive pulmonary disease may be taking many combined drugs to help them maintain effective respirations. These people should have an overall treatment plan involving complex pulmonary, toilet, positioning, fluids, nutrition, humidified air, rest and activity plans, as well as a complicated drug regimen to deal with the impact of this disease.

lacking, the alveoli collapse and gas exchange cannot occur. Pharmacological therapy for RDS involves instilling surfactant into the alveoli. Treatment of ARDS involves reversal of the underlying cause of the problem combined with ventilatory support. See Box 55.1 for the use of lower respiratory tract agents with different age groups.

BRONCHODILATORS/ANTIASTHMATICS

Bronchodilators (Table 55.1) are medications used to facilitate respiration by dilating the airways. They are helpful in symptomatic relief or prevention of bronchial asthma and for bronchospasm associated with COPD. Several of the bronchodilators are administered orally and absorbed systemically, giving them the potential for many systemic adverse effects. Other medications are administered directly into the airways by nebulisers. These medications have the advantage of fewer systemic adverse reactions. Bronchodilators include xanthines, sympathomimetics and anticholinergics.

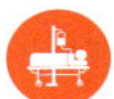 **Nursing management of the adult with asthma**

XANTHINES

The **xanthines**, including caffeine and theophylline, come from a variety of naturally occurring sources. These drugs were once the main treatment choices for asthma and bronchospasm. However, because they have a relatively narrow margin of safety and interact with many other drugs, they are no longer considered the first-choice bronchodilators. Xanthines used to treat

TABLE 55.1 DRUGS IN FOCUS Bronchodilators/antiasthmatics

Drug name	Dosage/route	Usual indications
Xanthines		
Ⓟ aminophylline (generic)	Loading dose: adult, paediatric (> 6 months): 6 mg/kg slow IV infusion over 20–30 minutes Maintenance: adult 0.7 mg/kg for next 12 hours then 0.5 mg/kg thereafter Young adult smokers and children (9–16 years): 1 mg/kg for next 12 hours then 0.8 mg/kg	Relief of symptoms or prevention of bronchial asthma and reversal of bronchospasm associated with COPD
caffeine (*Cafnea*)	Paediatric: 20 mg/kg IV followed by 5 mg/kg/day for neonatal apnoea Oral solution when enteral feeding established: 5 mg/kg once daily to a maximum of 10 mg/kg once daily	Short-term management of neonatal apnoea
theophylline (*Nuelin*)	Adult 200–300 mg q 12 hours Paediatric (2–12 years) 10 mg/kg q 12 hours	Relief of symptoms or prevention of bronchial asthma and reversal of bronchospasm associated with COPD
Sympathomimetics		
Ⓟ adrenaline (epinephrine) (*Adrenaline 1:10,000, Adrenaline 1:1000, Epipen, Epipen Jr*)	*Adrenaline 1:10,000: adjunct in the management of cardiac arrest* Adult: 1 mg (10 mL of 1:10,000) IV, preferably through a central line, and repeated every 3–5 minutes during CPR Paediatric: 10 micrograms (0.1 mL of 1:10,000 solution) per kilogram body weight IV. This may be repeated every 3–5 minutes *Adrenaline 1:1,000: emergency treatment of anaphylaxis* Adult: 100–500 micrograms (0.1–0.5 mL of 1:1,000 solution) SC or IM; SC doses may be repeated at 20 minute–4 hour intervals Paediatric: 10 micrograms (0.01 mL of 1:1,000 solution)/kg SC; maximum 500 micrograms/dose, repeated if necessary at intervals of 20 minutes to 4 hours *Epipen, Epipen Jr: emergency treatment of anaphylaxis* Adult (> 30 kg): Epipen Auto-Injector IM containing 0.3 mg adrenaline injection (0.3 mL, 1:1000) Paediatric: (15–30 kg): Epipen Jr Auto-Injector IM containing 0.15 mg adrenaline injection (0.3 mL, 1:2000)	Drug of choice for treatment of acute bronchospasm, emergency treatment of cardiac arrest, emergency treatment of anaphylaxis due to insect stings, bites, foods, drugs or other allergens
formoterol (eformoterol) (*Foradile, Oxis*)	*Foradile powder for inhalation, 12 microgram capsules through aeroliser:* Adult: 1–2 caps inhaled bd Paediatric: (> 5 years) 1 cap bd *Oxis Turbuhaler:* Adult: 6–12 micrograms bd; maximum 48 micrograms/day Paediatric ≥ 12 years: 24 micrograms/day	Maintenance treatment of asthma and prevention of bronchospasm in people ≥ 5 years of age with reversible obstructive airway disease; prevention of exercise-induced bronchospasm in people ≥ 12 years of age **Special considerations:** people taking the drug for asthma maintenance should not use additional doses of the drug for exercise-induced asthma

TABLE 55.1 DRUGS IN FOCUS Bronchodilators/antiasthmatics *(continued)*

Drug name	Dosage/route	Usual indications
Sympathomimetics *(continued)*		
indacaterol (*Onbrez*)	Adult: 150 micrograms (one inhalation capsule) once daily by inhalation; maximum 300 micrograms/day	Long-term maintenance of COPD
olodaterol (*Striverdi Respimat*)	Oral inhalation: 5 micrograms given as 2 puffs from the supplied inhaler once daily, at the same time of the day	Maintenance treatment of COPD
salbutamol (*Ventolin*)	Metered-dose inhaler, adult and paediatric: 1–2 inhalations; may repeat 4-hourly Nebuliser, adult: 5 mg q 4–6 hours Paediatric 4–12 years: 2.5 mg q 4–6 hours Elixir 2 mg/5 mL, adult: 5–10 mL (2–4 mg salbutamol) PO tid–qid; maximum single dose 20 mL (8 mg salbutamol) Paediatric: 2–6 years: 2.5–5 mL (1–2 mg salbutamol) PO tid–qid 6–12 years: 5 mL (2 mg salbutamol) PO tid–qid > 12 years: 5–10 mL (2–4 mg salbutamol) PO tid–qid	Treatment and prophylaxis of bronchospasm and acute asthma attacks
salmeterol (*Seretide, Serevent*)	Adult and paediatric > 12 years: 1–2 puffs q 12 hours Paediatric (4–12 years): one inhalation bd at least 12 hours apart	Prevention of exercise-induced asthma; prophylaxis of bronchospasm in selected people > 4 years of age
terbutaline (*Bricanyl*)	Turbuhaler 200 micrograms (which corresponds to a 250 microgram metered dose) Adult, paediatric > 12 years: 1–2 inhalations as required; maximum single dose 6 inhalations; maximum of 24 inhalations in 24 hours Paediatric 3–12 years: 1–2 inhalations as required; maximum single dose 4 inhalations; maximum of 16 inhalations in 24 hours	Treatment and prophylaxis of bronchospasm
Anticholinergics		
aclidinium (*Bretaris Genuair*)	Adult: 1 inhalation bid, 12 hours apart	Long-term maintenance treatment of COPD
(P) ipratropium (*Atrovent*)	Metered-dose inhaler, adult: 2 puffs tid–qid; paediatric 6–12 years: 1–2 puffs tid–qid; < 6 years: 1 puff tid Nebuliser, adult: 250–500 micrograms qid, to a maximum of 2 mg/day; paediatric 250 micrograms qid; maximum 1 mg/day Nasal spray, rhinitis, adult, paediatric > 12 years: 2–4 sprays bid–tid Nasal spray, common cold, adult, paediatric > 12 years: 4 sprays tid–qid for a maximum of 4 days	Maintenance and treatment of bronchospasm for adults with COPD; nasal spray for rhinorrhoea associated with seasonal and perennial rhinitis or the common cold
tiotropium (*Spiriva*)	Powder for inhalation: 18 micrograms/day (1 inhalation capsule) using the HandiHaler inhalation device Solution for inhalation: two 2.5 microgram inhalations once daily	Long-term, once-daily maintenance and treatment of bronchospasm associated with COPD in adults

respiratory disease include aminophylline (generic), caffeine (*Cafnea* and others) and theophylline (*Nuelin*).

Therapeutic actions and indications

The xanthines have a direct effect on the smooth muscles of the respiratory tract, both in the bronchi and in the blood vessels (Figure 55.3). Although the exact mechanism of action is not known, one theory suggests that xanthines work by directly affecting the mobilisation of calcium within the cell. They do this by stimulating two prostaglandins, resulting in smooth muscle relaxation, which increases the vital capacity that has been impaired by bronchospasm or air trapping. Xanthines also inhibit the release of inflammatory mediators and histamine, decreasing the bronchial swelling and narrowing that

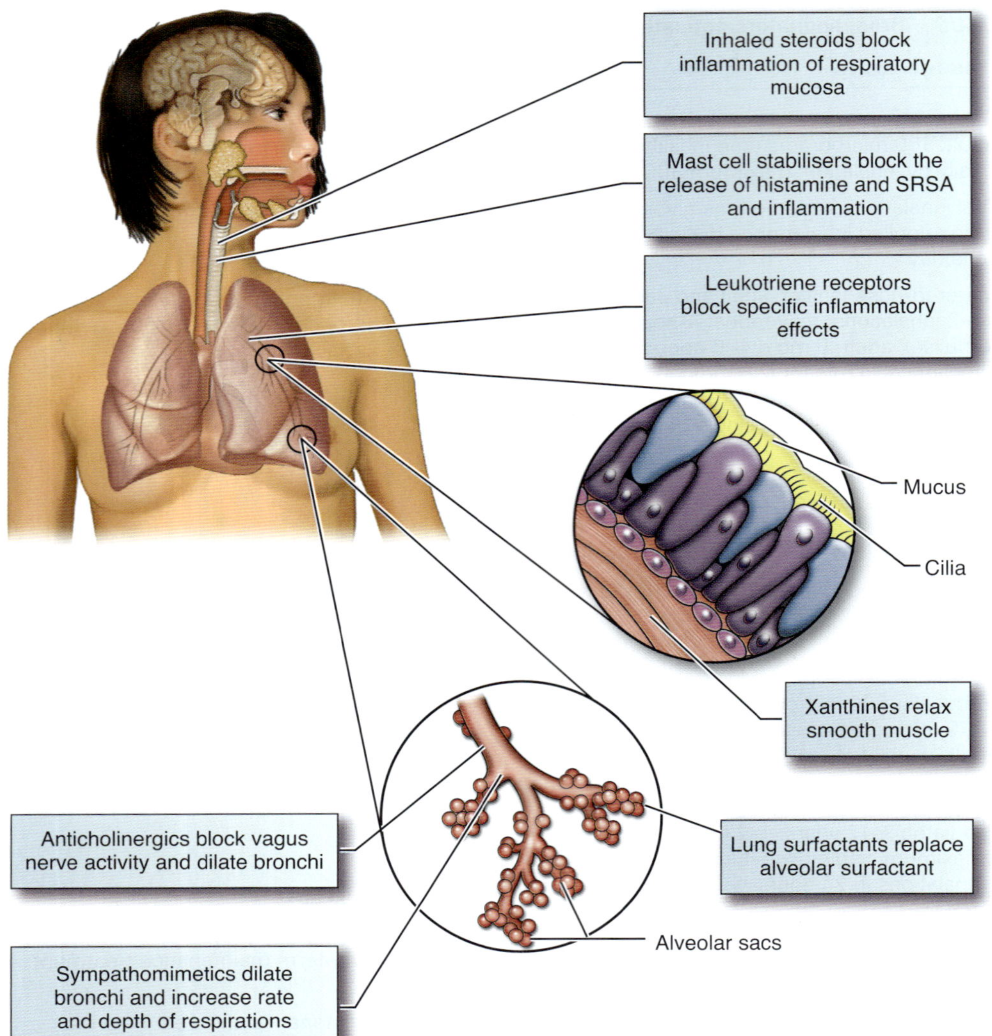

FIGURE 55.3 Sites of action of drugs used to treat obstructive pulmonary disorders. SRSA, slow-reacting substance of anaphylaxis.

occurs as a result of these two chemicals. See Table 55.1 for usual indications for these drugs. Unlabelled uses include stimulation of respirations in **Cheyne–Stokes respiration**, an abnormal pattern of breathing characterised by apnoeic periods followed by periods of tachypnoea that may reflect delayed blood flow through the brain, and the treatment of apnoea and bradycardia in premature infants.

Pharmacokinetics

The xanthines are rapidly absorbed from the gastrointestinal (GI) tract when given orally, reaching peak levels within 2 hours. They are also given IV, reaching peak effects within minutes. They are widely distributed and metabolised in the liver and excreted in urine. Xanthines cross the placenta and enter breast milk (see Contraindications and cautions).

Contraindications and cautions

Caution should be taken with any person with GI problems, coronary disease, respiratory dysfunction, renal or hepatic disease, alcoholism or hyperthyroidism *because these conditions can be exacerbated by the systemic effects of xanthines*. Xanthines are available for oral and parenteral use; the parenteral drug should be switched to the oral form as soon as possible *because the systemic effects of the oral form are less acute and more manageable*.

Although no clear studies of xanthines are available in human pregnancy, they have been associated with fetal abnormalities and breathing difficulties at birth in animal studies. Use should be limited to situations in which the benefit to the mother clearly outweighs the potential risk to the fetus. Because the xanthines enter breast milk and could affect the baby, another method of feeding the baby should be selected if these drugs are needed during breastfeeding.

Adverse effects

Adverse effects associated with xanthines are related to theophylline levels in the blood (*see the Critical thinking scenario for additional information on toxic reaction to theophylline*). Therapeutic theophylline levels are from 10 to 20 micrograms/mL. With increasing levels, predictable adverse effects are seen, ranging from GI upset, nausea, irritability and tachycardia to seizures, brain damage and even death (see Table 55.2).

Prototype summary: aminophylline

Indications: symptomatic relief or prevention of bronchial asthma and reversible bronchospasm associated with chronic bronchitis and emphysema.

Actions: directly relaxes bronchial smooth muscle, causing bronchodilation and increasing vital capacity; also inhibits the release of SRSA and histamine.

Pharmacokinetics:

Route	Onset	Peak	Duration
Oral	1–6 hours	4–6 hours	6–8 hours
IV	Immediate	30 min	4–8 hours

$T_{1/2}$: 3–15 hours (non-smoker), 4–5 hours (smoker); metabolised in the liver and excreted in urine.

Adverse effects: irritability, restlessness, dizziness, palpitations, life-threatening arrhythmias, loss of appetite, proteinuria, respiratory arrest, fever, flushing.

Clinically important drug–drug interactions

Because of the mechanism of xanthine metabolism in the liver, many drugs interact with xanthines. The list of interacting drugs should be checked whenever a drug is added to or removed from a drug regimen.

Nicotine increases the metabolism of xanthines in the liver; xanthine dose must be increased in people who continue to smoke while using xanthines. In addition, extreme caution must be used if the person decides to decrease or discontinue smoking, because severe xanthine toxicity can occur. Caffeine also contains xanthines so excessive intake of caffeine-containing foods may also increase levels.

TABLE 55.2 Adverse effects associated with various serum levels of theophylline

Serum level (micrograms/mL)	Adverse effects
≤ 20	Uncommon
> 20–25	Nausea, vomiting, diarrhoea, insomnia, headache, irritability
> 30–35	Hyperglycaemia, hypotension, cardiac arrhythmias, tachycardia, seizures, brain damage, death

Care considerations for people receiving xanthines

Assessment: history and examination

- Assess for *possible contraindications or cautions*: any known allergies *to prevent hypersensitivity reactions*; cigarette use, *which affects the metabolism of the drug*; peptic ulcer, gastritis, renal or hepatic dysfunction and coronary disease, *all of which could be exacerbated and require cautious use*; and pregnancy and breastfeeding, *which are contraindications because of the potential for adverse effects on the fetus or breastfeeding infant.*
- Perform a physical examination *to establish baseline data for assessing the effectiveness of the drug and the occurrence of any adverse effects associated with drug therapy.*
- Perform a skin examination, including colour and the presence of lesions, *to provide a baseline as a reference for drug effectiveness.*
- Monitor blood pressure, pulse, cardiac auscultation, peripheral perfusion and baseline electrocardiogram (ECG) *to provide a baseline for effects on the cardiovascular system.*
- Assess bowel sounds and do a liver evaluation, and monitor liver and renal function tests, *to provide a baseline for renal and liver function tests.*
- Evaluate serum theophylline levels *to provide a baseline reference and identify conditions that may require caution in the use of xanthines.*

Implementation with rationale

- Administer oral drug with food or milk *to relieve GI irritation if GI upset is a problem.*
- Monitor response to the drug (eg, relief of respiratory difficulty, improved airflow) *to determine the effectiveness of the drug dose and to adjust dose as needed.*
- Provide comfort measures, including rest periods, quiet environment, dietary control of caffeine and headache therapy as needed, *to help the person cope with the effects of drug therapy.*
- Provide periodic follow-up, including blood tests, *to monitor serum theophylline levels.*
- Provide thorough teaching, including the drug name and prescribed dosage, measures

to help avoid adverse effects, warning signs that may indicate problems and the need for periodic monitoring and evaluation, *to enhance knowledge about drug therapy and to promote compliance*.

- Monitor for smoking or excessive caffeine intake that may interfere with xanthine levels.

Evaluation

- Monitor response to the drug (improved airflow, ease of respirations).
- Monitor for adverse effects (CNS effects, cardiac arrhythmias, GI upset, local irritation).
- Monitor for potential drug–drug interactions; consult with the prescriber to adjust doses as appropriate.
- Evaluate the effectiveness of the teaching plan (person can name drug, dosage, adverse effects to watch for and specific measures to avoid adverse effects).
- Monitor the effectiveness of comfort measures and compliance with the regimen.

CRITICAL THINKING SCENARIO

Toxic reaction to theophylline

THE SITUATION

R.P. has a medical diagnosis of chronic bronchitis and has been stabilised on theophylline for the past 3 years. She has been labelled as non-compliant with medical therapy because she continues to smoke cigarettes (more than three packs per day), knowing that she has a progressive pulmonary disease. R.P. was referred to a nursing student for teaching. After several sessions in which the student presented posters and pictures and gave R.P. a great deal of personal attention and encouragement, it was determined that R.P. had a good understanding of her problem and would stop or at least cut down on her smoking. Three days later, R.P. presented to the emergency department with complaints of dizziness, nausea, vomiting, confusion, grouchiness and palpitations. Her admission heart rate was 96 beats/minute with occasional to frequent premature ventricular contractions.

CRITICAL THINKING

What probably happened to R.P.?
What information should the student have known before conducting the teaching program?
How could that information have been included in the teaching program?
What would the best approach be to R.P. now?

DISCUSSION

R.P. probably did cut down on her smoking. However, she was not aware that cigarette smoking increases the metabolism of theophylline and that she had been stabilised on a dose that took that information into account. When she cut down on smoking, theophylline was not metabolised as quickly and began to accumulate, leading to the toxic reaction that brought R.P. into the emergency department. This is a real nursing challenge. By following the teaching program and doing what she was asked to do, R.P. became sicker and felt awful. A careful teaching approach will be necessary to encourage R.P. to continue cutting down on cigarette smoking.

Staff should be educated on the numerous variables that affect drug therapy and encouraged to check drug interactions frequently when making any changes in a person's regimen. Regular follow-up and support will be important to help R.P. regain trust in her medical care providers and continue her progress in cutting down smoking. Frequent checks of theophylline levels should be done while R.P. is cutting back, and dose adjustments should be made by her prescriber to maintain therapeutic levels of theophylline and avoid toxic levels.

CARE GUIDE FOR R.P.: XANTHINES

Assessment: history and examination

Assessment parameters include a health history focused particularly on allergies, peptic ulcer, gastritis, renal or hepatic dysfunction, coronary disease, cigarette use, pregnancy and breastfeeding, as well as concurrent use of cimetidine, erythromycin, ciprofloxacin, hormonal contraceptives, ranitidine, rifampicin, barbiturates, phenytoin, benzodiazepines and beta blockers.

Focus the physical examination on the following areas:
Neurological: orientation, reflexes, affect, coordination
Respiratory: respiratory rate and character, adventitious sounds
Skin: colour, lesions
Cardiovascular: blood pressure, pulse, peripheral perfusion, baseline electrocardiogram
Gastrointestinal: bowel sounds, abdominal examination
Laboratory tests: serum theophylline levels, renal and liver function tests

Implementation

Provide supportive care with comfort and safety measures:

- Give drug with meals.
- Allow for rest periods.
- Provide a quiet environment.
- Ensure dietary control of caffeine.
- Provide headache therapy as needed.

Provide reassurance to deal with drug effects and lifestyle changes.

Provide teaching regarding drug name, dosage, adverse effects, precautions, warnings to report, dietary cautions and need for follow-up.

Evaluation

Evaluate drug effects: relief of respiratory difficulty, improvement of air movement.

Monitor for adverse effects: GI upset, CNS effects, cardiac arrhythmias; monitor for drug–drug interactions as appropriate.

Evaluate the effectiveness of the teaching program and comfort and safety measures.

TEACHING FOR R.P.

- The drug that has been prescribed for you, theophylline, is called a bronchodilator. Bronchodilators work by relaxing the airways, helping to make breathing easier and to decrease wheezes and shortness of breath. To be effective, this drug must be taken exactly as prescribed.
- This drug should be taken on an empty stomach with a full glass of water. If GI upset is severe, you can take the drug with food. Do not chew the enteric-coated or time-release capsules or tablets – they must be swallowed whole to be effective.
- Common effects of this drug include the following:
  - *Gastrointestinal upset, nausea, vomiting, heartburn:* taking the drug with food may help with these problems.
  - *Restlessness, nervousness, difficulty in sleeping:* the body often adjusts to these effects over time. Avoiding other stimulants such as caffeine, may help to decrease some of these symptoms.
  - *Headache:* this often goes away with time. If headaches persist or become worse, notify your health care provider.
- Report any of the following to your health care provider: *vomiting, severe abdominal pain, pounding or fast heartbeat, confusion, unusual tiredness, muscle twitching, skin rash or hives.*
- Many foods can change the way that your drug works; if you decide to change your diet, consult with your health care provider.
- Adverse effects of the drug can be avoided by avoiding foods that contain caffeine or other xanthine derivatives (coffee, cola, chocolate, tea) or by using them in moderate amounts. This is especially important if you experience nervousness, restlessness or sleeplessness.
- Cigarette smoking affects the way your body uses this drug. If you decide to change your smoking habits, such as increasing or decreasing the number of cigarettes you smoke each day, consult with your health care provider regarding the possible need to adjust your dose.
- Avoid the use of any OTC medication without first checking with your health care provider. Several of these medications can interfere with the effectiveness of this drug.
- Tell any doctor, nurse or other health care provider involved in your care that you are taking this drug.
- Keep this drug, and all medications, out of the reach of children.

SYMPATHOMIMETICS

Sympathomimetics are drugs that mimic the effects of the sympathetic nervous system. One of the actions of the sympathetic nervous system is dilation of the bronchi with increased rate and depth of respiration. This is the desired effect when selecting a sympathomimetic as a bronchodilator. Sympathomimetics that are used as bronchodilators include adrenaline (epinephrine) (*EpiPen*), formoterol (eformoterol) (*Foradile*, *Oxis*), ephedrine (generic), indacaterol (*Onbrez*), olodaterol (*Striverdi Respimat*), salbutamol (*Respigen*, *Salair*, *Ventolin*), salmeterol (*Serevent*) and terbutaline (*Bricanyl*).

Therapeutic actions and indications

Most of the sympathomimetics used as bronchodilators are beta-2-selective adrenergic agonists. That means that at therapeutic levels their actions are specific to the beta-2-receptors found in the bronchi (see Chapter 30). This specificity is lost at higher levels. Other systemic effects of sympathomimetics include increased blood pressure, increased heart rate, vasoconstriction and decreased renal and GI blood flow – all actions of the sympathetic nervous system. These overall effects limit the systemic usefulness of these drugs in certain people.

Salbutamol, the prototype drug, is the drug of choice in adults and children for the treatment of acute bronchospasm, including that caused by anaphylaxis; it is also available for inhalation. Because adrenaline is associated with systemic sympathomimetic effects, it is not the drug of choice for people with cardiac conditions. See Table 55.1 for usual indications for each of these agents.

Pharmacokinetics

Sympathomimetics available only as inhalants include formoterol, indacaterol and salmeterol.

Other sympathomimetics are available in various forms. Terbutaline and salbutamol can be used as inhalants and as oral and parenteral agents.

These drugs are rapidly distributed after injection; they are transformed in the liver to metabolites that are excreted in the urine. The half-life of these drugs is relatively short – less than 1 hour except for indacaterol whose half-life is 49 hours. They are known to cross the placenta and to enter breast milk (see Contraindications and cautions). The inhaled drugs are rapidly absorbed into the lung tissue. Although very little of the drug is absorbed systemically, any absorbed drug will still be metabolised in the liver and excreted in urine. Indacaterol, however, is eliminated predominantly (~90%) through the fecal route. About 54% of the drug is eliminated unchanged, and ~23% is excreted as hydoxylated indacaterol metabolite.

Contraindications and cautions

These drugs are contraindicated or should be used with caution, depending on the severity of the underlying condition, *in conditions that would be aggravated by the sympathetic stimulation*, including cardiac disease, vascular disease, arrhythmias, diabetes and hyperthyroidism. Indacaterol is indicated for people with COPD and not for people with asthma. Indacaterol should not be used for treatment of acute symptoms of COPD or administered more than once a day. Indacaterol should not be administered with other long-acting beta-2 agonists. These drugs should be used during pregnancy and breastfeeding only if the benefits to the mother clearly outweigh potential risks to the fetus or neonate.

Adverse effects

Adverse effects of these drugs, which can be attributed to sympathomimetic stimulation, include CNS stimulation, GI upset, cardiac arrhythmias, hypertension, bronchospasm, sweating, pallor and flushing. If the person is taking formoterol for asthma maintenance, additional doses of drug should not be used for exercise-induced asthma because the cumulative sympathomimetic effects can cause serious cardiovascular problems.

Clinically important drug–drug interactions

Special precautions should be taken to avoid the combination of sympathomimetic bronchodilators with the general anaesthetics cyclopropane and halogenated hydrocarbons. Because these drugs sensitise the myocardium to catecholamines, serious cardiac complications could occur. The therapeutic effect of indacaterol is blocked with the concomitant use of beta blockers. Hypokalaemic effects of indacaterol may be potentiated in individuals using diuretics, steroids or xanthine derivatives.

Prototype summary: adrenaline (epinephrine)

Indications: treatment of anaphylactic reactions, acute asthma attacks; relief from respiratory distress of COPD and bronchial asthma.

Actions: reacts at alpha- and beta-receptor sites in the sympathetic nervous system to cause bronchodilation, increased heart rate, increased respiratory rate and increased blood pressure.

Pharmacokinetics:

Route	Onset	Peak	Duration
SC	5–10 min	20 min	20–30 min
IM	5–10 min	20 min	20–30 min
IV	Instant	20 min	20–30 min
Inhalation	3–5 min	20 min	1–3 hours

$T_{1/2}$: unknown; metabolised by normal neural pathways.

Adverse effects: fear, anxiety, restlessness, headache, nausea, decreased renal formation, pallor, palpitation, tachycardia, local burning and stinging, rebound congestion with nasal inhalation.

Care considerations for people receiving sympathomimetics

Assessment: history and examination

- Assess for *possible contraindications or cautions*: any known allergies to any sympathomimetic or drug vehicle *to prevent hypersensitivity reactions*; cigarette use, *which affects the metabolism of the drug*; pregnancy or breastfeeding, *which require cautious use of the drug*; cardiac disease, vascular disease, arrhythmias, diabetes and hyperthyroidism, *which may be exacerbated by sympathomimetic effects*; and use of the general anaesthetics cyclopropane and halogenated hydrocarbons, *which sensitise the myocardium to catecholamines and could cause serious cardiac complications if used with these drugs.*

- Perform a physical examination *to establish baseline data for assessing the effectiveness of the drug and the occurrence of any adverse effects associated with drug therapy.*
- Assess reflexes and orientation *to evaluate CNS effects of the drug.*
- Monitor respirations and adventitious sounds *to establish a baseline for drug effectiveness and possible adverse effects.*
- Evaluate pulse, blood pressure and, in certain cases, a baseline ECG *to monitor the cardiovascular effects of sympathetic stimulation.*
- Evaluate liver function tests *to assess for changes that could interfere with metabolism of the drug and require dose adjustment.*

Implementation with rationale

- Reassure person that the drug of choice will vary with each individual. *These sympathomimetics are slightly different chemicals and are prepared in a variety of delivery systems.* A person may have to try several different sympathomimetics before the most effective one is found.
- Advise the person to use the minimal amount needed for the shortest period necessary *to prevent adverse effects and accumulation of drug levels.*
- Teach people who use one of these drugs for exercise-induced asthma to use it 30–60 minutes before exercising *to ensure peak therapeutic effects when they are needed.*
- Provide safety measures as needed if CNS effects become a problem *to prevent injury.*
- Provide small, frequent meals and nutritional consultation if GI effects interfere with eating *to ensure proper nutrition.*
- Provide thorough teaching, including the drug name and prescribed dosage, measures to help avoid adverse effects, warning signs that may indicate problems and the need for periodic monitoring and evaluation, *to enhance knowledge about drug therapy and to promote compliance.* Carefully teach the person about proper use of the prescribed delivery system. Review that procedure periodically *because improper use may result in ineffective therapy* (Box 55.2).
- Monitor vital signs closely.
- Offer support and encouragement *to help the person cope with the disease and the drug regimen.*

Evaluation

- Monitor response to the drug (improved breathing).
- Monitor for adverse effects (CNS effects, increased pulse and blood pressure, GI upset).
- Evaluate the effectiveness of the teaching plan (person can name drug, dosage, adverse effects to watch for, specific measures to avoid them and measures to take to increase the effectiveness of the drug).
- Monitor the effectiveness of other measures to ease breathing.

ANTICHOLINERGICS

People who cannot tolerate the sympathetic effects of the sympathomimetics might respond to the anticholinergic drugs aclidinium (*Bretaris Genuair*) ipratropium (*Atrovent*) and tiotropium (*Spiriva*). These drugs are not as effective as the sympathomimetics but can provide some relief to those people who cannot tolerate the other drugs.

Therapeutic actions and indications

Anticholinergics are used as bronchodilators because of their effect on the vagus nerve, which is to block or antagonise the action of the neurotransmitter acetylcholine at vagal-mediated receptor sites (see Figure 55.3). Normally, vagal stimulation results in a stimulating effect on smooth muscle, causing contraction. By blocking the vagal effect, relaxation of smooth muscle in the bronchi occurs, leading to bronchodilation. See Table 55.1 for usual indications for these drugs.

Pharmacokinetics

These drugs are available for inhalation, using an inhaler device. Ipratropium is also available as a nasal spray for seasonal rhinitis. Ipratropium has an onset of action of 15 minutes when inhaled. Its peak effects occur in 1–2 hours, and it has a duration of effect of 3–4 hours. Little is known about its fate in the body. It is generally not absorbed systemically.

Tiotropium has a rapid onset of action and a long duration, with a half-life of 5–6 days. It is excreted unchanged in urine.

Contraindications and cautions

Caution should be used in any condition *that would be aggravated by the anticholinergic or atropine-like effects of the drug*, such as narrow-angle glaucoma (*drainage of the vitreous humour can be blocked by smooth muscle relaxation*), bladder neck obstruction or prostatic hypertrophy (*relaxed muscle causes decreased bladder tone*) and conditions aggravated by dry mouth and throat. The use of ipratropium or tiotropium is contraindicated in the presence of known allergy to the drug or to soy products or peanuts (the vehicle used to make ipratropium into an aerosol contains a protein associated with peanut allergies) *to prevent hypersensitivity reactions*. These drugs are not usually absorbed systemically, but, as with all drugs, caution should be used in pregnancy and breastfeeding *because of the potential for adverse effects on the fetus or breastfeeding infant*.

Adverse effects

Adverse effects are related to the anticholinergic effects of the drug if it is absorbed systemically. These effects include dizziness, headache, fatigue, nervousness, dry mouth, sore throat, palpitations and urinary retention.

Clinically important drug–drug interactions

There is an increased risk of adverse effects if these drugs are combined with any other anticholinergics; this combination should be avoided.

 **Prototype summary: ipratropium**

Indications: maintenance treatment of bronchospasm associated with COPD; treatment of seasonal allergic rhinitis as a nasal spray.

Actions: anticholinergic that blocks vagally mediated reflexes by antagonising the action of acetylcholine.

Pharmacokinetics:

Route	Onset	Peak	Duration
Inhalation	15 min	1–2 hours	3–4 hours

$T_{1/2}$: unknown; metabolised by neural pathways.

Adverse effects: nervousness, dizziness, headache, nausea, GI distress, cough, palpitations.

Care considerations for people receiving anticholinergics

Assessment: history and examination

- Assess for *possible contraindications or cautions*: allergy to atropine or other anticholinergics or any component of the drug *to prevent hypersensitivity reactions*; acute bronchospasm, *which would be a contraindication*; narrow-angle glaucoma (*drainage of the vitreous humour can be blocked by smooth muscle relaxation*), bladder neck obstruction or prostatic hypertrophy (*relaxed muscle causes decreased bladder tone*) and conditions aggravated by dry mouth and throat, *all of which could be exacerbated by the use of this drug*; and pregnancy and breastfeeding, *which would require cautious use*.
- Perform a physical examination *to establish baseline data for assessing the effectiveness of the drug and the occurrence of any adverse effects associated with drug therapy*.
- Assess skin colour and lesions *to assess for dryness or allergic reaction and to evaluate oxygenation*.
- Evaluate orientation, affect and reflexes *to evaluate CNS effects*.
- Assess pulse and blood pressure *to monitor cardiovascular effects of the drug*.
- Evaluate respirations and adventitious sounds *to monitor drug effectiveness and possible adverse effects*.
- Evaluate urinary output and prostate palpation as appropriate *to monitor anticholinergic effects*.

Implementation with rationale

- Ensure adequate hydration and provide environmental controls, such as the use of a humidifier, *to make the person more comfortable*.
- Encourage the person to void before each dose of medication *to prevent urinary retention related to drug effects*.
- Provide safety measures if CNS effects occur *to prevent injury*.
- Provide small, frequent meals and sugarless lozenges *to relieve dry mouth and GI upset*.
- Advise the person not to drive or use hazardous machinery if nervousness, dizziness and drowsiness occur with this drug *to prevent injury*.
- Provide thorough teaching, including the drug name and prescribed dosage, measures to help avoid adverse effects, warning signs that may indicate problems and the need for periodic monitoring and evaluation, *to enhance knowledge about drug therapy and to promote compliance*.
- Review the use of the inhaler with the person; caution the person not to exceed 12 inhalations in 24 hours *to prevent serious adverse effects*.
- Offer support and encouragement *to help the person cope with the disease and the drug regimen*.

Evaluation

- Monitor response to the drug (improved breathing).
- Monitor for adverse effects (CNS effects, increased pulse or blood pressure, GI upset, dry skin and mucous membranes).

- Evaluate the effectiveness of the teaching plan (person can name drug, dosage, adverse effects to watch for, specific measures to avoid them and measures to take to increase the effectiveness of the drug).
- Monitor the effectiveness of other measures to ease breathing.

KEY POINTS

- Asthma, emphysema, chronic obstructive pulmonary disease (COPD) and respiratory distress syndrome (RDS) are pulmonary obstructive diseases. All but RDS involve obstruction of the major airways; RDS obstructs the alveoli.
- Drug treatment of asthma and COPD aims to relieve inflammation and promote bronchial dilation.
- Xanthine-derived drugs affect the smooth muscles of the respiratory tract – both in the bronchi and in the blood vessels. The effects of the xanthines are directly related to blood levels of theophylline. Excessive or toxic levels can lead to coma and death.
- Sympathomimetics replicate the effects of the sympathetic nervous system; they dilate the bronchi and increase the rate and depth of respiration.
- Anticholinergics affect the vagus nerve to relax the bronchial smooth muscle and thereby promote bronchodilation.

DRUGS AFFECTING INFLAMMATION

Bronchodilation is important in opening up the airway to allow air to flow into the alveoli. The second component of treating obstructive pulmonary disorders is to alter the inflammatory process that leads to swelling and further airway narrowing. Effective treatment of asthma and COPD targets both components. The drugs used to affect inflammation are the inhaled steroids, the leukotriene-receptor antagonists and a mast cell stabiliser, which can affect both bronchodilation and inflammation (Table 55.3).

INHALED STEROIDS

Inhaled steroids have been found to be a very effective treatment for bronchospasm. Agents approved for this use include beclometasone (*Qvar*), budesonide (*Pulmicort*), ciclesonide (*Alvesco, Omnaris*) and fluticasone (*Flixotide*). The drug of choice depends on the individual person's response; a person may have little response to one agent and do very well on another. It is usually useful to try another preparation if one is not effective within 2–3 weeks.

Fixed-dose combination drugs are also available using some of these drugs (Box 55.3).

Therapeutic actions and indications

Inhaled steroids are used to decrease the inflammatory response in the airway. In an airway that is swollen and narrowed by inflammation and swelling, this action will increase air flow and facilitate respiration. Inhaling the steroid tends to decrease the numerous systemic effects that are associated with steroid use. When administered into the lungs by inhalation, steroids decrease the effectiveness of the inflammatory cells. This has two effects: decreased swelling associated with inflammation and promotion of beta-adrenergic-receptor activity, which may promote smooth muscle relaxation and inhibit bronchoconstriction (see Figure 55.2). See Table 55.3 for usual indications.

Pharmacokinetics

These drugs are rapidly absorbed from the respiratory tract, but they take 2–3 weeks to reach effective levels, and so people must be encouraged to take them to reach and then maintain the effective levels. They are metabolised by natural systems, mostly within the liver, and are excreted in urine. The glucocorticoids are known to cross the placenta and to enter breast milk (see Contraindications and cautions).

Contraindications and cautions

Inhaled steroids are not for emergency use and not for use during an acute asthma attack or status asthmaticus. They should not be used during pregnancy or breastfeeding unless the benefit to the mother clearly

Prototype summary: budesonide

Indications: prevention and treatment of asthma; to treat chronic steroid-dependent bronchial asthma; as adjunct therapy for people whose asthma is not controlled by traditional bronchodilators.

Actions: decreases the inflammatory response in the airway; this action will increase airflow and facilitate respiration in an airway narrowed by inflammation.

Pharmacokinetics:

Route	Onset	Peak	Duration
Inhalation	Slow	Rapid	8–12 hours

$T_{1/2}$: 2–3 hours; metabolised in the liver and excreted in urine.

Adverse effects: irritability, headache, rebound congestion, epistaxis, local infection.

BOX 55.2 FOCUS ON **Individual and family teaching**

Teaching people to self-administer medication

It is important to deliver inhaled drugs into the lungs to achieve a rapid reaction and decrease the occurrence of systemic adverse effects. People who self-administer inhaled drugs may be using an inhaler or a nebuliser.

INHALERS

An inhaler is a device that allows a canister containing the drug to be inserted into a metered-dose inhaler (MDI) that will deliver a specific amount of the drug when the person compresses the canister. The inhaler has a mouthpiece and may also have a spacer, which is used to hold the dose of the drug while the person inhales. This is advantageous if the person has difficulty compressing the canister and inhaling at the same time or if inhaling is difficult. If a powder for inhalation is being administered, a spacer is not used.

Have the person shake the canister, exhale and place the spacer in their mouth. (If a spacer is not being used, they should hold the device about 2–3 centimetres from the open mouth.) The person should compress the canister while inhaling, hold their breath as long as possible and exhale through pursed lips. The person should then rinse their mouth and wash the spacer (if used). Some drugs come with a very specific inhaling device designed just for that drug. If the person is using one of those drugs, the manufacturer's instructions should be consulted.

NEBULISERS

A nebuliser uses compressed air to change a liquid drug into a fine mist for inhalation. If a person is using a handheld device or a mask, they should sit upright or in a semi-Fowler position and place the correct amount of liquid (drug dose) in the nebuliser chamber, which is attached to a compressed gas system. The person should breathe slowly and deeply during the treatment. After the liquid is gone, the person should rinse their mouth and clean the mask or device.

People may use these devices for several years. It is important to check their administration techniques periodically to ensure that the person is getting a therapeutic dose of the drug.

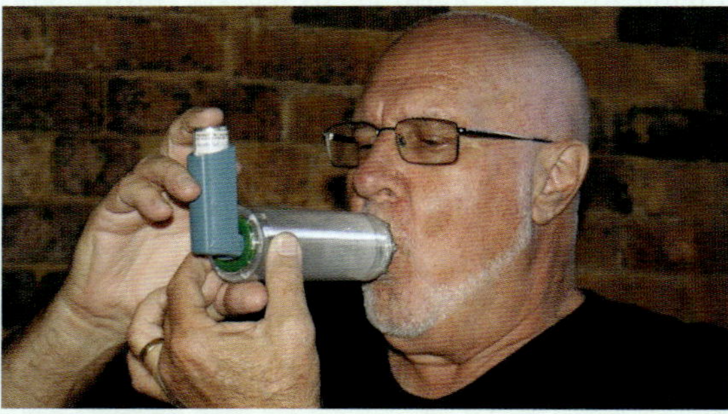

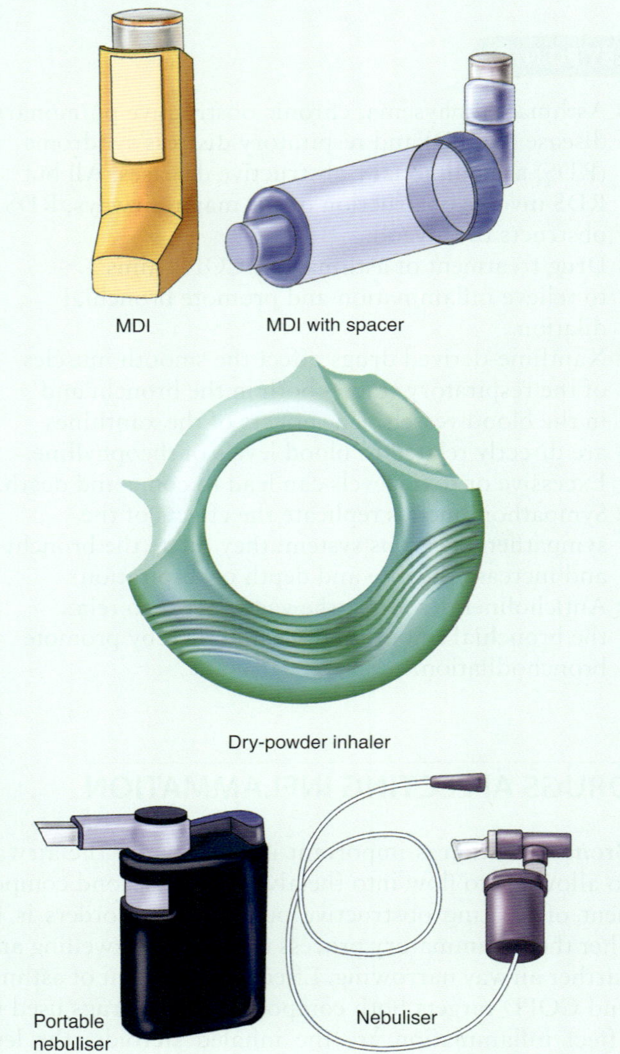

outweighs any potential risk to the fetus or breastfeeding infant. These preparations should be used with caution in any person who has an active infection of the respiratory system *because the depression of the inflammatory response could result in serious illness.*

Adverse effects

Adverse effects are limited because of the route of administration. Sore throat, hoarseness, coughing, dry mouth and pharyngeal and laryngeal fungal infections are the most common side effects encountered. If a person does not administer the drug appropriately or develops lesions that allow absorption of the drug, the systemic side effects associated with steroids may occur.

LEUKOTRIENE-RECEPTOR ANTAGONISTS

A newer class of drugs, the **leukotriene-receptor antagonists**, was developed to act more specifically at the site

TABLE 55.3 DRUGS IN FOCUS Drugs affecting inflammation

Drug name	Dosage/route	Usual indications
Inhaled steriods		
beclometasone (*Qvar*)	Adult: 50–200 micrograms bd Paediatric (5–12 years): 50 micrograms bd	Prevention and treatment of asthma; treatment of chronic steroid-dependent bronchial asthma; used as adjunctive therapy for people with asthma who do not respond to traditional bronchodilators
(P) budesonide (*Pulmicort*)	Inhaler, adults: usually 400–800 micrograms/day; maximum 2400 micrograms/day; Paediatric: usually 200–400 micrograms/day; maximum 800 micrograms/day Nebulising solution, adults: 1–2 mg bd; paediatric: 0.5–1 mg bd	Prevention and treatment of asthma; treatment of chronic steroid-dependent bronchial asthma; used as adjunctive therapy for people with asthma who do not respond to traditional bronchodilators
ciclesonide (*Alvesco, Omnaris*)	Adults and children ≥ 12 years: 80–320 micrograms/day; may increase to 320 micrograms bd in adults Children 6–11 years: 80–160 micrograms/day	Prevention and treatment of asthma; treatment of chronic steroid-dependent bronchial asthma; used as adjunctive therapy for people with asthma who do not respond to traditional bronchodilators
fluticasone (*Flixotide*)	Adult: 100–1000 micrograms bd Paediatric (1–16 years): 50–100 micrograms bd	Prevention and treatment of asthma; treatment of chronic steroid-dependent bronchial asthma; used as adjunctive therapy for people with asthma who do not respond to traditional bronchodilators
Leukotriene-receptor antagoists		
(P) montelukast (*Lukair, Montekast, Respikast, Singulair, T-Lukast*)	Adult and paediatric (> 14 years): 10 mg PO daily in the evening Paediatric: 2–5 years: 4 mg chewable tablet PO in the evening; 6–14 years: 5 mg chewable tablet PO in the evening	Prophylaxis and treatment of chronic bronchial asthma in adults and children 6 months and older
Mast cell stabilisers		
nedocromil sodium (*Tilade*)	Adult and paediatric (> 2 years): 4 mg qid	Prophylaxis of mild to moderate asthma, exercise-induced bronchospasm
(P) sodium cromoglycate (*Intal*)	Inhaler, 1 mg/dose: 2 inhalations qid; 5 mg/dose: 2 inhalations bd; maximum 4 inhalations qid	Prophylaxis of mild to moderate asthma, exercise-induced bronchospasm

BOX 55.3 Fixed-dose combination respiratory drugs

The benefit of combining different classes of drugs for the treatment of asthma has resulted in the development of fixed-dose combination drugs.

- *Breo Elipta, Relvar Elipta* are combinations of fluticasone (inhaled corticosteroid) and vilanterol (long-acting beta-2 agonist).
- *Duolin* is a combination of ipratropium (anticholinergic agent) and salbutamol (sympathetic agent, short-acting beta-2 agonist).
- *DuoResp Spiromax, Symbicort* are combinations of formoterol (eformoterol) (long-acting beta-2 agonist) and budesonide (inhaled corticosteroid).
- *Flutiform* is a combination of formoterol (long-acting beta-2 agonist) and fluticasone (inhaled corticosteroid).
- *Pavtide, Salplus F, Seretide Accuhaler and Seretide MDI* are combinations of fluticasone (inhaled corticosteroid) and salmeterol (sympathetic agent, long-acting beta-2 agonist).
- *Spiolto Respimat* is a combination of tiotropium (long-acting muscarinic antagonist) and olodaterol (long-acting beta-2 adrenergic agent).
- *Duolin* is a combination of ipratropium (anticholinergic agent) and salbutamol (sympathetic agent).

People should be stabilised on each drug separately before switching to the fixed-dose combination drug. Once the switch has been made, the dosing is cut in half, and most people find it easier to be compliant with drug therapy.

Care considerations for people receiving inhaled steroids

Assessment: history and examination

- Assess for *possible contraindications or cautions*: acute asthma attacks and allergy to the drugs, *which are contraindications*, and systemic infections, pregnancy or breastfeeding, *which require cautious use*.
- Perform a physical examination *to establish baseline data for assessing the effectiveness of the drug and the occurrence of any adverse effects associated with drug therapy*.
- Assess temperature *to monitor for possible infections*.
- Monitor blood pressure, pulse and auscultation *to evaluate cardiovascular response*.
- Assess respirations and adventitious sounds *to monitor drug effectiveness*.
- Examine the nares *to evaluate for any lesions that might lead to systemic absorption of the drug*.

Implementation with rationale

- Do not administer the drug to treat an acute asthma attack or status asthmaticus *because these drugs are not intended for treatment of acute attack and will not provide the immediate relief that is needed*.
- Taper systemic steroids carefully during the transfer to inhaled steroids; *deaths have occurred from adrenal insufficiency with sudden withdrawal*.
- Have the person use decongestant drops before using the inhaled steroid *to facilitate penetration of the drug if nasal congestion is a problem*.
- Have the person rinse the mouth after using the inhaler *because this will help to decrease systemic absorption and decrease GI upset, nausea and risk of fungal infection*.
- Monitor the person for any sign of respiratory infection; *continued use of steroids during an acute infection can lead to serious complications related to the depression of the inflammatory and immune responses*.
- Provide thorough teaching, including the drug name and prescribed dosage, measures to help avoid adverse effects, warning signs that may indicate problems and the need for periodic monitoring and evaluation, *to enhance knowledge about drug therapy and to promote compliance*.
- Instruct the person to continue to take the drug *to reach and then maintain effective levels (drug takes 2–3 weeks to reach effective levels)*.
- Offer support and encouragement *to help the person cope with the disease and the drug regimen*.

Evaluation

- Monitor response to the drug (improved breathing).
- Monitor for adverse effects (nasal irritation, fever, GI upset).
- Evaluate the effectiveness of the teaching plan (person can name drug, dosage, adverse effects to watch for, specific measures to avoid them and measures to take to increase the effectiveness of the drug).
- Monitor the effectiveness of other measures to ease breathing.

of the problem associated with asthma. Montelukast (*Lukair, Montekast, Respikast, Singulair, T-Lukast*) is the only drug currently available in this class in Australia and New Zealand.

Therapeutic actions and indications

Leukotriene-receptor antagonists selectively and competitively block receptors for the production of leukotrienes D_4 and E_4, components of slow-reacting substance of anaphylaxis (SRSA). As a result, these drugs block many of the signs and symptoms of asthma, such as neutrophil and eosinophil migration, neutrophil and monocyte aggregation, leukocyte adhesion, increased capillary permeability and smooth muscle contraction. These factors contribute to the inflammation, oedema, mucus secretion and bronchoconstriction seen in people with asthma. See Table 55.3 for usual indications of these drugs. They do not have immediate effects on the airways and are not indicated for treating acute asthma attacks.

Pharmacokinetics

These drugs are given orally. They are rapidly absorbed from the GI tract. Montelukast is extensively metabolised in the liver by the cytochrome P450 system and primarily excreted in faeces. The drug crosses the placenta and enters breast milk (see Contraindications and cautions).

Contraindications and cautions

These drugs should be used cautiously in people with hepatic or renal impairment *because these conditions can affect the drug's metabolism and excretion*. Fetal toxicity has been reported in animal studies, so montelukast should be used during pregnancy only if the benefit to the mother clearly outweighs the potential risks to the fetus. No adequate studies have been done on the effects on the baby if these drugs are used during breastfeeding; caution should be used.

The drug is not indicated for the treatment of acute asthma attacks; it does not provide any immediate effects on the airways. People need to be cautioned that they should not rely on this drug for relief from an acute asthma attacks.

Children may be at increased risk of neuropsychiatric adverse effects.

Adverse effects

Adverse effects associated with leukotriene-receptor antagonists include headache, dizziness, myalgia, nausea, diarrhoea, abdominal pain, thirst, headache, hyperkinesia (in young children); elevated liver enzyme levels, vomiting, generalised pain, fever and myalgia. Less common adverse effects include dry mouth, dyspepsia, oedema, dizziness, malaise, sleep disturbances, sleep-walking, abnormal dreams, anxiety, aggression, depression, paraesthesia, hypoaesthesia, seizures, agitation, arthralgia, myalgia, epistaxis, bruising, pruritus; rarely palpitation, tremor, bleeding; very rarely hepatic disorders, hallucinations, suicidal thoughts and behaviour, and Churg–Strauss syndrome. Because these drugs are relatively new, there is little information about their long-term effects. People should be advised to monitor their use of these drugs and to report any increase of acute episodes or lack of response to the drug, which could indicate a worsening problem or decreased responsiveness to drug therapy.

Clinically important drug–drug interactions

Use caution if propranolol, theophylline or warfarin is taken with these drugs because increased toxicity can occur. Toxicity may also occur if these drugs are combined with calcium channel blockers, ciclosporin or aspirin; decreased dose of either drug may be necessary.

MAST CELL STABILISERS

A **mast cell stabiliser** prevents the release of inflammatory and bronchoconstricting substances when the mast cells are stimulated to release these substances because of irritation or the presence of an antigen. The currently available mast cell stabilisers are sodium cromoglycate (*Intal*) and nedocromil sodium (*Tilade*).

Therapeutic actions and indications

These drugs are used for the treatment of asthma and allergies (see Table 55.3 for usual indications). They work at the cellular level to inhibit the release of histamine (released from mast cells in response to inflammation

Prototype summary: montelukast

Indications: prevention and long-term treatment of asthma in adults and children 12 years of age or older.

Actions: specifically blocks receptors for leukotrienes, which are components of SRSA, blocking airway oedema and processes of inflammation in the airway.

Pharmacokinetics:

Route	Onset	Peak	Duration
Oral	Rapid	3 hours	Unknown

$T_{1/2}$: 10 hours; metabolised in the liver and excreted in urine and faeces.

Adverse effects: headache, dizziness, nausea, generalised pain and fever, infection.

Care considerations for people receiving leukotriene-receptor antagonists

Assessment: history and examination

- Assess for *possible contraindications or cautions*: allergy to the drug and acute bronchospasm or asthma attacks, *all of which would be contraindications to the use of the drug*; impaired renal or hepatic function, *which could alter the metabolism and excretion of the drug and might require a dose adjustment*; and pregnancy or breastfeeding, *which require cautious use.*
- Perform a physical examination *to establish baseline data for assessing the effectiveness of the drug and the occurrence of any adverse effects associated with drug therapy.*
- Evaluate temperature *to monitor for underlying infection.*
- Assess orientation and affect *to monitor for CNS effects of the drug.*
- Evaluate respirations and adventitious breath sounds *to monitor the effectiveness of the drug.*
- Evaluate renal and liver function tests *to assess for impairments that could interfere with metabolism or excretion of the drugs.*
- Perform an abdominal evaluation *to monitor GI effects of the drug.*

Implementation with rationale

- Administer drug on an empty stomach, 1 hour before or 2 hours after meals; *the bioavailability of these drugs is decreased markedly by the presence of food.*

- Caution the person that these drugs are not to be used during an acute asthma attacks or bronchospasm; *instead, regular emergency measures will be needed.*
- Caution the person to take the drug continuously and not to stop the medication during symptom-free periods *to ensure that therapeutic levels are maintained.*
- Provide appropriate safety measures if dizziness occurs *to prevent injury.*
- Urge the person to avoid OTC preparations containing aspirin, *which might interfere with the effectiveness of these drugs.*
- Provide thorough teaching, including the drug name and prescribed dosage, measures to help avoid adverse effects, warning signs that may indicate problems and the need for periodic monitoring and evaluation, *to enhance knowledge about drug therapy and to promote compliance.*
- Offer support and encouragement *to help the person cope with the disease and the drug regimen.*

Evaluation

- Monitor response to the drug (improved breathing).
- Monitor for adverse effects (drowsiness, headache, abdominal pain, myalgia).
- Evaluate the effectiveness of the teaching plan (person can name drug, dosage, adverse effects to watch for, specific measures to avoid them and measures to take to increase the effectiveness of the drug).
- Monitor the effectiveness of other measures to ease breathing.

or irritation) and inhibit the release of inflammatory mediators (see Figure 55.3). By blocking these chemical mediators of the immune reaction, they prevent the allergic asthmatic response when the respiratory tract is exposed to the offending allergen. Sodium cromoglycate is also used as an ophthalmic solution for the treatment of eye-related allergic symptoms, as a nasal spray for seasonal allergic rhinitis and in an inhaled form for the treatment of allergies.

Pharmacokinetics

Sodium cromoglycate is inhaled from a capsule and may not reach its peak effect for 1 week. It is also available as a nasal spray and as an ophthalmic solution, both of which have little systemic absorption. Nedocromil sodium is administered via metered-dose inhaler. They are primarily active in the lungs, and most of the inhaled dose is excreted during exhalation or, if swallowed, excreted in urine and faeces.

Contraindications and cautions

Sodium cromoglycate and nedocromil sodium are contraindicated in the presence of known allergy to the drug *to prevent hypersensitivity reactions.* They cannot be used during an acute attack, and people need to be instructed in this precaution. As with all medications, caution should be exercised, especially during the first trimester of pregnancy. These drugs should be used in pregnancy only if the benefit to the mother outweighs the potential risk to the fetus.

Adverse effects

Few adverse effects have been reported with the use of sodium cromoglycate and nedocromil sodium; those that do occur on occasion include headache, dry mucosa, myalgia, abdominal pain and nausea. Careful management (avoidance of dry or smoky environments, analgesics, use of proper inhalation technique, use of a humidifier and pushing fluids as appropriate) can help to make drug-related discomfort tolerable.

Prototype summary: sodium cromoglycate

Indications: prophylaxis of severe bronchial asthma; prevention of exercise-induced asthma.

Actions: inhibits the allergen-triggered release of histamine, SRSA and leukotrienes from mast cells; decreases the overall allergic response in the airways.

Pharmacokinetics:

Route	Onset	Peak	Duration
Inhaled	Slow	15 min	6–8 hours

$T_{1/2}$: 80 minutes; metabolised in the liver and excreted via exhalation.

Adverse effects: headache, dizziness, nausea, sore throat, dysuria, coughing, wheezing, nasal congestion.

Care considerations for people receiving a mast cell stabiliser

Assessment: history and examination

- Assess for *possible contraindications or cautions*: allergy *to prevent hypersensitivity reactions*; impaired renal or hepatic function, *which could interfere with the metabolism or excretion of the drug, leading to a need for dose adjustment*; and pregnancy or breastfeeding, *which require very cautious administration.*
- Perform a physical examination *to establish baseline data for assessing the effectiveness of the*

drug and the occurrence of any adverse effects associated with drug therapy.

- Assess the skin colour and lesions *to monitor for adverse effects of the drug.*
- Monitor respirations and adventitious sounds *to evaluate drug effectiveness.*
- Assess the patency of the nares *to determine the efficacy of inhaled preparations.*
- Evaluate orientation *to monitor adverse effects and headache.*
- Evaluate renal and liver function tests *to assess for potential problems with drug metabolism or excretion.*

Implementation with rationale

- Review administration procedures with the person periodically; *proper use of the delivery device is important in maintaining the effectiveness of this drug.*
- Caution the person not to discontinue use abruptly; sodium cromoglycate should be tapered slowly if discontinuation is necessary *to prevent rebound adverse effects.*
- Instruct the person that the drug cannot be used during an acute attack *because it has no immediate effects on the airways.*
- Caution the person to continue taking this drug, even during symptom-free periods, *to ensure therapeutic levels of the drug.*
- Advise the person not to wear soft contact lenses; if sodium cromoglycate eye drops (used for allergic reactions) are used, *lenses can be stained or warped.*
- Provide thorough teaching, including the drug name and prescribed dosage, measures to help avoid adverse effects, warning signs that may indicate problems and the need for periodic monitoring and evaluation, *to enhance knowledge about drug therapy and to promote compliance.*
- Offer support and encouragement *to help the person cope with the disease and the drug regimen.*

Evaluation

- Monitor response to the drug (improved breathing, relief of signs of allergic disorders).
- Monitor for adverse effects (drowsiness, dizziness, headache, GI upset, local irritation).
- Evaluate the effectiveness of the teaching plan (person can name drug, dosage, adverse effects to watch for, specific measures to avoid them and measures to take to increase the effectiveness of the drug).
- Monitor the effectiveness of other measures to ease breathing.

KEY POINTS

- Corticosteroids decrease the inflammatory response. The inhalable form is associated with many fewer systemic effects than the other corticosteroid formulations.
- To block various signs and symptoms of asthma, the leukotriene-receptor antagonists block or antagonise receptors for the production of leukotrienes D_4 and E_4.
- Mast cell stabilisers block the release of histamine and other chemicals associated with an allergic reaction. This decreases the inflammatory reaction in the airways.

LUNG SURFACTANTS

Lung surfactants (Table 55.4) are naturally occurring compounds or lipoproteins containing lipids and apoproteins that reduce the surface tension within the alveoli, allowing expansion of the alveoli for gas exchange. Two lung surfactants available for use are beractant (*Survanta*) and poractant (*Curosurf*).

Therapeutic actions and indications

These drugs are used to replace the surfactant that is missing in the lungs of neonates with RDS (see Figure 55.2). See Table 55.4 for usual indications.

Pharmacokinetics

These drugs are instilled directly into the trachea and begin to act immediately on instillation. They are metabolised in the lungs by the normal surfactant metabolic pathways.

Contraindications and cautions

Because lung surfactants are used as emergency drugs in the newborn, there are no contraindications.

Adverse effects

Adverse effects that are associated with the use of lung surfactants include patent ductus arteriosus, bradycardia, hypotension, intraventricular haemorrhage, pneumothorax, pulmonary air leak, hyperbilirubinaemia and sepsis. These effects may be related to the immaturity of the neonate, the invasive procedures used or reactions to the lipoprotein.

TABLE 55.4 **DRUGS IN FOCUS** **Lung surfactants**

Drug name	Dosage/route	Usual indications
(P) beractant (*Survanta*)	4 mL/kg birth weight, instilled intratracheally, may repeat up to four times in 48 hours	Rescue treatment of infants who have respiratory distress syndrome (RDS); prophylactic treatment of infants at high risk of development of RDS (birth weight of < 1350 g; birth weight > 1350 g who have evidence of respiratory immaturity)
poractant (*Curosurf*)	2.5 mL/kg birth weight, intratracheally, half in each bronchus, may repeat with up to two 1.25 mL/kg doses at 12-hour intervals	Rescue treatment of infants who have RDS

(P) Prototype summary: beractant

Indications: prophylactic treatment of infants at high risk for developing RDS; rescue treatment of infants who have developed RDS.

Actions: natural bovine compound of lipoproteins that reduce the surface tension and allow expansion of the alveoli; replaces the surfactant that is missing in infants with RDS.

Pharmacokinetics:

Route	Onset	Peak
Intratracheal	Immediate	Hours

$T_{1/2}$: unknown; metabolised by surfactant pathways.

Adverse effects: patent ductus arteriosus, intraventricular haemorrhage, hypotension, bradycardia, pneumothorax, pulmonary air leak, pulmonary haemorrhage, apnoea, sepsis, infection.

Care considerations for neonates receiving lung surfactants

Assessment: history and examination

- Assess for *possible contraindications or cautions*: screen for time of birth and exact weight *to determine appropriate doses*. Because this drug is used as an emergency treatment, there are no contraindications to screen for.
- Perform a physical examination *to establish baseline data for assessing the effectiveness of the drug and the occurrence of any adverse effects associated with drug therapy*.
- Assess the skin temperature and colour *to evaluate perfusion*.
- Monitor respirations, adventitious sounds, endotracheal tube placement and patency and chest movements *to evaluate the effectiveness of the drug and drug delivery*.
- Evaluate blood pressure, pulse and arterial pressure *to monitor the status of the neonate*.
- Evaluate blood gases and oxygen saturation *to monitor drug effectiveness*.
- Assess temperature and full blood count *to monitor for sepsis*.

Implementation with rationale

- Monitor the neonate continuously during administration and until stable *to provide life support measures as needed*.
- Ensure proper placement of the endotracheal tube with bilateral chest movement and lung sounds *to provide adequate delivery of the drug*.
- Have staff view the manufacturer's teaching video before regular use *to review the specific technical aspects of administration*.
- Suction the infant immediately before administration, but do not suction for 2 hours after administration unless clinically necessary, *to allow the drug time to work*.
- Provide support and encouragement to parents, explaining the use of the drug in the teaching program, *to help them cope with the diagnosis and treatment of their baby*.
- Continue other supportive measures related to the immaturity of the neonate *because this is only one aspect of medical care needed for premature infants*.

Evaluation

- Monitor response to the drug (improved breathing, alveolar expansion).
- Monitor for adverse effects (pneumothorax, patent ductus arteriosus, bradycardia, sepsis).
- Evaluate the effectiveness of the teaching plan, and support parents as appropriate.
- Monitor the effectiveness of other measures to support breathing and stabilise the neonate.
- Evaluate the effectiveness of other supportive measures related to the immaturity of the neonate.

KEY POINTS

- Lung surfactants are naturally occurring compounds that reduce the surface tension in the alveoli, allowing them to expand. They are injected directly into the trachea of neonates who have RDS.
- Administration of lung surfactants requires proper placement of the endotracheal tube, suctioning of the neonate before administration (but not for 2 hours after administration unless necessary) and careful monitoring and support of the neonate to ensure lung expansion and proper oxygenation.

OTHER DRUGS USED TO TREAT LOWER RESPIRATORY TRACT DISORDERS

The other major pathophysiology that can affect the lower respiratory tract is infection. Infection can manifest as bronchitis or pneumonia. These infections occur when pathogens are able to enter the normally well-protected airways and surrounding tissue. Stress, age and concurrent respiratory dysfunction all increase the opportunities for these pathogens to invade the respiratory tract and cause problems. These infections can be viral, bacterial, fungal or protozoal in origin. They are treated using the appropriate agents to affect the specific pathogen that is involved. See Chapter 9 for drugs used to treat bacterial infections, Chapter 10 for drugs used to treat viral infections, Chapter 11 for drugs used to treat fungal infection and Chapter 12 for drugs used to treat protozoal infections. People with infections of the respiratory tract may have difficulty breathing, decreased oxygenation leading to fatigue and changes in abilities to carry on the activities of daily living, including eating. These people require support, assistance to maintain function, help with nutrition and support to deal with the uncomfortable feeling of having difficulty breathing.

CHAPTER SUMMARY

- Pulmonary obstructive diseases include asthma, emphysema and chronic obstructive pulmonary disease (COPD), which cause obstruction of the major airways, and respiratory distress syndrome (RDS), which causes obstruction at the alveolar level.
- Drugs used to treat asthma and COPD include drugs to block inflammation and drugs to dilate bronchi.
- The xanthine derivatives have a direct effect on the smooth muscle of the respiratory tract, both in the bronchi and in the blood vessels.
- The adverse effects of the xanthines are directly related to the theophylline concentration in the blood and can progress to coma and death.
- Sympathomimetics are drugs that mimic the effects of the sympathetic nervous system; they are used for dilation of the bronchi and to increase the rate and depth of respiration.
- Anticholinergics can be used as bronchodilators because of their effect on the vagus nerve, resulting in relaxation of smooth muscle in the bronchi, which leads to bronchodilation.
- Steroids are used to decrease the inflammatory response in the airway. Inhaling the steroid tends to decrease the numerous systemic effects that are associated with use of oral steroids.
- Leukotriene-receptor antagonists block or antagonise receptors for the production of leukotrienes D_4 and E_4, thus blocking many of the signs and symptoms of asthma.
- The mast cell stabilisers block mediators of inflammation and help to decrease swelling and blockage in the airways.
- Lung surfactants are instilled into the respiratory system of premature neonates who do not have enough surfactant to ensure alveolar expansion.

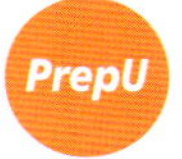

Knowing your strengths and weaknesses helps you to study more effectively. Take a PrepU Practice Quiz to find out how you measure up!

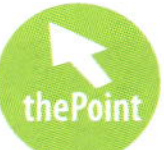

ONLINE RESOURCES

An extensive range of additional resources to enhance teaching and learning and to facilitate understanding of this chapter may be found online at the text's accompanying website, located on thePoint at http://thepoint.lww.com. These include Watch and Learn videos, Concepts in Action animations, journal articles, review questions, case studies, discussion topics and quizzes.

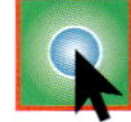

WEB LINKS

Health care providers and students may want to consult the following web resources:

www.aihw.gov.au/copd
Australian Institute of Health and Welfare information on COPD.

www.allergy.org.au
The Australasian Society of Clinical Immunology and Allergy.

www.asthmaaustralia.org.au
Asthma Australia.

www.asthmanz.co.nz
The Asthma Foundation of New Zealand.

www.nationalasthma.org.au
The National Asthma Council Australia.

http://nzformulary.org
The New Zealand formulary.

BIBLIOGRAPHY

Abramson, M., Glasgow, N. & McDonald, C. (2007). Managing chronic obstructive pulmonary disease. *Australian Prescriber, 30*, 64–67.

Bostock-Cox, B. (2013). Managing asthma in the community: A guide for nursing staff. *British Journal of Community Nursing, 18(3)*, 125–127.

Dandan, R. (2012). Indacaterol: *A Once-Daily Ultra-Long Acting β_2 Agonist for the Treatment of COPD*. Access Medicine from McGraw Hill. www.medscape.com/viewarticle/770762.

Dhand, R., Dolovich, M., Chipps, B., Myer, T. R., Restrepo, R. & Farrar, J. R. (2012). The role of nebulized therapy in the management of COPD: Evidence and recommendations. *COPD: Journal of Chronic Obstructive Pulmonary Disease, 9(1)*, 58–72.

Farrell, M. & Dempsey, J. (2014). *Smeltzer & Bare's Textbook of Medical-Surgical Nursing* (3rd edn). Sydney: Lippincott Williams & Wilkins.

Goodman, L. S., Brunton, L. L., Chabner, B. & Knollmann, B. C. (2011). *Goodman and Gilman's Pharmacological Basis of Therapeutics* (12th edn). New York: McGraw-Hill.

Jenkins, C. (2006). Starting steroids for asthma. *Australian Prescriber*, 29, 63–66.

Lim, A., Hussainy, S. Y. & Abramson, M. J. (2013). Asthma drugs in pregnancy and lactation. *Australian Prescriber, 36(5)*, 150–153.

McKenna, L. & Mirkov, S. (2019). *McKenna's Drug Handbook for Nursing and Midwifery* (8th edn). Sydney: Wolters Kluwer Health Australia.

National Asthma Council Australia. (2006). *Asthma Management Handbook 2006*. Melbourne: National Asthma Council Australia.

Porth, C. M. (2011). *Essentials of Pathophysiology: Concepts of Altered Health States* (3rd edn). Philadelphia: Lippincott Williams & Wilkins.

Porth, C. M. (2009). *Pathophysiology: Concepts of Altered Health States* (8th edn). Philadelphia: Lippincott Williams & Wilkins.

Reddel, H. (2012). Rational prescribing for ongoing management of asthma in adults. *Australian Prescriber, 35(2)*, 43–46.

Sin, D. D., Man, J., Sharpe, H., Gan, W. Q. & Man, S. F. (2004). Pharmacological management to reduce exacerbations in adults with asthma: A systematic review and meta-analysis. *JAMA, 293*, 367–376.

Sutherland, R. E. & Cherniak, R. M. (2004). Management of COPD. *New England Journal of Medicine, 350*, 2689–2697.

Van Asperen, P. (2012). Long-acting beta2 agonists for childhood asthma. *Australian Prescriber, 35(4)*, 111–113.

Worsnop, C. (2005). Combination inhalers for asthma. *Australian Prescriber, 28*, 26–28.

CHECK YOUR UNDERSTANDING

Answers to the questions in this chapter can be found in Appendix A at the back of this book.

MULTIPLE CHOICE

Select the best answer to the following.

1. Treatment of obstructive pulmonary disorders is aimed at:
   a. opening the conducting airways or decreasing the effects of inflammation.
   b. blocking the autonomic reflexes that alter respirations.
   c. blocking the effects of the immune and inflammatory systems.
   d. altering the respiratory membrane to increase the flow of oxygen and carbon dioxide.

2. The xanthines:
   a. block the sympathetic nervous system.
   b. stimulate the sympathetic nervous system.
   c. directly affect the smooth muscles of the respiratory tract.
   d. act in the CNS to cause bronchodilation.

3. A person has been maintained on theophylline for many years and has recently taken up smoking. The theophylline levels in this person would be expected to:
   a. rise, because nicotine prevents the breakdown of theophylline.
   b. stay the same, because smoking has no effect on theophylline.
   c. fall, because the nicotine stimulates liver metabolism of theophylline.
   d. rapidly reach toxic levels.

4. A person with hypertension and known heart disease has frequent bronchospasms and asthma attacks that are most responsive to sympathomimetic drugs. This person might be best treated with:
   a. an inhaled sympathomimetic to decrease systemic effects.
   b. a xanthine.
   c. no sympathomimetics because they would be contraindicated.
   d. an anticholinergic.

5. A person with many adverse reactions to drugs is tried on an inhaled steroid for treatment of bronchospasm. For the first 3 days, the person does not notice any improvement. You should:
   a. switch the person to a xanthine.
   b. encourage the person to continue the drug for 2–3 weeks.
   c. switch the person to a sympathomimetic.
   d. try the person on surfactant.

6. Leukotriene-receptor antagonists act to block production of a component of slow-reacting substance of anaphylaxis (SRSA). They are most beneficial in treating:
   a. seasonal rhinitis.
   b. pneumonia.
   c. COPD.
   d. asthma.

7. Respiratory distress syndrome occurs in:
   a. babies with frequent colds.
   b. babies with genetic allergies.
   c. premature and low-birth-weight babies.
   d. babies stressed during the pregnancy.

8. Lung surfactants used therapeutically are:
   a. injected into a developed muscle.
   b. instilled via a nasogastric tube.
   c. injected into the umbilical artery.
   d. instilled into an endotracheal tube properly placed in the baby's lungs.

MULTIPLE RESPONSE

Select all that apply.

1. People who are using inhalers require careful teaching about which of the following?
   a. avoiding food 1 hour before and 2 hours after dosing
   b. storage of the drug
   c. administration techniques to promote therapeutic effects and avoid adverse effects
   d. lying flat for as long as 2 hours after dosing
   e. timing of administration
   f. the difference between rescue treatment and prophylaxis

2. A child with repeated asthma attacks may be treated with which of the following drugs?
   a. a leukotriene-receptor antagonist
   b. a beta blocker
   c. an inhaled corticosteroid
   d. an inhaled beta-2 agonist
   e. a surfactant
   f. a mast cell stabiliser

PART 11

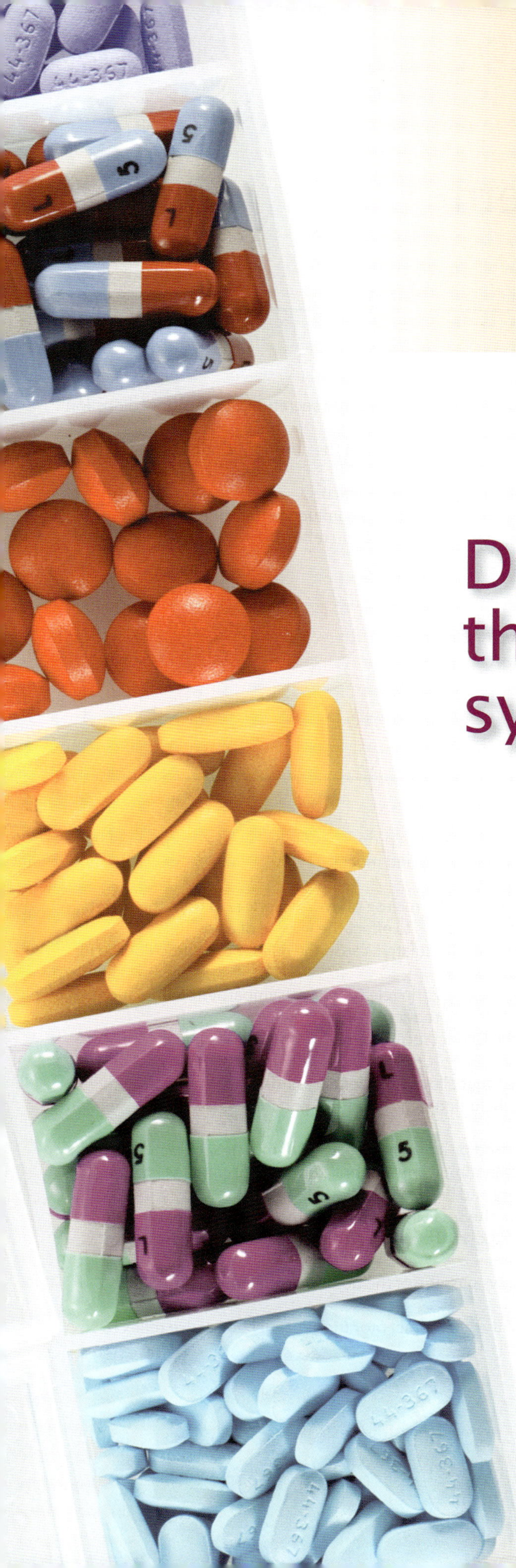

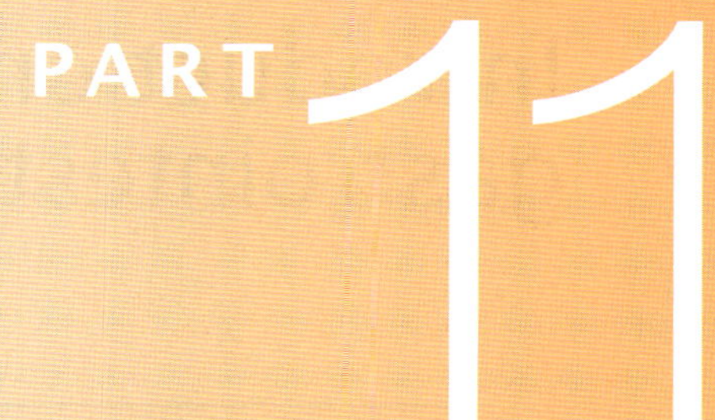

Drugs acting on the gastrointestinal system

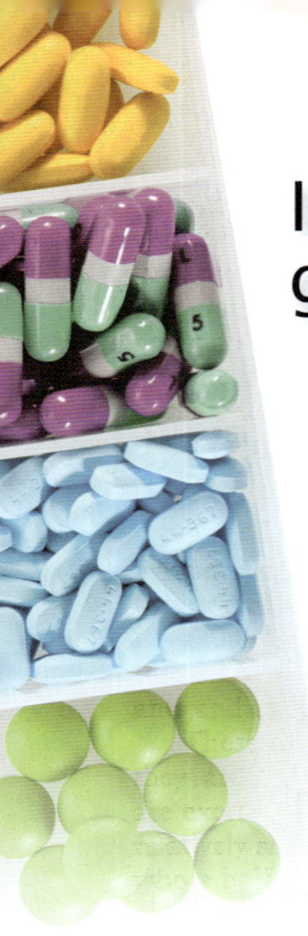

Introduction to the gastrointestinal system

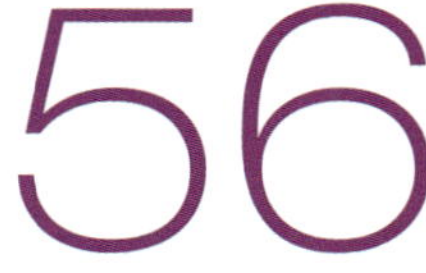

Learning objectives

On completing this chapter you should be able to:

1. Label the parts of the gastrointestinal (GI) tract on a diagram, describing the secretions, absorption, digestion and type of motility that occurs in each part.
2. Discuss the nervous system control of the GI tract, including influences of the autonomic nervous system on GI activity.
3. List three of the local GI reflexes and describe the clinical application of each.
4. Describe the steps involved in swallowing, including two factors that can influence this reflex.
5. Discuss the vomiting reflex, addressing three factors that can stimulate the reflex.

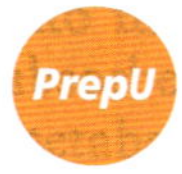

Test your current knowledge of the gastrointestinal system with a PrepU Practice Quiz!

Glossary of key terms

bile: fluid stored in the gallbladder that contains cholesterol and bile salts; essential for the proper breakdown and absorption of fats

chyme: contents of the stomach containing ingested food and secreted enzymes, water and mucus

gallstones: hard crystals formed in the gallbladder when the bile is concentrated

gastrin: substance secreted by the stomach in response to many stimuli; stimulates the release of hydrochloric acid from the parietal cells and pepsin from the chief cells; causes histamine release at histamine-2 receptors to effect the release of acid

histamine-2 (H_2) receptors: sites near the parietal cells of the stomach that, when stimulated, cause the release of hydrochloric acid into the lumen of the stomach; also found near cardiac cells

hydrochloric acid: acid released by the parietal cells of the stomach in response to gastrin release or parasympathetic stimulation; makes the stomach contents more acidic to aid digestion and breakdown of food products

local gastrointestinal reflex: reflex response to various stimuli that allows the GI tract local control of its secretions and movements based on the contents or activity of the whole GI system

nerve plexus: network of nerve fibres running through the wall of the GI tract that allows local reflexes and control

pancreatic enzymes: digestive enzymes secreted by the exocrine pancreas, including pancreatin and pancrelipase, which are needed for the proper digestion of fats, proteins and carbohydrates

peristalsis: type of GI movement that moves a food bolus forward; characterised by a progressive wave of muscle contraction

saliva: fluid produced by the salivary glands in the mouth in response to tactile stimuli and cerebral stimulation; contains enzymes to begin digestion, as well as water and mucus to make the food bolus slippery and easier to swallow

segmentation: GI movement characterised by contraction of one segment of the small intestine while the next segment is relaxed; the contracted segment then relaxes, and the relaxed segment contracts; exposes the chyme to a vast surface area to increase absorption

swallowing: complex reflex response to a bolus in the back of the throat; allows passage of the bolus into the oesophagus and movement of ingested contents into the GI tract

vomiting: complex reflex mediated through the medulla after stimulation of the chemoreceptor trigger zone; protective reflex to remove possibly toxic substances from the stomach

The gastrointestinal (GI) system is the only system in the body that is open to the external environment. It begins at the mouth and ends at the anus. The GI system is responsible for only a very small part of waste excretion. The kidneys and lungs are responsible for excreting most of the waste products of normal metabolism.

STRUCTURE AND FUNCTION OF THE GASTROINTESTINAL SYSTEM

The GI system is composed of one continuous tube that begins at the mouth, progresses through the oesophagus, stomach and small and large intestines and ends at the anus. The pancreas, liver and gallbladder are accessory organs that support the functions of the GI system (see Figure 56.1).

Structures

The tube that comprises the GI tract is continuous with the external environment, opening at the mouth and again at the anus. Because of this, the GI tract contains many foreign agents and bacteria that are not found in the rest of the body. The tube begins in the mouth, which has salivary glands that secrete digestive enzymes and lubricants to facilitate swallowing. The mouth leads to the oesophagus, which connects to the stomach. The stomach is responsible for mechanical and chemical breakdown of foods into usable nutrients. The stomach empties into the small intestine, where absorption of nutrients occurs. The pancreas deposits digestive enzymes and sodium bicarbonate into the beginning of the small intestine to neutralise the acid from the stomach and to further facilitate digestion. The liver produces bile, which is stored in the gallbladder. The bile is very important in the digestion of fats and is deposited into the small intestine when the gallbladder is stimulated to contract by the presence of fats. All of the nutrients absorbed from the small intestine pass into the liver, which is responsible for processing, storing or clearing them from the system. The small intestine leads to the large intestine, which is responsible for excreting any waste products that are in the GI system. The excretion occurs through the rectum and is an activity that one learns to control.

The peritoneum lines the abdominal wall and also the viscera, with a small 'free space' between the two layers. It helps to keep the GI tract in place and prevents a build-up of friction with movement. The greater and lesser omenta hang from the stomach over the lower GI tract and are full of lymph nodes, lymphocytes, monocytes and other

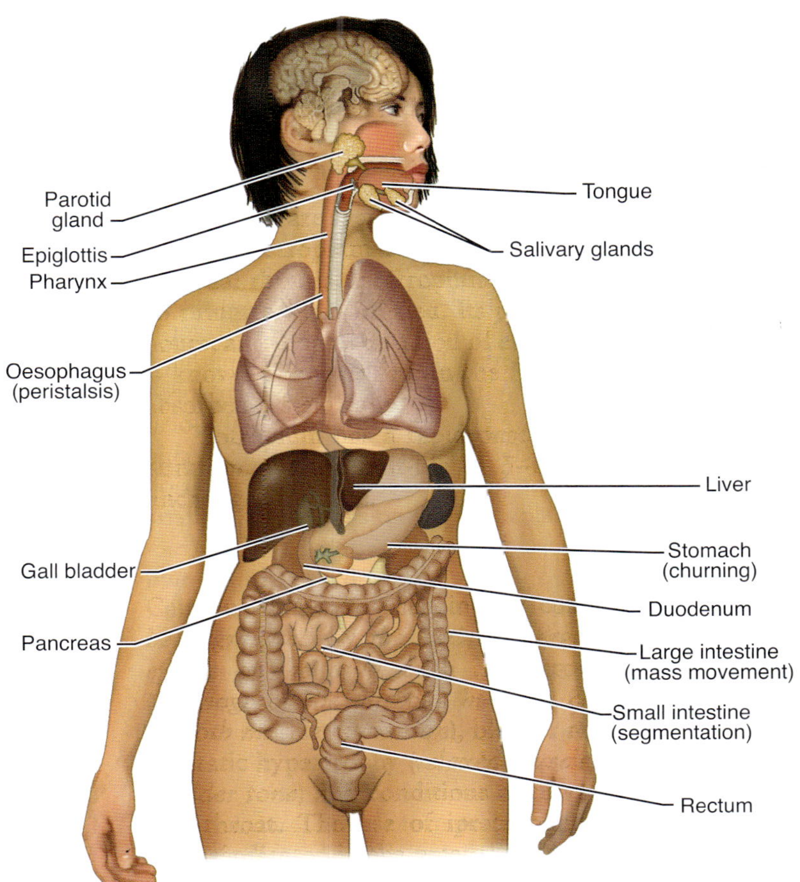

FIGURE 56.1 The gastrointestinal tract.

components of the mononuclear phagocyte system. This barrier provides rapid protection for the rest of the body if any of the bacteria or other foreign agents in the GI tract are absorbed into the body.

Layers of the GI tract

The GI tube is composed of four layers: the mucosa, the muscularis mucosa, the **nerve plexus** (a network of nerve fibres running through the wall of the GI tract that allows local reflexes and control) and the adventitia.

Mucosal layer

The mucosal layer provides the inner lining of the GI tract. It can be seen in the mouth and is fairly consistent throughout the tube. It is important to remember when assessing a person that if the mouth is very dry or full of lesions, that is a reflection of the state of the entire GI tract and may indicate that the person has difficulty digesting or absorbing nutrients. This layer has an epithelial component and a connective tissue component.

Muscularis mucosa layer

The muscularis mucosa layer is made up of muscles. Most of the GI tract has two muscle layers. One layer runs circularly around the tube, helping keep the tube open and squeezing the tube to aid digestion and motility. The other layer runs horizontally, which helps propel the gastrointestinal contents down the tract. The stomach has a third layer of muscle, which runs obliquely and gives the stomach the ability to move contents in a churning motion.

Nerve plexus layer

The nerve plexus has two layers of nerves – one submucosal layer and one myenteric layer. These nerves allow the GI tract local control over movement, secretions and digestion. The nerves respond to local stimuli and act on the contents of the GI tract accordingly. The GI tract is also innervated by the sympathetic and parasympathetic nervous systems. These systems can slow down or speed up the activity in the GI tract but cannot initiate local activity. The sympathetic system is stimulated during times of stress ('fight-or-flight' response) when digestion is not a priority. To slow the GI tract, the sympathetic system decreases muscle tone, secretions and contractions, and increases sphincter tone. By shutting down the GI activity, the body saves energy for other activities. In contrast, the parasympathetic system ('rest-and-digest' response) stimulates the GI tract, increasing muscle tone, secretions and contractions and decreasing sphincter tone, allowing easy movement.

Adventitia layer

The adventitia is the outer layer of the GI tract. It serves as a supportive layer and helps the tube maintain its shape and position (see Figure 56.2).

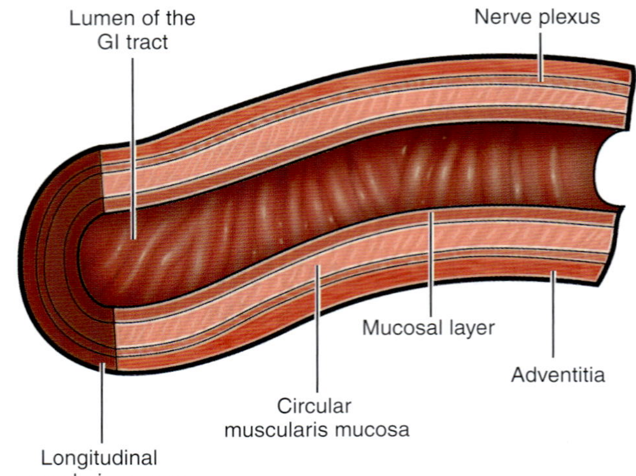

FIGURE 56.2 Layers of the gastrointestinal tract.

Gastrointestinal activities

The GI system has four major activities:

- *Secretion* of enzymes, acid, bicarbonate and mucus
- *Absorption* of water and almost all of the essential nutrients needed by the body
- *Digestion* of food into usable and absorbable components
- *Motility* (movement) of food and secretions through the system (what is not used is excreted in the form of faeces)

These functions are discussed in detail in the following sections.

Secretion

The GI tract secretes various compounds to aid the movement of the food bolus through the GI tube, to protect the inner layer of the GI tract from injury and to facilitate the digestion and absorption of nutrients (see Figure 56.1). Secretions begin in the mouth. **Saliva**, which contains water and digestive enzymes, is secreted from the salivary glands to begin the digestive process and to facilitate swallowing by making the bolus slippery.

Mucus is also produced in the mouth to protect the epithelial lining and to aid in swallowing. The oesophagus produces mucus to protect the inner lining of the GI tract and to further facilitate the movement of the bolus down the tube.

The stomach produces acid and digestive enzymes. In addition, it generates a large amount of mucus to protect the stomach lining from the acid and the enzymes. In the stomach, secretion begins with what is called the cephalic phase of digestion. The sight, smell or taste of food stimulates the stomach to begin secreting before any food reaches the stomach. Once the bolus of food arrives at the stomach, **gastrin** is secreted. Gastrin stimulates the stomach muscles to contract, the parietal cells to release **hydrochloric acid** and the chief cells to release pepsin. Parasympathetic stimulation also leads to acid release. Gastrin and the parasympathetic system stimulate **histamine-2 (H_2) receptors** near the parietal cells, causing the cells to release hydrochloric acid into the lumen of the stomach. Proteins, calcium, alcohol and caffeine in the stomach increase gastrin secretion. High levels of acid decrease the secretion of gastrin. Other digestive enzymes are released appropriately, in response to proteins and carbohydrates, to begin digestion. Peptic ulcers can develop when there is a decrease in the protective mucosal layer or an increase in acid production.

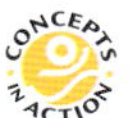
Digestive: Digestion of carbohydrates

As the now-acidic bolus leaves the stomach and enters the small intestine, secretin is released, which stimulates the pancreas to secrete large amounts of sodium bicarbonate (to neutralise the acid bolus), the **pancreatic enzymes** chymotrypsin and trypsin (to break down proteins to smaller amino acids), other lipases (to break down fat) and amylases (to break down sugars). These enzymes are delivered to the GI tract through the common bile duct, which is shared with the gallbladder.

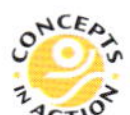
Digestive: Metabolism of amino acids

If fat is present in the bolus, the gallbladder contracts and releases **bile** into the small intestine. Bile contains a detergent-like substance that breaks apart fat molecules so that they can be processed and absorbed. The bile in the gallbladder is produced by the liver during normal metabolism. Once delivered to the gallbladder for storage, it is concentrated; water is removed by the walls of the gallbladder. Some people are prone to developing **gallstones** in the gallbladder when the concentrated bile crystallises. These stones can move down the duct and cause severe pain or even blockage of the bile duct.

In response to the presence of food, the small and large intestines may secrete various endocrine hormones, including growth hormone, aldosterone and glucagon. They also secrete large amounts of mucus to facilitate the movement of the bolus through the rest of the GI tract.

Digestion

Digestion is the process of breaking food into usable, absorbable nutrients. Digestion begins in the mouth, with the enzymes in the saliva starting the process of breaking down sugars and proteins. The stomach continues the digestion process with muscular churning, breaking down some foodstuffs while mixing them thoroughly with hydrochloric acid and enzymes. The acid and enzymes further break down sugars and proteins into building blocks and separate vitamins, electrolytes, minerals and other nutrients from ingested food for absorption. The beginning of the small intestine introduces bile to the food bolus, which is now called **chyme**. Bile breaks down fat molecules for processing and absorption into the bloodstream. Digestion is finished at this point, and absorption of the nutrients begins.

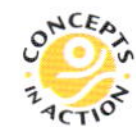
Digestive: General digestion

Absorption

Absorption is the active process of removing water, nutrients and other elements from the GI tract and delivering them to the bloodstream for use by the body. The portal system drains all of the lower GI tract, where absorption occurs, and delivers what is absorbed into the venous system directly to the liver. The liver filters, clears and further processes most of what is absorbed before it is delivered to the body (see Figure 56.1). Some absorption occurs in the lower end of the stomach, most commonly absorption of water and alcohol. The majority of absorption occurs in the small intestine. It about 8500 mL/day, including nutrients, drugs and anything that is taken into the GI tract, as well as any secretions. The small intestine mucosal layer is specially designed to facilitate this absorption, with long villi on the epithelial layer providing a vast surface area for absorption. The large intestine absorbs approximately 350 mL/day, mostly sodium and water.

Motility

The GI tract depends on an inherent motility to keep things moving through the system. The nerve plexus maintains a basic electrical rhythm (BER), much like the pacemaker rhythm in the heart. The cells within the plexus are somewhat unstable and leak electrolytes, leading to the regular firing of an action potential. This rhythm maintains the tone of the GI tract muscles and can be affected by local or autonomic stimuli to increase or decrease the rate of firing.

The basic movement seen in the oesophagus is **peristalsis**, a constant wave of contraction that moves from the top to the bottom of the oesophagus. The act of **swallowing**, a response to a food bolus in the back of the throat, stimulates the peristaltic movement that directs the food bolus into the stomach. The stomach uses its three muscle layers to produce a churning action. This action mixes the digestive enzymes and acid with the food to increase digestion. A contraction of the lower end of the stomach sends the chyme into the small intestine.

The small intestine uses a process of **segmentation** with an occasional peristaltic wave to clear the segment. Segmentation involves contraction of one segment of small intestine while the next segment is relaxed. The contracted segment then relaxes, and the relaxed segment contracts. This action exposes the chyme to a vast surface area to increase the absorption. The small intestine maintains a BER of 11 contractions per minute. This regular movement is assessed when listening for bowel sounds.

The large intestine uses a process of mass movement with an occasional peristaltic wave. When the beginning segment of the large intestine is stimulated, it contracts and sends a massive peristaltic movement throughout the entire large intestine. The end result of the mass movement is usually excretion of waste products.

Rectal distension after mass movement stimulates a defecation reflex that causes relaxation of the external and internal sphincters. Control of the external sphincter is a learned behaviour. The receptors in the external sphincter adapt relatively quickly and will stretch and require more and more distension to stimulate the reflex if the reflex is ignored.

KEY POINTS

- The GI system begins at the mouth and ends at the anus; a long tube extends between them and comprises the oesophagus, the stomach, the small intestine and the large intestine. Essential functions are digestion and absorption of nutrients.
- The GI system secretes enzymes, acid, bicarbonate and mucus to facilitate the digestion and absorption of nutrients.
- The small intestine is the organ where most absorption occurs. The veins of the small intestine carry the absorbed products to the liver for filtering, cleaning and metabolism, or the breaking down of absorbed products into usable substances.
- The nerve plexus controls the GI system by maintaining electrical rhythm and responding to local stimuli (increasing or decreasing activity). The autonomic nervous system influences GI activity, with the sympathetic system slowing and the parasympathetic system increasing activity.

GASTROINTESTINAL REFLEXES

To function effectively, several local and central reflexes occur. Local reflexes involve stimulation of the nerves in the GI tract and cause movement and secretion. Central reflexes, which include swallowing and vomiting, are controlled by the medulla.

Local reflexes

Stimulation of local nerves within the GI tract causes increased or decreased movement within the system, maintaining homeostasis. Loss of reflexes or stimulation can result in constipation and the lack of movement of the bolus along the GI tract or diarrhoea, with increased motility and excretion. The longer a faecal bolus remains in the large intestine, the more sodium and water are absorbed from it and the harder and less mobile it can become. There are many **local gastrointestinal reflexes.** Some knowledge of how these reflexes operate makes it easier to understand what happens when the reflexes are blocked or overstimulated and how therapeutic measures are often used to cause reflex activity.

- *Gastroenteric reflex*: stimulation of the stomach by stretching, the presence of food or cephalic stimulation (the body's response to smelling, seeing, tasting or thinking about food) causes an increase in activity in the small intestine. It is thought that this prepares the small intestine for the coming chyme.
- *Gastrocolic reflex*: stimulation of the stomach also causes increased activity in the colon, again preparing it to empty any contents to provide space for the new chyme.
- *Duodenal–colic reflex*: the presence of food or stretching in the duodenum stimulates colon activity and mass movement, again to empty the colon for the new chyme.

It is important to remember the gastroenteric, gastrocolic and duodenal reflexes when helping people to maintain GI movement. Taking advantage of stomach stimulation (eg, having the person drink prune juice or hot water or eat bran) and providing the opportunity of time and privacy for a bowel movement encourage normal reflexes to keep things in control.

Other local GI reflexes include the following:

- *Ileogastric reflex*: the introduction of chyme or stretch to the large intestine slows stomach activity, as does the introduction of chyme into the small and large intestine, allowing time for absorption. In part, this reflex explains why people who are constipated often have no appetite: the continued stretch on the ileum that comes with constipation continues to slow stomach activity and makes the introduction of new food into the stomach undesirable.
- *Intestinal–intestinal reflex*: excessive irritation to one section of the small intestine causes a cessation of activity above that section to prevent further irritation, and an increase in activity below that section, which leads to a flushing of the irritant. This reflex is active in 'Montezuma's revenge' (traveller's diarrhoea): local irritation of the intestine causes increased secretions and movement below that section, resulting in watery diarrhoea and a cessation of movement above that section. Loss of appetite or even nausea may occur. An extreme reaction to this reflex can be seen after abdominal surgery, when the handling of the intestines causes intense irritation and the reflex can cause the entire intestinal system to cease activity, leading to a paralytic ileus.

- *Peritoneointestinal reflex*: irritation of the peritoneum as a result of inflammation or injury leads to a cessation of GI activity, preventing continued movement of the GI tract and thus further irritation of the peritoneum.
- *Renointestinal reflex*: irritation or swelling of the renal capsule causes a cessation of movement in the GI tract, again to prevent further irritation to the capsule.
- *Vesicointestinal reflex*: irritation or overstretching of the bladder can cause a reflex cessation of movement in the GI tract, again to prevent further irritation to the bladder from the GI movement. Many people with cystitis or overstretched bladders from occupational constraints or neurological problems complain of constipation, which can be attributable to this reflex.
- *Somatointestinal reflex*: taut stretching of the skin and muscles over the abdomen irritates the nerve plexus and causes a slowing or cessation of GI activity to prevent further irritation. During the era when tight girdles were commonly worn, this reflex was often seen among women, and constipation was a serious problem for many women who wore such constraining garments. Tight-fitting clothing (eg, jeans) can have the same effect. People who complain of chronic constipation may be suffering from overactivity of the somatointestinal reflex.

Central reflexes

Two centrally mediated reflexes – swallowing and vomiting – are very important to the functioning of the GI tract.

Swallowing

The swallowing reflex is stimulated whenever a food bolus stimulates pressure receptors in the back of the throat and pharynx. These receptors send impulses to the medulla, which stimulates a series of nerves that cause the following actions: the soft palate elevates and seals off the nasal cavity; respirations cease in order to protect the lungs; the larynx rises and the glottis closes to seal off the airway; and the pharyngeal constrictor muscles contract and force the food bolus into the top of the oesophagus, where pairs of muscles contract in turn to move the bolus down the oesophagus into the stomach. This reflex is complex, involving more than 25 pairs of muscles.

This reflex can be facilitated in a number of ways if swallowing (food or medication) is a problem. Icing the tongue by sucking on ice cube blocks external nerve impulses and allows this more basic reflex to respond. Icing the sternal notch or the back of the neck, although not as appealing, has also proved effective in stimulating the swallowing reflex. In addition, keeping the head straight (not turned to one side) allows the muscle pairs to work together and helps the process. Providing stimulation of the receptors in the mouth through temperature variations and textured foods helps to initiate the reflex. People who do not produce their own saliva can be given artificial saliva to increase digestion and to lubricate the food bolus, which also helps the swallowing reflex.

Vomiting

The **vomiting** reflex is another basic reflex that is centrally mediated and important in protecting the system from unwanted irritants. The vomiting reflex is stimulated by two centres in the medulla. The more primitive centre is called the emetic zone. When stimulated, it initiates a projectile vomiting. This type of intense reaction is seen in young children and whenever increased pressure in the brain or brain damage allows the more primitive centre to override the more mature chemoreceptor trigger zone (CTZ). The CTZ is stimulated in several ways:

- tactile stimulation of the back of the throat, a reflex to get rid of something that is too big or too irritating to be swallowed
- excessive stomach distension
- increasing intracranial pressure by direct stimulation
- stimulation of the vestibular receptors in the inner ear (a reaction often seen with dizziness after 'wild' rides in amusement parks)
- stimulation of stretch receptors in the uterus and bladder (a possible explanation for vomiting in early pregnancy and before delivery)
- intense pain fibre stimulation
- direct stimulation by various chemicals, including fumes, certain drugs and debris from cellular death (a reason for vomiting after chemotherapy or radiation therapy that results in cell death).

Once the CTZ is stimulated, a series of reflexes occurs. Salivation increases, and there is a large increase in the production of mucus in the upper GI tract, which is accompanied by a decrease in gastric acid production. This action protects the lining of the GI tract from potential damage by the acidic stomach contents. (Nauseated people who start swallowing repeatedly or complain about secretions in their throat are in the process of preparing for vomiting.) The sympathetic system is stimulated, with a resultant increase in sweating, increased heart rate, deeper respirations and nausea. This prepares the body for fight or flight and the insult of vomiting. The oesophagus then relaxes and becomes distended and the gastric sphincter relaxes. The person takes one deep respiration; the glottis closes and the palate rises, trapping the air in the lungs and sealing off entry to the lungs. The abdominal and thoracic muscles contract, increasing intra-abdominal pressure. The stomach then relaxes, and the lower section of the stomach contracts in waves, approximately six times per minute. With nothing in the stomach, this movement is known as retching, and it can be quite tiring and uncomfortable. This action causes a backward peristalsis and movement of stomach contents up the oesophagus and out the mouth. The body thus rids itself of offending irritants.

The vomiting reflex is complex and protective, but it can be undesirable in certain clinical situations, when the stimulant is not something that can be vomited or when the various components of the vomiting reflex could be detrimental to a person's health status.

KEY POINTS

- Swallowing, a centrally mediated reflex important in delivering food to the GI tract for processing, is controlled by the medulla. It involves a complex series of timed reflexes.
- Vomiting is controlled by the chemoreceptor trigger zone (CTZ) in the medulla or by the emetic zone in immature or injured brains. The CTZ is stimulated by several different processes and initiates a complex series of responses that first prepare the system for vomiting and then cause a strong backward peristalsis to rid the stomach of its contents.

CHAPTER SUMMARY

- The gastrointestinal (GI) system is composed of one long tube that starts at the mouth, includes the oesophagus, the stomach, the small intestine and the large intestine, and ends at the anus. The GI system is responsible for digestion and absorption of nutrients.
- Secretion of digestive enzymes, acid, bicarbonate and mucus facilitates the digestion and absorption of nutrients.
- The GI system is controlled by a nerve plexus, which maintains a basic electrical rhythm and responds to local stimuli to increase or decrease activity. The sympathetic nervous system, if stimulated, slows GI activity; stimulation of the parasympathetic nervous system increases activity. Initiation of activity depends on local reflexes.
- A series of local reflexes within the GI tract helps to maintain homeostasis within the system. Overstimulation of any of these reflexes can result in constipation (underactivity) or diarrhoea (overactivity).

- Swallowing, a centrally mediated reflex important in delivering food to the GI tract for processing, is controlled by the medulla. It involves a complex series of timed reflexes.
- Vomiting is controlled by the chemoreceptor trigger zone (CTZ) in the medulla or by the emetic zone in immature or injured brains. The CTZ is stimulated by several different processes and initiates a complex series of responses that first prepare the system for vomiting and then cause a strong backward peristalsis to rid the stomach of its contents.

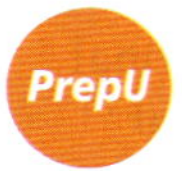

Knowing your strengths and weaknesses helps you to study more effectively. Take a PrepU Practice Quiz to find out how you measure up!

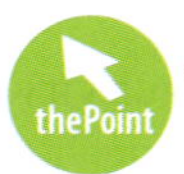

ONLINE RESOURCES

An extensive range of additional resources to enhance teaching and learning and to facilitate understanding of this chapter may be found online at the text's accompanying website, located on thePoint at http://thepoint.lww.com. These include Watch and Learn videos, Concepts in Action animations, journal articles, review questions, case studies, discussion topics and quizzes.

BIBLIOGRAPHY

Barrett, K. E. & Ganong, W. F. (2010). *Ganong's Review of Medical Physiology* (23rd edn). New York: McGraw-Hill.

Goodman, L. S., Brunton, L. L., Chabner, B. & Knollmann, B. C. (2011). *Goodman and Gilman's Pharmacological Basis of Therapeutics* (12th edn). New York: McGraw-Hill.

Guyton, A. & Hall, J. (2011). *Textbook of Medical Physiology* (12th edn). Philadelphia: Saunders Elsevier.

Johnson, L. R. (2007). *Gastrointestinal Physiology* (7th edn). St Louis, MO: Mosby.

Parkman, H. & Fisher, R. S. (2006). *The Clinician's Guide to Acid/Peptic Disorders and Motility Disorders of the GI Tract.* Thorofare, NJ: Slack.

Porth, C. M. (2011). *Essentials of Pathophysiology: Concepts of Altered Health States* (3rd edn). Philadelphia: Lippincott Williams & Wilkins.

Porth, C. M. (2009). *Pathophysiology: Concepts of Altered Health States* (8th edn). Philadelphia: Lippincott Williams & Wilkins.

Rhoades, R. A. & Bell, D. R. (2008). *Medical Physiology: Principles of Clinical Medicine.* Philadelphia: Lippincott Williams & Wilkins.

Seidel, E. (2006). *Crash Course: GI System.* St Louis, MO: Mosby.

Seifter, J., Rafnon, A. & Sloane, D. (2005). *Concepts in Medical Physiology.* Philadelphia: Lippincott Williams & Wilkins.

CHECK YOUR UNDERSTANDING

Answers to the questions in this chapter can be found in Appendix A at the back of this book.

MULTIPLE CHOICE

Select the best response to the following.

1. After teaching a group of students about GI activity and constipation, the instructor determines that the teaching was successful when the students state which of the following about constipation?
   a. It results from increased peristaltic activity in the intestinal tract.
   b. It occurs primarily when one does not have a daily bowel movement.
   c. It leads to decreased salt and water absorption from the large intestine.
   d. It can be artificially induced by increasing the volume of the large intestine.
2. In explaining the importance of the pancreas to a nursing or midwifery student, the instructor would explain that the pancreas:
   a. is primarily an endocrine gland.
   b. secretes enzymes in response to an increased plasma glucose concentration.
   c. neutralises the hydrochloric acid secreted by the stomach.
   d. produces bile.
3. Gastrin:
   a. stimulates acid secretion in the stomach.
   b. secretion is blocked by the products of protein digestion in the stomach.
   c. secretion is stimulated by acid in the duodenum.
   d. is responsible for the chemical or gastric phase of intestinal secretion.
4. When explaining control of movement and secretion activities of the GI tract, it would be most accurate to state that the GI is basically controlled by:
   a. the sympathetic nervous system.
   b. the parasympathetic nervous system.
   c. local nerve reflexes of the GI nerve plexus.
   d. the medulla in the brain stem.
5. The presence of fat in the duodenum causes:
   a. acid indigestion.
   b. decreased acid production.
   c. increased gastrin release.
   d. contraction of the gallbladder.
6. The basic type of movement that occurs in the small intestine is:
   a. peristalsis.
   b. mass movement.
   c. churning.
   d. segmentation.
7. Most of the nutrients absorbed from the GI tract pass immediately into the portal venous system and are processed by the liver. This is possible because almost all absorption occurs through:
   a. the lower section of the stomach.
   b. the top section of the large intestine.
   c. the small intestine.
   d. the ileum.

MULTIPLE RESPONSE

Select all that apply.

1. The chemoreceptor trigger zone in the brain is activated by which of the following?
   a. stretch of the uterus
   b. stretch of the bladder
   c. decreased GI activity
   d. radiation
   e. cell death
   f. extreme pain
2. Acid production in the stomach is stimulated by which of the following?
   a. protein in the stomach
   b. calcium products in the stomach
   c. high levels of acid in the stomach
   d. alcohol in the stomach
   e. low levels of acid in the stomach
   f. histamine-2 stimulation
3. When describing the action of pancreatic digestive enzymes in breaking down substances, which substances would the instructor include?
   a. gastric acid
   b. fats
   c. proteins
   d. sugars
   e. bile
   f. lipids

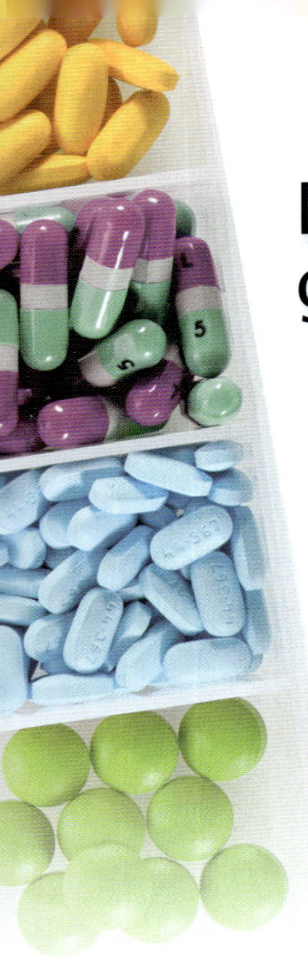

Drugs affecting gastrointestinal secretions

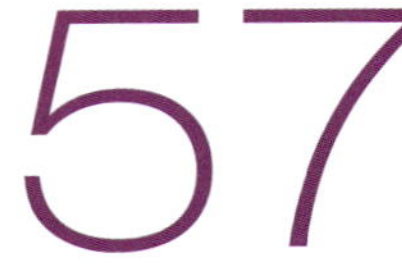

Learning objectives

On completing this chapter you should be able to:

1. Describe the current theories on the pathophysiological process responsible for the signs and symptoms of peptic ulcer disease.
2. Describe the therapeutic actions, indications, pharmacokinetics, contraindications and cautions, most common adverse reactions and important drug–drug interactions associated with drugs used to affect gastrointestinal (GI) secretions.
3. Discuss the drugs used to affect GI secretions across the lifespan.
4. Compare and contrast the prototype drugs used to affect GI secretions – cimetidine, omeprazole, sucralfate, misoprostol and pancrelipase – with other agents in their class and with other classes of drugs used to affect GI secretions.
5. Outline the care considerations, including important teaching points, for people receiving drugs used to affect GI secretions.

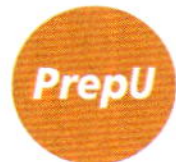

Test your current knowledge of drugs affecting gastrointestinal secretions with a PrepU Practice Quiz!

Glossary of key terms

acid rebound: reflex response of the stomach to lower-than-normal acid levels; when acid levels are lowered through the use of antacids, gastrin production and secretion are increased to return the stomach to its normal acidity

antacids: a group of inorganic chemicals that neutralise stomach acid

digestive enzymes: enzymes produced in the gastrointestinal (GI) tract to break down foods into usable nutrients

GI protectant: drug that coats any injured area in the stomach to prevent further injury from acid or pepsin

histamine-2 (H_2) antagonist: drug that blocks the H_2-receptor sites; used to decrease acid production in the stomach (H_2 sites are stimulated to cause the release of acid in response to gastrin or parasympathetic stimulation)

peptic ulcer: erosion of the lining of stomach or duodenum; results from imbalance between acid produced and the mucus protection of the GI lining, or possibly from infection by *Helicobacter pylori* bacteria

prostaglandin: any one of numerous tissue hormones that have local effects on various systems and organs of the body, including vasoconstriction, vasodilation, increased or decreased GI activity, and increased or decreased pancreatic enzyme release

proton pump inhibitor: drug that blocks the hydrogen–potassium–adenosine triphosphatase (H^+–K^+-ATPase) enzyme system on the secretory surface of the gastric parietal cells, thus interfering with the final step of acid production and lowering acid levels in the stomach

DRUGS USED TO TREAT GASTRO-OESOPHAGEAL REFLUX DISEASE AND ULCER DISEASE

Histamine-2 antagonists

(P) cimetidine
famotidine
nizatidine
ranitidine

Antacids

aluminium salts
calcium salts
magnesium salts
sodium bicarbonate

Proton pump inhibitors

esomeprazole
lansoprazole
(P) omeprazole
pantoprazole
rabeprazole

GI protectant

(P) sucralfate

Prostaglandin

(P) misoprostol

DRUGS USED TO TREAT DIGESTIVE ENZYME DYSFUNCTION

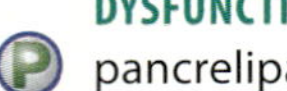
(P) pancrelipase

Gastrointestinal (GI) disorders are among the most common complaints seen in clinical practice. Many products are available for the self-treatment of upset stomach, heartburn or dyspepsia. The underlying causes of these disorders can range from dietary excess, stress, hiatus hernia, oesophageal reflux and adverse drug effects to the more serious peptic ulcer disease. This chapter addresses the major conditions often requiring drug therapy: peptic ulcer disease and disorders involving increased acid levels and digestive enzyme dysfunction (Box 57.1).

BOX 57.1 Major conditions for using drugs that affect GI secretions

ULCER DISEASE

Erosions in the lining of the stomach and adjacent areas of the GI tract are called **peptic ulcers**. People with ulcers present with a predictable description of gnawing, burning pain often occurring a few hours after meals. Many of the drugs that are used to affect GI secretions are designed to prevent, treat or aid in the healing of these ulcers. The cause of chronic peptic ulcers is not completely understood. For many years, it was believed that ulcers were caused by excessive acid production, and treatment was aimed at neutralising acid or blocking the parasympathetic system to decrease normal GI activity and secretions. Further research led many to believe that, because acid production was often normal in people with ulcers, ulcers were caused by a defect in the mucus lining that coats the inner lumen of the stomach to protect it from acid and digestive enzymes. Treatment was aimed at improving the balance between the acid produced and the mucus layer that protects the stomach lining. Research has shown that chronic ulcers may also be the result of infection by *Helicobacter pylori* bacteria. Combination antibiotics have been found to be quite effective in treating some people with chronic ulcers.

Acute ulcers, or 'stress ulcers', are often seen in situations that involve acute physiological stress, such as trauma, burns or prolonged illness. The activity of the sympathetic nervous system during stress decreases blood flow to the GI tract, leading to weakening of the mucosal layer of the stomach and erosion by acid in the stomach. Many of the drugs available for treating various peptic ulcers act to alter acid-producing activities of the stomach.

DIGESTIVE ENZYME DYSFUNCTION

Some people require a supplement to the production of digestive enzymes. People with strokes, salivary gland disorders, or extreme surgery of the head and neck may not be able to produce saliva. Saliva is important in beginning the digestion of sugars and proteins and is essential in initiating the swallowing reflex. People with common duct problems, pancreatic disease or cystic fibrosis may not be able to produce or secrete pancreatic enzymes. These enzymes may need to be administered to allow normal digestion and absorption of nutrients.

DRUGS USED TO TREAT GASTRO-OESOPHAGEAL REFLUX DISEASE AND ULCER DISEASE

Drugs typically used to affect GI secretions in treating peptic ulcer disease and disorders involving increased GI acid work to decrease GI secretory activity, block the action of GI secretions, or form protective coverings on the GI lining to prevent erosion from GI secretions. Recent research studies have begun questioning the effects that lowering acid levels might have on the homeostasis of the GI system and on total body homeostasis, including calcium levels (see Box 57.2).

The drugs used to treat gastro-oesophageal reflux disease (GORD) and ulcer disease include histamine-2 (H_2) antagonists, which block the release of hydrochloric acid in response to gastrin; antacids, which interact with acids at the chemical level to neutralise them; proton pump inhibitors, which suppress the secretion of hydrochloric acid into the lumen of the stomach; GI protectants, which coat any injured area in the stomach to prevent further injury from acid; and prostaglandins, which inhibit the secretion of gastrin and increase the secretion of the mucus lining of the stomach, providing a buffer. Figure 57.1 depicts sites of actions of these drugs used to treat GORD and ulcer disease. Box 57.3 highlights important considerations related to use of these drugs across the lifespan.

HISTAMINE-2 ANTAGONISTS

Histamine-2 (H_2) antagonists (Table 57.1) block the release of hydrochloric acid in response to gastrin. These drugs include cimetidine (*Magicul*), ranitidine (*Zantac*), famotidine (*Pepzan*) and nizatidine (*Nizac, Tazac*).

Therapeutic actions and indications

The H_2 antagonists selectively block H_2 receptors located on the parietal cells. Blocking these receptors prevents the release of gastrin, a hormone that causes local release of histamine (due to stimulation of histamine receptors), ultimately blocking the production of hydrochloric acid. This action also decreases pepsin production by the chief cells. H_2-receptor sites are also found in the heart, and high levels of these drugs can produce cardiac arrhythmias (see Adverse effects).

These drugs are used in:

- short-term treatment of active duodenal ulcer or benign gastric ulcer (reduction in the overall acid level can promote healing and decrease discomfort)
- treatment of pathological hypersecretory conditions such as Zollinger–Ellison syndrome (blocking the overproduction of hydrochloric acid that is associated with these conditions)

BOX 57.2 FOCUS ON The evidence

Drugs that decrease acid may affect more than acid levels

In December 2005, the *Journal of the American Medical Association* published a study that followed people taking proton pump inhibitors (*Nexium* and others) over a period of 10 years. The report showed that people using these drugs had *Clostridium difficile* infections leading to diarrhoea at three times the rate of people not using these drugs. There was also a reported twofold increase in these infections in people using histamine-2 (H_2) antagonists (*cimetidine*). *C. difficile* is a significant cause of diarrhoea in the community. Other studies have reported similar findings. Drugs that lower acid levels change the normal environment of the GI tract, perhaps allowing bacteria to thrive that would normally be destroyed by the acid. Most of these acid-lowering drugs are available in over-the-counter (OTC) preparations and may be used in excessive doses for prolonged periods of time without the health care provider's knowledge. This information should alert health care providers and people to the need for caution in using these drugs. If a person is complaining about diarrhoea, the health care provider should specifically ask about the use of acid-lowering products (sometimes people do not even think of these products as drugs because they can buy them without a prescription). During health care teaching sessions, it is important to remind people to read the labels of OTC drugs carefully and to follow instructions. If a person feels the need to take one of these products for a prolonged period of time, they should be advised to obtain a medical evaluation because the symptoms being treated with these drugs could have an underlying medical cause that should be evaluated.

When evaluating the data from the study, the researchers also noted a similar increase in these GI infections in people using non-steroidal anti-inflammatory drugs (NSAIDs) (ibuprofen, ketoprofen and others) for a prolonged period of time. The researchers suggested that further study be done on that group of people to verify the finding.

It is important to keep current with long-term studies on drugs and to remember that changing a normal function or environment in the body will change the balance of homeostasis in the body and could potentially cause other problems. In 2007, similar studies reported an increase in osteoporosis and bone fractures in people on long-term proton pump inhibitor use. Changing the acidity of the GI tract seems to affect calcium absorption. Further studies may show other changes in homeostasis with long-term use of these drugs.

Dial, S., Delaney, J. A., Barkun, A. N. & Suissa, S. (2005). Use of gastric acid suppressive agents and the risk of community acquired *Clostridium difficile* associated diarrhoea. *JAMA, 294*, 2898–2995.

Yu-Xiao, Y., Lewis, S. D, Epstein, S. & Metz, D. (2007). Long term proton pump inhibitor therapy and risk of hip fracture. *JAMA, 296*, 2947–2953.

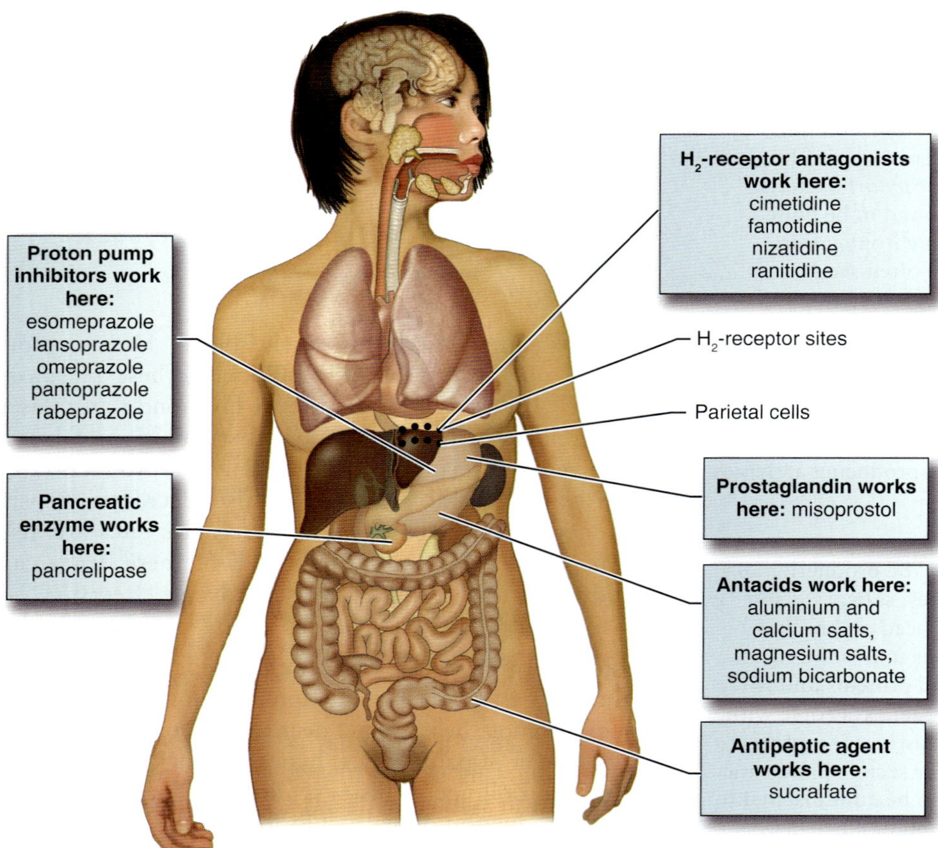

FIGURE 57.1 Sites of action of drugs affecting gastrointestinal secretions.

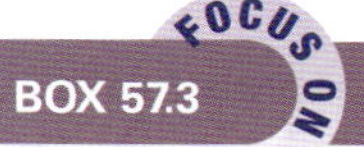

BOX 57.3 Drug therapy across the lifespan

Agents that affect gastrointestinal secretions

CHILDREN

Proton pump inhibitors have been very successfully used to decrease ulcer formation related to stress or drug therapy. Dose should be determined by the age and weight of the child.

Antacids may be used in children who complain of upset stomach or who are receiving therapy known to increase acid production.

Special caution should be used with any of these agents to prevent electrolyte disturbances or any interference with nutrition, which could be especially detrimental to children.

ADULTS

Adults should be cautioned not to overuse any of these agents and to check with their health care provider if GI discomfort continues after repeated use of any of these drugs. People should be monitored for any electrolyte disturbances or interference with the absorption or action of other drugs. If antacids are used, they should be spaced 1–2 hours before or after the use of other drugs. In 2005 and again in 2007, some studies were published that linked prolonged use of these agents with an increased incidence of colitis and other GI infections. Until further studies are done, people should be advised to limit the use of these agents.

PREGNANCY AND BREASTFEEDING

The safety of these drugs during pregnancy and breastfeeding has not been established, so they should be used with caution during pregnancy or breastfeeding.

Misoprostol is an abortifacient and should never be used during pregnancy. Women of childbearing age who use misoprostol should be advised to use barrier-type contraceptives. Use of the other agents should be reserved for those situations in which the benefit to the mother outweighs the potential risk to the fetus. The drugs may enter breast milk and also may alter electrolyte levels or gastric secretions in the neonate. It is advised that caution be used if one of these drugs is prescribed during breastfeeding.

OLDER ADULTS

Older adults frequently are prescribed one or more of these drugs. Older adults are more likely to develop adverse effects associated with the use of these drugs, including sedation, confusion, dizziness, urinary retention and cardiovascular effects. Safety measures may be needed if these effects occur and interfere with the person's mobility and balance. Because of changes that occur within the GI tract with age, absorption of nutrients can be affected when any of these drugs is used. The use of proton pump inhibitors and H_2 blockers in older adults has been associated with decreased absorption of vitamin B12 and the development of pernicious anaemia.

Older adults are also more likely to have renal and/or hepatic impairment related to underlying medical conditions, which could interfere with the metabolism and excretion of these drugs. The dose for older adults should be started at a lower level than recommended for younger adults. People should be monitored very closely, and dose adjustment should be made based on each individual's response.

These people also need to be alerted to the potential for toxic effects when using OTC preparations that may contain the same ingredients as many of these agents. They should be advised to check with their health care provider before beginning any OTC drug regimen.

Proton pump inhibitors may be the best choice for treating gastro-oesophageal reflux disease (GORD) in older people because of fewer adverse effects and better therapeutic response with these drugs.

TABLE 57.1 *DRUGS IN FOCUS* **Drugs used to treat gastro-oesophageal reflux disease and ulcer disease**

Drug name	Dosage/route	Usual indications
Histamine-2 antagonists		
(P) cimetidine (*Magicul*)	200 mg PO tds at meals and 400 mg at bedtime, or 800 mg PO at bedtime or 400 mg in the morning and at bedtime	Treatment of duodenal ulcer, benign gastric ulcer, pathological hypersecretory syndrome, GORD prophylaxis of stress ulcers; relief of symptoms of heartburn, acid indigestion, sour stomach **Special considerations:** not for children < 16 years old
famotidine (*Pepzan Pamacid*)	40 mg PO at bedtime; may reduce to 20 mg PO at bedtime	Treatment of duodenal ulcer, benign gastric ulcer, pathological hypersecretory syndrome, GORD; relief of symptoms of heartburn, acid indigestion, sour stomach

Continued on following page

TABLE 57.1 DRUGS IN FOCUS Drugs used to treat gastro-oesophageal reflux disease and ulcer disease *(continued)*

Drug name	Dosage/route	Usual indications
Histamine-2 antagonists *(continued)*		
nizatidine (*Nizac, Tazac*)	150–300 mg PO at bedtime or 150 mg PO bd; reduce dose in renally impaired or elderly people	Treatment of duodenal ulcer, benign gastric ulcer, pathological hypersecretory syndrome, GORD; relief of symptoms of heartburn, acid indigestion, sour stomach in adults **Special considerations:** not recommended for use in children
ranitidine (*Zantac*)	300 mg at bedtime or 150 mg daily to bd PO for 4–8 weeks; reduce dose in renally impaired or elderly people	Treatment of duodenal ulcer, benign gastric ulcer, pathological hypersecretory syndrome, GORD; relief of symptoms of heartburn, acid indigestion, sour stomach in adults **Special considerations:** not recommended for use in children
Antacids		
aluminium hydroxide (*Alu-Tab*)	600–1200 mg qid	Symptomatic relief of GI hyperacidity; treatment of hyperphosphatemia; prevention of formation of phosphate urinary stones
calcium salts (*Calci-Tab*)	0.5–2 g PO as needed as an antacid	Symptomatic relief of GI hyperacidity, treatment of calcium deficiency, prevention of hypocalcaemia
sodium bicarbonate (generic)	*De Witt's Antacid Powder* contains sodium bicarbonate. Dose is 5 g powder (2425 g sodium bicarbonate) in a half glass of water when required	Symptomatic relief of GI hyperacidity, minimisation of uric acid crystalluria, adjunctive treatment in severe diarrhoea
Proton pump inhibitors		
esomeprazole (*Nexium*)	Adult, paediatric > 12 years: initially 40 mg/day PO for 4–8 weeks, then maintenance: 20 mg/day PO	Treatment of GORD, severe erosive oesophagitis, duodenal ulcers and pathological hypersecretory conditions
lansoprazole (*Zopral, Zoton*)	Adult: 30 mg/day PO for 4 weeks, then maintenance 15 mg/day PO Paediatric 6–17 years: bodyweight ≤ 30 kg, 15 mg PO once daily; bodyweight > 30 kg, 30 mg PO once daily	Treatment of gastric ulcer, GORD, pathological hypersecretory syndromes; maintenance therapy for healing duodenal ulcers and oesophagitis; in combination therapy for the eradication of *Helicobacter pylori* infection; approved for use in children for treatment of GORD, peptic ulcer and Zollinger–Ellison syndrome
(P) omeprazole (*Losec*)	20–40 mg/day PO for 4–8 weeks, then maintenance 10–20 mg/day PO	Treatment of gastric ulcers, GORD, pathological hypersecretory syndromes; maintenance therapy for healing duodenal ulcers and oesophagitis; in combination therapy for the eradication of *H. pylori* infection; available over the counter (OTC) for relief of heartburn symptoms
pantoprazole (*Gastenz, Ozpan, Somac*)	40 mg PO daily to bd or 40 mg/day IV for 7–14 days; maintenance 20–40 mg/day PO	Treatment of GORD in adults; healing of erosive oesophagitis, treatment of hypersecretory syndromes
rabeprazole (*Pariet, Prabez*)	Adults: 20 mg/day for 4–8 weeks then maintenance 10 mg/day	Treatment and maintenance of GORD; treatment of duodenal ulcers, pathological hypersecretory conditions; used as combination therapy for the eradication of *H. pylori* infection

TABLE 57.1 DRUGS IN FOCUS Drugs used to treat gastro-oesophageal reflux disease and ulcer disease *(continued)*

Drug name	Dosage/route	Usual indications
GI protectant		
(P) sucralfate (*Carafate, Ulcyte*)	Initially 1 g qid for a maximum of 8 weeks, then 1 g bd maintenance	Short-term treatment of duodenal ulcers; maintenance of duodenal ulcers (at reduced dose) after healing in adults; treatment of oral and oesophageal ulcers due to radiation, chemotherapy or sclerotherapy; currently under investigation for treatment of gastric ulcers, gastric damage induced by NSAIDs, prevention of stress ulcers in acutely ill individuals
Prostaglandin		
(P) misoprostol (*Cytotec*)	200 micrograms PO qid for 4–8 weeks; reduce dose in people with renal impairment	Prevention of NSAID-induced ulcers in adults at high risk for development of these gastric ulcers; under investigation for treatment of duodenal ulcers in people who are not responsive to H_2 antagonists; used in combination therapy with mifepristone as an abortifacient

- prophylaxis of stress-induced ulcers and acute upper GI bleeding in critical people (blocking the production of acid protects the stomach lining, which is at risk because of decreased mucus production associated with extreme stress)
- treatment of erosive gastro-oesophageal reflux (decreasing the acid being regurgitated into the oesophagus will promote healing and decrease pain)
- relief of symptoms of heartburn, acid indigestion and dyspepsia.

See the Critical thinking scenario for additional information on H_2 antagonists.

Pharmacokinetics

Ranitidine is available in oral and parenteral forms. Nizatidine, cimetidine and famotidine are available only in oral form. Cimetidine was the first drug in this class to be developed. It has been associated with antiandrogenic effects, including gynaecomastia and galactorrhoea. It reaches peak levels in 1–1.5 hours and is metabolised mainly in the liver; it can slow the metabolism of many other drugs that use the same metabolising enzyme system. It is excreted in urine. It has a half-life of 2 hours and is known to cross the placenta and enter breast milk.

Ranitidine, which is longer acting and more potent than cimetidine, is not associated with the antiandrogenic adverse effects or the marked slowing of metabolism in the liver that cimetidine is. It reaches peak levels in 5–15 minutes when given parenterally and 1–3 hours when given orally. It has a duration of 8–12 hours and a half-life of 2–3 hours. Ranitidine is metabolised by the liver and excreted in urine. It crosses the placenta and enters breast milk.

Famotidine is similar to ranitidine, but it is much more potent than either cimetidine or ranitidine. It reaches peak effects in 1–3 hours and has a duration of 6–15 hours. Famotidine is metabolised in the liver and excreted in urine with a half-life of 2.5–3.5 hours. Famotidine crosses the placenta and enters breast milk.

Nizatidine, the newest drug in this class, is similar to ranitidine in its effectiveness and adverse effects. It differs from the other three drugs in that it is eliminated by the kidneys, with no first-pass metabolism in the liver. It is the drug of choice for people with liver dysfunction and for those who are taking other drugs whose metabolism is slowed by the hepatic activity of the other three H_2 antagonists. It reaches peak effects in 0.5–3 hours and has a half-life of 1–2 hours. Like the other three drugs, it crosses the placenta and enters the breast milk.

Contraindications and cautions

The H_2 antagonists should not be used with known allergy to any drugs of this class *to prevent hypersensitivity reactions.* Caution should be used during pregnancy or breastfeeding *because of the potential for adverse effects on the fetus or breastfeeding infant* and with hepatic or renal dysfunction, *which could interfere with drug metabolism and excretion.* (Hepatic dysfunction is not as much of a problem with nizatidine.) Care should also be taken if prolonged or continual use of these drugs is necessary *because they may be masking serious underlying conditions.*

Adverse effects

The adverse effects most commonly associated with H_2 antagonists include GI effects of diarrhoea or

CRITICAL THINKING SCENARIO

Histamine-2 antagonists

THE SITUATION

W.T., a 48-year-old travelling salesman, had experienced increasing epigastric discomfort during a 7-month period. When he finally sought medical care, the diagnosis was a peptic ulcer. He began taking Mylanta for relief of his immediate discomfort, as well as ranitidine (*Tagamet*), 150 mg b.i.d. W.T. was referred to the nurse for teaching and given an appointment for a follow-up visit in 3 weeks.

CRITICAL THINKING

Think about the physiology of duodenal ulcers and the various factors that can contribute to aggravating the problem. What teaching points should be covered with this person regarding diet, stress factors, and use of alcohol and tobacco?

What adverse effects of the drugs should this person be aware of?

What lifestyle changes may be necessary to ensure ulcer healing, and how can W.T. be assisted in making these changes fit into the demands of his job?

DISCUSSION

Further examination indicated that W.T. is a healthy man except for the ulcer. He admits to smoking cigarettes, drinking alcohol regularly at business lunches and dinners, and eating a great deal of fast food and drinking a lot of coffee when he is on the road. He states that his job has become increasingly stressful as the economy has worsened. Because he is basically healthy and does not seek medical care unless very uncomfortable (7 months of pain), he may find it difficult to comply with his drug therapy and any suggested lifestyle changes.

W.T. needs education, which for purposes of building trust, should preferably be with the same nurse. The instruction should include information on duodenal ulcer disease; ways to decrease acid production (such as avoiding cigarettes, acid-stimulating foods, alcohol and caffeine); and ways to improve the protective mucus layer of the stomach by decreasing stress and anxiety-causing situations. In addition, spacing of the ranitidine and antacid doses should be stressed. Ranitidine should be taken 1 hour before or 2 hours after any antacids because they can interfere with the absorption of ranitidine and the person may not receive a therapeutic dose. W.T. should be encouraged to avoid OTC medications and self-medication because several of these products contain ingredients that could aggravate his ulcer or interfere with the effectiveness of the drugs that have been prescribed. W.T. should be encouraged to return for regular medical evaluation of his drug therapy and his underlying condition.

Finally, W.T. should feel that he has some control over his situation. Because he does not routinely seek medical care, he may be more comfortable with a medical regimen that he has participated in planning. Allow him to suggest ways to decrease stress, ways to cut down on smoking or the use of alcohol without interfering with the demands of his job, and the best times to take the drugs in his schedule. He will learn in time which foods and situations irritate his condition. However, research has not shown that bland or restrictive diets are particularly effective in decreasing ulcer pain or spread, and they may actually increase anxiety. W.T. should be encouraged to jot down the situations or times of day that seem to cause him the most problems. This information can help to provide a guide for adjusting lifestyle and/or dietary patterns to aid ulcer healing and prevent further development of ulcers.

CARE GUIDE FOR W.T.: HISTAMINE-2 ANTAGONISTS

Assessment: history and examination

Assess W.T.'s health history for allergies to any of these drugs, renal or hepatic failure, and other drugs being taken, such as antimetabolites, alkylating agents, oral anticoagulants, phenytoin, beta blockers, alcohol, lidocaine (lignocaine), theophylline, benzodiazepines, nifedipine, tricyclic antidepressants (TCAs) and carbamazepine.

Focus the physical examination on the following areas:

Neurological: orientation, affect

Skin: colour, lesions

Cardiovascular: pulse, cardiac auscultation

GI: liver evaluation

Laboratory tests: full blood count, liver, renal function tests

Implementation

Administer with meals and at bedtime.

Provide comfort and safety measures: analgesics, access to bathroom, safety precautions.

Arrange for decreased dose in renal/hepatic disease.

Provide support and reassurance to deal with drug effects and lifestyle changes.

Provide teaching regarding drug name, dosage, adverse effects, precautions and warnings to report.

Evaluation

Evaluate drug effects: relief of GI symptoms, ulcer healing, prevention of ulcer progression.

Monitor for adverse effects: headache, dizziness, insomnia, gynaecomastia, arrhythmias, GI alterations.

Monitor for drug–drug interactions as listed.
Evaluate the effectiveness of the teaching program.
Evaluate the effectiveness of comfort and safety measures.

TEACHING FOR W.T.

- The drug that has been prescribed for you, ranitidine, is called a histamine-2 antagonist. A histamine-2 antagonist decreases the amount of acid that is produced in the stomach. It is used to treat conditions that are aggravated by excess acid.
- Some of the following adverse effects may occur with this drug:
  - *Diarrhoea*: have ready access to bathroom facilities. This usually becomes less severe over time.
  - *Dizziness, headache*: these usually lessen as your body adjusts to the drug. Change positions slowly. If you feel drowsy, avoid driving or dangerous activities.
  - (Report any of the following to your health care provider): *sore throat, unusual bleeding or bruising, confusion, muscle or joint pain, tarry stools.*
- Avoid taking any OTC medication without first checking with your health care provider. Several of these medications can interfere with the effectiveness of this drug.
- If an antacid has been ordered for you, take it exactly as prescribed, spaced apart from your ranitidine.
- Tell any doctor, nurse or other health care provider involved in your care that you are taking this drug.
- If you are taking any other medications, do not vary the drug schedules. Consult with your primary health care provider if anything should happen to change any of these drugs or your scheduled doses.
- It is important to have regular medical follow-up while you are taking this drug to evaluate your response to the drug and any possible underlying problems.
- Keep this drug, and all other medications, out of the reach of children.

constipation; central nervous system (CNS) effects of dizziness, headache, somnolence, confusion or even hallucinations (thought to be related to possible H_2-receptor effects in the CNS); cardiac arrhythmias and hypotension (related to H_2 cardiac-receptor blocking, more commonly seen with intravenous or intramuscular administration or with prolonged use); and gynaecomastia (more common with long-term use of cimetidine) and impotence.

Prototype summary: cimetidine

Indications: short-term treatment of active duodenal or benign gastric ulcers; treatment of pathological hypersecretory conditions; prophylaxis of stress-induced ulcers; treatment of erosive gastro-oesophageal reflux; relief of symptoms of heartburn and acid indigestion.

Actions: inhibits the actions of histamine at H_2-receptor sites of the stomach, inhibiting gastric acid secretion and reducing total pepsin output.

Pharmacokinetics:

Route	Onset	Peak	Duration
Oral	Varies	1–1.5 hours	4–5 hours
IM, IV	Rapid	1–1.5 hours	4–5 hours

$T_{1/2}$: 2 hours; metabolised in the liver and excreted in urine.

Adverse effects: dizziness, confusion, headache, somnolence, cardiac arrhythmias, cardiac arrest, diarrhoea, impotence, gynaecomastia, rash.

Clinically important drug–drug interactions

Cimetidine, famotidine and ranitidine can slow the metabolism of the following drugs, leading to increased serum levels and possible toxic reactions: warfarin anticoagulants, phenytoin, beta-adrenergic blockers, alcohol, lidocaine (lignocaine), theophylline, benzodiazepines, nifedipine, tricyclic antidepressants and carbamazepine. There is a risk of increased salicylate levels if nizatidine is taken with aspirin.

Care considerations for people receiving histamine-2 antagonists

Assessment: history and examination

- Assess for *possible contraindications or cautions*: history of allergy to any H_2 antagonists *to prevent potential allergic reactions*; impaired renal or hepatic function, *which could affect metabolism and excretion of the drug*; a detailed description of the GI problem, including length of time of the disorder and medical evaluation, *to evaluate the appropriate use of the drug and possibility of underlying medical problems*; and current status of pregnancy or breastfeeding *because of the potential for adverse effects on the fetus or newborn.*
- Perform a physical examination *to establish baseline data before beginning therapy, determine effectiveness of the therapy and evaluate for any adverse effects associated with drug therapy.*

- Inspect the skin for evidence of lesions or rash *to monitor for adverse reactions.*
- Evaluate neurological status, including orientation and affect, *to assess CNS effects of the drug and to plan for protective measures.*
- Assess cardiopulmonary status, including pulse, blood pressure and electrocardiogram (if intravenous use is needed), *to evaluate the cardiac effects of the drug.*
- Perform abdominal examination, including assessment of liver, *to establish a baseline and rule out underlying medical problems.*
- Monitor the results of laboratory tests, including liver and renal function tests, *to predict changes in metabolism or excretion of the drug that might require dose adjustment.*

Implementation with rationale

- Administer oral drug with or before meals and at bedtime (exact timing varies with product) *to ensure therapeutic levels when the drug is most needed.*
- Arrange for decreased dose in cases of hepatic or renal dysfunction *to prevent serious toxicity.*
- Monitor the person continually if giving intravenous doses *to allow early detection of potentially serious adverse effects, including cardiac arrhythmias.*
- Assess the person carefully for any potential drug–drug interactions if given in combination with other drugs *because of the drug effects on liver enzyme systems.*
- Provide comfort, including analgesics, ready access to bathroom facilities and assistance with ambulation, *to minimise possible adverse effects.*
- Periodically reorient the person and institute safety measures if CNS effects occur *to ensure safety and improve tolerance of the drug and drug effects.*
- Arrange for regular follow-up *to evaluate drug effects and the underlying problem.*
- Offer support and encouragement *to help people cope with the disease and the drug regimen.*
- Provide teaching regarding drug name, dosage, and schedule for administration; importance of spacing administration appropriately as ordered; need for readily available access to bathroom; signs and symptoms of adverse effects and measures to minimise or prevent them; danger signs that necessitate notifying the health care provider immediately; safety measures, such as avoiding driving and asking for assistance when ambulating, to deal with possible effects of dizziness, somnolence or confusion; the need for compliance with therapy to achieve the intended results; and the importance of periodic monitoring and evaluation, including laboratory testing, *to determine drug effectiveness and to enhance knowledge about drug therapy and to promote compliance.*

Evaluation

- Monitor response to the drug (relief of GI symptoms, ulcer healing, prevention of progression of ulcer).
- Monitor for adverse effects (dizziness, confusion, hallucinations, GI alterations, cardiac arrhythmias, hypotension, gynaecomastia).
- Evaluate the effectiveness of the teaching plan (person can name drug, dosage, adverse effects to watch for and specific measures to avoid them).
- Monitor the effectiveness of comfort measures and compliance with the regimen.

KEY POINTS

- Agents affecting GI secretion include H_2 antagonists, antacids, proton pump inhibitors, GI protectants and prostaglandins. Digestive enzymes replace missing GI enzymes.
- Among the most common complaints addressed in clinical practice are GI symptoms.
- Increased acid production, decrease in the protective mucus lining of the stomach, infection with *Helicobacter pylori* bacteria, or a combination of these is the likely cause of peptic ulcers.
- H_2 antagonists block the release of acid in response to gastrin or parasympathetic release; adverse effects can include dizziness, confusion, cardiac arrhythmias and galactorrhoea.

ANTACIDS

Antacids (Table 57.1) are a group of inorganic chemicals that neutralise stomach acid. Antacids are available over the counter, and many people use them to self-treat a variety of GI symptoms. There is no one perfect antacid (see Adverse effects). The choice of an antacid depends on adverse effect and absorption factors. Available agents are sodium bicarbonate, calcium carbonate, magnesium salts and aluminium salts.

Therapeutic actions and indications

Antacids neutralise stomach acid by direct chemical reaction (see Figure 57.1). They are recommended for the symptomatic relief of upset stomach associated with hyperacidity, as well as the hyperacidity associated with peptic ulcer, gastritis, peptic oesophagitis, gastric hyperacidity and hiatus hernia. See Table 57.1 for usual indications for each antacid.

Pharmacokinetics

Sodium bicarbonate, the oldest drug in this group, is readily available in many preparations, including baking soda powder, tablets, solutions and as an injectable for treating systemic acidosis. This drug is widely distributed when absorbed orally, reaching peak levels in 1–3 hours, crossing the placenta and entering breast milk. It is excreted in urine and can cause serious electrolyte imbalance in people with renal impairment.

Calcium carbonate is actually precipitated chalk and is available in tablet and powder forms. The main drawbacks to this agent are constipation and acid rebound. It has an onset of action in about 3–5 minutes. It can be absorbed systemically and cause calcium imbalance. When absorbed, it is metabolised in the liver and excreted in urine and faeces, with a half-life of 1–3 hours. Calcium carbonate is known to cross the placenta and enter breast milk.

Magnesium salts are very effective in buffering acid in the stomach but have been known to cause diarrhoea; they are sometimes used as laxatives. They are available as tablets, chewable tablets and capsules and in liquid forms. Although these agents are not generally absorbed systemically and are excreted in the faeces, absorbed magnesium can lead to nerve damage and even coma, if absorbed; they are excreted in the urine.

Aluminium salts, available as tablets, capsules, suspensions and in a liquid form, do not cause acid rebound but are not very effective in neutralising acid. They are bound in faeces for excretion. They have been related to severe constipation. Aluminium binds dietary phosphates and causes hypophosphataemia, which can then cause calcium imbalance throughout the system.

Aluminium and magnesium minimise the GI effects of constipation and diarrhoea by combining these two salts but may cause a rebound hyperacidity and alkalosis.

Many of these antacids are available in combination forms to take advantage of the acid-neutralising effect and block adverse effects. For example, a combination of calcium and aluminium salts (*Mylanta*) buffers acid and produces neither constipation nor diarrhoea.

Contraindications and cautions

The antacids are contraindicated in the presence of any known allergy to antacid products or any component of the drug *to prevent hypersensitivity reactions*. Caution should be used in the following instances: any condition that can be exacerbated by electrolyte or acid–base imbalance *to prevent exacerbations and serious adverse effects*; any electrolyte imbalance, *which could be exacerbated by the electrolyte-changing effects of these drugs*; GI obstruction, *which could cause systemic absorption of the drugs and increased adverse effects*; renal dysfunction, *which could lead to electrolyte disturbance if any absorbed antacid is not neutralised properly*; and pregnancy and breastfeeding *because of the potential for adverse effects on the fetus or neonate*.

Adverse effects

The adverse effects associated with these drugs relate to their effects on acid–base and electrolyte balance. Administering an antacid frequently causes **acid rebound**, in which the stomach produces more acid in response to the alkaline environment. Neutralising the stomach contents to an alkaline level stimulates gastrin production to cause an increase in acid production and return the stomach to its normal acidic state. In many cases, the acid rebound causes an increase in symptoms, which results in an increased intake of the antacid. This leads to more acid production and an ongoing cycle. When more and more antacid is used, the risk for systemic effects rises. Alkalosis with resultant metabolic changes (nausea, vomiting, neuromuscular changes, headache, irritability, muscle twitching and even coma) may occur. The use of calcium salts may lead to hypercalcaemia and milk-alkali syndrome (seen as alkalosis, renal calcium deposits or severe electrolyte disorders). Constipation or diarrhoea may result, depending on the antacid being used. Hypophosphataemia can occur with the use of aluminium salts. Finally, fluid retention and heart failure can occur with sodium bicarbonate because of its high sodium content.

Drug–drug interactions

Antacids can greatly affect the absorption of drugs from the GI tract. Most drugs are prepared for an acidic environment, and an alkaline environment can prevent them from being broken down for absorption or can actually neutralise them so that they cannot be absorbed. In addition, ion-containing antacids such as calcium, aluminium and magnesium can bind other medicines by chelation, reducing their absorption. For example, ciprofloxacin absorption is reduced by 20% in the presence of antacids. People taking antacids should be advised to separate them from any other medications by 1–2 hours.

If the pH of urine is affected by large doses of antacids, levels of salicylates may decrease.

Care considerations for people receiving antacids

Assessment: history and examination

- Assess for *possible contraindications or cautions*: any history of allergy to antacids *to prevent hypersensitivity reactions*; renal dysfunction, *which might interfere with the drug's excretion*; electrolyte disturbances, *which could be exacerbated by the effects of the drug*; and current status of pregnancy or breastfeeding *due to possible effects on the fetus or newborn.*

- Perform a physical examination *to establish baseline data before beginning therapy, determine the effectiveness of the therapy, and evaluate for any potential adverse effects associated with drug therapy.*
- Inspect the abdomen. Auscultate bowel sounds *to ensure GI motility.*
- Assess mucous membrane status *to evaluate potential problems with absorption and hydration.*
- Monitor laboratory test results, including serum electrolyte levels and renal function tests, *to monitor for adverse effects of the drug and potential alterations in excretion that may necessitate dose adjustment.*

Implementation with rationale

- Administer the drug apart from any other oral medications approximately 1 hour before or 2 hours after *to ensure adequate absorption of the other medications.*
- Have the person chew tablets thoroughly and follow with water *to ensure that therapeutic levels reach the stomach to decrease acid.*
- Obtain specimens for periodic monitoring of serum electrolytes *to evaluate drug effects.*
- Assess the person for any signs of acid–base or electrolyte imbalance *to ensure early detection and prompt intervention.*
- Monitor the person for diarrhoea or constipation *to institute a bowel program before severe effects occur.*
- Monitor the person's nutritional status if diarrhoea is severe or constipation leads to decreased food intake *to ensure adequate fluid and nutritional intake to promote healing and GI stability.*
- Offer support and encouragement *to help the person cope with the disease and the drug regimen.*
- Provide thorough teaching, including the drug name and prescribed dosage; schedule for administration; signs and symptoms of adverse effects and measures to minimise or prevent them; warning signs that may indicate possible problems and the need to notify the health care provider immediately; the importance of maintaining fluid and nutritional intake if diarrhoea or constipation occurs; possible bowel training programs to deal with constipation or diarrhoea if severe; cautions related to prolonged chronic use of drug and increased risk for acid rebound; the importance of checking with the health care provider before using any OTC medications; differences associated with the various OTC antacid formulations; and the need for periodic monitoring and evaluation *to enhance knowledge about drug therapy and to promote compliance.*

Evaluation

- Monitor response to the drug (relief of GI symptoms caused by hyperacidity).
- Monitor for adverse effects (GI effects, imbalances in serum electrolyte levels and acid–base status).
- Evaluate the effectiveness of the teaching plan (person can name the drug and dosage, as well as describe adverse effects to watch for, specific measures to avoid them and measures to take to increase the effectiveness of the drug).
- Monitor the effectiveness of comfort measures and compliance with the regimen.

KEY POINTS

- Antacids are used to chemically react with, and neutralise, acid in the stomach. They can provide rapid relief from increased acid levels. They are known to cause GI alterations such as diarrhoea or constipation and can alter the absorption of many drugs.
- Acid rebound occurs when the stomach produces more gastrin and more acid in response to lowered acid levels in the stomach, which commonly occurs with the use of antacids. Balancing the reduction of the stomach acid without increasing acid production is a clinical challenge.

PROTON PUMP INHIBITORS

Proton pump inhibitors (Table 57.1) suppress the secretion of hydrochloric acid into the lumen of the stomach. Five proton pump inhibitors are presently available: omeprazole (*Losec*), esomeprazole (*Nexium*), lansoprazole (*Zopral, Zoton*), pantoprazole (*Gastenz, Ozpan, Somac*) and rabeprazole (*Pariet, Prabez*).

Therapeutic actions and indications

The gastric acid pump or proton pump inhibitors suppress gastric acid secretion by specifically inhibiting the hydrogen–potassium–adenosine triphosphatase (H^+–K^+–ATPase) enzyme system on the secretory surface of the gastric parietal cells. This action blocks the final step of acid production, lowering the acid levels in the stomach (see Figure 57.1). They are recommended for the short-term treatment of active duodenal ulcers, GORD, erosive oesophagitis and benign active gastric ulcer; for the long-term treatment of pathological hypersecretory conditions; as maintenance therapy for healing of erosive oesophagitis and ulcers; and in combination with amoxicillin and clarithromycin for the treatment of *H. pylori* infection. See Table 57.1 for usual indications for each of these agents.

Pharmacokinetics

Esomeprazole, omeprazole and pantoprazole are available in oral forms and as IV preparations. Lansoprazole and rabeprazole are available only in delayed-release oral forms.

These drugs are acid labile and are rapidly absorbed from the GI tract, reaching peak levels in 3–5 hours. They undergo extensive metabolism in the liver and are excreted in urine. Omeprazole is faster acting and more quickly excreted than the other proton pump inhibitors. It has a half-life of 30–60 minutes. Esomeprazole is a longer-acting drug; it has a half-life of 60–90 minutes and a duration of 17 hours. It is not broken down as rapidly in the liver as the parent drug omeprazole. Lansoprazole has a half-life of 2 hours and duration of 12 hours.

Pantoprazole and rabeprazole have half-lives of 90 minutes and durations of 12–14 hours. There are no adequate studies about whether these drugs cross the placenta or enter breast milk.

Contraindications and cautions

These drugs are contraindicated in the presence of known allergy to either the drug or the drug components *to prevent hypersensitivity reactions*. Caution should be used in pregnant or breastfeeding women *because of the potential for adverse effects on the fetus or neonate*.

Monitoring of serum magnesium levels before and during treatment should be considered for:

- people expected to require long-term PPI treatment.
- people who take other medicines such as digoxin or medicines that may cause hypomagnesaemia (such as diuretics).

Adverse effects

The adverse effects associated with these drugs are related to their effects on the H^+–K^+–ATPase pump on the parietal and other cells. CNS effects of dizziness and headache are commonly seen; asthenia (loss of strength), vertigo, insomnia, apathy and dream abnormalities may also be observed. GI effects can include diarrhoea and increased risk of *Clostridium difficile* infection, abdominal pain, nausea, vomiting, dry mouth and tongue atrophy. Upper respiratory tract symptoms, including cough, stuffy nose, hoarseness and epistaxis, are frequently seen, as well as increased risk for community- and hospital-acquired pneumonia. Use of PPIs increases the risk of osteoporosis and fractures, vitamin B12 deficiency, acute interstitial nephritis and hypomagnesaemia. Other, less common adverse effects include rash, alopecia, pruritus, dry skin, back pain and fever. In preclinical studies, long-term effects of proton pump inhibitors included the development of gastric cancer.

Clinically important drug–drug interactions

There is a risk of increased serum levels and increased toxicity of benzodiazepines, phenytoin and warfarin if these are combined with these drugs; people should be monitored closely. Decreased levels of azole antifungals (eg, itraconazole, voriconazole [but not fluconazole]), antiviral agents (eg, atazanavir, sofosbuvir), theophylline and some oncology drugs (eg, sunitinib, erlotinib) have been reported when combined with these drugs, leading to loss of effectiveness. Sucralfate is not absorbed well in the presence of these drugs, and doses should be spaced at least 30 minutes apart if this combination is used.

Prototype summary: omeprazole

Indications: short-term treatment of active duodenal ulcer or active benign gastric ulcer; treatment of heartburn or symptoms of gastro-oesophageal reflux; treatment of pathological hypersecretory syndromes; eradication of *H. pylori* infection as part of combination therapy.

Actions: specifically inhibits the hydrogen–potassium–adenosine triphosphatase (H^+–K^+–ATPase) enzyme system on the secretory surface of the gastric parietal cells, blocking the final step in acid production and decreasing gastric acid levels.

Pharmacokinetics:

Route	Onset	Peak	Duration
Oral	Varies	0.5–3.5 hours	Varies

$T_{1/2}$: 30–60 min; metabolised in the liver and excreted in urine and bile.

Adverse effects: headache, dizziness, vertigo, insomnia, rash, diarrhoea, abdominal pain, nausea, vomiting, upper respiratory infection symptoms, cough.

Care considerations for people receiving proton pump inhibitors

Assessment: history and examination

- Assess for *possible contraindications or cautions*: history of allergy to a proton pump inhibitor *to reduce the risk of hypersensitivity reaction*; current status of pregnancy or breastfeeding *because of the potential for adverse effects on the fetus or infant.*

- Perform a physical examination to establish baseline data before beginning therapy *to determine the effectiveness of the therapy and to evaluate for the occurrence of any adverse effects associated with drug therapy.*
- Inspect the skin for lesions, rash, pruritus and dryness *to identify possible adverse effects.*
- Assess neurological status, including level of orientation, affect and reflexes, *to evaluate for CNS effects of the drug.*
- Inspect and palpate the abdomen *to determine potential underlying medical conditions*; assess for changes in bowel elimination and GI upset *to identify possible adverse effects.*
- Assess respiratory status, including respiratory rate and rhythm; note evidence of cough, hoarseness and epistaxis, *to monitor for potential adverse effects of the drug.*

Implementation with rationale

- Administer drug before meals to ensure that the person does not open, chew or crush capsules; they should be swallowed whole *to ensure the therapeutic effectiveness of the drug.*
- Provide appropriate safety and comfort measures if CNS effects occur *to prevent injury.*
- Monitor the person for diarrhoea or constipation *in order to institute an appropriate bowel program as needed.*
- Monitor the person's nutritional status; use of small frequent meals may be helpful *if GI upset is a problem.*
- Arrange for medical follow-up if symptoms are not resolved after 4–8 weeks of therapy *because serious underlying conditions could be causing the symptoms.*
- Offer support and encouragement *to help the person cope with the disease and the drug regimen.*
- Provide thorough teaching, including the drug name and prescribed dosage; the importance of taking the drug whole without opening, chewing or crushing it; signs and symptoms of possible adverse effects and measures to minimise or prevent them; danger signs that need to be reported to the health care provider immediately; nutritional measures, such as small, frequent meals; safety measures, such as avoiding driving and getting assistance with ambulation as needed; methods for dealing with constipation or diarrhoea; and the need for periodic monitoring and evaluation, *to enhance knowledge about drug therapy and to promote compliance.*

Evaluation

- Monitor response to the drug (relief of GI symptoms caused by hyperacidity; healing of erosive GI lesions).
- Monitor for adverse effects (GI effects, CNS changes, dermatological effects, respiratory effects).
- Monitor the effectiveness of comfort and safety measures and compliance with the regimen.
- Evaluate the effectiveness of the teaching plan (person can name the drug and dosage and describe adverse effects to watch for, specific measures to avoid them and measures to take to increase the effectiveness of the drug).

BOX 57.4 Proton pump inhibitors and interstitial nephritis

Acute renal impairment caused by interstitial nephritis is a recognised complication of treatment with omeprazole. Presenting symptoms may be non-specific and include malaise, fever, nausea, lethargy, weight loss, rash and eosinophilia. People known to be taking omeprazole who exhibit these symptoms should undergo urine microscopy and assessment of renal function. If either or both are abnormal, omeprazole should be withdrawn pending nephrology assessment.[1] Interstitial nephritis should also be considered if there is an unexpected rise in serum creatinine.

Proton pump inhibitors are now the commonest cause of interstitial nephritis in the Auckland region, perhaps due to their widespread use.[2] This suggests that prescribers should be vigilant for this adverse reaction when using omeprazole or other proton pump inhibitors.

References

1. Savage, R. (2001). Omeprazole-induced interstitial nephritis. *Prescriber Update, 20*(Feb), 11–13. www.medsafe.govt.nz/profs/PUarticles/omeprazole.htm.
2. Simpson, I. J., Marshall, M. R., Pilmore H., et al. (2006). Proton pump inhibitors and acute interstitial nephritis—report and analysis of 15 cases. *Nephrology, 11(5),* 381–385.

Source: MEDSAFE. (2006). *Prescriber Updates, 27(1)*, 3. www.medsafe.govt.nz/profs/PUarticles/watchingbriefsJune06.htm.

KEY POINTS

- The gastric acid pump, or proton pump, inhibitors suppress gastric acid secretion by specifically inhibiting the hydrogen–potassium–adenosine triphosphatase (H^+–K^+–ATPase) enzyme system on the secretory surface of the gastric parietal cells.

This action blocks the final step of acid production, lowering the acid levels in the stomach.

- Proton pump inhibitors are indicated for the short-term treatment of active duodenal ulcer or active benign gastric ulcer; treatment of heartburn or symptoms of gastro-oesophageal reflux; treatment of pathological hypersecretory syndromes; and eradication of *H. pylori* infection as part of combination therapy

GI PROTECTANTS

GI protectants (Table 57.1) coat any injured area in the stomach to prevent further injury from acid. Sucralfate (*Carafate*) is the only GI protectant currently available.

Therapeutic actions and indications

Sucralfate forms an ulcer-adherent complex at duodenal ulcer sites, protecting the sites against acid, pepsin and bile salts. This action prevents further breakdown of the area and promotes ulcer healing. The drug also inhibits pepsin activity in gastric juices, preventing further breakdown of proteins in the stomach, including the protein wall of the stomach (see Figure 57.1). See Table 57.1 for indications.

Pharmacokinetics

Sucralfate is rapidly absorbed after oral administration, metabolised in the liver and excreted in faeces. It crosses the placenta and may enter breast milk.

Contraindications and cautions

Sucralfate should not be given to any person with known allergy to the drug or any of its components *to prevent hypersensitivity reactions*. It should not be given to individuals with renal failure or undergoing dialysis *because a buildup of aluminium may occur if it is used with aluminium-containing products*. Caution should be used in women who are pregnant or breastfeeding *because of the potential adverse effects on the fetus or neonate*.

Adverse effects

The adverse effects associated with sucralfate are primarily related to its GI effects. Constipation is the most frequently seen adverse effect. Diarrhoea, nausea, indigestion, gastric discomfort and dry mouth may also occur. Other adverse effects that have been reported with this drug include dizziness, sleepiness, vertigo, skin rash and back pain.

Clinically important drug–drug interactions

If aluminium salts are combined with sucralfate, there is a risk of high aluminium levels and aluminium toxicity. Extreme care should be taken if this combination is used.

In addition, if phenytoin, fluoroquinolone antibiotics (eg, ciprofloxacin, norfloxacin), or penicillamine is combined with sucralfate, decreased serum levels and drug effectiveness may result. In such combinations, the individual agents should be administered separately, with at least 2 hours between drugs.

Prototype summary: sucralfate

Indications: short-term treatment and maintenance treatment of active duodenal ulcer; treatment of oral and oesophageal ulcers due to radiation, chemotherapy or sclerotherapy.

Actions: forms an ulcer-adherent complex at the duodenal ulcer site, protecting the ulcer from acid, bile salts and pepsin, promoting healing of the ulcer; also inhibits pepsin activity in gastric juices.

Pharmacokinetics:

Route	Onset	Duration
Oral	30 min	5 hours

$T_{1/2}$: 6–20 hours; metabolised in the liver and excreted in faeces.

Adverse effects: sleeplessness, dizziness, vertigo, insomnia, rash, constipation, diarrhoea, nausea, indigestion, dry mouth, back pain.

Care considerations for people receiving a GI protectant

Assessment: history and examination

- Assess for *possible contraindications or cautions*: any history of allergy to sucralfate *to prevent hypersensitivity reactions*; renal dysfunction or dialysis, *which can lead to a buildup of aluminium*; and current status of pregnancy or breastfeeding.
- Perform a physical examination *to establish baseline data before beginning therapy, to determine the effectiveness of therapy and to evaluate for any adverse effects associated with drug therapy*.
- Inspect the skin for colour and evidence of lesions or rash *that might indicate adverse drug effects*.

- Assess the person's neurological status, including level of orientation, affect and reflexes, *to monitor for CNS effects of the drug.*
- Examine the abdomen; auscultate bowel sounds *to evaluate GI motility*; evaluate bowel elimination pattern or changes *that could suggest possible adverse effects.*
- Assess mucous membrane status *to evaluate potential problems with absorption.*
- Monitor the results of laboratory tests such as renal function studies *to identify the need for possible dose adjustments and toxic effects.*

Implementation with rationale

- Administer the drug on an empty stomach, 1 hour before or 2 hours after meals and at bedtime, *to ensure the therapeutic effectiveness of the drug.*
- Monitor the person for GI pain, *and arrange to administer antacids to relieve pain if needed.*
- Administer antacids or antibiotics, if ordered, between doses of sucralfate, not within 30 minutes of a sucralfate dose, *because sucralfate can interfere with absorption of oral agents.*
- Provide comfort and safety measures if CNS effects occur *to prevent injury.*
- Provide frequent mouth care, including sugarless lozenges to suck, *to alleviate dry mouth.*
- Ensure ready access to bathroom facilities *if diarrhoea occurs*; institute bowel training as needed and provide small, frequent meals *if GI effects are uncomfortable.*
- Offer support and encouragement *to help the person cope with the disease and the drug regimen.*
- Provide thorough teaching, including the drug name and prescribed dosage; schedule for administration; importance of taking the drug on an empty stomach; use of antacids if ordered and the need to separate doses by at least 2 hours; signs and symptoms of possible adverse effects and measures to minimise or prevent their occurrence; danger signs that need to be reported to the health care provider immediately; safety measures, such as avoiding driving and asking for help with ambulation, *to minimise injury secondary to CNS effects*; dietary measures such as small, frequent meals *to minimise diarrhoea*; increased fluid and fibre in the diet *to reduce the risk of constipation*; small, frequent meals *to help with GI upset*; comfort measures, such as mouth care and use of sugarless lozenges, *to alleviate dry mouth*; the importance of compliance with therapy *to achieve the intended effects*; measures to help avoid adverse effects; warning signs that may indicate problems; and the need for periodic monitoring and evaluation *to evaluate the effectiveness of therapy, enhance knowledge about therapy and promote compliance.*

Evaluation

- Monitor the response to the drug (relief of GI symptoms; healing of erosive GI lesions).
- Monitor for adverse effects (GI effects, CNS changes, dermatological effects).
- Monitor the effectiveness of comfort and safety measures and compliance with the regimen.
- Evaluate the effectiveness of the teaching plan (person can name drug and dosage and describe the adverse effects to watch for, specific measures to avoid them and measures to take to increase the effectiveness of the drug).

KEY POINTS

- The GI protectant sucralfate forms a protective coating over the eroded stomach lining to protect it from acid and digestive enzymes to aid healing.
- Constipation is a common occurrence with this drug.

PROSTAGLANDINS

Prostaglandins are used to protect the stomach lining. The prostaglandin available for this use is the synthetic prostaglandin E_1 analogue misoprostol (*Cytotec*).

Therapeutic actions and indications

Prostaglandin E_1 inhibits gastric acid secretion and increases bicarbonate and mucus production in the stomach, thus protecting the stomach lining (see Figure 57.1). Misoprostol is primarily used to prevent NSAID-induced gastric ulcers in people who are at high risk for complications from a gastric ulcer (eg, elderly or debilitated people, people with a past history of ulcer). See Table 57.1 for more information and indications about this drug.

Pharmacokinetics

Miosprostol is given orally. It is rapidly absorbed from the GI tract, metabolised in the liver and excreted in urine. Misoprostol crosses the placenta and enters breast milk.

Contraindications and cautions

Misoprostol is contraindicated with allergy to any part of the drug *to prevent hypersensitivity reactions.* This drug is also contraindicated during pregnancy *because it is an abortifacient.* Women of childbearing age should be advised to have a negative serum pregnancy test within 2 weeks of beginning treatment, and they should begin the drug on the second or third day of their next menstrual cycle. In addition, they should be instructed to use barrier contraceptives during therapy. Caution should be used during breastfeeding *because of the potential for adverse effects on the newborn*. Caution also is necessary in people with hepatic or renal impairment, *which could interfere with the effective metabolism and excretion of the drug*.

Adverse effects

The adverse effects associated with this drug are primarily related to its GI effects – nausea, diarrhoea, abdominal pain, flatulence, vomiting, dyspepsia and constipation. Genitourinary effects, which are related to the actions of prostaglandins on the uterus, include miscarriages, excessive bleeding, spotting, cramping, hypermenorrhoea, dysmenorrhoea and other menstrual disorders. Women taking this drug should be notified, both in writing and verbally, of these potential effects of this drug.

Prototype summary: misoprostol

Indications: prevention of NSAID- or aspirin-induced gastric ulcers in people at risk for complications of gastric ulcers.

Actions: inhibits gastric acid secretion and increases bicarbonate and mucus production, protecting the lining of the stomach; increases stimulatory effects in the uterus.

Pharmacokinetics:

Route	Onset	Peak
Oral	Rapid	12–15 min

$T_{1/2}$: 20–40 minutes; metabolised in the liver and excreted in urine.

Adverse effects: nausea, diarrhoea, abdominal pain, flatulence, vomiting, excessive bleeding or spotting, hypermenorrhoea, dysmenorrhoea, miscarriage.

Care considerations for people receiving prostaglandin

Assessment: history and examination

- Assess for *possible contraindications or cautions*: any history of allergy to misoprostol *to prevent hypersensitivity reactions*, and current status of pregnancy or breastfeeding *because of the potential for adverse effects on the fetus or breastfeeding infant*.
- Perform a physical examination *to establish baseline data before beginning therapy, and during therapy to determine the effectiveness of the drug and to evaluate for the occurrence of any adverse effects associated with drug therapy*.
- Examine the abdomen for possible changes *to rule out medical conditions*.
- Perform a pregnancy test and assess normal menstrual activity *to make sure that the woman is not pregnant*.
- Monitor the results of laboratory tests, including renal and liver function tests, *to determine the need for possible dose adjustment and identify toxic effects*.

Implementation with rationale

- Administer to people at high risk for NSAID-induced ulcers during the full course of NSAID therapy *to prevent the development of gastric ulcers*. Administer four times a day, with meals and at bedtime, *to ensure maximum benefit of the drug*.
- Arrange for a serum pregnancy test within 2 weeks before beginning treatment, and begin therapy on the second or third day of the menstrual period, *to ensure that women of childbearing age are not pregnant and to prevent abortifacient effects associated with this drug*.
- Provide the woman with both written and oral information regarding the associated risks of pregnancy *to ensure that the woman understands the risks involved*; advise the use of barrier contraceptives during therapy *to ensure the prevention of pregnancy*.
- Evaluate nutritional status if GI effects are severe *to arrange for appropriate measures to relieve discomfort and ensure nutrition*, such as small, frequent meals, and increased fluid intake if appropriate.
- Explain the risk of menstrual disorders and pain, miscarriage and excessive bleeding *related to the drug effects on prostaglandin activity in the uterus*.
- Offer support and encouragement *to help the person cope with the disease and the drug regimen*.
- Provide thorough teaching, including the drug name and prescribed dosage; schedule for administration; the need to take the drug with meals and at bedtime; signs and symptoms of adverse effects and measures to minimise or prevent them; the importance of avoiding pregnancy while taking drug; the use of barrier contraceptives to prevent pregnancy; dietary

measures such as small, frequent meals and increased fluid intake to alleviate or minimise adverse GI effects; danger signs to report to the health care provider immediately; support to deal with changes in sexuality patterns that may occur; and the importance of periodic monitoring and evaluation *to enhance knowledge about drug therapy and to promote compliance.*

Evaluation

- Monitor the response to the drug (prevention of GI ulcers related to NSAIDs).
- Monitor for adverse effects (GI, genitourinary).
- Monitor the effectiveness of comfort and safety measures and compliance with the regimen.
- Evaluate the effectiveness of the teaching plan (person can name drug and dosage and describe adverse effects to watch for, specific measures to avoid them and measures to take to increase the effectiveness of the drug).

KEY POINTS

- The prostaglandin misoprostol is used to inhibit gastric acid secretion and increase bicarbonate and mucus production in the stomach; this action will protect the lining of the stomach.
- This drug increases prostaglandin effects in the uterus, causing increased contractions, excessive bleeding and cramping. This drug is pregnancy category X and cannot be used during pregnancy.

DIGESTIVE ENZYMES

Digestive enzymes (Table 57.2) are substances produced in the GI tract to break down foods into usable nutrients. Some people – with cystic fibrosis or pancreatic dysfunction resulting from surgery or illness – may require a supplement to the production of digestive enzymes. Pancrelipase (*Creon*, *Panzytrat*) is available for replacement in conditions that result in lower-than-normal levels of these enzymes.

Therapeutic actions and indications

The pancreatic enzymes are replacement enzymes that help the digestion and absorption of fats, proteins and carbohydrates (see Figure 57.1). See Table 57.2 for usual indications for each agent.

Pharmacokinetics

Pancrelipase, which is available in capsules and delayed-release capsules, is thought to be processed through normal metabolic systems in the body. Little is known about its pharmacokinetics.

Contraindications and cautions

Pancreatic enzymes should not be used with known allergy to the product or to pork products *to prevent hypersensitivity reactions.* In addition, pancreatic enzymes should be used cautiously in pregnancy and breastfeeding *because of the risk for adverse effects on the fetus or baby.*

Adverse effects

The adverse effects that most often occur with pancreatic enzymes are related to GI irritation and include nausea, abdominal cramps and diarrhoea.

Prototype summary: pancrelipase

Indications: replacement therapy in people with deficient exocrine pancreatic secretions.

Actions: replaces pancreatic enzymes to aid in the digestion and absorption of fats, proteins and carbohydrates.

Pharmacokinetics: generally not absorbed systemically.

$T_{1/2}$: generally not absorbed systemically.

Adverse effects: nausea, abdominal cramps, diarrhoea, hyperuricosuria.

TABLE 57.2 DRUGS IN FOCUS Drug used to treat digestive enzyme dysfunction

Drug name	Dosage/route	Usual indications
Digestive enzymes		
pancrelipase (*Creon*, *Panzytrat*)	Dosage varies with preparation and condition treated. See manufacturer's instructions	Aids digestion and absorption of fats, proteins and carbohydrates in conditions that result in a lack of this enzyme; used as replacement therapy in people with cystic fibrosis, chronic ductal obstruction, pancreatic insufficiency, steatorrhoea or malabsorption syndrome and after pancreatectomy or gastrectomy

Care considerations for people receiving digestive enzymes

Assessment: history and examination

- Assess for *possible contraindications or cautions*: any history of allergy to any of the drugs or to pork products *to prevent hypersensitivity reactions because there may be an abnormal absorption of electrolytes, including sodium, leading to increased cardiovascular load*; and current status of pregnancy or breastfeeding *because of the potential for adverse effects on the fetus or breastfeeding infant.*
- Perform a physical examination *to establish baseline data before beginning therapy and during therapy to evaluate the effectiveness of the drug and determine the occurrence of any adverse effects associated with drug therapy.*
- Perform an abdominal examination *to rule out underlying medical conditions and assess for adverse effects of the drug*; auscultate bowel sounds *to evaluate GI motility.*
- Assess cardiopulmonary status, including blood pressure and cardiac rate and rhythm, *to identify changes that may indicate electrolyte imbalances.*
- Monitor the results of laboratory tests, including renal function tests, *to determine the need for possible dose adjustment and identify toxic effects*, and pancreatic enzyme levels *to assure correct dose and to monitor response.*

Implementation with rationale

- Administer pancreatic enzymes with meals and snacks so that the enzyme is available when it is needed. Avoid spilling powder on the skin *because it may be irritating.* Do not crush the capsule or allow the person to chew it; it must be swallowed whole *to ensure full therapeutic effect.*
- Assess nutritional status if there are GI effects *to arrange for appropriate measures to relieve discomfort and ensure nutrition, such as frequent small meals.*
- Obtain laboratory specimens as indicated *to evaluate electrolyte levels and pancreatic enzyme levels.*
- Offer support and encouragement *to help the person cope with the disease and the drug regimen.*
- Provide thorough teaching, including the drug name and prescribed dosage; schedule for administration; the importance of taking pancreatic enzymes with meals and snacks; the need to take the pancreatic enzyme whole and not to crush or chew the capsule; dietary measures to follow; signs and symptoms of adverse effects and measures to minimise or prevent them; danger signs that need to be reported to the health care provider immediately; the need for periodic monitoring of pancreatic enzyme levels to evaluate the effectiveness of therapy; and the importance of complying with therapy and follow-up *to enhance knowledge about drug therapy and to promote compliance.*

Evaluation

- Monitor the response to the drug (eg, relief of dry mouth and throat; digestion of fats, proteins and carbohydrates).
- Monitor for adverse effects (eg, electrolyte imbalance, GI effects).
- Monitor the effectiveness of comfort and safety measures and compliance with the regimen.
- Evaluate the effectiveness of the teaching plan (person can name the drug and dosage and describe adverse effects to watch for, specific measures to avoid them and measures to take to increase the effectiveness of the drug).

KEY POINTS

- Digestive enzymes such as pancreatic enzymes may be needed if normal enzyme levels are very low and proper digestion cannot take place.
- People receiving replacement enzymes will need to be monitored to ensure that the dose is correct for their particular situation to avoid adverse effects.

CHAPTER SUMMARY

- GI complaints are some of the most common symptoms seen in clinical practice.
- Peptic ulcers may result from increased acid production, decrease in the protective mucus lining of the stomach, infection with *Helicobacter pylori* bacteria, or a combination of these.
- Agents used to decrease the acid content of the stomach include H_2 antagonists, which block the release of acid in response to gastrin or parasympathetic release; antacids, which chemically react with the acid to neutralise it; proton pump inhibitors, which block the last step of acid production to prevent release; and prostaglandins, which block gastric acid secretion and increase bicarbonate production.
- Acid rebound occurs when the stomach produces more gastrin and more acid in response to lowered acid levels in the stomach, which commonly occurs with the use of antacids. Balancing the reduction of

the stomach acid without increasing acid production is a clinical challenge.
- The GI protectant sucralfate forms a protective coating over the eroded stomach lining to protect it from acid and digestive enzymes to aid healing.
- The prostaglandin misoprostol blocks gastric acid secretion while increasing the production of bicarbonate and mucus lining in the stomach.
- Digestive enzymes such as pancreatic enzymes may be needed if normal enzyme levels are very low and proper digestion cannot take place.

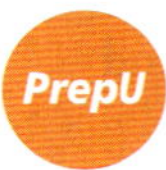

Knowing your strengths and weaknesses helps you to study more effectively. Take a PrepU Practice Quiz to find out how you measure up!

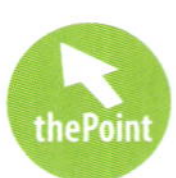

ONLINE RESOURCES

An extensive range of additional resources to enhance teaching and learning and to facilitate understanding of this chapter may be found online at the text's accompanying website, located on thePoint at http://thepoint.lww.com. These include Watch and Learn videos, Concepts in Action animations, journal articles, review questions, case studies, discussion topics and quizzes.

BIBLIOGRAPHY

Al-Sohaily, S. & Duggan, A. (2008) Long-term management of patients taking proton pump inhibitors. *Australian Prescriber, 31*, 5–7.

Dial, S., Delaney, J. A., Barkun, A. N. & Suissa, S. (2005). Use of gastric acid suppressive agents and the risk of community acquired *Clostridium difficile* associated diarrhea. *JAMA, 294*, 2898–2995.

Farrell, M. & Dempsey, J. (2014). *Smeltzer & Bare's Textbook of Medical-Surgical Nursing* (3rd edn). Sydney: Lippincott Williams & Wilkins.

Goodman, L. S., Brunton, L. L., Chabner, B. & Knollmann, B. C. (2011). *Goodman and Gilman's Pharmacological Basis of Therapeutics* (12th edn). New York: McGraw-Hill.

Green, C. (2010). Recommended management of GORD in general practice. *Prescriber, 21(1–2)*, 18–30.

McKenna, L. & Mirkov, S. (2019). *McKenna's Drug Handbook for Nursing and Midwifery* (8th edn). Sydney: Wolters Kluwer Health Australia.

MEDSAFE. (2006). Proton pump inhibitors and interstitial nephritis. *Prescriber Updates, 27(1)*, 3. www.medsafe.govt.nz/profs/PUarticles/watchingbriefsJune06.htm.

Morcom, J. (2008). Understanding GORD from a primary nurse perspective. *Gastrointestinal Nursing, 6(1)*, 12–20.

Pfizer New Zealand Ltd. (2005). Somac (pantoprazole) tablets data sheet. www.medsafe.govt.nz/profs/Datasheet/s/somacHeartBurnRelieftab.pdf.

Porth, C. M. (2011). *Essentials of Pathophysiology: Concepts of Altered Health States* (3rd edn). Philadelphia: Lippincott Williams & Wilkins.

Porth, C. M. (2009). *Pathophysiology: Concepts of Altered Health States* (8th edn). Philadelphia: Lippincott Williams & Wilkins.

Savage, R. (2001). Omeprazole-induced interstitial nephritis. *Prescriber Update, 20*(Feb), 11–13. www.medsafe.govt.nz/profs/PUarticles/omeprazole.htm.

Selby, M. (2010). GORD and dyspepsia...gastrooesophageal reflux disease. *Practice Nurse, 39(9)*, 19–22.

Simpson, I. J., Marshall, M. R., Pilmore H., et al. (2006). Proton pump inhibitors and acute interstitial nephritis—report and analysis of 15 cases. *Nephrology, 11(5)*, 381–385.

Wileman, S. M., McCann, S., Grant, A. M., Krukowski, Z. H. & Bruce, J. (2010). Medical versus surgical management for gastro-oesophageal reflux disease (GORD) in adults. *Cochrane Database of Systematic Reviews, 153*(3), JC3–JC10.

Wyeth (NZ) Limited. (2002). Zoton (lansoprazole) capsules data sheet. www.medsafe.govt.nz/profs/Datasheet/z/zotoncap.htm.

Yu-Xiao, Y., Lewis, S. D., Epstein, S. & Metz, D. (2007). Long term proton pump inhibitor therapy and risk of hip fracture. *JAMA, 296*, 2947–2953.

CHECK YOUR UNDERSTANDING

Answers to the questions in this chapter can be found in Appendix A at the back of this book.

MULTIPLE CHOICE

Select the best response to the following.

1. Which of the following would a nurse and midwife include when describing the action of histamine-2 antagonists to a person?
   a. They block the release of gastrin and pepsin, leading to a decrease in protein digestion.
   b. They selectively block histamine receptors, reducing swelling and inflammation at numerous sites.
   c. They selectively block specific histamine-receptor sites, leading to a reduction in gastric acid secretion.
   d. They are effective primarily for long-term use because of their slow onset of action.
2. H_2 receptors are found throughout the body, including:
   a. in the nasal passages, upper airways and stomach.
   b. in the CNS and upper airways.
   c. in the respiratory tract and the heart.
   d. in the heart, CNS and stomach.
3. Which H_2 antagonist would the nurse expect to be ordered for a person with known liver dysfunction?
   a. cimetidine
   b. famotidine
   c. nizatidine
   d. ranitidine
4. The nurse would monitor a person receiving intravenous cimetidine (*Magicul*) for an acute ulcer problem for:
   a. GI upset.
   b. gynaecomastia.
   c. cardiac arrhythmias.
   d. constipation.
5. Acid rebound is a condition that occurs when:
   a. lowering gastric acid to an alkaline level stimulates the release of gastric acid.
   b. raising gastric acid levels causes heartburn.
   c. combining protein, calcium and smoking greatly elevates gastric acid levels.
   d. eating citrus fruit neutralises gastric acid.
6. A nurse taking care of a person who is receiving a proton pump inhibitor should teach the person to:
   a. take the drug after every meal.
   b. chew or crush tablets to increase their absorption.
   c. swallow tablets or capsules whole.
   d. stop taking the drug after 3 weeks of therapy.
7. Misoprostol (*Cytotec*) is a prostaglandin that is used to:
   a. prevent uterine contractions.
   b. prevent NSAID-related gastric ulcers in people at high risk.
   c. decrease hyperacidity with meals and at bedtime.
   d. relieve the burning associated with hiatal hernia at night.
8. A nurse or midwife caring for a person receiving pancreatic enzymes as replacement therapy should be assessing the person for:
   a. hypertension.
   b. cardiac arrhythmias.
   c. excessive weight gain.
   d. signs of GI irritation.

MULTIPLE RESPONSE

Select all that apply.

1. People who use antacids frequently can be expected to experience which of the following adverse effects?
   a. systemic alkalosis
   b. electrolyte imbalances
   c. hypokalaemia
   d. metabolic acidosis
   e. constipation or diarrhoea
   f. muscular weakness

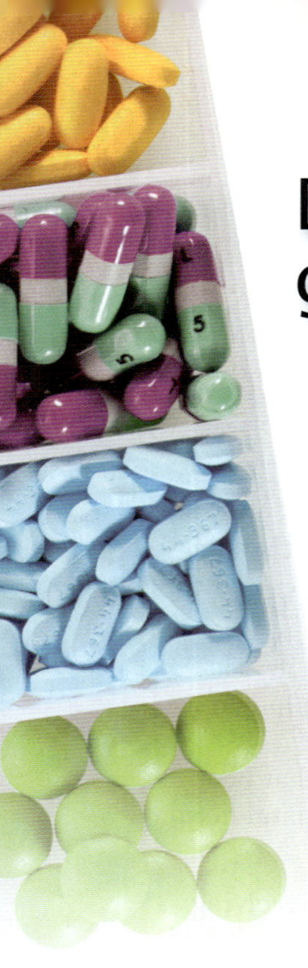

Drugs affecting gastrointestinal motility

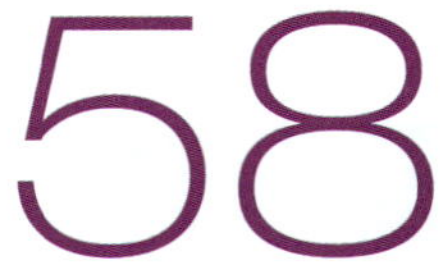

Learning objectives

On completing this chapter you should be able to:

1. Describe the underlying processes in diarrhoea and constipation and correlate them with the types of drugs used to treat these conditions.
2. Describe the therapeutic actions, indications, pharmacokinetics, contraindications and cautions, most common adverse reactions and important drug–drug interactions associated with laxatives and antidiarrhoeal drugs.
3. Discuss the use of laxatives and antidiarrhoeal agents across the lifespan.
4. Compare and contrast the prototype laxatives and antidiarrhoeals, liquid paraffin and loperamide, with other agents in their class and with other classes of laxatives and antidiarrhoeals.
5. Outline the care considerations, including important teaching points, for people receiving laxatives and antidiarrhoeal agents.

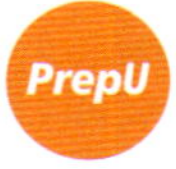

Test your current knowledge of drugs affecting gastrointestinal motility with a PrepU Practice Quiz!

Glossary of key terms

antidiarrhoeal drug: drug that blocks the stimulation of the gastrointestinal (GI) tract, leading to decreased activity and increased time for absorption of needed nutrients and water

bulk-forming laxative: agent that increases in bulk, frequently by osmotic pull of fluid into the faeces; the increased bulk stretches the GI wall, causing stimulation and increased GI movement

cathartic dependence: overuse of laxatives that can lead to the need for strong stimuli to initiate movement in the intestines; local reflexes become resistant to normal stimuli after prolonged use of harsher stimulants, leading to further laxative use

stimulant laxative: agent that stimulates the normal GI reflexes by chemically irritating the lining of the GI wall, leading to increased activity in the GI tract

constipation: slower-than-normal evacuation of the large intestine, which can result in increased water absorption from the faeces and can lead to impaction

diarrhoea: more-frequent-than-normal bowel movements, often characterised as fluid-like and watery because not enough time for absorption is allowed during the passage of food through the intestines

lubricant: agent that increases the viscosity of the faeces, making it difficult to absorb water from the bolus and easing movement of the bolus through the intestines

LAXATIVES

Stimulant laxatives
bisacodyl
senna

Bulk-forming laxatives
ispaghula (psyllium husk)
sterculia

Osmotic laxatives
glycerol
lactulose
macrogols
sodium chloride–sodium bicarbonate–potassium chloride solution

Lubricants (faecal softeners)
docusate
(P) liquid paraffin

Opioid-receptor antagonist
methylnaltrexone

ANTIDIARRHOEALS
bovine colostrum
(P) loperamide
opium derivatives

Ulcerative colitis drugs
balsalazide
mesalazine
olsalazine
sulfasalazine

IRRITABLE BOWEL SYNDROME DRUGS
hyoscine
mebeverine
peppermint oil

Drugs used to affect the motor activity or motility of the gastrointestinal (GI) tract can do so in several different ways. They can be used to speed up or improve the movement of intestinal contents along the GI tract when movement becomes too slow or sluggish, to allow for proper absorption of nutrients and excretion of wastes, as in **constipation**. Drugs are also used to increase the tone of the GI tract and to stimulate motility throughout the system. They can also be used to decrease movement along the GI tract when rapid movement decreases the time for the absorption of nutrients, leading to a loss of water and nutrients, and the discomfort of **diarrhoea**. This chapter addresses three major categories of drugs: laxatives, GI stimulants and antidiarrhoeal agents. See Figure 58.1 for sites of action of these drugs on GI motility. Box 58.1 highlights important considerations related to laxatives and other drugs affecting GI motility, based on the person's age.

LAXATIVES

Laxative, or cathartic, drugs (Table 58.1) are indicated for the short-term relief of constipation; to prevent straining when it is clinically undesirable (such as after surgery, myocardial infarction (MI) or after vaginal birth); to evacuate the bowel for diagnostic procedures; to remove ingested poisons from the lower GI tract; and as an adjunct in anthelmintic therapy when it is desirable to flush helminths (intestinal worms) from the GI tract (see Figure 58.1). Most laxatives are available in over-the-counter (OTC) preparations, and they are often abused by people who then become dependent on them for stimulation of GI movement. Such individuals may develop chronic intestinal disorders as a result. Measures such as instituting proper diet and exercise, and taking advantage of the actions of the intestinal reflexes have eliminated the need for laxatives in many situations; therefore, these agents are used less frequently than they once were in clinical practice.

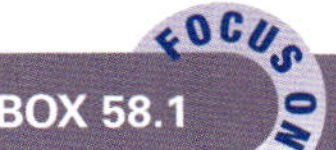

Drug therapy across the lifespan

Laxatives and antidiarrhoeal agents

CHILDREN

Laxatives should not be used in children routinely. Proper diet, including roughage, plenty of fluids and exercise, should be tried first if a child has a tendency to become constipated. Lubricants can be used in older children; harsh stimulants should be avoided. Children with encopresis, however, are often given senna preparations or liquid paraffin to help them to evacuate the massive stool.

Children receiving these agents should use them for only a short period and should be evaluated for potential underlying medical or nutritional problems if they are not able to return to normal function.

ADULTS

Adults who use laxatives need to be cautioned not to become dependent. Proper diet, exercise and adequate intake of fluids should keep the GI tract functioning normally. If an antidiarrhoeal is needed, adults should be carefully instructed in the proper dosing of the drug and monitoring of their total use to avoid excessive dose.

PREGNANCY AND BREASTFEEDING

The safety for the use of these drugs during pregnancy and breastfeeding has not been established. Use should be reserved for those situations in which the benefit to the mother outweighs the potential risk to the fetus. A mild stool softener is often used after delivery. The drugs may enter breast milk and also may affect GI activity in the neonate. It is advised that caution be used if one of these drugs is prescribed during breastfeeding.

OLDER ADULTS

Older adults are more likely to develop adverse effects associated with the use of these drugs, including sedation, confusion, dizziness, electrolyte disturbances, fluid imbalance and cardiovascular effects. Safety measures may be needed if these effects occur and interfere with the person's mobility and balance.

Older people also may be taking other drugs that are associated with constipation and may need help to prevent severe problems from developing.

Older adults are more likely to have renal and/or hepatic impairment related to underlying medical conditions, which could interfere with the metabolism and excretion of the antidiarrhoeal drugs. The dose for older adults should be started at a lower level than recommended for younger adults. The person should be monitored very closely, and dose adjustment should be made based on response.

These people also need to be alerted to the potential for toxic effects when using over-the-counter (OTC) preparations and should be advised to check with their health care provider before beginning any OTC drug regimen.

An ispaghula (psyllium husk) product is the agent of choice with older adults because there is less risk of adverse reactions. The person needs to be cautioned to drink plenty of fluid after taking one of these agents to prevent problems that can occur if the drug starts to pull in fluid while still in the oesophagus.

The older adult should be encouraged to drink plenty of fluids, to exercise every day and to get plenty of roughage in the diet. Many older adults have established routines, such as drinking warm water or prune juice at the same time each morning, that are disrupted with illness or hospitalisation. These people should be encouraged and helped to try to maintain their usual protocol as much as possible.

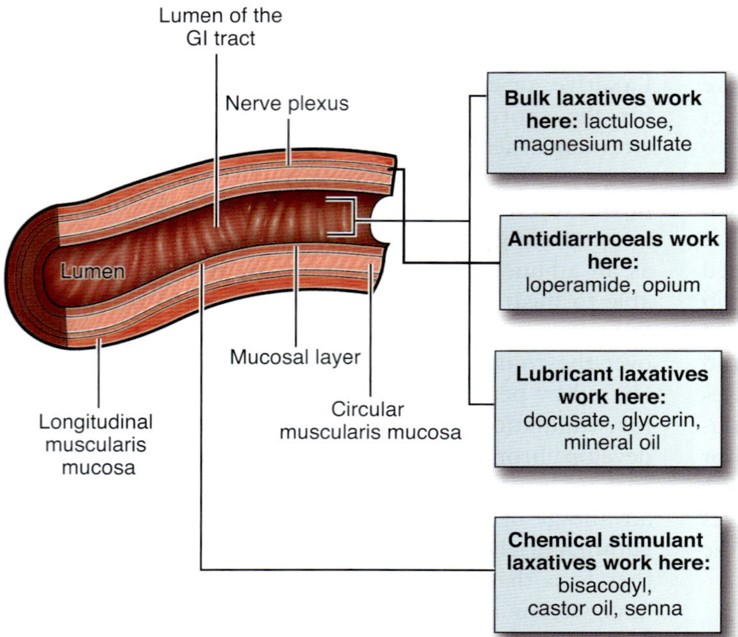

FIGURE 58.1 Sites of action of drugs affecting gastrointestinal motility.

Kinds of laxatives include chemical stimulants (which chemically irritate the lining of the GI tract), bulk stimulants (which cause faecal matter to increase in bulk) and lubricants (which help the intestinal contents move more slowly). Newer laxatives are available for very specific needs and alter sodium absorption or affect opioid receptors in the GI tract.

STIMULANT LAXATIVES

Stimulant laxatives directly stimulate the nerve plexus in the intestinal wall, causing increased movement and the stimulation of local reflexes. Laxatives classified as chemical stimulants include bisacodyl (*Dulcolax*), castor oil (generic) and senna (*Senokot*).

Therapeutic actions and indications

Castor oil is rarely used nowadays; however, it is still used in some countries. All of these agents begin working at the beginning of the small intestine and increase motility throughout the rest of the GI tract by irritating the nerve plexus. Bisacodyl can be given in rectal suppository and bowel preparation to stimulate the activity in the lower GI tract. Senna is available orally in tablet and powder forms.

Pharmacokinetics

Most of these agents are only minimally absorbed and exert their therapeutic effect directly in the GI tract. Changes in absorption, water balance and electrolytes resulting from GI changes can have adverse effects on people with underlying medical conditions that are affected by volume and electrolyte changes (see Adverse effects). They have an onset of action of 6–8 hours, making them preferable if one wants the drug to work overnight and see effects in the morning.

Contraindications and cautions

Laxatives are contraindicated with allergy to any component of the drug to prevent hypersensitivity reactions; in acute abdominal disorders, including appendicitis, diverticulitis and ulcerative colitis, when increased motility could lead to rupture or further exacerbation of the inflammation. Laxatives should be used with caution in heart block, coronary artery disease (CAD) or debilitation, which could be affected by the decrease in absorption and changes in electrolyte levels that can occur; with great caution during pregnancy and breastfeeding because in some cases, stimulation of the GI tract can precipitate labour, and many of these agents cross the placenta and are excreted in breast milk.

Castor oil should not be used during pregnancy because its irritant effect has been associated with induction of premature labour. Magnesium laxatives can cause diarrhoea in the neonate if used during breastfeeding.

Adverse effects

The adverse effects most commonly associated with laxatives are GI effects such as diarrhoea, abdominal cramping and nausea. Central nervous system (CNS) effects, including dizziness, headache and weakness, are not uncommon and may relate to loss of fluid and electrolyte imbalances that may accompany laxative use. Sweating, palpitations, flushing and even fainting have been reported after laxative use. These effects may be related to a sympathetic stress reaction to intense neurostimulation of the GI tract or to the loss of fluid and electrolyte imbalance.

A very common adverse effect that is seen with frequent laxative use or laxative abuse is **cathartic dependence**. This reaction occurs when people use laxatives over a long period of time and the GI tract becomes dependent on the vigorous stimulation of the laxative. Without this stimulation, the GI tract does not move for a period of time (i.e. several days), which could lead to constipation and drying of the stool, and ultimately to impaction.

Specifically related to chemical stimulants, cascara, although a reliable agent, may have a slow, steady effect or may cause severe cramping and rapid evacuation of the contents of the large intestine.

Clinically important drug–drug interactions

Because laxatives increase the motility of the GI tract and some interfere with the timing or process of absorption, it is advisable not to take laxatives at the same time as other prescribed medications. The administration of laxatives and other medications should be separated by at least 30 minutes.

BULK-FORMING LAXATIVES

Bulk-forming laxatives (also called mechanical stimulants) are rapid-acting, aggressive laxatives that cause the faecal matter to increase in bulk. They increase the motility of the GI tract by increasing the fluid in the intestinal contents, which enlarges bulk, stimulates local stretch receptors and activates local activity. The only currently available bulk-forming stimulant is ispaghula (psyllium) (*Consyl D, Mucilax, Metamucil*).

Therapeutic actions and indications

Bulk-forming laxatives increase the motility of the GI tract by increasing the fluid in the intestinal contents, which enlarges bulk, stimulates local stretch receptors and activates local activity.

Psyllium is a natural substance that forms a gelatine-like bulk out of the intestinal contents. It is milder and less irritating than many other bulk stimulants. People must use caution and drink plenty of water when taking it.

Pharmacokinetics

These drugs are all taken orally. They are directly effective within the GI tract and are not generally absorbed systemically. They are rapid acting, causing effects as they pass through the GI tract.

Contraindications and cautions

Bulk laxatives are contraindicated with allergy to any component of the drug *to prevent hypersensitivity reactions*; and in acute abdominal disorders, including appendicitis, diverticulitis and ulcerative colitis, *when increased motility could lead to rupture or further exacerbation of the inflammation*. Laxatives should be used with caution in heart block, CAD and debilitation, *which could be affected by the decrease in absorption and changes in electrolyte levels that can occur*; with great caution during pregnancy and breastfeeding *because in some cases, stimulation of the GI tract can precipitate labour, and many of these agents cross the placenta and are excreted in breast milk*. Sodium chloride–sodium bicarbonate–potassium chloride should be used with caution in any person with a history of seizures *because of the risk of electrolyte absorption causing neuronal instability and precipitating seizures*.

Adverse effects

The adverse effects most commonly associated with bulk laxatives are GI effects such as diarrhoea, abdominal cramping and nausea. CNS effects, including dizziness, headache and weakness, are not uncommon and may relate to loss of fluid and electrolyte imbalances that may accompany laxative use. Sweating, palpitations, flushing and even fainting have been reported after laxative use. These effects may be related to a sympathetic stress reaction to intense neurostimulation of the GI tract or to the loss of fluid and electrolyte imbalance. People must use caution and take bulk laxatives with plenty of water. If only a little water is used, the laxative may absorb enough fluid in the oesophagus to swell into a gelatine-like mass that can obstruct the oesophagus and cause severe problems.

Clinically important drug–drug interactions

Bulk laxatives increase the motility of the GI tract, and some interfere with the timing or process of absorption. It is advisable not to take laxatives with other prescribed medications. The administration of laxatives and other medications should be separated by at least 30 minutes.

TABLE 58.1 DRUGS IN FOCUS Laxatives

Drug name	Dosage/route	Usual indications
Stimulant laxatives		
bisacodyl (*Bisalax, Dulcolax*)	5–10 mg PO at night, or one suppository PR at night	Emptying of the GI tract before some surgeries or diagnostic tests (eg, barium enema); prevention of constipation and straining after GI surgery, MI, obstetrical delivery; short-term treatment of constipation
senna (*Senokot*)	Adults, paediatric > 12 years: 2–4 tablets daily; maximum 4 tablets/day without medical advice; divide doses > 4 tablets/day and take morning and night, or as prescribed	Short-term treatment of constipation; treatment of encopresis; found in many OTC preparations
Osmotic laxatives		
lactulose (*Actilax, Laevolac*)	Initially 30–45 mL tid-qid; maintenance 10–25 mL/day	Short-term treatment of constipation; alternative choice for people with cardiovascular disorders
sodium chloride–sodium bicarbonate–potassium chloride solution (*ColonLYTELY*)	Dosage: 2–4 L of oral solution on empty stomach in the evening before procedure	Stimulates bowel evacuation before GI examination (eg, colonoscopy, sigmoidoscopy)
sodium citrate dihydrate, sodium lauryl sulfoacetate and sorbitol (*Microlax*)	Adult: one microenema PR Children: half of the microenema PR	Treatment of constipation or in preparation for rectal examination
Sodium phosphate (*Fleet*)	Adult, paediatric ≥ 12 years, oral: single dose given once a day for a maximum of 3 days; enema: 1 bottle per day for a maximum for 3 days	Treatment of occasional constipation in adults
Bulk-forming laxatives		
ispaghula (psyllium) (*Metamucil*)	Refer to manufacturer instructions	Mild laxative; short-term treatment of constipation
Sterculia (*Normafibe, Normacol*)	Adult, 200 g or 500 g granules: 1–2 heaped teaspoons PO 1–2 times daily	Constipation
Lubricants (faecal softeners)		
docusate (*Coloxyl, Sennesoft*)	Adult, paediatric > 12 years: 100–240 mg PO	Prophylaxis for people who should not strain (such as after surgery, MI or obstetric delivery)
glycerol (generic)	One suppository PR. Allow to remain for 15–30 min	Short-term treatment of constipation
(P) liquid paraffin (*Agarol*)	Adults and paediatric > 6 years: 15–30 mL at bedtime Paediatric (3–6 years): 10–15 mL at bedtime	Short-term treatment of constipation

OSMOTIC LAXATIVES

Glycerol is a hyperosmolar laxative used in suppository form to gently evacuate the rectum without systemic effects higher in the GI tract.

Lactulose (*Actilax, Laevolac*) is a saltless osmotic laxative that pulls fluid out of the venous system and into the lumen of the small intestine. It needs to be taken with a large glass of water and takes at least 48 hours to work. The most common side effects are diarrhoea, bloating and wind. These are usually mild. Lactulose is a non-absorbable disaccharide but may contain small amounts of monosaccharide that can affect blood glucose levels. It is not suitable in people with lactose intolerance. In higher doses it is also used for the treatment of hepatic encephalopathy because it causes reduced urea production and reduced entry of ammonia into portal blood.

Macrogol (*Movicol*) is used in combination with electrolytes for treating chronic constipation and faecal impaction. It is contraindicated in people with intestinal perforation, ileus and severe inflammatory conditions of the intestinal tract, such as Crohn disease, ulcerative colitis and toxic megacolon.

Sodium chloride with sodium bicarbonate and potassium chloride (ColonLYTELY) contains many electrolytes that pull fluid out of the intestinal wall to increase the bulk of the intestinal contents.

Sodium phosphate (*Fleet*) is a saline laxative that works by pulling water from the body into the bowel, which helps to soften the stool and cause a bowel movement. The U.S. Food and Drug Administration (FDA) has warned that using more than one dose in 24 hours to treat constipation can cause severe dehydration and rare serious harm to the kidneys and heart, and even death. Enema produces a bowel movement in 1–5 minutes.

Microlax enema contains sodium citrate dihydrate, sodium lauryl sulfoacetate and sorbitol. It usually cause a bowel motion within 30 minutes.

LUBRICANTS (FAECAL SOFTENERS)

Sometimes it is desirable to make defecation easier without stimulating the movement of the GI tract. This is done using **lubricants**. People with haemorrhoids and those who have recently had rectal surgery may need lubrication of the stool. Some people who could be harmed by straining might also benefit from this type of laxative. The type of laxative recommended depends on the condition of the person, the speed of relief needed and the possible implication of various adverse effects. Lubricating laxatives include docusate (*Coloxyl*), and liquid paraffin (*Agarol*).

Therapeutic actions and indications

Docusate has a detergent action on the surface of the intestinal bolus, increasing the admixture of fat and water and making a softer stool.

Liquid paraffin is the oldest of these laxatives. It is not absorbed and forms a slippery coat on the contents of the intestinal tract. When the intestinal bolus is coated with liquid paraffin, less water is absorbed out of the bolus, and the bolus is less likely to become hard or impacted.

Pharmacokinetics

These drugs are not absorbed systemically and are excreted in the faeces. Docusate and liquid paraffin are given orally. Glycerol is available as a rectal suppository.

Contraindications and cautions

These laxatives are contraindicated with allergy to any component of the drug *to prevent hypersensitivity reactions*; and in acute abdominal disorders, including appendicitis, diverticulitis and ulcerative colitis, *when increased motility could lead to rupture or further exacerbation of the inflammation*. Laxatives should be used with caution in heart block, CAD and debilitation, *which could be affected by the decrease in absorption and changes in electrolyte levels that can occur*; caution should be used during pregnancy and breastfeeding *because in some cases, stimulation of the GI tract can precipitate labour, and many of these agents cross the placenta and are excreted in breast milk.*

Adverse effects

The adverse effects most commonly associated with lubricant laxatives are GI effects such as diarrhoea, abdominal cramping and nausea. In addition, leakage and staining may be a problem when liquid paraffin is used and the stool cannot be retained by the external sphincter. CNS effects, including dizziness, headache and weakness, are not uncommon and may relate to loss of fluid and electrolyte imbalances that may accompany laxative use. Sweating, palpitations, flushing and even fainting have been reported after laxative use. These effects are less likely to happen with the lubricant laxatives than with the chemical or mechanical stimulants.

Clinically important drug–drug interactions

Frequent use of liquid paraffin can interfere with absorption of the fat-soluble vitamins A, D, E and K.

(P) Prototype summary: liquid paraffin

Indications: short-term relief of constipation; to prevent straining when it is clinically undesirable; to remove ingested poisons from the lower GI tract; an adjunct in anthelmintic therapy when it is desirable to flush helminths from the GI tract.

Actions: forms a slippery coat on the contents of the intestinal tract; less water is absorbed out of the bolus, and the bolus is less likely to become hard or impacted.

Pharmacokinetics: not absorbed systemically.

$T_{1/2}$: not absorbed systemically.

Adverse effects: diarrhoea; abdominal cramps; bloating; perianal irritation; dizziness; interference with absorption of the fat-soluble vitamins A, D, E and K; leakage of stool and staining.

OTHER LAXATIVES

Another drug that does not fit into the categories usually used for laxatives has been approved recently for the treatment of opioid-induced constipation. This drug is discussed in Box 58.2.

BOX 58.2 Other laxatives

A drug that does not fit into the categories usually used for laxatives has been approved for the treatment of specific forms of constipation.

Methylnaltrexone (*Relistor*) was approved in 2008 for the treatment of opioid-induced constipation in people with advanced disease who are receiving palliative care and are no longer responsive to traditional laxatives. Opioids bind to various receptors in the body, including the μ (mu) opioid receptors, which leads to decreased GI motility and constipation. People on long-term opioid treatment frequently have a very difficult time with constipation. Methylnaltrexone is a selective antagonist to opioid binding at the mu opioid receptor. It does not cross the blood–brain barrier and therefore acts specifically at peripheral opioid receptor sites, like the GI tract, but does not affect the analgesic effects of opioids in the CNS. This drug is given by daily subcutaneous injections. It reaches peak levels in 30 minutes and is eliminated primarily unchanged in the urine. The half-life of the drug is about 8 hours. People may experience abdominal pain, flatulence, nausea, dizziness and diarrhoea. Severe or continued diarrhoea should be reported. Use of this drug beyond 4 months has not been studied.

Sterculia and frangula (*Normacol Plus*) is a combination laxative. Sterculia is a bulking agent; frangula is a stimulant.

Care considerations for people receiving laxatives

Assessment: history and examination

- Assess for *possible contraindications or cautions*: history of allergy to laxative *to prevent hypersensitivity reaction*; faecal impaction or intestinal obstruction, *which could be exacerbated by increased GI activity*; acute abdominal pain, nausea or vomiting, *which could represent an underlying medical condition*; and current status of pregnancy or breastfeeding, *which could be contraindications or require cautious use*.
- Perform a physical examination *to establish baseline data before beginning therapy and during therapy to determine the effectiveness of the drug and to evaluate for any adverse effects associated with drug therapy*.
- Inspect the skin for rash to *monitor for adverse reactions*.
- Assess the person's neurological status, including level of orientation and affect, *to evaluate any CNS effects of the drug*.
- Obtain a baseline pulse rate *to assess for any cardiovascular effects of the drug*.
- Assess bowel elimination patterns, including the person's perception of normal frequency, actual frequency and stool characteristics, *to determine the need for therapy*.
- Investigate the person's nutritional intake, including fluid intake and ingestion of fibre-containing foods, *to evaluate for possible contributing factors related to the need for the drug*.
- Assess the person's level of activity *to determine possible contributing factors for decreased bowel motility*.
- Perform an abdominal examination, including inspecting abdomen for distension, palpating for masses and auscultating for bowel sounds, *to establish adequate bowel function, rule out underlying medical conditions and assess the effectiveness of the drug*.
- Monitor results of laboratory tests, including serum electrolyte levels, *to detect any changes related to altered absorption*.

Implementation with rationale

- Administer a laxative only as a temporary measure *to prevent the development of cathartic dependence*.
- Arrange for appropriate dietary measures, exercise and environmental controls *to encourage the return of normal bowel function*.
- Administer the oral form with a full glass of water, and caution the person not to chew tablets, *to ensure that the laxative reaches the GI tract to allow for therapeutic effects*. Encourage fluid intake throughout the day as appropriate *to maintain fluid balance and improve GI movement*.
- Administer bulk laxatives with plenty of water. If only a little water is used, it may absorb enough fluid in the oesophagus to swell into a gelatine-like mass *that can obstruct the oesophagus and cause severe problems*.
- Insert rectal suppositories high into the rectum; encourage people to retain enemas or rectal solution as long as possible *to improve effectiveness*.
- Do not administer in the presence of acute abdominal pain, nausea or vomiting, *which might indicate a serious underlying medical problem that could be exacerbated by laxative use* due to potential risk of bowel perforation.
- Monitor bowel function *to evaluate drug effectiveness*. If diarrhoea or cramping occurs, discontinue the drug *to relieve discomfort and to prevent serious fluid and electrolyte imbalance*.
- Provide comfort and safety measures *to improve compliance and to ensure safety*, including ready access to bathroom facilities, assistance with

ambulation and periodic orientation if CNS effects occur.
- Offer support and encouragement *to help the person deal with the discomfort of the condition and drug therapy.*
- Offer support and encouragement *to help the person deal with the diagnosis and the drug regimen.*
- Provide thorough teaching, including the drug name, dosage and schedule for administration; method of administration, such as taking the oral form with a full glass of water, thoroughly mixing the powdered or granular form with water or juice *to ensure complete dissolution*, inserting the suppository form or using and retaining an enema; approximate time for achievement of results and importance of having bathroom facilities readily available; safety measures, such as changing positions slowly and using assistance with ambulation if dizziness or weakness occurs; signs and symptoms of possible adverse effects and measures *to minimise or prevent them*; possible leakage and staining when liquid paraffin is used and the stool cannot be retained by the external sphincter; danger signs and symptoms *to be reported to a health care provider immediately*; the importance of daily activity *to promote bowel function*; the need for the ingestion of high-fibre foods and adequate fluids *to stimulate GI motility*; the importance of avoiding the overuse of laxatives *to prevent chronic or long-term problems with elimination*; a bowel training program if indicated *to prevent dependence on laxatives*; and importance of periodic monitoring and evaluation *to evaluate the effectiveness of therapy, enhance knowledge about drug therapy and promote compliance.*

Evaluation

- Monitor response to the drug (relief of GI symptoms, absence of straining, evacuation of GI tract).
- Monitor for adverse effects (dizziness, confusion, GI alterations, sweating, electrolyte imbalance, cathartic dependence).
- Monitor the effectiveness of comfort measures and compliance with the regimen.
- Evaluate the effectiveness of the teaching plan (person can name the drug and dosage, describe adverse effects to watch for and specific measures to use to avoid them).

KEY POINTS

- Laxative drugs stimulate GI motility and assist in bowel elimination.
- Laxatives can be chemical or bulk stimulants or lubricants.
- In many cases, implementing diet and exercise strategies and promoting natural intestinal reflexes have decreased the need to use laxatives.
- Chronic use of laxatives can lead to dependence on them and on external stimuli for normal GI function.

ANTIDIARRHOEALS

Antidiarrhoeals block stimulation of the GI tract for symptomatic relief from diarrhoea. Available agents include loperamide (*Imodium*), kaolin, codeine and opium derivatives. Several antidiarrhoeal products are available in combination (Box 58.3). Other antidiarrhoeals are salicylate derivatives that are used to reduce inflammation and associated diarrhoea in individuals with inflammatory bowel disease, such as ulcerative colitis. These include balsalazide (*Colazide*), mesalazine (*Pentasa, Mesasal, Salofalk* and others), olsalazine (*Dipentum*) and sulfasalazine (*Pyralin EN, Salazopyrin*).

There is also a drug approved strictly for use in preventing traveller's diarrhoea (Box 58.4).

BOX 58.3 Combination antidiarrhoeal products

Some popular antidiarrhoeal agents combine different compounds.

codeine, kaolin, aluminium hydroxide, pectin (*Bis-Pectin*)	Adult and paediatric (> 12 years): 15 mL hourly for three doses, then q 3 hours Paediatric (8–11 years): 11 mL q 4 hours
diphenoxylate with atropine (*Lofenoxal, Lomotil*)	Adult: 5 mg PO tds or qid initially, reducing when controlled

BOX 58.4 Treating traveller's diarrhoea

Recently, bovine colostrum (*Travelan*) has been approved for use in prevention of traveller's diarrhoea. The preparation contains high levels of antibodies against *E. coli* to prevent infections caused by the bacteria, a common cause of traveller's diarrhoea. Other available products work to manage diarrhoea from *E. coli* infection after it has occurred. One capsule is taken before each meal, and additional capsules can be taken if needed in between meals when there may be increased risk of infection.

TABLE 58.2 DRUGS IN FOCUS Antidiarrhoeals*

Drug name	Dosage/route	Usual indications
bovine colostrum (*Travelan*)	200 mg PO tds on empty stomach at least 1 hour before food or 2 hours after	Management of traveller's diarrhoea
(P) loperamide (*Imodium*)	Adult: 4 mg PO, then 2 mg PO after each loose stool	Short-term treatment of diarrhoea associated with dietary problems, viral infections

*For information on drugs used to treat irritable bowel syndrome, see *Box 58.5 Treating irritable bowel syndrome*. For dosage, routes and indications of drugs used for ulcerative colitis, see *Chapter 16. Anti-inflammatory, antiarthritis and related agents*.

Therapeutic actions and indications

Antidiarrhoeal agents slow the motility of the GI tract through direct action on the muscles of the GI tract to slow activity (loperamide) or through action on CNS centres that cause GI spasm and slowing (opium derivatives; see Figure 58.1). These drugs are indicated for the relief of symptoms of acute and chronic diarrhoea, reduction of volume of discharge from ileostomies and prevention and treatment of traveller's diarrhoea (Table 58.2; Box 58.4). Bovine colostrum (*Travelan*) has been found to be very helpful in treating traveller's diarrhoea (*see the Critical thinking scenario for additional information*).

Pharmacokinetics

Loperamide is slowly absorbed after oral administration, metabolised in the liver and excreted in urine and faeces. It may cross the placenta and enter breast milk. Codeine, a controlled substance, is readily absorbed after oral administration, metabolised in the liver and excreted in urine. It crosses the placenta and enters breast milk.

Salicylates are readily absorbed directly from the stomach, reaching peak levels within 5–30 minutes. They are metabolised in the liver to salicylic acid, an active metabolite and excreted in the urine, with a half-life of 15 minutes to 12 hours, depending on the salicylate. Salicylates cross the placenta and enter breast milk; they are not indicated for use during pregnancy or breastfeeding because of the potential adverse effects on the neonate and associated bleeding risks for the mother.

Contraindications and cautions

Antidiarrhoeal drugs should not be given to anyone with known allergy to the drug or any of its components *to prevent hypersensitivity reactions*. Caution should be used in pregnancy and breastfeeding *because of the potential adverse effects to the fetus or baby*. Care should also be taken in individuals with any history of GI obstruction, acute abdominal conditions, *which could be exacerbated by the effects of the drugs*, or diarrhoea due to poisonings, *which could be worsened by slowing of the GI tract, allowing increased time for absorption of the poison;* or with hepatic impairment, *which could alter the metabolism of the drugs*.

Renal function should be monitored before starting treatment and during treatment (more frequent monitoring may be required in renal impairment); cardiac hypersensitivity reactions have been reported; caution is required if there is a previous history of myocarditis or pericarditis, irrespective of cause.

Adverse effects

The adverse effects associated with antidiarrhoeal drugs, such as constipation, distension, abdominal discomfort, nausea, vomiting, dry mouth and even toxic megacolon, are related to their effects on the GI tract. Other adverse effects that have been reported include fatigue, weakness, dizziness and skin rash. Opium derivatives are also associated with lightheadedness, sedation, euphoria, hallucinations and respiratory depression related to effect on the opioid receptors.

Drug–drug interactions

Drug interactions vary depending on the antidiarrhoeal agent. Consult the drug package insert for specific interactions.

KEY POINTS

- Antidiarrhoeal drugs are used to soothe irritation to the intestinal wall; block GI muscle activity to decrease movement; or affect CNS activity to cause GI spasm and stop movement.
- Antidiarrhoeal drugs can cause GI discomfort and constipation.

IRRITABLE BOWEL SYNDROME DRUGS

Irritable bowel syndrome (IBS) is a very common disorder. It is experienced by three times as many women as men and reportedly accounts for a large number of all referrals to GI specialists. The disorder is

Prototype summary: loperamide

Indications: control and symptomatic relief of acute, non-specific diarrhoea and chronic diarrhoea associated with irritable bowel syndrome; reduction of volume of discharge from ileostomies.

Actions: inhibits intestinal peristalsis through direct effects on the longitudinal and circular muscles of the intestinal wall, slowing motility and movement of water and electrolytes.

Pharmacokinetics:

Route	Onset	Peak
Oral (capsule)	Varies	5 hours

$T_{1/2}$: 10.8 hours; metabolised in the liver and excreted in urine and faeces.

Adverse effects: abdominal pain, distension or discomfort; dry mouth; nausea; constipation; dizziness; tiredness; drowsiness.

characterised by abdominal distress, bouts of diarrhoea or constipation, bloating, nausea, flatulence, headache, fatigue, depression and anxiety. No anatomical cause has been found for this disorder. Underlying causes might be stress-related. People with this disorder have often suffered for years, not enjoying meals or activities because of their GI pain and discomfort. Mebeverine (*Colese*, *Colofac*) is the most common drug used to treat this condition. Other drugs are discussed in Box 58.5.

CHAPTER SUMMARY

- Laxatives are drugs used to stimulate movement along the GI tract and to aid bowel evacuation. They may be used to prevent or treat constipation.
- Laxatives can be chemical stimulants, which directly irritate the local nerve plexus; bulk stimulants, which increase the size of the food bolus and stimulate stretch receptors in the wall of the intestine; or

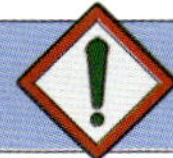

CRITICAL THINKING SCENARIO

Traveller's diarrhoea

THE SITUATION

P.F. received an all-expenses-paid trip to Thailand to celebrate his graduation from university. He was very excited about getting away for a week of sun and fun, and arranged to stay in the same hotel as two college friends who were also celebrating. The three men had a wonderful time visiting the beaches, bars and nightclubs in the area. On the third day of the trip, P.F. began experiencing nausea, some vomiting and a low-grade fever. Several hours later he began experiencing intense cramping and diarrhoea. For the next 2 days, P.F. felt so ill he was unable to leave his hotel room. The next morning, he arranged for an emergency trip home.

CRITICAL THINKING

What is probably happening to P.F.? *Think about the GI reflexes and explain the underlying cause for his signs and symptoms.*

What treatment should be started now?

What could have been done to prevent this problem from occurring?

What possible drug therapy might have been helpful for P.F.?

DISCUSSION

P.F. is probably experiencing the common disorder called traveller's diarrhoea. This disorder occurs when pathogens found in the food and water of a foreign environment are ingested. (Because these pathogens are commonly found in the environment, they do not normally cause problems for the people who live in the area.) When the pathogen, usually a strain of *Escherichia coli*, enters a host that is not accustomed to the bacteria, it releases enterotoxins and sets off an intestinal–intestinal reaction in the host.

The intestinal–intestinal reaction results in a reduction of activity above the point of irritation (which causes nausea and in some cases vomiting) and an increase in activity below the point of irritation. The body is trying to flush the invader from the body. A low-grade fever may occur as a reaction to the toxins released by the bacteria. Muscle aches and pains, malaise and fatigue are often common symptoms. It is important at this stage of the disease to maintain fluid intake to prevent dehydration from occurring.

P.F. may want to return home, but with intense cramping and diarrhoea it might not be a good idea. Bovine colostrum (*Travelan*) has been effective in preventing traveller's diarrhoea and associated problems. It is available OTC and is readily accessible for travellers. Taken during a course of traveller's diarrhoea, it may relieve the stomach upset and nausea, and some of the discomfort of the diarrhoea. It should not be used if the person has bloody diarrhoea or diarrhoea that worsens or persists for more than 48 hours.

The best course of action, however, is prevention. Several measures can be taken to avoid ingestion of the local bacteria: drinking only bottled or mineral water; avoiding fresh fruits and vegetables that may have been washed in the local water, unless they are peeled; avoiding ice cubes in drinks because the ice cubes are made from the local water; avoiding any food that might be undercooked or rare, including shellfish; and even being cautious about using water to brush teeth or gargle. People who have suffered a bout of traveller's diarrhoea are very cautious about exposure to local bacteria when they travel again, often combining prophylactic drug therapy with careful avoidance of local pathogens. P.F. can be reassured that in a few days the diarrhoea and associated signs and symptoms should pass and he will regain his strength and energy.

CARE GUIDE FOR P.F.: ANTIDIARRHOEALS

Assessment: history and examination

Assess the person's health history for allergies to any of these drugs, acute abdominal pain, concurrent use of aspirin products, methotrexate, sodium valproate, corticosteroids, oral tetracyclines, oral hypoglycaemic agents or sulfinpyrazone.

Focus the physical examination on the following:

Neurological: orientation, reflexes

GI: abdominal evaluation, bowel sounds

Respiratory: respiratory rate and depth

Laboratory tests: serum electrolyte levels

Genitourinary: renal function

Other: temperature

Implementation

Administer an antidiarrhoeal agent only as a temporary measure.

Provide comfort and safety measures, including assistance, access to bathroom and safety precautions if necessary.

Monitor bowel function.

Provide support and reassurance for coping with drug effects and discomfort.

Provide teaching regarding drug name and dosage, adverse effects and precautions, and warning signs of serious adverse effects to report.

Evaluation

Evaluate drug effects: relief of GI symptoms.

Monitor for adverse effects: GI alterations, dizziness, confusion, salicylate toxicity.

Monitor for drug–drug interactions as indicated.

Evaluate the effectiveness of teaching program and comfort and safety measures.

TEACHING FOR P.F.

- The drug you are taking is called bovine colostrum (*Travelan*). This drug is called an antidiarrhoeal agent. It forms a protective coating over the inner lining of the intestine and soothes the irritated areas.
- Take this drug exactly as indicated. Shake the bottle well before using the liquid preparation. If you are using tablets, make sure that you chew them thoroughly; do not swallow them whole.
- Common effects of this drug include:
  - *Darkening of the stools*: do not become concerned; this is a normal effect that will go away when you stop taking the drug.
  - Report any of the following conditions to your health care provider: *diarrhoea that does not stop within 2 days, ringing in the ears, rapid respirations, fever and/or intense abdominal pain.*
- Stay away from any food or beverage that may be contaminated with bacteria. Use bottled water for drinking, as well as for brushing your teeth. Do not wash fruit or vegetables with water from the local supply.
- Tell any doctor, nurse or other health care provider involved in your care that you are taking this drug.
- Keep this drug and all medications out of the reach of children.

Care considerations for people receiving antidiarrhoeals

Assessment: history and examination

- Assess for *possible contraindications or cautions*: any history of allergy to these drugs *to prevent hypersensitivity reactions*; acute abdominal conditions, *which could be exacerbated by these drugs*; poisoning, *which is a contraindication to slowing GI activity*; hepatic impairment, *which could alter the metabolism of the drug*; and current status of pregnancy or breastfeeding, *which require cautious use.*
- Perform a physical examination *to establish baseline data before beginning therapy and during therapy to determine the effectiveness of the drug and to evaluate for the occurrence of any adverse effects associated with drug therapy.*
- Inspect the skin for colour and evidence of lesions or rash *to monitor for potential hypersensitivity reactions.*
- Perform an abdominal examination, including inspecting for distension, palpating for masses and auscultating bowel sounds, *to evaluate GI function and to rule out potential underlying medical conditions.*

- Assess bowel elimination pattern, including frequency and characteristics of stool, *to assist in determining appropriateness for drug therapy.*
- Assess the person's neurological status, including level of orientation and affect, *to monitor for CNS effects of the drug.*

Implementation with rationale

- Administer the drug after each unformed stool *to ensure therapeutic effectiveness.* Keep track of the exact amount given *to ensure that the dose does not exceed the recommended daily maximum dose.*
- Monitor the response carefully; note the frequency and characteristics of the stool. If no response is seen within 48 hours, *the diarrhoea could be related to an underlying medical condition.* Arrange to discontinue the drug, and arrange for medical evaluation *to allow for the diagnosis of underlying medical conditions.*
- Provide appropriate safety and comfort measures if CNS effects occur *to prevent injury.*
- Offer support and encouragement *to help the person deal with the diagnosis and the drug regimen.*
- Provide thorough teaching, including the drug name and prescribed dosage; schedule for administration; use of drug after each loose stool; recommended daily maximum dose and the need not to exceed it; signs and symptoms of adverse effects, including measures to minimise or prevent them; safety measures, such as avoiding driving and obtaining assistance with ambulation as needed *to reduce the risk of injury due to weakness or dizziness*; danger signs and symptoms that need to be reported immediately; the importance of notifying health care provider if diarrhoea is not controlled within 48 hours; and the need for follow-up *to enhance knowledge about drug therapy and to promote compliance.*

Evaluation

- Monitor the response to the drug (relief of diarrhoea).
- Monitor for adverse effects (GI effects, CNS changes, dermatological effects).
- Monitor the effectiveness of comfort and safety measures and compliance with the regimen.
- Evaluate the effectiveness of the teaching plan (person can name the drug and dosage, as well as describe adverse effects to watch for, specific measures to use to avoid them and measures to take to increase the effectiveness of the drug).

BOX 58.5 Treating irritable bowel syndrome

Hyoscine

Hyoscine (*Buscopan*), an anticholinergic agent that was found to decrease GI spasm, was approved in 2001 as an adjunctive therapy for the treatment of IBS.

Support and symptomatic relief remain the mainstays of treating this disorder. Stress management and a consistent relationship with a health care provider may help to relieve some of the problems associated with this common, although not entirely understood, disorder.

Mebeverine

Mebeverine (*Colese*, *Colofac*) has become a key drug in managing IBS. It is an antispasmodic that relaxes vascular, cardiac and other smooth muscle, including that in the GI tract. It has some antimuscarinic activity, although much less than atropine. It needs to be used with caution in people with underlying cardiac, renal or liver impairment. Mebeverine is not recommended for use by women in the first trimester of pregnancy or during breastfeeding.

Peppermint oil

Peppermint oil (*Mintec*) is readily available over-the-counter and this preparation has been designed specifically for managing IBS. Peppermint oil acts as an antispasmodic, relaxing GI smooth muscle and reducing gas production that also contributes to discomfort.

lubricants, which facilitate movement of the bolus through the intestines.

- Using proper diet and exercise, as well as taking advantage of the actions of the intestinal reflexes, has eliminated the need for laxatives in many situations.
- Cathartic dependence can occur with the chronic use of laxatives, leading to a need for external stimuli for normal functioning of the GI tract.
- GI stimulants act to increase parasympathetic stimulation in the GI tract and to increase tone and general movement throughout the GI system.
- Antidiarrhoeal drugs are used to soothe irritation to the intestinal wall; block GI muscle activity to decrease movement; or affect CNS activity to cause GI spasm and stop movement.
- Drugs used to treat IBS are specific for the main underlying complaint, either diarrhoea or constipation, and a person's selection must be carefully matched to the effect of the drug.

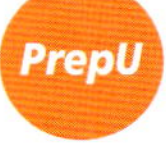

Knowing your strengths and weaknesses helps you to study more effectively. Take a PrepU Practice Quiz to find out how you measure up!

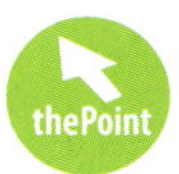

ONLINE RESOURCES

An extensive range of additional resources to enhance teaching and learning and to facilitate understanding of this chapter may be found online at the text's accompanying website, located on thePoint at http://thepoint.lww.com. These include Watch and Learn videos, Concepts in Action animations, journal articles, review questions, case studies, discussion topics and quizzes.

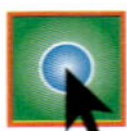

WEB LINKS

Health care providers and students may want to consult the following web resources:

www.gesa.org.au
The Gastroenterological Society of Australia. Information about a range of gastrointestinal conditions.

www.nlm.nih.gov/medlineplus/constipation.html
Information on constipation – causes, diagnosis, research, treatment and prevention across the lifespan.

www.racgp.org.au/afp/200504/200504kass.pdf
Information for health professionals about traveller's diarrhoea.

www.smartraveller.gov.au/tips/travelwell.html
Information for the traveller about maintaining good health.

BIBLIOGRAPHY

Bisanz, A. (2007). Chronic constipation. *American Journal of Nursing, 107(4)*, 72B–72H.

Farrell, M. & Dempsey, J. (2014). *Smeltzer & Bare's Textbook of Medical-Surgical Nursing* (3rd edn). Sydney: Lippincott Williams & Wilkins.

Gage, H., Goodman, C., Davies, S. L., Norton, C., Fader, M., Wells, M., Morris, J. & Williams, P. (2010). Laxative use in care homes. *Journal of Advanced Nursing, 66*, 1266–1272.

Goodman, L .S., Brunton, L. L., Chabner, B. & Knollmann, B. C. (2011). *Goodman and Gilman's Pharmacological Basis of Therapeutics* (12th edn). New York: McGraw-Hill.

McKenna, L. & Mirkov, S. (2019). *McKenna's Drug Handbook for Nursing and Midwifery* (8th edn). Sydney: Wolters Kluwer Health Australia.

Nazarko, L. (2007). Managing diarrhoea in the home to prevent admission. *British Journal of Community Nursing, 12(11)*, 508–512.

Paul, S. P., Dewdney, C. & Lam, C. (2012). Managing children with constipation in the community. *Nurse Prescribing, 10(6)*, 274–284.

Porth, C. M. (2011). *Essentials of Pathophysiology: Concepts of Altered Health States* (3rd edn). Philadelphia: Wolters Kluwer Health Australia.

Porth, C. M. (2009). *Pathophysiology: Concepts of Altered Health States* (8th edn). Philadelphia: Wolters Kluwer Health Australia.

Prynn, P. (2011). Managing adult constipation. *Practice Nurse, 41(17)*, 23–28.

Sarre, R. (2005). Bowel preparation. *Australian Prescriber, 28*, 16–17.

Selby, W. (2010). Managing constipation in adults. *Australian Prescriber, 33*, 116–119.

Shah, S. B. & Hanauer, S. B. (2007). Treatment of diarrhea in patients with inflammatory bowel disease: concepts and cautions. *Reviews in Gastroenterology Disorders, 7* (Suppl 3), S3–S10.

Tobias, N., Mason, D., Lutkenhoff, M., Stoops, M. & Ferguson, D. (2008). Management and principles of organic causes of childhood constipation. *Journal of Pediatric Health Care, 22(1)*, 12–23.

Wang, M., Szucs, T. D. & Steffen, R. (2008). Economic aspects of traveler's diarrhea. *Journal of Travel Medicine, 15(2)*, 110B.

CHECK YOUR UNDERSTANDING

Answers to the questions in this chapter can be found in Appendix A at the back of this book.

MULTIPLE CHOICE

Select the best response to the following.

1. Laxatives are drugs that are used to:
   a. increase the quantity of wastes excreted.
   b. speed the passage of the intestinal contents through the GI tract.
   c. increase digestion of intestinal contents.
   d. increase the water content of the intestinal contents.

2. The laxative of choice when mild stimulation is needed to prevent straining is:
   a. senna.
   b. castor oil.
   c. bisacodyl.
   d. magnesium sulphate.

3. Cathartic dependence can occur when:
   a. people do not use laxatives routinely and experience severe bouts of constipation.
   b. chronic laxative use leads to a reliance on the intense stimulation of laxatives.
   c. people maintain a nutritious high-fibre diet.
   d. people start an exercise program to promote bowel elimination.

4. Drugs that stimulate parasympathetic activity are used to increase GI activity and secretions. For which of the following would this group be most likely used?
   a. duodenal ulcers
   b. gastric ulcers
   c. gastro-oesophageal reflux disease
   d. poisoning, to induce nausea and vomiting

5. The drug of choice for treating traveller's diarrhoea is:
   a. loperamide.
   b. opium.
   c. bisacodyl.
   d. peppermint oil.

MULTIPLE RESPONSE

Select all that apply.

1. A nurse or midwife is preparing a teaching plan for a person who has been prescribed a laxative. The teaching plan should include which of the following?
   a. the importance of proper diet and fluid intake
   b. the need to take the drug for several weeks to get the full effect
   c. the importance of exercise
   d. the need to take advantage of natural reflexes by providing privacy and time to allow them to work
   e. the need to limit fluids
   f. the importance of limiting the duration of laxative use

2. A nurse or midwife might expect an order for liquid paraffin for which person?
   a. a debilitated person low on nutrients
   b. a person with haemorrhoids
   c. a person with recent rectal surgery
   d. a child with encopresis
   e. a postpartum woman
   f. a person with Crohn's disease

3. When explaining the actions of laxatives to a person, the nurse or midwife would state that they can work by:
   a. acting as chemical stimulants.
   b. acting as lubricants of the intestinal bolus.
   c. acting to increase bulk of the intestinal bolus and stimulate movement.
   d. stimulating CNS centres in the medulla to cause GI movement.
   e. blocking the parasympathetic nervous system.
   f. causing CNS depression.

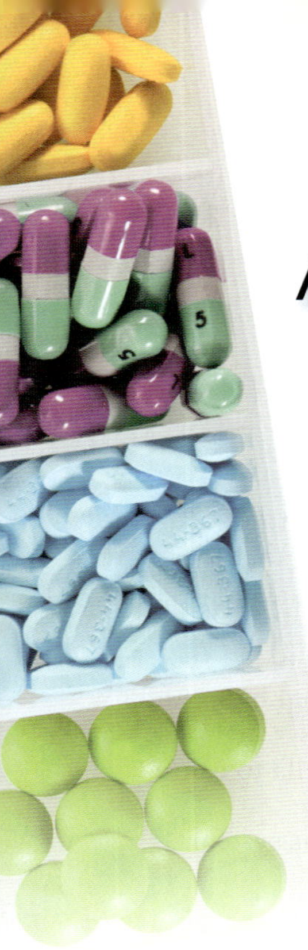

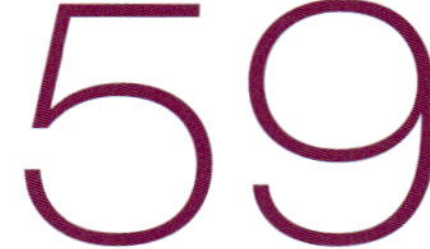

Antiemetic agents

Learning objectives

On completing this chapter you should be able to:

1. Outline how the vomiting reflex works, including factors that stimulate it and mechanisms for measures used to block it.
2. Describe the therapeutic actions, indications, pharmacokinetics, contraindications and cautions, most common adverse reactions and important drug–drug interactions associated with each of the classes of antiemetic agents.
3. Discuss the use of antiemetics across the lifespan.
4. Compare and contrast the prototype antiemetics prochlorperazine, metoclopramide, ondansetron and aprepitant with other agents in their class and with other classes of antiemetics.
5. Outline the care considerations, including important teaching points, for people receiving antiemetics.

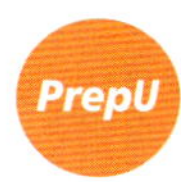

Test your current knowledge of antiemetic agents with a PrepU Practice Quiz!

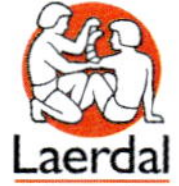

Simulation-based learning

On completion of the chapter, consider the scenario of Doris Bowman (Part 1) who arrives in the recovery room after undergoing major abdominal surgery and is complaining of nausea. Consider Doris' nausea management in this case. How might the concepts learnt in this chapter, apply more broadly to post-operative management of nausea?

Glossary of key terms

antiemetic: agent that blocks the hyperactive response of the chemoreceptor trigger zone (CTZ) to various stimuli, the response that produces non-beneficial nausea and vomiting

intractable hiccough: repetitive stimulation of the diaphragm that leads to hiccough, a diaphragmatic spasm that persists over time

phenothiazine: anti-anxiety drug that blocks the responsiveness of the CTZ to stimuli, leading to a decrease in nausea and vomiting

photosensitivity: hypersensitive reaction to the sun or ultraviolet light, seen as an adverse reaction to various drugs; can lead to severe skin rash and lesions, as well as damage to the eye

ANTIEMETIC AGENTS

Phenothiazines
- chlorpromazine
- (P) prochlorperazine
- promethazine

Non-phenothiazine
- domperidone
- (P) metoclopramide

5-HT$_3$-receptor blockers
- granisetron
- (P) ondansetron
- palonosetron
- tropisetron

Substance P / neurokinin 1–receptor antagonists
-  aprepitant
- fosaprepitant

One of the most common and most uncomfortable complaints encountered in clinical practice is that of nausea and vomiting. Vomiting is a complex reflex reaction to various stimuli (see Chapter 56). In some cases of overdose or poisoning, it may be desirable to induce vomiting to rapidly rid the body of a toxin. This can be accomplished by physical stimuli, often to the back of the throat. In some cases, gastric lavage is used to clear the contents of the stomach.

In many clinical conditions, the reflex reaction of vomiting is not beneficial in ridding the body of any toxins but is uncomfortable and even clinically hazardous to the person's condition. In such cases, an **antiemetic** is used to decrease or prevent nausea and vomiting. Antiemetic agents can be centrally acting or locally acting, and they have varying degrees of effectiveness. See Figure 59.1 for sites of action of antiemetics. Box 59.1 highlights important considerations related to use of antiemetics across the lifespan.

ANTIEMETIC AGENTS

Drugs used in managing nausea and vomiting are called antiemetics (Table 59.1). All of them work by reducing the hyperactivity of the vomiting reflex in one of two ways: locally, to decrease the local response to stimuli that are being sent to the medulla to induce vomiting, or centrally, to block the chemoreceptor trigger zone (CTZ) or suppress the vomiting centre directly. The locally acting antiemetics may be antacids, local anaesthetics, adsorbents, protective drugs that coat the GI mucosa, or drugs that prevent distension and stretch stimulation of the GI tract. These agents are often reserved for use in mild nausea. Many of these drugs are discussed in Chapter 57.

Centrally acting antiemetics can be classified into several groups: phenothiazines, non-phenothiazines, anticholinergics/antihistamines, serotonin (5-hydroxytryptamine [$5\text{-}HT_3$])-receptor blockers and substance P / neurokinin 1–receptor antagonists.

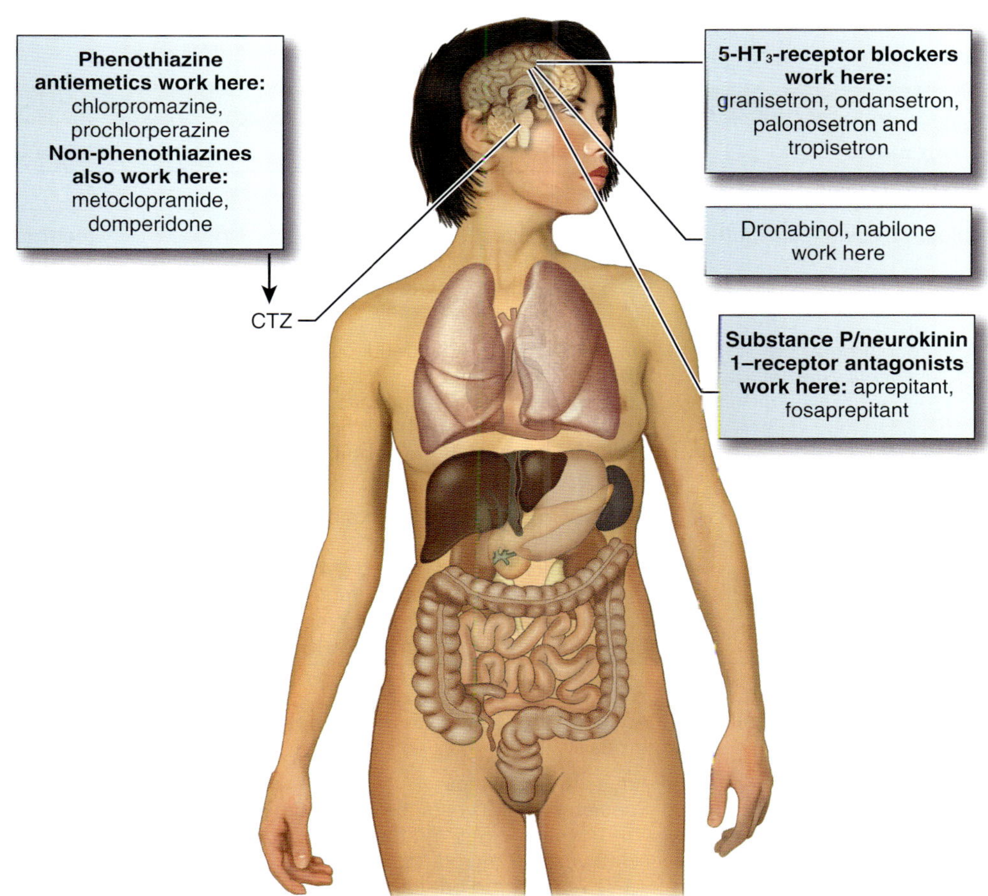

FIGURE 59.1 Sites of action of emetics/antiemetics, CTZ, chemoreceptor trigger zone.

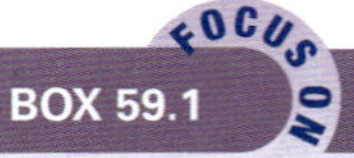

BOX 59.1 Drug therapy across the lifespan

Antiemetic agents

CHILDREN

Parents should be taught to call their health care provider or a local poison control centre if their child ingests potentially toxic substances. The health professional will advise them of the best treatment in each individual case.

Antiemetics should be used with caution in children who are at higher risk for adverse effects, including central nervous system (CNS) effects, as well as fluid and electrolyte disturbances.

Prochlorperazine is often a drug of choice with children, and it has established oral, rectal and parenteral doses. Promethazine often has fewer adverse effects, but it should not be used with children who have liver impairment, Reye syndrome or sleep apnoea. The serotonin 5-HT_3 agents have been used very successfully in children younger than 2 years of age. Care should be used when determining dose and timing of dose.

ADULTS

Antiemetics are often used after surgery or chemotherapy, and precautions should be used to ensure that CNS effects do not interfere with mobility or other activities.

PREGNANCY AND BREASTFEEDING

The safety of these drugs during pregnancy and breastfeeding has not been established. Use should be reserved for those situations in which the benefit to the mother outweighs the potential risk to the fetus. The drugs may enter breast milk and also may cause fluid imbalance that could interfere with milk production. It is advised that caution be used if one of these drugs is prescribed during breastfeeding.

OLDER ADULTS

Older adults are more likely to develop adverse effects associated with the use of these drugs, including sedation, confusion, dizziness, fluid imbalance and cardiovascular effects. Safety measures may be needed if these effects occur and interfere with the person's mobility and balance.

Older adults are also more likely to have renal and/or hepatic impairment related to underlying medical conditions, which could interfere with the metabolism and excretion of these drugs. The dose for older adults should be started at a lower level than that recommended for young adults. The person should be monitored very closely, and dose adjustment should be made based on the individual's response.

TABLE 59.1 DRUGS IN FOCUS Antiemetic agents

Drug name	Dosage/route	Usual indications
Phenothiazines		
chlorpromazine (*Largactil*)	Adult: 10–25 mg PO q 4–6 hours Paediatric: 0.5 mg/kg PO q 4–6 hours or 0.5 mg/kg IM q 6–8 hours	Treatment of nausea and vomiting, including that specifically associated with anaesthesia; severe vomiting; intractable hiccoughs
(P) prochlorperazine (*Nausetil, Stemetil*)	Oral, adult: 5–10 mg bid–tid; paediatric 0.25 mg/kg bid–tid Suppository, adult: 1 suppository (25 mg); may use oral preparation after 6 hours Injection, adult: 12.5 mg deep IM; may use oral preparation after 6 hours	Treatment of severe nausea and vomiting, including that specifically associated with anaesthesia
promethazine (*Avomine, Phenergan*)	Adult: 25 mg q 4–6 hours to a maximum daily dose of 100 mg Paediatric 6–12 years: 10 mg q 4–6 hours to a maximum daily dose of 25 mg Paediatric 2–5 years: 5 mg PO repeated q 4–6 hours to a maximum of 15 mg/day	Prevention and control of nausea and vomiting associated with anaesthesia and surgery
Non-phenothiazine		
domperidone (*Motilium*)	Adult: 10 mg PO tds 15–30 minutes before meals	Treatment of nausea and vomiting before meals
(P) metoclopramide (*Maxolon*)	Adult: 10 mg PO tds Paediatric 15–19 years: 5–10 mg tds; 5–14 years: 2.5–5 mg tds; 3–5 years: 2 mg bd–tds; 1–3 years: 1 mg bd–tds	Treatment of nausea and vomiting, especially related to chemical stimulation of the CTZ in adults

TABLE 59.1 **DRUGS IN FOCUS** **Antiemetic agents *(continued)***

Drug name	Dosage/route	Usual indications
5-HT$_3$-receptor blockers		
granisetron (*Kytril*)	Oral: 2 mg once a day; first dose < 1 hour before chemotherapy IV, adult, prophylaxis: 3 mg IV over 5 minutes within half an hour before chemotherapy; established nausea and vomiting: 1 mg IV; may repeat at ≥ 10 minute intervals; maximum 9 mg/day	Treatment of nausea and vomiting associated with emetogenic chemotherapy
Ⓟ ondansetron (*Zofran*)	Adult: 8 mg PO 1–2 hours before chemotherapy, followed by 8 mg orally 12 hours later, then 8 mg bd up to 5 days Paediatric 4–12 years: 4 mg PO twice daily; emetogenic chemotherapy dose: 5 mg/m^2 IV over 15 minutes immediately before chemotherapy, followed by oral therapy at doses of 4 mg bd for up to 5 days	Treatment of severe nausea and vomiting associat ed with emetogenic chemotherapy, radiation therapy, postoperative situations
palonosetron (*Aloxi*)	0.25 mg IV as a single dose over 30 seconds given 30 minutes before the start of chemotherapy	Treatment of acute and delayed vomiting associated with highly emetogenic chemotherapy
tropisetron (generic)	Postoperative nausea: 2 mg slowly IV Chemotherapy nausea: 5 mg/day for 6 days	Treatment of severe nausea and vomiting associated with emetogenic chemotherapy, radiation therapy, postoperative situations
Substance P / neurokinin 1–receptor antagonists		
Ⓟ aprepitant (*Emend*)	Postoperative nausea: 40 mg PO 3 hours before anaesthesia Chemotherapy nausea: dose complex, see manufacturer's instructions; taken PO 1 hour before chemotherapy with dexamethasone and a 5-HT$_3$ antagonist	Prevention of acute and delayed nausea and vomiting associated with highly emetogenic cancer chemotherapy
fosaprepitant (*Emend IV*)	150 mg IV infusion on day 1, 30 minutes before chemotherapy with dexamethasone and a 5HT$_3$ antagonist	Prevention of acute and delayed nausea and vomiting associated with highly emetogenic cancer chemotherapy

PHENOTHIAZINES

The two **phenothiazines** most commonly used as antiemetics are prochlorperazine (*Stemetil*) and promethazine (*Phenergan*), both of which have rapid onset and limited adverse effects. Other drugs in this group include chlorpromazine (*Largactil*). Chapter 22 discusses the phenothiazines in greater detail. (*See the Critical thinking scenario for additional information about caring for a person taking prochlorperazine.*)

Therapeutic actions and indications

Phenothiazines are centrally acting antiemetics that change the responsiveness or stimulation of the CTZ in the medulla (Figure 59.1). The phenothiazines are recommended for the treatment of nausea and vomiting, including that specifically associated with anaesthesia; severe vomiting; and **intractable hiccoughs**, which occur with repetitive stimulation of the diaphragm and lead to persistent diaphragm spasm. See Table 59.1 for usual indications for each of these agents.

Pharmacokinetics

These drugs are available as tablets or as syrup for oral administration, as rectal suppositories and as solution for intramuscular (IM) or intravenous (IV) use. Route of choice is determined by the condition of the person. These agents have a rapid onset of action of 5–20 minutes and duration of action of 3–12 hours, depending on route of administration. They are metabolised in the liver and excreted in the urine. They are known to cross the placenta and enter breast milk.

Contraindications and cautions

In general, antiemetics should not be used in people with coma or severe CNS depression or in those who have experienced brain damage or injury *because of the risk of further CNS depression*. Other contraindications include severe hypotension or hypertension and severe liver dysfunction, *which might interfere with the metabolism of the drug.* Caution should be used in individuals with renal dysfunction, moderate liver impairment, active peptic ulcer or during pregnancy and breastfeeding *because of the potential for adverse effects on the fetus or baby.* See Chapter 22 for details about the phenothiazines.

Adverse effects

Adverse effects associated with antiemetics are linked to their interference with normal CNS stimulation or response. Drowsiness, dizziness, weakness, tremor and headache are common adverse effects. Other, not uncommon adverse effects include hypotension, hypertension and cardiac arrhythmias. Autonomic effects such as dry mouth, nasal congestion, anorexia, pallor, sweating and urinary retention often occur with phenothiazines. Endocrine effects such as menstrual disorders, galactorrhoea and gynaecomastia have been reported with phenothiazine use. **Photosensitivity** (increased sensitivity to the sun and ultraviolet light) is a common adverse reaction with these antiemetics. People should be advised to use sunscreens and protective garments if exposure cannot be avoided. There is a risk of serious tissue injuries and amputation from the inadvertent arterial injection

CRITICAL THINKING SCENARIO

Handling postoperative nausea and vomiting

THE SITUATION

A.J. is a 16-year-old boy who has undergone reconstructive knee surgery after a football injury. After the surgery, A.J. complains of nausea and vomits three times in 2 hours. A.J. becomes increasingly agitated. Intravenous prochlorperazine (*Stemetil*) is ordered to relieve the nausea, to be followed by an oral dose when tolerated. The prochlorperazine is somewhat helpful in relieving the nausea.

CRITICAL THINKING

What are the important nursing implications in this case? What other measures could be taken to relieve A.J.'s nausea?

DISCUSSION

It is often impossible to pinpoint an exact cause of a person's nausea and vomiting in a hospital setting. For example, the underlying cause may be related to the pain, a reaction to the pain medication being given, or a response to what A.J. described as the 'awful hospital smell'. A combination of factors should be considered when dealing with nausea and vomiting. A.J., as a teenager, may become increasingly agitated by the discomfort and possible embarrassment of vomiting. The administration of prochlorperazine may 'take the edge off' the nausea. A.J. will have to be reminded that the drug he is being given may make him dizzy, weak or drowsy and that he should ask for assistance if he needs to move.

Once the nausea and vomiting diminish somewhat, it will be possible to try other interventions to help stop the vomiting reflex. One such intervention is removing the offending odour that A.J. described, if possible, because doing so may relieve a chemical stimulus to the CTZ. Administration of pain medication, as prescribed, may relieve the CTZ stimulus that comes with intense pain. Other interventions include providing a serene, quiet environment and encouraging A.J. to take slow, deep breaths, which stimulate the parasympathetic system (vagus nerve) and partially override the sympathetic activity stimulated by the CTZ to activate vomiting. For many people, mouth care, ice chips or small sips of water may also help to relieve the discomfort and ease the sensation of nausea.

CARE GUIDE FOR A.J.: ANTIEMETICS

Assessment: history and examination

Assess A.J.'s health history for allergies to any antiemetic, coma, CNS depression, severe hypotension, liver dysfunction, bone marrow depression, epilepsy and concurrent use of alcohol, anticholinergic drugs and barbiturate anaesthetics. Determine the type and amount of anaesthesia used.

Focus the physical examination on the following areas:

Neurological: orientation, affect

Skin: colour, lesions

Cardiovascular: pulse, blood pressure, orthostatic blood pressure

Gastrointestinal: abdominal and liver evaluation

Laboratory tests: haematological, full blood count, liver function tests

Implementation

Administer antiemetics only as a temporary measure.

Provide comfort and safety measures, including assistance with mobility, access to bathroom, safety precautions, mouth care and ice chips.

Monitor A.J. for dehydration and provide remedial measures as needed.

Provide support and reassurance for coping with drug effects and discomfort.

Provide teaching regarding drug name, dosage, adverse effects, precautions and warnings to report.

Evaluation

Evaluate drug effects, for example, relief of nausea and vomiting.

Monitor for adverse effects, including GI alterations, orthostatic hypotension, dizziness, confusion, sensitivity to sunlight and dehydration.

Monitor for drug–drug interactions as appropriate.

Evaluate the effectiveness of the teaching program and comfort and safety measures.

TEACHING FOR A.J.

- The drug that has been prescribed for you is called prochlorperazine. It belongs to a class of drugs called antiemetics. An antiemetic helps to prevent nausea and vomiting and the discomfort they cause.
- Common effects of this drug include:
  - *Dizziness, weakness*: change positions slowly. If you feel drowsy, avoid driving or dangerous activities for at least 24 hours after the last dose of this drug (such as the use of heavy machinery or tasks requiring coordination).
  - *Sensitivity to the sun*: avoid exposure to the sun and ultraviolet light because serious reactions may occur. If exposure cannot be prevented, use sunscreen and protective clothing to cover the skin.
  - *Dehydration*: avoid excessive heat exposure, and try to drink fluids as much as possible, because you will have an increased risk of heat stroke.
- Report any of the following conditions to your health care provider: *fever, rash, yellowing of the eyes or skin, dark urine, pale stools, easy bruising, rash and vision changes.*
- Avoid over-the-counter (OTC) medications. If you feel that you need one, check with your health care provider first.
- Tell any doctor, nurse or other health care provider that you are taking this drug.
- Keep this drug and all medications out of the reach of children.

or IV extravasation of injectable promethazine. Use of injectable promethazine is not recommended.

Clinically important drug–drug interactions

Additive CNS depression can be seen with any of the antiemetics if they are combined with other CNS depressants, including alcohol. People should be advised to avoid this combination and any OTC preparation unless they check with their health care provider. Other drug–drug interactions are specific to each drug (refer to a nursing or midwifery drug guide).

Prototype summary: prochlorperazine

Indications: control of severe nausea and vomiting.

Actions: mechanism of action not understood; depresses various areas of the CNS, including the CTZ in the medulla.

Pharmacokinetics:

Route	Onset	Peak	Duration
Oral	30–40 min	Unknown	3–4 hours
Rectal	60–90 min	Unknown	3–4 hours
IM	10–20 min	10–30 min	3–4 hours
IV	Immediate	10–30 min	3–4 hours

$T_{1/2}$: unknown; metabolised in the liver and excreted in urine.

Adverse effects: drowsiness, dystonia, photophobia, blurred vision.

OTHER DOPAMINE D_2 RECEPTOR ANTAGONISTS

Two other non-phenothiazine dopamine D_2 receptor antagonists currently available for use as antiemetics are metoclopramide (*Maxolon*) and domperidone (*Motilium*). These act to reduce the responsiveness of the nerve cells in the CTZ to circulating chemicals that induce vomiting. Chapter 58 discusses metoclopramide, which is also commonly used to treat gastroparesis, in greater detail.

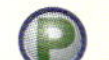 **Prototype summary: metoclopramide**

Indications: prevention of nausea and vomiting associated with emetogenic cancer chemotherapy; prevention of postoperative nausea and vomiting.

Actions: slows GI activity; sedating.

Pharmacokinetics:

Route	Onset	Peak	Duration
Oral	30–60 min	60–90 min	1–2 hours
IM	10–15 min	60–90 min	1–2 hours
IV	1–3 min	60–90 min	1–2 hours

$T_{1/2}$: 5–6 hours; metabolised in the liver and excreted in urine.

Adverse effects: drowsiness, fatigue, restlessness, extrapyramidal symptoms, diarrhoea.

5-HT_3-RECEPTOR BLOCKERS

The 5-HT_3-receptor blockers block those receptors associated with nausea and vomiting in the CTZ and locally. These drugs include granisetron (*Kytril*), ondansetron (*Zofran*), palonosetron (*Aloxi*) and tropisetron (generic).

Therapeutic actions and indications

The 5-HT_3-receptor blockers have proven especially helpful in treating the nausea and vomiting associated with antineoplastic chemotherapy, radiation therapy, and postoperative nausea and vomiting. They are specific for the treatment of nausea and vomiting associated with emetogenic chemotherapy.

Pharmacokinetics

The 5-HT_3-receptor blockers are rapidly absorbed, reaching peak levels within 1 hour. They are metabolised in the liver and excreted in urine. Ondansetron, granisetron and tropisetron are available in oral and IV forms; palonosetron is only available in an IV form.

Contraindications and cautions

These drugs are contraindicated with known allergy to any component of the drug *to prevent hypersensitivity reactions*. Caution should be used during pregnancy and breastfeeding *because of the potential for adverse effects on the fetus or nursing baby*.

Adverse effects

The adverse effects most frequently seen with these drugs are headache, dizziness and myalgia related to their CNS effects. Ondansetron can cause QT interval prolongation and dangerous *torsades de pointes*. Pain at the injection site, rash, constipation, hypotension and urinary retention have also been reported.

 **Prototype summary: ondansetron**

Indications: control of severe nausea and vomiting associated with emetogenic cancer chemotherapy, radiation therapy; treatment of postoperative nausea and vomiting.

Actions: blocks specific receptor sites associated with nausea and vomiting, peripherally and in the CTZ.

Pharmacokinetics:

Route	Onset	Peak	Duration
Oral	30–60 min	60–90 min	1.7–2.2 hours
IV	Immediate	60–90 min	Duration of infusion

$T_{1/2}$: 3.5–6 hours; metabolised in the liver and excreted in urine.

Adverse effects: headache, dizziness, drowsiness, myalgia, urinary retention, constipation, pain at injection site.

SUBSTANCE P / NEUROKININ 1–RECEPTOR ANTAGONISTS

Two drugs in the newest class of drugs for treating nausea and vomiting are the substance P / neurokinin 1–receptor antagonists aprepitant (*Emend*) and fosaprepitant (*Emend IV*). Aprepitant is available in oral form while fosaprepitant is given IV.

Therapeutic actions and indications

These drugs act directly in the CNS to block receptors associated with nausea and vomiting, with little to no effect on serotonin, dopamine or corticosteroid receptors. They are approved for use in treating the nausea and vomiting associated with highly emetogenic antineoplastic chemotherapy, including cisplatin therapy. They are given orally, in combination with dexamethasone.

Pharmacokinetics

They are metabolised in the liver and excreted in urine and faeces, and are known to cross the placenta and to enter breast milk.

Contraindications and cautions

Aprepitant and fosaprepitant should not be used during pregnancy and breastfeeding *because of the potential for adverse effects on the fetus or breastfeeding infant* or with known allergy to any component of the drug *to prevent hypersensitivity reactions*.

Adverse effects

The adverse effects associated with aprepitant and fosaprepitant include GI effects of diarrhoea, constipation, gastritis, nausea; anorexia; headache; and fatigue.

Clinically important drug–drug interactions

There is a risk of serious increase in serum levels of pimozide if these drugs are used together. There is a decrease in effectiveness of warfarin if it is combined with aprepitant or fosaprepitant, and the person must be monitored very closely and adjustments made in the warfarin dose if this combination must be used. There is a decrease in the effectiveness of hormonal contraceptives if they are taken concurrently with these drugs; use of a barrier contraceptive should be suggested.

Prototype summary: aprepitant

Indications: in combination with other agents for the prevention of acute and delayed nausea and vomiting associated with severely emetogenic cancer chemotherapy.

Actions: selectively blocks human substance P / neurokinin 1 (NK1) receptors in the CNS, blocking the nausea and vomiting caused by highly emetogenic chemotherapeutic agents.

Pharmacokinetics:

Route	Onset	Peak
Oral	Rapid	4 hours

$T_{1/2}$: 9–13 hours; metabolised in the liver and excreted in urine and faeces.

Adverse effects: anorexia, fatigue, constipation, diarrhoea, elevated liver enzyme levels, dehydration.

Care considerations for people receiving an antiemetic agent

Assessment: history and examination

- Assess for *possible contraindications or cautions*: history of allergy to antiemetic *to avoid potential hypersensitivity reactions*; impaired renal or hepatic function, *which could interfere with the metabolism or excretion of the drug*; coma or semiconscious state, CNS depression or CNS injury, *which could be exacerbated by the CNS-depressing effects of the drug*; hypotension or hypertension, *which could be affected by the CNS effects of the drug*; active peptic ulcer, *which could be exacerbated by the GI effects of the drug*; and current status of pregnancy and breastfeeding *because of the potential for adverse effects on the fetus or breastfeeding infant.*
- Perform a physical examination *to establish baseline data before beginning therapy and during therapy to determine the effectiveness of the drug and evaluate for the occurrence of any adverse effects associated with drug therapy.*
- Assess the person's neurological status, including level of orientation, affect and reflexes, *to monitor for CNS effects and to rule out underlying CNS problems that could be a contraindication.*
- Assess cardiopulmonary status, including baseline pulse and blood pressure, *to evaluate effects on the cardiovascular system.*
- Inspect the skin for colour and evidence of lesion or rash *to evaluate for photosensitivity and adverse effects of the drug.*
- Examine the abdomen, including the liver, and auscultate bowel sounds *to evaluate GI function and motility, rule out underlying medical problems and identify possible adverse drug effects.*
- Assess complaints of nausea and evaluate emesis; note colour, amount and frequency of vomiting episodes *to determine the need for therapy.*
- Monitor laboratory test results, including liver and renal function tests, *to monitor for potential problems with metabolism or excretion.*

Implementation with rationale

- Assure that route of administration is appropriate for each person *to ensure therapeutic effects and decrease adverse effects*: if used to prevent motion sickness, should be given 30 minutes before activity that involves motion; some oral tablets can be placed in the mouth and allowed to dissolve slowly; rectal suppositories should be inserted high into the rectum; IV infusions should be run slowly, monitoring the person for CNS depression.
- Assess the person carefully for any potential drug–drug interactions if giving antiemetics in combination with other drugs *to avert potentially serious drug–drug interactions.*
- Provide comfort and safety measures, including mouth care, ready access to bathroom facilities, assistance with ambulation and periodic orientation, ice chips to suck, protection from sun exposure and remedial measures to treat dehydration if it occurs, *to protect the person from injury and to increase comfort.*
- Provide support and encouragement, as well as other measures (quiet environment, carbonated drinks, deep breathing), *to help the person cope with the discomfort of nausea and vomiting and drug effects.*
- Provide thorough teaching, including the drug name and prescribed dosage; the schedule and method for administration; the need to avoid alcohol and other CNS depressants (if the person is not hospitalised); signs and symptoms of adverse effects and measures to minimise or prevent them; the use of sunscreen and protective clothing when outside; comfort measures to reduce feelings of nausea, such as adequate ventilation, deep breathing and a quiet environment; the importance of fluid intake and signs and symptoms of dehydration that should be reported to the health care provider; safety measures, such as assistance with ambulation and gradual position changes; the need to notify the health care provider before using any OTC medications; and the importance

of periodic monitoring and evaluation *to enhance knowledge about drug therapy and to promote compliance.*

Evaluation

- Monitor the response to the drug (relief of nausea and vomiting).
- Monitor for adverse effects (dizziness, confusion, GI alterations, cardiac arrhythmias, hypotension, gynaecomastia, pink- to red–brown-tinged urine, photosensitivity).
- Monitor the effectiveness of comfort measures and compliance with the regimen.
- Evaluate the effectiveness of the teaching plan (person can name the drug and dosage, as well as describe adverse effects to watch for and specific measures to avoid them).

KEY POINTS

- Antiemetics are used to manage nausea and vomiting in situations in which these actions are not beneficial and could cause harm to the person.
- Antiemetics act by depressing the hyperactive vomiting reflex, either locally or through alteration of CNS actions.
- The choice of an antiemetic depends on the cause of the nausea and vomiting, and the expected actions of the drug.
- Antiemetics include the phenothiazines and centrally acting non-phenothiazine metoclopramide; anticholinergic/antihistamines; the 5-HT_3-receptor blockers; and the newest class of antiemetic, the substance P / neurokinin 1–receptor antagonists.

CHAPTER SUMMARY

- Phenothiazines and the non-phenothiazine metoclopramide are used as antiemetics to depress the CNS, including the CTZ. People must be monitored for CNS depression. Photosensitivity is a common adverse effect of these drugs.
- Anticholinergic/antihistamine drugs are used to block the transmission of impulses within the CNS. They may be particularly effective in treating motion sickness. People receiving these drugs must be monitored for parasympathetic blocking effects, drowsiness and sedation.
- The 5-HT_3 blockers are antiemetics that directly block specific receptors in the CTZ to prevent nausea and vomiting. They are used in cases of nausea and vomiting associated with antineoplastic chemotherapy and radiation therapy as well as postoperative nausea and vomiting.
- Most antiemetics cause some CNS depression, with resultant dizziness, drowsiness and weakness. Care must be taken to protect the person and advise them to avoid dangerous situations.
- Photosensitivity is another common adverse effect with antiemetics. People should be protected from exposure to the sun and ultraviolet light. Sunscreens and protective clothing are essential if exposure cannot be prevented.

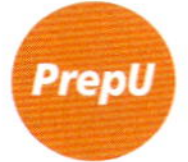

Knowing your strengths and weaknesses helps you to study more effectively. Take a PrepU Practice Quiz to find out how you measure up!

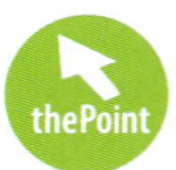

ONLINE RESOURCES

An extensive range of additional resources to enhance teaching and learning and to facilitate understanding of this chapter may be found online at the text's accompanying website, located on thePoint at http://thepoint.lww.com. These include Watch and Learn videos, Concepts in Action animations, journal articles, review questions, case studies, discussion topics and quizzes.

BIBLIOGRAPHY

Barrett, K. E. & Ganong, W. F. (2010). *Ganong's Review of Medical Physiology* (23rd edn). New York: McGraw-Hill.

Forbes, D. & Fairbrother, S. (2008). Cyclic nausea and vomiting in childhood. *Australian Family Physician, 27(1–2)*, 33–36.

Goel, R. & Wilkinson, M. (2013). Recommended assessment and treatment of nausea and vomiting. *Prescriber, 24(3)*, 23–27.

Goodman, L. S., Brunton, L. L., Chabner, B. & Knollmann, B. C. (2011). *Goodman and Gilman's Pharmacological Basis of Therapeutics* (12th edn). New York: McGraw-Hill.

Graudins, L. V. (2009). Preventing motion sickness in children. *Australian Prescriber, 32*, 61–63.

Gutierrez-Williams, G. & Goldman, M. (2008). Cost effective management of postoperative vomiting. *Connecticut Medicine, 72(1)*, 21–24.

Kelly, B. & Ward, K. (2013). Nausea and vomiting in palliative care. *Nursing Times, 109(39)*, 16–19.

Kerr, C. L. (2008). What goes in must come out. *Journal of Paediatric Health Care, 22(1)*, 44–48.

Kovac, A. (2013). Update on the management of postoperative nausea and vomiting. *Drugs, 73(14)*, 1525–1547.

McKenna, L. & Mirkov, S. (2019). *McKenna's Drug Handbook for Nursing and Midwifery* (8th edn). Sydney: Wolters Kluwer Health Australia.

Middleton, J. & Lennan, E. (2011). Managing chemotherapy-induced nausea and vomiting. *British Journal of Nursing, 22*(supp), S7–S15.

Porth, C. M. (2011). *Essentials of Pathophysiology: Concepts of Altered Health States* (3rd edn). Philadelphia: Lippincott Williams & Wilkins.

Porth, C. M. (2009). *Pathophysiology: Concepts of Altered Health States* (8th edn). Philadelphia: Lippincott Williams & Wilkins.

Raymond, S. H. (2013). A survey of prescribing for the management of nausea and vomiting in pregnancy in Australia. *Australian and New Zealand Journal of Obstetrics and Gynaecology, 53*, 358–362.

CHECK YOUR UNDERSTANDING

Answers to the questions in this chapter can be found in Appendix A at the back of this book.

MULTIPLE CHOICE

Select the best answer to the following.

1. The health care professional anticipates that prochlorperazine (*Stemetil*) would be the antiemetic of choice for which of the following?
   a. nausea and vomiting after anaesthesia
   b. nausea and vomiting due to cancer chemotherapy
   c. motion sickness
   d. intractable hiccoughs
2. Most antiemetics work with the CNS to decrease the activity of:
   a. the medulla.
   b. the CTZ.
   c. the respiratory centre.
   d. the sympathetic nervous system.
3. Which of the following instructions would be most appropriate to give to a person to reduce the risk of photosensitivity related to the use of antiemetic agents?
   a. Avoid having their picture taken.
   b. Cover the head at extremes of temperature.
   c. Take extra precautions to avoid heat stroke.
   d. Wear protective clothing when in the sun.
4. The 5-HT_3-receptor blockers, including ondansetron (*Zofran*) and granisetron (*Kytril*), are particularly effective in decreasing the nausea and vomiting associated with:
   a. vestibular problems.
   b. cancer chemotherapy.
   c. pregnancy.
   d. severe pain.
5. A parent calls with concerns that a 2-year-old child ate a full bottle of baby aspirin. The health care professional would advise the parent to:
   a. administer ipecac immediately.
   b. induce vomiting by inserting a finger against the back of the child's throat.
   c. force fluids as the parent brings the child in for evaluation.
   d. feed the child charcoal.

MULTIPLE RESPONSE

Select all that apply.

1. Care interventions for the person receiving an antiemetic drug would include which of the following?
   a. frequent mouth care
   b. bowel program to deal with constipation
   c. protection from falls or injury
   d. fluids to guard against dehydration
   e. protection from sun exposure
   f. quiet environment and temperature control
2. Palonosetron (*Aloxi*) would be a drug of choice for a person with which of the following problems?
   a. nausea and vomiting associated with cancer chemotherapy
   b. a prolonged QT interval
   c. delayed nausea and vomiting associated with antineoplastic chemotherapy
   d. difficulty swallowing
   e. hypokalaemia
   f. hypomagnesaemia

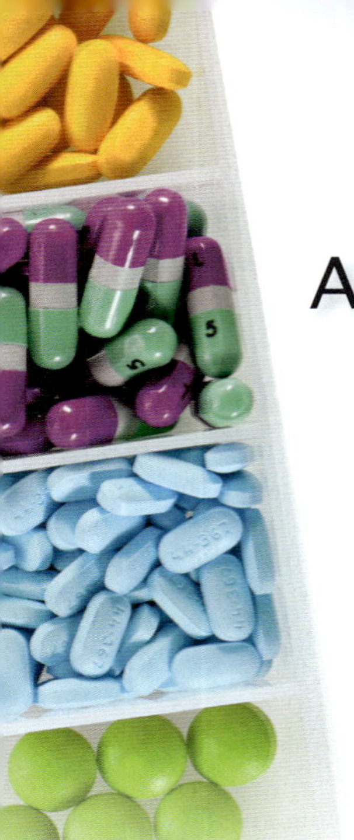

Appendix A

Answers to questions

Chapter 1

Multiple choice

1. b
2. d
3. a
4. c
5. a
6. b
7. c

Multiple response

1. c, d, e, f
2. a, c, d, f

Chapter 2

Multiple choice

1. c
2. b
3. d
4. b
5. c
6. a
7. b

Multiple response

1. c, d, e
2. a, d, e, f
3. b, e, f

Chapter 3

Multiple choice

1. c
2. d
3. b
4. d
5. b
6. c

Multiple response

1. a, b, f
2. a, b, c, d, e, f
3. a, b, e, f
4. b, c, d, e

Chapter 4

Multiple choice

1. c
2. a
3. c
4. a
5. d
6. c
7. a

Multiple response

1. a, b, c
2. b, c, d
3. a, b, d, e, f

Chapter 5

Multiple choice

1. b
2. d
3. b
4. b
5. d
6. b

Complete the problems

1. a. 0.1 g; b. 1.5 kg; c. 100 mL; d. 0.5 L
2. a. 1 tsp; b. 2 tbsp.
3. 11.25 mL
4. 0.65 mL
5. 0.58 (0.6) mL
6. 1.6 mL
7. 1.9 mL

Chapter 6

Multiple choice

1. b
2. a
3. c
4. b
5. c

Multiple response

1. c, e, f
2. b, d, e

Chapter 7

Multiple choice

1. d
2. a
3. b
4. c
5. b
6. c
7. b

Multiple response

1. b, e, f
2. b, d, e
3. a, d, f

Chapter 8

Multiple choice

1. c
2. c
3. a
4. c
5. b
6. c
7. b

Multiple response

1. a, b, c
2. a, c, d

Chapter 9

Multiple choice

1. d
2. c
3. b
4. a
5. c
6. c
7. b
8. c
9. c
10. b

Multiple response

1. b, d, f
2. a, b, c, f

Chapter 10

Multiple choice

1. c
2. b
3. c
4. d
5. c
6. b
7. a
8. b

Multiple response

1. a, d, e, f

Chapter 11

Multiple choice

1. b
2. c
3. d
4. c
5. b
6. c
7. b
8. c

Multiple response

1. a, d, f
2. a, c, f

Chapter 12

Multiple choice

1. d
2. b
3. d
4. b
5. c
6. d
7. c
8. a
9. c

Multiple response

1. c, d, f

Chapter 13

Multiple choice

1. b
2. a
3. c
4. d
5. a
6. b
7. a

Chapter 14

Multiple choice

1. c
2. d
3. a
4. c
5. b
6. b
7. b
8. b

Multiple response

1. a, b, c, e, f
2. a, b, d

Chapter 15

Multiple choice

1. d
2. b
3. a
4. b
5. d
6. b
7. b
8. d

Multiple response

1. a, b, c
2. a, b, d

Chapter 16

Multiple choice

1. d
2. c
3. d
4. b
5. d
6. a
7. c
8. c

Multiple response

1. a, b, c, f

Chapter 17

Multiple choice

1. d
2. d
3. a
4. d
5. c

Multiple response

1. a, b, d
2. a, c, d

Chapter 18

Multiple choice

1. b
2. a
3. d
4. b
5. d
6. b
7. a

Multiple response

1. a, b, c, [illegible]
2. c, e, f
3. b, c

Chapter 19

Multiple choice

1. b
2. b
3. c
4. a
5. b
6. c
7. a
8. b

Multiple response

1. a, b, c
2. a, c, f

Chapter 20

Multiple choice

1. d
2. a
3. a
4. c
5. c
6. d
7. a
8. c

Multiple response

1. a, b, c, e
2. a, b, c, f

Chapter 21

Multiple choice

1. c
2. c
3. d
4. b
5. d
6. b
7. d
8. c

Multiple response

1. a, c, d
2. a, c, d

Chapter 22

Multiple choice

1. d
2. c
3. b
4. c
5. b
6. a
7. d
8. a

Multiple response

1. a, b, c, d
2. a, b, d

Chapter 23

Multiple choice

1. c
2. d
3. b
4. a
5. d
6. c
7. a
8. b

Multiple response

1. b, e
2. b, c, d

Chapter 24

Multiple choice

1. d
2. c
3. c
4. a
5. b
6. c
7. b
8. c

Multiple response

1. a, b, c
2. b, c, f

Chapter 25

Multiple choice

1. c
2. d
3. d
4. c
5. d
6. c
7. c

Multiple response

1. a, b, d, f
2. a, c, d, e, f

Chapter 26

Multiple choice

1. b
2. c
3. c
4. c
5. b
6. d
7. b
8. c

Multiple response

1. b, c, d, e
2. a, c, f

Chapter 27

Multiple choice

1. b
2. c
3. b
4. c
5. a

Multiple response

1. a, b, d, f
2. a, b, d, e
3. a, b, c, f

Chapter 28

Multiple choice

1. a
2. c
3. c
4. b
5. c
6. b
7. a

Multiple response

1. a, b, c

Chapter 29

Multiple choice

1. c
2. b
3. d
4. c
5. d
6. b
7. d
8. a

Multiple response

1. a, b, f
2. a, b, d, f

Chapter 30

Multiple choice

1. c
2. b
3. c
4. d
5. c
6. a

Multiple response

1. b, c, d, e
2. b, c, e, f

Chapter 31

Multiple choice

1. d
2. c
3. b
4. a
5. c
6. d
7. c

Multiple response

1. a, b, d, f
2. a, b, d, f

Chapter 32

Multiple choice

1. b
2. c
3. a
4. c
5. b
6. d
7. b
8. c

Multiple response

1. a, b, d
2. a, b, d

Chapter 33

Multiple choice

1. a
2. c
3. b
4. d

Multiple response

1. a, b, c
2. a, e, f

Chapter 34

Multiple choice

1. d
2. b
3. a
4. c
5. d
6. d
7. c

Multiple response

1. a, b, e, f
2. a, b, d
3. c, e, f

Chapter 35

Multiple choice

1. a
2. c
3. d
4. b
5. c
6. c
7. d
8. b

Multiple response

1. d, e, f
2. c, e

Chapter 36

Multiple choice

1. b
2. c
3. d
4. a
5. a
6. d
7. a
8. c

Multiple response

1. a, b, c, f
2. a, b, d, f

Chapter 37

Multiple choice

1. b
2. c
3. c
4. b
5. d
6. b
7. c
8. b

Multiple response

1. b, d
2. a, b, d

Chapter 38

Multiple choice

1. c
2. c
3. a
4. b
5. b
6. c
7. a

Multiple response

1. a, b, c, e, f
2. a, b, d, f

Chapter 39

Multiple choice

1. a
2. b
3. b
4. c
5. b
6. c
7. d
8. a

Multiple response

1. a, b, c, f
2. a, c, d, e

Chapter 40

Multiple choice

1. b
2. c
3. a
4. b
5. b
6. c
7. c

Multiple response

1. b, c, e, f
2. a, b, c, e, f
3. a, b, d, e

Chapter 41

Multiple choice

1. a
2. d
3. c
4. b
5. c
6. a
7. c
8. d

Multiple response

1. a, b, d
2. b, d, e, f

Chapter 42

Multiple choice

1. c
2. c
3. d
4. c
5. a
6. b
7. a
8. c
9. c

Multiple response

1. a, b, c, e, f
2. a, b, c, f

Chapter 43

Multiple choice

1. b
2. b
3. d
4. c
5. b
6. c
7. d

Multiple response

1. a, b, c, e
2. a, b, d, e

Chapter 44

Multiple choice

1. b
2. c
3. a
4. c
5. d
6. b
7. c
8. b

Multiple response

1. a, b, c
2. a, c, d, e

Chapter 45

Multiple choice

1. d
2. c
3. d
4. d
5. a
6. c

Multiple answer

1. a, c, d, f
2. a, b, c, e, f

Chapter 46

Multiple choice

1. a
2. b
3. d
4. b
5. d
6. b

Multiple response

1. a, b, d, e, f
2. a, b, c, f
3. a, d, e
4. c, e, f

Chapter 47

Multiple choice

1. b
2. b
3. c
4. d
5. b
6. c
7. c
8. d

Multiple response

1. a, b, f
2. a, b, e, f

Chapter 48

Multiple choice

1. c
2. b
3. c
4. d
5. b
6. c

Multiple response

1. a, b, c
2. b, c, d
3. a, b, c, f
4. a, b, c, e, f

Chapter 49

Multiple choice

1. c
2. b
3. a
4. c
5. d
6. c
7. c
8. d

Multiple response

1. b, c, e, f
2. a, c, d

Chapter 50

Multiple choice

1. a
2. d
3. a
4. c
5. c
6. d
7. b

Multiple response

1. a, b, c, e, f
2. a, c, d, e, f
3. a, c, d, f

Chapter 51

Multiple choice

1. b
2. c
3. b
4. c
5. d
6. a
7. d
8. c

Multiple response

1. a, b, d, f
2. a, c, d, f

Chapter 52

Multiple choice

1. b
2. d
3. b
4. a
5. a
6. b
7. c

Multiple response

1. a, b, d, e
2. a, b, d, f

Chapter 53

Multiple choice

1. c
2. a
3. c
4. d
5. c
6. d
7. b

Multiple response

1. a, b, c
2. a, c, d, e, f
3. a, b, c, f

Chapter 54

Multiple choice

1. d
2. c
3. d
4. b
5. a
6. c
7. d

Multiple response

1. a, b, c, e
2. a, c, d, e
3. a, b, d, e, f

Chapter 55

Multiple choice

1. a
2. c
3. c
4. a
5. b
6. d
7. c
8. d

Multiple response

1. b, c, e, f
2. a, c, d, f

Chapter 56

Multiple choice

1. d
2. c
3. a
4. c
5. d
6. d
7. c

Multiple response

1. a, b, c, e, f
2. a, b, d, e, f
3. b, c, d, f

Chapter 57

Multiple choice

1. c
2. d
3. c
4. c
5. a
6. c
7. b
8. d

Multiple response

1. a, b, c, e, f

Chapter 58

Multiple choice

1. b
2. c
3. b
4. c
5. d

Multiple response

1. a, c, d, f
2. b, c, d
3. a, b, c

Chapter 59

Multiple choice

1. a
2. b
3. d
4. b
5. c

Multiple response

1. a, c, d, e, f
2. a, c

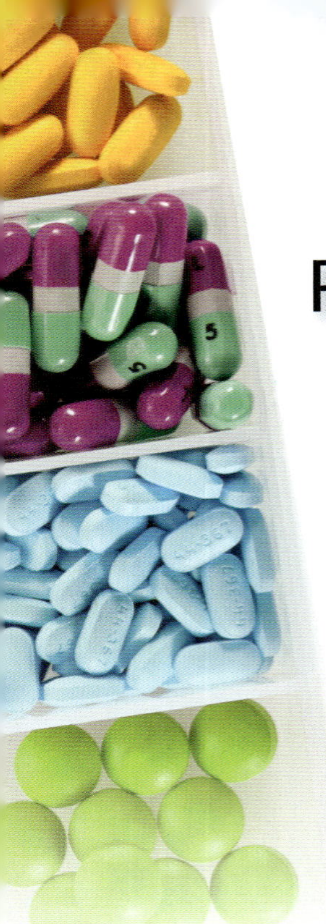

Appendix B

Parenteral agents

Parenteral preparations are fluids that are given either intravenously (IV) or through a central line (Box B.1).

Therapeutic actions and indications

Parenteral agents (Table B.1) are used to provide replacement fluids, sugars, electrolytes and nutrients to people who are unable to take them in orally; to provide ready access for administration of drugs in an emergency situation; to provide rehydration; and to restore electrolyte balance. The composition of the IV fluids needed for an individual depends on the person's fluid and electrolyte status.

Total parenteral nutrition

Total parenteral nutrition (TPN) is the administration of essential proteins, amino acids, carbohydrates, vitamins, minerals, trace elements, lipids and fluids. TPN is used to improve or stabilise the nutritional status of cachectic or debilitated people who cannot take in or absorb oral nutrition to the extent required to maintain their nutritional status. The exact composition of the TPN solution is determined after a nutritional assessment and must take into account the person's current health status, age and metabolic needs.

Contraindications and cautions

TPN is contraindicated in anyone with known allergies to any component of the solution. (Multiple combination products are available, so a suitable solution may be found.) TPN should be used with caution in individuals with unstable cardiovascular status because of the change in fluid volume that might occur and the resultant increased workload on the heart. These preparations also should be used with caution in individuals with unstable fluid and electrolyte status, who could react adversely to sudden changes in fluids and electrolytes. Multivitamins (*Cernevit*, *Souvit*, *Vitalipid*) and specially formulated IV preparations of trace elements can be added to the TPN. Do not add any other medications to the TPN.

BOX B.1 Types of venous lines

The type of the line is defined by the position of the distal catheter tip, not by initial point of entry into the vascular system.

Peripheral lines include peripheral, midline and midclavicular catheters. The tip position is outside of central vessels. Peripheral catheters should be changed every 48–72 hours. Peripheral lines are not appropriate to infuse hypertonic solutions with osmolality > 900 mOsm/L, concentrated antibiotics, vesicants, chemotherapy or parenteral nutrition exceeding 10% glucose and/or 5% protein, solutions or medications that are acidic (pH < 5) or alkaline (pH > 9).

Advantages of peripheral lines: simple, cheap, less trauma, easier for nurses.

Disadvantages of peripheral lines: insertion trauma, irritancy of drugs, block rapidly, infection.

Central lines are not limited by drug pH, osmolarity or volume, and the risk of extravasation is reduced. They are used for administration of chemotherapy, antibiotics and total parenteral nutrition (TPN). Central lines can be single or multiple lumen; open ended (eg, Broviac, Hickman) or valved (eg, Groshong); non-tunnelled or tunnelled catheters or implanted ports.

A **PICC line** is a peripherally inserted central catheter. It is placed percutaneously via a peripheral vein (basilic, cephalic, brachial). The location of the tip of PICC line is in the lower one-third of the superior vena cava. The central positioning of the PICC line is confirmed by X-ray before use.

Advantages of central lines: hypertonic fluid and irritants, rapid administration, multiple lumens (2–4) in one central line allow administration of multiple medications at the same time.

Disadvantages of central lines: high risk of infection, expensive, require time and skill to insert, associated with the risks of insertion (eg, air embolism, arrhythmias, haemothorax, pneumothorax, TPN-thorax, nerve injury), requires skilled nursing staff.

TABLE B.1 Parenterals

Solution	Kilojoule content (kJ/L)	Osmolarity (mOsm/L)	Usual indications
In solutions			
Glucose solutions			
5% (50 g/L)	835	278	Provides kJ and fluid, keeps vein open for administration of IV drugs; frequent choice for dilution of IV drugs
10% (100 g/L)	1670	556	Hypertonic solution used after admixture with other fluids; provides kJ and fluid
25% (250 g/L)	4175	1389	Hypertonic solution used after admixture with other fluids; provides kJ and fluid; treatment of acute hypoglycaemic episodes in infants to restore glucose levels and suppress symptoms; sclerosing agent for varicose veins
50% (500 g/L)	8350	2778	Hypertonic solution used after admixture with other fluids; provide kJ and fluid; treatment of hyperinsulinaemia; sclerosing agent for varicose veins
70% (700 g/L)	11690	3889	Hypertonic solution used after admixture with other fluids; provides kJ and fluid

Solution	Sodium content (mmol/L)	Chloride content (mmol/L)	Osmolarity (mOsm/L)	Usual indications
Saline solutions				
0.45% (½ normal saline)	77	77	155	Hydrating solution; may be used to evaluate kidney function; treatment of hyperosmolar diabetes
0.9% (normal)	154	154	310	Replacement of fluid, sodium and chloride; flushing lines and catheters; dilution of IV medications; priming of dialysis machines; neonatal blood transfusions
3%	513	513	1030	Hypertonic solution to treat sodium and chloride depletion; emergency treatment of water intoxication or severe salt depletion
5%	855	855	1710	Hypertonic solution to treat sodium and chloride depletion; emergency treatment of water intoxication or severe salt depletion

Commonly used combination fluids[a]

Solution	Na content (mmol/L)	K content (mmol/L)	Cl content (mmol/L)	Ca content (mmol/L)	Mg content (mmol/L)	Lactate (mEq/L)	Acetate (mEq/L)	Osmolarity (mOsm/L)
Plasma-lyte-56	40	13	40	—	1.5	—	18	111
Ringer injection	147	4	156	2	—	—	—	310
Lactated Ringer (Hartmann)	130	4	109	1.5	—	28	—	273
Normosol-R	140	5	96	—	1.5	—	27	295

Typical total parenteral nutrition solution[a,b] **for administration via central line only**

Component	Purpose	Availability	Special considerations
10% Amino acids	Provides 50 g protein for growth and healing	500 mL	Monitor blood pressure, cardiac output, blood chemistries and urine to determine the effect of intravascular protein pull
50% Glucose	Provides 3400 kJ for energy	500 mL	Monitor blood sugar; evaluate injection site for any sign of infection, irritation
10% Fat emulsion (*Intralipid*)	Provides 4600 kJ ready energy per 1000 mL	500 mL	Monitor for any sign of emboli (eg, shortness of breath, chest pain, deep leg pain, neurological changes); carefully monitor individual for any sign of increased vascular workload, especially very young and geriatric individuals

Continued on following page

TABLE B.1 Parenterals *(continued)*

Typical total parenteral nutrition solution[a,b] for administration via central line only *(continued)*

Component	Purpose	Availability	Special considerations
20% Fat emulsion (*Intralipid*)	Provides 8400 kJ ready energy per 1000 mL	100 mL, 500 mL, 1 L	Monitor for any sign of emboli (eg, shortness of breath, chest pain, deep leg pain, neurological changes); carefully monitor individuals for any sign of increased vascular workload, especially very young and elderly individuals
30% Fat emulsion (*Intralipid*)	Provides 12 600 kJ, ready energy per 1000 mL	250 mL, 333 mL, 500 mL, 1 L	Monitor for any sign of emboli (eg, shortness of breath, chest pain, deep leg pain, neurological changes); carefully monitor individuals for any sign of increased vascular workload, especially very young and elderly individuals
Sodium chloride	Provides sodium and chloride needed for various chemical reactions within the body	40 mmol	Monitor cardiac rhythm, serum electrolytes
Calcium gluconate	Provides essential calcium for muscle contraction, blood clotting, numerous chemical reactions	2.4 mmol	Monitor cardiac rhythm, muscle strength, serum electrolytes
Magnesium sulfate	Provides magnesium for various chemical reactions within the body	4 mmol	Monitor blood pressure, deep tendon reflexes and serum electrolytes
Potassium phosphate	Provides needed potassium for nerve functioning, muscle contractions, etc.	9 mmol	Monitor pulse, including rhythm, muscle function and serum electrolytes
Multivitamins	Provide a combination of essential vitamins to maintain cell integrity, promote healing	10 mL	Monitor for signs of vitamin deficiency or toxicity
Trace elements	Provide small amounts of elements essential for numerous chemical reactions in the body and maintenance of cell integrity and healing		Periodically monitor blood chemistries to determine adequacy of replacement
Zinc		3 mg	
Copper		1.2 mg	
Manganese		0.3 mg	
Chromium		12 micrograms	
Selenium		20 micrograms	

Typical peripheral total parenteral nutrition solution[a,b,c]

Component	Purpose	Availability	Special considerations
8.5% Amino acids	Provides 41 g protein for growth and healing	500 mL	Monitor blood pressure, cardiac output, blood chemistries, urine to determine effect of intravascular protein pull
20% Glucose	Provides 1360 kJ for energy	500 mL	Monitor blood sugar; evaluate injection site for any sign of infection or irritation
Sodium chloride	Provides sodium and chloride needed for various chemical reactions within the body	40 mmol	Monitor cardiac rhythm, serum electrolytes
Calcium gluconate	Provides essential calcium for muscle contraction, blood clotting, numerous chemical reactions	2.4 mmol	Monitor cardiac rhythm, muscle strength, serum electrolytes
Magnesium sulfate	Provides magnesium for various chemical reactions within the body	4 mmol	Monitor blood pressure, deep tendon reflexes and serum electrolytes

TABLE B.1 Parenterals *(continued)*

Component	Purpose	Availability	Special considerations
Typical peripheral total parenteral nutrition solution[a,b,c] *(continued)*			
Potassium phosphate	Provides needed potassium for nerve functioning, muscle function contractions, etc.	9 mmol	Monitor pulse, including rhythm, muscle function and serum electrolytes
Multivitamins	Provide a combination of essential vitamins to maintain cell integrity, promote healing, etc.	10 mL	Monitor for signs of vitamin deficiency or toxicity
Trace elements	Provide small amounts of elements essential for numerous chemical reactions in the body and maintenance of cell integrity and healing		Periodically monitor blood chemistries to determine adequacy of replacement
Zinc		3 mg	
Copper		1.2 mg	
Manganese		0.3 mg	
Chromium		12 micrograms	
Selenium		12 micrograms	

[a] Multiple combination preparations are available commercially. Each preparation varies in the concentration of one or more components and should be checked carefully before hanging.
[b] Actual concentration of solution and components of any particular solution will be determined by the assessment of the person's current status and nutritional needs.
[c] Solutions used for peripheral therapy are usually less concentrated and less irritating to the vessel.

Adverse effects

Adverse effects associated with the use of TPN include IV irritation, extravasation of the fluid into the tissues, infection of the insertion site, fluid volume overload, vascular problems related to fluid shifts and potential electrolyte imbalance related to dilution of the blood. TPN is also associated with mechanical problems related to insertion of the line, such as pneumothorax, infections or air emboli; emboli related to protein or lipid aggregation; infections related to nutrient-rich solution and invasive administration; metabolic imbalances related to the composition of the solution; gallstone development (especially in children); and nausea (especially related to the administration of lipids).

Clinically important drug–drug interactions

Some IV drugs can be diluted only with particular IV solutions to avoid precipitation or inactivation of the drug. A drug guide should be checked before diluting any IV drug in solution.

Care considerations

Assessment: history and examination

- Obtain a nutritional assessment. Screen for any medical conditions and drugs being taken.
- Evaluate the insertion site; skin hydration; orientation and affect; height and weight; pulse, blood pressure and respirations; and blood chemistries, full blood count with differential and glucose levels.

Implementation

- Assess the person's general physical condition before beginning test *to decrease the potential for adverse effects.*
- Monitor the IV insertion site or central line and regularly consult with the prescriber *to discontinue the site of infusion and treat any infection or extravasation as soon as it occurs.*
- Follow these administration guidelines *to provide the most therapeutic use of TPN with the fewest adverse effects:*
  - Refrigerate TPN solutions until ready to use.
  - Check contents before hanging to ensure that no precipitates are present.
  - Do not hang bag for longer than 24 hours.
  - Suggest the use of in-line filters to decrease bacterial invasion and infusion of aggregate.
- Discontinue TPN only after an alternative source of nutrition has been established *to ensure*

continued nutrition for the person; taper slowly *to avoid severe reactions.*

- Provide comfort measures *to help the person tolerate drug effects* (eg, provide skin care as needed, analgesics, hot soaks to extravasation sites).
- Include information about the solution being used in a test (eg, what to expect, adverse effects that may occur, follow-up tests that may be needed) *to enhance knowledge about drug therapy and promote compliance with the drug regimen.*

Evaluation

- Monitor response to the drug (stabilisation of nutritional state, fluid and electrolyte balance, laboratory values).
- Monitor for adverse effects (local irritation, infection, fluid and electrolyte imbalance).
- Evaluate the effectiveness of the teaching plan (person can name adverse effects to watch for and specific measures to avoid them; person understands the importance of follow-up that will be needed).
- Monitor the effectiveness of comfort measures and compliance with the regimen.

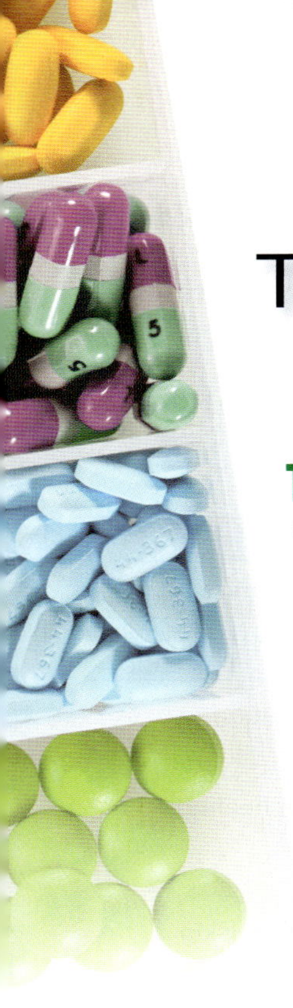

Appendix C

Topical agents

Topical agents are intended for surface use only and are not meant for ingestion or injection. They may be toxic if absorbed into the system, but they have several useful purposes when applied to the surface of the skin or mucous membranes. Some forms of drugs are prepared to be absorbed through the skin for systemic effects. These drugs may be prepared as transdermal patches (eg, glyceryl trinitrate, oestrogens, nicotine), which are designed to provide a slow release of the drug from the vehicle. Drugs prepared for this type of administration are discussed with the specific drug in the text and are not addressed in this appendix.

Therapeutic actions and indications

Topical agents are used to treat a variety of disorders in a localised area. Table C.1 describes the usual uses for the many different types of topical agents. Because these drugs are designed for topical application, they are minimally absorbed systemically and, if used properly, should have minimal systemic effects.

Contraindications and cautions

The use of topical agents is contraindicated *in cases of allergy to the drugs* and in the presence of open wounds or abrasions, *which could lead to the systemic absorption of the drugs*. Caution should be used during pregnancy *if there is any possibility that the agent might be absorbed*. Caution should also be used *in the presence of any known allergy to the vehicles of preparation (creams, lotions)*.

Adverse effects

Because these drugs are not intended to be absorbed systemically, the adverse effects usually associated with topical agents are local effects, including local irritation, stinging, burning or dermatitis. Toxic effects are associated with inadvertent systemic absorption.

Care considerations

Assessment: history and examination

- Screen for the presence of *any known allergy to the drug*, which would be a contraindication to its use.
- Include *screening for baseline status before beginning therapy and for any potential adverse effects*. Assess the following: condition of area to be treated.

Implementation

- Ensure proper administration of the drug *to provide best therapeutic effect and least adverse effects as follows*:
  - Apply sparingly. Some preparations come with applicators, some should be applied while wearing protective gloves and others are dropped onto the site with no direct contact. Consult information regarding the individual drug being used for specific procedures.
  - Do not use with open wounds or broken skin, *which could lead to systemic absorption and toxic effects*.
  - Avoid contact with the eyes, *which could be injured by the drug*.
  - Do not use with occlusive dressings, *which could increase the risk of systemic absorption*.
- Monitor the area being treated *to evaluate drug effects on the condition being treated*.
- Provide comfort measures *to help the person tolerate drug effects* (eg, analgesia as needed for local pain, itching).
- Provide teaching *to enhance knowledge about drug therapy and promote compliance with the drug regimen*:
  - Teach the person the proper administration technique for the topical agent ordered.
  - Caution the person that transient stinging or burning may occur.
  - Instruct the person to report severe irritation, allergic reaction or worsening of the condition being treated.

Evaluation

- Monitor response to the drug (improvement in condition being treated).

- Monitor for adverse effects (local stinging or inflammation).
- Evaluate the effectiveness of the teaching plan (person can name drug, dosage, adverse effects to watch for and specific measures to avoid them; individual understands the importance of continued follow-up).
- Monitor the effectiveness of comfort measures and compliance with the regimen.

TABLE C.1 Topical agents

Drug	Brand name	Dosage	Usual indications/special considerations
Emollients			
boric acid ointment	*Boric Acid, Olive Oil and Zinc Oxide Ointment*	Apply as needed	Relieves burns, itching, irritation
	Gold Cross B.O.Z. Ointment		Relieves itching and aids in healing for mild skin irritations
urea	*Calmurid, Nutraplus, Urecare, Urederm*	Apply bd to qid to area affected	Rub in completely
vitamins A and D	generic	Apply locally with gentle massage bd to qid	Relieves minor burns, chafing, skin irritations; consult health care provider if not improved within 7 days
zinc oxide	*Curash, Desitin, Prickly Heat Powder, Rectogesic Zinc Powder, Sudocrem*	Apply as needed	Relieves burns, abrasion, nappy and heat rash
Lotions and solutions			
aluminium acetate (Burrow's solution)	generic	Apply q 15–30 minutes for 4–8 hours	Astringent wet dressing for relief of inflammatory conditions, insect bites, athlete's foot, bruises, sores; do not use occlusive dressing
calamine lotion	generic	Apply to affected area tds to qid	Relieves itching, pain, insect bites and minor skin irritations
hamamelis water	*Witch Hazel*	Apply locally up to six times per day	Relieves itching and irritation of insect bites, haemorrhoids, postepisiotomy discomfort, posthaemorrhoidectomy care
Antiseptics			
benzalkonium chloride	*Bepanthen Antiseptic Cream*	Apply as directed	Thoroughly rinse detergents and soaps from skin before use
chlorhexidine gluconate	*Bepanthen First Aid Antiseptic Cream, Microshield*	Scrub or rinse; leave on for 15 seconds; for surgical scrub – 3 minutes	Use for surgical scrub, preoperative skin preparation, wound cleansing; preoperative bathing and showering
iodine	generic preparations	Wash affected area	Highly toxic; avoid occlusive dressings; some preparations stain skin and clothing; iodine allergy is common
povidone–iodine	*Betadine, Inadine Dressing, Microshield PVP Solution*	Apply as needed	Treated areas may be bandaged; HIV is inactivated in this solution; causes less irritation than iodine; less toxic

TABLE C.1 Topical agents *(continued)*

Drug	Brand name	Dosage	Usual indications/special considerations
Antibiotics			
ciprofloxacin/ hydrocortisone	*Ciloxan, Ciproxin HC Ear Drops*	Apply drops to ears or outer ear canal	Treatment of acute otitis media
mupirocin	*Mupider*	Apply small amount to affected area tds	Used to treat impetigo caused by *Staphylococcus aureus*, *Streptococcus* pathogens; may be covered with a gauze pad; monitor for signs of superinfection, re-evaluate if no clinical response in 3–5 days
mupirocin calcium	*Bactroban, Bactroban Nasal*	Apply small amount inside each nostril bd	Eradication of nasal colonisation of staphylococci
Antivirals			
aciclovir	*Blistex Antiviral Cold Sore Cream, Zovirax, ViruPOS eye ointment*	Apply to affected area six times per day for 5–14 days	Treatment of herpes simplex cold sores and fever blisters; eye ointment for treatment of herpes simplex keratitis
imiquimod	*Aldara*	Apply thin layer to warts and rub in three times per week at bedtime for 16 weeks	For treatment of genital warts and perianal warts; remove with soap and water after 6–10 hours
Antipsoriatics			
calcipotriol	*Daivobet, Daivonex*	Apply thin layer twice a day	Monitor serum calcium levels with extended use; use only for disorder prescribed; may cause local irritation; is a synthetic vitamin D_3
Antiseborrhoeics			
selenium sulfide	*Selsun Blue*	Massage 5–10 mL into scalp; rest 2–3 minutes, rinse	May damage jewellery, remove before use; discontinue if local irritation occurs
Antifungals			
ciclopirox	*Rejuvenail nail laquer*	Apply directly to affected fingernails or toenails	Treatment of onychomycosis of the fingernails and toenails
clotrimazole	*Canesten, Clonea, Clozole*	Gently massage into affected area bd to tds	Cleanse area before applying; use for up to 4 weeks; discontinue if irritation or worsening of condition occurs
econozole nitrate	*Pevaryl*	Apply locally daily to bd	Treatment of athlete's foot (intradigital pedia), tinea corporis, ringworm, tinea cruris; cleanse area before applying; treat for 2–4 weeks; for athlete's foot, change socks and shoes at least once a day
ketoconazole	*DaktaGOLD, Nizoral, Sebizole*	Apply shampoo daily Apply cream daily or bd	Reduction of scaling due to dandruff; burning may occur Tinea corporis, tinea cruris, tinea manus, tinea pedis, cutaneous candidiasis

Continued on following page

TABLE C.1 Topical agents *(continued)*

Drug	Brand name	Dosage	Usual indications/special considerations
Antifungals *(continued)*			
miconazole	*Daktarin, Eulactol, Resolve*	Apply to area bd for 2 weeks after clinical signs disappear	Treatment of various fungal infections
terbinafine	*Lamisil*	Apply to area bd until clinical signs are improved; 1–4 weeks	Do not use occlusive dressings; report local irritation; discontinue if local irritation occurs
tolnaftate	*Mycil, Tinaderm, Tineafax*	Apply small amount bd for 2–3 weeks; 4–6 weeks may be needed if skin is very thick	Cleanse skin with soap and water before applying drug, dry thoroughly; wear loose, well-fitting shoes if feet affected; change socks at least qid
Pediculocides/scabicides			
crotamiton	*Eurax*	Thoroughly massage into skin over entire body, repeat in 24 hours; person should take a cleansing bath or shower 48 hours after last application	Change all bed linens and clothing the next day; contaminated clothing can be dry cleaned or washed in hot water; shake well before using
permethrin	*Lyclear, Quellada*	Thoroughly massage into all skin areas; wash off after 8–14 hours; shampoo into freshly washed, rinsed and towel-dried hair, leave on for 10 minutes, rinse	Single application is usually curative; notify health care provider if rash, itch becomes worse; approved for prophylactic use during head lice epidemics
Keratolytics			
podophyllum resin	generic	Applied only by doctor	Do not use if wart is inflamed or irritated; very toxic; use minimum amount to avoid absorption
podophyllotoxin	*Condyline*	Apply q 12 hours for three consecutive days	Allow to dry before using area; dispose of used applicator; may cause burning and discomfort
Pain relief			
capsaicin	*Zostrix*	Do not apply more than three to four times per day	Provides temporary relief from the pain of osteoarthritis, rheumatoid arthritis, neuralgias; do not bandage tightly; stop use and seek medical help if condition worsens or persists after 14–28 days
Burn preparations			
silver sulfadiazine	*Flamazine*	Apply daily to bd to a clean, debrided wound; use 3–5 mm thickness	Bathe person in a whirlpool to aid debridement; dressings are not necessary but may be used; reapply when necessary; monitor for fungal infections
Oestrogens			
oestradiol	*Sandrena*	Applied once daily onto the skin of the trunk or thigh	Treatment of climacteric symptoms following menopause; attempt to taper every 3–6 months

TABLE C.1 Topical agents *(continued)*

Drug	Brand name	Dosage	Usual indications/special considerations
Acne products			
adapalene	*Differin*	Apply a thin film to affected area after washing	Do not use near cuts or open wounds; avoid sunburned areas; do not combine with other products; limit exposure to the sun; less drying than most acne products
azelaic acid	*Azclear, Finacea*	Wash and dry skin; massage thin layer into skin bd	Wash hands thoroughly after application; improvement usually seen within 4 weeks; initial irritation usually passes with time
clindamycin	*ClindaTech, Dalacin, Zindaclin*	Wash and dry area; massage into area morning and evening	Do not use occlusive dressings; may cause transient burning
clindamycin with benzoyl peroxide	*Duac Once Daily*	Apply to affected area	Wash and pat dry area before application once daily in the evening
erythromycin	*Eryacne*	Apply thin film bd	Treatment of acne vulgaris
isotretanoin	*Isotrex*	Apply thin layer to affected area once daily at night	Avoid contact with eyes, mouth and mucous membranes. Should not be applied to nose angles
metronidazole	*Rozex*	Apply cream to affected area bd	Treatment of rosacea
tazarotene	*Zorac*	Apply thin film daily in the evening	Avoid use in pregnancy; drying, causes photosensitivity; do not use with products containing alcohol
tretinoin, 0.025% cream	*Stieva-A*	Apply thin layer daily	Discomfort, peeling, redness and worsening of acne may occur for first 2–4 weeks
tretinoin, 0.05% cream	*Retin-A, ReTrieve, Stieva-A*	Apply thin coat in evening	Use for acne vulgaris, the removal of fine wrinkles
tretinoin, gel	*Retin-A Gel*	Apply to cover daily, after cleansing	Exacerbation of inflammation may occur at first; therapeutic effects usually seen in first 2 weeks
Antihistamine			
azelastine HCl	*Azep*	One spray per nostril bd	Avoid use of alcohol and over-the-counter (OTC) antihistamines; dizziness and sedation may occur
Hair removal			
eflornithine	*Vaniqa*	Apply to unwanted facial hair bd for up to 24 weeks	For use in women only
Topical corticosteroids			

These drugs enter cells and bind to cytoplasmic receptors, initiating complex reactions that are responsible for the anti-inflammatory, antipruritic and antiproliferative effects of these drugs. They are used to relieve the inflammation and pruritic manifestations of corticosteroid-sensitive dermatoses and for temporary relief of minor skin irritations and rashes. These agents should always be applied sparingly because of the risk of systemic corticosteroid effects if absorbed systemically. Occlusive dressings and tight coverings should be avoided. Prolonged use should also be avoided because of the risk of systemic effects and local irritation and breakdown. These agents are applied topically two to three times daily.

Drug	Brand name	Dosage
betamethasone dipropionate	*Diprosone, Eleuphrat*	Ointment, cream, lotion, aerosol: 0.05% concentration
betamethasone valerate	*Antroquoril, Betnovate, Celestone M, Cortival*	Ointment, cream, lotion: 0.01–0.05% concentration
ciclesonide	*Alvesco*	Inhalation: 80 micrograms, 160 micrograms per actuation
clobetasone butyrate	*Eumovate*	Cream: 0.05% concentration
desonide	*Desowen*	Lotion: 0.05% concentration

Continued on following page

TABLE C.1 Topical agents *(continued)*

Drug	Brand name	Dosage	Usual indications/special considerations
Topical corticosteroids *(continued)*			
dexamethasone	*Maxidex*	Eye drops: 0.1% concentration	
	Otodex, Sofradex	Ear drops: 8 mL bottle	
fluticasone propionate	*Flixonase Nasule Drops*	Nasule: 400 micrograms	
hydrocortisone	*DermAid, DermAssist*	Cream, lotion, ointment, aerosol: 0.5%, 1% concentration	
hydrocortisone acetate	*Colifoam Rectal Foam*	Foam: 10% concentration	
	Cortic-DS, Sigmacort	Cream: 1% concentration	
hydrocortisone butyrate	*Locoid, Locoid Lipocream, Locoid Crelo*	Cream: (*Locoid Lipocream*): 0.1% Ointment 0.1% Scalp lotion 0.1% Topical emulsion (*Locoid Crelo*): 0.1%	
mometasone furoate	*Elocon, Novasone*	Ointment, cream, lotion: 0.1% concentration	
	Nasonex	Nasal spray: 0.2% concentration	
triamcinolone acetonide	*Aristocort, Tricortone*	Ointment: 0.02% concentration	
	Aristocort, Tricortone	Cream: 0.02% concentration	
	Kenalog in Orabase	Oral paste: 0.1%	
	Telnase	Nasal spray: 55 micrograms/dose	

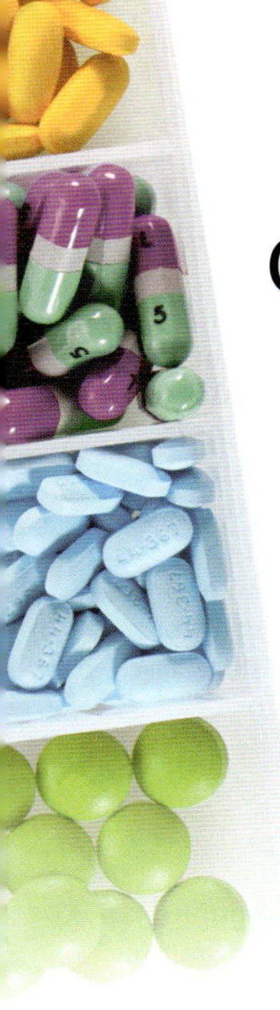

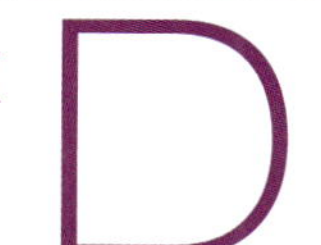

Appendix D

Ophthalmic agents

Ophthalmic agents are drugs that are intended for direct administration into the conjunctiva of the eye. These drugs are used to treat glaucoma (miotics constrict the pupil and decrease the resistance to aqueous flow); to aid in the diagnosis of eye problems (mydriatics dilate the pupil for examination of the retina; cycloplegics paralyse the muscles that control the lens to aid refraction); to treat local ophthalmic infections or inflammation; and to provide relief from the signs and symptoms of allergic reactions.

These drugs are not generally absorbed systemically because of their method of administration. Caution should always be used when giving drugs during pregnancy or breastfeeding.

Contraindications and cautions

These drugs are contraindicated in the presence of allergy to the specific drug or to any component of the product being used. Although they are seldom absorbed systemically, caution should be used in any person who would have problems with the systemic effects of the drugs if they were absorbed systemically.

Adverse effects

Adverse effects of these drugs include local irritation, stinging, burning, blurring of vision (prolonged when using ointments), tearing and headache.

Clinically important drug–drug interactions

Because of their actions on the eye or because of the components of the drug, many of these drugs cannot be given at the same time but should be spaced 1–2 hours apart. Check the specific drug being used for details.

Dosage

The usual dosage for any of these drugs is one to two drops in each eye or in the affected eye two to four times daily, or for ointment, 0.5–1 cm in the affected eye or eyes.

Care considerations

Assessment

- Screen for the following: allergy to the specific drug or components of the preparation; underlying medical conditions *that would be affected if the drug were absorbed systemically*.
- Evaluate eye, conjunctival colour; note any lesions. A vision examination may be appropriate.

Implementation

- Assess the person's general physical condition before beginning the test *to decrease the potential for adverse effects*.
- Follow these administration guidelines to *provide the most therapeutic use of the drug with the fewest adverse effects*:
  - Solution or drops: wash hands thoroughly before administering; do not touch the dropper to the person's eye or to any other surface. Have the person tilt the head backwards or lie down and stare upwards. Gently grasp the lower eyelid and pull the eyelid away from the eyeball; instil drops into the pouch formed by the eyelid. Release the lid slowly; have the person close the eye and look downwards. Apply gentle pressure to the inside corner of the eye for 3–5 minutes to retard drainage. Do not rub the eyes; do not rinse the eyedropper. Do not use eye drops that have changed colour; if more than one type of eye drop is used, wait at least 5 minutes between administrations. Refer to Figure D.1.
  - Ointment: wash hands thoroughly before administering; hold the tube between the hands for several minutes to warm the ointment; discard the first centimetre of ointment when opening the tube for the first time. Tilt the person's head backwards or have the person lie down and stare upwards. Gently pull out the lower lid to form a pouch; place 1–1.5 cm of ointment inside the lower lid. Have the person close the eye for 1–2 minutes and roll the eyeball in all directions; remove any excess ointment from around the eye. If using more than one kind of ointment, wait at least 10 minutes between administrations. Refer to Figure D.2.

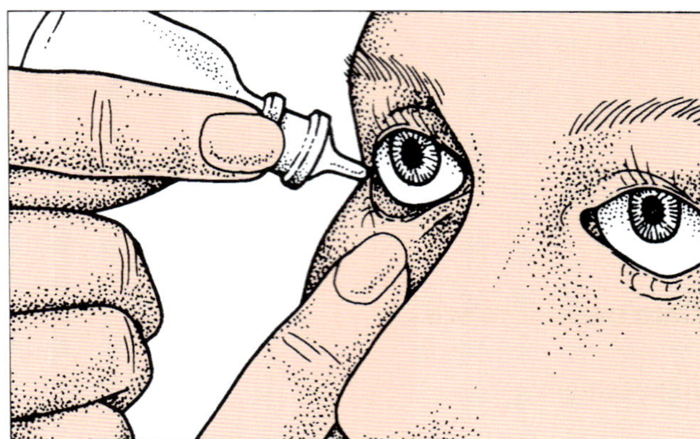

FIGURE D.1 Administration of ophthalmic drops.

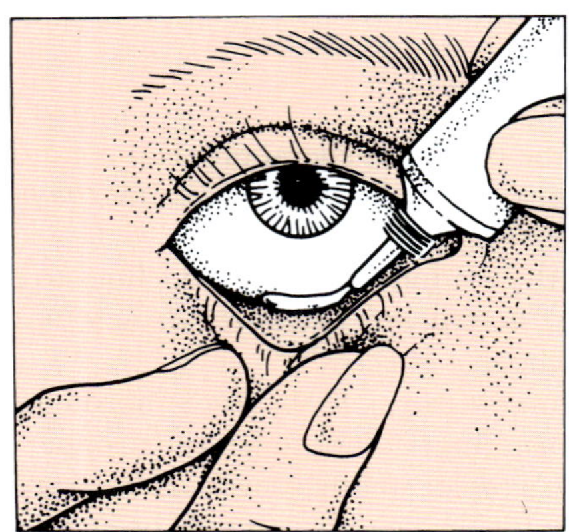

FIGURE D.2 Administration of ophthalmic ointment.

- *Provide comfort measures to help the person tolerate drug effects* (eg, control light, administer analgesics as needed).
- Include the following information – in addition to the proper administration technique for the drug – in the teaching program for the person *to improve compliance and provide safety and comfort measures as necessary*: safety measures may need to be taken if blurring of vision should occur; burning and stinging may occur on administration but should pass quickly; the pupils will dilate with mydriatic agents and the eyes may become very sensitive to light (the use of sunglasses is recommended); any severe eye discomfort, palpitations, nausea or headache should be reported to the health care provider.

Evaluation

- Monitor response to the drug (changes in pupil size, relief of pressure of glaucoma, relief of itching and tearing related to allergic reaction).
- Monitor for adverse effects (local irritation, blurring of vision, headache).
- Evaluate the effectiveness of the teaching plan (person can name adverse effects to watch for and specific measures to avoid them; the person understands the importance of the follow-up that will be needed).
- Monitor the effectiveness of comfort measures and compliance with the regimen.

TABLE D.1 Ophthalmic agents

Drug	Usage	Special considerations
aciclovir (*Zovirax Ophthalmic Ointment*)	Treatment of ocular herpes simplex	One centimetre into lower conjunctival sac five times daily for 14 days
apraclonidine (*Iopidine*)	To control or prevent postsurgical elevations of intraocular pressure (IOP) after argon-laser eye surgery	Monitor for the possibility of vasovagal attack; do not give to individuals with allergy to clonidine
atropine (*Atropt*)	Conditions necessitating pupil dilation and paralysis of accommodation	One drop into the eye as needed. Apply gentle pressure to tear duct for 1 minute after administration
azelastine (HCl) (*Eyezep*)	Treatment of ocular itching associated with allergic conjunctivitis	Antihistamine, mast cell stabiliser; dosage (≥ 3 years): 1 drop bd; rapid onset, 8 hours' duration
betaxolol (*Betoptic, Betoquin*)	Reduction of IOP with chronic open-angle glaucoma, ocular hypertension	One drop bd; may take up to 2 weeks to see results; do not combine with beta-adrenergics
bimatoprost (*Lumigan*)	Reduction of IOP in individuals with open-angle glaucoma or ocular hypertension	Used for people who are intolerant to other IOP-lowering drugs or who have failed to achieve optimal IOP with other IOP-lowering medications
brimonidine tartrate (*Alphagan, Alphagan P, Enidin*)	Treatment of open-angle glaucoma and ocular hypertension	Selective alpha$_2$-antagonist; minimal effects on cardiovascular and pulmonary systems; do not use with monoamine oxidase inhibitors; dosage: one drop tds
brimonidine with timolol (*Combigan*)	Treatment of IOP	One drop to the affected eye q 12 hours; do not use with contact lenses

TABLE D.1 Ophthalmic agents *(continued)*

Drug	Usage	Special considerations
brinzolamide (*Azopt, BrinzoQuin*)	To decrease intraocular pressure in open-angle glaucoma	May be given with other agents; dosage: one drop tds; give 10 minutes apart from any other agents
brinzolamide with timolol (*Azarga*)	To decrease intraocular pressure in open-angle glaucoma	Shake bottle well before use. Apply one drop to affected eye bd
carbachol (*Isopto, Miostat*)	Direct-acting miotic; for treatment of glaucoma; miosis during surgery	Surgical dose: a one-use-only portion; for glaucoma: 1–2 drops up to tds as needed
chloramphenicol (*Chloromycetin, Chlorsig*)	Treatment of bacterial conjunctivitis and other eye infections	Chronic use may result in toxicity
ciprofloxacin hydrochloride (*CiloQuin, Ciloxin*)	Treatment of severe bacterial conjunctivitis and corneal ulcers	May cause local burning or stinging, crystalline precipitate
cyclopentolate (*Cyclogyl*)	Mydriasis/cycloplegia in diagnostic procedures	Individuals with dark-pigmented irises may require higher doses; compress lacrimal sac for 1–2 minutes after administration to decrease any systemic absorption
dexamethasone (*Maxidex*)	Treatment of inflammation and allergic conditions	Apply 1–2 drops 4–6 times daily; not to be used with contact lenses
diclofenac sodium (*Voltaren Ophtha*)	Photophobia: for use in individuals undergoing incisional refractive surgery	Apply one drop qid beginning 24 hours after cataract surgery; continue through the first 2 weeks after surgery
dorzolamide (*Trusopt*)	Treatment of elevated IOP in open-angle glaucoma or ocular hypertension	A sulfonamide; monitor individuals taking parenteral sulfonamides for possible adverse effects
dorzolamide 2% and timolol 0.5% (*Cosopt*)	To decrease IOP in open-angle glaucoma or ocular hypertension in individuals who do not respond to beta blockers alone	Administer one drop in affected eye b.d; monitor for cardiac failure; if absorbed, may mask symptoms of hypoglycaemia or thyrotoxicosis
fluorescein sodium (generic)	Staining of the eye for ophthalmic examination	Care needs to be taken to ensure solution is kept sterile due to potential spread of eye infection
fluorometholone (*Flarex, Flucon, FML*)	Topical corticosteroid used for treatment of inflammatory conditions of the eye	Improvement should occur within several days; discontinue if no improvement is seen; discontinue if swelling of the eye occurs
framycetin sulfate (*Soframycin*)	Treatment of conjunctivitis, minor infections, corneal abrasion	Two drops q 1–2 hours decreasing to 2–3 drops tds
gentamicin (*Genoptic*)	Treatment of external eye infection	1–2 drops into affected eye q 4 hours; apply pressure to tear duct following administration
hydrocortisone (*Siguent Hycor Ointment*)	Treatment of inflammatory eye conditions	Apply to affected eye(s) bd to qid
ketorolac (*Acular*)	Temporary relief of symptoms of allergic conjunctivitis	One drop qid for up to 4 weeks
ketotifen (*Zaditen*)	Temporary relief of itching due to allergic conjunctivitis	Remove contact lenses before use – may be replaced 10 minutes after administration; an antihistamine/mast cell stabiliser
latanoprost (*Xalatan*)	Treatment of open-angle glaucoma or ocular hypertension in individuals intolerant or unresponsive to other agents	Remove contact lenses before use and for 15 minutes after use; allow at least 5 minutes between this and the use of any other agents; expect blurring of vision
latanoprost with timolol (*Xalacom*)	Treatment of open-angle glaucoma or ocular hypertension in individuals intolerant or unresponsive to other agents	Apply pressure to tear duct immediately after administration. Remove contact lenses before use and for 15 minutes after use
lodoxamide (*Lomide*)	Treatment of vernal conjunctivitis and keratitis	Individuals should not wear contact lenses while using this drug; discontinue if stinging or burning persists after instillation

Continued on following page

TABLE D.1 Ophthalmic agents *(continued)*

Drug	Usage	Special considerations
naphazoline hydrochloride (*Albalon, Murine Clear I, Naphcon Forte*)	Use as topical vasoconstrictor	1–2 drops up to qid
olopatadine hydrochloride (*Patanol*)	Mast cell stabiliser and antihistamine; provides fast onset of relief of itching due to conjunctivitis and has prolonged action	Not for use with contact lenses; headache is a common side effect
phenylephrine hydrochloride (*Albalon Relief*	Management of minor eye irritation in the absence of infection	1–2 drops to affected eye tds
phenylephrine hydrochloride with prednisolone acetate (*Prednefrin Forte*)	Treatment of non-infectious eye inflammation	Initially two drops hourly, then 1–2 drops bd– qid; apply pressure to tear duct after administration
pilocarpine (*Isopto Carpine*)	Chronic and acute glaucoma; treatment of mydriasis caused by drugs; direct-acting mitotic	Can be stored at room temperature for up to 8 weeks, then discard; may use 1–2 drops up to six times per day, based on individual response
propamidine isethionate (*Brolene*)	Treatment of mild conjunctivitis	1–2 drops into affected eye(s) tds or qid up to 1 week
proxymetacaine hydrochloride (*Alcaine*)	Eye anaesthesia	1–2 drops as needed
timolol (*Nyogel, Tenopt*)	Treatment of elevated IOP in ocular hypertension or open-angle glaucoma	One drop in affected eye(s) each day in the morning
tobramycin (*Tobrex*)	Treatment of external eye infections	1–2 drops qid or 1–1.5 cm ointment bd or tds
travoprost (*DuoTrav, Travatan*)	Reduction of intraocular pressure in individuals with open-angle glaucoma or ocular hypertension	Reserve for individuals who are intolerant of other IOP-lowering medications or who have failed to achieve optimal IOP with other IOP-lowering medications
tropicamide (*Mydriacyl*)	Mydriatic and cyclopegic for refraction	One to two drops, repeat in 5 minutes; may repeat in 30 minutes for prolonged effects

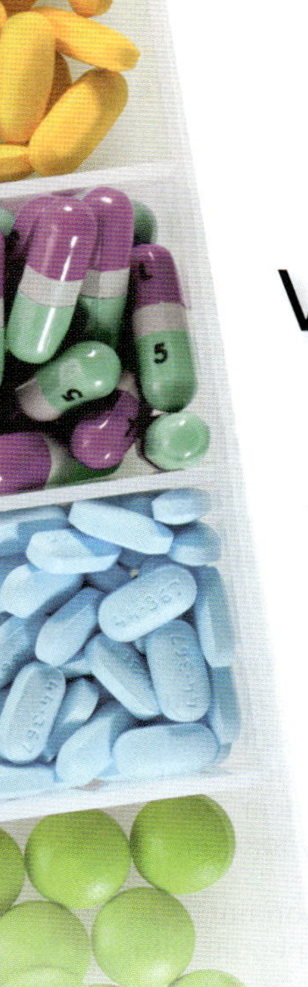

Appendix E

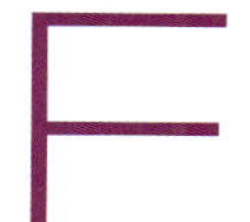

Vitamins

Vitamins are substances that the body requires for carrying out essential metabolic reactions. The body cannot synthesise enough of these components to meet all of its needs; therefore, they must be obtained from animal and vegetable tissues taken in as food. Vitamins are only needed in small amounts because they function as coenzymes that activate the protein portions of enzymes, which catalyse a great deal of biochemical activity. Vitamins are either water soluble and excreted in the urine or they are fat soluble and capable of being stored in adipose tissue in the body.

Therapeutic actions and indications

Vitamins act as coenzymes to activate a variety of proteins on enzymes that catalyse biochemical activity. They are indicated for the treatment of vitamin deficiencies, as dietary supplements when needed and as specific therapy related to the activity of the vitamin.

Contraindications and cautions

These drugs are contraindicated in the presence of any known allergy to the drug or the colourants, additives or preservatives used in the drug. Some are used to maintain adequate vitamin levels during pregnancy and breastfeeding.

Adverse effects

The adverse effects primarily associated with these drugs are related to gastrointestinal (GI) upset and irritation, which is caused by direct GI contact with the drugs.

Clinically important drug–drug interactions

Pyridoxine – vitamin B6 – interferes with the effectiveness of levodopa. Fat-soluble vitamins may not be absorbed if given concurrently with mineral oil, cholestyramine or colestipol.

Care considerations

Assessment

- Obtain a nutritional assessment. Screen for any medical conditions and drugs being taken and for any known allergies.
- Evaluate skin and mucous membranes, as well as pulse, respirations and blood pressure. Full blood count and clotting times may need to be evaluated with specific vitamins.

Implementation

- Assess the person's general physical condition before beginning test *to decrease the potential for adverse effects and ensure need for the drug.*
- Advise the person to avoid the use of over-the-counter preparations that contain the same vitamins *to prevent inadvertent overdose of the vitamin.*
- Provide comfort measures *to help the person tolerate drug effects* (eg, take drug with meals to alleviate GI distress).
- Include information about the solution being used in a test (eg, what to expect, adverse effects that may occur, follow-up tests that may be needed) *to enhance knowledge about drug therapy and promote compliance with drug regimen.*

Evaluation

- Monitor response to the drug (adequate vitamin intake).
- Monitor for adverse effects (GI upset).
- Evaluate the effectiveness of the teaching plan (person can name adverse effects to watch for and specific measures to avoid them; person understands the importance of follow-up that will be needed).
- Monitor the effectiveness of comfort measures and compliance with the regimen.

TABLE E.1 Vitamins

Vitamin	Solubility type	Recommended dietary intake (RDI)	Therapeutic uses/special considerations
retinol (vitamin A) (generic)*	Fat	900 micrograms (male) 700 micrograms (female) 700–800 micrograms (pregnancy) 1100 micrograms (breastfeeding) 300–700 micrograms (paediatric)	Hypervitaminosis A can occur, including cirrhotic-like liver syndrome with central nervous system effects; GI drying, rash and liver changes. Treat by discontinuing the vitamin and give saline, prednisone and calcitonin IV. Liver damage may be permanent
ascorbic acid (vitamin C) (generic)	Water	45 mg (male) 45 mg (female) 80–85 mg (breastfeeding) 55–60 mg (pregnancy) 35–40 mg (paediatric)	Treatment of scurvy: 300–1000 mg/day. Enhanced wound healing: 300–500 mg/day for 7–10 days. Burns: 1–2 g/day. Also being studied for treatment of common cold, asthma, coronary artery disease, cancer and schizophrenia. May be very toxic at high doses
biotin (vitamin B7) (contained in combined generic products)	Water	30 micrograms (male) 25 micrograms (female) 35 micrograms (breastfeeding) 30 micrograms (pregnancy) 8–25 micrograms (paediatric)	Biotin deficiency is uncommon but increased requirements in people with genetic biotinidase deficiency
cholecalciferol (vitamin D_3) (*Ostelin, OsteVit-D*)	Fat	5–15 micrograms (male) 5–15 micrograms (female) 5 micrograms (breastfeeding) 5 micrograms (pregnancy) 5 micrograms (paediatric)	Vitamin D deficiency: 25 micrograms/day. May be useful for the treatment of hypocalcaemic tetany and hypoparathyroidism
choline (contained in combined generic products)	Water	550 mg (male) 425 mg (female) 525 mg (breastfeeding) 415–440 mg (pregnancy) 200–400 mg (paediatric)	Vegetarians may experience choline deficiency
cyanocobalamin (B12) (generic)	Water	2.4 micrograms (male) 2.4 micrograms (female) 2.8 micrograms (breastfeeding) 2.6 micrograms (pregnancy) 0.9–2.4 micrograms (paediatric)	Deficiency: 25–250 micrograms/day. (Note: oral route is not for the treatment of pernicious anaemia.) Pernicious anaemia: 100 micrograms IM each month for life; given with folic acid; nasal route is preferable
alpha tocopherol (vitamin E) (generic)	Fat	10 mg (male) 7 mg (female) 11–12 mg (breastfeeding) 7–8 mg (pregnancy) 5–8 mg (paediatric)	Used in certain premature infants to reduce the toxic effects of oxygen on the lung and retina; report fatigue, weakness, nausea or headache
niacin (nicotinic acid, nicotinamide, vitamin B3) (generic)	Water	16 mg (male) 14 mg (female) 17 mg (breastfeeding) 18 mg (pregnancy) 6–16 mg (paediatric)	Prevention and treatment of pellagra: up to 500 mg/day. Niacin deficiency: up to 100 mg/day
bioflavonoids (contained in combined generic products)	Water	Unknown	Used to treat bleeding, abortion, poliomyelitis, diabetes and other conditions. There is little evidence these uses have any clinical efficacy
pantothenic acid (vitamin B5) (contained in combined generic products)	Water	6 mg (male) 4 mg (female) 6 mg (breastfeeding) 5 mg (pregnancy) 3.5–4 mg (paediatric)	Deficiency very uncommon; symptoms similar to those of other B-group vitamins

TABLE E.1 Vitamins *(continued)*

Vitamin	Solubility type	Recommended dietary intake (RDI)	Therapeutic uses/special considerations
phytonadione (vitamin K)	Fat	70 micrograms (male) 60 micrograms (female) 60 micrograms (breastfeeding) 60 micrograms (pregnancy) 25–55 micrograms (paediatric)	Hypoprothrombinaemia due to anticoagulant use: 2.5–10 mg PO, IM. Haemorrhagic disease of the newborn: 1 mg IM within 1 hour of birth. Hypoprothrombinaemia in adult: 2.5–25 mg PO or IM
pyridoxine HCl (vitamin B6) (Pyroxin)	Water	1.3–1.7 mg (male) 1.3–1.5 mg (female) 2.0 mg (breastfeeding) 1.9 mg (pregnancy) 0.5–1.2 mg (paediatric)	Deficiency: 10–20 mg/day PO or IM for 3 weeks. Vitamin B6 deficiency syndrome: up to 600 mg/day for life
riboflavin (vitamin B2) (contained in combined generic products)	Water	1.3–1.6 mg (male) 1.1–1.3 mg (female) 1.6 mg (breastfeeding) 1.4 mg (pregnancy) 0.5–1.1 mg (paediatric)	Treatment of deficiency: 5–15 mg/day. May cause a yellow or orange discolouration to the urine
thiamin (vitamin B1) (*B-Dose, Betamin*)	Water	1.2 mg (male) 1.1 mg (female) 1.4 mg (breastfeeding) 1.4 mg (pregnancy) 0.5–1.1 mg (paediatric)	Treatment of beriberi: 10–20 mg IM tds for 2 weeks with multivitamin containing 5–10 mg/day for 1 month. Do not mix in alkaline solutions. Used orally as a mosquito repellent, alters body sweat composition. Feeling of warmth and flushing may occur with administration but usually passes within 2 hours

* Comparison of various forms of vitamin A is by retinol equivalents (RE). 1 RE = 1 microgram retinol = 6 micrograms of trans beta carotene = 12 micrograms alpha carotene. Doses are expressed here as RE.

Reference: National Health and Medical Research Council (2017). *Nutrient Reference Values for Australia and New Zealand Including Recommended Dietary Intakes*. Commonwealth of Australia. Available at www.nhmrc.gov.au/sites/default/files/images/nutrient-refererence-dietary-intakes.pdf

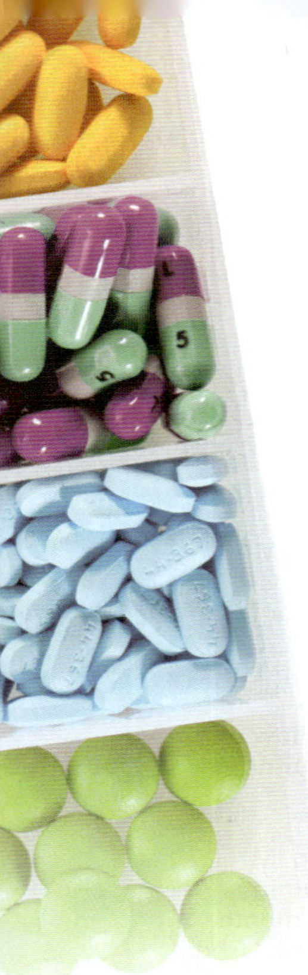

Appendix F

Drug interactions with complementary and alternative (CAM) therapies

Many dietary supplements and 'natural' remedies are used by the public for self-treatment. These substances, many derived from the folklore of various cultures, commonly contain ingredients that have been identified and that have known therapeutic activities. Some of these substances have unknown mechanisms of action but over the years have been reliably used to relieve specific symptoms. There is an element of the placebo effect in using some of these substances. The power of believing that something will work and that there is some control over the problem is often beneficial in achieving relief from pain or suffering. Some of these substances may contain yet-unidentified ingredients that eventually may prove useful in the modern field of pharmacology. Because these products are not regulated or monitored, there is always a possibility of toxic effects. Some of these products may contain ingredients that interact with prescription drugs. Historical use of these alternative therapies may explain unexpected reactions to some drugs.

TABLE F.1 Drug interactions of complementary and alternative therapies

Substance	Possible interactions
acidophilus (probiotics)	Decreased effectiveness of **warfarin**
alfalfa	Increased risk of bleeding with **warfarin**; increased photosensitivity with **chlorpromazine**; increased risk of hypoglycaemia with **oral hypoglycaemic agents**; loss of effectiveness with **hormonal contraceptives** or **hormone replacement**
allspice	Risk of seizures with excessive use; decreased **iron** absorption
aloe leaves	Caution: oral use may cause serious hypokalaemia; risk of spontaneous abortion if used in third trimester
androstenedione	Caution: may increase risk of cardiovascular disease and certain cancers
angelica	Risk of bleeding if combined with **anticoagulants**
anise	May increase **iron** absorption and cause toxicity
apple	May interfere with **oral hypoglycaemic agents**
arnica	May decrease effects of **antihypertensives** and increase effects of **anticoagulants** and **platelet drugs**; very toxic to children
ashwagandha	May increase bleeding with **anticoagulants**; may interfere with **thyroid replacement** therapy; discourage use during pregnancy and breastfeeding
astragalus	May increase effects of **antihypertensives**; caution against use during fever or acute infection
barberry	Risk of spontaneous abortion if taken during pregnancy May increase effects of **antihypertensives**, **antiarrhythmics**
basil	Risk of increased hypoglycaemic effects of **oral hypoglycaemic agents**
bayberry	May block effects of **antihypertensives**
bee pollen	Risk of hyperglycaemia; discourage use by patients with diabetes or with **oral hypoglycaemic agents**; may cause allergic reaction in individuals allergic to bees
betel palm	Increased risk of hypertensive crisis with **monoamine oxidase (MAO) inhibitors**; blocks heart-rate reduction of **beta blockers**, **digoxin**; alters effects of **antiglaucoma drugs**
bilberry	Increased risk of bleeding with **anticoagulants**; disulfiram-like reaction with **alcohol**
birch bark	Topical form very toxic to children
black cohosh root	Contains oestrogen-like components; caution against use with **hormone replacement therapy** or **hormonal contraceptives**; discourage use during pregnancy and breastfeeding; may lower blood pressure with **sedatives**, **antihypertensives**, **anaesthetics**; increased risk of fungal infection with **immunosuppressants**
blackberry	Risk of interaction with **oral hypoglycaemic agents**
bromelain	May cause nausea, vomiting, diarrhoea, menstrual disorders

■ **TABLE F.1 Drug interactions of complementary and alternative therapies *(continued)***

Substance	Possible interactions
burdock	May increase hypoglycaemic effects of **oral hypoglycaemic agents**
capsicum	May increase bleeding with **warfarin**, **aspirin**; increases cough with **angiotensin-converting-enzyme inhibitors (ACEIs)**; increases toxicity with **MAO inhibitors**; increases sedation with **sedatives**
catnip leaves	Discourage use during pregnancy and breastfeeding and use by transplant recipients; increased risk of bleeding episodes if taken with oral **anticoagulants**; increased hypotension with **antihypertensives**
cayenne pepper	Advise caution when taken with **oral hypoglycaemic agents**
chamomile	Contains coumarin – closely monitor individuals taking **anticoagulants**; may cause depression; monitor individuals on **antidepressants**; cross-reaction with ragweed allergies may occur; discourage use during pregnancy and breastfeeding
chaste-tree berry	Advise caution when taken with **hormone replacement therapy** and **hormonal contraceptives**
Chinese angelica (dong quai)	Use caution with the flu, haemorrhagic diseases; monitor people on **antihypertensives**, **vasodilators** or **anticoagulants** for toxic effects; advise caution when taken with **hormone replacement therapy**
chondroitin	Risk of increased bleeding if combined with **anticoagulants**
chong cao fungi	Discourage use by children
Coleus forskohlii	Urge caution when taken with **antihypertensives** or **antihistamines**; severe additive effects can occur; discourage use if individual has hypotension or peptic ulcer
comfrey	Warn against using with **eucalyptus**; monitor liver function
coriander	Advise caution when taken with **oral hypoglycaemic agents**
creatine monohydrate	Warn against using with **insulin**; do not use with caffeine
dandelion root	Advise caution when taken with **oral hypoglycaemic agents**, **antihypertensives** and **quinolone antibiotics**
DHEA (dehydro-epiandrosterone)	Risk of interactions with **alprazolam**, **calcium channel blockers** and **oral hypoglycaemic agents**; screen individuals older than 40 years for hormonally sensitive cancers before use
di huang	Risk of hypoglycaemia with **oral hypoglycaemic agents**
dried root bark of *Lycium chinense* Mill	Advise caution with **oral hypoglycaemic agents**
echinacea (cone flower)	May be liver toxic; discourage use longer than 12 weeks; caution against taking with **liver-toxic drugs** or **immunosuppressants**; discourage use with **antifungals**; serious liver injury could occur; advise against use by individuals with systemic lupus erythematosus, tuberculosis, AIDS
ephedra (ma huang)	May cause serious complications or even death; increased risk of hypertension, stroke, myocardial infarction; interacts with many drugs; **banned import into Australia**
ergot	Monitor individuals who take ergot with **antihypertensives**
eucalyptus	Warn against using with **comfrey**; very toxic in children
evening primrose	Discourage use with **phenothiazines**, **antidepressants**—increases risk of seizures; discourage use by those with epilepsy, schizophrenia
false unicorn root	Advise against use during pregnancy and breastfeeding
fennel	Significantly decreases levels of **ciprofloxacin**
fenugreek	Advise caution when taken with **oral hypoglycaemic agents**, **anticoagulants**
feverfew	Advise caution when taken with **anticoagulants**; may increase bleeding; discourage use before or immediately after surgery because of bleeding risk
garlic	Advise caution if person has diabetes or takes an **oral anticoagulant**; known to affect blood clotting; anaemia reported with long-term use
ginger	Affects blood clotting; warn against use with **anticoagulants**
ginkgo	Can inhibit blood clotting; seizures reported with high doses; warn against use with **anticoagulants**, **aspirin** or **non-steroidal anti-inflammatory drugs (NSAIDs)**; can interact with **phenytoin**, **carbamazepine**, **phenobarbitone**, **tricyclic antidepressants**, **MAO inhibitors** and **oral hypoglycaemic agents**; advise caution
ginseng	May cause irritability if combined with **caffeine**; inhibits clotting; warn against use with **anticoagulants**, **aspirin**, **NSAIDs**; warn against use for longer than 3 months; may cause headaches, manic episodes if used with **phenelzine**, **MAO inhibitors**; may interfere with additive effects of **oestrogens** and **corticosteroids**; may also interfere with cardiac effects of **digoxin**; monitor person closely if taking these drugs or an **antidiabetic drug**
glucosamine	Monitor glucose levels in individuals with diabetes
goldenrod leaves	May decrease effects of **diuretics** by increasing sodium retention; advise caution if the individual has a history of allergies
goldenseal	May cause false-negative test results in those who use such drugs as marijuana and cocaine; large amounts may cause paralysis; affects blood clotting; warn against use with **anticoagulants**; may interfere with **antihypertensives**, **acid blockers**, **barbiturates**; may increase effects of **sedatives**; death can result from overdose

Continued on following page

TABLE F.1 Drug interactions of complementary and alternative therapies *(continued)*

Substance	Possible interactions
gotu kola	Warn against using with **oral hypoglycaemic agents**, **cholesterol-lowering drugs**, **sedatives**
grape seed extract	Advise caution with **oral anticoagulants**; may increase bleeding
green tea leaf	Advise caution with **oral anticoagulants**; may increase bleeding; may increase blood pressure; caution against using with milk
guarana	Advise caution; increases blood pressure, risk of cardiovascular events
guayusa	Advise caution with **antihypertensives**; decreases absorption of **iron**; may decrease clearance of **lithium**
hawthorn	Advise caution with **digoxin**, **ACE inhibitors**, **central nervous system (CNS) depressants**; may potentiate effects
hop	Discourage use with **CNS depressants**, **antipsychotics**
horehound	Use caution with **oral hypoglycaemic agents**, **antihypertensives**
horse chestnut seed	Advise caution with oral **anticoagulants**; may increase bleeding
hyssop	Warn against use by pregnant women and those with seizures; toxic in children and pets
jambul	Use caution with **CNS depressants**
Java plum	Advise caution with **oral hypoglycaemic agents**
jojoba	Used topically; toxic if ingested
juniper berries	Advise caution when taken with **oral hypoglycaemic agents**; not for use in pregnancy
kava	Warn against use with **alprazolam**; may cause coma; advise against use for Parkinson disease or history of stroke; discourage use with **St John's wort**, **anxiolytics**, **alcohol**; risk of serious liver toxicity
kudzu	Interacts with **anticoagulants**, **aspirin**, **oral hypoglycaemic agents**, **cardiovascular drugs**
lavender	Advise caution with **CNS depressants**; oil is potentially poisonous
Ledum tincture liquorice	Acts like aldosterone; blocks **spironolactone** effects; can lead to **digoxin** toxicity because of effects of lowering aldosterone; advise extreme caution; contraindicated with renal or liver disease, hypertension, coronary artery disease, pregnancy, breastfeeding; warn against taking with **thyroid drugs**, **antihypertensives**, **hormonal contraceptives**
ma huang	Contains ephedrine; warn against use with **antihypertensives**, **oral hypoglycaemic agents**, **MAO inhibitors** or **digoxin**; serious adverse effects could occur; **banned import into Australia**
marigold leaves and flowers	Advise against use during pregnancy and breastfeeding
melatonin	Advise caution with **antihypertensives**, **benzodiazepines**, **beta blockers**, **methamphetamine**
milk thistle	May affect metabolism and increase toxicity of **drugs using cytochrome P450 (CYP450)**, **CYP3A4 and CYP2C9 systems**
mistletoe leaves	Advise caution with **antihypertensives**, **CNS depressants**, **immunosuppressants**
Momordica charantia (karela)	Advise caution when taken with **oral hypoglycaemic agents**
nettle	Advise against use during pregnancy and breastfeeding; increases effects of **diuretics**
octacosanol	Advise against use during pregnancy and breastfeeding; avoid use with **carbidopa–levodopa**
parsley seeds and leaves	Risk of serotonin syndrome with **selective serotonin reuptake inhibitors (SSRIs)**, **lithium**, **opioids**; increased hypotension with **antihypertensives**
passionflower vine	May increase sedation with other **CNS depressants**, **MAO inhibitors**; advise against drinking **alcohol** while taking this herb; advise person not to use with **anticoagulants**
psyllium	Can cause severe gas and stomach pain; may interfere with nutrient absorption; avoid use with **warfarin**, **digoxin**, **lithium**—absorption of drug may be blocked; do not combine with **laxatives**
raspberry	Advise caution with **oral hypoglycaemic agents**; disulfiram-like reaction with **alcohol**
red clover	Risk of bleeding with **anticoagulants**, **antiplatelets**; discourage use in pregnancy
red yeast rice	Increased risk of rhabdomyolysis with **ciclosporin**, **fibric acid**, **niacin**, **lovastatin**, **grapefruit juice**
rose hips	Advise caution with **oestrogens**, **iron**, **warfarin**
rosemary	Disulfiram-like reaction with **alcohol**
rue extract	Advise caution with **antihypertensive drugs**, **digoxin**, **warfarin**
sage	Advise caution with **oral hypoglycaemic agents**, **anticonvulsants**, **alcohol**
SAM-e (AdoMet)	May cause frequent gastrointestinal complaints and headache; risk of serotonin syndrome with **antidepressants**
sarsaparilla	Advise caution with **anticonvulsants**
sassafras	Oil may be toxic to fetus, children and adults when ingested; interacts with many drugs
saw palmetto	Warn against use with oestrogen-replacement or hormonal contraceptives—may greatly increase adverse effects; may decrease iron absorption; advise against use with **finasteride**; toxicity could occur

TABLE F.1 Drug interactions of complementary and alternative therapies *(continued)*

Substance	Possible interactions
schisandra	Warn against use during pregnancy; causes uterine stimulation; advise caution with all **drugs metabolised in the liver**
squaw vine	May cause liver toxicity; increased toxicity of **digoxin**; disulfiram-like reaction with **alcohol**
St John's wort	Discourage tyramine-containing foods; hypertensive crisis is possible; thrombocytopenia has been reported; can increase sensitivity to light; advise against taking with drugs that cause **photosensitivity**; severe photosensitivity can occur in light-skinned people; serious interactions have been reported with **SSRIs**, **MAO inhibitors**, **kava**, **digoxin**, **theophylline**, **AIDS antiviral drugs**, **sympathomimetics**, **antineoplastics**, **hormonal contraceptives**; advise against these combinations
sweet violet flowers	Increases effects of **laxatives**
tarragon	Advise caution with **oral hypoglycaemic agents**
thyme	May increase sensitivity to light; warn against combining with **photosensitivity-causing drugs**; also warn against combining with **MAO inhibitors**, **SSRIs**; may cause serious adverse effects
valerian	Can cause severe liver damage; warn against use with **barbiturates**, **alcohol**, **CNS depressants** or **antihistamines**; can cause serious sedation
went rice	Warn against use in pregnancy, liver disease, alcoholism, acute infection
white willow bark	Advise caution with **anticoagulants**, **NSAIDs**, **diuretics**
xuan shen	Advise caution when taken with **oral hypoglycaemic agents**
	Can affect blood pressure; CNS stimulant; has cardiac effects; manic episodes have been reported in individuals with psychiatric conditions; warn against use with **SSRIs**, **tyramine-containing foods**; advise caution with **tricyclic antidepressants**

From McKenna, L. & Mirkov, S. (2014). *McKenna's Drug Handbook for Nursing and Midwifery* (7th edn). Sydney: Lippincott Williams & Wilkins.

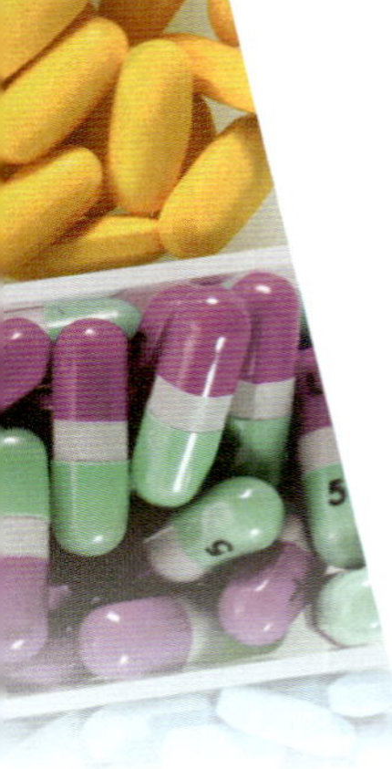

Index

E

F

J

K

Q

R

U